JL ABBAS • THOMAS ALBRECHT • G.G. ALTON • RAZA ALY • M. ZOUHAIR ATASSI • EDWAI
LISH • ALBERT BALOWS • LANE BARKSDALE • SAMUEL BAR   DERRIC
KBY • YECHIEL BECKER • L. JOE BERRY • NEIL R. BLACKLO   ENJAM
AVIDA • EDITH BOX • PHILIP BRACHMAN • DON J. BRENNER • JANET S. BUTEL • RICHAI
LDERONE • GILBERT CASTRO • JAN CERNY • MARY LOU CLEMENTS • JAY COHEN • FRANK
LINS • JOSE COSTA • ROBERT B. COUCH • JOHN P. CRAIG • JOHN H. CROSS • GEORGE CUKOI
DE G. CULBERTSON • JIM CUTLER • C. PATRICK DAVIS • FERDINANDO DIANZANI • J.P. DUBE'
ELA ENDERS • DOLORES G. EVANS • DOYLE J. EVANS • ADAM EWERT • JOHN L. FAHEY • JAM
EELEY • FRANK FENNER • SYDNEY M. FINEGOLD • HORST FINGER • RICHARD A. FINKELSTEII
MAS J. FITZGERALD • SAMUEL B. FORMAL • J.R.L. FORSYTH • SUBHASH C. GAUTAM • MAI
N GERENCSER • RALPH A. GIANNELLA • C.J. GIBBS, JR. • RANDALL GOLDBLUM • MART
LDFIELD • ARMOND S. GOLDMAN • SHERWOOD L. GORBACH • J. ANDREW GRANT, JR. • M. NE.
ENTZEL • DAVID J. HENTGES • DONALD HEYNEMAN • RANDALL K. HOLMES • HOPE E. HOPPS
CE S. HUANG • WALTER T. HUGHES • TONY E. HUGLI • BARBARA H. IGLEWSKI • RUSSELL
INSON • PETER JURTSHUK, JR. • ANAND G. KANTAK • ALBERT Z. KAPIKIAN • DORIS S. KELSE'
RALD T. KEUSCH • SIDNEY KIBRICK • KWANG-SHIN KIM • THOMAS J. KINDT • DAVID
GSBURY • JAN KLEIN • GARY R. KLIMPEL • GEORGE S. KOBAYASHI • CHIEN LIU • WALTER
ESCHE • JON T. MADER • HOWARD I. MAIBACH • JOHN R. MARTIN • CARL F.T. MATTERN
HAEL R. MCGINNIS • VIRGINIA A. MERCHANT • ERNEST A. MEYER • HARRY M. MEYER • STEPHI
MORSE • RICHARD MOXON • DANIEL M. MUSHER • ANDRE J. NAHMIAS • NEAL NATHANSON
WIN NETER • HAROLD C. NEU • LEROY J. OLSON • PAUL D. PARKMAN • M. JEVITZ PATTERSOI
WRENCE L. PELLETIER, JR. • RONALD P. PELLEY • JOHNNY PETERSON • CHARLES J. PFAU
INART PHILIPSON • ROBERT M. PIKE • DAVID D. PORTER • ROBIN D. POWELL • PAUL G. QUII
AN RABSON • SHMUEL RAZIN • SYLVIA E. REED • BERNARD ROIZMAN • PHILIP K. RUSSELI
TON R.J. SALTON • FRANK SCHMALSTEIG, JR. • NATHALIE J. SCHMIDT • GEORGE SCHREINEI
IN RICHARD SEED • JAMES G. SHAFFER • ROBERT E. SHOPE • WILLIAM A. SODEMAN • NORMA
LAL • GEORGE J. TODARO • JOHN P. UTZ • ALLAN WALKER • KENNETH S. WARREN • NORMAN
ATHERLY • WILLIAM O. WEIGLE • CAROL L. WELLS • SUSAN E.H. WEST • TRACY D. WILKINS
EODORE E. WOODWARD • RODRIGO A. ZELEDÓN • A.J. ZUCKERMAN • ABUL ABBAS • THOMA
BRECHT • G.G. ALTON • RAZA ALY • M. ZOUHAIR ATASSI • EDWARD BALISH • ALBERT BALOWS
NE BARKSDALE • SAMUEL BARON • JACK R. BATTISTO • DERRICK BAXBY • YECHIEL BECKER •
E BERRY • NEIL R. BLACKLOW • MARTIN J. BLASER • BENJAMIN BONAVIDA • EDITH BOX • PHIL
ACHMAN • DON J. BRENNER • JANET S. BUTEL • RICHARD CALDERONE • GILBERT CASTRO • JA
RNY • MARY LOU CLEMENTS • JAY COHEN • FRANK M. COLLINS • JOSE COSTA • ROBERT
UCH • JOHN P. CRAIG • JOHN H. CROSS • GEORGE CUKOR • CLYDE G. CULBERTSON • JIM CUTLI
PATRICK DAVIS • FERDINANDO DIANZANI • J.P. DUBEY • GISELA ENDERS • DOLORES G. EVANS
YLE J. EVANS • ADAM EWERT • JOHN L. FAHEY • JAMES C. FEELEY • FRANK FENNER • SYDNE
FINEGOLD • HORST FINGER • RICHARD A. FINKELSTEIN • THOMAS J. FITZGERALD • SAMUEL
RMAL • J.R.L. FORSYTH • SUBHASH C. GAUTAM • MARY ANN GERENCSER • RALPH A. GIANNELI
J. GIBBS, JR. • RANDALL GOLDBLUM • MARTIN GOLDFIELD • ARMOND S. GOLDMAN • SHERWOO
GORBACH • J. ANDREW GRANT, JR. • M. NEAL GUENTZEL • DAVID J. HENTGES • DONAI

Medical Microbiology

Second Edition

Jan Cerny, MD, PhD
Section Editor: Immunology
Professor
Department of Microbiology
University of Texas Medical Branch
Galveston, Texas

Johnny W. Peterson, PhD
Section Editor: Bacteriology, Mycology, and Organ Systems
Professor
Department of Microbiology
University of Texas Medical Branch
Galveston, Texas

Charles P. Davis, PhD
Section Editor: Bacteriology, Mycology, and Organ Systems
Associate Professor
Department of Microbiology
University of Texas Medical Branch
Galveston, Texas

Thomas B. Albrecht, PhD
Section Editor: Virology
Associate Professor
Department of Microbiology
University of Texas Medical Branch
Galveston, Texas

Ferdinando Dianzani, MD
Section Editor: Virology
Professor and Chairman
Institute of Virology
University of Rome
Rome, Italy

L. J. Olson, PhD
Section Editor: Parasitology
Professor
Department of Microbiology
University of Texas Medical Branch
Galveston, Texas

Medical Microbiology

Second Edition

SAMUEL BARON, MD
Editor
Chairman
Department of Microbiology
University of Texas Medical Branch
Galveston, Texas

Renee Robillard and
Diane Weigent
Assistant Editors

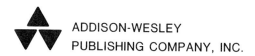
ADDISON-WESLEY
PUBLISHING COMPANY, INC.

Health Sciences Division, Menlo Park, California
Reading, Massachusetts • Don Mills, Ontario
Wokingham, UK • Amsterdam • Sydney • Singapore • Tokyo
Mexico City • Bogota • Santiago • San Juan

Sponsoring Editor: Katherine Pitcoff
Copyeditor: Lyn Dupré
Production Coordinator: Judith Hibbard
Cover and Book Design: Michael Rogondino
Cover: A computer-generated graphic of the structure of rosoxa-
cin, an antibacterial agent for urinary tract infections. Courtesy
of TAP Pharmaceuticals.

Library of Congress Cataloging in Publication Data
Main entry under title:

Medical microbiology.

  Includes bibliographies and index.
  1. Medical microbiology. I. Baron, Samuel, 1928–
[DNLM: 1. Microbiology. QW 4 M486]
QR46.M467 1986 616'.01   85-11153
ISBN 0-201-10146-7

    DEFGHIJ-MA-8987

The authors and publishers have exerted every effort to ensure that drug selection and dosage set forth in this text are in accord with current
recommendations and practice at the time of publication. However, in view of ongoing research, changes in government regulations and the
constant flow of information relating to drug therapy and drug reactions, the reader is urged to check the package insert for each drug for any
change in indications of dosage and for added warnings and precautions. This is particularly important where the recommended agent is a new
and/or infrequently employed drug.

Addison-Wesley Publishing Company
Health Sciences Division
2727 Sand Hill Road
Menlo Park, California 94025

Contents

*General chapters

Section II: Bacteriology

---

†Deceased

Section III: Mycology

Section IV: Virology

Section V: Parasitology

Section VI: Microbiology of Organ Systems

Consulting Editors

Jack B. Alperin, MD
Professor
Departments of Internal Medicine and Human
    Biological Chemistry and Genetics
University of Texas Medical Branch
Galveston, Texas

J. Edwin Blalock, PhD
Professor
Department of Microbiology
University of Texas Medical Branch
Galveston, Texas

Quellin T. Box, MD
Associate Professor
Departments of Pediatrics and Microbiology
University of Texas Medical Branch
Galveston, Texas

Teh-sheng Chan, MD, PhD
Associate Professor
Department of Microbiology
University of Texas Medical Branch
Galveston, Texas

William R. Fleischmann, Jr., PhD
Associate Professor
Department of Microbiology
University of Texas Medical Branch
Galveston, Texas

James Guckian, MD
Professor
Departments of Internal Medicine and Microbiology
University of Texas Medical Branch
Galveston, Texas

Michael T. Kelly, MD, PhD
Professor
Department of Pathology
University of Texas Medical Branch
Galveston, Texas

Garnett Kelsoe, DSc
Assistant Professor
Department of Microbiology
University of Texas Medical Branch
Galveston, Texas

Etta Mae Macdonald, MD, PhD
Associate Professor
Departments of Dermatology and Microbiology
University of Texas Medical Branch
Galveston, Texas

Richard B. Pollard, MD
Associate Professor
Department of Internal Medicine
University of Texas Medical Branch
Galveston, Texas

Edgar B. Smith, MD
Professor and Chairman
Department of Dermatology
University of Texas Medical Branch
Galveston, Texas

G. John Stanton, PhD
Professor
Department of Microbiology
University of Texas Medical Branch
Galveston, Texas

Allan L. Truant, PhD
Assistant Professor
Clinical Microbiology Division,
   Department of Pathology
University of Texas Medical Branch
Galveston, Texas

Douglas A. Weigent, PhD
Research Assistant Professor
Department of Microbiology
University of Texas Medical Branch
Galveston, Texas

Contributors

Abul Abbas, MD
Associate Professor
Department of Pathology
Harvard Medical School
Boston, Massachusetts

Thomas Albrecht, PhD
Associate Professor
Department of Microbiology
University of Texas Medical Branch
Galveston, Texas

G.G. Alton, DVM & S
New Friars, Mickley, Ripon
N. Yorkshire HG4 3JE
England

Raza Aly, PhD
Professor
Department of Dermatology
University of California
San Francisco, California

M. Zouhair Atassi, PhD, DSc
Robert A. Welch Professor
Department of Biochemistry
Baylor College of Medicine
Houston, Texas

Edward Balish, PhD
Professor
Departments of Surgery and Medical Microbiology
University of Wisconsin
Madison, Wisconsin

Albert Balows, PhD
Assistant Director for Laboratory Science
Center for Infectious Diseases
Centers for Disease Control
Atlanta, Georgia

Lane Barksdale, PhD
Professor
Department of Microbiology
New York University Medical Center
New York, New York

Samuel Baron, MD
Professor and Chairman
Department of Microbiology
University of Texas Medical Branch
Galveston, Texas

Jack R. Battisto, PhD
Staff Member
Department of Molecular and Cellular Biology
Cleveland Clinic Foundation
Cleveland, Ohio

Derrick Baxby, PhD
Senior Lecturer
Department of Medical Microbiology
Liverpool University
New Medical School
Liverpool, England

Yechiel Becker, PhD
Professor
Laboratory for Molecular Virology
Hebrew University
Hadassah Medical School
Jerusalem, Israel

L. Joe Berry, PhD
Professor
Department of Microbiology
University of Texas
Austin, Texas

Neil R. Blacklow, MD
Professor
Departments of Medicine and Microbiology
University of Massachusetts Medical School
Worcester, Massachusetts

Martin J. Blaser, MD
Associate Professor
Department of Medicine
University of Colorado School of Medicine
Denver, Colorado

Benjamin Bonavida, PhD
Professor
Department of Microbiology & Immunology
UCLA School of Medicine
University of California at Los Angeles
Los Angeles, California

Edith Box, ScD
Associate Professor Emeritus
Department of Microbiology
University of Texas Medical Branch
Galveston, Texas

Philip Brachman, MD
Director, Global EIS Program
Centers for Disease Control
Atlanta, Georgia

Don J. Brenner, PhD
Molecular Biology Laboratory
Division of Bacterial Diseases
Center for Infectious Diseases
Centers for Disease Control
Atlanta, Georgia

Janet S. Butel, PhD
Professor
Department of Virology and Epidemiology
Baylor College of Medicine
Houston, Texas

Richard Calderone, PhD
Associate Professor
Department of Microbiology
Georgetown University
School of Medicine
Washington, D.C.

Gilbert Castro, PhD
Professor
Department of Physiology
The University of Texas Health Science Center at
    Houston
Houston, Texas

Jan Cerny, MD, PhD
Professor
Department of Microbiology
University of Texas Medical Branch
Galveston, Texas

Mary Lou Clements, MD, MPH
Associate Professor
Department of International Health
Johns Hopkins University
School of Hygiene and Public Health
Baltimore, Maryland

Jay Cohen, PhD
Microbiologist
Host Factors Division
Center for Infectious Diseases
Centers for Disease Control
Atlanta, Georgia

Frank M. Collins, PhD, DSc
Member
Trudeau Institute
Saranac Lake, New York

Jose Costa, MD
Chairman
Institut de Pathologie VHUB
Rue du Bugnon 19
Lausanne, Switzerland

Robert B. Couch, MD
Professor
Departments of Microbiology and Immunology and
    Medicine
Baylor College of Medicine
Houston, Texas

John P. Craig, MD
Professor
Department of Microbiology and Immunology
State University of New York
Downstate Medical Center
Brooklyn, New York

John H. Cross, PhD
Professor, Tropical Public Health
Department of Preventive Medicine/Biometrics
Uniformed Services University of the Health Sciences
School of Medicine
Bethesda, Maryland

George Cukor, PhD
Associate Professor
Department of Medicine and Microbiology
University of Massachusetts
Medical School
Worcester, Massachusetts

Clyde G. Culbertson, MD
Professor Emeritus
Indiana University School of Medicine
Lilly Laboratory for Clinical Research
Indianapolis, Indiana

Jim Cutler, PhD
Associate Professor
Department of Microbiology
Montana State University
Bozeman, Montana

C. Patrick Davis, PhD
Associate Professor
Department of Microbiology
University of Texas Medical Branch
Galveston, Texas

Ferdinando Dianzani, MD
Professor and Chairman
Institute of Virology
University of Rome
Rome, Italy

J.P. Dubey, MVSc, PhD
Protozoan Diseases Laboratory
Animal Parasitology Institute
United States Department of Agriculture
Beltsville, Maryland

Gisela Enders, MD
Professor
Facharzt fur Mikrobiologie u.
Infektions-Epidemiologie
Virologisch-med. Diagnostisches Institut
Stuttgart, West Germany

Dolores G. Evans, PhD
Research Associate Professor
Department of Medicine
Baylor College of Medicine and
Veterans Administration Medical Center
Houston, Texas

Doyle J. Evans, Jr., PhD
Research Associate Professor
Department of Medicine
Baylor College of Medicine and
Veterans Administration Medical Center
Houston, Texas

Adam Ewert, PhD
Professor
Department of Microbiology
University of Texas Medical Branch
Galveston, Texas

John L. Fahey, MD
Professor
Departments of Microbiology and Immunology
University of California, Los Angeles
School of Medicine
Los Angeles, California

James C. Feeley, PhD
Chief, Field Investigations Section
Respiratory and Special Pathogens
Laboratory Branch
Center for Infectious Diseases
Centers for Disease Control
Atlanta, Georgia

Frank Fenner, MD
University Fellow
Professor, John Curtin School of
    Medical Research
Canberra, Australia

Sydney M. Finegold, MD
Chief, Infectious Disease Section
Veterans Administration
Wadsworth Medical Center
Los Angeles, California

Horst Finger, MD
Professor and Director
Stadt. Krankenanstalten Krefeld
Institut F. Hygiene U. Lab.-Medizin
Medizinaluntersuchungsamt
Krefeld, Federal Republic of Germany

Richard A. Finkelstein, PhD
Professor and Chairman
Department of Microbiology
University of Missouri
School of Medicine
Columbia, Missouri

Thomas J. Fitzgerald, PhD
Associate Professor
Department of Microbiology & Immunology
University of Minnesota at Duluth
Duluth, Minnesota

Samuel B. Formal, PhD
Chief
Department of Bacterial Diseases
Walter Reed Army Institute of Research
Washington, D.C.

J.R.L. Forsyth, MD
Microbiological Diagnostic Unit
University of Melbourne
Melbourne, Australia

Subhash C. Gautam, PhD
Project Scientist
Department of Molecular and Cellular Biology
Cleveland Clinic Foundation
Cleveland, Ohio

Mary Ann Gerencser, PhD
Research Associate
Department of Microbiology
West Virginia University Medical Center
Morgantown, West Virginia

Ralph A. Giannella, MD
Professor of Medicine
Director, Division of Digestive Diseases
University of Cincinnati College of Medicine
Cincinnati, Ohio

C.J. Gibbs, Jr., PhD
Deputy Chief
Laboratory of Central Nervous System Studies
National Institute of Neurological and Communicative
    Disorders and Stroke
National Institutes of Health
Bethesda, Maryland

Randall Goldblum, MD
Professor
Departments of Pediatrics and
Human Biological Chemistry and Genetics
University of Texas Medical Branch
Galveston, Texas

Martin Goldfield, MD
Professor
Department of Epidemiology
School of Public Health
University of South Carolina
Columbia, South Carolina

Armond S. Goldman, MD
Professor
Department of Pediatrics and Human Biological
  Chemistry and Genetics
University of Texas Medical Branch
Galveston, Texas

Sherwood L. Gorbach, MD
Professor
Infectious Diseases Division
Tufts University
New England Medical Center
Boston, Massachusetts

J. Andrew Grant, Jr., MD
Professor
Departments of Internal Medicine and Microbiology
University of Texas Medical Branch
Galveston, Texas

M. Neal Guentzel, PhD
Professor
Division of Life Sciences
University of Texas at San Antonio
San Antonio, Texas

David J. Hentges, PhD
Professor and Chairman
Department of Microbiology
School of Medicine
Texas Tech University Health Sciences Center
Lubbock, Texas

Donald Heyneman, PhD
Professor and Associate Chairman
Department of Epidemiology and International Health
University of California, San Francisco
San Francisco, California

Randall K. Holmes, MD, PhD
Associate Dean for Academic Affairs and Chairman
Department of Microbiology
Uniformed Services University of the Health Sciences
Bethesda, Maryland

Hope E. Hopps, MS
Consultant
National Center for Drugs and Biologics
Bethesda, Maryland

Alice S. Huang, PhD
Professor of Microbiology and Molecular Genetics
Harvard Medical School and
Children's Hospital
Boston, Massachusetts

Walter T. Hughes, MD
Director, Division of Infectious Diseases
St. Jude Children's Research Hospital
and Professor of Pediatrics
University of Tennessee
Center for Health Sciences
Memphis, Tennessee

Tony E. Hugli, PhD
Member
Department of Molecular Immunology
Scripps Clinic and Research Foundation
San Diego, California

Barbara H. Iglewski, PhD
Professor
Department of Microbiology and Immunology
Oregon Health Sciences University
Portland, Oregon

Russell C. Johnson, PhD
Professor
Department of Microbiology
University of Minnesota
Minneapolis, Minnesota

Peter Jurtshuk, Jr., PhD
Professor
College of Natural Sciences and
  Mathematics
University of Houston
Houston, Texas

Anand G. Kantak
Department of Pediatrics and
  Human Biological Chemistry and Genetics
University of Texas Medical Branch
Galveston, Texas

Albert Z. Kapikian, MD
Head
Epidemiology Section
Laboratory of Infectious Disease
National Institute of Allergy and
   Infectious Diseases
National Institutes of Health
Bethesda, Maryland

Doris S. Kelsey, MD
Associate Professor
Department of Pediatrics
Bowman Gray School of Medicine
Winston-Salem, North Carolina

Gerald T. Keusch, MD
Chief
Division of Geographic Medicine
Tufts University School of Medicine
Boston, Massachusetts

Sidney Kibrick, MD, PhD
Professor Emeritus
Departments of Microbiology and Pediatrics
Boston University Medical Center
Boston, Massachusetts

Kwang-Shin Kim, PhD
Associate Professor
Department of Microbiology
New York University School of Medicine
New York, New York

Thomas J. Kindt, PhD
Chief
Laboratory of Immunogenetics
National Institute of Allergy and Infectious Diseases
National Institutes of Health
Bethesda, Maryland

David W. Kingsbury, MD
Member
Department of Virology and Molecular Biology
St. Jude Children's Research Hospital
Memphis, Tennessee

George Klein, MA
Epidemiologic Investigations
Laboratory Branch
Bacterial Disease Division
Center for Disease Control
Atlanta, Georgia

Jan Klein, PhD
Professor and Director
Abteilung Immungenetik
Max Planck Institut fur Biologie
Tubingen, West Germany

Gary R. Klimpel, PhD
Associate Professor
Department of Microbiology
University of Texas Medical Branch
Galveston, Texas

George S. Kobayashi, PhD
Professor
Department of Medicine
Washington University
School of Medicine
St. Louis, Missouri

Jeffrey R. Lisse, MD
Assistant Professor
Department of Internal Medicine
University of Texas Medical Branch
Galveston, Texas

Chien Liu, MD
Professor
Departments of Medicine & Pediatrics
University of Kansas
College of Health Sciences and Hospital
Kansas City, Kansas

Walter J. Loesche, DMD, PhD
Professor
Departments of Dentistry and Microbiology
University of Michigan
School of Dentistry and Medicine
Ann Arbor, Michigan

Jon T. Mader, MD
Associate Professor
Department of Internal Medicine
Division of Infectious Diseases
Member, Marine Biomedical Institute
University of Texas Medical Branch
Galveston, Texas

Howard I. Maibach, MD
Professor
Department of Dermatology
University of California, San Francisco
School of Medicine
San Francisco, California

John R. Martin, MD
Senior Staff Fellow
Laboratory of Experimental Neuropathology
National Institute of Neurological and Communicative
   Disorders and Stroke
National Institutes of Health
Bethesda, Maryland

Carl F. T. Mattern, MD
Visiting Associate Professor
Department of Obstetrics and Gynecology
The Johns Hopkins University
School of Medicine
Baltimore, Maryland

Michael R. McGinnis, PhD
Director, Mycology and Mycobacteriology Laboratory
North Carolina Memorial Hospital
University of North Carolina
Chapel Hill, North Carolina

George Medoff, MD
Professor
Departments of Medicine and Microbiology and
   Immunology
Washington University
School of Medicine
St. Louis, Missouri

Virginia A. Merchant, DMD
Assistant Professor
Departments of Microbiology and Biochemistry
School of Dentistry
University of Detroit
Detroit, Michigan

Ernest A. Meyer, ScD
Professor
Department of Microbiology and Immunology
Oregon Health Sciences University
Portland, Oregon

Harry M. Meyer, Jr., MD
Director, Center for Drugs and Biologics
Food and Drug Administration
Bethesda, Maryland

Stephen A. Morse, PhD
Director
Sexually Transmitted Diseases Laboratory Program
Center for Infectious Diseases
Centers for Disease Control
Atlanta, Georgia

Richard Moxon, MD
Associate Professor
Department of Pediatrics
Johns Hopkins University
School of Medicine
Baltimore, Maryland

Daniel M. Musher, MD
Professor of Medicine, Microbiology and Immunology
Chief, Infectious Disease Section
Veterans Administration Hospital
Houston, Texas

Andre J. Nahmias, MD, MPH
Professor
Department of Pediatrics and Pathology
Emory University School of Medicine
Atlanta, Georgia

Neal Nathanson, MD
Chairman
Department of Microbiology
University of Pennsylvania School of Medicine
Philadelphia, Pennsylvania

Erwin Neter, MD
Deceased

Harold C. Neu, MD
Professor
Departments of Medicine and Pharmacology
Columbia University
New York, New York

Leroy J. Olson, PhD
Professor
Department of Microbiology
University of Texas Medical Branch
Galveston, Texas

Paul D. Parkman, MD
Deputy Director
Center for Drugs and Biologics
Food and Drug Administration
Bethesda, Maryland

Ethel Patten, MD
Director
Blood Bank
University of Texas Medical Branch
Galveston, Texas

M. Jevitz Patterson, MD, PhD
Associate Professor
Department of Microbiology and Public Health
Michigan State University
East Lansing, Michigan

Lawrence L. Pelletier, Jr., MD
Professor, Internal Medicine
University of Kansas Medical Service
Wichita, Kansas

Ronald P. Pelley, MD, PhD
Assistant Professor
Department of Pathology
University of Texas Medical Branch
Galveston, Texas

Johnny Peterson, PhD
Professor
Department of Microbiology
University of Texas Medical Branch
Galveston, Texas

Charles J. Pfau, PhD
Professor and Chairman
Department of Biology
Rensselaer Polytechnic Institute
Troy, New York

Lennart Philipson, MD, Dr Med Sci
Professor, Director General
European Molecular Biology Lab (EMBL)
6900 Heidelberg
Federal Republic of Germany

Robert M. Pike, PhD
Professor Emeritus
University of Texas Southwestern Medical School
Dallas, Texas

David D. Porter, MD
Professor
Department of Pathology
University of California, Los Angeles
School of Medicine
Los Angeles, California

Robin D. Powell, MD
Dean
College of Medicine
University of Kentucky
Albert B. Chandler Medical Center
Lexington, Kentucky

Paul G. Quie, MD
Professor
Department of Pediatrics
University of Minnesota
Minneapolis, Minnesota

Alan S. Rabson, MD
Director
Division of Cancer Biology and Diagnosis
National Cancer Institute
National Institutes of Health
Bethesda, Maryland

Shmuel Razin, PhD
Professor and Chairman
Department of Membrane and Ultrastructure Research
Hebrew University—Hadassah Medical School
Jerusalem, Israel

Sylvia E. Reed, MB
National Institute for Biological Standards and Control
Holly Hill, Hampstead
London, England

Bernard Roizman, ScD
Joseph Regenstein, Distinguished Service Professor
Department of Molecular Genetics and Cell Biology
University of Chicago
Chicago, Illinois

Philip K. Russell, MD
Commander
Fitzsimons Army Medical Center
Aurora, Colorado

Milton R. J. Salton, ScD
Professor and Chairman
Department of Microbiology
New York University School of Medicine
New York, New York

Frank Schmalstieg, Jr., MD
Associate Professor
Departments of Pediatrics and Human Biological
    Chemistry and Genetics
University of Texas Medical Branch
Galveston, Texas

Nathalie J. Schmidt, PhD
Research Specialist
Viral and Rickettsial Disease Laboratory
California Department of Health Services
Berkeley, California

George Schreiner, MD, PhD
Assistant Professor
Departments of Medicine and Pathology
Washington University School of Medicine
St. Louis, Missouri

John Richard Seed, PhD
Chairman
Department of Parasitology and Laboratory Practice
School of Public Health
University of North Carolina
Chapel Hill, North Carolina

James G. Shaffer, ScD
Deceased

Robert E. Shope, MD
Professor
Yale Arbovirus Research Unit
Department of Epidemiology and Public Health
Yale School of Medicine
New Haven, Connecticut

William A. Sodeman, Jr., MD
Professor and Chairman
Department of Comprehensive Medicine
University of South Florida
College of Medicine
Tampa, Florida

Norman Talal, MD
Professor
Departments of Medicine and Microbiology
University of Texas Health Science Center
San Antonio, Texas

George J. Todaro, MD
Scientific Director and CEO
Oncogen
Seattle, Washington

John P. Utz, MD
Professor
Department of Medicine
Georgetown University School of Medicine
Washington, D.C.

Allan Walker, MD
Professor
Department of Pediatrics
Harvard Medical School
Boston, Massachusetts

Kenneth S. Warren, MD
Director
Health Sciences
The Rockefeller Foundation
New York, New York

Norman F. Weatherly, PhD
Professor
Department of Parasitology and Laboratory Practice
School of Public Health
University of North Carolina
Chapel Hill, North Carolina

William O. Weigle, PhD
Member and Chairman
Department of Immunology
Scripps Clinic and Research Foundation
La Jolla, California

Carol L. Wells, PhD
Assistant Professor
Department of Laboratory Medicine and Pathology
University of Minnesota
Minneapolis, Minnesota

Susan E. H. West, MS
Department of Anaerobic Microbiology
Virginia Polytechnic Institute and State University
Blacksburg, Virginia

Tracy D. Wilkins, PhD
Department Head
Department of Anaerobic Microbiology
Virginia Polytechnic Institute and State University
Blacksburg, Virginia

Theodore E. Woodward, MD, MACP DSc (Hon)
Professor of Medicine Emeritus
University of Maryland
School of Medicine and Hospital: Baltimore Veterans
    Administration
Baltimore, Maryland

Rodrigo A. Zeledón, ScD
Professor
Escuela de Medicina Veterinaria
Universidad Nacional
Heredia, Costa Rica, Central America

A. J. Zuckerman, MD, DSc, FRCP, FRCPath
Professor and Director
Department of Medical Microbiology and the WHO
    Collaborating Centre for Reference and Research on
    Viral Hepatitis
London School of Hygiene and Tropical Medicine
University of London
London, England

Preface

Microbes in the Environment

Microbes may be the most significant life form sharing this planet with humans. Their ubiquitous presence in astronomic numbers gives rise to the many variants that account for rapid evolutionary adaptation. This adaptability has permitted microbes to utilize an enormous range of food sources. Depending on the food source used, microbes may play beneficial roles in maintaining life or undesirable roles in causing human disease.

Beneficial roles of microbes include recycling of organic matter through microbe-induced decay and through digestion and nutrition in animals and humans. In addition, natural microbial flora provide protection against more virulent microbes.

The microbes that cause infectious diseases may be virulent, although such diseases may also be caused by normally benign microbes either when the host defense mechanisms are impaired or when microbes are present in large numbers or in vulnerable body sites. Because death or severe impairment of an infected host is disadvantageous for the survival of the infecting microbe, natural selection favors predominance of less virulent microorganisms.

Understanding and employing the principles of microbiology enable the physician and medical scientist to control an increasing number of infectious diseases.

Rationale

Medical Microbiology grew out of our collective teaching experiences and educational studies of microbiology instruction. *It is specifically designed to meet the needs of students by achieving a balance of coverage without excessive detail.* Important basic concepts such as pathogenesis, host defenses, epidemiology, evolution, and replication are emphasized throughout the text as well as in introductory chapters.

The original philosophy of the book has been maintained in the second edition. The 115 chapters in this text cover comprehensively the principles and concepts of immunology, bacteriology, mycology, virology, and parasitology.

Organization

Medical Microbiology starts with an introduction to the basic principles of immunology so the student can understand the body's response to microorganisms.

Three new chapters have been added to this section and it has been completely reorganized. Next the bacteria are discussed, emphasizing the basic concepts and clinically important organisms. Sections III, IV, and V cover mycology, virology, and parasitology thoroughly; Section VI summarizes and provides clinical relevance by discussing diseases according to the organ system involved.

Almost half the chapters in this text are *general* chapters to help the student better understand subsequent discussions of specific microorganisms. By presenting the **mechanisms of infection,** these general chapters help prepare the student for later studies of clinical infectious diseases and advanced microbiology. **Emphasis on general principles** enables the student to deduce rather than memorize specifics and provides a theoretical framework on which to build as new knowledge of microbiology becomes available. General chapters, identified in the Table of Contents, do not follow a standardized outline; the diverse nature of their subjects has dictated their organization.

Each *specific* chapter is organized according to a common outline, beginning with a section entitled *"General Concepts,"* which orients the student and serves as a learning aid. The following sections discuss **distinctive properties** of the group of microorganisms, **pathogenesis** of the infection, **host defenses, epidemiology, diagnosis,** and **control.**

Coverage

Comprehensive and authoritative coverage is ensured because each chapter has been written by one or more scientists recognized for research contributions in the particular subject area. Twenty new contributors bring their expertise to this second edition. Each chapter has been carefully structured to provide a concise, digestible unit, offering the advantage of learnability.

Throughout the text, emphasis on general principles provides a mechanistic foundation for learning. **Balanced and complete coverage** of medical microbiology has been assured by section editors representing the relevant disciplines. An overview section on the microbiology of major organ systems offers a unique perspective to pave the way for the **transition from basic science to clinical medicine.**

Recognizing that no textbook can meet all needs, we have designed this text to offer optimal assistance to the student studying the principles of microbiology.

Acknowledgments

Primary acknowledgment must go to the many dedicated scientists who discovered the principles of microbiology. The scientific literature acknowledges individual contributions, but textbooks cannot adequately pay such tribute. Albert Einstein identified this problem, commenting that although "there are plenty of well-endowed (scientists) . . . it strikes me as unfair to select a few of them for recognition." We are indebted to all these unnamed investigators.

We are also grateful for the excellent cooperation and enthusiasm of our contributing authors and for the expertise provided by our consulting editors, who enhanced the thoroughness of our scientific review. Input from our students has been invaluable to the educational approach of this textbook. The support of the University of Texas Medical Branch administration in encouraging faculty participation in this endeavor has been outstanding.

The section editors deserve particular praise. They have processed many manuscripts with commendable dedication, attention to detail, scientific knowledge, and editorial skill.

Medical Microbiology provides material that is learnable, comprehensive, authoritative, and up to date. This second edition is current because of the unstinting efforts of the contributors and editors. Extensive reviews by students, colleagues at many schools, and journal reviewers have markedly improved this second edition through the addition of new chapters, expansion of others, and coordination of all.

Also, I acknowledge the essential participation of my wife, Phyllis G. Baron, in providing educational guidance and help with the organizational and editorial process. Indispensable administrative and secretarial help by our co-workers, especially Abbie Flood, Estella Hernandez, Charlene Huff, Louese McKerlie, Catherine Morrison, Linda Roberts, and Joyce Sabados, deserves grateful recognition. Audrey Hart, Hillary Heard, and Joanne Rose helped prepare the glossary.

Samuel Baron, MD

LIST OF REVIEWERS

L. J. Berry, PhD
University of Texas at Austin

S. H. Black, PhD
Texas A & M University
College of Medicine

Harold J. Blumenthal, PhD
Loyola University of Chicago
Stritch School of Medicine

Michael P. Cancro, PhD
University of Pennsylvania
School of Medicine

Gary Cashon, PhD
Philadelphia College of Osteopathic Medicine

Nyles Charon, PhD
West Virginia University
School of Medicine

James D. Folds, PhD
University of North Carolina at Chapel Hill
School of Medicine

Richard Fox, PhD
American University

Dolores Furtado, PhD
University of Kansas Medical Center
School of Medicine

Donald Heyneman, PhD
University of California, San Francisco
School of Medicine

Ted Johnson, PhD
St. Olaf College

Maurice Lefford, PhD
Wayne State University
School of Medicine

Alan Liss, PhD
State University of New York at Binghamton

Malcolm C. Modrzakowski, PhD
Ohio University

Paul C. Montgomery, PhD
Wayne State University
School of Medicine

Frederick L. Moolten, MD
Boston University
School of Medicine

Donald V. Moore, PhD
Southwestern Medical School
University of Texas
Health Science Center at Dallas

Richard S. Panush, MD
University of Florida
College of Medicine

Dianna Roberts, PhD
University of Texas at San Antonio

Leon T. Rosenberg, PhD
Stanford University

Gerald Schiffman, PhD
State University of New York
Downstate Medical Center
College of Medicine

William A. Summers, PhD
Indiana University
School of Medicine

Lucy Treagan, PhD
University of San Francisco

I

PRINCIPLES OF IMMUNOLOGY

Introduction

Jan Cerny, MD, PhD

Immunology is the study of the immune system and the immune mechanisms that have developed in the course of *evolution* to preserve the integrity of the body. The immune system protects an organism against invasion by foreign bodies—namely, microbial agents and their toxic products. The vital importance of immunity is best documented in cases of hereditary or acquired immune defects, because individuals with such defects die of multiple opportunistic infections. The other side of the coin is that the immune defense itself may have pathologic consequences because allergies, inflammatory tissue damage, and autoimmune diseases can result from the ongoing battle between the immune system and an invading agent. The efficiency of the immune system, as well as the balance between its protective and pathogenic effects, is influenced greatly by the individual makeup of the genes that regulate the immune response.

The substances to which the immune system responds are called **antigens.** An infectious agent such as virus may have a number of antigens. A molecule of antigen carries smaller, distinct **antigenic determinants** (also called **epitopes**). The immune system deals with antigens by using two kinds of interwoven mechanisms, specific and nonspecific.

The **specific** mechanisms begin with recognition of antigenic determinants by specific receptors on lymphocytes. The receptors on the B lymphocytes are immunoglobulin molecules (Ig); on the T lymphocytes, they are Iglike molecules. Each lymphocyte has receptors for only one epitope, which fits the receptor like a key into a lock. Lymphocytes that bear receptors for the same epitope compose an **immunologic clone.** Each clone reacts to its corresponding antigen by cell proliferation (clonal expansion) and functional differentiation. A human body may have cells with receptors for more than 10^7 epitopes. Many of these receptors recognize certain antigens within the body (i.e., self). The recognition of self-substances by the immune system is as important as the recognition of foreign antigens because it allows cooperation, regulation, and surveillance among the cells of the body.

The **nonspecific** immune mechanisms deal with all antigens regardless of their epitopes. The main nonspecific immune components are **phagocytes,** which engulf and destroy the infectious agents; **complement,** a system of enzymes that can be activated to attack foreign substances; and hormonelike substances called **lymphokines** and **monokines,** which are released by cells of the immune system in response to an antigen and which represent a functional communication system among the immune cells. Specific and nonspecific immune mechanisms are equally important; one cannot operate optimally without the other.

The harmonious action of the complex immune system in defense to an infectious agent is illustrated in Figure 1. Phagocytes (2) function as a first-line defense against foreign antigens (1). They also process the antigens and present the epitopes to the specific receptor-bearing B and T lymphocytes (3). Some **T lymphocytes** respond to the antigen by differentiation into **regulator cells** that help (4) or suppress (5) the actions of other branches of the immune reaction. Help and suppression are balanced according to the needs of the response. Other T cells become effector cells, which are responsible for the **cell-mediated** branch of the immune response that involves the cytotoxic T cells (6) (which specifically destroy body cells infected with the antigen) and the delayed hypersensitivity T cells (7) (which further activate phagocytic cells to kill microbes).

On the other hand, the **B lymphocytes** are responsible for the humoral branch of the immune response, which involves the production of **antibody** (8) (that is, immunoglobulin molecules secreted into circulation). Antibody is a powerful, specific effector mechanism. It may inactivate the antigen by neutralizing its infectivity (as with viruses) or toxicity (as with microbial toxin), and by removing the antigen from the system (9).

Both types of lymphocytes retain **immunologic memory** for the antigen (8). Thus, a second encounter with the same antigen results in a much faster and more vigorous (**secondary**) response.

In the final stage of the response, the specific effector T cells and the antibody activate and amplify various nonspecific accessory mechanisms that actually eliminate the foreign invader. The activated T cells use a variety of soluble factors (**lymphokines**) to activate macrophages for killing the ingested invader (10), to activate natural killer cells (11), and to increase the resistance of cells to virus infections (**interferon;** 12).

The antibody binds to the antigen, and the resulting complex is much more avidly phagocytosed (**opsonization**) than the free antigen (13). The antibody also binds to antigen on cell surfaces, which allows the antibody-dependent cytotoxic cells (14) (a variant of normal killer cells) to attack and destroy the infected cell. Activation of **complement** (15) by antigen–antibody complexes has many consequences in addition to the most obvious, cytolysis. The antibody also binds nonspecifically to **basophils** and **mast cells,** and when such "armed" cells encounter antigen, they release a number of biologically active substances (for example, histamine) that participate in the defense against infection (16).

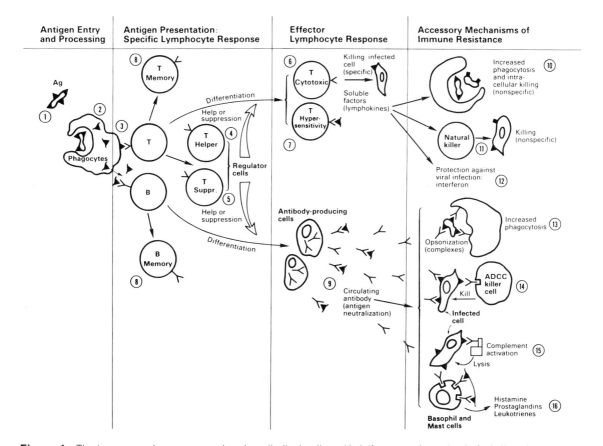

Figure 1. The immune system response to a hypothetical antigen (Ag) (for example, a virus). **1.** Antigen bearing an epitope ▲. **2.** Processing of antigen to fragments. **3.** Presentation of Ag to T cells (on the phagocyte surface) and B cells (free antigenic pieces). Regulator T cells help **(4)** or suppress **(5)** both B and T effector responses. **6.** Ag-specific cytotoxic (killer) T cells. **7.** T cells responsible for delayed hypersensitivity and resistance to microbes. **8.** Some lymphocytes (both T and B) activated by antigen differentiate into a long-lived pool of memory cells responsible for rapid, secondary response to the same antigen. **9.** Antibody (Ab) combines with antigen (neutralization, elimination). Products of T cells activate macrophages for killing of ingested microbes **(10)** and natural killer cells **(11)** for nonspecific cytotoxicity against tumor cells and virus-infected cells. **12.** Interferons are produced for protection of body cells against virus infection. **13.** Complexing of antibody with antigen (opsonization) increases the engulfment of the antigen by phagocytes. **14.** Binding of antibody to infected target cells activates the antibody-dependent cytotoxic cell (ADCC). **15.** Complement (C) enzymatic cascade is activated by antigen-antibody complex (in this case, the antigen is on the cell surface). **16.** Antibody binds to Ig receptors on basophils and mast cells.

Immunology has provided medicine with powerful preventive, therapeutic, and diagnostic tools. Specific immunization and blood transfusion still remain the best examples; however, immunology is moving rapidly into other areas of medicine because of the progress in basic immunology that has produced a better understanding of immune mechanisms. The prevention of fetal erythroblastosis, the advances in tissue transplantation, and the intervention with tumors are only a few examples of medical accomplishments that depend upon research in immunology. By the time you read this introduction, a battle with a hitherto unknown disease, the acquired immunodeficiency syndrome (AIDS), will probably be won or well advanced, an example of how immunology and virology together can overcome a new disease through an increase in basic knowledge of the immune system. We hope that the immunology section of this book will not only teach you the fundamentals of immunology, but will also ignite your interest in this fascinating medical and biological science.

1

Antibody (Immunoglobulin) Structure

Thomas J. Kindt, PhD

General Concepts
Immunoglobulin Classification
   Isotypes
   Allotypes
   Idiotypes
Immunoglobulin Structural Studies
Conclusion

General Concepts

Within the body of a normal individual is a diverse group of molecules called **antibodies, or immunoglobulins.** These molecules can bind to the numerous foreign substances (**antigens**) the individual may encounter in his or her lifetime. As free molecules in the blood, antibodies mediate humoral immunity. As molecules in the plasma membrane of B lymphocytes, antibodies serve as antigen receptors (see Chapter 4). Structural studies of antibody have revealed the molecular architecture that enables the antibodies to perform these functions. The basic structure of immunoglobulin molecules, the nature of the variations in this structure, and the relationship between the structure and the function of the antibody molecule are discussed in this chapter.

The complexity of the humoral immune system is illustrated by the fact that an individual can produce antibody molecules that bind nearly every class of chemical substance or microorganism. It is estimated that at least 1 million distinct binding functions can be synthesized in any individual. This immense diversity (the **antibody repertoire**) ensures that antibodies against virtually any invading pathogen will be

5

produced. In order to destroy or thwart the invader, the antibody may act alone or interact with several other molecular and cellular immune systems.

Several general terms are used in discussing antibody or immunoglobulin structure. The term **immunoglobulin** (abbreviated **Ig**) designates the entire group of immune molecules. **γ-globulin** may be used synonymously with immunoglobulin and, at other times, may be used specifically to designate the single immunoglobulin class, IgG.

This ambiguous notation comes from early studies in which most antigen-binding activity was associated with the serum proteins that migrated in the gamma electrophoretic region. Therefore, although IgG is the only true γ-globulin, the term is still sometimes used to mean all classes of antibodies. Although the term *antibody* is often used interchangeably with immunoglobulin, it is more properly reserved for situations in which the binding specificity of the molecules is known (for example, antirabies antibody or, less specifically, antiviral antibody).

All immunoglobulin molecules have the same basic structure, consisting of two pairs of polypeptide chains: the **heavy, or H, chains** are 440 to 550 amino acid molecules in length, and the **light, or L, chains** are about 220 amino acid molecules long. Figure 1-1 depicts a generalized Ig molecule. The H chain has one or more carbohydrate units associated with it, whereas the L chain is generally free of carbohydrate units. The chains are covalently linked to each other by disulfide bridges that form between cysteine molecules. The H chains are held together by one or more bonds; each L chain is bound to an H chain. Thus, the fundamental structure of the Ig molecule may be denoted by the formula, H_2L_2. In addition, there are regularly occurring intrachain disulfide bridges that allow the chains to be divided into repeating units of about 110 residues called **domains.** The L chains consist of two domains and the H chains of four or five, depending on the **isotype.** As we shall see later, the domain structures represent the specific sites where the antibody molecule binds antigen (the first domain of the heavy and light chain), fixes complement (the penultimate domain of the heavy chain), and arms certain cells (the terminal domain of the heavy chain).

Certain immunoglobulins occur normally in the blood serum as oligomers that consist of several of the basic four-chain units. These oligomers are created by joining

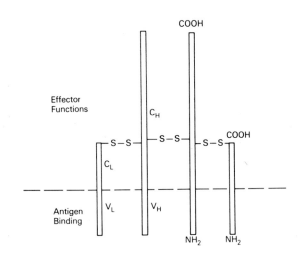

Figure 1-1 Generalized immunoglobulin molecule showing basic four-chain structure. The two long heavy (H) chains in the middle are flanked by two shorter light (L) chains. Each is composed of variable (V) and constant (C) regions. $H = V_H + C_H$. $L = V_L + C_L$.

Table 1-1   Molecular Characteristics of Human Immunoglobulin

Class or Subclass*		Structure	Mol. Wt.	Serum Half Life (days)	Adult Serum Level (mg/mL)
IgG 1	γ_4		146,000	21	9†
2	γ_2	$(\gamma_2 L_2)$	146,000	20	2.5
3	γ_3		170,000	7	1
4	γ_4		146,000	21	0.4
IgM§	μ	$(\mu_2 L_2)_5 J$	970,000	10	0.6–2.0
IgA 1	$\alpha 1$	$(\alpha_2 L_2)$	160,000	6	1.0–4.5
2	$\alpha 2$		160,000	6	
sIgA§		$(\alpha_2 L_2)_2 SJ$	385,000	—	—
IgD	δ	$(\delta_2 L_2)$	184,000	3	0.05
IgE	ϵ	$(\epsilon_2 L_2)$	185,000	2	0.003

*The greek letters are used to denote class or H chain; for example, IgM H chain may be called μ chain.
†Total IgG concentration may range from 8 to 18 mg/mL in a normal adult. The subclasses comprise relatively stable proportions of this value.
§IgM and sIgA include the J chain (○) (mol. wt. 15,000) designated J, and sIgA also contains the secretory component (mol. wt. 70,000) designated S.

the terminal domain of the H chains with a small protein, the **J chain.** (The J protein is not to be confused with the J segment involved in the Ig gene structure (see discussion that follows). For example, IgM occurs as a pentamer containing five H_2L_2 units (Table 1-1). IgA in serum has the basic H_2L_2 structure, but **secretory IgA,** which is found in milk, saliva and other secretions (see Chapter 10), occurs as a dimer consisting of two such units plus a **secretory piece.**

Figure 1-1 shows that each chain of the immunoglobulin molecule can be divided into two regions: the part above the dotted line is called the **constant, or C, region** and the portion below the line is called the **variable, or V, region.** This division calls attention to the fact that antibodies are bifunctional molecules that carry out two interrelated operations. First, the V region binds the antigen; second, the C region carries out effector functions. Effector functions include: complement fixation, binding to specific cells that release chemical substances, and signaling to phagocytic cells to engulf the antigen-antibody complex. The various functions are carried out by specialized portions of the Ig molecule called **domains** (Figure 1-2).

Immunoglobulin Classification

Immunoglobulins (Ig) are complex proteins that bear a number of antigenic determinants. These determinants are defined by specific antisera that are raised by the immunization of appropriate animals with purified Ig. These anti-Ig antisera are then used to classify Ig into groups according to their shared determinants, which in fact represent shared molecular structures. Three categories of determinants are used: isotypes, allotypes, and idiotypes.

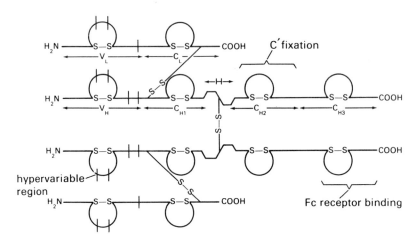

Figure 1-2 Immunoglobulin model showing the actual domain structure. The V_H/V_L domains contain the hypervariable regions (Figure 1-5) of antigen-binding site. The constant region domains (C_L and C_{H1-3}) are the sites for various effector functions such as complement (C') fixation (C_{H2}) and Fc receptor binding (C_{H3}).

Isotypes

Isotypes are the determinants that characterize the Ig molecules within each Ig class (five isotypes: IgM, IgD, IgG, IgE, and IgA). Isotypes are defined by unique antigenic determinants (molecular structure) associated with the C region of the H chains (C_H) of an Ig molecule. Thus, there are five H chain types corresponding to the five immunoglobulin classes: μ for IgM, δ for IgD, γ for IgG, ϵ for IgE, and α for IgA. Isotypes are shared by all individuals within a species, because each species utilizes a single genetic locus to encode each C_H region.

Each Ig class has distinguishing characteristics, and each is involved in a different facet of immunity. Response to an antigen usually follows an ordered sequence of isotype expression. The majority of antibodies directed against the antigen may be initially of the IgM class, but this will shift (through the process of **class switching**) to IgG, IgE, or IgA in the maturation phase of the response. The specificity of the antibody is precisely maintained during the switch by retention of the same V_H region and the same light chain. Although isotypes are defined serologically, they can readily be differentiated by physical and chemical procedures. Table 1-1 lists the classes of human immunoglobulins, and the molecular properties of each class.

IgG and IgM are the major components found in the circulation, whereas IgA is found in higher concentrations in saliva, milk, and secretions from mucosal surfaces. IgG is the most abundant immunoglobulin and may be present in the serum of healthy adults at levels up to 18 mg/mL. The least abundant species is IgE, the antibody involved in allergic reactions (**immediate hypersensitivity**); this immunoglobulin is present in serum at levels of about 0.003 mg/mL. Little is known about the primary function of IgD, which is present on surface membranes of B lymphocytes.

Some immunoglobulin classes may be further divided into subclasses. For example, in humans IgG occurs in four distinct forms. The most abundant of these subclasses,

IgG$_1$, comprises 70% of the IgG found in the circulation of a normal individual; the least abundant, IgG$_4$, makes up less than 3% of the total IgG. These subclasses, which can be differentiated by both serologic and structural techniques, also differ in functional properties, such as the ability to fix complement. IgA in the human also occurs in two distinct forms or subclasses. Table 1-2 lists biologic properties of the human Ig classes and subclasses.

There are two L chain isotypes, κ and λ, as well. Each isotype is determined by the C region of the L chain (C$_L$). L chain isotypes do not determine the class of an Ig molecule; that is, any Ig isotype may be associated with either κ or λ L chains. In the human, approximately 60% of all Ig molecules contain κ L chains and 40% contain λ L chains.

Allotypes

Allotypes are antigenic determinants present in some, but not all, individuals of an animal species. In other words, allotypes reflect genetically determined antigenic differences among immunoglobulins of the same isotype within a given species. Allotypic determinants are encoded by allelic forms of the C region gene segments that determine each Ig class. Thus, isotypic determinants identify the similarities between the genes specifying each Ig class, whereas allotypic determinants identify the differences between homologous C region gene segments (**alleles**). Allotypes are inherited as autosomal codominant alleles.

The principal allotypic groups in the human are the Gm markers, present on the H chain, and the Km (formerly Inv) markers, found on L chains. Allotypes have been valuable probes in studies of the genetic basis of antibody synthesis; for example, early allotype analysis determined that H and L chains are not genetically linked. Because allotypes represent allelic forms of the genes encoding the C region of the Ig chains, they have been employed as genetic markers in population studies. The presence of certain closely linked combinations of allotypes, called **haplotypes,** can characterize certain ethnic groups. The frequency of particular haplotypes within a population may be used to deduce migrations or the genetic relatedness among populations. Allotypes are not useful in determining paternity, because they lack the complexity of the blood group or the histocompatibility antigens.

Allotypes of experimental animals are detected by antisera raised by intraspecies injection of Igs. In the human, allotypic antisera are obtained from multiparous women

TABLE 1-2   Levels of Variation in Immunoglobulins

Variation	Examples	Occurrence
Isotype	Classes (IgG, IgA, etc.) L chain types (κ, λ)	All members of species
Allotype	Gm types on H chains Inv types on L chains	Some but not all members of species
Idiotype	V region of specific antibody (e.g., anti-A) of one individual	Single individual or genetically related group

whose Ig allotypes do not match those of their mates or from individuals who have received multiple blood transfusions.

Idiotypes

Idiotypes are unique determinants of specific antibody molecules. They are located on the V region of the antibody molecule, near or at the site that binds to the antigen. Idiotypes are generally thought to be created by the conformation of the V regions of the associated H and L chains (V_H and V_L). As an individual may synthesize many thousands of different V_H and V_L regions, the number of idiotypes that may be produced is immense, a reflection of the antibody repertoire. For this reason, idiotypes are often used to identify specific families of antibody (molecules bearing identical V_H and V_L regions but not necessarily identical C regions).

The term *idiotype* was coined by Oudin to identify a unique antigenic structure(s) shared by those antibody molecules of a single individual that were specific for a particular antigen. These determinants were discovered using intraspecies immunization of allotype-matched rabbits with antibodies of defined specificity. The resulting antisera (*antibody against antibody*) reacted with only the specific antibody used for immunization; that is, they were anti-idiotypic antisera. Similar studies with human myeloma proteins (identical Ig molecules produced by a malignant plasmacyte clone) demonstrated that the potential number of idiotypes present in any individual was vast, on the order of 10^6. It was also soon determined that antibodies with identical allotypic and isotypic markers could have entirely different idiotypes.

The most direct proof of the intimate relationship between the idiotype and the combining site was demonstrated when anti-idiotypic antisera (antibodies that specifically recognize and bind the idiotypic determinant) were used to block the antigen-combining site (the region defined by the V_H/V_L dimer). Only anti-idiotypic antibody inhibited antigen binding; antibodies specific for allotype or isotype were ineffective.

Early studies using rabbit antibodies directed against streptococcal carbohydrates indicated that idiotypes were inherited; more recent data, mainly from studies of antibodies in inbred mouse strains, have shown the genetic linkage of idiotypes to H chain allotypes (the molecular basis of this linkage will be explained later). It should be emphasized that even in genetically identical individuals (for example, twins or inbred mice), the antibody response to a particular antigen is unlikely to be idiotypically identical. Idiotypes that are produced by most members of a genetically restricted population are referred to as **cross-reactive** or **public idiotypes** (**IdX**). Those found in a very few individuals are referred to as **individual** or **private idiotypes** (**IdI**). The molecular architecture that defines an idiotype cannot be defined simply. Idiotypic determinants represent the tertiary structure of the V_H and V_L dimer; frequently, several similar but nonidentical amino acid sequences will produce serologically identical IdXs. This is in contrast to isotypes and allotypes that are based simply on different amino acid sequences.

Immunoglobulin Structural Studies

In early studies of antibody structure, proteolytic digestions were used to cleave the antibody molecule; the fragments were separated and their activities studied. The enzyme papain cleaved the molecule into a fragment that crystallized upon standing (**Fc**)

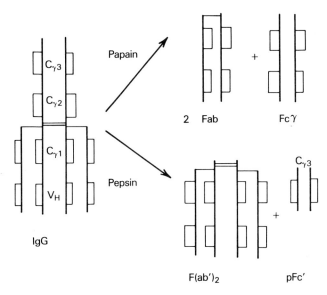

Figure 1-3 Cleavage of IgG with the proteolytic enzymes, papain or pepsin. The Fab fragment has antigen binding properties and Fc contains sites of effector function. Prolonged cleavage with papain will produce an additional cleavage between the γ_2 and γ_3 domains. The pepsin fragment pFc' includes residues 333 to the carboxy terminus (residues 440); the remainder of the molecule ($C_{\gamma 2}$ domain) is digested to small peptides by pepsin.

and another soluble fragment that included the L chains and had antigen-binding activity (**Fab**). Similar, but not identical, cleavage of the antibody molecule may be accomplished using pepsin proteolysis (Figure 1-3).

Because immunoglobulins, even within a given class or subclass, comprise a group of molecules directed against a multitude of different antigens, obtaining sufficient amounts of a single antibody from a normal individual to carry out detailed studies on amino acid sequence used to be difficult or impossible. This difficulty was circumvented by using immunoglobulins that occur in high concentrations in the serum of patients with multiple myeloma or related lymphoproliferative diseases. These proteins are the products of single clones of B cells and bind a single antigen, the identity of which may not be known. The electrophoretic pattern produced by serum from a myeloma patient is compared to normal serum in Figure 1-4.

The availability of such human myeloma molecules made it possible to unravel the structural details of the immunoglobulins. Myeloma proteins have also occurred in dogs, cats, and rats and have been experimentally induced in certain inbred mouse strains. An alternative successful means for obtaining homogeneous antibodies in species that do not produce myeloma proteins has been hyperimmunization with certain bacterial vaccines.

Another recently described method for producing homogeneous antibodies involves production of antibody-secreting cell lines by fusion of mouse myeloma cells to B lymphocytes obtained from an immunized mouse. The resulting cells, called **hybridomas,** can supply virtually unlimited supplies of monoclonal antibodies; their use is revolutionizing the field of immunology.

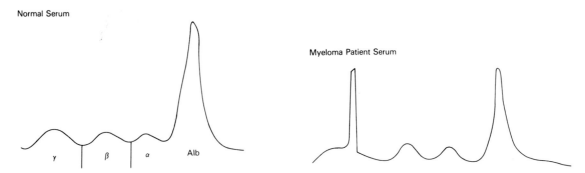

Figure 1-4 Electrophoretic analyses of normal serum and serum from patient with multiple myeloma. The homogeneous Ig (M-component) depicted here is of the IgG class.

Amino acid sequence studies of the homogeneous immunoglobulins obtained from humans quickly led to exciting findings. These studies showed that immunoglobulin light chains could be differentiated into constant and variable regions based on their primary structure. The amino terminal regions were found to vary considerably in amino acid sequence, whereas the carboxyl terminal portions of the light chains studied were similar in structure. In addition to the obvious correlation of these structural data to the known functions of the different regions of the antibody molecule, this information also gave rise to speculation on the nature of antibody genes. Two genes were postulated to be responsible for synthesis of a single polypeptide chain: a single gene encoding the constant region could interact with any one of a number of genes encoding one of numerous variable regions. This postulated deviation from classical genetic concepts was supported by studies of immunoglobulin allotypes and was recently verified by studies on the structure of immunoglobulin genes. These studies, carried out at the DNA level, have shown that the original two-gene–one-polypeptide-chain hypothesis is approximately correct and that several genes interact to encode the complete Ig chain.

As amino acid sequence data became available for a number of antibody-variable regions, a striking pattern began to emerge: certain amino acid residues within the V regions of both H and L chains showed far more variability than other residues; the residues exhibiting this extreme variability were clustered in several discrete groups, now called **hypervariable regions.** Figure 1-5 shows the location of the hypervariable regions in human H and L chains. These regions participate in antigen binding and provide much of the structural basis for idiotypic determinants. Variations in these

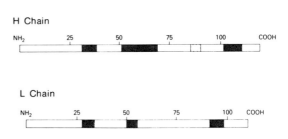

Figure 1-5 Hypervariable regions within V regions of human H and L chains are shown in black.

regions give rise to molecules capable of binding the multitude of antigens that have been tested in various natural and experimental circumstances.

Figure 1-6 depicts a simplified series of steps in the biosynthesis of an immunoglobulin L chain starting with the gene. The gene for the Ig chain exists in the genome as several separate DNA sequences (**coding segments**), each encoding some portion of the chain. The genomic sequences that encode proteins that are expressed are called **exons.** The DNA sequences that separate the coding segments are called *intervening sequences* or **introns.** The altered arrangement of exons, observed in the differentiated cell that produces an immunoglobulin chain, places the V region gene contiguous with the J gene and close to but not adjoining the C gene. The rearranged DNA is first directly transcribed into nuclear RNA, which maintains the complete rearranged sequence. A *splicing out* step then occurs to form the messenger RNA (**mRNA**), which is translated into the Ig chain. Before secretion, the Ig chain loses the hydrophobic NH_2 terminal portion encoded by the gene fragment designated L (**leader**).

Although H chain synthesis proceeds by the same general pathway as that of the L chain, there are several additional elements involved. First, in the synthesis of variable regions there is an additional gene segment designated D. The V_H region is therefore the product of interaction among V, D, and J segments. In addition to diversity gained by

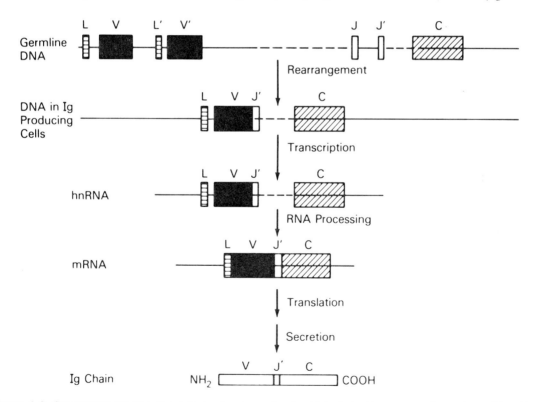

Figure 1-6 Generalized scheme of events leading to synthesis of IgL chain. V gene encodes amino acid residues 1–100; the J gene, residues 101–110; and the C gene, residues 111–220. L gene encodes a hydrophobic peptide that is removed from NH_2 terminus of chain before secretion.

flexibility in the use of 10 or more D segments, there is the further possibility of **junctional diversity** at the V-D and D-J interfaces. Junctional diversity occurs when the D-J and V-D joining mechanisms do not precisely splice the joined gene segments. Even when two cells join the same V and D segments, the coding sequence of the two resulting V genes could differ as the recombination mechanisms often introduce or delete nucleotides at these junctions.

Note that the first two hypervariable regions are encoded by the V_H and V_L gene segments. In V_L, the third hypervariable region is defined by the junctional diversity produced by the V-J interface, whereas in V_H the third and fourth hypervariable regions are formed by the V-D and D-J joinings, respectively. X-ray crystallographic studies indicate that the tertiary structure of the Ig molecule is such that the V region folds to produce a kind of pocket. This pocket is lined with the amino acids comprising the four V_H and three V_L hypervariable regions. Each particular combination of hypervariable regions thus produces a unique antigen-combining site.

A second feature of H chains is the process of class switching; that is, the appearance of the same antigen-combining site (or idiotype) on Ig molecules of different isotypes. This occurs when the VDJ gene complex is rearranged en bloc to a position adjacent to any of the C_H gene segments (the order of C_H genes in the human is $5'$ — μ/δ, γ_3, γ_1, γ_2, γ_4, ϵ, and α — $3'$). The initial gene rearrangement always brings the VDJ complex proximal to the μ/δ locus. Later rearrangements may join the VDJ complex to any C_H gene $3'$ to its location.

Third, the exon structure of all C_H genes encodes for two alternative carboxy-terminal sequences, one representing the secreted form of the Ig and the other the membrane-bound form. Membrane-bound Ig molecules are slightly longer than their secreted counterparts, as they terminate in hydrophobic transmembrane and cytoplasmic amino acids. Cells produce secreted or membrane-bound forms of Ig by either splicing out the membrane exon from the mRNA (produces secreted Ig) or retaining it (membrane-bound Ig).

Conclusion

The immunoglobulin molecule performs two basic roles: binding to an antigen and initiating a process aimed at eliminating or destroying the antigen. The binding function requires tremendous diversity in Ig structure, and this is generated by variations within defined regions of the variable portion of the molecule. The elimination/destruction function is accomplished by a small number of structures within the constant regions of the Ig molecule.

Evidence indicates that different H chain classes use the same variable regions, thereby economizing in the amount of genetic information needed to produce a large variety of antibodies. Furthermore, at least one hypervariable region of the H and L chains is encoded by small, separate gene segments (J and D genes), which can interact in different combinations to synthesize numerous variants of the variable region. Thus, the observed diversity in immunoglobulins appears to be generated, at least in part, by combinations involving a limited number of interacting structures: random associations of light chains with heavy chains, various assortments of variable regions with J or D region segments, the junctional diversity created by these interchain associations, and the effect of mutation on any of the involved genes.

Questions concerning the precise number of V region genes in an individual's genome and the role of somatic mutations in diversification of the genes are yet to be answered.

References

Capra, J.D., Kehoe, J.M.: Hypervariable regions, idiotypy and the antibody combining site. In: *Advances in Immunology*. Dixon F, Kunkel HG (editors): New York: Academic Press, 1975.

Fudenberg, H.H., Pink, J.R.L., Wang, A.C., Douglas, S.D.: *Basic Immunogenetics,* 2nd ed. New York: Oxford University Press, 1978.

Glynn, L.E., Steward, M.W. (editors): *Immunochemistry: An Advanced Textbook*. London: John Wiley and Sons, 1977.

Honjo, T.: Immunology genes. *Ann Rev Immunol* 1983; 1:499.

Kabat, E.A.: *Structural Concepts in Immunology and Immunochemistry,* 2nd ed. New York: Holt, Rinehart, and Winston, 1976.

Kennett, R.H., McKearn, T.J., Bechtol, K.B. (editors): *Monoclonal Antibodies: Hybridomas: A New Dimension in Biological Analysis*. New York: Plenum Press, 1980.

Kindt, T.J., Capra, J.D.: *The Antibody Enigma*. New York: Plenum Press, 1984.

Kunkel, H.G., Kindt, T.J.: Allotypes and idiotypes. In: *Immunogenetics and Immunodeficiency*. Benacerraf B (editor). Baltimore: University Park Press, 1975.

Natvig, J.B., Kunkel, H.G.: Human immunoglobulins: Classes, subclasses, genetic variants and idiotypes. In: *Advances in Immunology*. Dixon F, Kunkel HG (editors). New York: Academic Press, 1973.

Putnam, F.W.: *The Plasma Proteins,* Vol 3, 2nd ed. New York: Academic Press, 1977.

Weigert, M., et al: The joining of V and J gene segments creates antibody diversity. *Nature* 1980; 283:497.

2 The Major Histocompatibility Complex

Jan Klein, PhD

General Concepts
MHC Genes and Products
Immune Regulation
MHC-Related Diseases
Tissue Transplantation

General Concepts

Three principal types of genetic relationship can exist between two individuals:

1. **Syngeneic,** in which two individuals are genetically identical (monozygotic twins or mice of the same inbred strain)

2. **Allogeneic,** in which two individuals are genetically dissimilar but belong to the same species (two human beings or two wild mice)

3. **Xenogeneic,** in which two individuals are not only genetically dissimilar but also belong to two different species (a cat and a mouse)

In the allogeneic situation, the genetic difference is transcribed and translated into gene products that differentiate the two individuals biochemically. The major histocompatibility complex (MHC) antigens are those gene products which have a strong (major) effect on the incompatibility of tissues transplanted between allogeneic individuals. Each species has an MHC; human MHC is called the human leukocyte antigen (HLA) complex. The MHC antigens are involved in the regulation of the immune response. For the immune response to occur, antigens must be presented to the lymphocytes in context (association) with MHC products, since the collaboration between lymphocytes is based partially on recognition of these products on the cell surface. Because of their role in the control of immune response, the MHC genes have been called immune response (Ir) genes. Certain diseases are more likely to occur in individuals who carry certain HLA antigens.

MHC Genes and Products

The first step in a specific immune response is the recognition of an antigen by a T lymphocyte. This recognition occurs only if the antigen is offered to the T lymphocyte by a specialized cell, the **antigen-presenting cell (APC)**, in the context of a specialized molecule, the **major histocompatibility complex (MHC)** molecule. T lymphocytes have dual specificity in that they recognize simultaneously the foreign antigen (nonself) and the organism's own MHC molecule (self). It also can be said that the specificity of T lymphocytes is *restricted* by self MHC molecules.

The MHC has a strong (major) effect on the incompatibility of tissues transplanted between genetically disparate individuals. This effect occurs because different individuals often express different MHC molecules, which then act as antigens and trigger an allograft reaction responsible for the rejection of the transplanted tissues. **Minor histocompatibility (H) antigens** also can elicit allograft reaction, but they are not related to the MHC and their effect is weaker than that of the MHC antigens. The involvement of MHC molecules in the allograft reaction probably has nothing to do with their true function, which is to provide a context for antigen recognition, and such involvement is observed only in artificial situations in which transplantation is performed.

The name of the MHC varies according to species. In humans, it is called the **human leukocyte antigen (HLA) complex;** in mice (which are used often in MHC studies), it is referred to as the **histocompatibility-2 (H-2) complex** (all of the other mouse histocompatibility systems—*H-1, H-3, H-4*—are minor). Most of the MHC genes are located in a single region on chromosome 6 in humans and on chromosome 17 in mice. The MHC genes can be divided into two classes, which differ in their organization and function. **Class I genes** code for polypeptide chains that are each about 350 amino acids long and that have a molecular weight of about 39,000 daltons. Each chain has one or two carbohydrate side-chains, and the entire glycoprotein has a molecular weight of approximately 44,000 daltons. The polypeptide can be divided into five domains: three extracellular (α1 through α3) domains; one that spans the plasma membrane (the transmembrane domain); and one that protrudes into the cytoplasm (the cytoplasmic domain) (Figure 2-1). The domains are encoded in six to eight exons that are separated by intervening sequences (Figure 2-2). The third external domain (α3) associates noncovalently with a short polypeptide, β_2-**microglobulin**, which is controlled by a gene outside the MHC region (on chromosome 15 in humans and chromosome 2 in mice). Both the α3 domain and the β_2-microglobulin show structural homology with one domain of the immunoglobulin heavy-chain constant region.

The **class II polypeptide** chains are of two kinds, α and β, which have similar overall organization but differ in their primary structure. The chains consist of three to

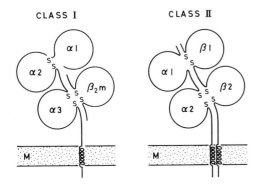

Figure 2-1 The domain organization of class I and class II MHC molecules.

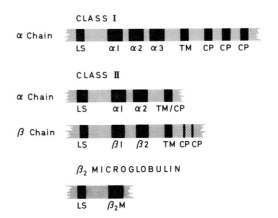

Figure 2-2 The exon-intron organization of the MHC genes. LS, leader sequence; TM, transmembrane region; CP, intracytoplasmic region.

five domains: two extracellular (α_1, α_2 and β_1, β_2), one transmembrane, and one or two cytoplasmic (see Figure 2-1). The α chains are about 230 and the β chains about 240 amino acids long, and each chain contains one or two carbohydrate side-chains. The molecular weights of the α and β glycoproteins are approximately 34,000 and 28,000 daltons, respectively. The domain organization of class II resembles that of the class I chains, except for the one extra external domain in class I chains. In the plasma membrane, one α chain associates noncovalently with one β chain. The α_2 and β_2 domains are structurally homologous to a constant domain of the immunoglobulin molecule.

The MHC consists of some 30 to 40 genes. About 36 class I and 8 class II genes exist in mice (Figure 2-3), humans have fewer class I but more class II genes (about 20). Only some of these genes are functional; others are either defective **pseudogenes** or they have no demonstrable function. The functional human class I genes are referred to as A, B, and C; the functional mouse class I genes are K, D, and L. The functional mouse class II genes are A_α, A_β and E_α, E_β. In humans, the situation with class II genes is more complex and not well known; the expressed human class II genes of the D region have been designated DR_α, DR_β, SB_α, SR_β, and DC_α, DC_β (Figure 2-4).

The functional difference between class I and class II molecules is that the class I genes provide the context for the recognition of antigens by cytolytic T lymphocytes that kill their target cells specifically. In contrast, class II molecules provide the context for antigen recognition by regulatory T lymphocytes (helper and suppressor cells that modulate the response of the other T or B lymphocytes).

Products of allelic MHC genes can be distinguished serologically. In mice, immunization of recipients with lymphocytes from MHC-disparate donors leads to the production of MHC-specific antibodies that can be used to kill (in the presence of complement) or to stain donor lymphocytes. The antibodies define individual H-2 **antigenic determinants** (antigens). Some of these determinants (called *public*) are shared by different mouse strains, whereas others (*private*) are restricted to strains with a

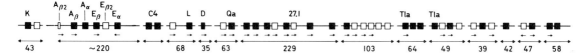

Figure 2-3 The genes of the mouse H-2 complex. Full rectangles represent expressed genes, empty rectangles nonexpressed genes or pseudogenes. Arrows indicate direction of transcription; numbers indicate the length of the segments in kilobase pairs. Breaks in the connecting line indicate that the segments have not yet been joined at the molecular level.

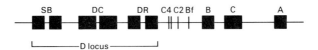

Figure 2-4 Some of the genes of the human HLA complex.

particular *H-2* haplotype. In humans, HLA-specific antibodies arise as a result of multiple blood transfusions, multiple pregnancies, or immunization. Antisera from any of these sources contain a multitude of antibodies; thus, to render them reasonably monospecific, some antibodies must be removed by absorption. Antisera produced in different laboratories are compared and evaluated by an international body of investigators, the *Histocompatibility Testing Workshop*, which also assigns tentative and definite designations to the individual determinants (Table 2-1). Antisera that define individual HLA determinants are then used by tissue-typing laboratories to match donors and recipients for organ transplantation. In both mice and humans, these antisera are now gradually being replaced by monoclonal antibodies.

Immune Regulation

Some of the functional class I and class II genes are highly **polymorphic;** that is, they occur in a number of allelic forms carried by different individuals. The polymorphic loci are K, D, A_β, and E_β in mice and A, B, DR_β, SB_β, and DC_β in humans. More than 100 alleles may exist at the K locus and another 100 at the D locus in mice, and they all occur in certain frequencies in natural populations. This extraordinary polymorphism is apparently unique to, and characteristic of, the MHC. Its significance is unclear, but it may represent a way of coping with MHC-associated **nonresponsiveness** to certain antigens. It has been established that certain combinations of antigen and MHC molecules are not recognized by T lymphocytes; thus, an individual carrying the MHC molecules in those combinations (alleles at a particular MHC locus) is unresponsive to the particular antigen. Because the nonresponsiveness depends on the presence of a particular MHC allele, when responders mate with nonresponders the ability to respond segregates in the progeny with the MHC. Outwardly, it appears that special immune response (Ir) genes are linked to the MHC but, in fact, the MHC themselves are the Ir genes.

Table 2-1   HLA Antigenic Determinants

*HLA-A**	*HLA-B*	*HLA-C*	*HLA-D†*
A1	B5	Cw1	Dw1
A2	B7	Cw2	Dw2
A3	B8	Cw3	Dw3
A9	B12	Cw4	Cw4
A10	B13	Cw5	Dw5
A11	B14	Cw6	Cw6
Aw19	B15	Cw7	Cw7
Aw23	B17	Cw8	Dw7
A25	B27		Cw9
A26	B37		Dw10
A28	B40		Dw11
A29	Bw4		DRw1
Aw30	Bw6		DRw2
Aw31	Bw16		DRw3
Aw32	Bw21		DRw4
Aw33	Bw22		DRw5
Aw34	Bw35		DRw6
Aw36	Bw38		DRw7
Aw43	Bw39		DRw8
	Bw41		DRw9
	Bw42		DRw10
	Bw44		
	Bw45		
	Bw46		
	Bw47		
	Bw48		
	Bw49		
	Bw50		
	Bw51		
	Bw52		
	Bw53		
	Bw54		
	Bw55		
	Bw56		
	Bw57		
	Bw58		
	Bw59		
	Bw60		
	Bw61		
	Bw62		
	Bw63		

*w, tentatively identified (workshop) determinants.
†D, determinants defined by mixed lymphocyte reaction; DR, determinants defined by serologic means.

The reasons for nonresponsiveness are not known, but two competing hypotheses are currently being tested. One hypothesis states that, as T lymphocytes express their MHC- and antigen-specific receptors during ontogeny, some of them recognize molecules in the individual's tissues (self molecules) and are functionally inactivated to prevent autoimmune reactions. Some of these inactivated T lymphocytes, however, also may recognize foreign antigens that resemble or mimic certain self molecules. The inactivation therefore creates *blind spots* in the T-cell repertoire of the individual, who is unable to respond to certain foreign antigens. In contrast, the second hypothesis states that MHC molecules interact with the antigen in the antigen-presenting cell and select which antigenic determinant will be offered to the T lymphocyte. In nonresponder individuals, according to this theory, the particular MHC molecule orients the antigen in such a way that the particular determinant remains hidden from the T lymphocyte.

Whatever the explanation, certain MHC molecules produce nonresponsiveness to certain antigens in some individuals, thus rendering them vulnerable to certain pathogens. The polymorphism of the MHC may be the consequence of selection for individuals that have survived past epidemics. Most of the variability responsible for the MHC polymorphism occurs at specific sites in the first external domain ($\alpha1$) and (in the case of class I molecules) in the $\alpha2$ domain.

MHC-Related Diseases

As stated, individuals who express certain MHC alleles are nonresponders to certain antigens; much evidence also indicates that certain diseases occur more often in individuals who carry certain HLA antigens. The most striking example of this association between HLA and disease is that between the HLA-B27 determinant and *ankylosing spondylitis,* an inflammatory disorder that causes stiffening of vertebrae and deformities of the spine. Approximately 90% of Caucasians with this disease carry the B27 determinant; among healthy individuals, the frequency of B27 is only 7%. This 15-fold increase in B27 frequency among patients with ankylosing spondylitis suggests that B27-bearing individuals are significantly more susceptible to the disease than individuals with other HLA determinants. Some of the other diseases that show a strong association with HLA are Reiter's syndrome, acute anterior uveitis, juvenile rheumatoid arthritis, celiac disease, and Graves' disease. The reasons for these associations are not known, although one possibility is that patients are unable to respond immunologically to an important disease-associated antigen because their T-cell repertoire contains a blind spot for the particular combination of that antigen and the HLA molecule.

Tissue Transplantation

The HLA antigens are the major obstacles to successful *organ transplantation.* Organs transplanted to a recipient from a donor with a different HLA are rejected by a complex immunological process called **allograft reaction.** The actual destruction of the graft is initiated primarily by T lymphocytes that recognize the donor HLA antigens as foreign. Three in vitro tests have been developed for monitoring HLA-incompatibility: serological HLA typing, mixed lymphocyte reaction (MLR), and cell-mediated lymphocytotoxicity (CML). Serological HLA typing was described earlier. The MLR occurs when two populations of allogeneic lymphocytes are cocultured in a single dish. The incompatible small lymphocytes are stimulated by the MHC alloantigens to enlarge into blast cells and to divide. Since the division is preceded by a period of DNA synthesis, this activation can be measured by the incorporation of radioactively labeled precursors into DNA. A simple mixing of two cell populations results in a two-way reaction in which both populations respond. To obtain a one-way reaction, the cells in one population must be inactivated by irradiation. The inactivated or **stimulator cells** cannot be activated themselves, but can activate the **responding cell** population. Of the many loci in the MHC, the strongest MLR stimulus is provided by the *A* and *E* loci of the mouse *H-2* complex and by the *D* loci of the human *HLA* system.

In the CML reaction, lymphocytes from a mixed culture are used to lyse target cells that share MHC antigens with the stimulator. The lysis is accomplished by **killer** or **effector cells,** into which some of the stimulated lymphocytes develop after their transformation into blast cells. The reaction is measured by the release of isotope bound in the cytoplasm of the target cells. Although CML also can be generated against antigens other than those controlled by the MHC (minor H antigens, viral antigens, tumor-specific antigens, and membrane-bound haptens), the specificity of such a reaction is restricted by the MHC complex. Cells that present a nonMHC molecule alone cannot generate the CML reaction. In contrast, MHC antigens stimulate strong CML response. The strongest CML is elicited by products of the *K* and *D* loci of the *H-2* complex, and of the *A* and *B* loci of the *HLA* complex.

Closely linked to the MHC of many species are the genes that code for certain components of the complement system (see Chapter 6). Although such genes have no functional or evolutionary relationship with the MHC, some investigators regard them as class III MHC genes.

References

Klein, J.: The major histocompatibility complex of the mouse. *Science* 1979; 203:516–521.

Klein, J.: *Immunology: The Science of Self-Nonself Discrimination.* New York: Wiley, 1982.

Parham, P., Strominger, J. (editors): *Histocompatibility Antigens.* London: Chapman and Hall, 1982.

Svejgaard, A.: *The HLA System.* Basel: Karger, 1979.

3 Cells and Tissues of Immune Responses

George F. Schreiner, MD, PhD

Abul K. Abbas, MD

General Concepts

The immune system consists of a complex mixture of interacting cell types, which include clones of lymphocytes committed to recognizing and responding to foreign antigens, as well as a variety of accessory cells whose primary function is to regulate the growth and maturation of lymphocytes. These cell types can be identified not only by their functions but also by their expression of unique markers. Moreover, lymphocytes and accessory cells are organized morphologically in lymphoid tissues in a manner that is most appropriate for their function. This chapter describes the cells and tissues of the immune system, with particular emphasis on structure-function relationships and the evolution of humoral immunity. The principal cells mentioned are *T lymphocytes, B lymphocytes,* and *accessory cells.* The primary lymphoid tissues discussed are *thymus* and *bone marrow;* the secondary tissues described are the *lymph nodes* and the *spleen.*

Kinetics of Antibody Responses and the Clonal Selection Hypothesis

The study of humoral immunity, defined as the protection against foreign moieties conferred by the production of specific antibodies, constituted the first investigations into the immune system. The most fundamental observation, that of primary and secondary antibody responses, is essentially quite simple.

The primary antibody response encompasses the kinetics of antibody production when an individual is exposed to an antigen for the first time. As seen in Figure 3-1, after a latent period of several days, antibody (largely IgM) with binding specificity to the particular antigen appears in the serum. The antibody level increases exponentially, peaks in 1 to 2 weeks, and then decreases rapidly. If the individual is then reexposed to the same antigen, the secondary antibody response occurs. This response is more rapid, the quantity of antibody produced is much greater, and the peak may be sustained for weeks or months. The secondary antibody response consists largely of IgG molecules; it is specific for the antigen and depends on previous exposure to that antigen. Thus, the response is said to have memory, or to be an **anamestic** response. During the course of the secondary antibody response, a dramatic increase occurs in the affinity of the antibodies for the antigen.

To explain both the anamestic aspects of the immune response and the changes in affinity, Niels Jerne and MacFarlane Burnet independently proposed the **clonal selection** theory of immunity in the 1950s. Since then, clonal selection has emerged as the fundamental principle of cellular immunology. The theory states that an organism contains numerous clones of lymphocytes, each of which is responsive to a unique antigenic determinant by virtue of the expression of a set of unique surface receptors. Administration of an antigen selects the appropriate clone, which responds by proliferating (**clonal expansion**) and differentiating (Figure 3-2). The expanded clone is responsible for immunologic memory; that is, the larger magnitude of the secondary immune response. Moreover, as the antigen is cleared from the circulation, it selects and activates cells with progressively greater affinity, which increases the affinity of antibody in secondary responses. The mammalian immune system has been found to be capable

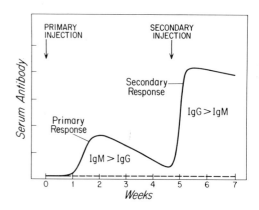

Figure 3-1 The primary and secondary immune response of an animal injected with two doses of the same antigen.

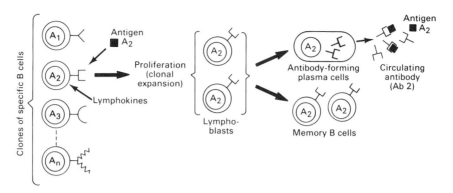

Figure 3-2 Clonal selection of B cells in response to an antigen. The antigen (A_2) binds only to the specific receptor of B lymphocytes of clone A_2; other clones have receptors of different specificities (A_1–A_n). The antigen binding activates the clone A_2 and, with the help from various nonspecific factors (lymphokines produced by other cells), the A_2 cells proliferate (clonal expansion), and differentiate into plasmacytes that produce and release antibodies of the original metabolically active lymphoblasts. Some blasts differentiate into specificity ($Ab_2 \rightarrow Ag_2$) and then die. Other cells of the expanded clone enter the pool of memory B lymphocytes specific for the antigen (A_2).

of producing about 10^7 antibody specifications, but only one in about 10^5 lymphocytes can respond to any one antigenic determinant. The genetic basis for this remarkable diversity, and the cellular events that lead to clonal expansion and differentiation, are discussed in Chapters 1 and 4.

Cells of the Immune Response

The cells that participate in immune responses are the antigen-specific lymphocytes, the nonspecific effector cells, and the accessory cells. Lymphocytes can be divided into two major classes: the B and the T lymphocytes, which are named after their tissue of differentiation (see sections on bone marrow and thymus below).

The **B lymphocyte** is the precursor of the antibody-secreting cell, the plasma cell. The resting B lymphocyte is a small cell (6 to 9 μm in diameter) with scanty cytoplasm surrounding a large, indented nucleus. It is defined by its antigen receptor, a membrane-bound antibody molecule known as surface immunoglobulin. As detailed later, the B cell can express different classes of immunoglobulin on its membrane (according to its state of differentiation or activation), but any individual B cell and its progeny recognize the same, single antigenic determinant.

When B lymphocytes encounter antigen in conjunction with factors released by adjacent T lymphocytes, they divide and become lymphoblasts. Part of the proliferating clone goes on to differentiate into plasma cells, which are a terminal differentiation form of B cells (Figure 3-2). The plasma cells are capable of releasing large quantities of antibody, all of the same specificity as the antigen receptor of the precursor B lymphocyte. They are short-lived and usually die in 7 to 10 days. Other cells in the antigen-stimulated clone do not evolve into plasma cells, but remain as small lymphocytes called **memory B cells.** Memory B cell generation occurs in germinal centers and may depend on the generation of complement (C3b)-associated immune complexes during the primary antibody response.

In addition to the surface immunoglobulin, other membrane proteins characterize the B cells, although they are not unique to them (Table 3-1). These cells bear receptors for the Fc portion of IgG when IgG is complexed with antigen. The capacity to bind immune complexes is thought to represent a feedback mechanism that may inhibit B cell stimulation. B cells also express receptors for C3b and C3d, which are cleavage products of C3, and Ia antigens, which are membrane proteins encoded in the immune response region of the major histocompatibility complex. The function of Ia in B cell activation is discussed in Chapter 4. During the last 5 years, several B cell–specific surface molecules have been described in humans as well as in experimental animals. Some of these (such as Lyb2 and Lyb3 in mice) are lineage-specific differentiation antigens that also may be involved in B cell activation, but their physiologic function has not yet been established definitively.

B cells are functionally distinct from T cells by sensitivity to mitogens that induce proliferation, especially lipopolysaccharide (LPS), an endotoxin of *Escherichia coli* to which T cells will not respond. LPS, a polyclonal mitogen for murine B cells, activates all clones of B cells, regardless of their antigen specificity.

T lymphocytes, which differentiate within the thymus, are the second major class of lymphocytes. Their antigen receptor is not an immunoglobulin, but has been identified recently as a heterodimer that has limited homology to immunoglobulin at the nucleotide level and may have a genetic organization similar to antibody genes. Within the class of T lymphocytes are additional subdivisions relating to effector functions. **Helper** or **inducer cells** are the T lymphocytes that, when stimulated by

Table 3-1   Membrane Markers and Functional Characteristics of Immune Cells*

	B Lymphocytes	*Helper*	*Suppressor*	*Cytotoxic*	*Killer Cells*	*Macrophages*
		T Lymphocytes				
Surface Ig	+	−	−	−	−	−
Sheep RBC binding†	−	+	+	+	−	−
Fc-IgG	+	−	+†	−	+	+
Fc-IgM	−	+†	−	−	−	+
C3b receptor	+	−	−	−	+	+
Thy-1‡	−	+	+	+	±	−
Ia antigens (MHC, class II)	+	−	+‡	−	−	+
Lyl‡§	−	+	−	−	−	−
Ly2,3‡‖	−	−	+	+	−	−
Lipopolysaccharide stimulation	+	−	−	−	−	−
Concanavalin A stimulation	−	+	?	?	−	−

*For more details on human T cell markers, see Table 7-1.
†In humans only.
‡In mice only.
§In humans, T4 is a similar marker for this subset.
‖In humans, T8 is a similar marker for this subset.

antigen, promote the differentiation of B cells and other T lymphocytes. T lymphocytes also mediate delayed hypersensitivity reactions by secreting factors (lymphokines) in response to antigenic stimulation that recruit and activate macrophages. The first membrane protein discovered that served to distinguish T lymphocytes from B lymphocytes was **Thy-1 antigen,** also known as Θ antigen. The Thy-1 antigen is expressed by all rodent thymus-derived cells, and by some brain cells and epithelial cells, but not by B lymphocytes. T lymphocytes express a number of other surface molecules that can be recognized by specific monoclonal antibodies. In human T cells, the T3 antigen is associated with the antigen receptor. Human T lymphocytes also have a receptor for sheep erythrocytes (termed the T11 molecule) whose function is unknown, but which is often used to separate T and B lymphocytes. Helper T cells are further characterized by the Lyt 1 alloantigen in the mouse and by T4 in man and its analogue, L3T4, in the mouse. On a functional basis, T lymphocytes are preferentially stimulated by polyclonal activators such as Concanavalin A, a plant-derived lectin that stimulates T, but not B, lymphocytes to proliferate.

A second class of T lymphocytes is composed of **suppressor T cells.** Suppressor T cells recognize the antigen or antigen-binding receptors (idiotypes) on other lymphoid cells but, instead of boosting the immune response, they act to inhibit it. In most experimental systems, suppressor T cells block the activity of helper cells by the release of factors that have not yet been characterized completely. Like all T cells, suppressor T cells are Thy 1 positive. Together with the cytotoxic T lymphocytes discussed below, murine suppressor cells express Ly2,3 antigens; in humans, they bear an antigenic marker known as T8.

A third class of T lymphocytes is the **cytotoxic T lymphocytes.** These lymphocytes, on becoming immunized to cell-associated viruses or intact cells (such as tumor cells), can bind to those cells directly and kill them. Cytotoxic T lymphocytes bear the Ly1,2,3, antigen in mice. In humans, most of them are T8-positive. These cells, which are believed to play a major role in surveillance against viruses and tumors, are discussed in Chapters 7 and 15. It should be emphasized that cytotoxic and helper cells recognize foreign antigens in association with class I and class II histocompatibility determinants (Chapters 2 and 7).

In addition to classic B and T lymphocytes, lymphoid cells exist which express surface markers that are not characteristic of either B or T cells. Such cells, often classified as **null cells,** include two functionally important groups: **killer (K) cells** and **natural killer (NK) cells.** The K cells bind and lyse antibody-coated cells in a reaction called antibody-dependent, cell-mediated cytotoxicity (ADCC). Killer cells are different from cytotoxic T lymphocytes in that they do not depend upon previous immunization and they require antibody as a cofactor. K cells express Fc receptors for IgG, but less than half of them express T cell markers such as Thy-1 and none express surface immunoglobulin. About one-half do express receptors for C3b. Although K cells resist easy classification, they are extremely potent as effector cells of humoral immunity.

Natural killer cells, which also are not induced by overt immunization, are capable of lysing hemopoietic cells and tumors. This group may consist of a heterogeneous population of some cells with Fc receptors and others with T cell markers (Chapter 7).

Accessory Cells

Cells of the mononuclear phagocyte system (previously termed the "reticuloendothelial system") are composed of **monocytes** and **macrophages** and their derivatives. These cells play a major role as scavengers that actively phagocytose foreign substances (such as microbes) and altered host proteins (such as aged red blood cells and necrotic tissue). Macrophages are larger than lymphocytes (15 to 30 μm in diameter) and have active cytoplasm filled with lysosomes that contain numerous enzymes capable of digesting proteins, polysaccharides, nucleic acids, and lipids. In addition to their phagocytic and degradative capacities, macrophages secrete a variety of materials, including collagenase and elastase, which can digest connective tissue components; plasminogen activators, which promote fibrinolysis; a variety of complement proteins; and lysozyme, a bactericidal peptidoglycan. Bone marrow–derived phagocytes circulate as monocytes and settle in tissues as resident phagocytes. In the peripheral tissue, these cells are known by different names, depending on their location. Thus, they are alveolar macrophages in the lung, Kuppfer cells in the liver, and peritoneal macrophages in the peritoneum. Both free and fixed macrophages are distributed throughout the lymph nodes and spleen. Inflammation results in the accumulation of monocytes and their differentiation at the site of inflammation into activated macrophages.

In addition to their nonimmunologic phagocytic functions, macrophages are the prototype *accessory cells* of the immune system. They bind, process, and present foreign protein antigens to helper T lymphocytes in order to initiate immune responses, and secrete factors (notably interleukin-1) that promote lymphocyte growth and differentiation (Chapter 7). Macrophages also secrete growth factors for mesenchymal cells (fibroblasts, endothelium, and smooth muscle) and factors that induce hemopoietic differentiation. Whether macrophage-processed antigen is required for stimulating B cells is not yet known.

Macrophages display a characteristic constellation of membrane proteins that enhance the efficiency of binding and thus of phagocytosis (see Table 3-1). They express Fc receptors, as well as receptors for both C3b and C3bi (a breakdown product of C3b) and all these receptors contribute to the binding of opsonized particles. Macrophages can also express Ia antigens and they play a crucial role in the presentation of antigens to histocompatibility (Ia)-restricted T lymphocytes. Activated T lymphocytes release a variety of factors that cause the macrophages to become larger, to be more phagocytic and bactericidal, and to display additional Ia antigens. This involves an amplifying loop, because such activated macrophages are even more stimulatory to T lymphocytes. Activated macrophages are also the effector cells of delayed hypersensitivity (Chapter 7).

In addition to macrophages, other cells have been defined recently as accessory cells in immune responses. Known as **dendritic cells,** they are found in the spleen and in the deep cortex of lymph nodes, and are quite similar to the Langerhans cells in the skin. Dendritic cells do not exhibit Fc or C3 receptors, but they do display class II histocompatibility (Ia) antigens on their membranes; they are capable of binding antigen and displaying it on their membranes for long periods of time. These cells are not to be confused with the follicular dendritic cells that form the core of the lymphoid follicles. The follicular dendritic cells are Ia-negative; they bind immune complexes coated with complement proteins and display them on their membranes for the stimulation of B lymphocytes, and they may be critical for the generation or activation of memory B cells.

Functional Anatomy of Lymphoid Tissues

The tissues in which the network of immunologically responsive cells appear are called lymphoid because of the primary immune cells, the lymphocytes. Lymphoid tissues, however, can contain other cell types (most important, accessory cells) and lymphocytes and antigen-processing cells are important constituents of nonlymphoid tissues such as those in the respiratory and gastrointestinal tracts. The principal lymphoid tissues are bone marrow, thymus, lymph nodes, and spleen. Lymphoid tissues have been divided by their functions into two categories: *primary* and *secondary*. The primary lymphoid organs are the thymus and bone marrow, in which proliferation and differentiation of lymphocytes take place independently of antigen stimulation. In the tissues of these organs, the evolution of stem cell progeny into mature lymphocytes takes place. The mature lymphocytes then seed into the periphery, where exposure to antigen and appropriate immune responses occur.

Thymus

The **thymus** is a small organ in the anterior mediastinum. It is derived from the third and fourth branchial pouches and is divided into two parts: an outer **cortex** and an inner **medulla.** Immature cells called **prothymocytes,** which are derived from stem cells in the bone marrow, migrate through the circulation into the cortex where they proliferate and acquire membrane proteins characteristic of mature T lymphocytes. During this phase, the cells are termed **thymocytes.** T lymphocyte maturation is most vigorous during fetal and neonatal development and proceeds actively until puberty, after which the thymus atrophies. As the immune response becomes capable of generating long-lived memory cells to react against antigens to which it has been previously exposed, the need for newly derived thymocytes decreases. Thus, surgical removal of the thymus in adulthood causes little, if any, immune impairment, whereas its absence during neonatal life can produce a profound immunodeficiency.

The blood capillaries in the cortex of the thymus are impermeable to proteins, like blood vessels in the brain, but unlike capillaries elsewhere in the body; the maturing thymocytes are isolated from contact with any circulating protein, and thus with any potential antigens. This is important because an immature T cell that encounters an antigen actually turns itself off rather than becoming activated.

Other cells in the specialized microenvironment of the thymic cortex include epithelial cells and scattered macrophages. The function of the epithelial cells is understood poorly, although it is known that they synthesize peptide hormones that can induce in vitro differentiation of stem cell precursors into thymocytes, and that they also may play a role in promoting the differentiation of thymocytes in vivo. In addition, both epithelial cells and macrophages in the cortex display, on their membranes, high quantities of Ia proteins, which may be critical for "educating" maturing T lymphocytes to distinguish between self and nonself on the basis of major histocompatibility products.

The thymocytes in the cortex are small-to-medium in size, although a few large blast cells are dispersed throughout the cortex. The thymocytes leave the cortex in the first stage of their differentiation and then migrate into the medulla, where they become progressively smaller and functionally mature. The medulla is completely permeable to circulating antigens and contains many more macrophages than does the cortex; they are concentrated near the cortical medullary area. Epithelial cells in the medulla are organized into whorled structures called **Hassal's corpuscles,** which may represent the degenerating cells. In the medulla, the thymocytes complete their maturation process and migrate into the blood as mature T lymphocytes capable of responding to antigenic exposure.

Bone Marrow

In birds, B lymphocytes differentiate in the Bursa of Fabricius, a primary lymphoid organ associated with the gastrointestinal tract. No corresponding organ for B cells exists in mammals and current evidence suggests that the bone marrow is the site for both stem cell proliferation and the origin of pre-B cells, as well as the maturation of pre-B cells into functionally mature B lymphocytes. We do know that, as B cells leave the bone marrow and settle into the secondary lymphoid organs, they are completely mature lymphocytes that are capable of responding to antigen by proliferation and differentiation into plasma cells.

The membrane protein that defines the B lymphocyte is its antigen receptor, membrane-associated immunoglobulin (Ig). B cells, in their earliest stages of maturation, express IgM as their principal antigen receptor. These cells lack both the C3 and the Fc receptors. As they mature, B cells acquire IgD, in addition to IgM, on their membranes. Both molecules share the function of antigen receptor and, although they belong to different classes of immunoglobulins, both recognize the same antigenic epitope and thus share idiotypes. Acquisition of C3 and Fc receptors marks the entrance of the B cell into its mature phase; the cell now also acquires receptors for immunoregulatory factors and hormones. Later, in the context of antigen stimulation, some B cells make additional switches in the class of their antigen receptor and display either IgG or IgA on their membranes. Immature B lymphocytes are unable to proliferate in response to antigen that binds their surface immunoglobulin; mature B lymphocytes will proliferate when given additional signals derived from T cells.

Secondary Lymphoid Organs

The life cycle of a B or T lymphocyte can be seen as occurring in two phases, separated by a plateau. In the first phase, the lymphocyte acquires receptors for antigen and for hormones or factors derived from other cells that permit it to respond to antigen as part of a modulatable network of intercommunicating cells. This takes place in a primary lymphoid organ, the thymus, or bone marrow. The second phase concerns the encounter of these cells with an antigen and with other cells that are also reacting to that antigen. The encounter takes place in the secondary lymph organs, primarily the lymph nodes and spleen. These organs are subdivided into regions for the specialized accumulation of the different cellular components of the immune reaction (T and B lymphocytes and accessory cells). During the course of the immune response, considerable traffic occurs between these regions of the organs, as well as between all the secondary organs.

The secondary lymphoid organs are interconnected by both the vascular system and the lymphatic system. The **lymphatics,** which are found throughout the body, are vessels organized in networks that parallel the blood circulation (Figure 3-3). They function to absorb circulating proteins and fluid that have extravasated from permeable capillary beds. This material, **lymph,** is restored to the circulation after being percolated through the lymph nodes. Thus, when the integrity of peripheral tissues is broken by invasion of pathogens, the resulting mixture of antigens and extravasated proteins that arises from the disruption of blood vessels is absorbed by the lymphatic system.

Situated along the lymphatics are **lymph nodes,** collections of secondary lymphoid tissue with a complex internal organization. The lymphatic vessels that carry lymph into a node are called the **afferent** lymphatics; those that drain the node are **efferent.** The lymphatics get larger as networks that drain different beds of lymph nodes fuse, and

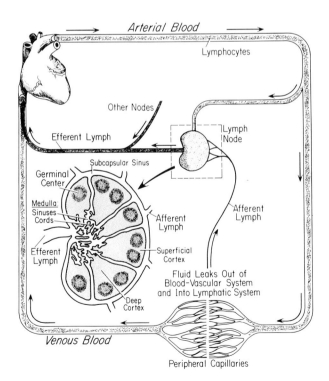

Figure 3-3 The circulation of lymphocytes and an enlargement of a lymph node. Lymph enters from the afferent lymphatic and percolates through the deep cortex to the medullary sinus and then into the efferent lymphatic. Lymphocytes enter the node from the circulation through the postcapillary venules in the cortex and exit via the efferent lymphatics. Antigen is taken up by macrophages in the sinuses and the cortex and by dendritic cells in the deep cortex. Immune complexes localize to the follicles.

eventually major lymphatic vessels (such as the thoracic duct) are formed, which drain into the venous circulation (see Figure 3-3).

Lymph Nodes

The lymph nodes are the arena in which the encounter between an antigen and a naive immune system takes place. Macrophages line the sinuses into which the afferent lymphatic channels break up on entering the lymph node. Lymph percolates through the subcapillary sinus and through the lymphoid region of the cortex. The cortex is filled with macrophages and with interdigitating dendritic cells. The sinuses reanastomose in the core of the lymph nodes, the medulla. The medullary sinuses are broken up by islands of cells consisting of macrophages and plasma cells.

The lymphoid cortex can be subdivided further into areas in which either B lymphocytes or T lymphocytes predominate. In the outer or superficial cortex are clusters (**follicles**) of lymphocytes, which consist predominantly of B lymphocytes in close apposition to multibranched cells known as **follicular dendritic cells.** The follicular dendritic cells are believed to be sites at which B cell proliferation takes place within the lymph node. The area between the follicles, within the deep cortex (intermediate between the superficial cortex and the medullary sinuses), contains mostly T lymphocytes.

The tendency for the subclasses of lymphocytes to reside chiefly in different areas of lymph nodes provided early clues to the division of the lymphocyte system into two classes. In the 1950s, pediatricians observed that children without thymuses lacked lymphocytes in the deep cortex, which thus became known as the **thymus-dependent area.** The same children, however, were found to have persistent follicles in the superficial cortex, which was thus called the **thymus-independent area.** In other immune deficiency states, both clinical and experimental, in which loss or depletion of B lymphocytes has occurred, no follicles have been observed in the superficial cortex and the deep cortex has been found to be normal.

Spleen

The architecture of the **spleen** reflects a compartmentalization which is analogous, but not identical, to that of the lymph nodes. Located beneath the rib cage, the spleen is the largest collection of lymph tissue in the body. It has two segregated areas: the **red pulp** and the **white pulp.** The red pulp consists of cords of cells that divide venous sinuses. These cords are composed of a reticular connective tissue lined with fixed macrophages. The white pulp, the lymphoid portion of the spleen, consists of sheaths of lymphocytes organized around penetrating, or **trabecular, arteries.** At branch points of the trabecular arteries, the white pulp expands into larger structures known as **splenic follicles.** The follicles, the T-independent areas, consist of collections of B lymphocytes in varying stages of activation. The sheath of lymphocytes that surrounds the artery leading into the follicle consists of T cells. Unlike the lymph nodes, the spleen has no lymphatic drainage; it is primarily an organ for responding to blood-borne antigens.

Tissue Response to Antigens

A lymph node is not a static tissue. In addition to the continuous percolation of lymph through its sinuses, various types of immune cells pass constantly in and out of it. Lymphocytes can enter a lymph node either by migration through the afferent lymphatics (after leaving a more distal node in the same lymphatic chain), or from the systemic circulation via a specialized area in the pericortical region, the **postcapillary venules.** The venules are blood vessels that consist of specialized endothelium bearing receptors for polysaccharide moieties on the lymphocyte membrane. On attachment to the endothelium, the lymphocytes migrate through to the deep cortex where they localize; this is not unexpected, since 80%–90% of circulating lymphocytes are thymus-derived. In an inactive lymph node, approximately 90% of the lymphocyte traffic occurs via the postcapillary venules.

When antigens enter a lymph node and induce a priming reaction, lymph bearing antigenic molecules enters the subcapsular sinus from the afferent lymphatics and then diffuses through the deep cortex via the intrafollicular sinuses. The antigens then are taken by antigen-presenting cells in the deep cortex and the number of lymphocytes in this area increases rapidly. A concomitant reduction occurs in the number of all lymphocytes leaving by the efferent lymphatics, regardless of their antigen specificity. Two to five days later, a marked increase occurs in the number of lymphocytes migrating through the medulla and out of the lymph node via the efferent lymphatics. At the same time, the influx of lymphocytes from the systemic circulation increases. Most of these lymphocytes do not have specificity for the antigen that is being processed in the deep cortex. The lymphocytes with specificity for the immunogen become concentrated in the deep cortex as a result of their interaction with the antigen-presenting cells. A substantial proliferation of the lymphocytes takes place in the deep cortex and scattered, antibody-synthesizing cells appear in the superficial cortex and in the medullary sinus region. After 5 days, antigen-specific lymphocytes begin to exit the node via the efferent lymphatics. These primed T lymphocytes, which have arisen from clonal expansion in response to the antigen, will disseminate to lymph nodes along the lymphatic chain and then to other lymphoid structures via the systemic circulation. As these cells disseminate, the host becomes prepared systemically for further antigenic challenge.

As lymphocytes disseminate, antigen reappears in the lymph, now complexed to the antibodies that were synthesized during the early phase of the reaction. These antigen-antibody complexes have particular affinity for the follicular dendritic cells that constitute the core of the superficial cortical follicles. Such cells display the complexes for long periods (up to months) without phagocytosing them. The uptake of antigen-antibody complexes by the follicular dendritic cells is followed by the rapid expansion of the follicles into large nodules, **germinal centers,** of actively proliferating B lymphocytes. The process of germinal center formation and the production of activated B cells contributes both to the appearance of plasma cells throughout the lymph node (particularly in the medullary sinuses) and to the generation of memory B cells.

References

Cantor, H., Boyse, E.: Regulation of cellular and humoral responses by T cell subclasses. *Cold Spring Harbor Symp Quant Biol* 1977; 41:23-32.

Kincade, P.W.: Formation of B lymphocytes in fetal and adult life. *Adv Immunol* 1981; 31:177.

Nossal, G., et al: Antigens in immunity. XV. Ultrastructural features of antigen capture in primary and secondary lymphoid follicles. *J Exp Med* 1968; 127:277.

Reinherz, E., Schlossman, S.: The differentiation and function of human T lymphocytes. *Cell* 1980; 19:821.

Unanue, E.R.: Cooperation between mononuclear phagocytes and lymphocytes in immunity. *N Engl J Med* 1980; 303:977.

4 Humoral Immunity: Cellular Events and Regulation

Abul K. Abbas, MD

General Concepts

The mammalian immune system consists of phenotypically and functionally distinct cells that interact with each other to determine the magnitude, duration, and nature of the total immune response. Immune responses can be divided into two distinct classes: antibody (humoral) immunity, which is mediated by B lymphocytes and their antibody-producing progeny cells, and cell-mediated immunity (for example, delayed hypersensitivity and lymphocyte-mediated cytotoxicity), in which the effector cells are T lymphocytes. The most extensive studies of how immunity is regulated have been done on antibody responses. In general, all immune responses consist of three phases: **induction**, in which an antigen first interacts with clones of B and/or T lymphocytes that express specific membrane receptors; **expansion** and **differentiation**, during which the induced lymphocyte clones proliferate and mature to a functional stage; and the **effector phase,** in which antibodies or differentiated T cells exert their biologic effects, often with the participation of other cell types (such as macrophages and other leukocytes) or effector systems (for example, complement). The process of immune induction involves the presentation of antigen to specific receptor-bearing lymphocytes, usually by Ia-bearing cells that have the same histocompatibility determinants as the recipient lymphocyte. Before and after the encounter with antigen, the lymphocytes undergo a series of events that are best defined by the differentiation of B cells. In fact, the sequence of B cell differentiation can now be related precisely to patterns of immunoglobulin production and can be explained, in molecular terms, as alterations in immunoglobulin gene expression. Moreover, the maturation and function of immunocompetent lymphocytes are finely tuned by other lymphoid cells with regulatory roles, including helper T lymphocytes, which provide necessary activating and amplification signals for many different immune responses; and suppressor T cells, whose inhibitory effects may serve as negative feedback loops to ensure the maintenance of immunologic homeostasis.

In this chapter, the induction, differentiation, and regulation of lymphocytes will be outlined, with particular emphasis on humoral immunity (antibody production). The cell types that participate in immune responses are described in Chapter 3, and cell-mediated immunity is discussed in Chapter 7.

Immune Induction: Role of Antigen-Presenting Cells

It has been known for 20 years that macrophage-associated foreign proteins are more immunogenic than soluble proteins. This basic observation led to the development of the concept that one function of macrophages is to present antigens in an immunogenic form to lymphocytes that are identical at the major histocompatibility complex (MHC). However, B and T lymphocytes differ in their requirement for the antigen presentation. B lymphocytes may be capable of responding to some soluble antigens (antigens not associated with presenting cells). For example, they respond to polysaccharide antigens that cannot be degraded by mammalian enzymes and thus cannot be processed by antigen-presenting cells (APC). Helper T lymphocytes, on the other hand, recognize foreign antigens only in association with class II MHC molecules (Ia determinants), and this associative recognition is the basis for the **MHC restriction** (the requirement for histocompatibility) that is characteristic of T-cell–macrophage interactions.

We now know that cells of the monocyte-macrophage lineage are the prototype, but not the only cells capable of presenting foreign antigens to immunocompetent lymphocytes. A variety of cell types that express membrane Ia can perform this function: dendritic cells, epidermal Langerhans cells, B lymphocytes, and (possibly) some endothelial cells and fibroblasts. Foreign protein antigens bind to macrophages, are interiorized and degraded enzymatically, and antigen fragments are presumably reexpressed on the surface of APC where they are recognized by Ia-restricted, antigen-specific T cells in association with Ia molecules. This description clearly applies to Ia-restricted T cells (helper cells and T lymphocytes that mediate delayed hypersensitivity). On the other hand, the role of APC in stimulating precursors of cytolytic T lymphocytes and suppressor T cells is unclear.

In addition to antigen processing and presentation, many APC, particularly macrophages, actively secrete a factor with a molecular weight of about 15,000 daltons, **interleukin 1,** that enhances the differentiation of helper T lymphocytes. Activated T cells, in turn, produce γ-interferon, which induces Ia expression on a variety of cells and thus sets up an amplification loop that enhances the ability of APC to stimulate Ia-restricted T cells.

Differentiation of B Lymphocytes and Induction of Humoral Immune Responses

With the advent of recombinant DNA technology for the analysis of immunoglobulin (Ig) genes and RNA, we have achieved remarkable progress in our understanding of B lymphocyte differentiation during the past few years. We can now divide the sequence of B cell differentiation into a series of antigen-independent stages and events induced by antigens. These stages (illustrated in Table 4-1) each correspond to a defined alteration in Ig genes or mRNA and Ig biosynthesis and secretion.

Antigen-Independent Differentiation

The commitment of bone marrow stem cells to the B lymphocyte lineage involves a rearrangement of Ig genes; probably the heavy-chain genes go first, and are followed by κ light chain and λ genes. In the embryonic stage, all these genes (which are located on different chromosomes; see Chapter 1) are split genes; that is, they consist of several exons separated by intervening DNA sequences (introns) that are not transcribed. Thus, one each of several V (variable), D (diversity), and J (joining) segment genes of heavy chains rearrange in each B cell to give a V-D-J segment that is separated from the Cμ (constant) region DNA by an intron. The primary RNA transcript has this same configuration.

Subsequently, the Cμ RNA is brought adjacent to the V-D-J segment by splicing, and the mature mRNA generated is translated to form the μ polypeptide. At this stage,

Table 4-1   B Lymphocyte Differentiation

		Antigen-Independent			Antigen-Induced	
		Bone Marrow	Periphery			
Cell type:	Stem cell	Pre-B cell	Immature B lymphocyte	Mature B lymphocyte	Activated B lymphocyte	Antibody-secreting cell (plasmacyte)
Ig genes/RNA:	?	Rearranged H chain*	Rearranged H + L chain genes*	Alternative splicing of H chain RNA	1. From membrane-bound to secreted IgM, by RNA splicing 2. Expression of other H chain genes	
Ig production, function:	? none	Cytoplasmic μ only; not antigen-reactive	Surface IgM$^+$; tolerance-sensitive	Surface IgM$^+$; IgD$^+$; antigen-responsive	1. Low rate Ig secretion 2. H chain class switching	High rate Ig secretion, reduction of membrane Ig

*H and L refer to immunoglobulin (Ig) heavy and light chains, respectively.

no light chains are synthesized and, since isolated heavy chains cannot be exteriorized, the cell contains only cytoplasmic μ, the *pre-B cell,* which is located in the bone marrow. The next step is V-J rearrangement of κ light chain DNA followed by RNA splicing to produce a κ mRNA, which is then translated. The λ DNA probably is rearranged only in cells that have undergone an abortive or aberrant, nonfunctional κ gene rearrangement, since only one light chain is present in each B cell.

Once the light chains are synthesized, the assembled IgM molecules are expressed on the cell surface. These are **immature B cells:** they bear readily detectable membrane IgM; they exit from the bone marrow; and they are highly susceptible to tolerance induction so that the usual result of an encounter with antigen is unresponsiveness or **tolerance** (Chapter 11). The next stage of differentiation is the *mature B lymphocyte,* which expresses both IgM and IgD molecules on the cell surface; both forms of Ig have the same light chains and V regions (antigen specificity and idiotype). The association of the same V region with $C\mu$ or $C\delta$ is a result of alternative splicing of the V-D-J RNA to either $C\mu$ or to $C\delta$, which is located 3′ to $C\mu$ and separated from it by an intron. It is not known whether IgM and IgD receptors for antigens serve different functions. The mature B cell responds to antigen by undergoing a series of alterations that lead to the humoral immune response.

Antigen-Induced Differentiation

Similar molecular events are believed to occur after the encounter of mature B lymphocytes with thymus-dependent antigens (together with helper T lymphocytes), thymus-independent antigens, or polyclonal B cell activators (such as *Escherichia coli* lipopolysaccharide, pokeweed mitogen, and anti-Ig antibodies). Two basic changes in Ig expression take place. First, cells with predominantly membrane IgM (and IgD) begin to secrete IgM. The mRNA determines whether the expressed Ig in a B lymphocyte is membrane-bound or secretory, through the presence of the message for a hydrophobic protein segment at the 3′ end of the $C\mu$ mRNA. If the message is included, the IgM is membrane-bound; if it is omitted, the IgM is secreted by the cell. Such IgM secretion is detected as the primary antibody response.

The second event is *heavy chain class (isotype) switching,* in which the rearranged V-D-J DNA is transcribed with various $C\gamma$, $C\alpha$, or $C\epsilon$ DNAs that are located 3′ to $C\mu$, are separated by introns, and that bear switch sites at their 5′ ends, which regulate joining of V-D-J with C regions. Deletion of genes for intervening C regions (that is, the regions closest to V-D-J) probably leads to expression of more distal C regions, thus explaining the appearance of $C\gamma$ after $C\mu$, a characteristic of most secondary antibody responses. As B cells differentiate, they secrete more Ig and express progressively less membrane Ig. Plasma cells (plasmacytes) are the morphologically defined, terminally differentiated stage of this maturational sequence.

The antigen-driven maturation and heavy chain class switching is controlled not only by helper T cells, but also by the nature of the antigen. For example, polysaccharide antigens tend to induce IgM antibody and not the other isotypes. The tissue microenvironment also influences the isotype switch; for example, B cells at mucosal sites differentiate predominately into producers of IgA (Chapter 10).

B cells that express membrane or secretory forms of IgG, IgA, or IgE are the memory cells that arise after antigen priming, and thus are the major contributors to secondary immune responses. Secondary responses are characterized by higher amounts of antibody (because of the expansion of relevant B cell clones induced by priming) and by higher affinity antibody (because of the selection of appropriate B cells).

Helper Function in Humoral Immunity

In the 1960s, Claman and Chaperon showed that optimal responses to protein antigens were obtained from mixtures of thymus and bone marrow cells, although the antibody-secreting cells themselves were derived entirely from bone marrow. More convincing proof for the obligatory role of cellular cooperation in immunity derived from studies done by Mitchison and coworkers on antihapten antibody production in response to immunization with hapten-carrier conjugates (see Chapter 5 for the definition of hapten). For example, in one such experiment, mice immunized with a hapten conjugated to one protein (the carrier) made antihapten antibody only when challenged with the same conjugate (Table 4-2).

Later studies demonstrated that hapten-carrier immunization induced the expansion and functional differentiation of hapten-specific B cell clones and carrier-specific T cell clones. In order to elicit the antihapten response, the carrier and hapten molecules must be linked physically (see Table 4-2). Thus, carrier-primed T cells and hapten-specific B cells must be *bridged* together with the antigen complex for T cells to stimulate the B cell antibody response (Figure 4-1A). The T lymphocytes in this process are *helper* cells. It should be emphasized that the concepts that developed from studies of hapten-carrier conjugates apply to all multideterminant protein antigens in which one determinant (epitope) may function as a hapten and another may be analogous to the carrier. Moreover, some antigens (thymus-independent) stimulate antibody production even if few or no helper T cells are present.

The demonstration of a critical role for helper T lymphocytes in antibody responses was soon followed by studies that showed such T cells recognized protein antigens not by themselves, but in association with products of the major histocompatibility gene complex (MHC) on antigen-presenting cells. Moreover, Katz and Benacerraf found that optimal cooperation between carrier-primed helper cells and hapten-specific B lymphocytes required that the two be histocompatible, and, in particular, have identical Ia (class II) MHC determinants. Therefore, a hypothesis was developed that helper cells

Table 4-2 Antibody Response to Hapten-Carrier Conjugates*

Group	Primary Immunization	Challenge	Anti-Hapten (DNP) Antibody Response
1	DNP-A	DNP-A	Yes
2	DNP-A	DNP-B	No
3	DNP-A	DNP-B plus free A	No

*Mice immunized with a hapten, 2,4-dinitrophenol (DNP), linked to a protein carrier, A, and challenged with DNP-A (group 1) give a good anti-DNP antibody response, but they do not respond to challenge with DNP linked to a different carrier, B (group 2), even if unhaptenated A is administered simultaneously (group 3). The results from group 3 are explained by postulating that hapten-specific lymphocytes (B cells) and carrier-specific lymphocytes (helper T cells) need to be in contact or in close proximity, and this is achieved only by providing a hapten-carrier bridge between these two cell types.

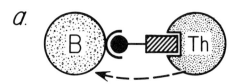

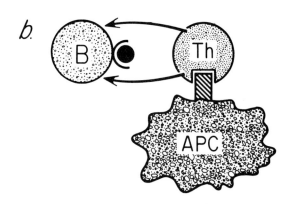

Figure 4-1 Mechanisms of T lymphocyte-mediated help for B cells. **A**, MHC-restricted T–B interaction: hapten-specific B cells and carrier-specific helper T lymphocytes (Th) interact via the hapten-carrier bridge. This interaction is Ia-restricted (that is, in the physiologic situation, Th and B cells must be syngeneic in I region of MHC). The mechanism of the helper effect is unknown; broken arrows indicate the possibility that Th may secrete helper factors. **B**, Factor-mediated help: Th recognize antigen on any APC and secrete helper factors (such as BCGF, BCDF) that act on antigen-stimulated B cells. Linked hapten-carrier recognition is not required. Th and B cells are not in contact and do not have to share MHC. In this case, the Th–APC interaction is Ia-restricted.

recognize hapten-carrier conjugates in association with Ia determinants on B lymphocytes. This concept implied an obligatory role for direct cell–cell contact and accounted for the necessity of linked hapten-carrier recognition (see Table 4-2).

In apparent contradiction to these findings was the observation that during an immune response in vitro against one antigen, B lymphocytes that were specific for an unrelated antigen but present in the same culture could be induced to secrete antibody in the absence of relevant helper cells. This stimulation of **bystander** B cells without specific T cell help could be explained only by postulating a role for mediators or factors secreted by helper cells of one specificity that could act on bystander B lymphocytes. In these cases, direct T–B contact would not be required.

We know now that helper T lymphocytes may function in two ways that are not mutually exclusive (see Figure 4-1). First, they may participate in MHC (Ia)-restricted cell–cell interaction. In this situation, an antigen that binds to immunoglobulin (Ig) receptors on the relevant clone of B cells is expressed on the cell surface *in association with* Ia determinants, and is recognized by Ia-restricted helper T cells that are specific for a carrierlike epitope of the antigen (see Figure 4-1A). Thus, the B cell functions much like an APC to activate helper cells, which then deliver (thus far undefined) signals that stimulate the B cells clone to expand and differentiate.

Helper T cells also may offer MHC unrestricted, soluble factor-mediated help. Here, B lymphocytes are stimulated by antigen to enter the cell cycle and presumably express membrane receptors for helper T-cell-derived factors. The helper cells are activated by antigen on any APC to secrete factors that induce the B cells to proliferate and differentiate (see Figure 4-1B). The only MHC-restricted interactions are between

Table 4-3   Helper Factors for Immune Responses

Factor	Molecular Weight (Daltons)	Function and Bioassay Results
T cell lymphokines		
B cell growth factor (BCGF)	11,000–20,000 (? two species)	Proliferation of B cells
B cell differentiation factor (BCDF)	?30,000–40,000	Induction of IgM secretion: (1) synergizes with anti-Ig and BCGF in B cell activation; (2) different BCGFs may preferentially induce antibodies of different H chain class
Thymus replacing factor(s) (TRF)	30,000–40,000	Induction of Ig secretion (may be identical to BCDF); replaces helper T cells in antibody responses of unprimed cells to particulate antigens and of primed cells to hapten-carriers
Interleukin 2	14,000–18,000	Stimulates proliferation of T lymphocytes; may have some effect on B cells
γ-interferon (IFNγ)	$\approx$40,000	Required for B cell activation
Antigen-specific helper factors	?	Promote B cell proliferation and differentiation, but only in presence of relevant antigen
Monokines		
Interleukin 1 (IL 1)	$\approx$15,000	Promotes B cell proliferation and T lymphocyte differentiation

the helper T cells and APC, since once helper factors are secreted they can act on any B lymphocytes that bear appropriate receptors for these mediators.

A large number of helper factors that are known to act on B lymphocytes have been identified biologically, and some have been purified to homogeneity (Table 4-3). These factors include B cell growth factor, B cell differentiation factors (which induce membrane IgM$^+$ cells to secrete IgM and undergo heavy chain class switching so that they express other Ig isotypes), and thymus-replacing factors (which replace T cells in antibody responses, and may be similar or identical to the differentiation factors mentioned above). In addition, macrophage-derived interleukin 1 and T-cell–derived interleukin 2 and γ-interferon also may be involved in proliferation and differentiation of a B cell. None of these soluble lymphokines have antigen specificity. We know that B cells have receptors to which the helper factors bind. The subsequent biochemical events that lead to proliferation and alterations in the expression of B cell immunoglobulin genes are not known.

The Role of Surface Ig in B Lymphocyte Activation

Researchers agree that the interaction between an antigen and its specific Ig receptor on B cells has two main consequences. First, it activates the cells to undergo a G0 to G1 switch (that is, enter the cell cycle) and express functional receptors for helper factors.

Second, the receptor/antigen complex is interiorized and processed so that some antigenic determinants reappear on the B cell surface in association with Ia molecules. The antigen and Ia are then recognized by the Ia-restricted, antigen-specific helper T cells. This mechanism may serve as a focusing device for B–T cell collaboration.

T Cell Help for Primary Versus Secondary Antibody Responses and Responses to Thymus-Independent Antigens

Both primary and secondary responses to most protein antigens of the *thymus-dependent* class require functional helper T cells. Primed (memory) B lymphocytes, however, may need less help for activation than unprimed cells. Moreover, unique subsets of T lymphocytes, helper factors, or both may induce heavy chain class switches (for example, to μ, γ, α) that result frequently from immunization. Finally, some experimental evidence indicates that helper T cells can themselves discriminate between B lymphocytes that have different membrane Ig heavy chains; for example, some helper T cells have specificity for antigen and others are specific for immunoglobulin itself.

There is a long-established notion that certain antigens can induce the entire spectrum of antibody responses without the overt participation of helper T lymphocytes. This idea has been challenged as cell purification techniques have improved. Thus, apparent *thymus independence* may be merely a quantitative phenomenon, and the activation of B lymphocytes by all antigens may require some helper T cells or T-cell–derived factors. It seems likely, however, that MHC-restricted T cells do not play a role in antibody responses to most or all thymus-independent antigens (especially the polysaccharides that constitute the largest group of such antigens) and that only helper factors are important in these responses.

Helper Function in Cell-Mediated Immunity

The general principles that have been developed from studies of antibody responses also are applicable to cell-mediated immunity. Precursors of cytolytic T lymphocytes (CTL) clearly require Ia-restricted helper T cells to develop into mature CTL. These events, as well as the cellular cooperation during delayed hypersensitivity, are described in Chapter 7.

Regulation of Antibody Responses by Suppressor T Lymphocytes

Gershon and coworkers discovered that experimentally induced tolerance (unresponsiveness) to an antigen could be transferred by lymphocytes from tolerant to normal animals so that the recipients of the cells became unresponsive to the antigen. We now know that the cells responsible for inhibiting immune responses are **suppressor T lymphocytes** (T_s). Such T_s are phenotypically distinct from helper T cells, they can suppress both humoral and cell-mediated immune responses, and they may play a major role in physiologic control of immune responses as well as in the production of disorders of the immune system.

Induction of Suppressor T Lymphocytes

From the many diverse experimental systems for studying T_s, a few basic concepts have emerged. First, a direct presentation of antigens to T cells in the absence of Ia determinants may induce T_s rather than helper cells. Alternatively, the T_s may respond to antigens in association with MHC determinants that are different from those that stimulate helper cells.

Second, the cells involved in immune suppression may be heterogeneous and composed of different cell subsets. Thus, the differentiation of T_s may depend on inducer T lymphocytes, which perform a role much like that played by helper T cells in effector immunity. Moreover, the development of T_s may involve a series of receptor–antireceptor (or idiotype–antiidiotype) interactions between different T cells. In other words, a T cell of the suppressor subset that is induced by, and that recognizes, an antigen may first stimulate a second-order cell that is specific for the antigen-binding receptor (idiotype) of the first cell, and then an effector T_s which is also antigen-specific.

A third basic observation is that many forms of immunization preferentially induce T_s, including large amounts of weakly immunogenic antigens (or antigens administered without potent adjuvants), as well as multiple, small doses of antigens. Moreover, neonates may be particularly prone to develop T_s in response to immunization regimens that would stimulate immune responses in adults.

Mode of Action of Suppressor T Lymphocytes

Most early studies showed that T_s inhibit the function of helper T cells, although it has become clear recently that some effector T_s can also inhibit directly the function of effector cells such as antibody-producing lymphocytes and delayed hypersensitivity-mediating T cells. The biologic effects of T_s appear to be mediated by secreted suppressor factors that may be antigen- or idiotype-specific. In certain situations, these factors interact with the antigen bound to macrophages, which then secrete the final suppressive molecules. Such macrophage-derived immunosuppressants (which may be products of arachidonic acid or oxidative metabolism) are themselves not antigen- or idiotype-specific; the specificity in the system results because the antigen activates only the relevant T_s. Despite intensive investigation, the biochemical structure of suppressive factors, the nature of their interaction with target cells, and the subcellular events that lead to inhibition of immune responses remain largely unknown.

It should be emphasized that although much experimental work supports the view that T_s can be induced by a variety of immunization protocols, and that they inhibit humoral or cell-mediated immune responses, few data indicate what role these cells play in physiologic immune regulation. Thus, the hypothesis that the magnitude and duration of immune responses is mediated by T_s has not been confirmed by direct experimentation. Similarly, it is possible that unresponsiveness to some self antigens may be maintained by T_s but so far no cells specific for autologous antigens have been identified. The possible roles of T_s in tolerance to self and in autoimmunity are discussed in Chapters 11 and 12.

Idiotypic Regulation of Immune Responses

In 1974, Niels Jerne proposed that the immune system consisted of a network of cells in which combining sites of antibodies (and cellular receptors for antigen) themselves functioned as unique antigens (idiotypes) that were capable of stimulating regulatory antiidiotypic responses. Thus, administration of a foreign antigen would stimulate expansion of specific lymphocyte clones and production of specific antibodies. Because these antibodies were not present earlier, their idiotypes were analogous to a new set of antigenic determinants to which the host would respond. Since antiidiotypic antibodies could bind to receptors on these first antigen-responsive clones, they could inhibit the function of these clones and thereby provide a negative feedback loop.

Many studies have assessed the validity of Jerne's **network theory,** and three of its major points are now well-established. First, antiidiotypic antibodies can, under different situations, inactivate or stimulate specific receptor-bearing B cells (Figure 4-2) as well as T lymphocytes; this indicates that antigen receptors on B and T cells share the idiotype. Since the recent demonstration that the receptor for antigen on MHC-restricted T cells is not Ig, the effects of antibodies raised against Ig idiotypes on such T cells are difficult to explain. Nucleotide sequence data do indicate, however, that significant homology exists between Ig and T cell receptors, so that idiotypic cross-reactivity between B and T cells is certainly possible. Administration of antiidiotypic antibodies is becoming a powerful tool for specific regulation of immune response. Second, after adminstration of some antigens, waves of antibodies (idiotypes), followed by antiidiotypes, can be detected. Such autologous antiidiotypic immunity may be critical for regulating the response to the antigen. Third, functional idiotype-recognizing T cells of the helper and suppressor class have been identified (see Figure 4-2); therefore, the idiotype network may consist of regulatory T lymphocytes as well as antibodies.

In summary, antireceptor immunity probably does play a role in regulating immune responses. The factors that determine the importance of idiotypic regulation in different immune responses, and the reasons why antiidiotypic antibodies or T cells are inhibitory

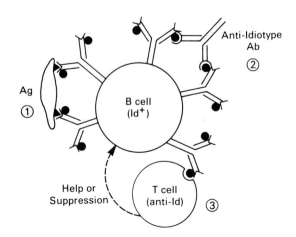

Figure 4-2 Idiotypic regulation. A B lymphocyte with immunoglobulin receptors for an antigen is shown (①). The receptor has a unique determinant, idiotype (Id, ●). An antiidiotypic antibody may cross-link the receptors (②) and thereby activate or inhibit the B cell. Similarly, a T cell with a receptor for Id may interact with the B cell (③) and provide help or suppression. In this case, the bridge between the two cells is formed by receptors and not the antigen (compare with Figure 4-1).

or stimulatory in different situations, have not yet been defined. As understanding of immunoregulatory mechanisms in experimental animals has increased, attempts have been made to determine if aberrations in regulatory pathways can lead to disease. Congenital and acquired defects of immune regulations are described in Chapters 12 and 13, respectively.

References

Howard, M., Paul, W.E.: Regulation of B cell growth and differentiation by soluble factors. *Ann Rev Immunol* 1983; 1:307-333.

Rajewsky, K, Takemori, T.: Genetics, expression and function of idiotypes. *Ann Rev Immunol* 1983; 1:569-607.

Singer, A., Hodes, R.J.: Mechanisms of T cell-B cell interaction. *Ann Rev Immunol* 1983; 1:211-241.

Unanue, E.R.: The regulatory role of marcophages in antigenic stimulation. *Adv Immunol* 1982; 31:1-136.

5 Antigen-Antibody Reactions and Their Biologic Consequences

M. Zouhair Atassi, PhD, DSc

R. P. Pelley, PhD, MD

General Concepts

The immune system is distinguished as a unique biologic entity by its ability to respond to an apparently limitless variety of antigens. The antibody, or humoral, immune response is a central part of the process. Chapters 1 and 4 on antibody structure and formation mentioned that the humoral response to an antigen, when it occurs, is usually characterized by production of a heterogeneous collection of antibody molecules that differ in their classes (G,.M, A, D, or E) as well as in the affinities (that is, the tenacity) with which they combine with the antigen. These antibodies, however, share the common ability to bind specifically with the particular antigen.

Antigen-antibody reactions are highly specific. Only occasionally do antibodies combine with antigens other than those against which they were made or those that are closely related to them. The exquisite specificity of antibodies enables them to discriminate among various antigens and permits the immune system to respond simultaneously to many different antigens without confusing their identities. This is a vital capability of the immune system and one for which it was specifically selected. Understanding the chemical principles that underlie the nature and specificity of antigen-antibody reactions is, therefore, of utmost importance to our comprehension of immunologic processes.

The physiologic consequences of the humoral response depend largely on the amounts and isotypes of antibodies that are elicited, and the amount and structure of the antigens that are encountered. Thus, knowing the amounts of antibodies, their specificity for antigen and their affinities for the antigen(s) in question is important in developing diagnoses and prognoses for patients.

This chapter is concerned primarily with the chemical principles on which antigen-antibody reactions are based, and with their biological consequences. Recent research in immunology, biochemistry, and related areas of study has provided intriguing details on the molecular design of antibodies and antigens. Besides shedding light on immunologic reactions, these details have suggested therapeutic approaches for beneficial manipulation of immune responses in persons with certain diseases.

Antibodies react with antigens at a molecular level through specialized regions of their respective structures: antibody-combining sites on the antibody molecule, and antigenic sites (determinants or epitopes) on the antigen. The following descriptions of antibodies and antigens focus on these specialized regions.

Antibodies

All **antibodies (Ab)** belong to the class of proteins known as **immunoglobulins.** In general, Ab are T- or Y-shaped structures, with two identical combining sites; one is located on each of the two arms of the molecule. These combining sites have characteristic shapes and can be visualized as cavities or grooves into which fit the antigenic sites. The overall shape of the antibody-combining site is determined by the manner in which certain portions of the heavy and light chains are folded and, in finer detail, by the specific amino acid residues that line the surface of the site. The particular shape of an antibody-combining site is a major factor in the ability of the antibody to combine with a specific antigen (see Chapter 1).

Nonantigen-binding domains of the antibody molecule maintain the proper shape of the combining sites and perform many other biologic (effector) functions. These effector functions, which include the binding to cell surfaces and interactions with other classes of serum proteins such as complement, are extremely important in the immune system.

Antigens

In contrast to antibodies, **antigens (Ag)** are not exclusively proteins. We have already defined an antigen operationally as that substance which binds to an antibody. More properly, an antigen is a molecule, a portion of which binds to the site of an antibody molecule that is specified by the genes that determine the complementarity region. Antigens may belong to virtually almost any class of molecule (proteins, polysaccharides, nucleic acids) or to a combination of classes. They may exist in chemical forms that are freely soluble in physiologic fluids or as components of particulate and more complex structures such as bacterial cells.

At the molecular level, each antigen possesses unique three-dimensional and chemical characteristics that distinguish it from other molecules encountered by the immune system. Because antigens have such varied chemical compositions, antigenic sites (epitopes) are somewhat harder to define than antibody-combining sites. Nevertheless, they may be thought of as the smallest portion of the antigen molecule capable of combining, specifically and optimally, with its corresponding antibody molecule. Antigen molecules that possess only one antigenic site (such as haptens) are **monovalent antigens.** Those antigens that have more than one antigenic site (for example, polysaccharides and proteins) are **multivalent antigens.** Most macromolecular antigens are multivalent.

Most of our knowledge of the molecular characteristics of antigenic sites is derived from studies on three classes of antigens: haptens, polysaccharides, and proteins.

Haptens

A **hapten** is one of an assortment of relatively small chemical compounds that, by themselves, usually do not elicit an antibody response; however, when linked to larger *carrier* molecules such as proteins, they act as effective immunogens. Penicillin (Figure 5-1) is a hapten that elicits antibody when coupled to a carrier molecule (usually a host protein). Some of the antibodies made against these penicillin-protein conjugates will react only with the haptenic group and not with the carrier protein. The specificity of these antibodies is seen readily in their reaction with penicillin itself. When it reacts with antibody, the entire hapten molecule is thought to be engulfed by the antigen-combining site on the antibody. Haptens are probably the smallest molecular compounds that will optimally and specifically bind to Ab.

Polysaccharide Antigens

The antigenic sites of **polysaccharides** (for example, dextrans), which are long-chain carbohydrate polymers of monosaccharide units, have been studied extensively. These polymers have large molecular weights, and their antigenic sites consist of relatively small portions of the polymer, encompassing from five to seven monosaccharide units. The repetitious structure of such polysaccharides enables them to possess many antigenic sites, some of which are identical to one another in the antibodies they elicit. Carbohydrates and carbohydrate polymers are essential for the antigenic specificity of a variety of natural antigens, such as those of bacterial cell walls and those of blood group substances. In glycoproteins, the carbohydrate may contribute to the antigenic properties of the molecule.

Studies of polysaccharide antigens provided the first insights into the approximate dimensions of antibody-combining sites. The size of polysaccharide antigenic sites led researchers to infer that the corresponding antibodies must possess complementary combining sites capable of accommodating five to seven monosaccharide units.

Penicillin G **Penicilloic Acid-Protein Complex** **Penicillinic Acid-Protein Complex**

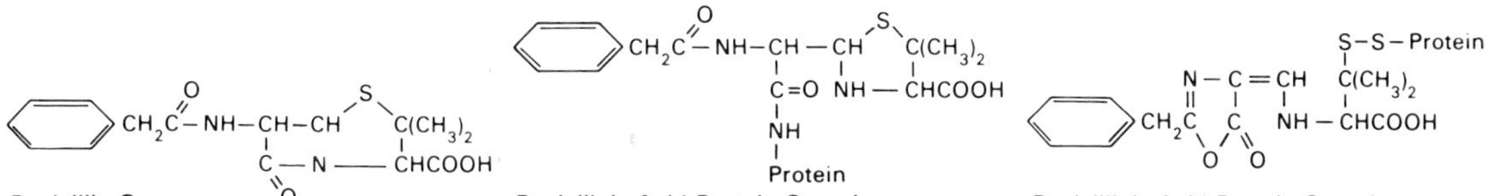

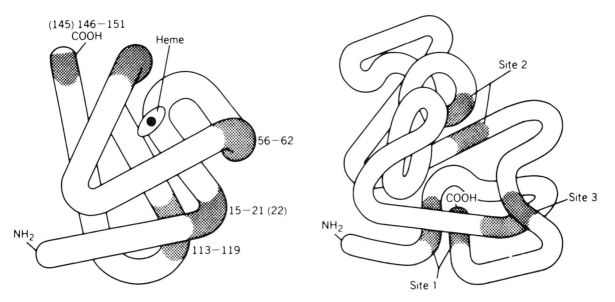

Figure 5-1 Chemical structure of the hapten penicillin and the chemical forms in which it is coupled to host protein.

Figure 5-2 Very schematic diagrams showing distribution of antigenic sites on protein molecules. Left, Sperm whale myoglobin. Right, Hen eggwhite lysozyme. Shading indicates position of antigenic sites (reactive regions); numbers show positions of amino acid residues constituting antigenic sites. (Myoglobin diagram is adapted from Atassi MZ: *Immunochemistry* 1975; 12:423; lysozyme diagram is adapted from Atassi MZ, Lee CL. *Biochem J* 1978; 171:429).

Interestingly, when molecular descriptions of the antigenic sites of proteins first became available (Figure 5-2), their molecular dimensions (in contrast to their chemical compositions) were comparable to those of polysaccharides. Thus, some uniformity appears not only in the sizes of the antigenic sites of complex macromolecules such as polysaccharides and proteins, but also, by inference, in the sizes of the corresponding antibody-combining sites.

Protein Antigens

Although immune responses to haptens and polysaccharides have been studied in detail, **protein antigens** have received such attention only recently because of their chemical complexity. Protein antigens are often associated with pathologic responses (for example, responses to invasive agents such as viral and bacterial antigens, toxins, and allergens) and immune regulation and disturbances of this regulation (such as occurs in autoimmune response). Although proteins vary greatly in structure, certain generalizations may be made about their antigenic properties. The first two proteins for which the complete antigenic structures were elucidated were myoglobin and lysozyme (see Figure 5-2). The antigenic sites of these two proteins consist of discrete surface areas of the respective three-dimensional structures. It appears that a surface localization of antigenic determinants is typical for protein molecules. This location facilitates rapid and efficient reaction with antibodies, which is an important advantage to the immune system, especially when circulating antibodies are called on to combat immediately the harmful effects of substances such as toxins.

The number of antibody-binding sites on an antigen is another important feature. Myoglobin and lysozyme (and most other proteins) are multivalent, possessing five and three independent antigenic sites, respectively. Multivalency increases the opportunity for antibodies to recognize an antigen and react with it. The factors that determine the location of an antigenic site on an antigen are probably complex and are not known. Thus, we have no reliable method to predict the number or locations of the antigenic sites of a protein; such factors must be determined independently for each protein.

The molecular dimensions of the antigenic sites of myoglobin and lysozyme also may be considered representative for all proteins. Each site is relatively small and consists of five to seven amino acid residues in close proximity to one another on the surface of the molecule. These dimensions coincide with the dimensions of polysaccharide antigenic sites.

The antigenic sites of these two proteins, however, differ in their architecture. The amino acid residues that constitute each antigenic site of myoglobin (see Figure 5-2B) are linked directly by peptide bonds and therefore represent continuous segments of the primary structure of the protein; these are called **continuous antigenic sites.** In contrast, residues of the antigenic sites of lysozyme (see Figure 5-2D) are not linked directly but are located at different parts of the primary structure. The residues of each site are brought into close proximity on the protein surface from distant parts of the primary structure by the specific manner in which the polypeptide chain of lysozyme is folded; these are called **discontinuous antigenic sites.** At present, the factors that determine whether a protein possesses continous or discontinuous antigenic sites are not fully understood; however, both of these structural alternatives for antigenic sites have been observed in proteins other than myoglobin and lysozyme, and continuous and discontinuous sites have been found to coexist in the same protein.

Although these generalizations apply to all protein antigens, each antigenic site has its own particular chemical and three-dimensional properties. These properties account for the specificity of the antigen's reaction with antibodies. Even very subtle distortions or changes in the antigenic site or in its chemical environment within the protein may prevent the protein from reacting with specific antibodies. Occasionally, however, antibodies to a particular site will crossreact with a site on a related protein that is structurally similar although not identical (see section on crossreactivity). In such situations, the two sites must resemble one another closely.

Structural and Chemical Basis of Antigen-Antibody Reactions

The immune system distinguishes among various antigens, specifically and selectively. The structural and chemical factors responsible for the highly specific interactions that occur between antigens and antibodies are no different that those that govern and direct most molecular interactions in all biologic systems. The principles for understanding antigen-antibody reactions, therefore, are also useful for formulating generalized concepts about all molecular interactions.

One prerequisite for the specific combination of an antibody with its antigen is that the regions through which they combine (antibody-combining sites) must exhibit an overall complementarity in their shapes. This complementarity has been referred to as a lock-and-key relationship. For example, a protrusion on the antigen is matched by a cavity on the antibody. The lock-and-key relationship is depicted schematically in Figure 5-3, which is an oversimplification. Antigens and antibodies are extremely complex molecules (see Figure 5-2) and do not have smoothly contoured surfaces; the structural and chemical complementarity between them is far more intricate than the illustration indicates.

In addition to a complementarity in their shapes, the binding between an antibody-combining site and an antigenic site depends on their ability to attract one another; that is, their ability to interact chemically. The chemical interactions that play a role in antigen-antibody reactions are all noncovalent. Primary apposition is established by ionic interactions between oppositely charged groups; hydrophobic interactions caused by the tendency of nonpolar groups to associate with one another; and hydrogen bonds that occur between hydrogen atoms such as those of the $-OH$ and $-NH$ groups (the *donor* group), and of atoms such as oxygen and nitrogen, which are present on acceptor groups (for example, $-N-H \ldots O; O-H \ldots N$). Once the antigenic site (epitope) and the antigen-combining site are brought into close proximity, **Van der Waals interactions** occur. These are weak attractive forces that exist between virtually all atoms or chemical groups that come within a certain distance of one another. The Van der Waals interactions serve to further stabilize the Ag-Ab bond.

Individually, these interactions are weak compared to covalent bonds, and are easily disrupted. Only when many such interactions can be formed between the antigen and antibody does sufficient strength exist to keep them together. In addition, these weak noncovalent attractive forces exert their effects only very short distances. Therefore, the antibody and antigen must come into close contact and mutually provide the

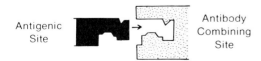

Antigenic Site → Antibody Combining Site

Figure 5-3 Lock-and-key complementarity between antigenic site and antibody-combining site. Only when overall shapes and electrostatic charge properties complement one another can binding occur. Molecular surfaces of antigen and antibody that come into contact during binding are extremely complex and require precise complementarity (see Figure 5-2B).

opportunity for forming the many interactions necessary. This requires a careful juxtapositioning of the complementary chemical groups on the antigen and antibody that will interact. In other words, a precise complementarity in their three-dimensional shapes, as well as in their respective hydrophobic and electrostatic or charge properties, provides the basis for the highly specific nature of antigen-antibody interactions.

Equilibrium in Antigen-Antibody Reactions

The types of interactions involved in the reaction of an antigenic site (epitope) with an antibody molecule are fragile and are broken easily under certain physiologic conditions. At any instant, some of these noncovalent interactions are forming while others are breaking. For a single antigen-antibody complex to exist, a certain minimum number of interactions must occur. These interactions are reversible processes in which complexes can coexist with unbound antigen and antibody molecules. At equilibrium, the rate at which complexes form equals the rate at which they dissociate, so that no net change occurs in the concentrations of either the reactants or products. For the simplest case of one antibody-combining site binding to one antigenic site, this equilibrium is represented by Figure 5-4. An antibody molecule that contains two combining sites (in the Fab portion) reacts with an antigen epitope and yields an Ag-Ab complex. This reaction, like all other chemical reactions, obeys the law of mass action so that the concentration of product [Ab · Ag], formed at equilibrium, depends on the concentrations of reactants [Ab] and [Ag] present initially. The equilibrium constant (K) of this reaction is represented by the following mathematical equation:

$$K_a = \frac{[Ab \cdot Ag]}{[Ab][Ag]}$$

This equilibrium constant is a measure of the affinity the antibody has for the antigen and is also known as the **affinity constant (K_a).**

The magnitude of the affinity constant reflects the strength with which the antigen-antibody complex is held together. High affinity constants indicate tightly held complexes. Also, as indicated earlier, the affinity with which an antibody and antigen combine is proportional to the maximum number of interactions possible between the two. Although little information is available on the specific number of interactions that occur between various antigen-antibody complexes, it is known that their affinities can range over several orders (10^4 to 10^{12} L/mole) of magnitude. Thus, the number and types of interactions that can form between an antibody and its antigen may be variable, and they depend on the particular antigen-antibody reaction involved.

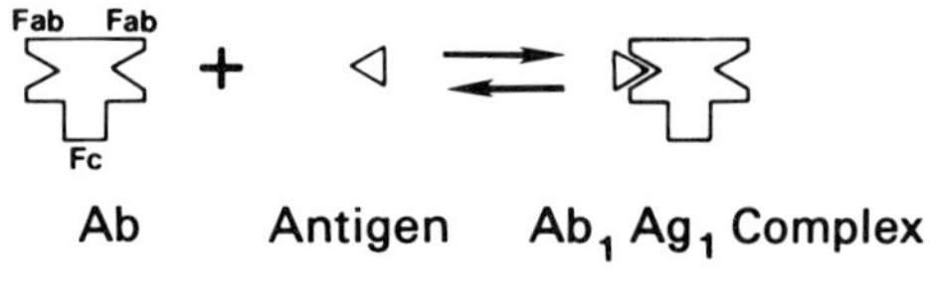

Figure 5-4 Reversible interaction of antigen and antibody.

Fab   Fab

Fc

Ab   Antigen   Ab$_1$ Ag$_1$ Complex

Ratios of Antigen to Antibody: The Bridge to Biologic Activity

The ratio of antigen to antibody is crucial in determining the ultimate outcome of the reaction. The result can range from neutralization (antibody excess), through optimal precipitation (at antigen-antibody equivalent), to antigen excess. These relationships can be visualized in the classic precipitin curve illustrated in Figure 5-5. Each of these relationships has a unique biologic impact. In high concentrations, antibodies can bind to virus, toxins, or hormones, and, by obscuring the attachment or active site of the antigen, inactivate it (**antibody excess**). In some amounts, antibody can bind to cellular antigen and trigger eventual lysis of the cell when complement binds to a crosslinked patch of antibody. When the ratio of antibody and antigen in a fluid is optimal; the lattice or complex that forms gives the largest amount of precipitate. This ratio is called the **equivalence** point. Finally, if the amount of antibody is small relative to the amount of antigen, small, soluble complexes will form (**antigen excess**) and less or no precipitate will be produced.

Although the ratio of Ag to Ab is critical to biologic activity, other factors also play a role. The exact pathophysiologic effect of antibody excess, equivalence, or antigen

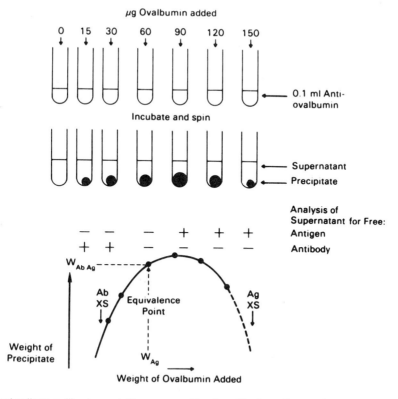

Figure 5-5 Typical antigen-antibody precipitin curve resulting from titration of increasing antigen concentration plotted against amount of immune precipitate formed. Amount of antibody is kept constant throughout.

excess depends on the class (isotype) of antibody, because some antibodies (like IgE) bind to cells, whereas others activate complement. In addition, the site in the body at which the reaction occurs can alter the clinical picture, because of the lack or availability of receptors and amplification systems such as complement. The size and stability of the lattice is influenced profoundly by antigen size, heterogeneity and density of antigenic sites, and antibody affinity. The ratio of antigen to antibody, however, is the crucial variable in the production of a lattice that can trigger tissue injury. We will now explore various permutations of antigen-antibody interactions in terms of their biologic consequences and role in immunologic tests.

Antibody Excess

When an individual who has received several doses of influenza vaccine is exposed moderately to influenze virus, each virus (viewed simplistically as a single antigen molecule bearing multiple antibody attachment sites) encounters a large number of antibodies and is neutralized; this is an example of a reaction in antibody excess (Figure 5-6). The receptors on the virus for cell surface absorption (the first step in infection) all are occupied by antibody. The virus cannot bind and the patient is protected. In antibody excess, most antibodies are bound univalently to antigenic sites (epitopes) and a rigid lattice does not form. In the absence of crosslinking, biologic amplification systems will not be triggered and the immunopathologic effects will be minimal. In toxin or virus neutralization, the selective advantage of producing high affinity antibody is obvious: dissociation of antigen from the complex at a later time (which would free toxin or virus) is prevented. The isotype of the antibody is not critical, since the biologic effect (masking a determinant) is not dependent upon activating complement or binding to a cell. Therefore, IgA or IgG_4, which activate complement only weakly, can be quite efficient in preventing the adherence of gonococci to mucosal surfaces or in neutralizing tetanus toxin.

Antigen Excess and Circulating Complexes

The region of antigen excess that constitutes the opposite end of the spectrum of Ag-Ab ratio should also be examined. Early in the course of a bacterial or viral infection, antibody is made in only minute quantities. In this situation, for example, large amounts of bacterial polysaccharide may be released into the circulation. A single antibody molecule may crosslink two molecules of antigen (or perhaps two viruses), but too little antibody is present to form a crosslinked matrix (Figure 5-7).

If these complexes are in the circulation, they will not be removed rapidly by phagocytic cells, perhaps because a rigid lattice of Fc pieces may not be established. When circulating Ag-Ab complexes are not removed by phagocytes, they may lodge in tissues. Later in the infection, as larger quantities of antibody are produced, these tissue-fixed complexes may grow. When the complexes reach equivalence, certain biologic events can be triggered. Some of the most striking examples of circulating immune complexes are manifested in autoimmune diseases. As will be discussed in Chapter 12, many of these diseases remain quiescent as long as the complexes are in Ag

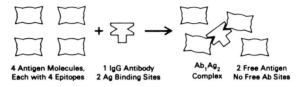

Figure 5-6 Formation of an antigen-antibody complex in antibody excess.

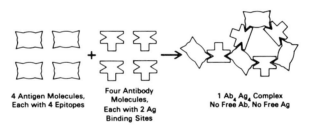

Figure 5-7 Formation of an antigen-antibody complex in antigen excess.

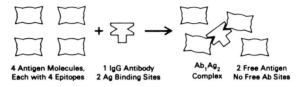

Figure 5-8 Formation of an antigen-antibody complex at equivalence.

excess. If the rate of antibody production increases, however, complexes at equivalence will form and illness will result.

Antigen-Antibody Equivalence—Lattice Formation

When antigen and antibody molecules interact in approximately equivalent amounts (that is, the amount necessary for mutual saturation) they can crosslink each other into a rigid matrix. If this lattice grows large enough, it will no longer by soluble and a precipitate will form (Figure 5-8). Several factors—number of antigenic sites (antigen valency) and their heterogeneity, as well as amount and heterogeneity of antibodies—are involved in forming these large complexes. These factors influence the stability of the lattice and determine the exact molecular Ag-Ab ratio at which equivalence (optimal precipitation) occurs. When the antigens reacting with antibody are univalent, both binding sites on the antibody will be occupied, antibodies cannot be crosslinked by

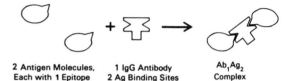

Figure 5-9 Reaction of antibody with a monovalent antigen does not lead to lattice formation.

2 Antigen Molecules, Each with 1 Epitope   1 IgG Antibody 2 Ag Binding Sites   Ab₁Ag₂ Complex

antigen, and the lattice cannot grow (Figure 5-9). The reaction is similar to the interaction of hapten and antibody.

The effect of antigen multivalency can be seen in the idealized diagram shown in Figure 5-7. It should be noted that the antigen, although tetravalent, has only a single type of homogeneous determinant. As was mentioned earlier, this homogeneous multivalency exists in many carbohydrate and protein antigens. For example, the capsule of type 3 pneumococcus contains numerous repeating units of the same disaccharide. Most protein antigens have dissimilar antigenic sites (epitopes); in the myoglobin molecule in Figure 5-2, no two sites are similar. If antibody were directed toward only one site (for example, monoclonal antibody), a lattice and precipitate would not form. For myoglobin to form a lattice and precipitate, for example, antibodies directed toward at least two different epitopes must be present. Typically, antibody diversity is large, and most immune responses recognize several site (epitopes) on an antigen. It should be noted that the response to each site is known to be under separate genetic control. Production of antibodies directed toward different antigenic sites is therefore related to the dissimilarity of these sites. These two processes assist in lattice formation, because the lower-affinity antibodies can stabilize a complex crosslinked initially by smaller amounts of high-affinity antibodies.

In summary, antigen size influences lattice formation in several ways. Simplistically, the number of antigenic sites is a function of the size of the antigen: a larger molecule provides more epitopes. These factors increase the chance that one Ab molecule will crosslink two antigen molecules.

For optimal lattice formation, a large antigen with several distinct epitopes is required. Each of these epitopes is present at several locations on the surface of the antigen; in Figure 5-10, a mixture of antibodies appears and the concentration of antibody is adjusted so that the numbers of antibody-combining sites and antigenic sites are about the same.

Equivalence and Immunologic Tests.   Many diagnostic tests are precipitation assays, which are based on unamplified lattice formation. In precipitation tests, optimal Ag-Ab ratio is critical, and most of these tests use antibody to measure and analyze relatively large, complicated antigens (such as serum proteins). Some tests (Table 5-1) use diffusion through agar to ensure that the functional ratio of antibody to antigen is equivalent. In other assays, complex kinetic methods are employed to achieve the same goal—optimal lattice formation.

Lattice Formation and Biologic Activity.   The biologic significance of lattice formation lies in orienting multiple antibody molecules into a matrix. The antigen crosslinks these Ab molecules so that the Fc portions of the immunoglobulins form a

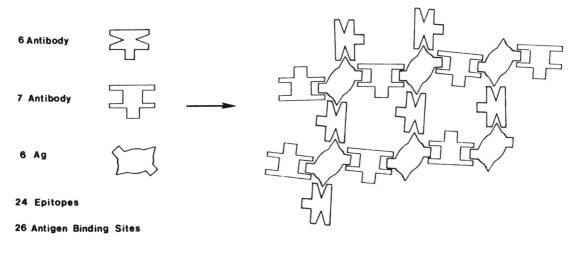

6 Antibody

7 Antibody

6 Ag

24 Epitopes

26 Antigen Binding Sites

1 Ab$_{13}$ Ag$_6$ Complex
No Free Ab, No Free Ag

Figure 5-10 Reaction of antibodies (directed against several antigenic sites) with antigens bearing two dissimilar but repeating antigenic sites (epitopes) leads to the formation of a large, solid complex when the number of antibody combining sites is at equivalence with the number of antigenic sites (epitopes).

Table 5-1   Clinical Tests Used to Detect Antigen-Antibody Reactions

Assay	Principle	Sensitivity (mg Ab/mL)
Immunofluorescence	Antibody bound to tissues is visualized by use of an anti-immunoglobulin antisera tagged with a fluorescent dye	100 ±
Precipitation	Antibody crosslinks soluble antigen to form a visible, insoluble complex (generally done in agar)	20-60
Complement fixation	If antibody is present, it reacts with antigen to form a complement-activating lattice; if complement is activated (fixed), no complement will be detected when the indicator system (erythrocytes coated with anti-erythrocyte antibody) is added	1
Agglutination	Antibody crosslinks organisms that have antigen on their surface to form a visible clump	0.1
Passive agglutination	Antibody crosslinks particles coated with antigen to form a visible clump	0.01
Radioimmunoassay	Antibody reacts with radiolabelled antigen; the immunoglobulin in the serum is then insolubilized and tested for bound labelled antigen	0.001
Enzyme-linked immunoassay	Insolubilized antigen is mixed with serum and washed; the presence of antigen-bound antibody is detected by an enzyme-tagged anti-immunoglobulin	0.001

lattice. CIq can bind to this array, provided that the immunoglobulin is of an isotype (IgM, IgG_1, IgG_2, or IgG_3) capable of activating complement. Once complement is activated, the consequence of forming an equivalence Ag-Ab lattice is to activate mediators of inflammation (see Chapter 6).

Enhancement of phagocytosis by antibody (opsonization) also results from lattice formation. Phagocytes such as macrophages and neutrophils have difficulty adhering to, and phagocytosing, bacterial capsules, but they do have receptors for the Fc portion of immunoglobulins. When phagocytes encounter a lattice, these Fc receptors can engage the antibody molecules in the complex. Although each individual Fc-phagocyte bond is weak, the multivalent nature of the lattice helps the phagocyte to gain a firm hold. Opsonization is enhanced further when complement is activated.

Ag-Ab Interaction on a Surface.   If small amounts of antigen or antibody are fixed on a cell surface, the effect of Ag-Ab lattice formation can be profound, because it may activate cellular functions, crosslink (agglutinate) cells, or activate complement and cell lysis.

In situations in which antibody is on the surface of a cell, at least two immunoglobulin molecules must be bridged to trigger the cell. If the cell is a B lymphocyte, the immunoglobulin is produced endogenously. Antigen binding to B cell receptors leads to the first step in B cell activation and is required for antibody production. If the cell is a mast cell or basophil, the IgE antibodies on its surface were produced by a plasma cell and bound to the IgE-specific receptor on that surface (Chapter 9; Figure 9-1). The result of an antigen crosslinking two IgE molecules on a basophil is the activation of the cell leading to the production and release of mediators of immediate hypersensitivity. The exact relationship between the linking of two antibody molecules on the surface and activation of the cell has not yet been determined, but it is known that the same factors that are important in fluid-phase lattice formation (antigen valence and antibody affinity) are also important in cellular activation.

When antigen is present on the surface of a cell, antibodies can crosslink two cells together (Figure 5-11). Because of the large size of the cells, Ab multivalency and large Ab molecular dimension becomes critical; thus, IgM is more efficient at this agglutination than is IgG.

Many common laboratory assays for detecting infection (looking for Ab produced in response to infection), or for classifying infectious agents (typing bacteria by their antigens), involve agglutination tests. The range of these tests has been expanded by coupling antigens chemically either to red blood cells or to plastic spheres, and using these visible substrates to detect antibodies. Many of these tests are discussed in Chapter 25.

As mentioned earlier, complement binding to Ag-Ab complexes is involved in the production of mediators of inflammation, and complement aids in opsonization of Ag by phagocytes. The role of complement that has been characterized best, however, is the damaging of the membrane of a cell *identified* by bound Ag-Ab complexes. This reaction requires the proper orientation of crosslinked antibody molecules that present their Fc domains as a matrix to which CIq can bind. Because pentameric IgM already has five Fc domains, the complement cascade will begin when IgM binds to the cell. Researchers have shown that a single IgM molecule is enough to trigger lysis of a red

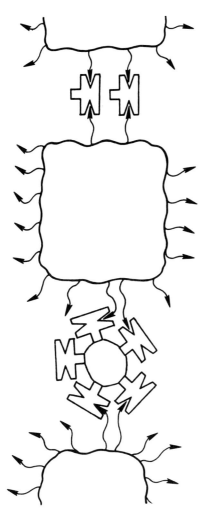

Figure 5-11 IgM is more efficient at agglutinating cells than is IgG.

blood cell. For IgG to be effective, however, several molecules must bind in close proximity.

Crossreactivity

Thus far, our examination of the interaction of antigen with antibody has assumed that Ag-Ab interactions are absolutely specific, but, of course, **crossreactions** occur often. In crossreactivity, antibody reacts not only with the specific antigen, but also with a different antigen, which, nevertheless, carries an antigenic site. Crossreactivity results from similarity of antigenic sites or from the reaction of antibodies of two different fine specificities with the same antigenic site (or alternatively, reaction of two antigenic sites of different fine specificity with the antibody). The appearance of identical or similar sites (epitopes) on different antigens is the basis for many serologic tests for infectious diseases. Perhaps the best known example is the test for syphilis (Chapter 51). Infection of humans with *Treponema pallidum* gives rise to antibodies against the membrane of the spirochete, particularly against its phospholipid, diphosphatidyl-glycerol. This epitope also is present in mammalian mitochondrial membranes as a cardiolipin. Since antigen prepared from treponemes is extremely expensive, cardiolipin prepared from mammalian sources is used in the agglutination screening test for syphilis infections (Table 5-1). Thus, antibody induced against an antigenic site (epitope) on the surface of a microorganism is assayed with the same epitope, prepared from another source.

Similar epitope sharing is seen between *Rickettsia* (the organism responsible for various forms of typhus) and *Proteus* (a common gram-negative bacteria). Antibodies from patients with primary louse-borne typhus (*R prowazekii*) strongly agglutinate *Proteus* OX-19 because the organisms probably have identical, or very similar, oligosaccharides in their surface polysaccharide antigens. Patients with scrub typhus (*R rickettsii*) have antibodies that react best with *Proteus* OXK. Thus, a high degree of serologic specificity in serologic tests is achieved because of sharing of antigenic sites.

A second form of crossreactivity occurs when an antibody that is raised against one molecular configuration encounters a similar, but not identical, molecular configuration (Figure 5-12). For example, in the polysaccharide antigens of the pneumococcal capsule, the core repeating units of two common types are:

Streptococcus   type 3   glucuronic-glucose-glucuronic-glucose
                        acid   acid
pneumoniae   type 8   glucuronic-glucose-glucose-galactose
                        acid

Heidelberger raised horse antisera to each of these and studied the interaction of each antiserum with each of the two polysaccharides. Antisera to type 8 precipitated type 3 polysaccharide (related epitope), but only 28% as well as it precipitated type 8 (identical epitope). Similarly, anti-type 3 precipitated type 8, but only 22% as well as it precipitated the homologous type 3 Ag. These crossreactions occur because a single antibody can recognize similar (nonidentical) structures. The strength of recognition is related to the closeness of fit. Since the fit of anti 8 Ab with type 3 is better than the fit with type 8, the reaction with S3 will have a lower affinity than with S8. Lower affinity will result in a weaker lattice structure (and therefore less precipitation).

This example shows that, although the binding groove or cavity on an antibody molecule accommodates four to six sugars, an antibody can discriminate single sugar (or single amino acid) differences. This ability is the basis for the human ABO blood group system, since the difference between the two major blood groups is the difference

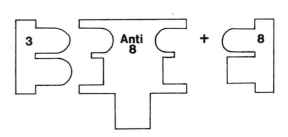

Figure 5-12 Although antibody to type 8 pneumococci will react with type 3 pneumococcal polysaccharide because of fine specificity crossreactivity, the reaction is energetically less favorable than the reaction of antibody to type 8 with type 8 pneumococcal polysaccharide.

between N acetyl galactosamine and galactose (Chapter 14, Figure 14-2). In addition, the serotyping of *Salmonella* depends on the ability of antibodies to recognize subtle differences in the side chain of lipopolysaccharides. Protein allotypes may vary by only a single amino acid, but they can often be differentiated by antibodies. As another example, in patients sensitized to penicillin, administration of a cephalosporin antibiotic (although produced by a different fungus from penicillin) can lead to death, because of the chemical resemblance between the two agents.

References

Atassi, M.Z.: Precise determination of protein antigen structures has unravelled the molecular immune recognition of proteins and provided a prototype for synthetic mimicking of other protein binding sites. *Mol Cell Biochem* 1980; 32:21–43.

Eisen, H.N.: Antibody-antigen reactions. In: *Microbiology Including Immunology and Molecular Genetics*, 3rd ed. Davis BD et al (editors). New York: Harper and Row, 1980.

Klein, J.: *Immunology, the Science of Self-Nonself Discrimination.* New York: Wiley-Interscience, 1982.

Stites, D.P.: Clinical laboratory methods for detection of antigens and antibodies. In: *Basic and Clinical Immunology*, 4th ed. Stites DP et al (editors). Los Altos: Lange Medical Publishers, 1982.

Weir, D.M., (editor): *Handbook of Experimental Immunology*, 3rd ed. Oxford: Blackwell Scientific Publishers, 1978.

6 Complement

Tony E. Hugli, PhD

General Concepts

Complement, a multicomponent system in the blood of all higher mammals, is composed of heat-labile substances that combine with antibodies to lyse microorganisms and viruses. In 1900, Paul Ehrlich originally observed that these serum components interact independently with cell-bound antibodies to enhance lysis of the bacteria, a process that complements the initial complexing of antibody to the cellular antigens. Thus, Ehrlich coined the term **complement** for the assorted serum protein components that play an integral role in the immune process by enhancing or intensifying reactions initiated by antigen-antibody complexes. Von Buchner specifically demonstrated the bactericidal activity of sera by killing typhoid bacilli with fresh rabbit serum; he also showed that sera heated at 56 C lost their bactericidal activity.

Complement function is limited by temperature. Heating fresh serum for 15 min at 56 C destroys lytic action and some other functions of complement; therefore heating is frequently used to deactivate complement's activity. Simply keeping serum at room temperature for 2-3 hours precludes activation of complement in freshly drawn blood; however, at 4 C, complement's activity lasts for several days and serum frozen soon after collection maintains full function months after storage at -70 C. Additionally, divalent metal ions—calcium or magnesium or both—are required to activate the complement pathways. Sonication or extremely acidic or alkaline conditions produce an irreversible loss of complement activity; however, inactivation caused by exposure to hypertonic salt solution or to ions, including citrate, EDTA, $SO_4^=$, Ba^{++} or Sr^{++}, is readily reversible.

Although complement is ascribed a primary role in immune surveillance and host defense, the complement system seems biosynthetically unrelated to the immune response in higher mammals. Accordingly, hypercatabolism of complement and significant anabolic rate changes in levels of its components are apparently independent of changes in immunoglobulin biosynthesis. The absence of conclusive evidence linking complement activation to an initiation of immunoglobulin synthesis is a paradox considering the presumed role of complement in supporting or intensifying immunologic mechanisms. Furthermore, the popular hypothesis that complement and the immunoglobulin systems share a common genetic origin remains more speculation than fact. Nonetheless, recent progress in understanding the genetic processes involved promises to uncover subtle biosynthetic relationships between complement and the immune system.

From species to species within the animal kingdom, concentrations of the individual complement components vary, as does total complement activity. Hemolytic activities of mammalian sera are generally greater than those of birds, reptiles, amphibians, and fish. An exception may be the turtle, which has an unusually high complement titer when measured by the CH_{50} hemolytic assay (for CH_{50}, see page 77); however, turtle serum is virtually void of activity when assessed for hemolysis induced by cobra venom (see discussion of the classical pathway on page 64).

On the other hand, complement components isolated from a wide variety of higher animals are functionally interchangeable. For example, guinea pig or rabbit complement components can restore function to complement-deficient human serum. Furthermore, a given animal's serum may lyse erythrocytes from a wide variety of animal sources. In general laboratory practice, sheep erythrocytes have become the favored cellular reagent for quantifying hemolytic activity of the human complement system and, because bacteriolysis is difficult to perform, hemolytic assays have become the preferred method to detect and quantify individual complement components.

Nature of Complement Components

In the past 10 years, understanding of the complement system at the molecular level has progressed remarkably. At least 20 macromolecular components have been identified (Table 6-1). These components act as recognition factors, proteolytic factors, modulators or stabilizers, biologically active cleavage products, or inactivators. The complement proteins interact in sequences that constitute two distinct activation pathways. Since complement activation involving the C1, C2, and C4 components was the first to be described, the pathway that consists of these components is called the **classical pathway,** and the remaining course of activation is called the **alternative pathway** (Figure 6-1).

Table 6-1 Serum Components of the Complement System

Intact Protein Component	Function	Mol. Wt.	Number of Chains	Electro-phoretic Mobility	Serum Concentration (µg/mL)
Classical Pathway Components					
C1	Recognition	774,000	22	γ	130–140
C1q	Recognition	410,000	6 × 3	γ 2	70
C1r	Enzyme precursor	190,000	2	β 1	34
C1s	Enzyme precursor	180,000	2	α	31
C2	Enzyme precursor	115,000	1	β 1	25
C3	Modulator	180,000	2	β 1	1200–600
C4	Modulator	206,000	3	β 1	450
Alternative Pathway Components					
Factor D (PAase, GBGase)*	Enzyme	24,000	1	α	1–5
Factor B (PA or GBG)*	Enzyme precursor	93,000	1	β 2	140–225
Components of Lytic Complex					
C5	Lytic complex	180,000	2	β 1	75
C6	Lytic complex	120,000	1	β 2	60
C7	Lytic complex	120,000	1	β 2	60
C8	Lytic complex	154,000	3	γ 1	80
C9	Lytic complex	80,000	1	α	150
Regulators and Control Factors					
C4b-binding protein (C4bp)	Modulator	570,000	6–8	NA	275
Properdin (P)	Modulator	212,000	4	γ 2	25
Factor H (β1H)	Modulator	150,000	1	β	560
$\overline{C1}$ INH*	Inhibitor	105,000	1	α 2	180
Factor I (C3b INA* KAF)	Enzyme	88,000	2	β	35
S-protein (MAC inhibitor)*	Inhibitor	90,000	1	α 2	350–500
SCPN (KININASE I)*	Enzyme	310,000	4	α 1	30–40

*C3 proactivator convertase or glycine-rich β glycoprotein convertase (factor D); C3 proactivator or glycine-rich β glycoprotein (factor B); membrane attack complex inhibitor (MAC inhibitor); C1 esterase inhibitor (C1 INH); C3b inactivator (C3b INA); and serum carboxypeptidase N (SCPN). N.A., not available. The current nomenclature uses a numerical system for the classical pathway components and an alphabetical system to identify components of the alternative pathway (e.g., Factors B, D, H, and I).

The Classical Pathway

Immunoglobulins (antibodies) in the form of single molecules do not function efficiently as complement activators; however, when numerous immunoglobulin molecules cluster on the surface of a particle or cell, or associate through specific interactions with an antigen, conformational changes are believed to occur in the structure of the immunoglobulin molecules. This conformational change, which can be artificially induced by heat to promote aggregation of the immunoglobulin molecules, presumably enables the immunoglobulin to interact with the first component of complement (C1); thus the classical pathway becomes activated by immunologic means (Figure 6-2). However, it is not yet established whether activation is transmitted via the C1q subcomponent of C1 as a result of conformational changes in the immunoglobulin molecule or because cooperative binding occurs between aggregated immunoglobulin molecules and the multiple Fc binding sites on C1q. The major activators of the classical

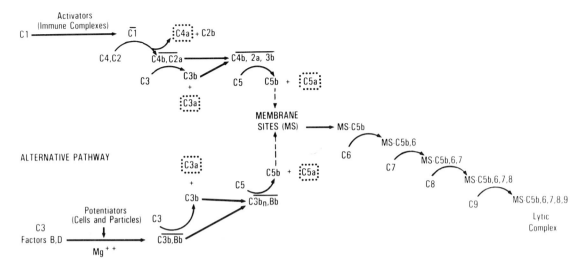

CLASSICAL PATHWAY

ALTERNATIVE PATHWAY

Figure 6-1 Summary of complement activation via the classical and alternative pathways. The classical pathway is initiated when component C1 is activated to C1. A subcomponent of C1, C1s, is an enzyme that cleaves components C3 and C4. The complex C4b, 2a, an enzyme that converts component C3, is called C3 convertase. Association of C3b to this complex constitutes the C5 convertase. When C3 is converted by factor B of the alternative pathway, C3b, Bb complex is formed. This complex is an efficient C3 convertase; addition of C3b molecules to this complex produces a C5 convertase. Beyond the C5 conversion step, both pathways merge into a single cascade. The C5b component anchored to a membrane surface (MS) initiates assembly of the terminal membrane attack or lytic complex. The bioactive factors C3a, C4a, and C5a are called anaphylatoxins.

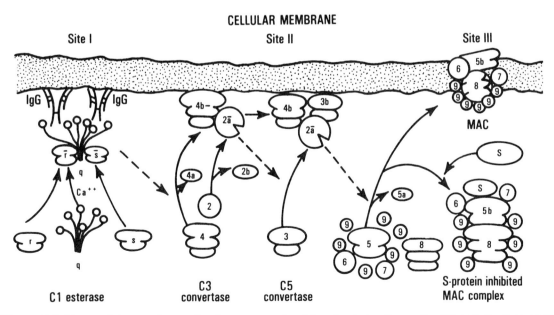

Figure 6-2 Three cellular membrane sites for components of the classical pathway. The C1 complex is reversibly bound to antibody molecules at site I through the C1q subunit. C3 and C5 convertases are assembled on site II. C5b-9 complex (MAC) is assembled via C5b attachment to site III. Modified from Müller-Eberhard, HJ: Complement. In *Annual Review of Biochemistry*, Vol. 44. Snell EE (editor). Palo Alto, Calif.: Annual Reviews, 1975.

pathway are IgM and IgG antibody. The beauty of the complement system, however, is that various other compounds, such as staphylococcal microorganisms, DNA, plasmin, and streptokinase, can also be activators (Table 6-2).

C1, the first component of the classical pathway, serves as a recognition component, sensing activators that modify C1 to an activated form. C1 is a Ca^{++}-dependent complex that consists of 22 polypeptide chains in the form of three subunits ($C1q$, $C1r_2$, and $C1s_2$).

C1q, the true recognition portion of the component and perhaps the most interesting subunit of C1, is unique. A glycoprotein, C1q contains small amounts of the rare amino acids hydroxylysine and hydroxyproline. Generally, these two amino acids are found only in connective tissues such as collagen. In fact, a collagenlike domain exists in the multichained N-terminal region of the C1q molecule. The C1q structure is composed of 18 chains (six A chains, six B chains, and six C chains) that progressively diminish in size from A, the longest, to C, the shortest. (See Figure 6-3). These chains form six bundles, each of which contains an A, B, and C chain; the carboxyl ends of the six bundles that comprise C1q look like six globes connected to a common stalk by triple-helical, collagenlike threads. In electron microscopic pictures, the C1q molecule resembles a bouquet of flowers.

C1r is a proenzyme subunit of C1. A proenzyme is an inactive precursor form of the active enzyme. $C1r_2$ consists of two identical, noncovalently linked polypeptide chains. C1r is cleaved into $\overline{C1r}$ during activation—the bar denotes an active enzyme (protease). The mechanism of this conversion is unknown, although we believe that C1r may undergo autoactivation (one chain cleaves another chain). When C1q is perturbed by an activator, one C1r subunit or monomer cleaves a neighboring C1r subunit in the C1 complex.

C1s is also a proenzyme. Much like C1r, $C1s_2$ consists of two identical, noncovalently linked polypeptide chains. C1s is cleaved into a two-chain $\overline{C1s}$ form by $\overline{C1r}$. Together, C1q, C1r, and C1s compose the precursor C1. Activated C1 (for example, $\overline{C1}$) is thus composed of C1q, $\overline{C1r_2}$, and $\overline{C1s_2}$. Consequently, two forms of C1 exist: C1 in its resting or precursor state and the activated C1, denoted $\overline{C1}$. When C1 combines with antibodies attached to a surface such as on an erythrocyte, the C1 becomes activated to $\overline{C1}$ (summarized in Figure 6-4).

C1 esterase inhibitor (C1 INH) is a regulatory component consisting of a single polypeptide chain. It forms a stable complex with $\overline{C1s}$ and physically neutralizes $\overline{C1}$ activity, thereby terminating participation of $\overline{C1}$ in the activation process.

C2 is the next enzyme precursor in the classical component cascade and consists of a single polypeptide chain. C2 is selectively cleaved by $\overline{C1s}$ into C2a and C2b. C2a at 80,000 molecular weight (mol. wt.) has only marginal enzymatic activity, a function that is greatly enhanced when C2a combines with C4b on a membrane site or in serum; however, C2b (34,000 mol. wt.) has no known function except perhaps a kininlike activity, a claim that requires further verification.

C4 was discovered after C3, but was found to participate before C3 in the stepwise pathway of activation. Activated C4 acts as a modulator in that it enhances the enzymatic activity of C2. C4 consists of three polypeptide chains. C4, like C2, is selectively cleaved by the $\overline{C1s}$ subunit of $\overline{C1}$ into two fragments: C4a and C4b. C4a is a 9000 mol. wt. fragment consisting of a single chain. Recently, C4a was accorded

Table 6-2   Activators of the Human Blood Complement System

Activator	Classical Pathway	Alternative Pathway
Immunologic activators	IgM >> IgG1, IgG3 > IgG2	IgA, IgE, and some IgG subclasses
Nonimmunologic activators	Trypsinlike proteases (plasmin, streptokinase, and lysosomal proteases)	Trypsinlike proteases (plasmin, streptokinase, etc.)
	Deoxyribonucleic acid polyinosinic acid	Lipopolysaccharides, damaged mammalian cell walls
	Staphlococcal protein A	Plant or bacterial polysaccharides (inulin and zymosan)
	C-reactive protein, polyanion/ polycation complexes	Cobra venom factor (A C3b analog)

POLYPEPTIDE CHAINS

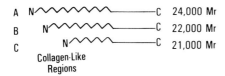

SUBUNIT ORGANIZATION

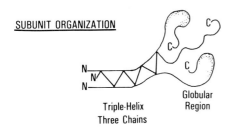

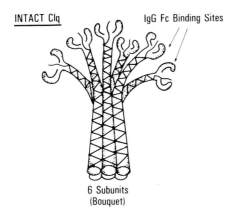

Figure 6-3 Molecular organization of the recognition component C1q. Three separate polypeptide chains comprise the C1q molecule. Chains A, B, and C each contain collagenlike *N*-terminal sequences complete with hydroxyl amino acids. Chains of the C1q molecule range in size from 21,000–24,000 mol. wt. Subunit structure is characterized by a triple helical arrangement of the *N*-terminal regions of an A, B, and C chain, a conformation usually found in proteins of connective tissue. *C*-terminal portions of the three-chain subunit assume a globular conformation. Intact C1q appears as a bouquet containing six of the subunits aligned in parallel fashion. Extended globular regions of C1q recognize the Fc region of immunoglobulin molecules.

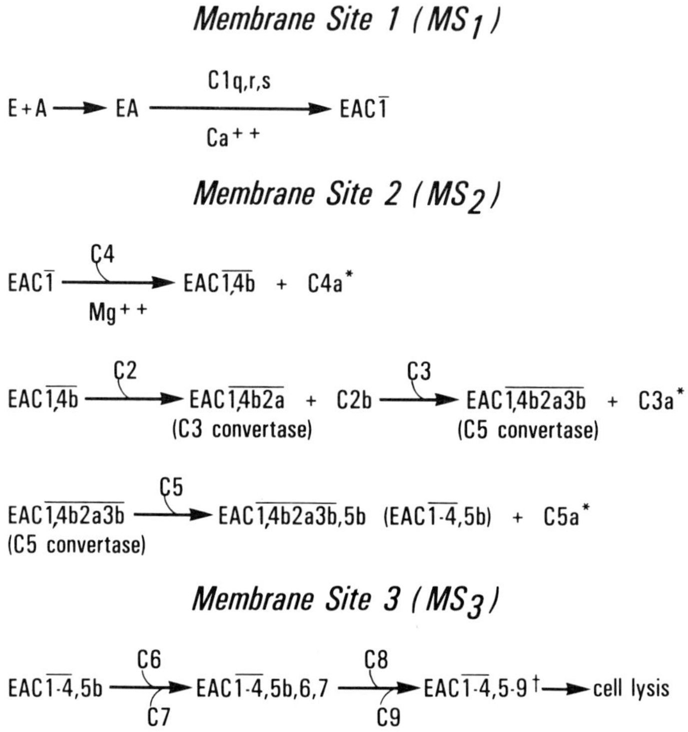

Membrane Site 1 (MS$_1$)

$$E + A \longrightarrow EA \xrightarrow[\text{Ca}^{++}]{\text{C1q,r,s}} EA\overline{C1}$$

Membrane Site 2 (MS$_2$)

$$EA\overline{C1} \xrightarrow[\text{Mg}^{++}]{\text{C4}} EA\overline{C1,4b} + C4a^{*}$$

$$EA\overline{C1,4b} \xrightarrow{\text{C2}} EA\overline{C1,4b2a} + C2b \xrightarrow{\text{C3}} EA\overline{C1,4b2a3b} + C3a^{*}$$
$$\text{(C3 convertase)} \qquad\qquad \text{(C5 convertase)}$$

$$EA\overline{C1,4b2a3b} \xrightarrow{\text{C5}} EA\overline{C1,4b2a3b,5b} \; (EA\overline{C1\text{-}4},5b) + C5a^{*}$$
$$\text{(C5 convertase)}$$

Membrane Site 3 (MS$_3$)

$$EA\overline{C1\text{-}4},5b \xrightarrow[\text{C7}]{\text{C6}} EA\overline{C1\text{-}4},5b,6,7 \xrightarrow[\text{C9}]{\text{C8}} EA\overline{C1\text{-}4},5\text{-}9\dagger \longrightarrow \text{cell lysis}$$

Figure 6-4 Reaction sequence of classical pathway of complement activation. Erythrocytes (E) combine with antibody (A) directed toward cell surface antigens to form EA complex. C1q, r, and s with Ca^{++} and a complement (C) activator (see Table 6-2) generate $\overline{C1}$ esterase activity. C4 and C2 are then cleaved by C1 esterase to form EAC1,4b,2a complex. Enzyme complex EAC1,4b,2a is specific for cleaving C3 and is known as C3 convertase. Addition of product C3b to EAC1,4b,2a complex modifies specificity of complex to that of C5 convertase, and C5 is then cleaved. C5b attaches to independent site on E; lytic complex (MAC, membrane attack complex) is formed by the sequential binding of C6, C7, C8, and C9 into a complex, and lysis occurs immediately. C3a*, C4a*, and C5a* are low-molecular-weight fragments (anaphylatoxins) that mediate inflammatory reactions.

activities similar to, although not as strong as, those of the C3a and C5a anaphylatoxins. The activities incited by purified C4a include contraction of isolated strips of guinea pig small intestine (spasmogenic) and an inflammatory response, including wheals (edema) and a localized red discoloration (erythema) in injected skin. C4b, the 196,000 mol. wt. modulator fragment of C4, consists of three polypeptide chains. In combination with C2a, C4b forms the C3-cleaving enzyme known as the C3 convertase (see Figures 6-3 and 6-4).

C3, also a modulator that functions only after activation, is composed of two polypeptide chains. C3 is selectively converted into C3a and C3b fragments by the protease C4b,2a. The C3a fragment is a 9000 mol. wt. polypeptide chain that is a potent anaphylatoxin; C3b is a 171,000 mol. wt. fragment consisting of two chains. This fragment modifies the activity of C3 convertase (C4b,2a). When C3b combines with the C3 convertase to form the complex C4b,2a,3b, a C5 convertase is generated. C3b also binds to various cells (for example, bacterial cells, damaged mammalian cells, and yeast cells) to make them more susceptible to ingestion by white blood cells (a process known as phagocytosis). The C3 molecule and its fragments are directly associated with such phenomena as immunoregulation, immunoagglutination, immune adherence, opsonization, phagocytosis, histamine release, smooth muscle contraction, and enhanced vascular permeability (see discussion of alternate pathway on this page.)

C5 is composed of two polypeptide chains and is selectively cleaved into C5a and C5b by the C5 convertase (C4b,2a,3b). Human C5a (11,000 mol. wt.) consists of a single glycoprotein chain. This fragment is a potent spasmogen and chemotaxin. The two-chain C5b (170,000 mol. wt.) functions as an anchor at the cell surface, where the lytic membrane attack complex (MAC), C5-9, attaches. C5a, like C3a and C4a, is associated with anaphylatoxic reactions (histamine release, smooth muscle contraction, and enhanced vascular permeability) and in addition promotes chemotaxis and the release of enzymes, oxygen, and arachidonate metabolites from leukocytes. Recently, C5a was shown to enhance the cellular immune response.

Four complement components, in addition to C5b, function as that part of the MAC that actually promotes lysis of cells: C6, C7, C8 and C9. C6, a lytic component, is a single-chain polypeptide that forms a stable, noncovalent complex with C5b either on the surface of a cell or in the serum. C7, also a lytic component, exists as a single chain. It also binds by autoassociation to the C5b and C6 complex, forming a solid or fluid phase C5b-7 complex. C8, composed of three polypeptide chains, is the next to last component of the lytic complex. Association of C8 with the C5b-7 complex on the erythrocyte promotes a slow lysis. C9 is a single polypeptide chain that completes the lytic or MAC complex; C9's association with C5b-8 produces rapid lysis (see Figure 6-2).

Thus, the classical pathway has two sets of components: those present in the precursor or resting state are C1 (q,r,s), C2, C3, C4, and C5; those present in the activated state are C$\overline{1}$ ($\overline{q,r,s}$), C2a, C2b, C3a, C3b, C4a, C4b, C5a, C5b. Components C6–C9 do not undergo covalent structural changes but do participate in a noncovalent complex with C5b, thereby completing the activation cascade.

The Alternate Pathway

An alternative pathway of complement activation may be initiated by immunologic or nonimmunologic means. Although immunoglobulins of the IgA, IgE, and IgG classes serve as functional initiators of this pathway, far more commonly nonimmunologic agents such as complex polysaccharides from plant and bacterial cell walls or cellular membrane components serve as potent alternative pathway activators. Cobra venom has long been known as an efficient complement activator, which is not surprising because the venom factor is apparently a structural analog of the C3b molecule. Cobra venom factor acts by entering the alternative pathway as a functional substitute for endogenous C3b.

The initial step of the alternative pathway has remained the least understood of all the complement reactions. Presumably, trace quantities of autoantibodies fulfill a recognition function; however, a component found in sera of patients with glomerulonephritis exerts a more specific action. This component, referred to as **nephritic factor,** is a four-chain polypeptide that resembles the IgG molecule and presumably is an autoantibody directed toward the C3b,Bb complex. Binding of nephritic factor to

$\overline{\text{C3b,Bb}}$ enhances the activity of the convertase, presumably by stabilizing the complex. Nephritic factor was originally mistaken as an initiating factor of activation.

Factor D, an enzyme consisting of a single polypeptide, is a serine esterase that cleaves factor B at a precise scission site. The specific mechanism by which factor D activates B is also unknown; however, substances that are recognized as foreign to an organism (see Table 6-2), or endogenous factors such as autoantibodies, may be involved in promoting the attack of D on B. The possibility also exists that factor D requires no special activation process but rather is normally present in an active enzyme form. The first step in the activation of the alternative pathway (Figure 6-5) assumes that factor D exists in serum in an active and not a precursor form. Factor D is also referred to in the literature as C3PAase (C3 proactivator convertase) or as GBGase (glycine-rich β-globulin convertase).

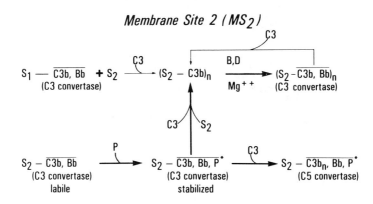

Figure 6-5 Activators and factor D, in conjunction with a cell surface, are prerequisite for factor B conversion. Activating factor B leads to conversion of C3 molecule and deposition of C3b at first membrane site (MS_1). Low levels of C3 convertase are produced in this manner; however, as C3b becomes available, it deposits at a separate site (MS_2), and C3 convertase S_2-C3b,Bb accumulates further. This cycle of C3b deposition leading to enzyme formation, which in turn produces more C3b for deposition on the membrane, is known as an amplification or "feedback" loop of the alternative pathway. Properdin stabilizes C3 convertase, thereby producing enzyme complex S_2-C3b,Bb,P*, which participates in amplification process. As multiple C3b molecules attach to MS_2-C3b,Bb,P* complex, specificity of C3 convertase changes to that of C5 convertase. C5b attaches to membrane site 3 (MS_3), and lytic complex assembles by sequential association of C6, C7, C8, and C9.

Factor B is a proenzyme with a single-chain polypeptide structure. When cleaved by factor D, factor B is fragmented into Ba and Bb, both of which consist of a single polypeptide chain structure. The smaller Ba fragment (30,000 mol. wt.) has no well-defined function; however, Bb (62,000 mol. wt.) is an active enzyme that contains the active site of the C3 convertase (see MS_1 in Figure 6-5).

C3 serves a prominent role in both activation pathways and is the pivotal component in activating complement. Not only is C3 the pivotal protein during activation, but it is produced in higher levels than any of the other complement proteins; this is probably more than a fortuitous phenomenon and may be related to the important physiologic role that C3 plays. Recently it was shown that small quantities of the modulator C3b spontaneously form in blood and then combine with Bb to generate C3 convertase. Autoactivation of C3 occurs when an intramolecular thioester linkage

$$
\begin{array}{l}
R{-}OH \rightarrow \\
\\
R{-}NH_2 \rightarrow
\end{array}
\left[\begin{array}{c} \\ \overset{O}{\underset{\parallel}{-}}S{-}\overset{}{C}{-} \\ \end{array} \right]
\begin{array}{l}
\rightarrow -SH + \overset{\overset{\textstyle O}{\parallel}}{-}C{:}O{-}R \\
\\
\rightarrow -SH + \overset{\overset{\textstyle O}{\parallel}\;H}{-}C{:}N{-}R
\end{array}
$$

is ruptured by nucleophiles such as hydroxyl or amino groups. A transesterification of the thioester in C3 with a donor nucleophile on a cell or particle will "fix" small quantities of C3 capable of binding Bb. This spontaneous chemical reaction may account for initiation of the alternative pathway of activation. Further details of this relatively novel mechanism are available in articles by Pangburn and Müller-Eberhard and by Tack et al. Membrane-bound C3b,Bb at MS_1 (MS_1 indicates first site on a membrane) converts a small portion of C3 into C3a and C3b. (C3a is the anaphylatoxin discussed in detail on page 68). The C3b,Bb complex is not usually formed in the fluid phase but rather at the MS_1 site on a membrane. This C3b,Bb complex initiates further C3 conversion, and the major portion of C3b is deposited on additional membrane sites (see Figure 6-5, MS_2). Once the C3b,Bb enzyme forms at the second membrane site, more C3 is cleaved. That is, the C3b,Bb complex generates more S_2-C3b sites. Thus, this phenomenon is called the **feedback, or amplification, loop.** Once the C3b,Bb complex on the secondary membrane site is constituted, it decays spontaneously and rapidly to S_2-C3b and Bb, or it becomes stabilized by the uptake of the component properdin. The difference between MS_1 and MS_2 sites appear to be only quantitative.

Properdin, perhaps the best known and most controversial of the complement proteins, is a cationic glycoprotein composed of four chains; it plays a modulating role in the activation process. The four subunit chains are free of interchain covalent linkages such as disulfide bonds. In 1954, Pillemer hypothesized that complement could be activated by a process entirely independent of antibody or immunoglobulin. He conjectured that activation of a pathway other than the classical route was based on the action of properdin; therefore, he called this separate pathway the **properdin pathway.** His theory was widely disputed, and recent molecular analyses of the complement system have established that properdin is not central to activation of the alternative pathway. Rather, properdin exerts a stabilizing influence on the C3 convertase (C3b,Bb), an enzyme with transient activity. Two physically distinct forms of properdin exist, P and P*; the P* form accounts for properdin's behavior as a promoter or an enhancer of complement activation. P* stabilizes the labile, surface-bound C3 convertase, Ms_2-C3b,Bb, and the C5 convertase, MS_2-C3b$_n$,Bb, thus prolonging their functional lifetimes by approximately tenfold (see Figure 6-5, MS_3). The nature of the differences between P and P* is unknown, except that the covalent structure is apparently unaffected during the conversion.

C3b inactivator (also referred to as factor I, C3b INA or KAF) is an 88,000 mol. wt. enzyme composed of two polypeptide chains. This protease controls the rate of alternative pathway activation by cleaving the C3b molecule of the C3b,Bb complex into two nonfunctional fragments called C3c and C3d. The C3b INA activity is itself modulated by an association of the C3b molecule with a nonproteolytic glycoprotein called β1H or Factor H.

β1H is a single-chain polypeptide that binds to the same site on the C3b molecule that otherwise binds factor Bb. Once β1H binds to MS_2-C3b, forming MS_2-C3b,β1H, the C3b molecule becomes as much as thirtyfold more susceptible to inactivation by C3b INA and fails to bind Bb. Therefore, β1H modulates or facilitates C3b inactivation, thereby dampening the rate of complement activation. The primary purpose of β1H is to preserve sufficient complement levels in circulation for combating recurrent infections.

The final enzyme of the alternative activation pathway is the C5 convertase. This protease is selective for C5 and is composed of C3b and factor Bb, similar to that of the C3 convertase. The difference between C3 and C5 convertases is that the C5 converting enzyme complex contains multiple C3b molecules, whereas C3 convertase contains one C3b molecule. Hence, the C5 convertase is identified as C3b$_n$,Bb and it exists only in the membrane-bound form MS_2-C3b$_n$,Bb. The remainder of the alternative pathway sequence beyond the C5 convertase step is identical to that described for the classical pathway (see Figures 6-4 and 6-5). The C5b-C9 lytic complex (MAC) assembles at a separate membrane site (MS_3) being formed by a sequential autoassociation of components C5b, C6, C7, C8, and C9. Assembly of the C5b–C9 complex completes the alternative pathway's function.

The alternative pathway has two sets of components, much like the classical pathway. The components present in a precursor form are factors B, P, C3, and C5; those present in an activated state are factors D, Bb, P*, C3a, C3b, C5a, and C5b. Auxilliary control factors such as β1H and C3b INA also constitute a dynamic part of the activated alternative pathway.

Control of the Pathways

Control factors regulate the rate and extent of complement activation; they also destroy pharmacologically potent fragments that are produced in the course of the activation. C1 inactivator or inhibitor (C1 INH) inhibits C1 as well as enzymes of the kinin-forming, coagulation, and fibrinolytic systems in plasma. C1 INH performs its inhibitory action by combining with the active site of the C1s subunit of C1 and blocking its enzymatic capability. The stable C1:C1 INH complex is consequently inactive as a C2 or C4 convertase. Therefore, C1 INH represents a major control factor of the classical pathway.

C4b-binding protein (C4bp) participates in regulation of the classical pathway by interacting with C4b in the C4b,2a complex and accelerates decay. The C4bp is a large, spiderlike molecule with 7 tentacles extending from a single central body. The C4b molecules bind to the ends of the C4bp tentacles causing C4b to dissociate from C2a, which renders the C3 convertase inactive. In addition, the C4b in complex with C4bp is particularly susceptible to C3b INA, which cleaves C4b to C4c and C4d. Further details concerning the C4bp protein are given in an article by Dahlbäck et al.

Primary control of the alternative pathway resides with C3b INA, a selective protease that inactivates C3b by cleaving it into C3c and C3d fragments (Figure 6-6). The component β1H is involved importantly in alternative pathway control by binding to C3b and thereby increasing the rate of C3b cleavage by C3b INA. In this sense, the β1H protein functions in the complement system as a modulator.

The S-protein, a control factor, prevents attachment of the MAC to cell surfaces. This inhibitory glycoprotein binds to the autoassociated complex C5b-9 and competes with the cellular receptor site for C5b-9 binding. The S-protein interacts at the site on C5b-9 that normally serves as the cellular attachment site and thereby inhibits indiscriminant or excessive lysis by the MAC.

Serum carboxypeptidase N is an enzyme that controls the activities of anaphylatoxins (see page 76). As mediators of allergic, muscular, and inflammatory responses, these complement factors must be precisely monitored in vivo to avoid lethal systemic effects that resemble anaphylactic shock. This enzymatic control mechanism involves simply the removal of an essential arginyl residue from the COOH-terminus of the polypeptide chains of C3a, C4a, and C5a anaphylatoxins.

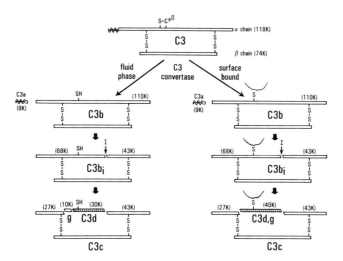

Figure 6-6 A scheme portraying the breakdown of component C3 in blood. The activation fragment C3a is cleaved from the α chain of C3 by convertase as a first step in the degradation process. Then either the thiolester bond is ruptured to generate a free sulphydryl group (fluid phase), or a nucleophile on a particle or cellular surface attacks the labile ester bond to form a covalent linkage between C3b and this surface (solid phase). Factor I (see Table 6-1) then cleaves the α' chain of C3b to form iC3b, inactivating C3b for future participation in convertase formation. Finally, an undefined enzyme cleaves the 68K portion of C3bi to generate C3c (144K), C3d (30K) and C3g (10K) from the fluid phase C3bi. Alternatively, C3c and C3d,g are generated from the particle-bound iC3b. The component C4 is processed in a similar manner in blood.

Biologic Activities of Complement

Numerous biologic activities (for example, immunoagglutination, immune adherence, and opsonization, as well as hemolysis, virolysis, and bacteriolysis) are associated with complement components and their fragments (Figure 6-7). Immunoagglutination, adherence, and opsonization deal with the deposition or fixation of C3b on either a cell or a particle surface. Bactericidal, bacteriolytic, and hemolytic mechanisms are much more complex and involve a sequence of events that ultimately leads to cell death or lysis. In general, only gram-negative bacteria are lysed by antibody and complement; gram-positive bacteria are relatively resistant to complement lysis. The microorganisms most susceptible to antibody/complement lysis include those from the genera *Escherichia, Salmonella,* and *Shigella*. Cell death results from a physical attachment, first of antibody and then of complement, at the cell surface to produce loss of cell associated enzymes, inhibition of active transport, and structural changes such as the loss of phospholipids from the cell envelope. Figure 6-8 shows a representative scheme of the bactericidal and bacteriolytic reaction. Bacteriolytic mechanisms and the exact role of complement in this process are unclear. Nevertheless, this basic function of complement is graphically portrayed in the scanning electron micrographs of lysed *E coli* K12 (Figure 6-9). It has been suggested that the primary role of the interaction of antibody and complement on the surface of a bacterium is to enhance phagocytosis, and that the bactericidal and bacteriolytic events may be of minor importance. Phagocytosis, the phenomenon in which granulocytes ingest cells or cellular debris, is markedly facilitated whenever C3b fixes to the target's surface.

Unlike complement-mediated bacteriolysis, which usually involves gram-negative bacteria and participation by the classical activation pathway, phagocytosis seems to involve predominantly gram-positive bacteria and the alternative pathway of activation. *Staphylococcus aureus, E coli, Streptococcus pneumoniae* type 25, and the yeast *Candida albicans* undergo complement-dependent phagocytosis in C4-deficient serum, indicat-

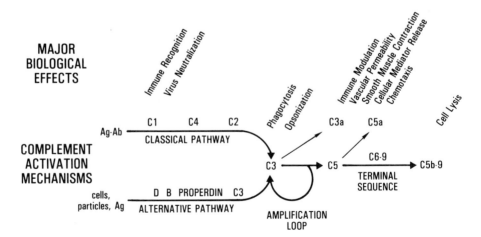

Figure 6-7 Functional attributes of various components of the complement cascade. (Modified from a figure provided by Dr. J. Andrew Grant, University of Texas Medical Branch, Galveston, Texas.)

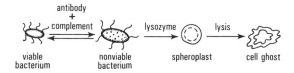

Figure 6-8 Proposed sequence of events in complement-induced bacteriolysis.

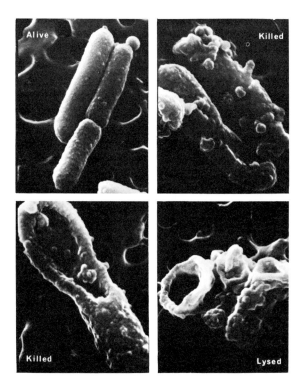

Figure 6-9 Scanning electron microscopic view of bacteria killed and then lysed by action of complement. Upper left view shows viable bacterium *E coli* K12 W1485 under normal conditions. Upper right and lower left views illustrate bactericidal action of complement. These bacteria were killed by incubation with isolated complement components of the alternative pathway plus components C5–C9. Lower right view shows extensive bacteriolysis of complement killed cells once egg white lysozyme was added. From Schreiber et al: *J Exp Med* 1979; 149:870–882.

ing alternative pathway activity. Consequently, the C3 molecule, common to both pathways, acts both as a recognition factor and as bridging ligands that greatly amplify and intensify the phagocytic process. Clearly, antibodies (immunoglobulins) attached to cells or particles promote complement-mediated phagocytosis, but are not absolutely required for this process.

Complement can neutralize virus by interacting with antibody-sensitized virus particles (**virions**); this interaction either lyses the virions or prevents their penetration into cells, thereby interfering with viral replication. Details concerning the exact components and the molecular processes of neutralization are sketchy; however, we know that T2 bacteriophage inactivation by specific antibody is enhanced 1000-fold in the presence of a complement source. A similar effect has been observed with herpes simplex and polyoma viruses.

Complement receptors specific for C3b, C3d, and C4b have now been identified on human lymphocytes. Therefore, complement components may bind to these cells, and this binding may trigger other mechanisms of cellular immunity. One of the most active areas in complement research today concerns the demonstration of such lymphocyte receptors and their importance. Much interest has focused on the possibility that complement provides a signal for antibody synthesis. If complement activation does stimulate or signal antibody synthesis, this activating mechanism would fill an obvious missing link between complement and the immune response in host defense mechanisms. Recent evidence shows that C5a enhances lymphocyte proliferation in cell cultures, whereas C3a suppresses the T-cell-dependent antibody response. These findings, along with the identification of another fragment from C3 (for example, C3d-K) with immunosuppressive activities, support the hypothesis that complement factors play an important role in immunoregulation.

Bradykinin is one of the most potent vasodilators known. C3a, C4a, and C5a, however, may be even more potent vasodilators as demonstrated by the dramatic wheal and erythema that is visible in mammalian skin injected subcutaneously with the anaphylatoxins. As little as 10^{-9} moles of C4a, 10^{-11} moles of C3a, or 10^{-13} moles of C5a produce a clearly visible wheal. This dermatologic response is primarily attributed to mast cell degranulation (Figure 6-10). The C5a molecule is also the primary humoral factor responsible for chemotactic activity (directional migration of leukocytes) that is detected in complement-activated serum. Purified human C5a stimulates chemotaxis of human neutrophils under in vitro conditions at concentrations well below potential levels generated in blood after complement is activated. C3a, if active, is much less active than C5a as a chemotaxin and is therefore not considered a humoral chemotactic factor of primary physiologic importance.

Numerous genetic deficiencies in the human complement system have now been reported, yielding the consensus that critical deficiencies in pivotal components such as C3 or C5 greatly reduce or eliminate the capacities for chemotaxis, phagocytosis, and immune adherence, and thereby render an individual more susceptible to infection and less able to combat disease. Deficiency of the first two or three (early acting) components of either pathway, however, does not have a serious physiologic effect on an individual, because the remaining pathway, with its own set of components, can essentially overcome these deficiencies. In other words, an alternative route for

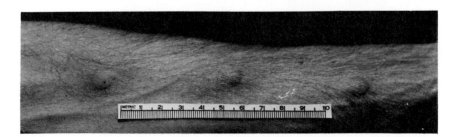

Figure 6-10 Anaphylatoxins injected subcutaneously produce local skin reaction called wheal and flare (erythema). As illustrated, complement-derived fragments C3a, C4a, and C5a injected into human forearm produced raised areas (wheal) and radial red streaks (flare, or erythema) in response to enhanced vascular permeability and histamine released by the anaphylatoxins. From left to right: response to injection of 10^{-13} moles human C5a, 10^{-7} moles human C4a, and 10^{-10} moles human C3a.

activation still exists. Deficiency in any one of the MAC components (C6–C9) does not result in serious clinical disorders, probably because other host defense mechanisms such as immune adherence and phagocytosis remain unimpaired and nullify any loss of blood's lytic capacity.

Complement Assays

The complement-fixation assay requires a known antigen, or an antibody directed to a known antigen, plus a complement source for detection of a given antigen or antibody (Figure 6-11). Because trace quantities of antigen-antibody complexes fix complement, test serum containing an antibody must be heated to deplete it of endogenous complement before assaying. The heated serum is then combined with test samples suspected of containing antigen. Complement is added to the test mixture and fixes to or is consumed by preformed antigen-antibody complexes. Antibody-sensitized sheep red cells (EA) are then added to the assay mixture; the extent to which they are lysed by complement indicates the residual complement level. If the reaction mixture does not lyse the EA, indications are that complement has been consumed, thereby confirming that the unidentified antigen or antibody is present. This test has long been the basis of the clinical Wassermann test for syphilis.

Another hemolytic assay used to quantify the individual complement components is based on the relationship between the percent of hemolysis and the amount of complement added, which is usually valid over the range of 25%–75% lysis. Since the midrange of the dose-response curve is nearly linear, the quantity causing 50% lysis has been chosen as a reference point; hence, the term CH_{50} signifies a 50% hemolysis by complement. A CH_{50} unit of complement activity is an arbitrary unit, since variables include the concentration of red blood cells, cell fragility, antibody used to sensitize the red blood cells, ionic strength, metal ion concentrations, pH, temperature, and reaction time. If these factors are carefully controlled, reliable titrations of complement

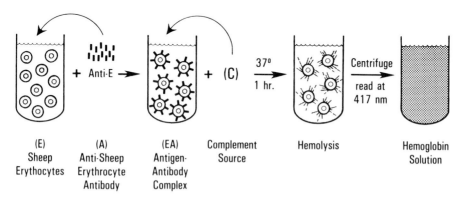

(E)   (A)   (EA)   Complement   Hemolysis   Hemoglobin
Sheep   Anti-Sheep   Antigen-   Source   Solution
Erythocytes   Erythrocyte   Antibody
              Antibody   Complex

Figure 6-11 The complement fixation assay depends on complement (C) for lysis of the sensitized sheep red cells. Therefore, in a usual test system the complement source is incubated with the test solution prior to addition of the EA. If the complement is consumed by antigen-antibody (immune) complexes in the test sample, then hemolysis fails to occur when the C and EA are combined. Inhibition of the lysis reaction indicates that the antigen or antibody being analyzed was indeed present, and thus is a positive test result.

components are possible utilizing the hemolytic assay. This procedure employs serum deficient in the particular component being estimated; the extent of the deficiency in the test serum is judged according to the amount of component that must be added to reconstitute hemolytic activity.

More recently, radioimmunoassays have been developed for a number of the complement components. In particular, radioimmunoassays for activation fragments such as the anaphylatoxins offer a more sensitive means of detecting complement activation than is possible using hemolytic assays.

In summary, both pathways of the complement system are crucial facets in the immune defense mechanism of all higher mammals and offer a variety of intricate ways to combat invasive agents. Despite the tremendous amount of information amassed concerning the nature of the complement system, the role of this sophisticated humoral system in various disease processes is just being realized. Indeed, the status of the complement system promises to be a valuable measure of a patient's well-being and will find wider clinical utilization in the future as a monitor of good health or as an indicator of disease.

References

Cooper, N.R., Ziccardi, R.J.: The nature and reactions of complement enzymes; proteolysis and physiological regulations. In: *Miami Winter Symposia* 11. Ribbons, D.W., Breed, K. (editors): New York: Academic Press, 1976.

Dahlbäck, B., Smith, C.A., Müller-Eberhard, H.J.: Visualization of human C4b-binding protein and its complexes with vitamin K-dependent protein S and complement protein C4b. *Proc Natl Acad Sci USA* 1983; 80:3461.

Ehrlich, P., Morgenroth, J.: Über Haemolysin dritte Mitteilung. *Berl Klin Wschr* 1900; 37: 453.

Götze, O., Müller-Eberhard, H.J.: The alternative pathway of complement activation. *Adv Immunol* 1976; 24:1.

Hugli, T.E., Müller-Eberhard, H.J.: Anaphylatoxins: C3a and C5a. *Adv Immunol* 1978; 26:1-53.

Ingram, D.G.: Biological activities of complement. In: *5th International Symposium of the Canadian Society of Immunology*. Ingram, D.G., (editor): Basel: Karger, 1972.

Kabat, E.A., and Mayer, M.M.: *Experimental immunochemistry*, 2nd ed. Springfield, Ill.: Charles C Thomas, Publisher, 1961.

Müller-Eberhard, H.J.: The serum complement system. In: *Textbook of Immunopathology*. Miescher, P.A., Müller-Eberhard, H.J., (editors). New York: Grune and Stratton, 1976.

Müller-Eberhard, H.J.: Chemistry and function of the complement system. *Hosp Practice* 1977; 12: 33.

Müller-Eberhard, H.J.: The membrane attack complex. *Springer Semin Immunopathol* 1984; 7(2-3):93.

Müller-Eberhard, H.A., Schreiber, R.D.: Molecular biology and chemistry of the alternative pathway of complement. *Adv Immunol* 1980; 29:1.

Osler, A.G.: *Complement: mechanisms and functions*. Englewood Cliffs, N.J.: Prentice-Hall, 1976.

Pangburn, M.K., Müller-Eberhard, H.J.: Relation of a putative thioester bond in C3 to activation of the alternative pathway and the binding of C3b to biological targets of complement. *J Exp Med* 1980; 152: 1102.

Pillemer, L., et al: The properdin system and immunity. I. Demonstration and isolation of a new serum protein, properdin, and its role in immune phenomena. *Science* 1954; 120:279.

Porter, R.R., Reid, K.B.M.: Activation of the complement system by antibody-antigen complexes: The classical pathway. In: *Advances in protein chemistry*, Vol. 33. Anfinsen, C.R., Edsall, J.T., Richards, F.M., (editors). New York: Academic Press, 1979.

Tack, B.F. et al. Evidence for presence of an internal thioester bond in third component of human complement. *Proc Nat Acad Sci USA* 1980; 77: 5764.

von Buchner, H.: *Arch F Hyg* 1893; 17: 179.

Ziccardi, R.J.: The first component of human complement (C1): activation and control. *Springer Semin Immunopathol* 1983; 6:213.

7 Cell-Mediated Immunity and Mediators

Jack R. Battisto, PhD

Subhash C. Gautam, PhD

General Concepts

Cell-mediated immunity (CMI), as conceived originally by Eli Metchnikoff, was the province of cells that engulfed invading microorganisms and presumably destroyed them. Today, these cells are identified as any of the phagocytic series, which includes neutrophils and macrophages. In his attempts to differentiate cellular immunity from humoral immunity, Metchnikoff showed that phagocytosis (at least of certain organisms) did not require the presence of serum. Today, the phagocytic process is known to be assisted by antibody directed toward the microorganism; indeed, some bacteria are not engulfed at all without the presence of a specific antibody. Nevertheless, phagocytosis with or without the assistance of antibody is a most important aspect of the body's defense against disease (Chapter 8).

The current definition of cell-mediated immunity, however, goes beyond a general description of phagocytosis in that it focuses on resistance to disease that is mediated by specific T lymphocytes, as well as by phagocytes and their products. T lymphocytes (T cells) arise from progenitor stem cells in bone marrow. They then migrate to the thymus where, in several days, they mature under the influence of thymic hormones. During the maturation process, the T cells acquire cell-surface markers that distinguish them from B cells, and they also develop specific receptors for antigens. After maturation, the T cells leave the thymus and come to reside in the cortical regions of lymph nodes or in the spleen, or they circulate continually in peripheral lymph and blood (Chapter 3). Upon contact with an antigen, T cells divide and become differentiated into clones of effector cells with different functions.

One group of T cells involved in attacking and lysing other cells is the **cytolytic T lymphocytes (CTL)**. Another group is composed of those cells that mediate delayed hypersensitivity (**T$_{DH}$ effectors**) in conjunction with macrophages. Other T cells regulate the immune response. Separate sets of **helper T cells** assist both T and B lymphocytes to become effector cells by elaborating helper factors. On the other hand, **suppressor T cells** make factors that suppress the development or function of effector T and B cells.

The CMI process also encompasses cytolytic reactions that are mediated by cells other than T lymphocytes. Some of these cytolytic reactions require synergy between a cytotoxic cell and antibody that is specific for the target cell.

This chapter provides a brief description of each of the aspects of CMI, as they are viewed currently. Of course, viewpoints on the subject are changing continually as research increases and becomes more sophisticated. For example, much new knowledge about the many cell products that mediate the CMI process is now being derived from various investigations.

T Lymphocyte Subpopulations

T lymphocytes (T cells) constitute a heterogeneous population of cells that have vastly different functions. The origins of these cells and their localization in the lymphatic system was described in Chapter 3. The diverse activities of T cells are carried out by two distinct, functionally specialized, subpopulations (Table 7-1), which can be classified as the regulator T cells and the effector T cells.

The two major types of **regulator T cells** are **helper** and **suppressor T cells**. Helper T cells participate in activation, proliferation, and differentiation of other lymphocytes that respond to an antigen and thereby help B lymphocytes to produce antibody (Chapter 4). They also help in the development of T$_{DH}$ effector and cytolytic (killer) T cells. Suppressor T cells, on the other hand, inhibit the responses of other

Table 7-1   Subpopulations of T Lymphocytes

| Group | Surface Antigens in | | Conventional Symbol |
	Mice	Human	
All T cells	Thy-1 (θ)	Leu 4,OKT3 EA receptors (E-rosettes)	T
Effector cells			
Delayed hypersensitivity	Lyt 1$^+$	?	T_{DH}
Cytolytic (killer)	Lyt 2$^+$,3$^+$	Leu 2b,OKT8,OKT5	T_{CTL} (T_K)
Regulatory cells			
Helper (inducer)	Lyt 1$^+$	Leu 3,OKT4	T_H
Suppressor	Lyt 2$^+$,3$^+$ I-J$^+$	Leu 2a,OKT8	T_S

lymphocytes to antigen. The balance between helper and suppressor T cells ensures that the immune system functions properly. Other types of regulator cells may also exist. For example, recent experiments in mice have suggested the presence of *contrasuppressor* T cells that prevent the suppressor T cells from inhibiting responses to antigens.

The **effector T cells** class includes several subpopulations involved in the manifestation of the various aspects of CMI, including **delayed hypersensitivity (DH), contact sensitivity** (from dermal exposure to chemicals, metals, or plant extracts), and **rejection** of tissue allografts and infected cells (cell-mediated cytotoxicity, carried out by cytolytic T cells).

All T cells share a surface antigen which is called Thy in mice and Leu 4,OKT3 in humans (see Table 7-1). In addition, all T cells have a receptor for sheep erythrocyte antigen. Although it is not clear why it occurs, the binding of sheep erythrocytes (E) results in the formation of clusters of E around the T cells (E rosettes). The E rosettes then can be separated easily from the remaining non-T cell leukocytes, a process that has been a useful tool for purification of T cells from peripheral blood.

Recent studies of lymphocyte surface antigens have revealed the existence of differentiation determinants that serve as markers of the functionally distinct T cell subpopulations. In mice, the lymphocyte differentiation antigens that have been analyzed most extensively are Lyt antigens 1, 2, and 3. These antigens are present only on the surface of T cells. Analyses of peripheral T cells by using alloantisera against Lyt antigens have identified at least three separate T cell subpopulations, which are referred to as Lyt 1$^+$; Lyt 2$^+$, 3$^+$; and Lyt 1$^+$, 2$^+$, 3$^+$. Lyt surface phenotypes of various subpopulations of T cells correlate well with their functional activities (see Table 7-1). T cells that bear the Lyt 1$^+$ antigen are helper cells and the cells responsible for DH. On the other hand, Lyt 2$^+$, 3$^+$ cells are programmed to develop into alloreactive cytotoxic cells and suppressor cells. The role of Lyt 1$^+$, 2$^+$, 3$^+$ cells is not clear. Ontogenically, such cells are more primitive than either Lyt 1$^+$ and Lyt 2$^+$, 3$^+$ cells; thus, they are probably precursor cells from which the Lyt 1$^+$ and Lyt 2$^+$, 3$^+$ cells are derived.

The availability of monoclonal antibodies to cell surface antigens of human T cells has facilitated the dissection of human T cell populatons into distinct subsets with unique functional properties. The human counterparts of murine T cell surface antigens Lyt 1, 2, and 3 are Leu 3, 2a, 2b, and OKT4, OKT5, and OKT8. The Leu 3 and OKT4 antigens occur most often on a subpopulation of T cells that serve as helpers for both T and B lymphocytes. Leu 2a and 2b and T-5 and T-8 are found on cytotoxic and suppressor T lymphocytes (see Table 7-1).

Other determinants are also expressed on lymphocyte surfaces, and these may eventually help us to define the functional subsets of T cells more thoroughly. An example is the I-J determinant (see Table 7-1), an antigen appears to be expressed on suppressor T cells.

Cellular Immunity in Infection

Entry into the body of an infectious agent triggers a series of immunologic reactions in an attempt to ward off the infection. In general, antimicrobial immunity mechanisms involve the production of antibodies (humoral immunity), the activation of T cells and macrophages, or both. Although resistance to certain microorganisms may depend primarily on only one of these mechanisms, protection results most often from a combination of several mechanisms (Figure 7-1A). For example, humoral immunity is important in acute infections caused by several pyogenic and gram-positive microorganisms that can multiply extracellularly. These organisms (*Streptococci, Staphylococci*) cause the production of specific antibodies which, when the antibodies are bound to the antigens, often results in the fixation of complement. The antibody-antigen complex is then rapidly phagocytized by polymorphonuclear neutrophils and macrophages. Once engulfed, the organisms are usually killed in the intracellular milieu of the phagocytic cells. Thus, a critical step in resistance to such infections is the production of specific antibodies that facilitate phagocytosis of the bacteria.

Humoral immunity also offers protection against pathogens that produce exotoxins (diphtheria, tetanus). The antibodies can neutralize the toxins efficiently and prevent them from affecting target organs. Antibodies can also neutralize some viruses, especially if viremia is present.

Although humoral immunity is important in resistance against infections caused by bacteria that can multiply extracellularly, it is ineffective against many organisms (viruses, bacteria, fungi, and protozoa) that can multiply intracellularly in normal phagocytes and leukocytes (Figure 7-1B). Although most of these microorganisms are taken up by the phagocytic cells, they may not be killed even if they are bound to antibody and complement. Protection against such organisms can be achieved only by measures that alter the intracellular environments of phagocytes drastically from one in which the parasite normally prospers to one that will not support its multiplication. Thus, cellular immunity that requires T cell–macrophage interaction has been recognized widely as the mechanism of resistance against such microorganisms.

The classic example of cellular immunity in infection is **Koch's phenomenon,** in which delayed hypersensitivy and acquired resistance occurs simultaneously in guinea pigs infected with *Mycobacterium tuberculosis.* In the experiments that established this

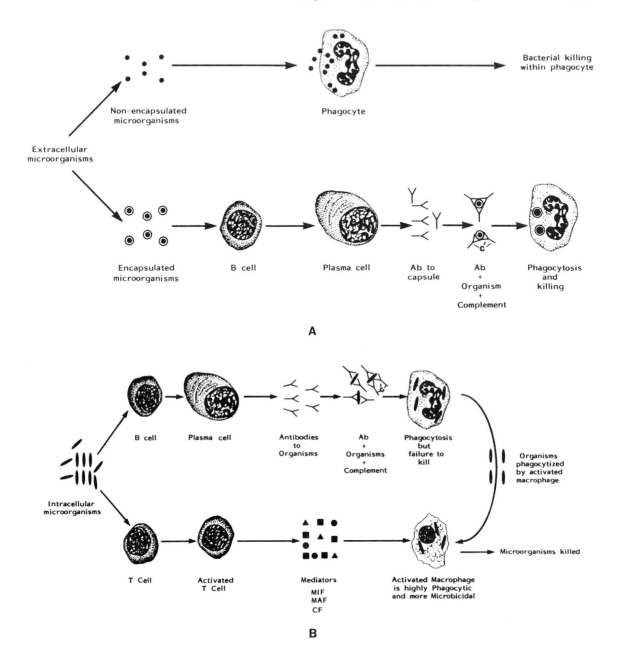

Figure 7-1 A, Killing of extracellular microorganisms by phagocytes. Certain nonencapsulated microbes are phagocytized by polymorphonuclear leukocytes without any enhancing process. The encapsulated microbes usually are engulfed only in the presence of specific antibody and complement. Once phagocytosed, the microbes are killed readily inside the phagocytic cells. **B,** Microbes phagocytized by polymorphonuclear leukocytes in the presence of antibody and complement may not be killed, but keep multiplying inside the cell. Protection against these organisms is provided by macrophages activated by several mediators produced by specifically sensitized T lymphocytes.

principle, subcutaneous injection of tubercle bacilli in unimmunized guinea pigs led to severe systemic infection and death. On the other hand, inoculation of previously infected immune guinea pigs resulted in the formation of a localized indurated nodule in the skin, but no systemic dissemination of the bacteria. The infective foci or granuloma consisted largely of phagocytic cells; few lymphocytes were present. The bacilli that had been engulfed by those phagocytic cells were unable to grow and multiply.

Skin lesions similar in nature to the granulomas produced in the experiments described above have also appeared 24 to 48 hours after intradermal injection with a soluble boiled product of tubercle bacilli (tuberculin) in the immune host. This **delayed hypersensitivity (DH)** reaction denotes a state of cellular immunity to the tubercle bacilli. Thus, the granuloma produced in the skin by infection with live tubercle bacilli and the DH lesion induced by injection with tuberculin resulted from the same mechanisms.

A systematic study of the mechanisms of cellular immunity was done by Mackaness in mice infected with a bacillus that causes intracellular infection, *Listeria monocytogenes*. Cellular immunity against this organism involves two steps: (1) a specific reaction, in which the T lymphocytes interact specifically with the organism; and (2) a nonspecific reaction, in which macrophages are localized rapidly to the site of infection and activated. Early during *Listeria* infection, short-lived small lymphocytes undergo intense proliferation in the spleens of infected mice. Then, the interaction between bacteria and the specifically reactive lymphocytes initiates events that lead to the activation of macrophages (see Figure 7-1B). The most important function of the activated macrophages is their enhanced microbicidal activity. The action of these macrophages is nonspecific in that they will inactivate *any* bacteria or viruses, and not only the organism that induced the infection. This state of heightened activity of macrophages usually lasts for several weeks. On the other hand, the specific memory of sensitized T cells may last for months or years, and is responsible for the lasting resistance to repeated infection (challenge) with the same agent. This principle is illustrated in Table 7-2. Mice immunized to *L monocytogenes* are specifically resistant to this bacteria, but not to an unrelated *M tuberculosis*. However, the animals will resist the *M tuberculosis* injected simultaneously with *L monocytogenes*, as the latter will rapidly activate the nonspecific macrophage resistance. Thus, cellular immunity to infections is an immunologically specific mechanism that induces a population of defensive phagocytic cells with nonspecific microbicidal properties.

Table 7-2   Demonstration of Specific and Nonspecific Aspects of Delayed Hypersensitivity

Mice Immunized With	Mice Become Infected When Challenged With		
	L monocytogenes	*M tuberculosis*	*L monocytogenes and M tuberculosis*
Listeria monocytogenes	0	+	0
Mycobacterium tuberculosis	+	0	0

Cellular immunity to a viral infection involves the activation of cytolytic T cells (T_{CTL}) that recognize viral antigens on the infected cells and destroy them (Figure 7-2). This effector arm of CMI will be discussed later.

Delayed Hypersensitivity

Induction of Delayed Hypersensitivity

As stated in the previous section, DH skin reaction is one of the manifestations of T cell immunity. The term *delayed hypersensitivity* was coined originally to distinguish this cell-mediated skin reaction from the much faster *immediate hypersensitivity* (IH) that occurs when an antigen is administered to an individual with certain types of antibodies (Table 7-3; see also Chapter 9).

Table 7-3   Some Features That Differentiate DH From IH

Distinguishing Characteristic	Type of Hypersensitivity	
	Immediate	Delayed
The Afferent Limb		
Inciting antigens	T cell-independent and T cell-dependent antigens	T cell-dependent antigens (also conjugates of simple chemicals, metals, and plant products to dermal self-antigens)
Route of administration of antigen	Intraperitoneal, subcutaneous, intramuscular	Intradermal
Minimal immunization interval	10–14 days	5–6 days
Enhancers	Alum adjuvant; Freund's incomplete adjuvant	Freund's complete adjuvant; pretreat host with cyclophosphamide
The Efferent Limb		
Dermal reaction in sensitive host		
Time of onset (from antigen injection)	Minutes	Several hours
Macroscopic appearance	Wheal, flare, edema	Erythema, induration, desquamation
Microscopic appearance	Eosinophils	Macrophages
Systemic reaction in sensitive host	Anaphylactic shock within 10 minutes	Endotoxinlike death within 72 hours
Transfer accomplished with	Homocytotropic antibodies, such as IgE, operate in conjunction with host's mast or basophilic cells	T cells (Lyt 1^+) operate in conjunction with host's macrophages

The types of antigens that induce DH best are generally complex proteins, glycoproteins, and lipoproteins, which are referred to as T cell–dependent antigens (see Table 7-3). The antigens that are found on the surfaces of cells are particularly efficient at initiating DH. T cell–independent antigens are molecules with repetitious moieties, such as polysaccharides, and they generally do not provoke DH unless they are conjugated with peptides or bound to cell surfaces. Simple chemicals such as picryl chloride, and metals like nickel or beryllium that have the ability to conjugate, adhere to, or alter the chemical structure of proteins or cell surface molecules in another way, also initiate DH.

Unless the antigen is microbial, the route by which it is introduced to induce DH must be intradermal; introducing an antigen via the intravenous, intraperitoneal, intramuscular, or subcutaneous routes does not normally cause DH. When a simple chemical such as picryl chloride is painted on the skin, it conjugates spontaneously to dermal elements and enters the lymphatic system to initiate DH. A DH that is specific for the hapten picryl chloride is not detectable for 5 to 6 days. This inductive phase of DH is the **afferent limb** of the response. The elicitation of dermal or systemic reactions at any time after this interval is the **efferent limb** of the response (see Table 7-3). Any DH engendered in this manner is long lived; that is, although the degree of sensitivity may decrease slightly with time, the individual generally remains hypersensitive to the antigen until death. A heightened level of DH can be achieved (particularly in an experimental situation) by incorporating the antigen into Freund's adjuvant, which is a mixture of oils and killed mycobacteria.

Nature of Delayed Hypersensitivity

DH skin reactions have distinct characteristics that differ substantially from those that occur in IH (Table 7-3). In humans, for example, the DH dermal reaction to tuberculin or its purified protein derivative (PPD) is characterized by erythema and induration. In severe DH reactions, the center may be white because of an accumulation of white blood cells, and discoloration of the entire area, as well as desquamation, may persist for 1 week or more. Scarring may occur in extreme reactions. The typical DH reaction reaches its maximum intensity 48 to 72 hours after exposure. Macrophages predominate in the reaction site at these times. In contrast, local IH responses are characterized by wheal, flare, and edema that generally start within minutes, reach a peak in 1 to 2 hours, and fade within 6 to 8 hours. Microscopic examination of tissue samples collected during the maximal response reveals a predominance of eosinophils.

The systemic DH reaction is best observed in experimental animals, such as guinea pigs, that have been sensitized to mycobacteria and then injected intraperitoneally with a suitable amount of PPD. The animals experience an endotoxinlike reaction that is characterized by a dramatic fall in body temperature, lassitude, distress and, usually, death within 72 hours. Huge cellular infiltrates in the peritoneum and along the needle track are observed at autopsy. In contrast with this reaction, the systemic response in IH is a rapid anaphylactic shock; the animal dies within 10 minutes.

The fact that DH is a manifestation of T cell immunity was established in experiments involving the transfer of cells between animals. First, DH was induced in an animal by immunization. T cells (Lyt-1$^+$ subset) from that animal were then isolated and

Table 7-4   Mediators of Cellular Immunity

Target of Factor	Cell-Derived Substance*	Remarks
Macrophages (MØ)	Migration inhibition factor (MIF)	First hinders movement, then activates the MØ
	Macrophage activation factor (MAF)	Indistinguishable from MIF
	Macrophage chemotactic factor (MCF)	Attracts MØ into a reactive site
	Colony stimulating factor (CSF)	Helps MØ elaborate IL-1 and DF; helps bone marrow cells to differentiate
T lymphocytes	Interleukin 1 (IL-1)	An MØ product required by helper T cells
	Interleukin 2 (IL-2)	A helper T cell product that is needed by T cells for replication
	Interleukin 3 (IL-3)	Promotes differentiation of helper T cells
	Differentiation factor (DF)	A second signal for precursor CTLs
	Transfer factor (TF)	Transfers DH by an unknown mechanism
	Interferon(s) (IF)	Protects against viral infections, has antitumor action and is immunoregulatory
Neutrophils, basophils, eosinophils	Chemotactic factor(s)	Attracts these cells to reactive site
	Leukocyte inhibitory factor (LIF)	Analogous to, but different from, MIF

*Factors are from antigen- or mitogen-stimulated T cells except where noted.

injected into an unimmunized animal. The recipient of the cells was found to display the DH reaction upon challenge with the antigen (the experiment requires histocompatibility between the animals; see Chapter 2). These experiments also revealed that the DH reaction site contained only a few antigen-reactive T cells, but a great number of macrophages and monocytes. Thus, the thesis has emerged that specific, antigen-triggered T cells release a number of biologically active substances that, in turn, attract macrophages into the site of the reaction. The macrophages are then activated by these substances to phagocytose and kill the microorganisms. This intense activity causes the histopathologic manifestation in DH. The nature of the soluble substances released by activated T cells is discussed in the next section.

Soluble Mediators Seen in Cell-Mediated Immunity

The first lymphokine, **migration inhibition factor (MIF)** (Table 7-4), was detected by isolating peritoneal exudate cells (using cell separation techniques) and inserting them into capillary tubes that allowed their migration. MIF is a product of T cells (and perhaps B cells) that have been sensitized and reexposed to an antigen. In the presence of antigen, lymphocytes have been observed to produce MIF within a few hours and for as long as 5 days. MIF from guinea pigs appears to consist of three molecules of different sizes (mol. wt. 28,000, 43,000, and 65,000 daltons). The two largest molecules are thought to be dimers and trimers of the smaller molecule.

Macrophage activating factor (MAF) was originally thought to be a separate lymphokine, especially since macrophages were found to become highly mobile and phagocytic long after exposure to the substance. Now, however, MAF is thought to be MIF (Table 7-4). Macrophages exposed to MIF first become sticky and immobile, but after internalizing or catabolizing MIF, they become hyperactive.

Since the detection of MIF, antigen-activated T lymphocytes have been shown to elaborate a host of lymphokines. **Macrophage chemotactic factor (MCF)** is known to attract macrophages toward the reactive site. The cells travel over a concentration gradient of MCF toward the greatest amount of the factor. **Colony-stimulating factor (CSF)** apparently possesses two functions: it causes immature bone marrow cells to differentiate into more mature cell types such as granulocytes; and it assists macrophages to elaborate interleukin 1 (IL-1) and a differentiation factor (DF) needed by precursors of CTL cells.

Three apparently distinct interleukins (IL) have been described. IL-3 is required by precursor cells that become established as helper T cells in vitro (see Table 7-4 and Figure 7-2). Helper T cells must be stimulated with IL-1, which is produced by macrophages before they can produce IL-2. IL-2 is needed by such cells as CTL precursors to multiply after they have had a separate input from a DF.

One of the earliest mediators of cellular immunity, **transfer factor (TF)**, was described by Lawrence as being a product from circulating DH-reactive human leukocytes. TF is able to transfer DH reactivity for a particular antigen to nonsensitive recipients. Found in sonicates of white blood cells, the low-molecular-weight TF molecule possesses a polypeptide component. TF has been used to produce reactivity in individuals with immunodeficiencies.

The three interferons, α, β, and γ, have several biologic actions; the most important are antiviral, antitumor, and immunoregulatory. Immune interferon (γ) exerts a greater antitumor reactivity than do the others, and it also exerts an immunosuppressive effect on antibody production. Recently, interferon γ also has been shown to have an MAFlike activity; in fact, MAF may be interferon γ.

Discoveries of separate chemotactic factors for neutrophils, basophils, and eosinophils have also been reported. A **leukocyte inhibitory factor (LIF)** that is analogous to MIF is thought to attract basophils to a reactive site.

Regulation of Delayed Hypersensitivity

Concomitant with the induction of T_{DH} effector cells by the antigen is the activation of suppressor cells, which, at a certain point, begin down-regulation of the immune response. Recent data indicate that several different types of T suppressor cells (T_S) and their products, suppressor factors (T_SF), interact in the termination of the CMI. Some of the T_S are specific for the inducing antigen, whereas others appear to be antiidiotypic; that is, they recognize the unique determinants on the antigen receptor borne by T_{DH}.

Further studies of the process should produce tools and methods for regulation of CMI. For instance, one of the T_S populations has been found to be particularly sensitive to cyclophosphamide. Treatment with this agent therefore enhances the degree of DH induction in experimental mice. Other drugs such as glucocorticoids have been shown to suppress DH response through their inhibitory effect on the lymphokine-macrophage activation pathway.

In Vitro Correlates of Delayed Hypersensitivity

Various methods allow us to determine the hypersensitive state of T_{DH} from peripheral blood in vitro. Some of these methods are based on the fact that T_{DH}, when reexposed to a specific antigen, release various biologically active soluble factors. The assessment of these activities in a test tube containing T_{DH} and antigen may provide an in vitro correlate of DH. For example, in a classical test of this sort, the release of MIF by T_{DH}, which inhibits migration of macrophages and monocytes in a capillary tube, can be observed.

The most commonly used test for T_{DH} is the **blast transformation assay,** which is based on the fact that an early reaction of T_{DH} to an antigen involves DNA synthesis, mitotic cell division, and enlargement of T cells into lymphoblasts. The cell proliferation peaks within 3 to 5 days after addition of appropriate (homologous) antigen to the culture of lymphocytes from a sensitized donor. The proliferation is detected by incorporating a radioactive DNA precursor, H^3-thymidine, into the culture approximately 8 hours before harvesting the cells and measuring their radioactivity. Increased uptake of H^3-thymidine above the background level indicates the response of T_{DH} to the antigen.

Allograft Rejection and Graft Versus Host Reaction

When tissue from one member of a species is transplanted to an unrelated member of the same species, the allograft becomes vascularized within a week and then is rejected in a time interval that depends on the degree of antigenic foreignness of the graft as well as the immunological capability of the host. In mice, the rejection of a primary skin allograft usually occurs within 12 days. If the donor and recipient are related, however, and thus share some antigens, or if the host's immunological response is compromised (by, for instance, immunosuppressive drugs), the interval of rejection may be considerably prolonged. Rejection of the graft is a T cell-mediated event (as has been shown by adoptive cell transfer experiments). The main effector cells are CTL, which kill the allogeneic cells directly. Whether these cells function alone or are joined by cells that mediate DH is still unclear.

When a graft contains immunologically competent cells or their precursors (for instance, bone marrow cells), the host may be the target of rejection. This **graft versus host (GVH)** response, which can lead to death, generally causes an enlargement of the host's spleen (in experimental situations, the spleen is used as an assay system).

The allogeneic (transplantation) CMI is manifested in vitro as a **mixed lymphocyte reaction (MLR).** When lymphocytes from two allogeneic individuals are cocultured, the T cells from each population will recognize the class II histoincompatible antigens

(H2-AE in mice and HLA-D in humans) on the other set of cells. The T cells are triggered into proliferation and blastogenic differentiation (much like in antigen-triggered T_{DH}). This is called **two-way MLR**, since the reaction is mutual. The MLR can be monitored conveniently by assessment of the uptake of H^3-thymidine by the cells in culture. CTL that are specific for the stimulating alloantigen also are generated during a MLR. The reaction can be made one directional by preventing the replication of one set of cells through prior treatment with irradiation or mitomycin C. The intensity of MLR is a measure of strength of tissue incompatibility between two individuals.

Recent studies indicate that a recognition of class II MHC antigens that leads to cell stimulation may occur in cultures of T cells with non–T cells (for example, leukocytes other than T cells) from the same individual. This **autologous lymphocyte reaction** may be of a great theoretical importance in analyses of immune regulation, but it will not be discussed here. It should not be confused with the MLR.

Cell-Mediated Cytotoxicity

Cell-mediated cytotoxicity is involved in the rejection of foreign grafts and neoplastic and virus-infected cells (Table 7-5). In this reaction, various lymphoid effector cells display the ability to lyse target cells. The effector cells can be CTL, which are antigen-specific and MHC-restricted (MHC, major histocompatibility complex; this term will be explained later); natural killer cells (NK), which are not T cells; killer (K) cells involved in antibody-dependent cell cytotoxicity; or activated macrophages.

Table 7-5   Effector Cells Involved in Cell-Mediated Cytotoxicity

Effector Cell	*Surface Markers*						*Antibody to Target Cell Required*	*Probably Participate in:*
	Thy 1	*Ly*	*Ig*	*Ia*	*Fc*	*C3*		
Cytolytic T lymphocyte (CTL)	+	2, 3⁺	−	−	+	−	−	Rejection of tissue and organ transplants; rejection of tumors, viral infections; autoimmune diseases
Natural killer (NK) cell	−	−	−	−	±	−	−	Rejection of tumors; viral and parasitic infections
Null (K) cell	−	−	−	−	+	?	+	Surveillance against tumors and viral infections (ADCC)
Macrophage (after activation with T cell products)	−	−	−	+	+	+	−	Rejection of tumors; chronic bacterial and viral infections

Cytolytic T Lymphocytes

Cytolytic T lymphocytes are involved in the rejection of foreign tissues such as skin grafts, organ transplants, certain tumors, and virally infected autologous cells. In 1960, Goverts showed that thoracic-duct lymphocytes from dogs that had rejected kidney allografts killed donor kidney cells in vitro. Cytotoxic cells have been detected in the draining lymph nodes, spleen, and peripheral blood during allograft rejection. T cells with cytotoxic activity can be generated in MLR in vitro by culturing lymphoid cells from two genetically disparate strains of mice or from two persons with different human leukocyte antigens (HLA). Responding and stimulating cells are usually incubated for 5 to 7 days at 37 C and the viable cells are recovered from cultures to be assayed for cytotoxicity. Stimulating cells are not always allogeneic, since syngeneic tumor cells that bear tumor-specific antigens, or syngeneic cells that are infected with virus or are modified chemically, can also stimulate responding lymphoid cells to generate CTL.

CTL are detected with the ^{51}chromium-release assay. The target cells are labeled by using radioactive ^{51}Cr ions. When the CTL damage the membrane of the target cells, the ^{51}Cr is released into the culture fluid. The ratio of cell-free to cell-bound radioactivity indicates the CTL activity.

Cellular Cooperation and the Role of Major Histocompatibility Complex Products in the Generation of Cytolytic T Lymphocytes

The development of techniques for generating and measuring CTL activity in vitro, as well as the availability of alloantisera against various cell markers on lymphoid cells, has permitted identification of cell populations that interact during the generation of the CTL response against alloantigens. CTL are derived from precursor cells called **preCTL (CTL-P)**, which are present in the spleen and lymph nodes, as well as in the peripheral blood (see Figure 7-2). CTL-P have no detectable cytolytic activity, but they do differentiate into mature cytotoxic cells when stimulated with antigen if they receive an additional stimulus from helper T cells. Analyses of different lymphoid cell populations have demonstrated a complex series of collaborative events that occur among various T cell subpopulations and accessory cells. In mice, CTL-P directed toward alloantigens have been found to belong to the Lyt 1^-, 2^+, 3^+ subset; MHC-restricted CTL-P are Lyt 1^+, 2^+, 3^+. Amplifier or helper T cells have been identified as Lyt 1^+, 2^-, 3^-. In studies that used monoclonal antibodies to human T cell differentiation antigens, the T cells that produce helper factors for the induction of alloreactive CTL have been identified as OT 4^+, and the CTL-P have been found to be OKT 4^+, 5^+, 8^+. The role of macrophages and, perhaps, of other antigen-presenting cells is also important. The accessory cells appear to participate by presenting processed antigenic determinants (in context with class II MHC products on their surface) to CTL-P and helper T cells.

Examination of the nature of alloantigens that stimulate production of CTLs against MHC products has revealed that class I antigens stimulate CTL-P in both mice (antigens coded largely by the K, D, and L regions of the mouse H-2) and humans (coded by the A, B, and, to a lesser extent, C regions of the human HLA). The amplifier-helper T cells, on the other hand, are activated by class II antigens encoded primarily by genes of the I region in mice and the D region in humans. The acquisition of cytotoxic activity by the lymphoid cells is preceded by proliferation of the responding cells, a response that peaks 48 to 72 hours after initiation of the culture. Most of the proliferating T cells have a helper function. The CTL activity becomes detectable 24 to 48 hours later. The precise nature of the molecular events that lead to the generation of CTL is unclear, but evidence suggests that differentiation of CTL-P to become mature, functional CTL requires two signals (see Figure 7-2). Signal 1 involves the binding of class I antigens to specific receptors on CTL-P; this signal renders the antigen-selected CTL-P responsive to signal 2, which is provided by the interleukins (IL). The IL-1 produced by macrophages in the presence of antigen activates appropriate helper T cells (Lyt 1^{+}) to produce IL-2, which is responsible for proliferation of antigen-activated CTL-P. Other factors that are distinct from IL-1 and IL-2—for example, immune interferon (IIF) and DF—are also known to participate in the activation and maturation of CTL-P.

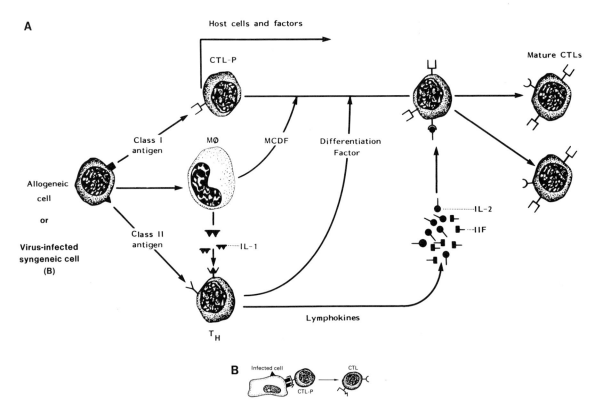

Figure 7-2 A, Cellular interactions involved in the induction of cytolytic T cells (CTL) in response to allogeneic cells (*alloreactive* CTL). Recognition of class I antigens (signal 1) on the allogeneic cell by precursors of CTL (CTL-P) renders them sensitive to inductive signal (signal 2) provided by various lymphokines (IL-2, IIF, MCDF, DF). When both signals 1 and 2 are present, CTL-P differentiates into mature effector CTL. IL-1, interleukin-1; IL-2, interleukin-2; IL-3, interleukin-3; IIF, immune interferon; MCDF, macrophage-derived cytotoxic T cell differentiation factor; DF, differentiation factor; ⊏, class I antigen receptor on CTL; ≺, receptor for IL-2 on CTL; ≺, receptor for class II molecules on T$_{H}$. Note: CTL against *virus-infected cells* develop along the same pathway, **B.** They are also *class I antigen restricted,* so that the receptors on both CTL-P and mature CTL recognize both class I (■) and viral (◼) antigen on the target cell.

Mechanism of Lysis

The CTL-mediated lysis of target cells occurs in at least two discrete steps. The first involves the recognition of specific antigens on the target cell surface by specific receptors on the CTL. The two cells establish an intimate contact that is stable upon subjection to physical forces. The binding, which requires Mg^{+2}, is enhanced linearly as the temperature increases from 4 C to 25 C. It can be inhibited by metabolic inhibitors that affect the cytoskeleton. The target cell is not damaged following binding; it can be recovered by disrupting the bond between it and the CTL.

The second step in the lytic process involves programming of the target cell for lysis or the "lethal hit." During this stage, the CTL causes irreversible damage to the target. The process requires Ca^{+2}, and it is even more temperature-sensitive than the binding stage. This step is completed within 3 to 10 minutes after the initial contact (the CTL can be detached or inactivated after this time without affecting subsequent lysis of the target cell). Depending on the nature of target cells, complete lysis may take one to several hours. The CTL remains unharmed by the encounter with the target cell; in fact, it can lyse another target cell without loss of its own viability. The molecular mechanisms of lysis are not clearly understood.

Major Histocompatibility Complex–Restricted Cytotoxicity

As has been indicated, specific CTL can be generated against syngeneic cells that are infected by viruses or chemically modified, or against minor histocompatibility antigens. Doherty and Zinkernagel originally observed that mice infected with the lymphocytic choriomeningitis (LCM) virus develop CTL that will kill syngeneic target cells infected with the same virus. Syngeneic target cells not infected, or infected with an unrelated virus, will not be killed. Most important, *allogeneic* cells infected with the *same* sensitizing virus will not be killed. These findings support the view that the killing depends on viral antigenic structures as well as on MHC-coded antigens. It has also been shown that syngeneity between the CTL and the target cell at the K, or D regions (class I antigens) but not at the I region, is required for cytolysis. This phenomenon, *MHC restriction*, has been reproduced with other viruses and several hapten-modified syngeneic cells. For CTL to develop against syngeneic cells that are either infected with viruses or hapten-modified, the CTL-P must recognize the foreign antigen in context with the appropriate MHC determinants.

A close physical association has been found between virus or hapten and MHC determinants on the membranes of cells infected with virus or hapten modified. Based on the evidence available, two hypotheses of MHC restriction have been proposed. The dual recognition hypothesis states that the self-MHC determinants and the extrinsic antigen (viral, haptenic, or other nonMHC antigen) on target cells are recognized separately by two receptors on the same reactive T cell. The altered-self hypothesis, on the other hand, proposes that a single T cell receptor recognizes the entire ligand and MHC complex. The latter theory is currently gaining more support.

Regulation of Cytolytic T Lymphocyte Response

Information on the control of the CTL response is not as extensive as that on the DH response, partly because the suppressor T cell circuits that control the CTL response are not as well defined as those that have been shown to down-regulate the in vivo DH response. However, suppressor cells capable of inhibiting proliferative and cytotoxic responses do appear to be generated in murine and human MLR. Some of these suppressor cells are antigen-specific, whereas others cause suppression by nonspecific means. The exact modes of action of these suppressor cells remain to be determined. Suppressor cells, or the soluble suppressor factors produced by them, may inhibit the generation of CTL by affecting CTL-P, the function of helper T cells, or both.

Memory in Cytolytic T Lymphocyte Responses

Evidence for the existence of memory in CTL responses comes from both in vitro and in vivo studies. CTL tend to lose their cytolytic activity when maintained in culture for a protracted period; however, their cytolytic activity reappears quickly when they are restimulated with the sensitizing antigens. This secondary CTL response differs from the primary CTL response in the kinetics and magnitude of the cytolytic activity. Similarly, the magnitude of the CTL response in vitro can be increased substantially by prior sensitization of lymphoid cells in vivo by the relevant antigen. In fact, priming in vivo must be performed to generate an in vitro response to virally infected cells, minor histocompatibility antigens, and certain hapten-modified syngeneic cells. Recent studies have provided evidence that secondary CTL responses result, at least in part, from the expansion of CTL-P. The number of CTL-P may increase up to 20 times after priming with the antigen. These findings suggest that the memory for CTL may reside in CTL-P and the generation of CTL follows a CTL-P to CTL to "memory" CTL-P pattern.

Spontaneous Cell-Mediated Cytotoxicity (NK Cells)

Spontaneous cell-mediated cytotoxicity or **natural killing** is the capacity of naive or virgin lymphoid cells to display cytotoxicity for a variety of normal and neoplastic cells unrestricted by MHC. Cells with this type of cytotoxicity, **natural killer (NK) cells,** lack the properties of classical macrophages, granulocytes, or cytotoxic T cells. NK are present in appreciable numbers in human peripheral blood and in the spleens of normal and nude mice (see Table 7-5). The cell populations are extremely heterogeneous with regard to cell-surface markers, biophysical properties, and range of cytotoxic reactivity. Considerable NK activity has been found in cell populations that lack typical T and B cell markers but display varying proportions of Fc or complement (C3) receptors. Some NK cells do display surface markers that are usually present on T lymphocytes, whereas others express antigens that are specific for NK cells. Since both human and murine NK cells have prominent azurophilic cytoplasmic granules, they are described as **large granular lymphocytes (LGL).** The variations in NK cells reflect either clonal heterogeneity of the cells or differences in the stage of cell differentiation.

Generally, the cytotoxicity of NK cells is nonselective, and the extent of killing depends upon susceptibility of the target cells and on the cytotoxic efficiency of the cell populations. Unlike antigen-specific CTL, NK cells are inactivated after interaction with one target cell. In addition, NK cells lack classic immunological memory. Interferon and interleukin-2 both enhance NK activity, whereas treatment of animals with cyclophosphamide and corticosteroids abrogates such activity. Evidence that indicates that NK cells are active in resistance against neoplastic growth and metastatic spread of tumors is increasing. NK cells also have been implicated in resistance to certain viral infections and in the regulation of hematopoiesis.

Antibody-Dependent Cell-Mediated Cytotoxicity

Antibody-dependent cell-mediated cytotoxicity (ADCC) is a cell-mediated cytolysis that requires the presence of target-specific antibody. It was first described in systems that employed antibody-coated chicken erythrocytes or xenogeneic cells as targets. The precise identity and ontogeny of ADCC effector cells are unclear. Since such cells have Fc receptors for IgG on their surface but lack C3 receptors and surface immunoglobulin, they are called null or K cells (see Table 7-5). These cells require conventional antibody for the recognition of target-cell antigens and do not show antigen specificity. Specific immunization is not required for expression of ADCC activity by K cells when exogenous antitarget antibody is present. Antibody of the IgG class appears to form a bridge between the target cell and the effector cell; presumably, the antibody binds to the target antigen and the K cell binds to the Fc portion of the antibody via its Fc receptor. The mechanism of ADCC-mediated lysis is not clear, although complement does not appear to be required. ADCC is believed to participate in immunologic surveillance and to provide protection against viral infections and tumors.

Macrophage Cytotoxicity

Macrophages that have been activated by various immunologic and nonimmunologic procedures have been shown to be cytotoxic for several allogeneic tumor cells. Activated macrophages obtained from mice injected with infectious agents such as Bacillus Calmette Guerin (BCG), toxoplasma, or *Listeria* exhibit direct cytotoxicity for tumor cells (see Table 7-5). Additionally, normal macrophages activated by T cell-mediators such as MIF (interferon γ) also acquire cytotoxic capacity. The cytotoxic function of macrophages is mostly nonspecific, and may be involved in rejection of tumors growing in vivo and in destroying cells infected with viruses.

Diseases Associated With Cell-Mediated Immunity

In some instances, exposure to certain antigens leads to a state of hypersensitivity; subsequent contact with the same antigen elicits a complex set of events that are harmful, and sometimes fatal, to the host. Some of these immunologic reactions are mediated by sensitized T lymphocytes and are referred to as *immunologic diseases associated with delayed hypersensitivity*. Injuries produced by these reactions may result from the direct cytotoxic effects of sensitized T lymphocytes, the production of cytotoxic substances such as lymphotoxins, or the elaboration of lymphokines that then recruit and activate macrophages.

Delayed hypersensitivity occurs concomitantly with autoantibodies in several autoimmune diseases in humans and experimental animals. For example, T lymphocytes that are directly cytotoxic for thyroid cells have been found in patients with Hashimoto's thyroiditis, and T cells that display DH occur in patients with Hashimoto's and Graves' syndromes. In addition, one of the complications following immunization with rabies vaccine in humans is the occurrence of allergic encephalomyelitis. This disease occurs because the host responds to the antigens of central nervous system tissues rather than to the antigens of the virus. A similar disorder, experimental allergic encephalomyelitis (EAE), can be induced in mice, rats, guinea pigs, and monkeys by injecting brain or spinal-cord tissue with adjuvant. Specific antibodies and cytotoxic T cells are found in the peripheral blood of such animals 14 to 21 days after sensitization. DH responses to CNS antigens also may be involved in the pathogenesis of multiple sclerosis, a chronic demyelinating disease of humans that shares several clinical features with EAE. DH also is suspected in chronic disease of the liver and kidney as well as in rheumatoid arthritis. Whether cell-mediated immune responses that are associated with various autoimmune diseases are the cause or consequence of these disorders is not clear (see Chapter 12).

References

Asherson, G.L.: The control of the immune response. *Ann Allergy* 1984 (Dec); 53 (6, Pt 2): 557-62.

Battisto, J.R., Claman, H.N., Scott, D.W., (editors): Immunological tolerance to self and nonself. *Ann NY Acad Sci* 1982; 392.

Germain, R.N., Benaceraff, B.: A single major pathway of T-lymphocyte interactions in antigen-specific immune suppression. *Scand J Immunol* 1981; 13:1-10.

Goldstein, A.L., Chirigos, M.A. (editors): Lymphokines and thymic hormones. Their potential utilization in cancer therapeutics. *Progress in Cancer Research and Therapy,* Vol. 20. New York: Raven Press, 1981.

Moller, G., (editor): Natural killer cells. *Immunological Reviews,* Vol. 44. Copenhagen: Munksgaard, 1979.

Moller, G., (editor): Interleukins and lymphocyte activation. *Immunological Reviews,* Vol. 63. Copenhagen: Munksgaard, 1982.

Mackaness, G.B.: Resistance to intracellular infection. *J Inf Dis* 1971; 123:439-445.

Riethmuller, G., Wernet, P., Cudkowicz, G. (editors): *Natural and Induced Cell-Mediated Cytotoxicity: Effector and Regulatory Mechanisms.* New York: Academic Press, 1979.

8 Functions of Phagocytes

Paul G. Quie, MD
Armond S. Goldman, MD

General Concepts
Locomotion of Phagocytes
Antimicrobial Mechanisms of Polymorphonuclear Neutrophil Leukocytes
Defective Phagocyte Function
Role of Phagocytic Cells in Disease

General Concepts

Neutrophils and monocytes are highly mobile, phagocytic leukocytes that are exceptionally important in host defense against antigens and in the production of inflammatory disorders, including many that are immunologically mediated. Neutrophils are the most numerous phagocytic cells in the peripheral blood. They are released from the bone marrow, circulate for approximately 8 hours, then adhere to endothelial cells and migrate into tissues in which they engulf and destroy microbial pathogens or other foreign particles. Their life span in extravascular tissues is approximately 4 to 5 days. A large pool (50 to 100 times the number that circulate) is available in the bone marrow to respond to inflammatory stimuli.

Neutrophils have specialized functions for their role in host defense. They are characterized by a large number of (a) primary or azurophilic granules (lysosymes) that contain acid hydrolases and (b) specific granules that contain lactoferrin and lysozyme. Their deformability allows them to pass between endothelial cells and through narrow tissue spaces (diapedesis), and to orient rapidly and move toward gradients of attractant chemotactic factors. They are able to recognize foreign particles and then attach them to their outer surface membranes by various attachment mechanisms, including hydrophobicity, surface charge, and specific receptors for the opsonins, the C3b and IgG antibodies. Opsonized bacteria, for example, attach by receptors for the Fc portion of antibody opsonin or by receptors for complement opsonins. The neutrophils are the earliest and the most prominent cells in acute inflammation.

Mononuclear phagocytes (monocytes) also are released from the bone marrow. They circulate for a short time and then "home" to selected organ systems (the vascular and lymph channels of the spleen, liver, skin, lymph nodes, lungs, and gastrointestinal tract), where they mature to become macrophages. The system of macrophages is the **reticuloendothelial system.** Macrophages often acquire highly specialized characteristics according to the microenvironment of the organ in which they reside, but they also have certain common features, including C3b or IgG receptors and efficient microbial mechanisms. In addition, mononuclear phagocytes play an important role in the production of chronic inflammation and in those reactions that are due to T cell sensitization (see Chapter 7).

The stimulation of neutrophils and mononuclear phagocytic cells may lead to protection or to disease. These cells are affected strongly by antibodies, activated complement components, and T cell products. Their role in protection and the mechanisms responsible for their functions are particularly highlighted in patients with hereditary defects in these cells. Phagocytic cells often are recruited and activated to participate in inflammation by immune complexes and the production of active complement fragments.

Locomotion of Phagocytes

In addition to receptors for IgG antibodies and C3b, neutrophils and monocytes have receptors for bacterial N-formylated peptides and for activated serum complement, C5a for example. These agents are potent chemoattractants for neutrophils (Figure 8-1) and monocytes and stimulate the secretion of granular constituents from these cells.

The leading front or **hyaloplasm** of phagocytic cells is the "motor" that propels the cell (see Figure 8-1). The hyaloplasm is rich in actin and myosin. The polymerization of actin into filaments is controlled by ionized calcium; thus, shifts in calcium within

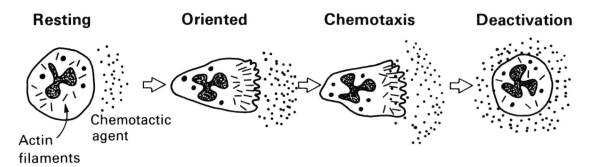

Resting   **Oriented**   **Chemotaxis**   **Deactivation**

Chemotactic agent

Actin filaments

Figure 8-1 Sequence of cellular response to chemotactic agent. The direction of movement is indicated by the arrow.

cellular compartments are involved in the regulation of both phagocytosis and locomotion. Once a cell is surrounded by equal concentrations of a chemotaxin, it ceases to move and becomes rounded.

Neutrophils are also secretory cells. The contents of specific and azurophilic granules are released when a neutrophil is stimulated by particle attachment or by other stimuli, including bacterial endotoxin and the products of inflammation. Certain other major activities of neutrophils (adherence to endothelial cells, directed movement, and secretion of mediators) depend upon the same stimuli, and, therefore, the activities are integrated.

Phagocytic cell receptors for C3b and the Fc portion of antibody act as a *lock* for the opsonic *key* that coats opsonized bacteria. Attachment of an opsonic ligand to the phagocytic membrane modifies an actin binding protein that stimulates polymerization of actin and a cytoplasmic sol-gel reaction (Figure 8-2). As a consequence, the neutrophil membrane surrounds opsonized particles by a zipperlike action. The opsonized particle is surrounded rapidly by the neutrophil membrane and becomes a newly formed intracellular organelle, called a **phagocytic vacuole** or **phagosome** (Figure 8-3). Both granules (azurophilic and specific) migrate toward, fuse with, and discharge their contents into the vacuole to form a **phagolysosome.**

Antimicrobial Mechanisms of Polymorphonuclear Neutrophil Leukocytes

When neutrophils are stimulated by phagocytosis, a membrane-associated, metal-dependent nonmitochondrial enzyme, cytochrome B, is activated. Molecular oxygen is reduced to the reactive radical superoxide by the oxidase activity of the phagocyte membrane. Hydrogen peroxide is then formed by the action of superoxide dismutase. Reactive oxygen radicals that result from oxidase activity, acting with contents from cytoplasmic granules, contribute to potent, broad-spectrum microbicidal activity in phagosomes (see Figure 8-3). Reactions between hydrogen peroxide and superoxide that

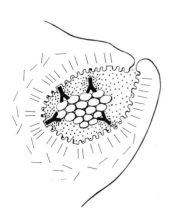

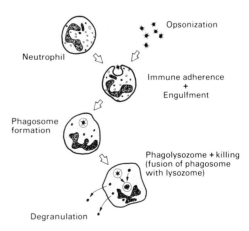

Figure 8-2 Phagocytosis of bacteria opsonized by specific antibody (γ).

Figure 8-3 Principal events of phagocytosis.

are catalyzed by lactoferrin (contributed by specific granules) result in the formation of hydroxyl radicals. Myeloperoxidase (contributed by azurophilic granules) combines with hydrogen peroxide and halides to form the principal microbicidal system in these cells. Hydroxyl radicals and similar agents formed in this manner are likely to be the primary microbicidal factors in neutrophils.

The control mechanisms for these reactive radicals include superoxide dismutase, catalase, and the glutathione system. Superoxide, hydrogen peroxide, and other radicals that diffuse from phagosomes are detoxified so that autolysis is prevented.

Defective Phagocyte Function

Patients with decreased numbers or reserves of granulocytes are especially susceptible to bacterial and fungal infections. These infections usually manifest as abscesses in soft tissue or in bones (osteomyelitis), since the primary function of granulocytes is surveillance of tissue spaces and the scavenging of invading microbes. *Staphylococcus aureus* often causes these disorders; however, infections with other opportunistic agents, such as gram-negative enteric species (*E coli, Pseudomonas aeruginosa, Serratia marcescens,* and *Klebsiella pneumoniae*) and the fungal species (*Candida albicans* and *Aspergillus fumigatus*), also occur frequently.

Similar types of infections take place in patients with disorders of phagocyte function. Abnormalities of phagocyte function include defects in adherence to endothelium, chemotaxis, deformability, the attachment of opsonized particles, phagocytosis, degranulation, oxidative metabolic response, and microbial killing. Abnormality of adherence may be present in patients receiving corticosteroid drugs, since those agents inhibit adherence of phagocytic cells to endothelial cells. In several patients, defective adherence of neutrophils has been found to be caused by a deficiency of specific glycoproteins on the surface of the neutrophils. The failure of adherence diminishes the phagocytic and chemotactic activities of the neutrophils and the patients experience recurrent bacterial infections.

Patients with disorders of phagocyte locomotion and response to chemotactic stimulation have frequent severe abscesses of soft tissue. In these disorders, a delay in accumulation of phagocytic cells during the early stages of bacterial invasion contributes to the pathogenesis of the abscesses. *Staphylococcus aureus* is the most frequent cause of infection in these cases; however, infections with gram-negative enteric bacteria and fungal species, as well as with *Staphylococcus epidermidis,* may occur. Patients with clinical and laboratory findings that include eczematoid skin lesions, "cold" subcutaneous abscesses, greatly increased serum levels of IgE, and intermittently defective granulocyte chemotaxis probably have Job's syndrome (also referred to as the hyperimmunoglobulin E, Hill-Quie, or Buckley syndrome). In patients with this disorder, lung abscesses, suppurative lymphadenitis, and subcutaneous abscesses may occur, and prolonged treatment with antistaphylococcal antibiotics is often necessary.

Neutrophils and other phagocytic cells from many patients with chronic granulomatous disease of childhood (CGD) lack cytochrome B and therefore are unable to generate oxygen radicals during phagocytosis. As a result, intracellular bacteria remain viable in the neutrophils. Catalase-negative (and, thus, hydrogen peroxide-positive) bacterial species such as *Streptococcus pyogenes, Streptococcus pneumoniae,* and other species of streptococci, as well as *Hemophilus influenzae,* are killed in vitro by neutrophils from patients with CGD, because these organisms provide their own lethal oxygen metabolites within the phagocytic vacuole.

Patients with a total lack of glucose 6-phosphate dehydrogenase (G-6-PD) have a neutrophil dysfunction that is phenotypically similar to that found in patients with CGD. Since G-6-PD is necessary for maintaining adequate cellular levels of the reduced pyridine nucleotide NADPH (the source of electrons for conversion of oxygen to superoxide during phagocytosis), patients without G-6-PD have no respiratory oxidative response during phagocytosis. The role of glutathione reductase in detoxifying reactive oxygen radicals is highlighted in patients who lack that enzyme; they develop profound neutropenia during infections.

Role of Phagocytic Cells in Disease

The presence of neutrophils is the hallmark of nonspecific acute inflammation, and they are prevalent in lesions caused by immune complex diseases such as serum sickness, acute poststreptococcal glomerulonephritis, and systemic lupus erythematosus. The pathogenesis of the vasculitis and other tissue injuries in these disorders involves the following process. As immune complexes are deposited in tissues, complement is activated to produce opsonic and chemotactic agents. Neutrophils then migrate into the tissue and attempt to phagocytize the immune complexes. These complexes then are stimulated to degranulate and to produce the toxic oxygen radials that injure the host tissue (see Chapter 9).

In contrast with neutrophils, monocytes and macrophages are responsible for chronic inflammation. Recruitment and activation of these cells is stimulated chiefly by the release of lymphokines from stimulated T lymphocytes (see Chapter 7).

References

Babior, B.M.: Oxidants from phagocytes: agents of defense and destruction. *Blood* 1984 (Nov); 64(5):959–66.

Badwey, J.A., Karnovsky, M.L.: Active oxygen species and the functions of phagocyte leukocytes. *Ann Rev Biochem* 1980; 49:695–726.

Fearon, D.T.: Identification of the membrane glycoprotein that is the C3b receptor of the human erythrocyte, polymorphonuclear leukocyte, B lymphocyte and monocyte. *J Exp Med* 1980; 152:20.

Klebanoff, S.J.: Myeloperoxidase-halide-hydrogen peroxide antibacterial system. *J Bacteriol* 1968; 95:2131–2138.

Quie, P.G., et al: In vitro bactericidal capacity of human polymorphonuclear leukocytes: Diminished activity in chronic granulomatis disease of childhood. *J Clin Invest* 1967; 46:668–679.

Root, R.K., Cohen, M.S.: The microbicidal mechanisms of human neutrophils and eosinophils. *Rev Infect Dis* 1981; 3:565–598.

Stossel, T.P.: How do phagocytes eat? *Ann Int Med* 1978; 89:398.

9 Hypersensitivity

J. Andrew Grant, Jr., MD

Jeffrey R. Lisse, MD

General Concepts
Background
Immediate Hypersensitivity Reactions (Type I)
Cytotoxic Hypersensitivity (Type II)
Immune Complex Hypersensitivity (Type III)
Delayed Hypersensitivity (Type IV)

General Concepts

An intact immune system is essential for defending an organism against microorganisms and thus for survival; however, inappropriate or excessive activation of the immune system can be harmful to the host. These detrimental responses are referred to as **hypersensitivity reactions.** When such reactions occur within minutes after exposure to an antigen, antibodies of the IgE class may be involved. Three additional processes that initiate hypersensitivity reactions have been described: production of antibodies against tissue antigens, formation of circulating antigen-antibody complexes and subsequent tissue deposition, and antigen activation of T lymphocytes.

Background

During the nineteenth century, researchers identified the protective role of the immune system. Early in this century, they described the potentially harmful elements of immunity. While attempting to protect dogs against a sea anemone toxin by repeated immunizations with small doses of the toxin, investigators observed that some animals developed fatal shock after challenge with a dose much lower than the toxic dose for an unimmunized dog. They coined the term **anaphylaxis,** the opposite of protection, to describe this reaction. About the same time, the protective value of serum from animals immunized with diphtheria and tetanus toxins was being investigated. Although most human recipients responded favorably, some developed fever, rash, and arthralgias within 1 to 2 weeks after receiving animal serum. This illness was called **serum sickness.** In 1906, the altered reactivity of the host after exposure to a foreign substance (**allergen**) was defined as an **allergy.** These studies made it possible to distinguish between the protective and harmful potential of immune responses. Since then, various models have been developed to explore the mechanisms of allergic or hypersensitivity reactions and to correlate these with specific human disease states. The most widely utilized classification, introduced by Gell and Coombs in 1963, describes four types of hypersensitivity (Figure 9-1).

Type I immediate hypersensitivity reactions tend to occur quickly following the interaction of antigens with IgE antibodies on the surface of tissue mast cells and blood basophils. A variety of potent mediators are released that increase vascular permeability and constrict smooth muscle tissue.

Type II cytotoxic hypersensitivity reactions are initiated by antibodies combining with the surface of cells or with antigens attached to tissues. Secondary damage

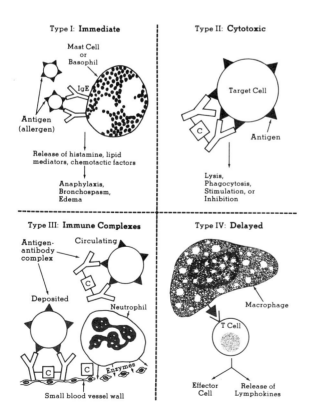

Figure 9-1 Types of hypersensitivity responses. C, complement; ▲, antigen.

to cells may result from activation of the serum complement system or effector mononuclear cells (T lymphocytes and macrophages).

Type III immune complex hypersensitivity reactions occur when antigens combine with antibodies in the circulation, forming aggregates referred to as immune complexes. If these complexes are deposited in the microcirculation, they may induce intense inflammatory responses through complement activation.

Type IV delayed hypersensitivity occurs when T lymphocytes respond to appropriate antigens by releasing various lymphokines. These lymphokines secondarily activate other cells to induce delayed hypersensitivity reactions. Antibody is not required.

The Gell and Coombs classification is clearly an oversimplification, since most human illnesses have features of more than one type of reaction. Nevertheless, this classification facilitates the effort to distinguish the mechanisms causing hypersensitivity responses.

Immediate Hypersensitivity Reactions (Type I)

About 75 years ago, investigators recognized similarities between hay fever and asthma in humans and the anaphylactic reaction described earlier in dogs. In 1921, serum from an allergic individual was used to transfer passively sensitivity to the skin of a normal individual. The serum factor responsible for transferring allergic sensitivity was called **reagin.** About 45 years later, reaginic antibody was isolated from allergic serum. Almost simultaneously, a similar protein was discovered in the blood of a patient with multiple myeloma. These discoveries established a unique class of reaginic antibodies, which were subsequently called **immunoglobulin E (IgE).**

IgE antibodies are similar to other immunoglobulin classes in their protein structure. Each molecule consists of two identical heavy and two identical light chains, but the ϵ heavy chain of IgE distinguishes it from other classes. IgE concentration is the lowest of any of the five classes in normal human serum (about 1/100,000 the level of IgG), and it is synthesized by plasma cells in the regional lymph nodes surrounding the respiratory and gastrointestinal tracts. IgE synthesis is regulated by specialized T helper and T suppressor cells. Both the absolute level of IgE synthesized and the ability to make IgE antibodies against specific antigens appear to be genetically controlled.

Immunoglobulins express their antibody function through the Fab portion of the molecule and their unique isotype functions through the Fc portion. IgE antibodies are tightly bound to the plasma membrane of blood basophils and tissue mast cells. A unique receptor for the Fc region of IgE antibodies has been identified on the surface of these cells.

Immediate hypersensitivity reactions are triggered when an appropriate antigen (or allergen) combines with the Fab portion of two adjacent IgE molecules on the surface of a mast cell or basophil (see Figure 9-1). In patients with allergic rhinitis, the allergens are typically proteins (frequently about 30,000 daltons in size) released from pollen granules. Other allergens are derived from molds, insects, or animal disorders. Following exposure to an allergen, persons with a genetic predisposition to develop allergies will synthesize IgE antibodies against this protein. Subsequent exposure leads to activation of mast cells and basophils. The bridging of two IgE antibodies by an allergen triggers a series of intracellular events, including activation of serine proesterase, augmented phospholipid turnover, increased calcium flux across the plasma membrane, changes in cyclic-AMP levels, and assembly of microtubules. Although the precise connection between these events is unknown, the result is the release of numerous preformed mediators and the synthesis of new ones (Table 9-1). These substances in turn induce an intense inflammatory response.

Histamine, the first mediator identified, is confined almost exclusively to lysosomal granules of the basophil and mast cell. Within these granules, preformed histamine is bound to heparinlike molecules. Once an appropriate antigen triggers the cells, the granules are extruded from the cell. Histamine is subsequently released into the extracellular space and is responsible for many of the events occurring during the first minutes after onset of hypersensitivity reactions.

Two separate receptors, designated H1 and H2, have been identified for histamine. H1 receptors are blocked by the classical antihistamines, such as diphenhydramine. The vascular effects of H1 stimulation include dilatation of terminal arterioles, increased capillary permeability, and constriction of postcapillary venules. The combined effects of these actions produce edema, a major feature of most type I hypersensitivity reactions (allergic rhinitis, urticaria, and bronchial asthma). More extensive loss of intravascular fluid can cause shock, as seen in anaphylaxis. H1 receptors also cause constriction of bronchial smooth muscle, as observed in bronchial asthma.

Understanding of the diverse actions of histamine has increased with the recent discovery of specific inhibitors of H2 receptors such as cimetidine. H2 receptors have long been recognized in stimulation of gastric acid secretion. More recently, evidence has accumulated that some vascular responses to histamine (vasodilation with flushing, headache and hypotension) may be a combination of H1 and H2 effects. H2 receptors have also been identified on a number of inflammatory cells. Paradoxically, stimulation of H2 receptors on these cells may have profound antiinflammatory effects. Release of lysosomal granules by basophils, neutrophils, and mast cells is retarded. The function of T lymphocytes may be inhibited, as shown by reduced proliferation, synthesis of lymphokines, and diminished cytotoxicity.

Table 9-1   Factors Involved in Immediate Hypersensitivity Reactions

Factor	Biologic Properties
Histamine	Smooth muscle contraction; increased vascular permeability; increased mucus production; vasodilation; pruritus
Prostaglandin D_2	Bronchoconstriction; vasodilation
Leukotrienes C4, D4	Smooth muscle contraction; increased vascular permeability; increased mucus production
Leukotriene B4	Increased migration of neutrophils and eosinophils
Platelet activating factor	Aggregates platelets with release of platelet mediators
Enzymes	A number of proteases, acid hydrolases, and oxidative enzymes have been described that can activate the complement and kinin systems and otherwise modulate the inflammatory response
Chemotactic factors	Several proteins, peptides, and lipids have been described that attract each type of leukocyte

Some of the most potent mediators of hypersensitivity reactions are not preformed, but are newly synthesized by metabolism of arachidonic acid (Figure 9-2). This lipid is released from the plasma membrane shortly after cell activation. Subsequently arachidonic acid is metabolized by two different enzymatic pathways. The cyclooxygenase pathway leads to the production of a diverse family of compounds: the prostaglandins, prostacyclins, and thromboxanes. Practically all cell types can synthesize cyclooxygenase products, but the mixture varies from cell to cell depending on which enzymes are present. For example, prostaglandin D2 is released by lung mast cells and causes bronchoconstriction and vasodilation. Synthesis of several prostaglandins is stimulated by histamine.

The lipoxygenase products of arachidonic acid metabolism seem to play an important role in immediate hypersensitivity, especially in bronchial asthma. The leukotrienes C4 and D4 are the most potent constrictors of bronchial smooth muscle, especially in the small airways, and also cause increased vascular permeability and mucus production. The leukotrienes are more potent than histamine in causing all of these effects. Another lipoxygenase product, leukotriene B4, is a potent stimulant of neutrophil and eosinophil migration.

A number of additional chemotactic factors that direct the migration of leukocytes have been described. Eosinophils commonly accumulate locally several hours after onset of a hypersensitivity response, and probably prolong the reaction. These cells often are attracted to sites of parasitic infestations, and a major basic protein released from the granules of these cells may be important for killing helminths. Eosinophils also are seen in secretions produced during bronchial asthma and allergic rhinitis. Recently it has been observed that eosinophils' major basic protein is present in the sputum of asthmatic patients, and that this compound is toxic to respiratory tract cells. Thus, eosinophils may have both a beneficial and a harmful role.

Platelet activating factor (PAF) also is derived from membrane phospholipids (see Figure 9-2). This mediator causes margination and activation of platelets, and may have additional effects on the cardiorespiratory system. The role of PAF in human hypersensitivity responses remains to be elucidated.

A number of enzymes, released by basophils and mast cells, have secondary effects on inflammation, especially by activation of the complement and kinin pathways.

The type of symptoms experienced in type I reactions is dependent upon many

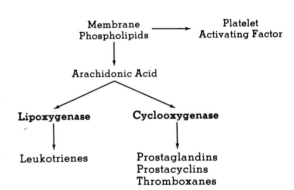

Figure 9-2 Metabolism of arachidonic acid.

factors, especially the nature of the allergen and the route of exposure. For example, pollens tend to induce allergic reactions of the upper (rhinitis) or lower (asthma) respiratory system. Insect venoms and injected drugs are associated with systemic reactions involving the cardiovascular system (anaphylactic shock).

Type I hypersensitivity to an antigen is tested by determining the cutaneous reactivity. A drop of solution containing the antigen is placed on the skin and the epidermis is pricked with a needle. A more sensitive test can be performed by injecting the antigen intradermally. The wheal and flare response is determined after 15 minutes. The reaction is caused by mediators, especially histamine released from skin mast cells, and is correlated with sensitivity to the antigen. Type I hypersensitivity also can be demonstrated by measurement of increased serum IgE antibodies against the antigen.

The goal of therapy for type I reactions is to decrease exposure to offending antigens, reduce synthesis of IgE antibodies, prevent the binding of antigen to cellular IgE, block the release of mediators from basophils and mast cells, and inhibit the effects of the mediators.

Clearly, then, it is possible to identify IgE, basophils, mast cells, and a number of small molecules as principal participants in immediate hypersensitivity reactions (anaphylaxis, rhinitis, urticaria, and bronchial asthma). Philosophically, it is hard to conceive how this elaborate orchestra of inflammatory participants could have evolved without a beneficial purpose. It has been proposed that this system acts as a gatekeeper. Harmful exogenous toxins or parasites stimulate production of small quantities of IgE antibodies that sensitize mast cells and basophils lining the respiratory and gastrointestinal tracts. The presence of these toxins or parasites induces an intense inflammatory response, initiated by mast cells and basophils, with the secondary appearance of phagocytic cells and protective antibodies of other classes. This regulatory role of IgE antibodies may assure that host defenses are mounted in an appropriate fashion. Perhaps the best proof of this theory is found in the extremely high levels of IgE antibodies seen in persons infected with parasites.

Cytotoxic Hypersensitivity (Type II)

During cytotoxic hypersensitivity reactions, circulating antibodies—usually IgG or IgM—may develop against antigens on the surface of one or more cell types in the body, and cause tissue damage. Two of the most straightforward illnesses involving this type of hypersensitivity are pemphigus and bullous pemphigoid, diseases characterized by mucocutaneous blisters. In the former, there are circulating IgG antibodies to the intercellular substance between epidermal cells. This antibody also can be deposited between the epidermal cells in the skin lesions. Additionally, it has been possible to reproduce the changes by treating skin cells in culture with the antibody. In bullous pemphigoid, most patients have circulating antibody (usually IgG) to the basement membrane zone (BMZ) of the epidermis, and a linear deposition of this antibody in the BMZ of the skin lesions. In bullous pemphigoid, the complement system is essential for evolution of the lesions. Cells are damaged both through the direct effects of the complement cascade, and also by neutrophils attracted by C5a released during complement activation. A variety of enzymes and other products liberated from neutrophils potentiate the inflammatory reaction.

The diversity of antibodies that may be produced in type II reactions is illustrated by the entity known as autoimmune hemolytic anemia (AHA), in which antibodies are formed against the red blood cell surface. Although this may occur in systemic lupus erythematosus and other autoimmune diseases, probably the most relevant conditions for this discussion are those induced by drugs. Quinine and quinidine, as well as hydralazine, combine with antidrug antibodies. The resulting complex may settle onto the surface of the red cell. These antibodies, usually IgM, fix and activate complement avidly, which in turn punches a hole in the red cell membrane. The ensuing intravascular hemolysis may be quite fulminant.

Another type of AHA occurs with penicillin. This drug becomes inserted into the proteins of the red cell membrane. IgG is formed against the penicillin hapten and through this interaction damages the membrane. Complement usually is not activated and hemolysis is more mild.

The last type of AHA is caused by methyldopa and involves a drug-induced antibody to the native red cell surface. The drug is not itself antigenic, but may cause a decrease in suppressor T cell function with escape of autoantibody-producing cells. This same mechanism may lead to destruction of platelets or white blood cells.

Another disease classically involving type II hypersensitivity is Goodpasture's syndrome, in which hemoptysis, hematuria, and progressive glomerulonephritis are frequently seen. Virtually 100% of patients have circulating antiglomerular basement membrane IgG antibodies detected by radioimmunoassay. These antibodies also may be seen as linear deposits in the basement membrane of the lung and kidney. Plasmapheresis, a therapeutic measure that removes plasma, and along with it the offending antibody, may lead to preservation of renal function and resolution of symptoms, with eventual recovery from an otherwise fatal disease.

Autoantibodies may be directed against cellular receptors and cause either inhibition or activation of the receptors. A unique consequence occurs in Graves' disease, in which an antibody is made against the thyroid-stimulating hormone receptor with activation of thyroid cells and subsequent overproduction of thyroxine. In myasthenia gravis, which is characterized by muscular weakness, autoantibodies directed against the acetylcholine receptor of the neuromuscular junction impair muscular contraction. Finally, antibodies to insulin receptors are recovered from the blood of certain patients with insulin-resistant diabetes mellitus; they block the action of insulin on its target cells.

Therapy for type II reactions is directed toward blocking the production and, if possible, increasing the removal of the offending antibody.

Immune Complex Hypersensitivity (Type III)

Immune complex hypersensitivity reactions begin a few hours after exposure to an antigen. A localized version of this is the Arthus reaction, which is caused by the local injection of antigen (usually into the skin) in an animal with circulating antibody to that antigen. Within a few hours swelling and redness are noted, but most signs disappear within 1 or 2 days. When examined by immunofluorescent microscopy, immune complexes are seen to form early by the antigen and antibody, and complement fragments subsequently are deposited as a result of complement activation. Chemotactic factors that attract neutrophils, especially C5a, are formed. These cells release a variety of enzymes, superoxides, and arachidonic acid metabolites (see Figure 9-2) that amplify the inflammatory response by direct tissue damage and by recruitment of other cellular and humoral immunologic elements. Finally mononuclear cells appear with removal of the immune complexes and subsequent resolution of most of the evidence of inflammation. With more prolonged antigen accumulation, a chronic lesion develops with signs of tissue necrosis.

Immune complex hypersensitivity also can develop as a result of systemic exposure to antigens. As mentioned earlier, it was observed at the end of the last century that injections of animal serum are sometimes followed by serum sickness. One or 2 weeks after injection, antibodies are formed, first of the IgM class, then IgG. These combine with circulating antigens to form immune complexes. The size of the complex is related to the type of antigen and antibody as well as to the molecular ratio of each. Smaller complexes tend to pass directly through the glomerulus and larger complexes usually are removed by the reticuloendothelial system. Neither of these clearance mechanisms results in tissue damage. In contrast, complexes of intermediate size may become trapped in smaller vessels, producing a vasculitis characteristic of immune complex hypersensitivity reactions. The pathogenesis of this lesion shares the same sequence of events described above for the Arthus reaction: local deposition of antigen-antibody complexes, complement activation, attraction of neutrophils, release of inflammatory mediators, and tissue injury. The microvasculature of the renal glomerulus, periarticular tissues, and the skin are common sites where immune complexes become localized; glomerulonephritis, arthritis, and cutaneous vasculitis are the types of injury noted.

Many additional factors probably influence the evolution of immune complex injury. Histamine released from blood basophils and tissue mast cells has been implicated, since this mediator increases vascular permeability and since antihistamines have been shown to reduce the incidence of glomerulonephritis in human serum sickness. Platelets and serotonin may also be involved in type II hypersensitivity.

A wide variety of antigens have been linked to human type III hypersensitivity disorders (Table 9-2). Many of these antigens are related to microorganisms. Poststreptococcal glomerulonephritis is an excellent example. The antigen (derived from the bacterial cell wall) and antibody become deposited in the kidney and activate the complement system. Polyarthritis, vasculitis, and glomerulonephritis have been described after hepatitis B virus infection. Hepatitis B surface antigen, as well as antibody to it, have been detected in some lesions. A number of drugs have been implicated, especially penicillin and animal serum proteins. Certain autoimmune and neoplastic disorders are associated with immune complexes. In systemic lupus erythematosus, antibodies against nuclear antigens are found. The levels of the antibodies in the circulation, as well as the degree of complement activation, may correlate with the severity of the disease, especially the renal and skin lesions.

Though some organ systems are more prone to disease resulting from the deposition of immune complexes, almost any organ can be involved. The symptoms and physical findings of type III hypersensitivity reactions vary widely depending on the area involved. The proper diagnosis of immune complex hypersensitivity is based upon demonstrating the classic pathologic findings in affected organs. A number of tests can be used to demonstrate the presence of circulating complexes, and serum complement

Table 9-2   Sources of Antigens Associated With Immune Complex Hypersensitivity

Microorganisms	*Autologous antigens*
Bacteria	Systemic lupus erythematosus
Poststreptococcal glomerulonephritis	Rheumatoid arthritis
Subacute bacterial endocarditis	Cryoglobulinemia
Vascular shunts	*Neoplasms*
Spirochetes	Solid tumors
Syphilis	Lung
Viruses	Colon
Hepatitis B	Kidney
Rubella	Leukemia
Infectious mononucleosis	Lymphoma
Parasites	
Malaria	
Toxoplasmosis	
Schistosomiasis	
Drugs	
Serum proteins	
Antitoxins	
Antilymphocyte globulin	
Penicillin	
Quinine	
Vaccines	

levels are often lowered. Treatment varies depending upon the organ systems involved. If possible, therapy is directed toward reducing the level of antigen and/or antibody, facilitating the removal of the complexes, and inhibiting the inflammatory response.

Delayed Hypersensitivity (Type IV)

The cutaneous response to tuberculin (antigenic material derived from *Mycobacterium tuberculosis*) is delayed longer than type I and III reactions and typically peaks at 2 days. The reaction is independent of antibody and is controlled by T lymphocytes. Microscopic examination of the reaction reveals a predominance of mononuclear cells, and an absence of the neutrophils that characterize type II and III hypersensitivity reactions.

The mechanism of delayed hypersensitivity is identical to normal (cellular) immunity mediated by T cells. T cells function in two ways in delayed hypersensitivity. The first is to release a host of factors, lymphokines, that modulate the immune response by other effector cells such as macrophages, neutrophils, basophils, and other lymphocytes. The second role of T lymphocytes is to function directly as effector cells, especially in the role as cytotoxic cells. Macrophages play an essential role in delayed hypersensitivity at all stages, including processing of antigens and phagocytosis. The details of these cellular reactions are described in Chapter 7.

Delayed hypersensitivity reactions are seen in several infectious diseases, and the antigens involved come from the infecting organism. *Mycobacterium tuberculosis*, *M leprae* (leprosy), and the deep fungal infections (e.g., coccidioidomycosis, histoplasmosis, blastomycosis) induce a cellular immune response essential for host defense. However, the reaction also may cause considerable damage to host tissues.

Contact dermatitis is another example of delayed hypersensitivity. The antigens commonly implicated are derived from plants (poison ivy), metals (nickel), drugs, preservatives and rubber compounds. The reaction to these antigens is usually maximal at about 2 days, as it is in the tuberculin response. Sensitivity is diagnosed clinically by placing small amounts of the antigen on the skin and observing a typical response after 2 days. The microscopic examination of the reaction reveals a predominance of mononuclear cells and often a transient increase in basophils. The role of basophils in contact dermatitis is unclear.

Cell-mediated immunity is thought to play a role in the pathogenesis of certain autoimmune disorders. Lymphocytic and histiocytic infiltrates are seen in Hashimoto's thyroiditis, a disease characterized in its later stages by hypothyroidism. Similar infiltrates are seen in the destructive joint lesions of rheumatoid arthritis.

The presence of normal cellular immunity is most easily confirmed by demonstrating delayed cutaneous hypersensitivity. The antigens used frequently are derived from microorganisms and cause sensitivity in most of the population. The absence of a significant response to this panel of ubiquitous antigens at 2 days suggests a deficiency in cellular immunity, which is known as **anergy.** This condition is often seen in chronic illnesses such as renal and hepatic failure, malnutrition, and neoplasms.

References

Hokama, Y., Nakamura, R.M.: 1982. Mechanisms of immunological injury, hypersensitivity and cellular toxicity. In: *Immunology and Immunopathology: Basic Concepts.* Boston: Little, Brown and Co., 1982.

Middleton, E., Reed, C.E., Ellis, E.F.: *Allergy: Principles and Practice.* St. Louis: the C.V. Mosby Co, 1983.

Parker, C.: *Clinical Immunology.* Philadelphia: W.B. Saunders Co, 1980.

Smith, H.R., Steinberg, A.D.: Autoimmunity—a perspective. *Ann Rev Immunol* 1983; 1:75-210.

Theofilopoulos, A.N.: Evaluation and clinical significance of circulating immune complexes. *Prog Clin Immunol* 1980; 4:63.

Wasserman, S.: The mast cell. *Clin Rev Allergy* 1983; 1:309-448.

10 Local Immunity

W. Allan Walker, MD

General Concepts

The ability of epithelial surfaces exposed to the external environment to defend against foreign substances has been well established for the respiratory and genitourinary tracts, as well as for the intestine. The defense common to all these sites is **secretory IgA** (SIgA) produced by plasma cells located close to the epithelial surface. These cells deliver the immunologublin (antibodies) by a transport system unique to the cells composing the epithelial surface. As they come in contact with the epithelial cells, these antibodies are specifically adapted to resist degradation by the proteolytic enzymes in the gut. Antibody is most likely produced at epithelial surfaces such as the lamina propria of the gut by contact between underlying sensitized lymphoid cells and antigens that penetrate the epithelium to stimulate proliferation and differentiation of these cells into antibody-secreting plasma cells. This process is distinct from those at other sites such as the mammary gland and salivary glands, where secretory immunoglobulin is present, but where direct antigen contact with lymphoid tissue is unlikely.

Much experimental evidence supports these observations. Enteral immunization in humans and experimental animals with enteropathogenic *E coli* and *Salmonella* protects the neonate against colonization by these organisms. Specific enterally induced immunity also includes protection against various other foreign antigens such as enterotoxins (cholera toxin) and viruses (polio viruses). This chapter develops the concept of local epithelial immunity, particularly migration of enterically stimulated lymphocytes to other epithelial surfaces such as the mammary gland, lung, and genitourinary tract, where they provide immunologic protection.

Studies that use the intestinal tract as a prototype epithelial surface suggest that cells in the gut-associated lymphoid tissue (GALT) are stimulated by intestinal antigens to proliferate and differentiate into IgA-secreting plasma cells lining epithelial surfaces. The transport process for polymeric (carrier-mediated) and monomeric (passive diffusion) intestinal antibodies underscores the relative importance of these antibodies in intestinal defense as discussed in detail later. Current evidence supports the concept that antibodies on epithelial surfaces function primarily as a barrier against penetration by pathologic organisms and toxins within the environment. Insufficient levels of secretory antibodies appear to be associated with a number of important local epithelial and systemic clinical disorders.

Origin and Distribution of Epithelial Surface Plasma Cells and Their Immunoglobulins

Local Antibody Production

Several lines of evidence suggest that production of secretory immunoglobulins, particularly secretory IgA, is mediated by plasma cells located at submucosal sites close to epithelial surfaces. Since the gastrointestinal tract has been studied most extensively, events occurring at this epithelial surface provide a prototype for local antibody production on other epithelial surfaces.

IgA-producing plasma cells in the lamina propria of the small intestine are apparently stimulated to proliferate and differentiate into antibody-secreting cells by contact with intestinal antigens that penetrate the epithelium. In fact, studies suggest that antigens crossing the mucosal barrier interact directly with lymphoid cells localized in the submucosa adjacent to the site of penetration. Studies involving inactivated polio virus introduced into the intestine demonstrate that specific IgA antiviral antibody levels were greatest in secretions obtained from those sites where direct contact with the virus occurred. The importance of local antigenic stimulation for secretory antibody production was also emphasized in studies showing a striking absence of mucosal antibody-producing cells in the intestines of germ-free animals and of newborn infants, both of which are associated with decreased concentrations of intestinal antigens.

Origin of IgA-Producing Plasma Cells

The events in the mucosal plasma cell cycle that precede local antibody production are less well understood than antibody production itself. Specifically, there is a lack of information concerning the site of origin of precursors to IgA-producing cells and the factors that contribute to the redistribution of these cells along epithelial surfaces. Recent studies, however, have suggested a working hypothesis to explain these processes. Reports from several laboratories have corroborated the observation that lymphoblasts populating the lamina propria are probably derived from GALT, primarily Peyer's patches, and are precommitted to IgA production before becoming distributed along the mucosal surface (Figure 10-1). Cells from Peyer's patches of rabbits, when isolated and injected into irradiated, allogeneic recipients, are distributed within the lamina propria of the small intestine and produce primarily IgA antibodies in response to

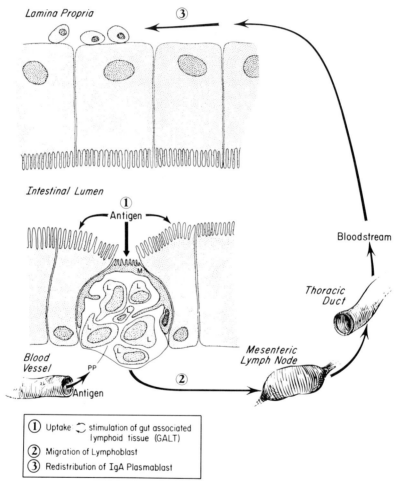

Figure 10-1 Lymphocytes within gut-associated lymphoid tissues (GALT), primarily Peyer's patches (PP) of the ileum, are stimulated by antigens (1) entering from intestinal lumen via specialized epithelium (M cells) across conventional absorptive cells or from systemic circulation. Stimulated lymphoblasts (L) migrate to mesenteric nodes for further maturation (2), then enter systemic circulation as plasmablasts to redistribute along intestinal mucosal surfaces and (3) produce secretory IgA antibodies in response to intestinally absorbed antigens. Blood-borne antigen also may sensitize GALT. Reprinted by permission from Walker, W.A., Isselbacher, K.J.: *New Engl J Med* 1977; 297:768.

stimulation. In contrast, cells isolated from peripheral lymph nodes of donor rabbits are found in the peripheral lymphoid tissue of irradiated recipients and produce primarily IgG antibodies on stimulation. Similar studies in mice have shown that large lymphoblasts isolated from mesenteric nodes and from thoracic lymph rapidly "home" to intestinal mucosal sites and then produce IgA antibodies. Thus, cells from Peyer's patches and mesenteric nodes appear to be precursors of IgA-producing plasma cells.

Maturation of Epithelial Plasma Cells

The access of GALT to the intestinal lumen may be an important determinant in its production of IgA precursor cells. Lymphoid cells in Peyer's patches appear to depend on intestinal antigens or nonspecific intestinal factors such as mitogens, for example, bacterial lipopolysaccharides, for the initial step of the activation process. Access to intestinal contents seems to be facilitated by a specialized epithelium overlying GALT in the ileum. These clusters of specialized epithelial cells, called **membranous epithelial cells (M cells)**, have been recognized in several species, including humans, and may be an important pathway for the direct access of intestinal antigens to lymphoid tissues.

Morphologic features of M cells, including a paucity of microvilli, a poorly developed mucus coating (glycocalyx), and an absence of lysosomal organelles, support the view that these cells are especially adapted for antigen transport. After the gut is exposed to small quantities of a substance such as horseradish peroxidase antigen, uptake of that antigen into M cells occurs. Exposure to larger amounts of the antigen results in uptake not only in M cells but in all epithelial cells, suggesting that the mode of antigen access to GALT may depend on the antigen concentration in the intestinal lumen. At physiologic or lower levels of luminal antigen, the specialized uptake pathway is preferred; at increased antigen levels, a more generalized uptake of antigen takes place. After uptake into M cells, horseradish peroxidase is rapidly released into the interstitial space and processed by lymphoid cells circulating through Peyer's patches.

These studies provide histochemical confirmation of the passage of luminal proteins into GALT. Although these observations suggest that intestinal antigens are important determinants in the proliferation and maturation of local plasma cells, the activation of IgA-producing cells may also be initiated by parenteral administration of antigen. Therefore, the presence of antigen at the site of lymphoid-cell activation, rather than the mode of transport of antigens, may be the primary determinant in activating the precursor cell of IgA plasma cells.

When incubated in vitro, cells isolated from Peyer's patches do not mature spontaneously into plasma cells capable of secreting antibodies; this suggests that other factors in addition to antigens from the intestinal lumen are involved in the differentiation process. These additional steps in the differentiation of cells bearing specific immunoglobulins on their surface, particularly IgA, probably include the helper effect of T cells. These helper T cells are present in Peyer's patches and, in all likelihood, contribute in situ to the lymphoid cell maturation process. The observation that congenitally thymus-deficient (nude) mice have decreased levels of circulating IgA supports the belief that the maturation process of IgA-producing plasma cells depends on T cells. Furthermore, patients with T cell defects (for example those with *ataxia telangiectasia*) also have an increased incidence of associated IgA deficiency.

Mucosal Redistribution of Plasma Cells

After initial activation of IgA precursors in Peyer's patches, lymphoblasts bearing IgA on their surfaces pass to mesenteric lymph nodes, where IgA may also be found within their cytoplasm. The increased synthesis of IgA within the cytoplasm may represent a change from monomeric to dimeric production of IgA. Lymphoblasts committed to IgA synthesis and bearing IgA on the cell surface and within the cytoplasm enter the thoracic-duct lymph and systemic circulation, where they become circulating plasma-blasts. Although these cells continually migrate between the circulation and tissue spaces, they ultimately home to epithelial surfaces such as the lamina propria of the small intestine and the submucosa of pulmonary bronchi.

The factors that control homing are not known. One possibility involves the presence of secretory component, a specific glycoprotein present on and in virtually all epithelial cells. This glycoprotein has a specific affinity for polymeric immunoglobulins, particularly IgA, and may facilitate transport of antibodies into the intestinal secretions. Previous studies have suggested that the interaction of secretory component with IgA on the surface of migratory plasmablasts entering and leaving the lamina propria may mediate the homing process and may govern the distribution of these cells along the intestinal epithelial surface.

Against this hypothesis is the lack of evidence that free secretory component is present in the lamina propria to interact with plasma cells bearing dimeric IgA on their surface. Another possibility is that homing depends on the presence of antigen in the lamina propria. Committed IgA lymphoblasts may localize in segments of the intestine containing the appropriate antigens. IgA-producing plasma cells that presumably synthesize cholera antitoxins can home to the small intestine after an intraluminal challenge with the toxin; however, homing is not entirely dependent on the presence of antigens, since plasma cell distribution in the lamina propria has been noted in germ-free animals and in fetal intestine explanted to sites free of antigen exposure. It seems likely that additional and as yet unknown microenvironmental factors contribute to the homing process and participate in the maturation process of precommitted IgA plasmablasts to produce IgA-secreting plasma cells.

Antigen and lymphoid follicles underlying their specialized epithelium interact to generate cells capable of secreting IgA. Specialized M cells bring antigen into contact with the lymphocytes and macrophages within Peyer's patches. Intact bacteria as well as synthetic particles have been shown to traverse this epithelium and be present in the follicular region. The antigens are in some way processed, and cells are sensitized and released, leading to the presence in thoracic duct lymph of cells that stain for specific IgA antibody. Antibody-producing cells are not normally detectable in Peyer's patches, as was indicated in a study using cholera toxin and toxoid in rats in which antitoxin-containing cells were demonstrated in thoracic duct lymph following intra-duodenal presentation of toxin. These lymphoid cells were eventually found in the lamina propria, particularly at sites in which the antigen was first presented. These findings imply that cells are stimulated by antigen to differentiate into IgA producers and are attracted back, or "home back," to the site where the antigen was originally present. This traffic pattern of cells migrating from the gut back to a mucosal surface occurs also between the gut and mammary gland in the lactating animal. Direct labeling of mesenteric node and Peyer's patch cells have confirmed this pathway, both by immunofluorescence and radioautography. To what extent a similar traffic pattern exists between brochi antigen stimulated cells and the breast remains to be studied.

During late pregnancy and early lactation, the mammary alveoli, which at other times are only sparsely populated by lymphocytes, become engorged with these cells. Hormonal influences apparently are important in causing the increase (up to sixfold) in the number of immunocytes per unit area of breast tissue. Although insulin, aldosterone, progesterone, estrogen, and prolactin have all been shown to be influential, the exact mechanism of these hormonal effects remains to be determined. Lymphocytes and mononuclear cells often exhibit pseudopodia oriented toward the alveolar luminal surface from which they are excluded by apical junctional complexes of the epithelial cells. Some lymphocytes also are associated with myoepithelial cells. These contractile myoepithelial cells may aid in the extrusion of immunocytes into the mammary secretions. The principal immunoglobulin of breast milk is SIgA, and studies in mice, rats, and humans have supported the concept that SIgA synthesis most likely occurs locally within the breast and is not transported from serum into colostrum.

Both immunologically active cells and antibody are secreted in breast milk and then ingested by the newborn. Maternal SIgA presumably acts within the newborn intestine much as endogenously produced SIgA acts, that is, by excluding foreign antigen from the systemic circulation by preventing its penetration through gut epithelium (Figure 10-2). These foreign antigens include bacteria, viruses, and other macromolecules such as those proteins present in food. It has been shown, at least in the newborn animal, that specific sites exist in the proximal third of the small intestine where maternal SIgA binds to the glycocalyx of epithelial cells of the microvilli, localizing maternal SIgA, much as endogenously produced SIgA remains localized and serves the same function as in the mature animal.

T cells, which are present in highest concentration in breast milk between the first and fourth postpartum days, exhibit the full range of T cell activities in vitro but often react to antigen differently than do peripheral blood lymphocytes, suggesting that they are not randomly passing from serum through breast tissue and into colostrum. In vitro, colostral T cells of some women proliferate in response to enteric antigenic substances such as those on *E coli* K-1, mumps, measles, rubella, and cytomegalovirus and yet proliferate poorly in response to systemic antigen such as those on *Candida*, tetanus toxoid, or streptokinase. Peripheral lymphocytes from the same donor respond to each of the systemic antigens with higher degrees of reactivity than the colostral cells. Studies during the last several years indicate that tuberculin sensitivity can be transferred to newborn infants from sensitized mothers whose colostrum contains cells reactive in vitro to PPD. These studies suggest that T cells in colostrum are activated by enteric-associated antigens rather than by systemic stimulation and probably derive from epithelial sites. Furthermore, T cells appear to encounter favorable conditions for survival in the gastrointestinal tract when gastric acidity is buffered to pH 6 following ingestion of colostrum. These properties of breast milk and the relative acid resistance of colostral lymphocytes allow T cells to survive and perhaps even take up residence in the lamina propria of the newborn intestinal tract, although evidence for this is still lacking. In addition to T lymphocytes in colostrum/breast milk, other cellular elements exist, including macrophages (antigen processing cells) and neutrophils, the function of which remain to be determined. Furthermore, a number of soluble factors, including lysozyme and bifidius factor, exist to control bacterial proliferation and penetration.

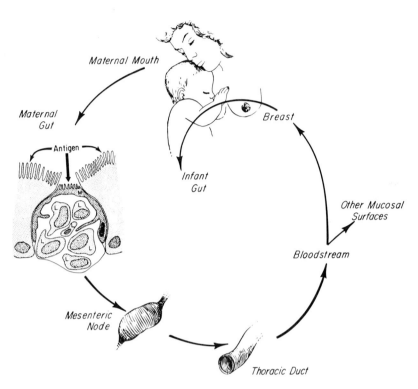

Figure 10-2 Antigen presented to maternal gut is brought into proximity to lymphoid follicles by specialized transport cells (M). Presence of antigen commits lymphoblasts (L) to specific IgA production; lymphoblasts then migrate via mesenteric nodes and thoracic duct into systemic circulation. During periods of proper hormonal stimulation, these cells populate the breast and secrete SIgA, which is ingested by the infant and functions in infant gut much as endogenous IgA. T cells, B cells, and macrophages are also extruded into breast milk and are immunologically active. Reprinted by permission from Kleinman, R.E., Walker, W.A.: *Dig Dis Sci* 1979; 24:880.

Transport of Intestinal Antibodies

Although all classes of immunoglobulins are present in intestinal secretions, the predominant secretory immunoglobulin is IgA, which exists in a dimeric form. In the absence of IgA (as in selective IgA deficiency), a compensatory increase occurs in the luminal secretion of another polymeric immunoglobulin, namely, IgM. This process suggests that polymeric immunoglobulins are the preferred form of secretory antibody. Polymeric antibodies in association with the secretory component may represent a unique adaptation of immunoglobulins for optimum function and survival in the complicated proteolytic milieu of the external environment and are the first line of defense against penetration of the intestinal mucosal barrier. Other immunoglobulins (IgG, IgD, IgE) are also present in secretions and vary in concentrations, depending on the type of secretion samples (saliva, tears, intestinal secretions). These monomeric antibodies appear to function in a secondary capacity as secretory antibodies, since their concentrations in secretions reach protective levels only with intestinal inflammation. From these observations, it is not surprising that two distinct transport processes are present within the gastrointestinal tract for delivery of polymeric and monomeric immunoglobulins into secretions (Figure 10-3).

Transport of Polymeric Antibodies

The delivery of **polymeric antibodies** into intestinal secretions has been carefully studied with immunofluorescent and histochemical techniques. These immunoglobulins are transported through the intestinal epithelium by a specific intracellular glycoprotein-carrier system localized to secretory columnar cells in the crypt region of the intestinal villus. Secretory antibodies are apparently not present in goblet cells. Strong evidence suggests that dimeric IgA and polymeric IgM are completely assembled within local plasma cells and that joining chain (J chain) participates in the formation of

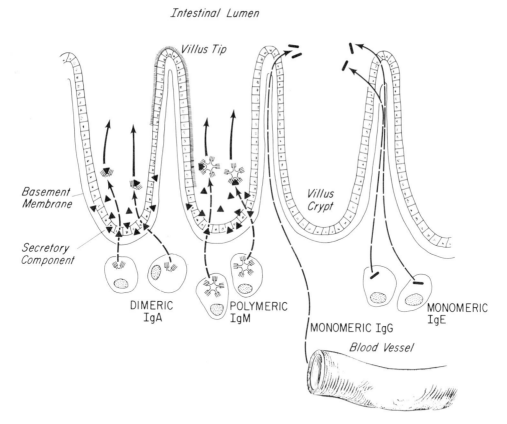

Figure 10-3 Polymeric immunoglobulins (IgA and IgM) are assembled and secreted in polymeric form by local plasma cells adjacent to crypt secretory cells. After diffusion across basement membrane, these molecules interact with a receptor, secretory component, on the surface of or within intestinal cells and are transported as complete secretory antibodies by a specific carrier process through the cell onto the intestinal surface. Monomeric immunoglobulins are synthesized locally (IgE) or transported to the lamina propria via circulation (IgG and IgD) and diffuse across villus epithelial cells by nonspecific mechanism common to other plasma proteins entering the intestinal lumen. Reprinted by permission from Walker, W.A., Isselbacher, K.J.: *New Engl J Med* 1977; 297:770.

polymeric immunoglobulins. After release from the plasma cells in the crypt region of intestinal villi and diffusion across the basement membrane, these antibodies are linked to secretory components, either during contact with this protein on the basal-lateral surface of the epithelial cells or during passage through the epithelial cell. After combining with secretory component, the completed secretory immunoglobulin is released from the epithelial cell by reverse pinocytosis.

The role of secretory component in immunoglobulin transport is unclear. Studies suggest that this glycoprotein is a specific and essential receptor site for uptake by and transport of polymeric immunoglobulins through intestinal epithelial cells. Another suggested role is the protection of secretory IgA against proteolysis. Linkage of secretory component to the IgA dimer protects IgA against breakdown by lysosomal enzymes during passage through the epithelial cell and against other enzymes on the intestinal surface. The cooperation between plasma cells producing the IgA dimer and epithelial cells producing secretory component is an unusual cellular interaction to provide most mammals with antibody molecules that can coexist with the proteolytic enzymes of intestinal secretions.

The inclusion of the liver and biliary tract as an integral part of the enteric mucosal immune defense has come about in the past 5 years as a result of experimental studies in laboratory animals. The importance of secretory IgA and IgA immune complexes in the generation of an immune response, and their participation in the immune exclusion of potentially pathogenic molecules and organisms, are areas of active investigation. The transport of IgA and IgA immune complexes by the liver from serum to bile may provide another means of immune-mediated host defense against enteric pathogens (Figure 10-4).

Transport of Monomeric Antibodies

In contrast to polymeric intestinal antibodies, **monomeric antibodies** are transported into secretions by a nonspecific process shared by other proteins entering the intestinal lumen from the systemic circulation. When injected intravenously, proteins with a molecular weight similar to that of monomeric immunoglobulins can readily pass from capillaries into the lamina propria of villi and can then be taken up by a pinocytotic mechanism into epithelial absorptive cells. These proteins are partially degraded by intracellular lysosomal enzymes and are then extruded by reverse pinocytosis into the intestinal lumen. IgG and IgD antibodies, which are synthesized by peripheral lymphoid tissues, and local lymphoid cells can be delivered to the gut by the same transudation process described for other proteins in serum or can enter by direct diffusion across the epithelial surface; however, IgE antibodies are produced locally by the IgE-producing plasma cells along epithelial surfaces. Regardless of the site of synthesis, all monomeric immunoglobulins are transported across epithelial surfaces at the villous tip. These antibodies do not interact with secretory component and therefore are not protected from intracellular and intraluminal degradation as are polymeric immunoglobulins.

As a result of nonspecific transport and degradation, minimal monomeric immunoglobulin can be detected in secretions. As yet, investigators do not know whether the decreased levels of monomeric antibodies result from extensive degradation, minimal transport, or a combination of these events. When the gastrointestinal tract becomes

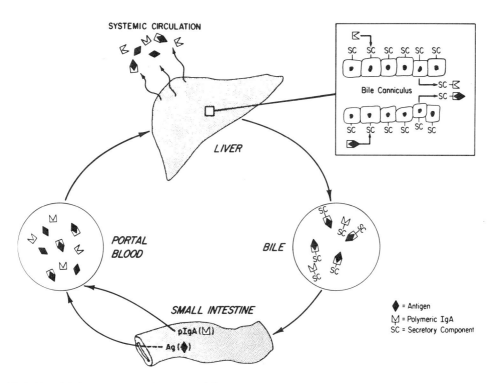

Figure 10-4 Hepatobiliary transport of pIgA and SC-IgA-antigen complexes. Enteric antigen which escapes digestion may complex with pIgA in the lamina propria or in the portal circulation, be transported into biliary secretions, and return to the intestinal lumen. With compromise of hepatic circulation or obstruction of the extrahepatic bile ducts, pIgA, antigen, or complexes of pIgA and antigen may return to the systemic circulation. Reprinted by permission from Kleinman, R.E., Harmatz, P.R., Walker W.A.: *Hepatology* 1982; 2:379–384.

inflamed, increased quantities of monomeric immunoglobulin, particularly IgG, appear in secretions. This increase in secondary secretory antibodies probably results from chemotactic factors that are released by inflammatory cells and that enhance exudation of immunoglobulins from the intravascular space. This process has been referred to as the **secondary line of defense** of intestinal epithelial surfaces.

Intestinal Antibodies and Immune Exclusion

From the foregoing discussion, it seems evident that the primary function of the secretory immune system is to protect the intestinal epithelial surface against harmful invasion of the host. Since antibodies in intestinal secretions were first described, investigators have sought to determine their mechanism of biologic action. Although numerous mechanisms of action, including opsonization and complement fixation, have been suggested, substantial evidence now shows that a major function of intestinal antibodies is the immune exclusion of antigen at the mucosal surface. Figure 10-5 shows one concept of this phenomenon.

BEFORE IMMUNIZATION   AFTER IMMUNIZATION

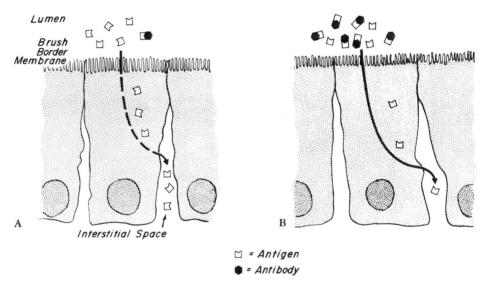

Figure 10-5 Diagrammatic representation of antigen absorption in the small intestine before and after immunization. **A,** Before immunization, antigens are continuously absorbed by enterocytes and transported into intercellular space. **B,** After a specific local immune response resulting in specific antibodies within gastrointestinal lumen, antigen absorption is inhibited by interaction of antibody with antigen within gut lumen or at epithelial cell surface (after immunization). Reprinted by permission from Walker W.A., Hong, R.: *J Pediatr* 1973; 85:517.

Specific Properties of Secretory Antibodies

Several specific properties of primary secretory antibodies enhance their effectiveness within the gastrointestinal tract. After transport from the lamina propria onto the intestinal surface, secretory antibodies are retained within the mucous coat on the surface of epithelial cells by interaction with cystine residues contained in mucins within the glycocalyx. This stationary juxtaposition of antibodies to the intestinal epithelial cell allows for more effective interaction with intestinal antigens that come in contact with the mucosal barrier. The extensive adherence of antibodies to the intestinal surface was substantiated experimentally in perfusion studies designed to wash the intestinal surface free of antibodies. Intestinal surface antibody activity was reduced only after extensive washing with dithiothreitol, an agent known to solubilize the mucous coat of the intestine. This property of secretory antibodies has led to the term antiseptic paint to describe the mucous barrier of gastrointestinal tract.

In addition to IgA's affinity for secretory component, the unique polymeric structure of primary secretory antibodies renders them much more efficient in agglutinating intestinal antigens. The agglutinating capacity of dimeric IgA has been estimated to be several times greater than comparable amounts of monomeric IgA obtained from serum. The agglutinating capacity of pentameric IgM is even greater than that of secretory IgA. As a result, fewer secretory antibodies are needed to contain intestinal antigens, thus enhancing the efficiency of protection provided for the epithelial surface.

Mechanism for Immune Exclusion

Several investigators have recently provided direct evidence for the immune exclusion function of intestinal antibodies. One study examined the adherence properties of oral pathogens such as viridans streptococci to epithelial cell surfaces before and after exposure of these organisms to specific secretory IgA antibodies. The investigators found a definite decrease in adhesion of these bacteria to the cell membrane after exposure to secretory antibodies. They concluded that secretory IgA antibodies block specific binding sites on the bacterial cell wall and thus interfere with bacterial adherence to epithelial surfaces. A decrease in adherence results in decreased colonization as well as enhanced clearance of the bacteria by oral secretions. Additional studies have shown interference in the attachment of *Vibrio cholerae* to intestinal mucosa by secretory IgA intestinal antibodies. The presence or absence of intestinal antibodies capable of interfering with specific bacterial adherence may also be important in determining the nature of indigenous bacterial flora in the gut.

Intestinal antibodies can also protect against the effects of toxic bacterial by-products such as enterotoxins. Secretory antitoxins complexing with cholera toxin can prevent toxin binding to receptors on intestinal microvillus membranes and thereby interfere with the activation of adenyl cyclase, a necessary step in the active secretion associated with toxigenic diarrhea. In like manner, intestinal antibodies interfere with the uptake of nonviable antigens introduced directly into the gastrointestinal tract. As previously mentioned, intestinal antigens become rapidly associated with antibodies in the glycocalyx. Antigen-antibody complex formation at that site appears to prevent migration of antigen to the cellular membrane surface and to interfere with pinocytosis by enterocytes. Other investigators have demonstrated that IgA myeloma antibodies injected into the respiratory tract of laboratory animals interfere with the uptake of human serum albumin by respiratory epithelium.

Immune Exclusion and Nonimmunologic Host Defenses

In addition to the direct effect of mucosal antibodies on intestinal antigens, the formation of immune complexes on the intestinal surface may facilitate other important nonimmunologic protective mechanisms that can further contribute to immune exclusion of antigen from the mucosal surface. The formation of antigen-antibody complexes on the gut surface results in enhanced degradation of antigens retained within the glycocalyx. The enhanced breakdown of antigen-antibody complexes is mediated by pancreatic enzymes adsorbed to the mucous coat lining the surface of the gut. Complexing of antigens by antibodies present in the mucous layer that coats the cell surface allows prolonged retention of antigen. At that site, degradation of antigen by pancreatic enzymes adherent to the mucous coat can then proceed. Recently, antigen-antibody complexes formed in antibody excess have been shown to stimulate the release of mucus from goblet cells of the mucosa. Release of mucus may in turn "wash" the intestinal surface free of complexes and thereby further interfere with the access of antigen to the epithelial cell.

Clinical Consequences of Disrupted Local Immune Systems

Once established, the IgA system of local immunity provides a barrier in the normal individual against a variety of potentially toxic substances. When absent or not fully developed, as in the neonatal period, the individual is at risk for various diseases, some of which may show immediate manifestations and others whose symptoms may be delayed until later in life. The following diseases are associated with disrupted local immunity: necrotizing enterocolitis; food/milk allergy; immune complex disease (chronic active hepatitis, nephrosis, and dermatitis); and inflammatory bowel disease.

Necrotizing enterocolitis, a disease seen in low-birth-weight or premature infants who have been formula fed, is a classical example of altered host defense. The essential components in the pathogenesis of necrotizing enterocolitis are availability of a metabolic substrate such as a formula feeding, bacterial colonization of the intestinal tract, and injury to the mucosa. Several reviews of large series of patients with necrotizing enterocolitis have shown that no specific bacterial species can be implicated in this condition, but that normal bowel flora enter the peritoneum and bloodstream through an altered intestinal mucosa. Although the mucosa can be damaged by various insults, such as ischemia secondary to altered perfusion or directly by hyperosmolar elemental feedings, the final common pathway may be the disruption of the mucosal barrier in an individual whose local immune defense is largely inadequate. This disruption allows penetration of toxic substances such as enteric organisms or endotoxin that lead to necrotizing enterocolitis or even food antigens such as soy or milk protein causing neonatal enterocolitis.

Gastrointestinal allergy requires prior sensitization to allergens. During the neonatal period, an increased uptake by the intestine of macromolecules and, in particular, cow's milk proteins occurs. Although the mechanisms of allergy are yet to be worked out, the result of neonatal sensitization may lead to an immediate intestinal allergic reaction with changes in the mucosal epithelium resulting in diarrhea and protein-losing enteropathy. Even after the mucosal barrier (including local immune defense) has matured, minute amounts of intact protein are still able to cross into the circulation, causing an allergic reaction in the previously sensitized individual.

Adult consequences of disrupted local immunity may play a role in pathogenesis of inflammatory bowel disease (IBD). Investigators have suggested that the lesions of IBD are due to a local hypersensitivity reaction from passage of macromolecules and enteric organisms through a gut wall that has been acutely insulted, perhaps by an acute gastroenteritis. The initial sensitization takes place during the neonatal period, a time when local immune defenses are decreased, and the same antigens can pass readily through the mucosal barrier to immunize the gut-associated lymphoid tissue. The reexposure in later life may lead to a local, cell-mediated hypersensitivity reaction with destruction of mucosal constituents and further sensitization to substances present in the mucosal cell membrane. This break in self tolerance is supported by the production of cytotoxic antibodies and T cells directed against colonic cells in patients with IBD.

The liver is another organ that may be a target for antigen or antigen-antibody complexes that have escaped the mucosal barrier and been absorbed into the portal system. Deposition of these substances within the parenchyma may then cause acute and chronic inflammatory changes in the liver. α-1-antitrypsin deficiency and cystic fibrosis, which are associated with cirrhosis in infancy and childhood, occur with an inadequate or disrupted mucosal barrier, and may represent diseases in which absorbed endotoxin is important in the pathogenesis of hepatic cell injury.

References

Bienenstock, J.: The mucosal immunologic network. *Ann Allergy* 1984(Dec); 53(6, Pt 2):535-40.

Bienenstock, J., Bejus, A.D.: Mucosal immunology. *Immunology* 1980; 41:249.

Kleinman, R.E., Harmatz, P.R., Walker, W.A.: The Liver: An integral part of the enteric mucosal immune system. *Hepatology* 1982; 3:379.

Ogra, P.L., Dayton, D.H.: *Immunology of Breast Milk*. New York: Raven Press, 1979.

Pierce, N.F., Gowans, J.L.: Cellular kinetics of the intestinal immune response to cholera toxoid in rats. *J Exp Med* 1975; 142:1550-63.

Tomasi, T.B., Jr.: *The Immune System of Secretions*. Englewood Cliffs, N.J.: Prentice-Hall, 1976.

Udall, J.N., Walker, W.A.: The physiologic and pathologic basis for the transport of macromolecules across the intestinal tract. *J Ped Gastro Nutr* 1982; 1:295.

Walker, W.A.: Host defense mechanisms in the gastrointestinal tract. *Pediatrics* 1976; 57:901-16.

Walker, W.A., Isselbacher, K.J.: Intestinal antibodies. *N Engl J Med* 1977; 297:767-73.

11 Tolerance*

William O. Weigle, PhD

General Concepts
Historical Background
Conditions of Tolerance Induction
Types of Tolerant States
    Peripheral Inhibition
    Central Unresponsiveness
    Role of Cellular Receptors in Tolerance Induction
Self-Tolerance and Autoimmunity

General Concepts

Normally an antigen is thought of as a substance that stimulates a specific immune response. Under certain conditions, an antigen specifically blocks an immune response; this state is defined as tolerance. Immunologic-tolerant states induced experimentally result from blockage of the immune response by competent cells (**peripheral inhibition**) or elimination of competent cells (**central unresponsiveness**). The latter best represents tolerance directed to the body's own self-antigens. Although tolerance can be induced in T and B cells, it is more stable and requires less antigen for induction in T cells. Macrophages appear to play a role in some cases as nonspecific handlers of antigen. Tolerance is more readily induced before maturation of the immune system than in mature animals; however, tolerance can be induced in adult animals under conditions that temporarily restrict their ability to make an immune response. The in

*Publication no. 1736 from the Department of Immunopathology, Scripps Clinic and Research Foundation, La Jolla, California.

vivo immune status of lymphocytes to self-antigens can be such that the T cells are tolerant, whereas the B cells are competent; this situation can lend itself to the circumvention of self-tolerance, possibly accompanied by autoimmune disease. With other self-constituents that are more completely sequestered from the body fluids, both T and B cells may be competent and both can be stimulated on appropriate contact with self-antigens.

Historical Background

That an unresponsive (tolerant) state as well as immunity can be induced in animals was first predicted by Burnet (1959), who suggested that unresponsiveness to foreign antigens could be induced in animals if these antigens were injected during early life. This suggestion originated in part from the work of Owens (1945), who first demonstrated that contact with foreign antigenic substances during early life resulted in immunologic tolerance. He observed that mature, dizygotic twin cows tolerated each other's body tissues; that is, they did not reject mutual grafts. Undoubtedly, the tolerance resulted from embryonic parabiosis (the union of two individuals, as of joined twins), in which blood was exchanged between the twins. Subsequently, Billingham and coworkers (1953) demonstrated that adult mice of an inbred strain would tolerate skin grafts of a second inbred strain if, as newborns, animals of the first strain had been injected with living replicating cells of the second strain. Subsequent studies have shown that immunologic tolerance can be induced in various animals to numerous nonliving antigens. Furthermore, the induction and maintenance of tolerant states in experimental situations have shown that specialized and distinctly different cellular events may be involved in different tolerant states.

Conditions of Tolerance Induction

Depending on the conditions, injecting an antigen into experimental animals results in antibody production, priming of lymphoid cells with no antibody production, cell-mediated hypersensitivity, or immunologic tolerance. This chapter concerns some basic cellular mechanisms involved in the induction, maintenance, and termination of **immunologic tolerance,** which can be defined as a specific refractory state to a given antigen. This state is antigen directed, in that it develops only when an animal has prior contact with that antigen. The degree and duration of tolerance induced with exogenous antigens depends on the nature of the antigen, immunologic competency of the host, dose of antigen, route of injection, and species of the host.

Tolerance is most readily induced in neonatal animals before the immune system matures, or in adult animals in which the immune systems have been temporarily suppressed. Furthermore, serum protein antigens, which equilibrate between the intravascular and extravascular spaces and persist in the body fluids, are better inducers of tolerance than complex, particulate antigens such as bacteria, viruses, tissue antigens, or red blood cells, which do not equilibrate and are rapidly eliminated from the body fluids. Although some experimentalists claim that exceptionally low and high doses of antigen induce tolerance while intermediate doses produce immunity, this low-high zone tolerance phenomenon is unusual and limited to only a small number of antigens.

In general, once a tolerance-inducing dose of antigen is established, all higher doses also induce tolerance and any lower dose fails to do so. Although the site of antigen injection is unimportant for inducing tolerance to serum protein antigens, tolerance to particulate antigens is more easily induced by antigen injected intravenously than antigen injected at sites draining into the lymph nodes.

Types of Tolerant States

Immunologic tolerance can be genetically determined or acquired. Since overwhelming evidence indicates that an animal's tolerance of its own body components is acquired during early life rather than genetically, this chapter concerns only acquired states of immunologic tolerance. The two categories of acquired tolerance are peripheral inhibition and central unresponsiveness.

Peripheral Inhibition

In **peripheral inhibition,** immunocompetent cells are present but blocked. Cells of the tolerant individual can bind specific antigen, and the tolerant state of these cells vanishes when they are transferred to a neutral host (irradiated recipients). This type of unresponsiveness may not be a true tolerant state, but it may represent suppression induced by regulatory mechanisms normally at play in controlling the immune response. Such regulatory mechanisms include antigen blockade, antibody (including antiidiotype) suppression, or suppressor cells as explained in Chapter 4. A classical example of peripheral inhibition is the immunologic paralysis that can be induced in adult mice by using pneumococcal polysaccharide, an antigen that persists in the host for many months because animals lack specific depolymerases to break it down. The tolerant state induced with this antigen is due to antigen blockade. Injection of small amounts (0.5-5 μg) results in immunity, whereas injection of larger amounts (10-25 μg) results in an unresponsive state, even though antibody-producing cells are present. The apparent tolerant state probably results from a "treadmill" neutralization of antibody by the persisting antigen. Thus, as antibody is complexed to the antigen persisting in the tissue, it is catabolized, freeing the antigen to react with additional antibody. When significantly larger amounts (over 250 μg) of the polysaccharide are injected, tolerance is induced, but no antibody-forming cells appear; however, the tolerant mice contain specific antigen-reactive cells. When transferred to a neutral host, these cells are triggered to differentiate into antibody-producing cells.

Specific suppressor cell activity has been associated with numerous models of experimentally induced tolerance over the past 9 to 10 years. Although such suppressor activity plays a major role in regulating the antibody response, its role in the induction and maintenance of tolerant states is less clear. In many cases, suppressor activity is obviously the major contributory factor, while at other times it is only a transient event and not responsible for maintaining the tolerant state.

The supposed tolerance of patients and animals with malignancies to progressive tumors appears also to be a peripheral tolerant state. In most cases, the animal tolerating the tumor possesses lymphocytes capable of killing the tumor in vitro. The killer cells, however, are blocked by a factor present in the sera. A similar mechanism has been suggested in certain cases of tolerance induced to allogeneic (genetically dissimilar) grafts in neonatal mice.

Central Unresponsiveness

Central unresponsiveness is a tolerant state in which competent cells specific for a given antigen are absent. Specific antigen-binding cells are not detectable, and no antibody-producing cells appear even transiently. Although suppressor activity may at times be associated with this tolerant state, such activity is not required for induction or maintenance of tolerance. Antigen blockade is not involved, and spleen cells transferred from the tolerant donor to a neutral host remain unresponsive. Central unresponsiveness can be induced in adult animals with nonimmunogenic forms of the antigen or after temporary inhibition of the immune mechanisms; however, it is best induced during early life before the immune mechanisms mature. The cellular and subcellular events involved in this type of tolerance are probably identical to those involved in tolerance to self.

The best examples of central unresponsiveness are tolerance induced by injecting neonatal animals with purified heterologous serum proteins and tolerance induced in adults to deaggregated (nonimmunogenic) γ-globulins. Commercial preparations of γ-globulin owe their antigenicity to small amounts of aggregated protein. If the aggregates are removed, the deaggregated (monomeric) preparations no longer incite an immune response. When a preparation such as tolerogen is injected into adult mice, a tolerant state is induced to subsequent injections of the aggregated form (immunogen). Injection of adult A/J strain mice with deaggregated human γ-globulin (DHGG) results in a tolerant state that is complete and of long duration. In these mice, DHGG induces tolerance in the T and B lymphocytes, which are responsible for most immune responses; however, the tolerant state lasts considerably longer in the T cells than in the B cells. The kinetics of tolerance induction in both bone marrow B cells and peripheral B cells are slower than in T cells. Furthermore, the tolerant state induced in T cells is of long duration, whereas tolerance induced in B cells is of short duration (Figure 11-1 and Table 11-1). Note also that the amount of tolerogen required to induce tolerance in B cells is approximately 1000 times higher than that required in T cells. This observation has considerable practical implications for tolerance to self, since tolerance to self-antigens in low concentration in the body fluids (for example, growth hormones) seems to occur only in T cells and not in B cells, although tolerance to self-antigens in high concentration (as in serum albumin) occurs in both T and B cells. Although tolerance induced by a single injection of tolerogen is finite in either T cells or B cells, periodic injections of the tolerogen should perpetuate the tolerant state indefinitely, mimicking life-long tolerance to self.

Several groups of workers have proposed that T cell tolerance—including that enjoyed to our own body constituents—is solely a result of specific suppressor T cell activity. This concept has been put in doubt recently by the demonstration that an immunologic-tolerant state to protein antigens can be induced in antigen-specific T cell clones. Such a clone is a homogenous population of effector T cells and does not contain any regulator cells. Thus, it is obvious that tolerance has been induced directly, rather than through activation of suppressor cells. The possible role of suppressor T cells in the maintainence of tolerance to self will be discussed further in Chapter 12.

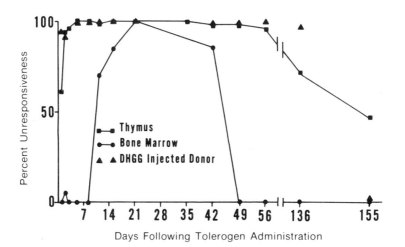

Days Following Tolerogen Administration

Figure 11-1 Kinetics of tolerance induction in thymus and bone marrow cells. Immunological tolerance to deaggregated human γ-globulin (DHGG) is rapidly induced in the thymus (or peripheral T cells) and is of relatively long duration, reflecting the pattern of tolerance induction in the intact donor. On the other hand, tolerance is more slowly induced in bone marrow cells (also peripheral B cells) and is of a relatively short duration.

Table 11-1 Temporal Patterns of Immunologic Unresponsiveness to HGG in A/J Mice*

Site	Induction (days)	Maintenance (days)
Thymus	1	120–135
Bone marrow	8–15	40–50
Spleen		
T Cells	1	100–150
B Cells	2–4	50–60
Whole animal	1	130–150

*Injected with 2.5 mg DHGG on day 0.

Role of Cellular Receptors in Tolerance Induction

One of the most intriguing questions about tolerance induction concerns the cellular and/or subcellular events that determine whether immunity or tolerance is induced. Theoretically, two signals (receptor recognition and mitogenesis) are required to trigger antibody production; it has been suggested that if the B cell receives only the first of the two signals, tolerance rather than antibody production results. In line with this suggestion, it may be the nature of receptors for antigen on B cells that determines whether tolerance or immunity results. Since, in the ontogeny of immunoglobulin receptors for antigen on B cells, IgM appears first and IgD does not appear until later, IgM may be a tolerance-inducing signal that IgD then converts to one of immunity. This concept is compatible with the parallel ontogeny of **thymus-dependent (TD)**

immune responses, in which neonatal mice are immunoincompetent, and optimal immune reactivity does not peak until early adult life. The immune responses to most antigenic substances require T cells and depend on the thymus, whereas the responses to certain polymeric antigens do not require T cells and do not depend on the thymus. IgD receptors for antigen are not required for thymus-independent responses. The dual receptor concept may explain the ability to induce tolerance in vitro in young B cells but not in adult B cells; however, if mature B cells were treated so that IgD receptors were preferentially removed from the B cells, tolerance could be as readily induced in these adult cells as in cells from newborn animals.

If both IgM and IgD receptors must react with antigen to trigger a thymus-dependent response, the two-signal theory appears to apply to B cell triggering in TD antibody responses. It then follows, as suggested previously, that if the B cells receive only the first of these two signals through the IgM receptors, tolerance results. Since the IgD receptors are not involved in **thymus-independent (TI) immune responses,** the ease of tolerance induction to TI antigens is the same in neonatal and adult animals.

Whether a similar two-signal model is responsible for T cell immunity and T cell tolerance is not clear. Before T cells can function in TD responses, they must be activated by antigen-reactive macrophages. Antigen-pulsed macrophages, in the absence of any apparent cell-free antigen, can activate specific helper T cells. Whether such presentation of antigen by macrophages involves one or two signals is not clear; however, significant documentation indicates that nonspecific handling of antigen by macrophages plays a determining role in inducing tolerance to deaggregated γ-globulins. Studies also show that genetically determined susceptibility to tolerance induction in different mouse strains is dependent on macrophages. Thus, when T cells are exposed directly to antigen with no participation by macrophages, a tolerance-inducing signal may result, whereas presentation of antigen associated with macrophages may give an additional signal, resulting in generation of helper T cell activity and, consequently, an effective immune response. It would thus not be surprising if the subcellular mechanisms responsible for inducing tolerance in T and B cells differ since the concentrations of antigen required to maintain tolerance in the two types of cells differ so markedly.

Some researchers believe that tolerance induced in B cells results from antigen blockade rather than from a central unresponsive state. This hypothesis is testable, since stimulation of B cells with the B cell mitogen, lipopolysaccharide (LPS), causes polyclonal activation in the absence of specific T cell helpers. If B cells are competent but blocked in tolerant mice, treating these B cells in culture with LPS should nonspecifically activate them to produce antibody to the tolerated antigen. Such in vitro activation of B cells from tolerant mice has been reported with TD antigens; however, no evidence was presented that the B cells were tolerant. Furthermore, in vitro activation of B cells can be achieved readily with a specific TD antigen and LPS in the absence of specific T cell help. Such activation occurs in B cells of specifically tolerant mice when the B cells are immunologically competent (60 days after administration of tolerogen) but not when the B cells are tolerant (10 days after administration of tolerogen). Along with this observation, the lack of specific antigen reactive cells in mice whose T cells and B cells both express tolerance and the association of IgM, but not IgD, receptors with induction strongly suggest that central unresponsiveness can be induced in B cells as well as in T cells. Again, remember that the mechanisms responsible for the central unresponsive state in T and B cells may differ at the subcellular level.

Self-Tolerance and Autoimmunity

Immunologic tolerance can develop through two different general pathways and thus may play two major biologic roles. First, tolerance sometimes results from regulatory mechanisms that normally control the immune response. Therefore, immunologic tolerance may involve suppression of the normal immune response to exogenous antigens such as infectious agents or tumors. This role would not be beneficial and, because of the antigens involved and the maturity of the host, the tolerance would be of peripheral inhibition rather than of central unresponsiveness. The second, more important role of immunologic tolerance is in self–nonself recognition. This capacity is obviously necessary for survival; the responsive pathway is that of central unresponsiveness.

The relationship between experimentally induced tolerance to exogenous antigens and acquired tolerance to self has both practical and theoretical implications. Burnet's original hypothesis (1959) assumed that tolerance induced to foreign antigens is the same as tolerance to an animal's or human's own body constituents. For an animal to make an immune response to foreign substances such as bacteria, viruses, and tumor antigens and still not respond to its own body constituents, the immune mechanisms must discriminate between endogenous and foreign antigens. This ability must be acquired early in life, before the immune mechanisms mature. Thus, during prenatal or neonatal life or both, animals develop an immunologically unresponsive state to their own body constituents that does not interfere with their ability to respond to foreign antigens as adults. Development of tolerance to self is not genetically determined, but rather results from direct contact between self-components and specific antigen reactive cells. To demonstrate this assumption, the hypophysis (buccal component of the pituitary gland) was removed from a tree frog during early life, allowed to differentiate away from its donor, and then returned to the donor at maturity; the gland was then rejected by a normal immune response. Similarly, animals make an immune response to body constituents that they lack as a result of a genetic deficiency.

Once tolerance to self is acquired, it usually persists throughout the animal's life, since a concentration of self-antigen sufficient to maintain this state is constantly present. Experimental models indicate that when self-antigens are present in high concentrations in the body fluids, tolerance is expected in T cells and B cells; however, when little self-antigen is present, only T cells are tolerant, and the animal's B cells are capable of reacting with that self-antigen. In the latter situation, the tolerant state to self is jeopardized because stimulation of immunologically competent B cells by a combination of signals that bypass the requirements of specific T cell activation could result in an autoantibody response and subsequent disease.

Such appears to be the case in experimental autoimmune thyroiditis, a disease resulting from a humoral autoimmune response to thyroglobulin. The body fluid of normal animals contains amounts of thyroglobulin sufficient to maintain tolerance at the T cell level but not in the B cells, and B cells reactive with autologous thyroglobulin can be detected (Figure 11-2). Autoantibodies and thyroiditis can be induced in

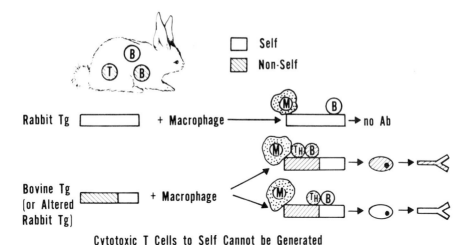

Rabbit Tg + Macrophage → no Ab

Bovine Tg (or Altered Rabbit Tg) + Macrophage

Cytotoxic T Cells to Self Cannot be Generated

Figure 11-2 Cellular events following injection of rabbits with homologous or heterologous thyroglobulin (Tg). The rabbit possesses antigen-specific T and B cells for nonself Tg, but possesses only antigen-specific B cells to self Tg. Thus, when self Tg is presented by macrophages (M) to lymphocytes, B cells but not T cells are able to recognize this protein and, since T cell help (T_H) is not present, no antibody is produced. On the other hand, when either altered self or nonself Tg is presented by macrophages to lymphocytes, the T helper cells recognize the nonself portion of the molecule, and self-competent B cells recognize the self portion. Thus, T cell help is now available to the B cells and the B cells are activated to produce antibody to self determinants, resulting in antibody reactive with rabbit Tg.

laboratory animals by immunizing them with aqueous preparations of heterologous thyroglobulin, which cross-react with the animals' own thyroglobulin. Apparently, T cells in the immunized animal react with structures on the heterologous thryoglobulin that are unrelated to those on the autologous thyroglobulin. Thus, T cells (nonspecific for self) become activated and collaborate with specific B cells, which then produce antibody reactive with self. The same sequence of events occurs when chemically or enzymatically altered preparations of autologous thyroblogulin are injected.

A similar phenomenon is observed in an experimental model of myasthenia gravis, an autoimmune disease that results when an antibody response to the acetylcholine receptors in skeletal muscle impairs neuromuscular transmission. These receptors are a normal constituent of the body, but it seems likely that tolerance to these self antigens occurs at both the T and B cells. Injecting a rabbit with acetylcholine receptors isolated from the electric eel causes the rabbit to make antibody cross-reactive with its own acetylcholine receptors, resulting in a disease that closely resembles myasthenia gravis of humans. Again, the disease appears to be caused by autoantibody produced by competent B cells triggered by nonspecifically activated T cells.

In other situations, the concentration of self-constituents may be so low in body fluids that a complete tolerant state is not maintained in either T or B cells. Thus, both the T and B cells can be activated by self-constituents. An example is experimental autoimmune encephalomyelitis, which has some features in common with multiple sclerosis. This disease can be induced in laboratory animals by immunization with either homologous or heterologous basic protein of myelin. Both T cells and B cells reactive with autologous basic protein of myelin can be detected in the spleen, and both cell types are activated by immunization with autologous basic protein; however, in this case, the activated T cells rather than antibody are responsible for the lesions and clinical symptoms.

Note that these autoimmune diseases represent only two of numerous examples of immune tolerance-related diseases. Such diseases include various abnormalities in the complex regulatory mechanisms that govern normal immune responses.

Although it is unlikely that suppressor T cells are responsible for the induction of tolerance to our own body constituents, these cells certainly are involved in the severity and regulation of autoimmune responses once they are initiated. They regulate these responses in the same manner as they do other immune responses. Furthermore, suppressor cell abnormalities may result in subtle autoimmune reactivities developing into progressive overt autoimmune diseases (see also Chapter 12).

References

Billingham, R.E., Brent, L., and Medawar, P.B.: Actively acquired tolerance to foreign cells. *Nature* 1953;172:603-606.

Burnet, F.M.: The clonal selection theory of acquired immunity. Cambridge: Cambridge University Press, 1959.

Fernandez, C., et al: Immunological tolerance affects only a subpopulation of the antigen-specific B lymphocytes: Evidence against clonal deletion as the mechanism of tolerance induction. *Immunol Rev* 1979;43:3-41.

Häsek, M., Hraba, T.: Active mechanisms of immunological tolerance. *Surv Immunol Res* 1984; 3(4):253-8.

Hellström, J.E., Hellström, I.: Immunological enhancement as studied by cell culture techniques. *Ann Rev Microbiol* 1970;24:383-98.

Howard, J.G., Mitchison, N.A.: Immunological tolerance. *Progr Allergy* 1975;18:43-96.

Kettman, J.R., et al: The role of receptor IgM and IgD in determining triggering and induction of tolerance in murine B cells. *Immunol Rev* 1979;43:69-95.

Metcalf, E.S., Schrater, A.F., Klinman, N.R.: Murine models of tolerance induction in developing and mature B cells. *Immunol Rev* 1979;43:143-83.

Owens, R.D.: Immunogenetic consequence of vascular anostomoses between bovine twins. *Science* 1945;102:400-01.

Weigle, W.O.: Immunological unresponsiveness. *Adv Immunol* 1973;16:61-121.

Weigle, W.O.: Cellular events in experimental autoimmune thyroiditis, allergic encephalomyelitis and tolerance to self. In: *Autoimmunity*. Talal, N.T. (editor). New York: Academic Press, 1978.

12 Autoimmunity

Norman Talal, MD

General Concepts
Self-Recognition
Autoimmune Disease

General Concepts

Autoimmunity represents an immunologic attack on the body's own tissues, which often but not necessarily leads to tissue injury. This attack occurs when self-antigens are recognized as foreign by the individual. An immune response to self-antigens (self-tissues) is triggered by several mechanisms, which are described later.

Autoimmunity appears in many clinical situations: aging, response to infections, organ-specific immunologic diseases such as thyroiditis, and generalized systemic diseases such as systemic lupus erythematosus. Autoimmunity also provides an important clue to normal immunologic mechanisms.

Regulation of immune reactivity involves complex interactions between specialized populations of cells such as lymphocytes and macrophages. Autoimmunity is characterized by the inappropriate activity of immune effector mechanisms. Examples are B lymphocytes that begin to synthesize autoantibodies (antibodies to self) and T lymphocytes that infiltrate and destroy tissues. The clearance of immune complexes may be impaired, and the complement system may activate phagocytic mononuclear cells. This abnormal activity is due to disordered immunologic regulation rather than to problems with the effector cells themselves.

The potential for autoimmunity is present in all individuals. Autoimmune disease is prevented because of the normal functioning of immunologic regulatory mechanisms. The interactions between various T lymphocyte subpopulations are chiefly responsible for this regulation (Figure 12-1). A disequilibrium resulting either in the generation of

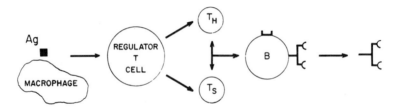

Figure 12-1 Normal regulation of the immune response by the immunologic network. The combination of antigen and macrophage activates the regulator T cell population and differentiation of effector helper (T_H) and suppressor (T_S) cells. The equilibrium established between the helper and suppressor T cells determines whether the B cell is activated. Depending on the regulatory equilibrium established, either antibody synthesis or immunologic unresponsiveness may result.

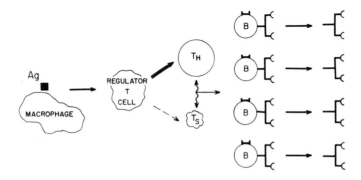

EXAMPLES : I) NZB AND NZB/NZW MICE

2) SYSTEMIC LUPUS ERYTHEMATOSUS

Figure 12-2 Immunologic network as it functions abnormally, creating a state of disordered immunologic control and autoimmune disease. A defect in the population of regulator T cells leads to an imbalance between T_H and T_S cells. The overproduction of T_H cells and deficiency of T_S cells result in B cell activation and the production of autoantibodies. This may represent the situation in NZB and NZB/NZW mice and in patients with systemic lupus erythematosus.

helper T cells or in a deficiency of suppressor T cells could trigger these potentially autoreactive B cell clones to autoantibody production (Figure 12-2). Intrinsic abnormalities in the B cells themselves also could be responsible, as can abnormalities in macrophages (particularly those expressing Ia antigens).

Self-Recognition

Recent developments in immunobiology suggest a distinction between self-recognition and autoimmune disease. Recognition of self (or **autologous**) antigens on cell surfaces, far from being a forbidden event, now appears to be a major, fundamental principle of the immune system. At least two groups of self-antigens are recognized actively by immunocompetent cells: idiotypes (Chapter 1) and major histocompatibility gene complex (MHC) products (Chapter 2).

Idiotypes are unique determinants that are located within or near the antigen-binding portion of lymphocyte receptors. Both B and T cells express idiotypes. Solid evidence now indicates that, for each idiotype, a clone of the antiidiotypic lymphocytes exists that may react with the idiotype-bearing cells. This network of complementary cells may function as a fundamental self-regulatory mechanism of the immune system (Chapter 4).

Self-recognition is not limited to idiotypic receptors. Many examples of immune response to modified self-antigens specified by genes contained within the MHC exist. Cellular interactions based on recognition of self-MHC antigens on cell membranes often constitute a necessary prerequisite for an immune response to foreign materials (for example, viral or chemical antigens). These interactions occur between different T lymphocyte populations and also between lymphocytes and macrophages.

Thus, self-recognition of membrane idiotypic receptors and MHC antigens appears to be a fundamental principle in immunobiology. This self-recognition may facilitate regulatory interactions between cells. Whether the response to any given antigen will be expressed as immunity or tolerance probably is determined by the regulatory equilibrium established by these cells. This equilibrium appears to be controlled by immune response genes linked to the MHC.

The immune system, however, does remain in a state of **tolerance** (immunologic unresponsiveness) to most of the body's own tissues. The mechanisms by which such tolerance is maintained, and may break down, are discussed in Chapter 11. The view put forward in that chapter holds that tolerance to self does not depend primarily on suppressor T cells (T_s). Here we will discuss some experimental animal models of autoimmune diseases that *do* suggest that a defect in the T_s population may lead to an autoimmune disease. The two seemingly opposing views reflect the present status of immunology as a developing experimental science. The next section explores the pathologic consequences of tolerance breakdown and the appearance of autoreactivity.

Autoimmune Disease

Autoimmunity may exist with or without autoimmune disease. Infectious diseases tending to chronicity, several drugs, and the process of aging are associated with a limited form of autoimmunity. The manifestations of autoimmunity disappear on successful eradication of the infection or discontinuation of the offending drug.

Two main categories of environmental factors are involved in autoimmunity: drugs and infectious agents. Numerous drugs can induce autoantibodies in large segments of the normal population. These autoantibodies often react against nuclear or erythrocyte antigens.

Drug-induced autoimmunity is often asymptomatic and is usually reversible. Symptoms generally disappear rapidly upon discontinuation of the offending agent, although serologic abnormalities may persist. For example, approximately 60% of individuals treated with procainamide for cardiac arrhythmias will develop serum antinuclear antibodies. Only 1%–2% of these individuals actually go on to develop arthralgias, skin rashes, fever, and pleurisy (features characteristic of drug-induced lupus). Upon discontinuation of procainamide, the clinical symptoms usually disappear in a matter of days or, at most, 2 to 3 weeks. The antinuclear antibodies frequently persist for several months.

Many chronic infections caused by bacteria, viruses, fungi, or parasites can lead to the production of autoantibodies, particularly rheumatoid factor and antinuclear factor.

Acute viral infections also may be associated with autoimmunity, as in the infectious mononucleosis that develops in association with Epstein-Barr (EB) virus. EB virus and bacterial lipopolysaccharide are examples of polyclonal B cell activators that can nonspecifically trigger autoantibody production. Autoimmunity associated with infection is usually reversible and disappears upon eradication of the infection.

The thymus is involved in tolerance and autoimmunity. Even before the discovery of suppressor T cells it was known that thymectomy predisposed to autoimmunity in experimental animals. Nude mice (born without a thymus and deficient in T lymphocytes) sometimes develop autoantibodies or even mild forms of glomerulonephritis.

The thymus is an epithelial organ that produces thymic differentiation hormones. The association of autoimmunity with thymic deficiency, therefore, could reflect a lack of thymus factors as well as a deficiency of suppressor T cells.

Autoantibody formation is a feature of aging both in humans and in animals. The incidence of rheumatoid factor and antinuclear factor may be as high as 40% in people over the age of 80 years. Although these individuals do not have rheumatoid arthritis or lupus, they nevertheless manifest the serologic abnormalities associated with these disorders.

Many autoimmune disorders are associated with specific histocompatibility antigens. For example, the presence of HLA-B8 and DRw3 predisposes to several autoimmune diseases, including thyroiditis, Addison's disease, juvenile-onset diabetes mellitus, myasthenia gravis, chronic active hepatitis, Sjögren's syndrome, celiac disease, and dermatitis herpetiformis. DRw2 is associated with multiple sclerosis, and DRw4 with rheumatoid arthritis.

Autoimmunity can also be associated with several immunodeficiency disorders involving humoral or cellular immunity, phagocytosis, or the complement system. Antibody deficiency is present in conditions such as chronic deforming arthritis, systemic lupus erythematosus, hemolytic anemia, and pernicious anemia. Cellular immunodeficiency often is accompanied by endocrinopathies (particularly Addison's disease and hypoparathyoidism) and chronic mucocutaneous candidiasis. Patients with these disorders may have autoantibodies directed against endocrine organs, even in the absence of endocrinopathy. A selective deficiency of certain complement components, particularly C2, may be present in patients who develop a lupuslike disorder. These clinical observations suggest that several different immune defects can lead to a common autoimmune pathway.

Animal models for human illness provide an unusual opportunity to study preclinical disease, which is only rarely possible in human medicine. Such studies afford valuable insights into pathogenetic mechanisms underlying early events in disease and offer the hope of finding more specific and effective modes of prophylaxis or therapy.

Systemic lupus erythematosus has been studied using animal models. This autoimmune disease involves primarily the joints, kidney, central nervous system, and serosal surfaces. It occurs more commonly in females than in males. Several animal models for human lupus now exist, including some new mouse strains and a lupuslike illness in dogs. The best known and most widely studied animal model for lupus is the NZB/NZW F_1 mouse, a hybrid of NZB and NZW.

The parent NZB mouse develops a spontaneous autoimmune disease characterized predominantly by Coombs' positive hemolytic anemia. In this anemia, erythrocytes are coated by immunoglobulin or complement and rendered insensitive to lysis. The parent NZW mouse is clinically normal for most of its life. Genetic, viral, immunologic, and hormonal factors are all involved in the pathogenesis of autoimmunity in the NZB and NZB/NZW strains. The genetic predisposition of NZB mice to develop autoimmune hemolytic anemia was appreciated more than two decades ago. Despite fairly extensive genetic analysis in several laboratories, precise information regarding the number of genes involved and how they might function is still lacking.

As for viral factors, NZB and NZB/NZW mice contain abundant type C viral particles. High concentrations of gp70, the major envelope glycoprotein of this virus, are present in serum and tissues. Immune complexes containing gp70 are found in the serum and glomerular deposits of NZB/NZW mice along with DNA–anti-DNA immune complexes.

Much evidence suggests that normal mechanisms of immunologic regulation are disordered in NZB and NZB/NZW mice. Abnormalities of B cells, T cells, and macrophages have been described, as well as abnormalities of thymic epithelial function. Major interest has focused on a loss of suppressor T cells, with consequent escape of autoantibody-producing B cell clones (see Figures 12-1 and 12-2), and on intrinsic defects in the B cells. A defect of splenic macrophages has been observed using in vitro immunization to foreign erythrocytes.

Female NZB/NZW mice develop severe lupus earlier than males. Prepubertal castration of male mice results in a female pattern of disease, characterized by earlier formation of high-titered antibodies to nucleic acids, more severe immune complex glomerulonephritis, and increased mortality. Prepubertal castration of female mice combined with androgen administration results in less autoantibody formation, reduced nephritis, and prolonged survival. Even if androgen therapy is delayed to an age when disease is already established, again less immune complex nephritis and prolonged survival occur. These results demonstrate the ability of sex hormones to modulate autoimmune disease and offer an explanation for the marked female predominance of autoimmunity.

Two new mouse strains (BXSB, MRL/1) that spontaneously develop a lupuslike disorder with glomerulonephritis have recently been developed. BXSB mice develop a spontaneous autoimmune disease characterized by hemolytic anemia, LE cells (polymorphonuclear cells ingesting cellular debris), immune complex glomerulonephritis, and necrotizing arteritis. Male BXSB mice die at a mean age of 5 months; females develop a similar high incidence of the disease but generally die after 1 year of age.

The F_1 hybrids between BXSB fathers and NZB mothers develop accelerated autoimmunity and immune complex nephritis, with death occurring at 5 months of age. By contrast, F_1 hybrids between BXSB mothers and NZB fathers survive at least one year. These results suggest that the disease may be influenced by the Y chromosome through mechanisms not yet understood.

The MRL/1 mice begin to develop a massive generalized lymph node enlargement at 2 months of age. At the same time, they demonstrate LE cells and a severe and rapidly progressive immune complex glomerulonephritis, with death in both sexes occurring between 4 and 5 months of age. Lymphadenopathy in the MRL/1 is massive, but no clear evidence exists that the proliferation is malignant. A single autosomal recessive gene is responsible for this massive proliferation. The cells in the enlarged lymph nodes are primarily T cells. A syndrome resembling systemic lupus erythematosus also occurs in dogs. Clinical and laboratory features of the canine disease include autoimmune hemolytic anemia, glomerulonephritis, polyarthritis, thyroiditis, thrombocytopenic purpura, LE cells, and antibodies to nuclear antigens.

A wide variety of autoimmune disorders can be induced experimentally by immunization with tissue antigens and Freund's adjuvant. The number of animal species susceptible to these illnesses and the variety of different syndromes that can be produced suggest that only minimal constraints exist against the development of experimental autoimmunity. These induced models for human diseases include experimental thyroiditis, experimental allergic encephalomyelitis, and experimental myasthenia gravis.

An important recent development in the study of autoimmunity is the demonstration of the antireceptor autoimmune diseases in humans. The three best-documented examples are Graves' disease, diabetes mellitus, and myasthenia gravis. In Graves' disease, many patients have a serum antireceptor autoantibody that stimulates the thyroid-stimulating hormone (TSH) receptor on thyroid cells and mimics the action of thyrotropic hormone, thus leading to hyperthyroidism. In certain patients with extreme insulin-resistant diabetes mellitus, serum autoantibodies to the insulin receptor are present. These antibodies significantly interfere with the association of insulin and its receptor. The antibody can also modulate the receptor off the cell surface.

From a clinical standpoint, the most important antireceptor autoantibody interferes with neuromuscular transmission at the motor end plate, and is found in 87% of patients with myasthenia gravis. This antibody effectively blocks the receptor, leading to an actual disappearance of the number of receptors that can be seen by electron microscopy. The antibody is detected because of its ability to interfere with the binding of radioactive bungarotoxin to the acetylcholine receptor. This autoantibody can also modulate the receptor from the surface and increase the rate of receptor destruction. Bivalent antibody is required, probably because the antibodies must cross-link the acetylcholine receptor to accelerate degradation.

References

Allison, A.C.: The roles of T and B lymphocytes in self-tolerance and autoimmunity. *Contemp Top Immunobiol* 1974; 3: 227-242.

Jerne, N.K.: Toward a network theory of the immune system. *Ann Immunol* (Paris) 1974; 125C: 373-389.

Moller, B. (editor): *Immunol reviews,* Vol. 55. Copenhagen: Munksgaard, 1981.

Talal, N. Natural history of murine lupus: Modulation by sex hormones. *Arthritis Rheum* 1978; 21: S58-S63.

Talal, N.: Autoimmunity and the immunologic network. *Arthritis Rheum* 1978; 21: 853-861.

Rose, N.R., Mackay, I.R. (editors): *The Autoimmune Diseases.* New York: Academic Press, 1984.

Talal, N. (editor): *Autoimmunity: Genetic, Immunologic, Virologic and Clinical Aspects.* New York: Academic Press, 1977.

13 Defects in Immunity

Armond S. Goldman, MD

Randall M. Goldblum, MD

Anand G. Kantak, MD

Frank Schmalstieg, MD, PhD

General Concepts
Congenital–Hereditary Defects
    B Lymphocytes
    T Lymphocytes
    Complement System
    Neutrophils
    Reticuloendothelial System
Acquired Defects

General Concepts

The fact that the immunologic system plays a decisive role in defending an organism against infection is highlighted by what is known about genetic-congenital immunodeficiencies. With the advent of antimicrobial agents to treat common bacterial infections, affected patients survived long enough to permit study of their increased susceptibility to infections. These studies led to a more fundamental understanding of the workings of the immune system and the role of each segment of the system in the defense against bacteria, fungi, and viruses, in the modulation of hypersensitivities, and in surveillance against neoplastic cells.

This chapter examines the characteristics and clinical consequences of major genetic-congenital defects involving B lymphocytes, T lymphocytes, the complement system, neutrophils, and the reticuloendothelial system. The discussion includes the molecular and acquired bases of certain deficiencies, the nature of the defects, the types of infections caused by the deficiencies, and treatment of the deficiency states.

Congenital–Hereditary Defects

B Lymphocytes

Hypo-γ-Globulinemias.   Defects in the formation or function of B lymphocytes were the first hereditary immunologic disorders discovered. The prototype of these B cell disorders, X-linked hypo-γ-globulinemia, is a disease that mimics the avian bursectomy model (Figure 13-1). In this condition, the thymus, T lymphocytes, and cellular immunity are normal, whereas circulating B cells bearing immunoglobulins, immunoglobulin-producing cells, and all classes of immunoglobulins are greatly diminished. Individuals with this disease are repeatedly infected by virulent bacteria that inhabit the respiratory tract (such as *Streptococcus pneumoniae, Haemophilus influenza*, and β-hemolytic streptococci). Otitis media, sinusitis, pneumonia, septicemia, and meningitis commonly occur. The importance of IgG deficiency in the genesis of these bacterial infections is shown by a decrease in these complications by passive immunizations by parenteral administration of pooled human γ-globulin, which primarily contain IgG.

Although hypo-γ-globulinemic patients recover from most viral infections normally, those with enteroviruses do not. Live, attenuated polioviruses used in immunization, for example, are prone to produce paralytic disease in hypo-γ-globulinemic subjects;

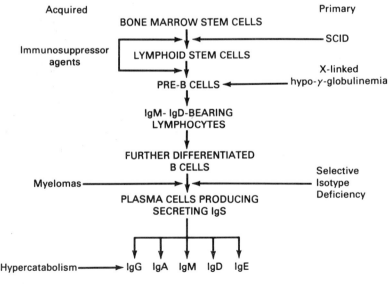

Figure 13-1 A general orientation to the pathogenesis of certain defects in B lymphocytes. Comparatively little is known about the molecular basis of these defects.

chronic echovirus infections of the central nervous system occur frequently in this same group of patients. These infections probably are due to the comparatively low titers of IgG antibodies to the viruses in γ-globulin preparations used to treat these patients prophylactically.

Recently, evidence has been presented that suggests that the basic fault in X chromosome-linked hypo-γ-globulinemia is a defect in V_H genes that are required to initiate the synthesis of antibody molecules. Pre-B cells in these patients express $C\mu$ but no V_H regions. This or similar molecular genetic defects appear to be responsible for this disorder. It is likely that future molecular probes will elucidate the genetic bases of inherent defects in antibody formation.

Several other types of hypo-γ-globulinemias occur, including common variable immunodeficiency, an autosomal recessive type, a type associated with a deficiency of T helper cells and a transient form in infancy. The most prevalent of these, common variable immunodeficiency, appears to be distinct from the X chromosome-linked hypo-γ-globulinemia. Circulating B cells usually are present. T cell suppression of immunoglobulin production by B cells has been demonstrated in some of these patients; in others, immunoglobulins are synthesized but are not secreted because the immunoglobulins are not glycosylated.

Selective Immunoglobulin Deficiencies.   Studies of selective immunoglobulin deficiencies have further elucidated the role of different classes of immunoglobulin in defense. The most common selective immunoglobulin deficiency, IgA deficiency, usually occurs sporadically (one in 700 of the general population). However, it has been found that in 20% of the cases the deficiency is due to an autosomal dominant defect that is linked to the inheritance of the major histocompatibility antigen, B8 (see Chapter 2). The deficiency appears to be caused by a failure in the terminal differentiation of IgA-producing B cells (see Figure 13-1), but the exact nature of the defect is not known. Both secretory and serum IgA are deficient in most cases and the production of secretory component is usually normal.

The many clinical problems in IgA deficiency exemplify the role of IgA, particularly of secretory IgA, in protecting mucosal surfaces. These problems include frequent viral respiratory infections, severe allergic rhinitis, asthma, collagen–vascular diseases, bacterial sinusitis and bronchitis, intestinal giardiasis, intestinal malabsorption, and epithelial malignancies. It is peculiar, however, that the types and severity of the clinical problems vary greatly in IgA deficiency. One possible explanation is the recent discovery that about 15%-20% of these patients lack IgG_2 and IgG_4 isotypes. Thus, it is possible that the frequency and severity of complications may also depend upon associated immunologic defects.

Patients with selective IgM deficiencies present not only with recurrent or chronic bacterial respiratory infections but also with sudden unexpected septicemias. This supports the concept that IgM antibodies are important in protecting the vascular compartment from bacterial infections.

Special replacement therapy for IgA or IgM deficiencies has not been possible for several reasons. First, the available quantities of IgA or IgM are insufficient. Second, the short biologic half-life of these immunoglobulins precludes their use. In addition, little if any injected serum type IgA reaches mucous membrane surfaces. Finally, the use of IgA in IgA-deficient individuals is contraindicated because of the frequent presence of antibodies to IgA in these patients. On injection, IgA complexes with these antibodies, and the resultant circulating immune complexes may produce anaphylaxis.

T Lymphocytes

Severe Combined Immunodeficiency (SCID).   The discovery of patients with severe combined immunodeficiency advanced the concept that the lymphocytes responsible for humoral and cellular immunity originated from common stem cells. In contrast to X-linked hypo-γ-globulinemia, severe combined immunodeficiency is characterized by lymphopenia, hypoplasia of all lymphoid organs, and deficiencies of cellular and humoral immunity. These patients are susceptible to devastating infections with highly virulent bacteria (for example, *Salmonella*) and with poorly virulent organisms (for example, *Candida albicans,* cytomegaloviruses, and *Pneumocystis carinii*).

Studies show that severe combined immunodeficiency is a syndrome consisting of different genetic diseases that display similar clinical and immunologic abnormalities. Although the number of blood lymphocytes and B cells may be normal or reduced, deficiencies in the number of T cells and the functions of B and T cells are consistently found.

The lymphocyte abnormalities in some cases are caused by an autosomal recessive deficiency of adenosine deaminase (ADA), an enzyme that catalyzes the deamination of adenosine to inosine. Some affected patients have been immunologically improved by enzyme replacement therapy with transfusions of normal human red blood cells, but others have not been helped.

In most patients with severe combined deficiency, enzyme deficiencies have not been demonstrated. Transplantation of histocompatible bone marrow cells has produced immunologic reconstitution in many patients. This success supports the concept that the disease is caused by a defect in the formation or maturation of lymphocyte stem cells (Figure 13-2).

Purine Nucleoside Phosphorylase Deficiency.   Purine nucleoside phosphorylase (PNP) is an enzyme that catalyzes the conversion of inosine to hypoxanthine. An autosomal recessive deficiency of this enzyme has been demonstrated in a number of patients with T cell deficiency but normal B cells. This deficiency culminates in an absence of cellular immunity and in severe infections similar to those that occur in other profound T cell deficiencies.

Congenital Thymic Hypoplasia (Di George's Syndrome).   The second major type of T cell deficiency that helped to demonstrate the separate pathways of development of B and T lymphocytes was found in the disease congenital thymic hypoplasia (see Figure 13-2). In this nongenetic disease, B lymphocytes develop into immunoglobulin-producing cells, whereas the development of T cells and cellular immunity is greatly impaired. This disease mimics the effects of neonatal thymectomy or the thymic hypoplasia produced by thymotropic virus in certain strains of mice. Affected patients have infections similar to those with severe combined immunodeficiency.

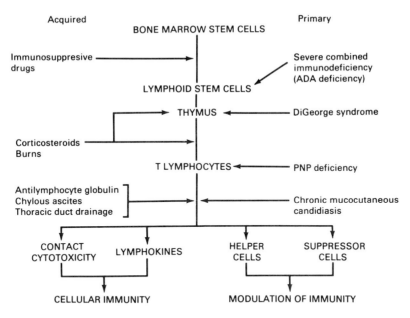

Figure 13-2 A general orientation to the pathogenesis of defects in T lymphocytes.

Congenital thymic hypoplasia is commonly associated with congenital hypoparathyroidism and anomalies of the face and aortic arch. It has been postulated that these abnormalities are caused by a defect in the development of the third and fourth pharyngeal pouches. Some affected patients have been treated with apparent success with transplants of human fetal thymus, but this treatment is difficult to evaluate, since T cell immunity spontaneously improves in some cases.

T Lymphocyte Subpopulations.   Recent evidence indicates that the balance between T helper and suppressor cells is altered in a number of autoimmune disorders including systemic lupus erythematosus. Further details regarding that information may be found in Chapter 12. There are also recent reports that some cases of defective antibody formation may be due to defects in T helper cells, and that transient hypo-γ-globulinemia in infancy may be due to a relative preponderance of T suppressor cells. As methods to characterize these lymphocyte subpopulations are refined, it would seem likely that the pathogenesis of T and B lymphocyte defects will be better understood.

Complement System

The genetic defects in the complement system are summarized in Table 13-1.

Deficiency of C1 Inhibitor.   The first genetic defect to be recognized in the complement system was the deficiency of C1 inhibitor. The disease involving this defect, hereditary angioneurotic edema, is transmitted by an autosomal dominant gene.

Table 13-1 Complement System Deficiencies

Complement Component Defect	Clinical Abnormalities			
	Collagen-Vascular Diseases; Glomerulonephritis	Pyogenic Bacterial Infections	Systemic Neisserial Infections	Angioedema
Afferent Pathways				
C1q	+	+		
C1r	+			
C4	+	+		
C2	+	+		
C3	+	+		
Membrane Attack Complex				
C5	+		+	
C6			+	
C7			+	
C8	+		+	
Inhibitors				
C1 Inhibitor	+			+
C3 Inactivator		+		
B-1H	+	+		

Repeated bouts of angioedema of the skin, respiratory tract, and intestines occur. Edema of the larynx may lead to a fatal respiratory obstruction.

Defects in the Recognition Phase of the Classical Pathway. Genetic defects in formation of the components of the classical pathways are due to autosomal recessive genes. Patients with deficiencies of C1q, C1r, C1s, C2, or C4 have been found to have systemic vasculities such as systemic lupus erythematosus. The associations are unexplained, but they suggest that the recognition phase of the classical pathway plays a major role in the defense against autoimmune processes. The comparatively few serious infections in these defects seems paradoxical, but the observations suggest that the alternative pathway is of great importance in activating the effector limb of the complement system, and in protecting the host against certain bacterial infections.

C3 Deficiency. Two types of C3 deficiency have been reported. One type is caused by inheritance of the null gene, C3⁻. In the homozygous state, the serum level of C3 is below 10 mg/dL, whereas the serum C3 level in heterozygous carriers is one-half of normal. Because of the failure to form the opsonin C3b and the chemotaxins C3a and C5a, affected patients have an increased susceptibility to infections, particularly with encapsulated bacteria. Limited data suggest that these patients benefit from infusions of human plasma containing normal levels of C3.

In the second type of C3 deficiency, synthesis of C3 is normal, but the catabolism of C3 is remarkably increased because of a deficiency in the modulating enzyme C3b inactivator. Because C3b is not inactivated, an unregulated feedback to the alternative pathway results, causing activation and degradation of factor B, which in turn enhances the degradation of nascent C3. Although similar infections occur in both types of C3 deficiency, infected patients with the second type of C3 deficiency are not helped by plasma infusions, since infused C3 is promptly catabolized.

Deficiencies of Components of the Attack Complex.   The membrane attack complex consists of activated components of C5–C8. Deficiencies of each of these components have been found. C5 deficiency presents with systemic lupus erythematosus, whereas deficiencies in the other components of the attack complex (C6–C8) present with sudden episodes of systemic neisserial infections (*N gonorrhoeae* and *N meningiditis*). This susceptibility to neisserial infections is supported by a low bactericidal capacity of the serum in C6-, C7-, C8-deficient individuals.

Neutrophils

Neutrophils are essential for the defense of the host. Any block in the development or function of these cells may lead to serious recurrent or indolent infections. The most frequent infections are caused by fungi (*C albicans*) and bacteria (*E coli, Pseudomonas aeruginosa,* and *S aureus*). Defects in production, deployment, adherence, motility, chemotaxis, phagocytosis, granule constituents, degranulation, and intracellular killing have been recognized (Figure 13-3).

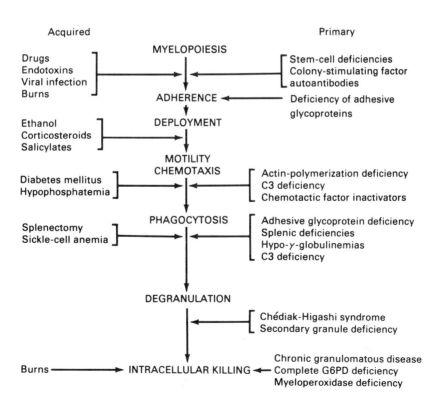

Figure 13-3 A general orientation to the pathogenesis of defects in neutrophils.

One disorder of neutrophil function deserves special emphasis, because investigations of the defect help explain how phagocytized microorganisms are killed. In chronic granulomatous disease, usually an X-linked recessive disorder, susceptibility to infections with catalase-positive microorganisms (*S aureus*, *E coli*, *P aeruginosa*, and *C albicans*) is greatly increased, whereas the defense against catalase-negative organisms (*S pneumoniae*, β-hemolytic streptococci, and *H influenza*) is normal. The reasons for this pattern of susceptibility became clear with the discovery of the myeloperoxidase-hydrogen peroxide (H_2O_2)-halide system of intracellular killing. Normally, when the surface of the neutrophil is perturbed during phagocytosis, the hexose monophosphate shunt is activated. Oxygen (O_2), by reacting with NADPH in the presence of an oxidase, is then converted to superoxide ($O_2^{\cdot -}$):

$$NADPH + O_2 \xrightarrow{\text{oxidase}} NADP^+ + O_2^{\cdot -}$$

Superoxide dismutase (SOD) then catalyzes the conversion of $O_2^{\cdot -}$ to H_2O_2:

$$2O_2^{\cdot -} + 2H \xrightarrow{+ \text{ SOD}} H_2O_2 + O_2$$

H_2O_2 then reacts with the heme protein enzyme myeloperoxidase (MPO) and halide ions (chloride or iodide) to form microbicidal agents.

$$H_2O_2 + \xrightarrow{- \text{MPO}} \text{microbicidal agents}$$

There is evidence that the failure to generate toxic oxygen compounds in granulomatous disease is due to a deficiency in b-245 cytochrome. Catalase-positive organisms are not killed by neutrophils from patients with chronic granulomatous disease because H_2O_2 is not produced, whereas catalase-negative organisms are killed because they produce the H_2O_2 needed for the microbicidal event. In addition, a similar defect in intracellular killing has been found in patients with complete deficiency of glucose-6-phosphate dehydrogenase (G6PD).

Two other diseases that aid in our understanding of the molecular basis of neutrophil function have been described. First, defective neutrophil movement was found to be associated with a failure of actin polymerization in one patient. More recently, a group of patients with defective neutrophil adherence were found to be deficient in a family of adhesive membrane glycoproteins. At least three high m.w. glycoproteins were absent from the cell surface of these patients. Significantly, one of the proteins appears to be part of the C3bi receptor, which is important in phagocytosis of opsonized particles. At least some of the patients appeared to have inherited the disease in an autosomal recessive manner.

Reticuloendothelial System

The reticuloendothelial system (RES) is a group of highly phagocytic, sessile macrophages that are principally found in the lung, liver, spleen, and lymph nodes. One of the major functions of these cells is to remove effete cells and foreign particles from the circulation. Comparatively little is known about defects in the RES. Some consequences of abnormalities of one RES organ, the spleen, are well known, however. After splenectomy, in congenital asplenia, or in hyposplenia accompanying sickle-cell anemia, the removal of certain encapsulated bacteria from the blood is greatly diminished. These patients are therefore prone to septicemias, particularly from *S pneumoniae*. Because of this susceptibility, these patients should be treated prophylactically with penicillin. Active immunizations to the most common infecting types of pneumococci also have been found to be beneficial.

Acquired Defects

A new development in the study of immunodeficiency has been an epidemic of a fatal T cell dysfunction (acquired immune deficiency syndrome, AIDS), found principally among homosexual men, drug abusers, Haitian immigrants, and hemophiliac patients who receive large numbers of blood transfusions. The types of infections are the same as those found in severe combined immunodeficiency. In addition, the patients are quite susceptible to Kaposi's sarcoma. The epidemiologic and experimental data support the hypothesis that the defect is due to an infectious agent, retrovirus (Human T cell leukemia virus type III), which may selectively attack T helper cells. The changing ratio of T helper (T_4) to T suppressor (T_8) cells is useful in early diagnosis of these cases.

The deleterious effect of infectious agents upon the immune system is more precisely known in other situations. For example, in many systemic viral infections, including rubella and rubeola, cellular immunity is transiently decreased. In addition, in malaria and certain other protozoan infections, complex changes that may lead to a failure of antibody production occur in the immunologic system.

Finally, there is growing evidence that tumor cells may abrogate the functions of certain parts of the immune system, such as T helper cells, and stimulate others, such as T suppressor cells. These alterations may lead not only to unregulated tumor growth but also to increased susceptibility to infections.

References

Anderson, D.C., et al: Abnormalities of polymorphonuclear leukocyte function associated with a heritable deficiency of a high molecular weight glycoprotein (GP 138). Common relationship to diminished cell adherence. *J Clin Invest* 1984; 74:536.

Crowley, C.A., et al: An inherited abnormality of neutrophil adhesion. Its genetic transmission and its association with a missing protein. *N Eng J Med* 1980; 302:1163.

Horowitz, S.D., Hong, R.: The pathogenesis and treatment of immunodeficiency. In *Monographs in Allergy*, Vol. 10. New York: S. Karger, 1977.

McLean, R.H., Winkelstein, J.A.: Genetically determined variation in the complement system. *J Pediatr* 1984; 105:179.

Mildvan, D., et al: Opportunistic infections and immune deficiency in homosexual men. *Ann Int Med* 1982; 96:705.

Popovic, M., et al: Detection, isolation and continuous production of cytopathic retroviruses (HTLV-III) from patients with AIDS and pre-AIDS. *Science* 1984; 224:497.

Schwaber, G., et al: Early pre-B cells from normal and X-linked hypogammaglobulinemia produce Cμ without an attached V_H region. *Nature* 1983; 304:355.

Segal, A.W., et al: Absence of cytochrome b-245 in chronic granulomatous disease. *N Eng J Med* 1983; 308:245.

14 Blood Group Antigens

Jan Klein, PhD
Ethel Patten, MD

General Concepts
ABO System
Rh System
Other Blood Group Systems
Hemolytic Transfusion Reactions

General Concepts

Blood group antigens are either alloantigens, which are detected on erythrocytes by antibodies from other individuals of the same species (**alloantibodies**), or xenoantigens, which are detected by antibodies from members of other species (**xeno antibodies**) (see also Chapter 2). In humans, some 400 erythrocytes antigens are currently recognized; many additional blood group antigens are known in various other species of mammals and in birds.

Most human blood group antigens are poorly immunogenic, do not stimulate antibody response upon blood transfusion, and are therefore of little clinical significance. However, certain blood group antigens, particularly those in the **ABO** and **Rh** blood group systems, are strongly immunogenic and clinically important. Testing for blood group antigens has application in transfusion medicine, transplantation, disputed paternity, forensic pathology, and anthropology.

ABO System

The best known and most important of the human blood group antigens belong to the ABO system. The two main antigens (A and B) of the ABO system are detected with the corresponding antibodies (anti-A and anti-B) obtained from the sera of normal individuals. The two antigens divide humans into four groups:

1. **Group A** individuals carry the A antigen on their erythrocytes and anti-B in their sera.

2. **Group B** individuals carry the B antigen on their erythrocytes and anti-A in their sera.

3. **Group AB** individuals possess both A and B antigens on their erythrocytes and no anti-A or anti-B in their sera.

4. **Group O** individuals lack both A and B antigens on erythrocytes and have both anti-A and anti-B in their sera.

Anti-A and anti-B are found in normal individuals who have never been exposed to foreign erythrocytes either by transfusion or pregnancy. Experiments in animals suggest that these antibodies are elicited by certain bacteria known to carry A- and B-like antigens. Whenever serum containing anti-A or anti-B antibodies is mixed with erythrocytes carrying the corresponding A or B antigen, **agglutination** (clumping) of the blood corpuscles results (Figure 14-1). Thus, only certain ABO blood groups are compatible with certain other groups, a fact that restricts which blood can be used in a transfusion.

In humans, the A and B antigens reside in a complex molecule consisting of a lipid or protein backbone and linear or branched polysaccharide side-chains (Figure 14-2A).

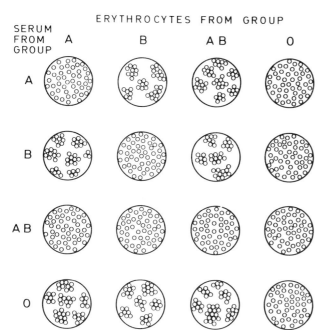

ERYTHROCYTES FROM GROUP

SERUM FROM GROUP   A   B   AB   O

Figure 14-1 Mixing sera and erythrocytes from individuals carrying different ABO blood groups. Whenever serum contains antibodies to antigens present on erythrocytes, the latter are agglutinated.

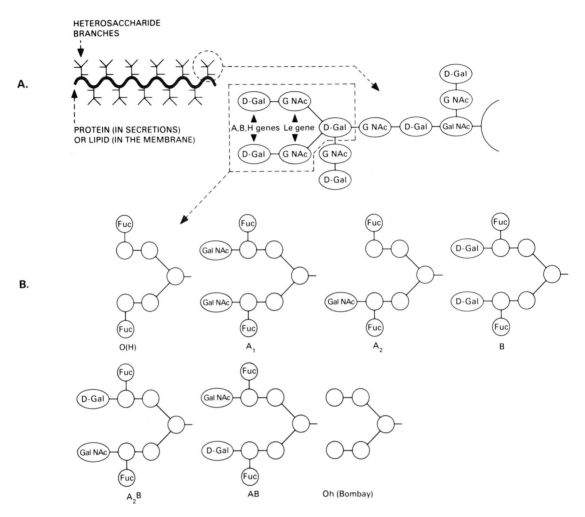

Figure 14-2 Chemical structure of ABH antigens. **A,** The ABH blood group antigens reside in a complex molecule consisting of a backbone (protein or lipid) with bifurcated polysaccharide side chains (heterosaccharide branches). **B,** The H antigen, which is inherited independently of the ABO system, serves as a precursor of the ABO antigens. Unconverted H substance is recognized as blood group O. The addition of terminal N-acetylgalactosamine (GalNAc) conveys A specificity; addition of terminal D-galactose (D-Gal) conveys B specificity; and if both are added, AB specificity occurs. Failure to inherit H leads to the rare phenotype known as Bombay (Oh) and the inability to express either A or B antigens.

For this discussion, the side-chains can be thought of as bifurcated, like a two-pronged fork. Each prong of the fork contains two sugars, terminal D-galactose (D-Gal) and penultimate N-acetylglucosamine (GNAc). The blood group antigens are generated by the attachment of additional sugars to this basic disaccharide unit: attachment of N-acetylgalactosamine (GalNAc) to the prongs generates antigen A. When GalNAc is added to both prongs of each fork, the resulting antigen is referred to as A_1; addition of GalNAc to only one prong results in antigen A_2. The variant A_2 is present in 20% of group A and AB individuals. (Other rare subtypes, such as A_3, A_x, A_m, and A_{el}, exist but are beyond the scope of this discussion.) Attachment of D-Gal to both prongs generates antigen B. Attachment of GalNAc to one prong and D-Gal to the other prong results in the AB phenotype. Failure to attach either D-Gal or GalNAc to the prongs leaves the precursor, H, unchanged and generates the O phenotype (Figure 14-2B).

The attachment of D-Gal or GalNAc is catalyzed by the glycosyltransferase enzymes as D-Gal and GalNAc transferase. These enzymes are controlled by a genetic locus that exists in the following four most common forms, or alleles:

A_1: coding for GalNAc transferase I, which places GalNAc on both prongs of the fork

A_2: coding for GalNAc transferase II, which places GalNAc on only one prong of the fork

B: coding for D-Gal transferase, which places D-Gal on both prongs of the fork

O: coding for nonfunctional enzyme that can add neither GalNAc nor D-Gal to the forks

A and B are codominant, and expression of both alleles leads to blood group AB. O appears to be recessive because it is a silent allele that does not produce any new antigen on the erythrocytes. However, it is now possible to detect the nonfunctional transferase in the serum of persons heterozygous for O and to distinguish between the homozygous (AA or BB) and the heterozyous (AO or BO) genotypes. It is also possible to determine which alleles have been inherited by a person with the Bombay (Oh) phenotype (see below) by demonstrating the GalNAC or D-Gal serum transferases that are encoded in the A or B gene(s), respectively.

The transferases encoded for by the ABO locus can only add GalNAc and D-Gal when the terminal D-Gal also has fucose (Fuc) attached to it (Figure 14-2B). The attachment of Fuc is catalyzed by another enzyme, fucosyltransferase, encoded by the H gene, which is distinct from ABO. The antigen produced, known as H, is recognized as a heterogenetic antigen, so designated because it is present in many phylogenetically unrelated species. An allele of the H gene coding for a nonfunctional Fuc transferase results in the so-called Bombay phenotype (discovered first in Bombay), characterized by the absence of Fuc on the terminal D-Gal and, thus, the absence of ABH antigens. Bombay erythrocytes have a normal life span.

The penultimate GNAc in the prongs may or may not have Fuc attached to them, depending on the product of a third gene, Le (named for Lewis, in whom the gene was discovered). Lewis antigens are soluble. They are not intrinsic to the erythrocyte but are adsorbed onto the red cell membrane from the plasma. The expression of the Le antigen is influenced by another gene, Se, or secretor (see below). Persons who are Le and lack Se produce the antigen Le[a]. Persons who are Le and Se produce the antigen Le[b].

Besides being present in erythrocytes, ABH substances are also found in body fluids (saliva, seminal fluid, gastric juice, sweat); however, these substances appear only in some 75%–80% of individuals who are referred to as secretors. The secretion or nonsecretion of ABH substances into body fluids is determined by the gene Se.

Rh System

Another human blood group system of great clinical importance is Rh, or Rhesus, so named because it was discovered with the aid of rabbit antibodies to rhesus monkey erythrocytes. The Rh antigens, unlike the ABO antigens, are proteins and are an integral part of the erythrocyte membrane. The red blood cells that lack Rh antigens (Rh null phenotype) have a shortened life span. The Rh system consists of antigens C, D and E, which are encoded in three closely linked allelic genes: *C* or *c*, *D* or *d*, and *E* or *e*. The most important antigen of the Rh system is D because it is most immunogenic. Over 80% of individuals who lack the D antigen will develop anti-D antibody after a transfusion of a single unit of red blood cells that contain the D antigen. Therefore, in addition to determining the ABO group of all blood donors and transfusion recipients, it is important to type their red blood cells for the D antigen. Persons having the D antigen on their red blood cells are considered Rh positive, and persons lacking the D antigen are considered Rh negative. Patients who are Rh negative should receive blood transfusions only from donors who are also Rh negative.

The D antigen is the major cause of *erythroblastosis fetalis,* also known as hemolytic disease of the newborn. During pregnancy and particularly at the time of delivery, fetal red blood cells may enter the maternal circulation. If the fetus has inherited the D antigen from an Rh-positive father and if the mother is Rh-negative, the fetal erythrocytes may stimulate the formation of anti-D antibody in the mother. In subsequent pregnancies, the maternal anti-D antibody of IgG class can cross the placenta and cause hemolysis of the fetal Rh-positive erythrocytes, leading to anemia, congestive heart failure, and death. While the fetus is in utero, the maternal liver can metabolize the bilirubin produced by the breakdown of fetal red blood cells. However, after birth the baby's bilirubin level rises. If bilirubin is deposited in the brain, a condition known as kernicterus develops, causing movement disorders, deafness, mental retardation, and death. Treatments of erythroblastosis fetalis include transfusion of the fetus in utero, plasma exchange of the mother to reduce the levels of anti-D antibody, early delivery of the fetus, and exchange transfusion of the newborn after birth. Exchange transfusion serves to remove maternal antibody, bilirubin, and antibody-coated erythrocytes that otherwise would be destroyed in the baby's spleen, and it provides the compatible red blood cells for correction of anemia. Fortunately, the disease can be prevented by the passive administration of specific antibody, which will block the antibody response to the antigen. Therefore, an administration of Rh immune globulin to the mother in late pregnancy and again just after the birth prevents the development of maternal antibody against the Rh-positive fetal erythrocytes. The Rh immune globulin must be given at every pregnancy; its preventive value is lost once the woman becomes actively sensitized and develops antibody.

Other Blood Group Systems

Over 400 different human erythrocyte antigens and over 20 different blood group systems have been described, the most important of which appear in Table 14-1. As stated earlier, most of these antigens are poorly immunogenic. However, once

Table 14-1   Blood Group Systems and Their Commonly Encountered Antigens

System	*Antigen*
ABO	A, B, AB, O (H)
H	H, h*
Lewis	Le^a, Le^b
I	I, i
P	P, P$_1$, p^k
Rhesus	C, c, D, d*, E, e
Kell	K, k, Kp^a, Kp^b, Js^a, Js^b
Duffy	Fy^a, Fy^b
Kidd	JK^a, Jk^b
MN	M, N, S, s, U
Lutheran	Lu^a, Lu^b
Xg	Xg^a

*No h or d antigens have ever been observed, and the lower case letters indicate the absence of the H and D antigens, respectively.

antibodies have been stimulated by either transfusion, pregnancy, or other means, any subsequent transfusion must use blood lacking the particular antigen. IgG antibodies against the ABO, Rhesus, Kell, Duffy, Kidd, MN, and other antigens can cause alloimmune hemolytic disease of the newborn.

Hemolytic Transfusion Reactions

The consequences of giving an incompatible transfusion to a sensitized individual may vary from no ill effect to death. The outcome is determined by factors intrinsic to the antibody response, the transfused erythrocytes, and the host. The critical properties of the antibody are the class, subclass, temperature dependence, titer, affinity, and ability to fix complement. Secondly, the number and distribution of antigenic sites on erythrocyte, as well as the dose (volume) of transfused blood, play an important role. Among the host factors, the function of the reticuloendothelial (RES) and complement systems must be considered.

It is convenient to think of antibodies as causing intravascular or extravascular hemolysis. Intravascular hemolysis is complement mediated. The entire complement cascade is triggered, punching holes in the erythrocyte membrane and leading to osmotic rupture of the cell. The resulting antigen (red cell stroma)-antibody complexes are capable of activating Hageman factor (clotting factor XII), which serves as the initiator of both the coagulation cascade and the kallikrein-bradykinin system. The activation of complement also results in the production of the anaphylotoxins C3a and C5a. In essence, an inflammatory reaction is produced within the blood vessels that involves blood cells, vascular mediators, and clotting factors. The final outcome can be hypotension, renal failure, diffuse intravascular coagulation, bleeding, and death. Anti-A and anti-B antibodies, capable of causing complement-mediated intravascular hemolysis, are the antibodies most commonly responsible for fatal hemolytic transfusion reactions.

Conversely, extravascular hemolysis is mediated by mononuclear phagocytic cells (MPC) of the RES. These MPC have receptors for IgG_1, IgG_3 and the C3b fragment of complement. Red cells that have been sensitized by antibody or complement (**opsonized**) adhere to and are phagocytized by MPC. These erythrocytes may be lysed within the MPC or they may be injured leading to the production of a rigid spherocyte, which can subsequently be trapped and destroyed in the spleen. Alternatively, such erythrocytes may be destroyed by antibody-dependent, cell-mediated cytotoxicity (ADCC—see Chapter 7). When incompatibility is due to an antibody that causes extravascular hemolysis, such as anti-D, the symptoms usually are less severe and are characterized by fever, anemia, and jaundice.

References

Garratty, G.: Mechanisms of immune red cell destruction and red cell compatibility testing. *Human Pathol* 1983; 14:204-212.

Mollison, P.L.: *Blood Transfusio*. *in Clinical Medicine,* 7th ed. Oxford, England: Blackwell Scientific Publications, 1983.

Race, R.R., and Sanger, R.: *Blood Groups in Man,* 6th ed. Oxford, England: Blackwell Scientific Publications, 1975.

Widman, F.K., (editor): *Technical Manual of the American Association of Blood Banks,* 8th ed. Washington, D.C.: American Association of Blood Banks, 1981.

15 Tumor Immunology

Benjamin Bonavida, PhD
John L. Fahey, MD

General Concepts

Tumor cells differ from normal cells in their ability to proliferate in an abnormal fashion, to invade normal tissues, and to metastasize. Furthermore, malignant cells can be transplanted into appropriate hosts of the same species and develop into tumors identical to those from which they were derived. These essential features reflect several changes in surface properties. In **primary tumors,** alterations of the surface properties of tumor cells exempt them from many of the restrictions to which normal cells are subject. Proliferation is no longer effectively regulated by cell-to-cell contact. Changes in membrane transport activities, membrane lipid composition and fluidity, and membrane glycoproteins and glycolipids also may be observed. A further and important difference between cancerous and normal cells is in the new antigens on the surface of the tumor cells. New antigens are recognized by the immune system and elicit a specific immune response capable of destroying the tumor (Figure 15-1). The concept that

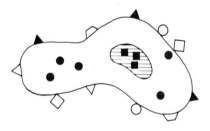

△ HISTOCOMPATIBILITY ANTIGENS (HLA or H-2, MINOR TRANSPLANTATION ANTIGENS)
○ TUMOR SPECIFIC TRANSPLANTATION ANTIGEN (TSTA)
◇ ONCOFETAL ANTIGENS (FETAL or EMBRYONIC)
⌒ ORGAN SPECIFIC ANTIGEN
● CYTOPLASMIC ANTIGEN
■ NUCLEAR ANTIGEN
▲ COAT PROTEIN ANTIGEN OF VIRUS

Figure 15-1 Cell-surface membrane and intracellular antigens found in a variety of malignant cells.

tumors bear antigens distinct from those of normal host tissue has stimulated a great deal of effort to determine the nature of the tumor antigens and to find means to manipulate the host response to overcome tumor growth.

Many tumors in humans emerge and become clinically detectable but do not appear to have antigens or have antigens of low immunogenicity, that is, antigens that do not elicit evident rejection reactions. Antibodies to such tumors, however, may be detected using sensitive immunologic methods. These antigens may be characteristic of the tumors and often are oncofetal antigens or those shared with other tissues. In animal systems, strongly antigenic tumors can be elicited with viral or chemical carcinogens. Some tumors induced by chemicals, however, are poorly immunogenic or are nonimmunogenic; these have not been studied as extensively as tumors that elicit readily discernible immune responses. Most available information concerns the way the immune system can recognize and respond to strong tumor-associated antigens. These data, however, may not apply to all tumors that arise in humans or animals.

Tumor immunotherapy is now being studied in animals and humans. The three major considerations in tumor immunotherapy are immunogenicity and quantity of tumor; the organism's capacity to mount an intense T cell–mediated delayed hypersensitivity reaction in the vicinity of the tumor (which may be stimulated specifically by tumor antigens or nonspecifically); and manipulation of the immune response to abrogate inappropriate suppression mechanisms, allowing the immune system to respond effectively to immunogenic tumors.

Tumor Antigens

The exact molecular structure of most tumor antigens is unknown, but several terms adopted over the years provide a functional and qualitative definition of tumor antigens. **Tumor-specific antigens (TSA)** are present only on tumor cells and are qualitatively different from antigens on normal cells. The specificity underlying this definition, however, is difficult to prove because the available techniques are relatively insensitive. Until molecular and biochemical methods of characterizing such antigens are available, this term should be used with caution. A more appropriate term is **tumor-associated antigens (TAA)**. These antigens are found on tumor cells and are undetectable on the cells of normal adult individuals, but may be found on normal cells under special circumstances. Antigens on tumor cells that can induce resistance to tumor growth in the autochthonous (same) host or in a genetically compatible host are called **tumor-associated** or **tumor-specific transplantation antigens (TATA and TSTA)**. These are operational definitions based on in vivo testing.

Chemically Induced Tumors

Chemically induced tumors (for example, methylcholanthrene-induced tumors) were the first shown to produce syngeneic immunity in highly inbred mice. Cross-immunization and transplantation experiments show that each tumor induced by a carcinogenic chemical is antigenically distinct from all others. Thus, tumors induced in the same animal by the same chemical are immunologically distinct from one another in transplantation tests. The uniqueness of the tumor-specific transplantation antigen in carcinogen-induced tumors suggests that these tumors arise from mutational events. Studies with carcinogen-induced tumors prove the existence of tumor-specific transplantation antigens.

Virus-Induced Tumors

Virus-induced tumors possess tumor-associated antigens capable of eliciting transplantation rejection responses. Three types of virus-specific antigens have been characterized.

Tumor Surface Antigens.   Tumor surface antigens are determined by the viral genome, are present on the membrane of neoplastic cells, and act as transplantation antigens. All tumors induced by one virus, such as polyoma, induce a virus-specific group of common antigens capable of provoking a specific immune response. Thus, animals inoculated with polyoma-induced tumors of syngeneic, allogeneic, or xenogeneic origin will develop immunologic resistance to subsequent challenge with any tumor induced by the polyoma virus. Tumor surface antigens are not present on the virion itself, although they are encoded by the DNA of the virus.

Virus-Specific Antigens.   Antigens of the virion are not transplantation antigens. Antibodies to the virion do not affect the growth of the tumor but neutralize virus infectivity.

Intracellular Antigens.   Intracellular antigens are denoted as T antigens, are encoded by the viral genome, and are shared by all cells infected by the same virus. T antigens may contribute to malignant transformation of normal cells and appear to be of little importance in host resistance to tumors.

Spontaneous Tumors

Spontaneous tumors arise in humans and in animals at relatively high frequencies. In general, it has been difficult to detect tumor antigens on spontaneous tumors. Investigations with several histologic types have emphasized the considerable differences in immunogenicity between spontaneous tumors and tumors induced by chemical, physical, or viral agents.

Oncofetal Antigens

In addition to the transplantation type of antigens described above, tumors also possess other types of tumor-associated antigens. Several tumors have oncofetal antigens on the surface, which are normally expressed in embryonic or fetal stages of development but are reexpressed in malignant cells. Examples of such antigens in humans include α-fetoprotein (α-FP), an α-globulin secreted in large amounts by hepatocarcinoma cells, and carcinoembryonic antigens (CEA), produced by tumors of the gastrointestinal tract, especially the colonic adenocarcinoma. These oncofetal antigens are not known to participate in the host antitumor response; however, when secreted in large quantities, they can serve as a marker for tumor load and recurrence of metastasis after therapy.

Immune Response to Tumor Antigens

In Vivo Studies

The concept that host defense mechanisms may play an important role in the development, growth, metastasis, regression, or recurrence of tumors in humans was first proposed at the end of the nineteenth century. In 1909, Ehrlich hypothesized that host defense may prevent neoplastic cells from developing into tumors. In experimental tumor systems, tumor rejection is mediated primarily by the cellular rather than by the humoral compartment of the immune system, a fact that has been demonstrated by the in vivo experiments described in the following sections.

Transplantation Resistance.   Various techniques can generate immunity to tumors. They include surgical removal of primary tumors or immunization with viral antigens, membrane fractions derived from the tumor, chemically modified tumor cells, or irradiated cells. Studies show that animals sensitized with tumor cells resist a subsequent challenge with a lethal dose of tumor cells. Such experiments also demonstrate that the immune response to chemically induced tumors is highly specific (Figure 15-2).

Adoptive Transfer of Immunity.   T lymphocytes derived from immune animals and transferred into normal animals have been shown to protect the recipient against subsequent challenge with the same tumor.

Neutralization of Tumors.   The assay for neutralization of tumors was developed by Winn and is used to test the immune potential of various cell populations and to evaluate directly their ability to inhibit tumor growth in vivo. Lymphoid cells from

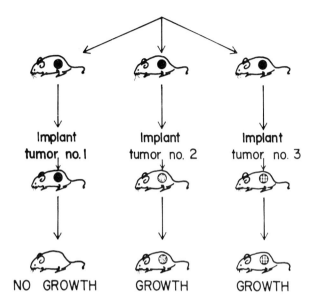

Implant
tumor no. 1

Implant
tumor no. 2

Implant
tumor no. 3

NO GROWTH

GROWTH

GROWTH

Figure 15-2 Transplantation resistance. Chemically induced tumors have distinct tumor-specific transplantation antigens (TSTAs). When mice immunized to the methylcholanthrene fibrosarcoma No. 1 are challenged with appropriate number of viable cells from tumors 1–3, tumor growth is observed. Mice immune to tumor No. 1 reject tumor No. 1; tumors No. 2 and No. 3 grow. These experiments show that immunity is antigen-specific.

animals immune to a tumor are mixed with a graded number of the same tumor cells, and the mixture is injected subcutaneously into normal syngeneic animals. If the lymphoid cells are immune, this fact is reflected by a decreased rate of tumor growth compared to that of control animals that receive normal cells with the same number of tumor cells.

Delayed Type Hypersensitivity.   The delayed type hypersensitivity (DTH) reaction is assayed using tumor cells or extracts. Animals immunized with tumor cells and subsequently challenged by subcutaneous injection of extracts from the same cells elicit a DTH reaction in the skin that involves a perivascular accumulation of mononuclear cells.

DTH reactions have also been observed with a variety of human tumors, including breast cancer, Burkitt's lymphoma, acute leukemia, intestinal cancer, and melanoma.

Cell-Mediated Immunity

Detection of Cell-Mediated Immune Reactions.   There are indirect and direct methods of determining cytotoxicity. In the direct method, immune lymphocytes are added to individual wells of microtest plates in which monolayers of tumor target cells have formed. The plates are incubated for 2 to 3 days, and the number of tumor cells adhering to the bottom of the wells is counted. The percent reduction compared to a culture with normal lymphocytes provides an index of cytoxicity (Figure 15-3). Direct cytotoxicity against tumor target cells is measured by the uptake of dye or by the release of radioactivity from labeled target cells. ^{51}Cr and ^{125}I are the two major isotopes used in this procedure (Figure 15-4).

Monolayers of Tumor Target Cells

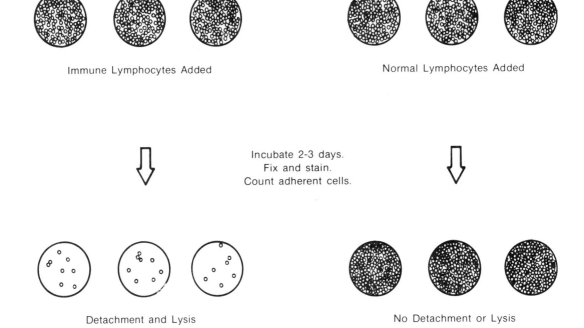

Figure 15-3 Microcytotoxicity test. A predetermined number of tumor target cells are plated and left to adhere overnight. Plates are washed, and immune lymphocytes or normal control lymphocytes are added to each well. Plates are incubated for 2–3 days, fixed, and stained. Remaining cells are counted. Cytotoxicity is determined by estimating percent of cells killed or detached.

Exposure of lymphocytes to tumor cells or to extracts from tumor cells results in the activation and proliferation of these lymphoid cells. This proliferative response can be assessed by enumerating lymphoblasts or by incorporating tritiated thymidine into the DNA. The index of stimulation (the number of lymphoblasts and incorporation of ³H-thymidine compared to control) reflects the response of lymphocytes to the tumor antigen.

Immune lymphocytes exposed to tumor antigens release lymphokines, some of which provide a direct measure of immunity. The migration inhibition factor, which inhibits the movement of macrophages, and the chemotactic factor are two lymphokines that can be readily measured.

Cells Involved in Cell-Mediated Immune Responses.   Five different types of cells have been shown to play a role in tumor immunity: T lymphocytes, B lymphocytes, K cells, NK cells, and macrophages (see also Chapter 7).

T lymphocytes play a major role in immunity and mediate several immune functions. Cytotoxic T lymphocytes appear to be directly involved in killing tumor cells (see Figure 15-4). The precise nature of the antigens recognized by the tumor-specific

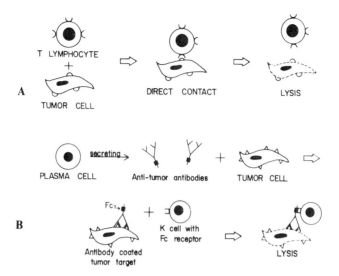

Figure 15-4 Mechanisms of cell-mediated cytotoxicity to tumor cells. **A,** T cell cytotoxicity. Cytotoxic T cells bind to the corresponding target and mediate lysis. Cytotoxicity is antigen-specific. **B,** Antibody-dependent cellular cytotoxicity (ADCC). The cytotoxic effector cell is a K cell, characterized as a non–T-or-B lymphocyte but bearing a receptor specific for the Fc fragment of immunoglobulin. Antitumor antibodies bind to tumor target; K cells bind to the target antibody complex through the Fc receptor. Lysis specificity is mediated by an antibody molecule.

cytotoxic T lymphocyte has not been determined. Studies with viruses and tumors have led to the development of the important concept that killing is restricted. Cytotoxic lymphocytes kill only viral-modified syngeneic tumor target cells that share with the lymphocytes the same gene products of the major histocompatibility complex (MHC) (HLA in humans and H-2 in the mouse).

B lymphocytes may produce specific antibodies to tumor-associated antigens. These antibodies may be cytotoxic for tumor cells in the presence of complement, or may mediate antibody-dependent cellular cytotoxicity (ADCC) by K cells. Antibodies also are involved in regulating the cellular immune response. In viral-induced tumors, antibodies may be effective in neutralizing viruses that are released, and thus reduce cell transformation and limit tumor growth.

K cells lack the characteristic antigens present on either T cells or B cells; however, they possess membrane-bound Fc receptors that can bind to the Fc portion of immunoglobulins. In the presence of tumor target cell and antitumor antibody complex, K cells can kill the tumor target via the ADCC reaction. These cells need not be sensitized to express cytotoxicity (see Figure 15-4). Although the role of ADCC is well defined in in vitro systems, it is not known if these cells affect tumor growth in vivo.

Natural killer (NK) cells are morphologically indistinguishable from most lymphocytes, but lack easily detectable T or B cell surface antigens. Both in animals and in humans, these cells are cytotoxic to certain susceptible target cells. For example, spleen cells from normal mice are cytotoxic against several virally transformed cells. In humans, NK cells also have been shown to kill several transformed lines such as K562 and MOLT; however, certain activating agents such as interferon allow the expression of NK cytotoxic cells directed to syngeneic leukemia cells. Furthermore, in animal model systems a correlation exists between the in vivo resistance to tumor and the presence of NK activity, suggesting that NK cells may play a role in vivo in controlling tumor growth.

Macrophages are important nonlymphoid effector cells in tumor immunity, since they are cytotoxic for tumor cells. Various stimuli such as endotoxin transform resting macrophages into cytotoxic macrophages that preferentially kill tumor cells. In addition to direct cytotoxicity, macrophages can become armed with antitumor antibodies and specifically kill tumor cells. Macrophages also are essential accessory cells in the induction of T and B cell immune responses.

Humoral Antibody Response

Tumor specific antibody can cause tumor-cell killing by different mechanisms: (1) by interacting with complement, (2) by arming K cells for antibody-dependent cellular cytotoxicity (ADCC), and (3) by arming macrophages leading to phagocytosis or opsonization.

Regulation of the Immune Response

Besides effector cells, the immune system includes regulatory cells and other factors that determine the dimensions of immune responses. The regulatory T cells may function as helper cells to assist maturation and proliferation of effector cells or as suppressor cells, which inhibit immune responses. Suppressor T cells can be antigen-specific or nonspecific. They can mediate suppression by cell-to-cell contact or by soluble factors derived from the suppressor cells. Suppressor cells have been found in animals with growing tumors. Such suppressor cells or their soluble factors actively inhibit the development of cell-mediated immune responses by normal cells. This is shown by adoptive transfer of cells from tumor-bearing mice into normal mice, which indirectly promotes the subsequent growth of the implanted tumor cells. The increased tumor growth occurs because the transferred suppressor cells inhibit the normal immune response against the tumor.

Genetic factors, as well as suppressor cells, determine whether an immune response to particular antigens is strong or weak. Genes that control immune responses to numerous antigens have been mapped to the MHC. Genetic factors regulate the antitumor immune response to viral-induced murine tumors and possibly to other types of tumors.

Immune Surveillance

According to the theory of immune surveillance, the immune system has evolved to distinguish self from nonself, and tumors are transformed cells bearing tumor-associated (nonself) antigens. Therefore, the immune system maintains a surveillance mechanism that operates effectively throughout the body to reject small clones of malignant cells as they arise. Initially, T cell immunity was believed to mediate surveillance, but the evidence for this is less strong now and the possible role of natural immunity is receiving increased attention.

Proponents of the theory argue that immunosuppressed animals are more susceptible to tumor development by oncogenic viruses. Also, humans with immunodeficiencies have shown increased frequency of tumor development; however, a distinction seems to exist between viral-induced tumors and chemically induced or spontaneous tumors. In viral-induced tumors, a correlation may exist between the response and immunity. The interaction of H-2 products with virus leads to an altered self and provides a strong stimulus for immune response. This is compatible with the concept of immune surveillance distinguishing self from nonself. Further experiments, however, are needed to provide direct evidence for the existence of this immunosurveillance mechanism in spontaneously arising tumors.

The immunosurveillance theory predicts that tumors produced in the absence of immunoselection, such as in vitro, would be strongly antigenic. Yet, transformation of cells in culture generates tumors that are only weakly immunogenic in animals. Also contrary to the expectations of this theory, the frequency of tumors induced chemically, virally, or arising spontaneously in mice treated with antilymphocyte serum (which abrogates cell-mediated immunity) or in nude mice (with functionally deficient thymus) is no different from the frequency in immunologically competent control mice. Thus, if T cell-mediated immunity were critical, the loss of immune surveillance should result in increased frequency of tumors. Natural killer activity, however, remains normal in these mice and appears to correlate with tumor resistance.

Escape of Tumors From the Host Immune Response

Despite the fact that several means are at the animal's disposal to destroy tumor cells, some tumors escape immune destruction and grow until the host dies. Several mechanisms may explain the escape of tumors from the host immune defenses.

Poor Immunogenicity of Tumors

The immune response to some tumors is nonexistent or too weak to destroy tumor cells. This may be because the tumor cells are similar to normal cells or the exposed antigens are not immunogenic. In some instances, the immune response genes are not functional for a particular tumor-associated antigen. Thus, the failure is quantitative rather than qualitative. In adoptive-transfer and neutralization experiments, the number of effector cells in relation to the number of tumor cells is critical, and there seems to be a threshold for the number of effector cells needed to kill a given number of tumor cells. Deviation from this threshold results in tumor growth.

Antigenic Modulation of Tumor Cells

Tumor cells may undergo modulation of their surface antigens as a natural circumstance of their growth or as a result of exposure to antibody.

Generation of Suppressor Cells

Suppressor cells generated by the tumor have been shown to inhibit antitumor immune responses and to influence tumor growth in vivo (see page 164).

Blocking Factors

Blocking factors in the serum of tumor-bearing hosts may interfere with in vitro cytotoxic responses and may enhance tumor growth in vivo. Blocking factors consist of antigen-antibody complexes and, sometimes, antigens. The complexes inhibit the function of the K cells in ADCC reactions by blocking the Fc receptor. Moreover, antibody has been shown to block cytotoxic T lymphocytes by interfering with the target antigenic sites for cytolysis. In a few instances, soluble antigens have been shown to block effector cells by competitively binding to the lymphocyte antigenic receptor.

Clinical Immunology

Several standard and specific tests can be done to assess general immunologic competence and for diagnostic purposes. For instance, the levels of immunoglobulins correlate with various diseases and in particular with the monoclonal gammopathies usually observed in myeloma patients and patients with chronic lymphocytic leukemia.

Immunocompetent cells, including lymphocytes, macrophages, and granulocytes, are all involved in delayed hypersensitivity reactions that are important in tumor immunity. Several tests that are of value in assessing cellular function are available for clinical use. The major tests include: (1) delayed hypersensitivity skin tests, (2) tests of lymphocyte activation, (3) assays for T and B lymphocytes, and (4) neutrophil function tests.

Delayed hypersensitivity skin tests detect cutaneous hypersensitivity to an antigen or group of antigens. These tests are important in assessing the overall immune competence of an individual. The inability to react to a battery of skin sensitizing antigens is **anergy.** Antigens used in vivo include the sensitizing antigens dinitrochlorobenzene and croton oil.

Lymphocyte activation is an in vitro correlate of an in vivo process that results from antigen activation or sensitization. Several **lymphocyte activation tests** are performed and include mitogenic activation by a battery of mitogens such as phytohemagglutinin (PHA), which stimulates T cells, and pokeweed mitogen (PWM), which stimulates B cells. Since mitogens stimulate large numbers of lymphocytes, antigen stimulation stimulates fewer cells that are specifically sensitized to the antigen. Such specific antigens include PPD, candida, tetanus toxoid, and tumor antigens. The mixed lymphocyte culture and cell-mediated lympholysis are special cases of antigen stimulation by foreign histocompatibility antigens or tumor-associated antigens. These tests measure T cell proliferation and the generation of cytotoxic cells.

In the **T lymphocyte assay,** the E rosette-forming cells measure T cells that bind to sheep red blood cells (SRBC). This assay enumerates the frequency of T cells. In addition, subpopulations of T cells are measured by immunofluorescence using class-specific monoclonal antibodies.

The **B lymphocyte assay** is based on the fact that lymphocytes that readily express surface immunoglobulins are B cells. In addition, B cells bear Fc receptors that can be measured by antigen-antibody complexes or anti-Fc receptor antibody. The clinical applications of B and T cells assays include diagnosis and classification of immunodeficiency diseases, determination of the origin of malignant lymphocytes in lymphocytic leukemia and lymphoma, and evaluation of immunocompetence and detection of changes of cellular immune competence in cancer, which might be of prognostic value.

There are several methods for determining neutrophil activity, including **neutrophil function tests** for motility, ingestion, degranulation, and intracellular killing.

Immunotherapy

Immunotherapy attempts to develop immune rejection reactions against tumor antigens (**specific immunotherapy**) or to modify components of the immune system (**nonspecific immunotherapy**). Approaches to immunotherapy may thus be active, passive, or adoptive.

Active immunotherapy requires a functionally intact immune system that is capable of being stimulated and participating in vigorous immunologic reactions. This type of therapy is successful with immunogenic animal tumors when small amounts of tumor are inoculated and then removed. The immune system is thus sensitized to the tumor antigens, and subsequent challenge by the tumor is met by an altered immune system (immunologic memory), which produces a vigorous tumor rejection.

Passive immunotherapy usually involves the transfer of an active immunologic end product, such as specific antibody.

A recent breakthrough in this area is the discovery of monoclonal antibody technology (see Kennett et al., 1980). Antibody-producing cells are immortalized by fusion with non-producing myeloma cells and the resulting hybridoma cells are cloned in vitro until a stable cell line producing antibody of a single specificity (i.e., against a single antigenic determinant) is obtained. Monoclonal antibodies reactive with specific determinants on tumor cells but not on normal cells may thus be prepared. There is a great hope for the use of such antibody in the diagnosis and therapy of tumors. In particular, a tumor-specific monoclonal antibody has been chemically conjugated with bacterial toxins. Because the resulting complex retains both antibody and toxin activities, it binds specifically to the tumor cells and destroys them. A successful experimental application of this technology in tumor-bearing animals may open a new era in human tumor therapy.

Adoptive immunotherapy involves the transfer of histocompatible, competent, and previously sensitized lymphoid cells to an unsensitized recipient, thus conferring immune competence. This technique has been used to demonstrate the cellular basis (T cells) of most tumor immunity in animal systems.

For most animal systems, 10^5 tumor cells seems to be the highest tumor burden that immunotherapy can control. Attempts to initiate immunotherapy in animals or humans with established tumors, especially those of poor immunogenicity, generally have been unsuccessful. However, combining immunotherapy with reduction of existing tumor load may provide an effective approach.

Nonspecific stimulation of immune amplification mechanisms, particularly the inflammatory processes, has been achieved with agents such as BCG (bacille Calmette Guerin) and *Corynebacterium parvum*. These agents have improved resistance to tumor growth in some animals, but these approaches to nonspecific immunotherapy are not transferable to human tumors, except for readily accessible tumors—usually basal cell and squamous cell carcinomas of the skin. Intense delayed hypersensitivity reactions are induced in the vicinity of the tumor by repeated local administration of dinitrochlorobenzene, 5-fluorouracil, or similar compounds. Factors released during the resultant inflammatory reactions are lethal to the tumor cells and to some normal cells; however, the normal cells are replaced by normal tissue repair processes when immunostimulation ends. This technique currently is the most effective form of immunotherapy in humans.

One of the more promising antitumor therapies is the use of interferons (IFNs) (see Chapter 68). Although they were originally discovered as antiviral agents, IFNs have a strong inhibitory effect on tumor cell growth in tissue culture as well as in an animal bearing a tumor mass. IFNs are also known to activate the natural killer cells that may represent a normal tumor surveillance mechanism (see above). Finally, IFNs are potent regulators of lymphocyte and macrophage functions. With the synthetic (recombinant) IFN now available, clinical trials on cancer patients should provide a definitive assessment of efficacy of IFN therapy.

Immune rejection of tumors may fail to occur because an excessive T suppressor response blocks the normal immune rejection mechanisms. The T suppressor arm of the immune reaction may be decreased by radiation or chemotherapy aimed at reducing the number of sensitive T suppressor cells, as well as by serologic attack (for example, anti-I-J antisera specific for suppressor cells) designed to damage these cells selectively. These approaches have restored effective immune tumor rejection in selected animal tumor systems.

References

Bloom, B.R., David, J.R., (editors): *In Vitro Methods in Cell-Mediated and Tumor Immunity.* New York: Academic Press, 1976.

Coggen, J.H., Jr., Anderson, N.G.: Cancer differentiation and embryonic antigens: Some central problems. *Adv Cancer Res* 1974; 19:105.

Fidler, I.J., Gersten, D.M., Hart, I.R.: The biology of cancer invasion and metastasis. *Adv Cancer Res* 1978; 149:250.

Fudenberg, H.H. et al: *Basic and Clinical Immunology.* Palo Alto, CA: Lange Medical Publications, 1980.

Goodwright, J.E., Morton, D.C.: Immunotherapy of malignant disease. *Ann Rev Med* 1978; 29:231.

Hellstrom, K.E., Hellstrom, I.: Lymphocyte mediated cytotoxicity and blocking serum activity to tumor antigens. *Adv Immunol* 1974; 18:209.

Herberman, R.B., (editor): *Natural Cell-Mediated Immunity.* New York: Academic Press, 1983.

Introna, M., Mantovani, A.: Natural killer cells in human solid tumors. *Cancer Metastasis Rev* 1983; 2(4):337-50.

Kennett, A.H., McKearn, T.J., Bechtol, K.B., (editors): *Monoclonal Antibodies.* New York and London: Plenum Press, 1980.

Lipschitz, D.A., et al: Cancer in the elderly: Basic science and clinical aspects. *Ann Intern Med* 1985 (Feb); 102(2):218-28.

Mitchison, N.A., Landy, M., (editors): *Manipulation of the Immune Response in Cancer.* New York: Academic Press, 1978.

Ross, D.S., Steele, G., Jr.: Experimental models in cancer immunotherapy. *J Surg Res* 1984 (Nov); 37(5):415-30.

Ruddon, R.W., (editor): *Biological Markers of Neoplasia: Basic and Applied Aspects.* New York: Elsevier, 1978.

Singhar, S.K., Sinclair, N.R., St. C.: *Suppressor Cells in Immunity.* Ontario: University of Western Ontario, 1975.

Stutman, O.: Immunodepression and malignancy. *Adv Cancer Res* 1975; 22:281.

Terry, W.D., Windhorst, D.: *Immunotherapy of Cancer: Present Status of Trials in Man.* New York: Raven Press, 1978.

Winn, J.H.: Immune mechanisms in homotransplantation II quantitative assay of the immunologic activity of lymphoid cells stimulated by tumor homografts. *J Immunol* 1961; 86:228.

BACTERIOLOGY

Introduction

Johnny W. Peterson, PhD
C. P. Davis, PhD

Bacteria are single-celled microorganisms that lack a nuclear membrane but are metabolically active and divide by binary fission. Superficially, bacteria appear to be relatively simple forms of life; in fact, they are highly adaptable, sophisticated life forms. These organisms exist everywhere in both parasitic and free-living forms. Because they are ubiquitous and have a remarkable capacity to adapt to changing environments, the importance of bacteria in every field of medicine cannot be overstated.

Although bacteriology is the study of all bacteria, Section II emphasizes only those genera and species of bacteria that have medical relevance. Pathogenic bacteria constitute only a small proportion of the total bacterial population; many nonpathogens are beneficial to humans and participate in essential processes such as nitrogen fixation, waste disposal, food production, and drug preparation.

In some situations, a disease state of a host may be viewed as a failure of a bacterium to adapt, since a well-adapted parasite ideally lives in close association with its host, perhaps to gain nutritional advantage, without causing significant damage to the host. Inducing disease or death of its host lessens a bacterium's chance for survival. In other situations, nonvirulent microorganisms cause disease if present in unusually large numbers, if the host's defenses are impaired, or if anaerobic conditions exist.

In developed countries, 90% of documented infections in hospitalized patients are caused by bacteria. These cases probably reflect only a small percentage of the actual number of bacterial infections occurring in the general population, and usually represent the most severe cases. In developing countries, bacterial infections often exert a devastating effect on the health of the inhabitants, who become infected with a large variety and number of bacteria. Malnutrition, parasitic infections, and poor sanitation are a few of the factors contributing to the increased susceptibility of these individuals to bacterial pathogens. Bacterial infections continue to be responsible for much morbidity and mortality as well as a major portion of health-care costs worldwide.

Although the advent of antibiotics has substantially improved the clinical course of many bacterial infections, and has often diminished the number of bacterial infections by limiting dissemination of the bacteria, chemotherapy has not eradicated even a single bacterial disease in any population. Likewise, only a few bacterial vaccines (for example, diphtheria toxoid, tetanus toxoid, and pneumococcal) have been shown to be highly effective in altering the number and severity of these few bacterial infections. In contrast, improved sanitation and water purification often have a greater effect on the number of bacterial infections than does availability of antibiotics or bacterial vaccines. Thus, the old adage "Cleanliness is next to godliness" is a sound medical principle.

Most diseases now known to have a bacteriologic etiology have been recognized for hundreds of years. Some of these diseases were described in the writings of the ancient Chinese, centuries prior to the first descriptions of bacteria by Antony van Leeuwenhoek in 1677. We believe that most bacterial diseases and their etiologic agents now have been described. However, a few diseases (such as chronic ulcerative colitis) are thought to be caused by bacteria, although no microbial etiologic agent has yet been described. Occasionally, previously unrecognized diseases are associated with a new group of bacteria. A recent example is the acute respiratory infection (Legionnaire's disease) caused by a previously unrecognized bacterial pathogen (*Legionella*). Another example, less dramatic but of immense importance in understanding the etiology of venereal diseases, was the association of at least 50% of the cases of nongonococcal urethritis with *Ureaplasma urealyticum* and *Chlamydia trachomatis*. In addition, only within the last 10 years have studies shown that many diarrheal diseases are caused by strains of *Escherichia coli* that acquire special virulence plasmids (extrachromsomal DNA), which code for enterotoxins, adherence, and invasive properties.

In recent years, medical scientists have concentrated on the study of pathogenic mechanisms and host defenses. Understanding host-parasite relationships involving specific pathogens requires familiarity with the fundamental characteristics of the parasite, the host, and their interactions. Therefore, the first third of this section deals with the basic concepts of bacterial structure, taxonomy, metabolism, genetics, and cultivation; knowledge of these concepts is essential to an understanding of both growth and virulence potential. Subsequent chapters emphasize normal relationships among bacteria on external surfaces; mechanisms by which microorganisms damage the host; host defense mechanisms; source and distribution of pathogens (epidemiology); principles of diagnosis; and mechanisms of action of antimicrobial drugs, antiseptics, and disinfectants. These chapters provide the basis for subsequent discussions of specific bacterial pathogens and the diseases they cause.

Within the text, bacteria are grouped on the basis of similar physical, chemical, and biologic characteristics; these similarities do not necessarily indicate close evolutionary or disease relationships. Thus, widely divergent diseases may be caused by bacteria within the same group. Chapters on specific microorganisms begin with the most commonly encountered bacteria and are followed by chapters on more unusual bacteria. The latter group includes the spiral-shaped bacteria; the *Mycoplasma,* which lack a bacterial cell wall; the rickettsiae and chlamydiae, which grow within host cells; and *Legionella,* a newly recognized pathogen.

16 Structure

Milton R. J. Salton, ScD
Kwang-Shin Kim, PhD

General Concepts
The Nucleoid
Surface Appendages
  Flagella
  Pili
Surface Layers
  Capsules or Loose Slime

Cell Wall and Gram-Negative Cell Envelope
Outer Membrane of Gram-Negative Bacteria
Intracellular Components
  Plasma (Cytoplasmic) Membranes
  Mesosomes
Other Intracellular Components

General Concepts

All bacteria, both pathogenic and saprophytic, are unicellular organisms that reproduce by binary fission. Most possess all genetic information, biosynthetic capabilities, and energy-yielding systems necessary for growth, replication, and biosynthesis and assembly of their macromolecular constituents and structure. The organization of the major functions and structures of bacterial cells distinguishes prokaryotic cells from the eukaryotic cells of microbial, protozoal, plant, and animal origins. The essential structural features of most **prokaryotic cells** are: a nucleoid (nuclear body) that is devoid of an enveloping membrane and undergoes amitotic replication; a rigid cell wall or envelope structure containing the peptidoglycan; a plasma or cytoplasmic membrane performing transport, energy-transducing, and certain biosynthetic functions; absence of intracellular membranous organelles (such as mitochondria, endoplasmic reticulum, golgi apparatus, and lysosomes); and organs of locomotion that are simple, flagellar structures.

Bacteria can be subdivided on the basis of Gram's stain into two major groups: gram-positive and gram-negative. The major difference between the two groups relates to the chemical nature and organization of the cell envelope. Bacteria also can be classified into two principal forms by their cellular morphology: bacilli for cylindrical, rod-shaped organisms and cocci for spherical ones. There are no relations between the bacterial forms and Gram stain reaction.

Figure 16-1 depicts the typical organization of a prokaryotic bacterial cell. This electron micrograph shows a thin section of the gram-negative diplococcus, *Neisseria gonorrhoeae*, the causal organism of gonorrhea.

The Nucleoid

Prokaryotic cells and eukaryotic cells were initially distinguished on the basis of structure: the prokaryotic nucleus is structurally simple compared to the eukaryote's true nucleus with its complex mitotic apparatus and surrounding nuclear membrane. As the electron micrograph in Figure 16-1 shows, the bacterial nucleoid containing DNA fibrils lacks a limiting membrane. In the light microscope, the nuclear body of the bacterial cell can be seen with the aid of the Feulgen stain; a positive reaction indicates the presence of DNA. By gentle lysis of most bacterial cells, it is possible to isolate the nucleoid and see a single, continuous, "giant" circular molecule, approximately 3×10^9 daltons in molecular weight (see Chapter 20). If displayed as an unfolded structure, the nuclear DNA is about 1 mm long (compare with an average length of 1–2 μm for the bacterial cell). The bacterial nucleoid, then, is a structure containing a single chromosome. The number of copies per cell is dependent on the stages of the cell cycle, including

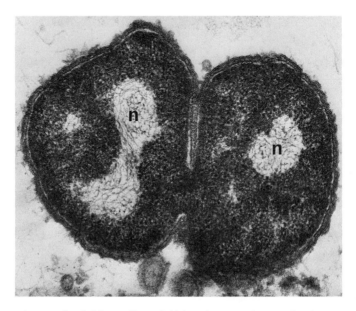

Figure 16-1 Electron micrograph of thin section of *Neisseria gonorrhoeae* showing organizational features of prokaryotic cells. Note electron-transparent nuclear region (n) packed with DNA fibrils, dense distribution of ribosomal particles in the cytoplasmic compartment of the cell, and absence of intracellular membranous organelles.

initiation of chromosome replication, cell enlargement, and chromosome segregation. Although the mechanism of segregation of the two sister chromosomes following replication is not fully understood, all of the models proposed require permanent attachment of the chromosomes to the membranes throughout the various stages of the cell division cycle.

Although basic histones are not present in bacterial chromatin, low-molecular-weight polyamines and magnesium ions may fulfill a similar function to the histones of eukaryotic chromatin. Despite these differences, prokaryotic DNA from bacteriophage λ-infected cells, when visualized by electron microscopy, has a beaded, condensed appearance not unlike that of eukaryotic chromatin.

Surface Appendages

Two types of surface appendages can be recognized on certain bacterial species: the **flagella** (organs of locomotion) and **pili** (L. *hairs*) or **fimbriae** (L. *fringes*). Flagella may be found in gram-positive or gram-negative bacteria; their presence, which permits motility of certain groups of organisms, can have taxonomic significance. For example, flagella are found on many species of bacilli but rarely on cocci. In contrast, pili (fimbriae) are almost exclusively found in gram-negative bacteria and only in a few gram-positive organisms (for example, *Corynebacterium renale* and *Streptococcus pyogenes*).

Some bacteria possess both flagella and pili. The electron micrograph in Figure 16-2 shows the characteristic wavy appearance of flagella and two types of pili on the surface of *Escherichia coli*.

Flagella

Structurally, bacterial flagella are long (3-12 μm), filamentous, surface appendages about 12-30 nm in diameter; the subunits of the flagellum (a singular filament or appendage) are assembled in the form of a cylindrical structure with a hollow core. Flagella consist of three parts: (1) the long **filaments,** which are appendages external to the cell surface; (2) the **hook** structure at the end of the filaments; (3) and the **basal body,** to which the hook is anchored, which consists of a rod and one or two pairs of discs and traverses the outer wall and membrane structures. The thrust for the propulsion or swimming movement of the bacterial cell is provided by the counterclockwise rotation of the basal body of the flagella applied to the helically twisted filament. It is driven by the proton motive force, not by ATP directly. The ability of bacteria to swim by means of the propellerlike action of their flagella provides them with the mechanical means to respond to attractant and repellent substances in their environment and thereby allows them to exhibit **chemotactic behavior.** Response to chemical stimuli involves a sophisticated sensory system of receptors in the cell surface and/or periplasm, which transmits information to methyl-accepting chemotaxis proteins that control the flagella motor. Genetic studies have revealed the existence of mutants that have alterations in flagella-motility and chemotaxis pathways.

Chemically, flagella are composed of subunits of a class of proteins called **flagellins.** The hooks and ring structures consist of different proteins, which are

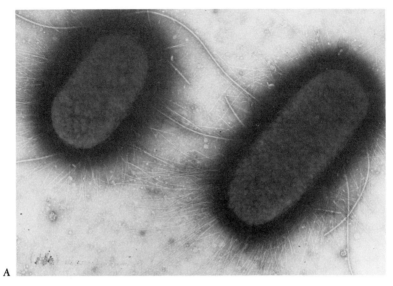

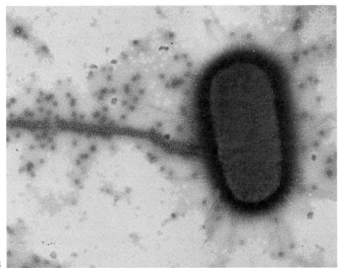

Figure 16-2 Electron micrograph of negatively stained *E coli* in **A** shows wavy flagella appendages and numerous short, thinner, and more rigid hairlike structures, the pili. In **B,** long sex pilus is distinguishable from shorter common type of pili by mixing *E coli* cells with male phage that binds specifically to sex pili.

distinctive for each part of the system responsible for flagella rotation. Mutations affecting any of these gene products may result in loss or impairment of motility. Flagellins are immunogenic and constitute a group of protein antigens (H antigens) characteristic of a given species, strain, or variant of an organism. Species specificity of the flagellins reflects differences in the primary structure of the proteins.

Numbers and distribution of flagella on the bacterial surface are characteristic for a given species and thus have value in identifying and classifying bacterial species. For example, *Vibrio cholerae*, which possesses a single flagellum at one pole of the cell, is **monotrichous**; *Proteus vulgaris*, which has many flagella distributed over its entire surface, is a **peritrichous** organism. The flagella of a peritrichous bacterium must aggregate as a posterior bundle to propel the cell in a forward direction.

Flagella can be sheared from the cell surface without affecting cell viability. The cells then become immobile, but they retain the capacity to resynthesize flagella and restore motility. The protein synthesis inhibitor, chloramphenicol, blocks regeneration.

Pili

The terms pili and fimbriae have been used interchangeably to describe the thin, hairlike appendages on the surfaces of many gram-negative bacteria. The pili are more rigid in appearance than flagella (Figure 16-2) and in some organisms, such as *Shigella* sp and *E coli*, the pili are profusely distributed over the cell surfaces with as many as 200 per cell. In strains of *E coli*, two types of pili are easily recognized: the short, abundant common pili and a small number (1–6) of very long pili, known as the sex pili. These sex pili can be identified (Fig 16-2B) by their ability to bind male-specific bacteriophages (the sex pilus acts as a specific receptor for the bacteriophages). The sex pili are essential for bacterial attachment during conjugation.

Pili in many enteric bacteria confer adhesive properties to the bacterial cells, enabling them to adhere to various epithelial surfaces, to red blood cells causing hemagglutination, and to surfaces of yeast and fungal cells. These adhesive properties play an important role in bacterial colonization of epithelial surfaces; thus these properties of piliated cells are referred to as colonization factors. The common type of pili found on *E coli* exhibits a sugar specificity analogous to phytohemagglutinins and lectins in that its adhesion and hemagglutinating capacity is inhibited specifically by mannose. Thus organisms possessing this type of pili hemagglutination are said to be mannose-sensitive. Other piliated organisms, such as gonococcus, are adhesive and hemagglutinating but insensitive to the inhibitory effects of mannose.

Pili can be sheared from the cell surface and isolated in pure form. The pili of *E coli* and *N gonorrhoeae* are composed of proteins, called pilins, which have subunit molecular weights of about 19,000. Enteric pili of the common type and those of the gonococci are antigenically distinct; evidence exists for antigenic heterogeneity within species. Indeed, some bacterial cells may possess more than one antigenic type of pili.

The term fimbriae has been applied to the very short, hairlike net of M protein on the surface of the gram-positive *S pyogenes* (group A streptococci). These fibrils are much shorter and finer than the pili usually seen on the surface of gram-negative bacteria.

Surface Layers

Surface layers of the bacterial cell have been identified by various techniques: light microscopy and staining; electron microscopy of thin-sectioned, freeze-fractured and negatively stained cells; and isolation and biochemical characterization of individual morphologic entities of the cell. The principal surface layers are capsules and loose slime, the cell wall of gram-positive bacteria and complex cell envelope of gram-negative organisms, plasma or cytoplasmic membranes, and mesosomal membrane vesicles that arise from invaginations of the plasma membrane.

Capsules or Loose Slime

Some bacteria form capsules, which constitute the outermost layer of the bacterial cell and surround the cell with a relatively thick, viscous gel that may be up to 10 μm in thickness. Organisms possessing a less well-defined capsule may have amorphous, loose slime layers external to the cell wall or cell envelope. In gram-negative bacteria, the cell wall forms a rigid structure of uniform thickness around the cell and is responsible for the characteristic shape of the cell (rod, coccus, or spiral). Below the cell wall (or rigid

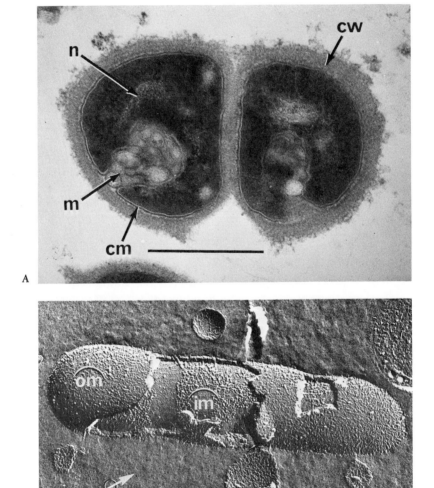

Figure 16-3 Electron micrograph of thin section of gram-positive *Micrococcus lysodeikticus* in **A** shows thick peptidoglycan cell wall (cw), underlying cytoplasmic (plasma) membrane (cm), mesosome (m), and nucleus (n). In **B**, freeze-fractured *Bacteroides* cell shows typical major convex fracture faces through inner (im) and outer (om) membranes. Bars = 1 μm; circled arrow in **B** indicates direction of shadowing.

peptidoglycan layer) is the plasma, or cytoplasmic, membrane; this is usually closely apposed to the wall layer. The topographic relationships of the cell wall and envelope layers to the plasma membrane are indicated in the thin section of a gram-positive organism (*Micrococcus lysodeikticus*) in Figure 16-3A, and in the freeze-fractured cell of the gram-negative *Bacteroides melaninogenicus* shown in Figure 16-3B. The latter shows the typical fracture planes seen in most gram-negative bacteria, which are weak cleavage planes through the outer membrane of the envelope and extensive fracture planes through the bilayer region of the underlying plasma membrane.

Not all bacterial species produce capsules; however, when pathogens form capsules, they are frequently important determinants of virulence. Encapsulated species are found in gram-positive and gram-negative groups of bacteria. In both, most capsules are composed of high-molecular-weight viscous polysaccharides that are retained as a thick gel external to the cell walls or envelopes. The capsule of *Bacillus anthracis* (the causal organism of anthrax) is unusual in that it is composed of a γ-glutamyl polypeptide. Table 16-1 presents the various capsular substances formed by a selection of gram-positive and gram-negative bacteria. A plasma membrane stage is involved in the biosynthesis and assembly of the capsular substances, which are extruded or secreted through the outer wall or envelope structures. Mutational loss of enzymes involved in the biosynthesis of the capsular polysaccharides can result in the smooth-to-rough variation seen in the pneumococcus.

The capsule is not an essential structure for bacterial cell viability. Capsular polysaccharides can be removed enzymatically from the cell surface without loss of viability. The exact functions of capsules are not fully understood, but they do confer resistance to phagocytosis and thus provide the bacterial cell with protection against host defenses to invasion.

Cell Wall and Gram-Negative Cell Envelope

The Gram stain broadly differentiates bacteria into gram-positive and gram-negative groups; a few organisms are consistently gram-variable. Gram-stain differentiation

Table 16-1   Nature of Capsular Substances Formed by Various Bacteria

Genus and Species	Capsular Substances
Gram-positive Bacteria	
S pneumoniae	Polysaccharides: e.g., type III, glucose, glucuronic acid (cellobiuronic acid); other types, various sugars and amino sugars
Streptococcus sp	Polysaccharides: e.g., hyaluronic acid (group A), others containing amino sugars, uronic acids
B anthracis	γ-glutamyl polypeptide
Gram-negative Bacteria	
H influenzae	Polyribosephosphate
Klebsiella sp	Polysaccharides: sugars such as hexoses, fucose, uronic acids
N meningitidis	Polysaccharides: N-acetylmannosamine phosphate polymer (group A); sialic acid polymers (groups B and C)

resides in the nature and organization of the cell wall structures of the two groups of organisms; it is not due to a particular macromolecular substance conferring gram-positivity. Because of essential differences in the organization and complexity of the surface layers of gram-negative bacteria, the term cell envelope (instead of cell wall) is a more acceptable description of their surface structure.

Most gram-positive bacteria have a relatively thick (about 20-80 nm), continuous cell wall (often referred to as the sacculus), which is largely composed of peptidoglycan (synonyms: mucopeptide, murein). When thick cell walls occur, other cell wall polymers (such as the teichoic acids, polysaccharides, and peptidoglycolipids) are covalently attached to the peptidoglycan. In contrast, the peptidoglycan layer in gram-negative bacteria is thin (about 5-10 nm); in *E coli*, the peptidoglycan is probably only a monolayer thick. External to the peptidoglycan layer in the gram-negative envelope is an outer membrane structure (about 7.5-10 nm in cross-section profile). In most gram-negative bacteria, this membrane structure is anchored noncovalently to lipoprotein (Braun's lipoprotein) molecules that are, however, covalently linked to the peptidoglycan. The lipopolysaccharides of the gram-negative envelope form part of the outer leaflet of the outer membrane structure.

The organization and overall dimensions of the outer membrane of the gram-negative envelope are similar to those of the plasma membranes (about 7.5 nm thick). Moreover, in gram-negative bacteria such as *E coli*, several hundred sites of adhesion exist between the outer and inner membranes (Bayer's patches); these sites can break up the continuity of the peptidoglycan layer. Differences in organization of the cell wall and of cell envelope layers of gram-positive and gram-negative bacteria are depicted diagrammatically in Figure 16-4. Table 16-2 summarizes the major classes of chemical constituents in the walls and envelopes of the two groups.

Table 16-2 Major Classes of Chemical Components in Bacterial Walls and Envelopes

Chemical Component	*Examples*
Gram-positive Cell Walls	
Peptidoglycan	All species
Polysaccharides	*Streptococcus* sp group A, B, C substances
Teichoic acid	
Ribitol	*S aureus, B subtilis, Lactobacillus* sp
Glycerol	*S epidermidis, Lactobacillus* sp
Teichuronic acids (aminogalacturonic or aminoman- nuronic acid polymers)	*B licheniformis, M. lysodeikticus*
Peptidoglycolipids (muramylpeptide-polysaccharide- mycolates)	*Corynebacterium* sp , *Mycobacterium* sp , *Nocardia* sp
Glycolipids ("waxes") (polysaccharide-mycolates)	
Gram-negative Envelopes	
Lipopolysaccharides	All species
Lipoprotein	*E coli* and many enteric bacteria, *P aeruginosa*
Porins (major outer membrane proteins)	*E coli, Salmonella typhimurium*
Phospholipids and proteins	All species
Peptidoglycan	Almost all species

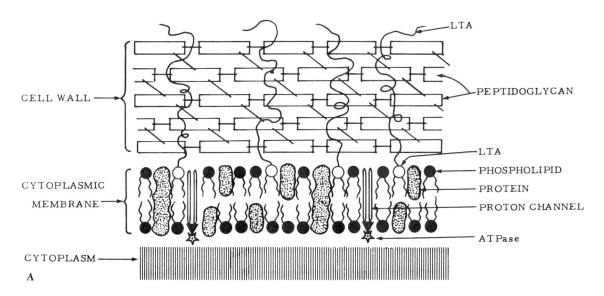

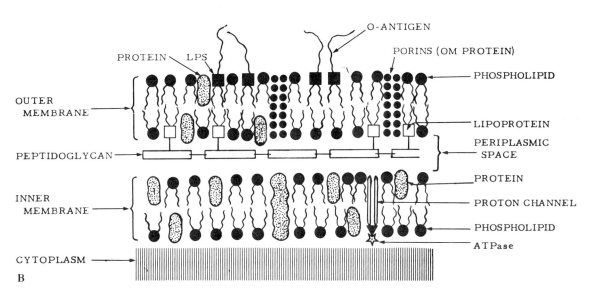

Figure 16-4 A, Diagrammatic representation of surface profile of a gram-positive organism shows thick peptidoglycan cell wall structure, with chains of membrane-bound lipoteichoic acid (LTA) emerging at the cell surface. Organization of underlying cytoplasmic membrane shows bilayer phospholipids, transmembrane and inner and outer leaflet proteins, proton channel, and inner face H^+-ATPase of the energy-transducing system. **B,** Profile through the gram-negative envelope diagrammatically depicts lipopolysaccharides (LPS) of the outer leaflet of the outer membrane (OM) organized to form a bilayer with phospholipids and the porin OM proteins. These OM proteins form a pore, allowing passage of small molecules (up to about 600–700 molecular weight). Other OM proteins are indicated; lipoprotein attached to the underlying peptidoglycan forms an anchor with OM lipids. Essential features of the cytoplasmic membrane are similar to those of gram-positive membrane structures.

The basic differences in surface structures of gram-positive and gram-negative bacteria (Figure 16-4) elucidate the mechanism of the Gram stain differentiation. Both gram-positive and gram-negative bacteria take up the same amounts of crystal violet (CV) and iodine (I). The CV-I complex, however, is trapped inside the gram-positive cell by the dehydration and reduced porosity of the thick cell wall that occurs during the differential washing step with 95% ethanol or other solvent mixture. In contrast, the thin peptidoglycan layer and probable discontinuities at the membrane adhesion sites do not impede solvent extraction of the CV-I complex from the gram-negative cell. Moreover, mechanical disruption of the cell wall of gram-positive organisms or its enzymatic removal with lysozyme results in complete extraction of the CV-I complex and conversion to a gram-negative reaction. Thus, autolytic wall-degrading enzymes that cause cell wall breakage may account for gram-negative or variable reactions in cultures of gram-positive organisms (such as *Staphylococcus aureus*, *Clostridium perfringens*, *Corynebacterium diphtheriae*, and some *Bacillus* sp).

Peptidoglycan.   Unique features of almost all prokaryotic cells (except for *Halobacterium halobium* and mycoplasmas) are cell wall peptidoglycan and the specific enzymes involved in its biosynthesis. These enzymes are target sites for inhibition of peptidoglycan synthesis by specific antibiotics. The primary chemical structures of peptidoglycans of both gram-positive and gram-negative bacteria have been established; they consist of a glycan backbone of repeating groups of β1,4-linked disaccharides of β1,4-N-acetylmuramyl-N-acetylglucosamine. Tetrapeptides of L-alanine-D-iso-glutamic acid-L-lysine (or diaminopimelic acid)-D-alanine are linked through the carboxyl group by amide linkage of muramic acid residues of the glycan chains; the D-alanine residues are directly cross-linked to the ϵ-amino group of lysine or diaminopimelic acid on a neighboring tetrapeptide, or they are linked by a peptide bridge. In *S aureus* peptidoglycan, a glycine pentapeptide bridge links the two adjacent peptide structures. The extent of direct or peptide-bridge cross-linking varies from one peptidoglycan to another. The staphylococcal peptidoglycan is highly cross-linked, whereas that of *E coli* is much less so, and has a more open peptidoglycan mesh. The diamino acid providing the ϵ-amino group for cross-linking is lysine or diaminopimelic acid, the latter being uniformly present in gram-negative peptidoglycans. The structure of the peptidoglycan is illustrated in Figure 16-5. A peptidoglycan with a chemical structure substantially different from that of all *Eubacteria* has been discovered in certain *Archaebacteria*. Instead of muramic acid, this peptidoglycan contains talosaminuronic acid and lacks the D-amino acids found in the eubacterial peptidoglycans. Interestingly, organisms containing this wall polymer (referred to as pseudomurein) are insensitive to penicillin, an inhibitor of the transpeptidases involved in peptidoglycan biosynthesis in *Eubacteria*.

The β-1,4 glycosidic bond between N-acetylmuramic acid and N-acetylglucosamine is specifically cleaved by the bacteriolytic enzyme, lysozyme. Widely distributed in nature, this enzyme is present in human tissues and secretions and can cause complete digestion of the peptidoglycan walls of sensitive organisms. When lysozyme is allowed to digest the cell wall of gram-positive bacteria suspended in an osmotic stabilizer (such as sucrose), protoplasts are formed. These protoplasts are able to survive and continue to grow on suitable media in the wall-less state. Gram-negative bacteria treated similarly produce spheroplasts, which retain much of the outer membrane structure. The

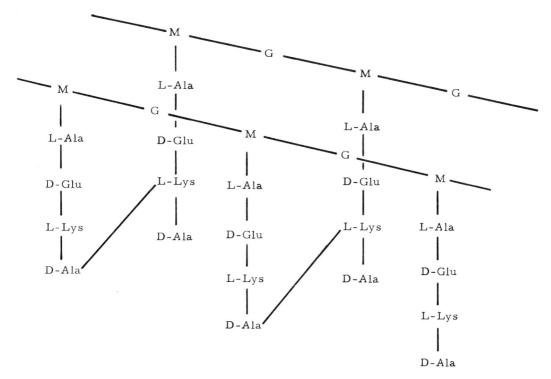

Figure 16-5 Diagrammatic representation of peptidoglycan structure with two adjacent glycan strands cross-linked from carboxyl terminal D-alanine to the ε-amino group of L-lysine in adjacent tetrapeptide. M, N-acetylmuramic acid; G, N-acetylglucosamine.

dependence of bacterial shape on the peptidoglycan is shown by the transformation of rod-shaped bacteria to spherical protoplasts or spheroplasts after enzymatic breakdown of the peptidoglycan. The mechanical protection afforded by the wall peptidoglycan layer is evident in the osmotic fragility of both protoplasts and spheroplasts. L-forms arising "spontaneously" in cultures or isolated from infections are structurally related to protoplasts and spheroplasts; all three forms, protoplasts, spheroplasts, and L-forms, revert infrequently and only under special conditions.

Teichoic Acids.   Wall teichoic acids are found only in certain gram-positive bacteria (such as staphylococci, streptococci, lactobacilli, and *Bacillus* sp); so far, they have not been found in gram-negative organisms. Teichoic acids are polyol phosphate polymers, with either ribitol or glycerol linked by phosphodiester bonds, and their structures are illustrated in Figure 16-6. Substituent groups on the polyol chains can include D-alanine (ester linked), N-acetylglucosamine, N-acetylgalactosamine, and glucose; the substituent is characteristic for the teichoic acid from a particular bacterial species and can act as a specific antigenic determinant. Teichoic acids are covalently linked to the peptidoglycan. These highly negatively charged polymers of the bacterial wall can serve as a cation-sequestering mechanism.

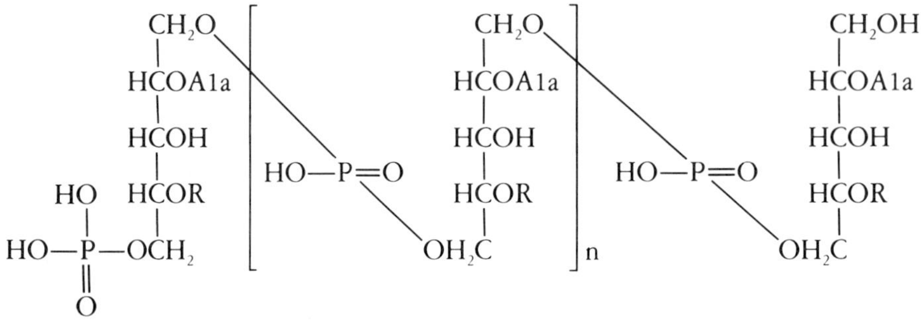

A RIBITOL TEICHOIC ACID

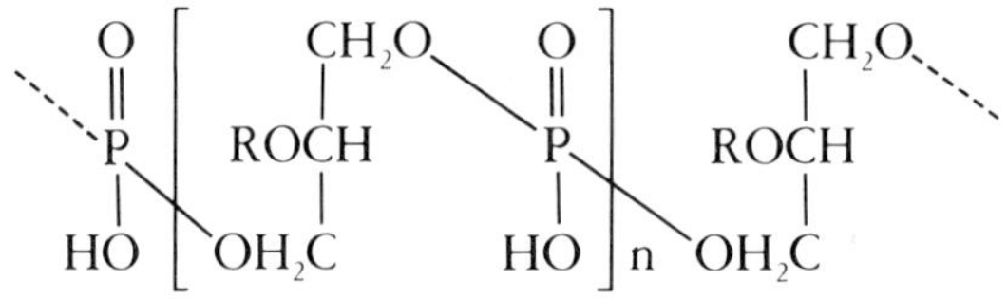

B GLYCEROL TEICHOIC ACID

Figure 16-6 Structures of cell wall teichoic acids. **A,** ribitol teichoic acid with repeating units of 1,5-phosphodiester linkages of D-ribitol and D-alanyl ester on position 2 and glycosyl substituents (R) on 4. Glycosyl groups may be N-acetylglucosaminyl (α or β) as in *Staphylococcus aureus* or α-glucosyl as in *Bacillus subtilis* strain W23. **B,** glycerol teichoic acid with 1,3-phosphodiester linkages of glycerol repeating units (1,2 linkages in some species). In the glycerol teichoic acid structure shown, the polymer may be unsubstituted (R = H) or substituted (R = D-alanyl or glycosyl).

Accessory Wall Polymers.   In addition to the principal cell wall polymers, the walls of certain gram-positive bacteria may possess polysaccharide molecules linked to the peptidoglycan. For example, the C polysaccharide of streptococci confers group specificity. Acidic polysaccharides attached to the peptidoglycan are called teichuronic acids. Mycobacteria have peptidoglycolipids, glycolipids, and waxes associated with the cell wall.

Lipopolysaccharides.   A characteristic feature of gram-negative bacteria is possession of the complex macromolecular lipopolysaccharides (LPS). So far, only one gram-positive organism, *Listeria monocytogenes,* has been found to contain an authentic lipopolysaccharide. The LPS of it and all gram-negative lipopolysaccharides are called **endotoxins,** thereby distinguishing these cell-bound, heat-stable toxins from heat-labile, protein **exotoxins** secreted into culture media. Endotoxins possess an array of powerful biological activities and play an important role in the pathogenesis of many gram-negative bacterial infections. In addition to causing endotoxic shock, LPS are **pyrogenic,** they can activate **macrophages** and **complement,** are mitogenic for B-lymphocytes, induce interferon production, cause tissue necrosis and tumor regression, and possess **adjuvant** properties. The endotoxic properties of LPS reside largely in the **lipid A** components. Usually, the lipopolysaccharide molecules have three regions: the lipid A structure required for insertion in the outer leaflet of the outer membrane bilayer; a covalently attached core composed of 2-keto-3-deoxyoctonic acid (KDO), heptose, ethanolamine, N-acetylglucosamine, glucose, and galactose; and polysaccharide chains linked to the core. The polysaccharide chains constitute the O-antigens of the gram-negative bacteria, and the individual monosaccharide constituents confer serologic specificity on these components. Figure 16-7 depicts the structure of lipopolysaccharide. Although it has been known that lipid A is composed of β-1,6-linked D-glucosamine disaccharide, substituted with phosphomonester groups at positions 4' and 1, uncertainties have existed about the attachment positions of the six fatty acid acyl and KDO groups on the disaccharide. The demonstration of the structure of lipid A of LPS of a heptoseless mutant of *Salmonella typhimurium* has established that amide-linked hydroxymyristoyl and lauroxymyristoyl groups are attached to the nitrogen of the 2- and 2'-carbons, respectively, and that hydroxymyristoyl and myristoxymyristoyl groups are attached to the oxygen of the 3- and 3'-carbons of the disaccharide, respectively. Thus, only position 6' is left for attachment of KDO units.

Lipopolysaccharides and phospholipids help confer asymmetry to the outer membrane of the gram-negative bacteria, with the hydrophilic polysaccharide chains outermost. The lipopolysaccharides are held in the outer membrane by relatively weak cohesive forces (ionic and hydrophobic interactions) and can be dissociated from the cell surface with surface-active agents.

As in peptidoglycan biosynthesis, lipopolysaccharide molecules are assembled at the plasma or inner membrane. These newly formed molecules are initially inserted into the outer-inner membrane adhesion sites.

Outer Membrane of Gram-Negative Bacteria

In thin sections, outer membranes of gram-negative bacteria have a similar overall appearance to that of plasma or inner membranes; however, they differ from the inner

LIPID A ———	——— CORE ———	——— O ANTIGEN
Glucosamine β-hydroxymyristate Fatty acids	Ketodeoxyoctonate Phosphoethanolamine Heptose Glucose, Galactose, N-acetylglucosamine	Polysaccharide chains: repeating units of species-specific monosaccharides, e.g., galactose, rhamnose, mannose and abequose in *S. typhimurium* LPS

Figure 16-7 The three major regions covalently linked to form typical lipopolysaccharide (LPS).

membranes and walls of gram-positive bacteria in numerous respects. The lipid A of lipopolysaccharide is inserted with phospholipids to create the outer leaflet of the bilayer structure; the lipid portion of the lipoprotein and phospholipid form the inner leaflet of the outer membrane bilayer of most gram-negative bacteria (Figure 16-4B).

In addition to these components, the outer membrane possesses several major outer membrane proteins; the most abundant is called **porin.** The assembled subunits of porin form a channel that limits passage of hydrophilic molecules across the outer membrane barrier to those having molecular weights that are usually less than 600–700. Evidence also suggests that hydrophobic pathways exist across the outer membrane and are partly responsible for the differential penetration and effectiveness of certain β-lactam antibiotics (ampicillin, cephalosporins) that are active against various gram-negative bacteria. Although the outer membranes act as a permeability barrier or molecular sieve, they do not appear to possess energy transducing systems to drive active transport. Several outer membrane proteins, however, are involved in the specific uptake of metabolites (maltose, vitamin B_{12}, nucleosides) and iron from the medium. Thus, outer membranes of the gram-negative bacteria provide a selective barrier to external molecules and thereby prevent loss of metabolite-binding proteins and hydrolytic enzymes (nucleases, alkaline phosphatase) found in the periplasmic space. The periplasmic space is defined as the region between the outer surface of the inner (plasma) membrane and the inner surface of the outer membrane (Figure 16-4B). Thus, gram-negative bacteria have a cellular compartment that does not appear to have an equivalent in gram-positive organisms. In addition to the hydrolytic enzymes, the periplasmic space acts as a compartment for the functioning of binding proteins (specifically binding sugars, amino acids, and inorganic ions) involved in membrane transport and chemotactic receptor activities. Moreover, plasmid-encoded β-lactamases in the periplasmic space produce resistance by degrading an antibiotic in transit to its target sites on the membrane (penicillin-binding proteins). These periplasmic proteins can be released by subjecting the cells to osmotic shock after treatment with the chelating agent ethylenediamine-tetraacetic acid.

Intracellular Components

Plasma (Cytoplasmic) Membranes

Bacterial plasma membranes, the functional equivalents of eukaryotic plasma membranes, are referred to variously as cytoplasmic, protoplast, or inner membranes (in gram-negative organisms). Similar in overall dimensions and appearance in thin sections to biomembranes from eukaryotic cells, they are composed primarily of proteins and lipids, principally phospholipids. Protein-to-lipid ratios of bacterial plasma membranes are approximately 3:1 and are thus close to those for mitochondrial membranes. Unlike eukaryotic cell membranes, the bacterial membrane (except for *Mycoplasma*) is devoid of sterols, and bacteria lack the enzymes required for sterol biosynthesis.

Although their composition is similar to that of inner membranes of gram-negative species, cytoplasmic membranes from gram-positive bacteria possess a class of macromolecules not present in the gram-negative membranes. Many gram-positive bacterial membranes contain membrane-bound lipoteichoic acid, and those species lacking this component (such as *Micrococcus* and *Sarcina* sp) contain an analogous membrane-bound succinylated lipomannan. Lipoteichoic acids are structurally similar to the cell wall glycerol teichoic acids in that they have basal, polyglycerol phosphodiester 1-3 linked chains (Figure 16-6). These chains terminate with the phosphomonester end of the polymer, which is linked covalently to either a glycolipid or phosphatidyl glycolipid moiety. Thus, a hydrophobic tail is provided for anchoring in the membrane lipid layers (Figure 16-4A). As in the cell wall glycerol teichoic acid, the lipoteichoic acids can have glycosidic and D-alanyl ester substituents on the C-2 position of the glycerol.

Both membrane-bound lipoteichoic acid and membrane-bound succinylated lipomannan can be detected as antigens on the cell surface, and the glycerol-phosphate and succinylated mannan chains appear to extend through the cell wall structure (see Figure 16-4A). This class of polymer has not yet been found in the cytoplasmic membranes of gram-negative organisms. In both instances, the lipoteichoic acids and the lipomannans are negatively charged components and can sequester positively charged substances. They have been implicated in adhesion to host cells, but their functions remain to be elucidated.

Multiple functions are performed by the plasma membranes of both gram-positive and gram-negative bacteria. Plasma membranes are the site of active transport, respiratory chain components, energy-transducing systems, the H^+-ATPase of the proton pump (see Chapter 19), and membrane stages in the biosynthesis of phospholipids, peptidoglycan, lipopolysaccharides, and capsular polysaccharides. In essence, the bacterial cytoplasmic membrane is a multifunction structure that combines the mitochondrial transport and biosynthetic functions that are usually compartmentalized in discrete membranous organelles in eukaryotic cells. The plasma membrane is also the anchoring site for DNA and provides the cell with a mechanism (as yet unknown) for separation of sister chromosomes.

Mesosomes

Thin sections of gram-positive bacteria reveal the presence of vesicular or tubular vesicular membrane structures called **mesosomes,** which are apparently formed by an invagination of the plasma membrane. These structures are much more prominent in gram-positive than in gram-negative organisms. At one time, the mesosomal vesicles were thought to be equivalent to bacterial mitochondria; however, many other membrane functions have also been attributed to the mesosomes. At present, no satisfactory evidence suggests that they have a unique biochemical or physiologic function. Indeed, electron microscope studies have suggested that the mesosomes, as usually seen in thin sections, may arise from membrane perturbation and fixation artifacts. No general agreement exists about this theory, however, and some evidence indicates that mesosomes may be related to events in the cell division cycle.

Other Intracellular Components

In addition to the nucleoid and cytoplasm (cytosol), the intracellular compartment of the bacterial cell is densely packed with ribosomes (Figure 16-1) of the 70S type. These ribonucleoprotein particles, which have diameters of 18 nm, are not arranged on a membranous rough endoplasmic reticulum as they are in eukaryotic cells. Other granular inclusions randomly distributed in the cytoplasm of various species include metabolic reserve particles such as poly-β-hydroxybutyrate (PHB), polysaccharide and glycogenlike granules, and polymetaphosphate or metachromatic granules.

Endospores are highly heat-resistant, dehydrated resting cells formed intracellularly in members of the genera *Bacillus* and *Clostridium*. *Sporulation*, the ability to form endospores, is an unusual property of certain bacteria. The series of biochemical and morphological changes that occur during this process represent true differentiation within the cycle of the bacterial cell. The process of sporulation, which usually begins in the stationary phase of the vegetative cell cycle, is initiated by depletion of nutrients (usually readily utilizable sources of carbon, nitrogen, or both). The cell then undergoes a highly complex, well-defined sequence of morphologic and biochemical events that ultimately lead to the formation of mature endospores. As many as seven distinct stages have been recognized by morphologic and biochemical studies of sporulating *Bacillus* species: *Stage 0*, vegetative cells with two chromosomes at the end of exponential growth; *Stage I*, formation of axial chromatin filament and excretion of exoenzymes, including proteases; *Stage II*, forespore septum formation and segregation of nuclear material into two compartments; *Stage III*, spore protoplast formation and elevation of TCA and glyoxylate cycle enzyme levels; *Stage IV*, cortex formation and refractile appearance of spore; *Stage V*, spore coat protein formation; *Stage VI*, spore maturation, modification of cortical peptidoglycan, uptake of dipicolinic acid (a unique endospore

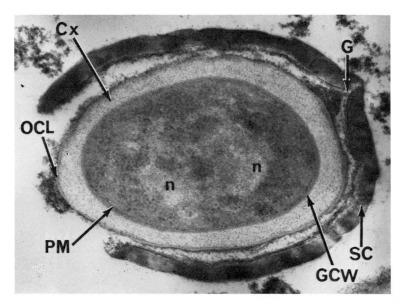

Figure 16-8 Electron micrograph of a thin section of *Bacillus megaterium* spore shows thick spore coat (SC), germinal groove (G) in the spore coat, outer cortex layer (OCL) and cortex (Cx), germinal cell wall layer (GCW), underlying spore protoplast membrane (PM), and regions where the nucleoid (n) is visible. (Courtesy John H. Freer.)

product) and calcium, and development of resistance to heat and organic solvents; and *Stage VII*, final maturation and liberation of endospores from mother cells (in some species).

When newly formed, endospores appear as round, highly refractile cells within the vegetative cell wall, or sporangium. Some strains produce autolysins that digest the walls and liberate free endospores. The spore protoplast, or core, contains a complete nucleus, ribosomes, and energy-generating components that are enclosed within a modified cytoplasmic membrane. The peptidoglycan spore wall surrounds the spore membrane and, on germination, this wall becomes the vegetative cell wall. Surrounding the spore wall is a thick cortex that contains an unusual type of peptidoglycan, which is rapidly released on germination. A spore coat of keratinlike protein encases the spore contained within a membrane (the exosporium). During maturation, the spore protoplast dehydrates, and the spore becomes refractile and resistant to heat, dessication, and chemicals; these properties correlate with the cortical peptidoglycan and the presence of large amounts of calcium dipicolinate. Figure 16-8 illustrates the principal structural features of a typical endospore (*B megaterium*) on initiation of the germination process. The thin section of the spore shows the ruptured, thick spore coat and the cortex surrounding the spore protoplast with the germinal cell wall that becomes the vegetative wall on outgrowth.

References

Costeron, J.W., Ingram, J.M., Cheng, K.J.: Structure and function of the cell envelope of gram-negative bacteria. *Bacteriol Rev* 1974; 38:87-110.

Di Rienzo, J.M., Nakamura, K., Inouye, M.: The outer membrane proteins of gram-negative bacteria: Biosynthesis, assembly, and functions. *Ann Rev Biochem* 1978; 47:481-532.

Gould, G.W., Hurst, A., (editors): *The bacterial spore*. New York: Academic Press, 1969.

Jawetz, E., Melnick, J.L., Adelberg, E.A.: *Review of Medical Microbiology*. Los Altos, Calif.: Lange, 1978.

Rogers, H.J.: *Bacterial Cell Structure, Aspects of Microbiology*. Washington, DC: American Society for Microbiology, 1983.

Salton, M.R.J., Owen, P.: Bacterial membrane structure. *Ann Rev Microbiol* 1976; 30:451-482.

Wright, A., Tipper, D.J.: The outer membrane of gram-negative bacteria. In: *The bacteria*, Vol 7. Sokatch, J.R., Ornston, L.N., (editors). New York: Academic Press, 1979.

17 Classification

Don J. Brenner, PhD

General Concepts

Bacteria are classified and identified to distinguish one organism from another and to group similar organisms by criteria of interest to all microbiologists, or to other groups of scientists. Bacteria are named in a certain way so that an organism can be defined without listing its characteristics. The most important level of this type of communication is the species level. A species name should mean the same thing to everyone; effective communication about bacteria cannot occur if strains of the same species are given different names on the basis of source of isolation, serotype, presence or absence of a converting bacteriophage, or the ability to perform a specific function, such as cause a disease or produce an antibiotic. Formerly, species were created on the basis of such criteria, which may be extremely important for clinical microbiologists and physicians, but which are not a sufficient basis for establishing a species. Now, verification of existing species and creation of new species should use a polyphasic approach that involves general biochemical and other phenotypic criteria, as well as DNA relatedness. In numerical or phenetic approaches to classification, strains are grouped on the basis of a large number of phenotypic characteristics. DNA relatedness is used to group strains on the basis of overall genetic similarity.

Identification of species in the clinical laboratory is done by biochemical tests, some of which have been supplemented by serologic assessments (for example, identification of *Salmonella* and *Shigella*). Because of differences in pathogenicity (*Escherichia coli, Yersinia enterocolitica*), or the necessity to characterize a disease outbreak (*Enterobacteriaceae, Vibrio cholerae, Clostridium, Campylobacter, Staphylococcus, Streptococcus, Pseudomonas aeruginosa*), strains of medical interest are often classified below the species level by serology, bacteriophage typing, or identification of toxins. Pathogenic or epidemic strains also can be classified by the presence of a specific plasmid, or by their plasmid profile (the number and sizes of plasmids). Newer molecular biologic techniques have made it possible to identify some species directly (without the use of biochemical tests) by identifying a specific gene or genetic sequence, sometimes without even isolating the organism.

Because of the commercial availability of biochemical identification systems and probabilistic computer programs, few laboratories have difficulty identifying typical strains of common bacteria. Problems do arise, however, if it is necessary to identify atypical strains of an existing species, a rare species, or a newly described species. Coping with these problems requires that laboratory personnel physicians (at least infectious disease specialists) be familiar with taxonomic reference texts and journals that publish papers on new species. In the past, changes in bacterial nomenclature at the species and genus levels occurred often. Such changes still occur occasionally. In addition one species may acquire more than one name. It is important to understand why these changes and synonyms exist in taxonomy to minimize confusion.

The primary clinical laboratory is concerned with the rapid, sensitive, and accurate identification of pathogenic bacteria. The number and types of tests done in such a laboratory depend on its size, and the population it serves. Tests that are highly specialized or done rarely should be performed by only state and reference laboratories. Physicians, the primary laboratory, and the reference laboratory must have a good working relationship if patients are to receive first-rate care. In addition, the physician and the primary laboratory must know which diseases are reportable to state and federal health laboratories, and how to report them.

Definitions

Taxonomy

Taxonomy is the science of classification. For eukaryotes, the species definition usually stresses the ability of similar organisms to reproduce sexually with the formation of a zygote, and to produce fertile offspring. In bacteria, however, sexual reproduction does not occur in the eukaryotic sense. Taxonomy involves classification, identification, and nomenclature.

Classification

Classification is the orderly arrangement of bacteria into groups. There is nothing inherently scientific about classification, and different groups of scientists may classify the same organisms in a different manner. For example, clinical microbiologists are interested in the serotype, antimicrobial resistance pattern, and toxin and invasiveness factors in *E coli,* whereas geneticists are interested in specific mutations and plasmids.

Identification

Identification is the practical use of a classification to isolate and distinguish certain organisms from others, to verify the authenticity or utility of a culture or a particular reaction, or to isolate and identify the causative organism of a disease or condition. Often, different groups of scientists identify organisms below the species level on the basis of the criteria of particular interest to them.

Nomenclature

Nomenclature is the means by which the characteristics of a species are defined and communicated among microbiologists. *A species name should mean the same thing to all microbiologists,* yet some names are defined differently in different parts of the world or by different microbiological specialty groups. *Klebsiella pneumoniae* is defined differently in England than in most other parts of the world, and *Vibrio cholerae* often has been equated with a single serotype by epidemiologists and clinical microbiologists.

Species

A bacterial species is a distinct kind of organism with certain distinguishing features, or a group of organisms that, in general, resemble one another closely in terms of the most important features of their organization. Unfortunately, various interpretations exist about the definition of a close resemblance, the most important features of an organism, and the number of distinguishing features necessary to distinguish a species. In the past, species were often defined solely on the basis of such criteria as host range, pathogenicity, ability or inability to produce gas in the fermentation of a given sugar, and rapid or delayed fermentation of sugars. Because no method was available for devising a single species definition that all researchers could use, criteria reflected the interests of the investigators who described a particular species. For example, bacteria that caused plant diseases were often defined by the plant from which they were isolated; also, each new serotype of *Salmonella* that was discovered was given species status. These practices have been replaced by a single series of genetic criteria that can be used to define species in all groups of bacteria.

Approaches to Taxonomy

Numerical Approach

In their studies on *Enterobacteriaceae,* Edwards and Ewing established the following principles for characterizing, classifying, and identifying organisms.

> Classification and identification of an organism should be based on its overall morphologic and biochemical pattern. A single characteristic (pathogenicity, host range, or biochemical reaction), regardless of its importance, is not a sufficient basis for classifying or identifying an organism.

> A large and diverse strain sample must be tested to determine accurately the number of biochemical characteristics used to distinguish a given species.

> Atypical strains often are perfectly typical members of a given biogroup within an existing species, but sometimes they are typical members of an unrecognized new species.

In numerical taxonomy (also called computer or phenetic taxonomy), a large number (50-200) of biochemical, morphologic, and cultural characteristics, as well as susceptibilities to antibiotics and inorganic compounds, are used to determine the degrees of similarity between organisms. In the numerical studies, investigators often calculate the coefficient of similarity or percentage of similarity between strains (we refer to strain as a single isolate from a specimen). A dendrogram or a similarity matrix is constructed that joins individual strains into groups and joins one group with other groups on the basis of their percentage of similarity. In the hypothetical dendrogram in Figure 17-1, group 1 represents three strains that are about 95% similar and join with a fourth strain at the level of 90% similarity. Group 2 is composed of three strains that are 95% similar, and group 3 contains two strains that are 95% similar, as well as a third strain

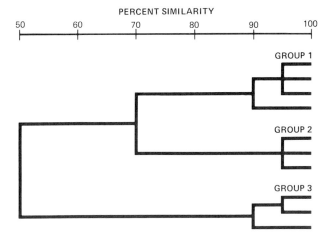

Figure 17-1 Hypothetical example of a dendrogram.

to which they are 90% similar. Similarity between groups 1 and 2 occurs at the 70% level, and group 3 is about 50% similar to groups 1 and 2.

Either all the characteristics included in the similarity matrix are given equal weight or certain characters may be weighted more heavily; for example, the presence of spores in *Clostridium* might be weighted more heavily than the organism's ability to use a given carbon source. A given level of similarity can be equated with relatedness at the species, genus, and sometimes, the subspecies level. For instance, strains of a given species may cluster at a 90% similarity level, and species within a given genus may cluster at a 70% level. If these values were applied to Figure 17-1, the strains in groups 1, 2, and 3 would each represent a separate species. The species in groups 1 and 2 would be placed in the same genus, and the species in group 3 would be in a separate genus.

When this approach is used as the only basis for defining a species, it is difficult to know how many and which tests should be chosen; whether the tests should be weighted and, if so, how; what level of similarity should be chosen to reflect relatedness at the species and genus levels; and whether the same level of similarity is applicable to all groups.

Most bacteria have enough DNA to specify some 1500 to 6000 average-sized genes. Therefore, even a battery of 300 tests would assay only 5%–20% of the genetic potential of a bacterium. Tests that are comparatively simple to conduct (such as those for carbohydrate utilization and for enzymes whose presence can be assayed colorimetrically) are performed more often than tests for structural, reproductive, and regulatory genes whose presence is difficult to assay.

Other types of errors may occur when speciating solely on the basis of phenotype. For example, different enzymes (specified by different genes) may catalyze the same reaction. Also, even if a metabolic gene is functional, negative reactions can occur because of the inability of the substrate to enter the cell, or because of a mutation in a regulatory gene. A negative reaction also can occur if the gene is present but not functional, because of a mutation that produces an inactive protein. The correlation between a reaction and the number of genes necessary to carry out that reaction is not necessarily one-to-one. For instance, six enzymatic steps may be involved in a given pathway. If an assay for the end product is performed, a positive reaction indicates six similar enzymes, whereas a negative reaction can mean the absence or nonfunction of from one to six enzymes. Fastidious strains will not cluster with nonfastidious strains from the same species. Several other strain characteristics can affect phenotypic characterization, including growth rate, temperature of incubation, salt requirement, and pH. Plasmids that carry metabolic genes can enable strains to carry out reactions that rarely, if ever, occur in the absence of the plasmids.

The same set of "definitive" reactions cannot be used to classify all groups of organisms, and there is no standard number of specific reactions that allows identification of a species. Organisms are identified on the basis of phenotype but, from the taxonomic standpoint, definition of species based solely on phenotype is subject to error.

Genetic Approach

The ideal means of identifying and classifying bacteria would be to compare each gene sequence in a given strain with the gene sequences for every known species. This cannot be done yet, but the total DNA of one organism can be compared with that of any other organism, by using a method pioneered by Marmur and Doty; Speigelman, Bolton, and McCarthy; and Britten and Kohne. The method, **nucleic acid hybridization** or **DNA hybridization,** can be used to measure the number of DNA sequences that any two organisms have in common, and to estimate the percentage of divergence or unpaired nucleotide bases within related, but not identical, DNA sequences. DNA-relatedness studies have been done in yeasts, viruses, bacteriophages, and many groups of bacteria, including members of the family *Enterobacteriaceae, Brucella, Bacillus, Pseudomonas, Lactobacillus, Haemophilus, Mycobacterium, Vibrio, Campylobacter, Staphylococcus, Streptococcus, Neisseria, Bacteroides* and other anaerobic groups, and *Legionella.*

Five factors are now used to determine DNA relatedness: genome size, guanine plus cytosine (G + C) content, DNA relatedness under conditions optimal for DNA reassociation, thermal stability of related DNA sequences, and DNA relatedness under supraoptimal conditions for DNA reassociation. Because it is not practical to conduct these genetic evaluations in clinical laboratories, the results of biochemical tests usually must be correlated with any known genetic data. For example, yellow-pigmented strains of *Enterobacter cloacae* were shown to be a separate species by genetic assessments, but were not designated as such (*Enterobacter sakazakii*) until practical tests were performed whose results correlated with the genetic data. The same procedure was followed before a number of new species in *Campylobacter, Yersinia,* and *Serratia* were designated.

Genome Size.   True bacterial DNAs have molecular weights between 1×10^9 and 8×10^9 daltons (genome size). Genome size determinations sometimes can distinguish between groups that have very different genome sizes. They were used to distinguish *Legionella pneumophila* (the Legionnaires' disease bacterium) from *Rochalimaea (Rickettsia) quintana. L pneumophila* has a genome size of about 3×10^9 daltons; that of *R quintana* is about 1×10^9 daltons.

Guanine Plus Cytosine (G + C) Content.   The G + C content in bacterial DNA ranges from about 25%-75%. This percentage is specific for a given species, but is not exclusive for that species. For example, *E coli, Salmonella,* and *Shigella* have 50%-52% G + C, as do *Bacillus subtilis* and *Pasteurella.* Therefore, two strains with a similar G + C percentage may or may not belong to the same species. If the G + C content is very different, however, then the strains cannot be members of the same species. Assessments of G + C content are especially useful for grouping strains for further testing. For instance, biochemical tests of a recently isolated organism indicated that it could have been either *Vibrio* or *Aeromonas.* It was placed in the *Vibrio* genus because its G + C content was 50%, which is within the range of that of *Vibrio* sp, but is significantly less than the 57%-60% G + C found in *Aeromonas* sp.

DNA Relatedness Under Conditions Optimal for DNA Reassociation.   DNA relatedness is determined by allowing single-stranded DNA from one strain to reassociate with single-stranded DNA from a second strain, to form a double-stranded DNA molecule. It is a specific, temperature-dependent reaction. The optimal temperature for DNA reassociation is 25 C-30 C below the temperature at which native double-stranded DNA is denatured into single strands. Many studies indicate that a bacterial species is composed of strains that are usually 70%-100% related. In contrast, relatedness between species is 0% to about 65%. It is important to emphasize that the term "related" does not mean "identical" or "homologous." Similar nucleic acid sequences can reassociate.

Thermal Stability of Related DNA Sequences. Each 1% of unpaired nucleotide bases in a double-stranded DNA sequence causes a 1% decrease in the thermal stability of that DNA duplex. Thus, a comparison between the thermal stability of a control double-stranded molecule (in which both strands of DNA are from the same organism) and that of a heteroduplex (DNA strands from two different organisms), allows assessment of differences in thermal stability. Decreased thermal stability reflects divergence in related nucleotide sequences. Strains that are 70% or more related show 0% to about 5% divergence in related sequences, whereas sequences held in common between different species show 6%-20% divergence. The amount of divergence is especially important to assess when strains are 60%-70% related.

DNA Relatedness Under Supraoptimal Conditions for DNA Reassociation. When the incubation temperature used for DNA reassociation is raised from 25 C-30 C below the renaturation temperature to only 10 C-15 C below the denaturation temperature, only very closely related (and therefore highly thermally stable) DNA sequences can reassociate. Strains from the same species are 55%-100% related at these supraoptimal incubation temperatures. Strains from different species are 50% or less related. High-temperature reactions are especially important in distinguishing between strains that are 60%-70% related under optimal reassociation conditions.

Application of these five assessments allows a species definition based on DNA to be generated. Thus, *E coli* can be defined as a series of strains with a G + C content of 49%-52%, a genome size of 2.3×10^9 to 3.0×10^9 daltons, relatedness of 70% or more at an optimal reassociation temperature with 0%-4% divergence in related sequences, and relatedness of 60% or more at a supraoptimal reassociation temperature. Experience with more than 100 species has produced an arbitrary molecular definition of a species as *a group of strains with similar G + C content that are 70% or more related and that have 0%-5% divergence among related sequences, and in which relatedness remains at 55% or more at supraoptimal incubation temperature.* Investigators agree that 70% or more indicates relatedness at the species level. The 70% species relatedness rule has been ignored occasionally when the existing nomenclature is both deeply ingrained and useful, as is that for *E coli* and the four species of *Shigella*. Because these organisms are all 70% or more related, genetic studies indicate that they should be grouped into a single species, instead of the present five species in two genera. This change has not been made because of the confusion that would be created among the medical community. Another example is *Yersinia pestis* and *Yersinia pseudotuberculosis* which, by genetic criteria, are the same species. It has been proposed that they be treated as two subspecies of a single species, but it is extremely important clinically to continue to report *Y pestis* and to distinguish it from *Y pseudotuberculosis*.

DNA relatedness provides one species definition that can be applied equally to all organisms. Moreover, it cannot be affected by phenotypic variation, mutations, or the presence or absence of metabolic or other plasmids. It measures overall relatedness and these factors affect only a very small percentage of the total DNA.

Polyphasic Approach

In practice, the approach to bacterial taxonomy should be polyphasic. The first step is phenotypic grouping of strains by biochemical reactions and any other characteristics of interest. The phenotypic groups are then tested for DNA relatedness to determine whether the observed phenotypic homogeneity (or heterogeneity) is reflected by genetic homogeneity or heterogeneity. The third and most important step for identification is reexamination of the biochemical characteristics of the DNA relatedness groups. This allows determination of the biochemical borders of each group, and of those reactions that are of diagnostic value for the group. For identification of a given organism, the importance of specific tests is weighted on the basis of correlation with DNA results. Occasionally, the reactions commonly used will not distinguish completely between two distinct DNA relatedness groups. In these cases, other biochemical tests that are of diagnostic value must be sought.

Phenotypic Characteristics Useful in Classification and Identification

Morphologic Characteristics

Wet-mounted and properly stained specimens can yield a great deal of information. Simple tests can indicate the Gram reaction of the organism, whether it is acid fast, its motility, the arrangement of its flagella, the presence of spores, capsules, and inclusion bodies and, of course, the shape of the organism. This information often can allow identification of an organism to the level of genus, or can minimize the possibility that it belongs to one or another group. Colonial characteristics and pigmentation are also quite helpful. For example, colonies of several *Legionella* sp autofluoresce under long-wave-length ultraviolet light, and *Proteus* sp swarm on appropriate media.

Growth Characteristics

Whether an organism grows aerobically, anaerobically, facultatively (either in the presence or absence of oxygen), or microaerophilically (in the presence of less than atmospheric oxygen) is a primary distinguishing characteristic. The proper atmospheric conditions are essential for isolating and identifying bacteria. Other important growth assessments include the temperature of incubation, pH value, nutrients required, and resistance to antibiotics. For example, one diarrheal disease agent, *Campylobacter jejuni*, grows well at 42 C in the presence of several antibiotics; another, *Yersinia enterocolitica*, grows better than most other bacteria at 4 C. *Legionella, Haemophilus,* and some other pathogens require specific growth factors, whereas *E coli* and most other enterobacteria can grow on minimal media.

Structural Genes

Cell wall (0), flagellar (H), and capsular (K) antigens are used in the classification of certain organisms at the species level to serotype strains of medically important species for epidemiologic purposes or to identify serotypes of public health importance. Some species for which serotyping is used for epidemiologic reasons are shigellae, *E coli*, salmonellae, legionellae, klebsiellae, *Vibrio cholerae*, *Yersinia enterocolitica*, *Campylobacter jejuni*, streptococci, *Listeria monocytogenes*, *Haemophilus influenzae*, and leptospires. Serotyping to distinguish strains of exceptional virulence or public health importance is done with *V cholerae* (01 is the pandemic strain), *S dysenteriae* (01 is highly virulent), *Salmonella* (*S typhi*), and *E coli* (enterotoxigenic, enteroinvasive, enteropathogenic serotypes).

Phage typing (the susceptibility pattern of a species to a set of specific bacteriophages) is used primarily as an aid in epidemiologic surveillance of diseases caused by *Staphylococcus aureus*, mycobacteria, *Pseudomonas aeruginosa*, *V cholerae*, and *S typhi*. Phage susceptibility also can be a valuable aid in classification and identification. For example, virtually all strains of *Hafnia* are sensitive to a *Hafnia*-specific bacteriophage, and almost all clinically significant salmonellae are susceptible to *Salmonella* phage 01. Susceptibility to bacteriocins sometimes is used as an epidemiologic strain marker.

Table 17-1   Biochemical Tests Used Routinely in the Identification of *Enterobacteriaceae**

Test	Enteric Laboratory Section, Centers for Disease Control	API 20E Analytab Products	Enterotube II Roche Diagnostics	Enteric-Tek Flow Laboratories	MICRO-ID General Diagnostics	Rapid E DMS Laboratories	Minitek BBL
Indole	+	+	+	+	+	+	+
Methyl red	+	−	−	−	−	−	−
Voges–Proskauer	+	+	+	−	+	+	+
Citrate (Simmons)	+	+	+	+	−	+	+
H₂S production	+	+	+	+	+	−	+
Urea	+	+	+	+	+	+	+
Phenylalanine deaminase	+	−	+	−	+	+	+
Tryptophan deaminase	−	+	−	+	−	−	−
Lysine decarboxylase	+	+	+	+	+	+	+
Arginine dihydrolase	+	+	−	−	−	−	+
Ornithine decarboxylase	+	+	+	+	+	+	+
Motility	+	−	−	−	−	−	−
Gelatin liquefaction	+	+	−	−	−	−	−
KCN (growth on)	+	−	−	−	−	−	−
Malonate	+	−	−	+	+	+	+
D-glucose (gas)	+	−	+	−	−	−	−
D-glucose (acid)	+	+	+	+	+	+	+
Lactose	+	−	+	+	−	−	+
Sucrose	+	+	−	−	−	+	+
D-mannitol	+	+	−	−	−	−	−
Dulcitol	+	−	+	−	−	−	−
Salicin	+	−	−	−	−	−	−
Adonitol	+	−	+	+	+	+	+

*+, available; −, not available.

Biochemical Characteristics

Most bacteria are identified and classified largely on the basis of their reactions in a series of biochemical tests. Some tests are used routinely in many groups of bacteria (oxidase, nitrate reduction, amino acid degrading enzymes, fermentation or utilization of carbohydrates); others are restricted to a single family, genus, or species (coagulase for staphylococci, arylsulfatase for mycobacteria, tyrosine clearing for *Proteus*, sensitivity to 0129 for *Vibrio*).

A strong argument has been made for identifying species in the clinical laboratory. However, such identification depends on the number of tests done. Both the number of tests and the specific tests used vary from one group of organisms to another. Thus, how far a laboratory should go in identifying organisms and for which organisms they should screen are decisions that must be made in each laboratory on the basis of the type of population it serves and the function of the laboratory. The tests for *Enterobacteriaceae* available in a reference laboratory and from commercial systems are shown in Table 17-1.

Table 17-1   (*Continued*)

Test	Enteric Laboratory Section, Centers for Disease Control	API 20E Analytab Products	Enterotube II Roche Diagnostics	Enteric-Tek Flow Laboratories	MICRO-ID General Diagnostics	Rapid E DMS Laboratories	Minitek BBL
i-inositol	+	+	–	–	+	–	+
D-sorbitol	+	+	+	+	+	–	+
L-arabinose	+	+	+	+	+	+	+
Raffinose	+	–	–	–	–	+	+
L-rhamnose	+	+	–	+	–	+	+
Maltose	+	–	–	–	–	–	–
D-xylose	+	–	–	–	–	+	–
Trehalose	+	–	–	–	–	+	–
Cellobiose	+	–	–	–	–	+	–
Alpha-CH$_3$-D-glucoside	+	–	–	–	–	–	–
Erythritol	+	–	–	–	–	–	–
Esculin	+	–	–	–	+	+	–
Melibiose	+	+	–	–	–	+	–
D-arabitol	+	–	–	–	–	–	–
Glycerol	+	–	–	–	–	–	–
Mucate	+	–	–	–	–	–	–
Tartrate (Jordans)	+	–	–	–	–	–	–
Acetate	+	–	–	–	–	–	–
Lipase (corn oil)	+	–	–	–	–	–	–
Deoxyribonuclease	+	–	–	–	–	–	–
Nitrate reduction	+	–	–	–	+	–	+
Oxidase	+	+	–	–	–	+	–
ONPG	+	+	–	–	+	+	+
D-mannose	+	–	–	–	–	–	–
Amygdalin	–	+	–	–	–	–	–

Classification Below and Above the Species Level

Below the Species Level

Clinical microbiologists must often distinguish strains with particular traits from other strains in the same species but, as stated above, this cannot be done at the species level. Occasionally, a subspecies designation is convenient, although subspecies are not commonly used clinically. Examples of subspecies designations are five subspecies in the single species of *Salmonella*. Salmonellae are reported clinically by serotype: *Salmonella*, serotype *typhi* (*S typhi*), *Salmonella*, serotype *typhimurium* (*S typhimurium*); *Klebsiella pneumoniae* ssp *pneumoniae*, *K pneumoniae* ssp *ozaenae*, and *K pneumoniae* ssp *rhinoscleromatis* (reported as *K pneumoniae, K ozaenae*, and *K rhinoscleromatis*); *Yersinia pseudotuberculosis* ssp *pseudotuberculosis*, and *Y pseudotuberculosis* ssp *pestis* (reported as *Y pseudotuberculosis* and *Y pestis*).

The communication needs of clinical microbiologists should be met by designations below the species level as "groups" or "types" on the basis of common serologic or biochemical reactions, phage or bacteriocin sensitivity, pathogenicity, or other characteristics. Many of these characteristics are already used and accepted: serotype, phage type, colicin type, biotype, bioserotype (a group of strains from the same species with common biochemical and serologic characteristics that set them apart from other members of the species), and pathotype (toxigenic *E coli*, invasive *E coli*, toxigenic *V cholerae*, and β-hemolytic streptococci are expressions of pathotype).

Above the Species Level

In addition to species and subspecies designations, clinical microbiologists must be familiar with genera and families. A **genus** is a group of related species, and a **family** is a group of related genera (some groups have **tribe** designations between the level of family and genus, but these are used infrequently). Some families that contain medically important genera are *Enterobacteriaceae* (for example, *Escherichia, Shigella, Salmonella, Klebsiella, Serratia,* and *Proteus*), *Vibrionaceae* (*Vibrio, Aeromonas,* and *Plesiomonas*), *Spirochaetales* (*Borrelia, Treponema, Leptospira*), *Pseudomonadaceae* (*Pseudomonas*), *Bacteroidaceae* (*Bacteroides*), *Neisseriaceae* (*Neisseria*), *Micrococcaceae* (*Staphylococcus*), *Streptococcaceae* (*Streptococcus*), *Bacillaceae* (*Clostridium*), *Mycobacteriaceae* (*Mycobacterium*), *Pasteurellaceae* (*Pasteurella, Haemophilus*), and *Legionellaceae* (*Legionella*).

A genus is not defined genetically. If it were, an ideal genus would be composed of species with similar phenotypic and genetic characteristics. Some genera that contain species that are phenotypically similar approach this criterion (*Citrobacter, Yersinia,* and *Serratia*). More often, however, the phenotypic similarity is present, but the genetic relatedness is not. *Bacillus, Clostridium, Vibrio, Campylobacter, Pseudomonas,* and *Legionella* are accepted phenotypic genera in which genetic relatedness between species is not 50%-65% but is 0%-65%. When both phenotypic similarity and genetic similarity are not present, phenotypic similarity generally should be given priority in establishing genera. When organisms are identified as the bench, it is convenient to have the most phenotypically similar species in the same genus. The primary consideration for a genus is that it contains biochemically similar species that are convenient or important to consider as a group, and that must be separated from one another.

Designation of New Species and Nomenclature Changes

Species are named according to principles and rules of nomenclature set forth in the Bacteriological Code. Scientific names usually are taken from Latin or Greek. The correct name of a species or higher taxonomic designation is determined by three criteria: valid publication, legitimacy of the name with regard to the rules of nomenclature, and priority of publication (that is, it is the first validly published name for the taxon).

To be published validly, a new species proposal must contain the species name, a description of the species, and the designation of a type strain for the species; and the name must be published in the *International Journal for Systematic Bacteriology (IJSB)*. Once proposed, a name does not go through a formal process to be accepted officially; in fact, the opposite is true—a validly published name is assumed to be correct unless and until it is challenged officially. A challenge is initiated by publishing a request for an opinion (to the Judicial Commission of the International Association of Microbiological Societies) in the *IJSB*. This occurs only in cases in which the validity of a name is questioned with respect to compliance with the rules of the Bacteriological Code. A question of classification that is based on scientific data (for example, whether a species, on the basis of its biochemical or genetic characteristics, or both, should be placed in a new genus or an existing genus) is not settled by the Judicial Commission, but by the preference and usage of the scientific community. This is why there are pairs of names such as *Citrobacter diversus/Levinea malonatica, Providencia rettgeri/Proteus rettgeri, Legionella dumoffii/Fluoribacter dumoffii,* and *Legionella micdadei/Tatlockia micdadei*. It is often necessary to be familiar with more than one name for a single organism. This is not, however, restricted to bacterial nomenclature. Multiple names exist for many antibiotics and other drugs and enzymes.

The best place to read about new species proposals and nomenclatural changes is the *IJSB*. In addition, the *Journal of Clinical Microbiology* often publishes descriptions of newly described bacteria isolated from clinical sources. Information, including biochemical reactions and sources of isolation about new organisms of clinical importance, disease outbreaks caused by newer species, and reviews of clinical significance of certain organisms may be found in the *Annals of Internal Medicine,* the *Journal of Infectious Diseases,* and *Reviews of Infectious Diseases*. The data provided in these publications supplement and update *Bergey's Manual of Systematic Bacteriology,* the definitive taxonomic reference text.

Assessing Newly Described Bacteria

Since the 8th edition of *Bergey's Manual* was published in 1974, the number of species in *Enterobacteriaceae* has almost tripled from 12 genera with 42 species to 25 genera and almost 130 species, some of which have not yet been named. Similar "explosions" have occurred in other genera. In 1974, five species were listed in the genus *Vibrio,* and the genus *Legionella* was unknown. Today, there are 31 species in *Vibrio,* and 11 species in *Legionella*. Work is in progress on more than 20 "enteric groups" and 22 *Legionella*like groups, many or all of which may represent additional new species. Since 1980, about 40 genus and 200 species name proposals have been made; most represent previously undescribed genera and species, not changes in nomenclature.

The clinical significance of the agent of Legionnaires' disease was well known long before it was isolated, characterized, and classified as *Legionella pneumophila.* In most cases, little is known about the clinical significance of a new species at the time that it is described. Usually, only after a species description has been published, and the organism has been isolated and identified, do assessments of clinical significance begin.

New species will continue to be described. Some of them will be pathogens and most, if not all, will be able to infect humans under the right conditions (infrequent opportunistic pathogens).

Role of the Clinical Laboratory

Clinical laboratories should be able to isolate, identify, and determine the antimicrobial susceptibility pattern of the vast majority of human disease agents, so that physicians can initiate appropriate treatment as soon as possible, and so that the source and means of transmission can be ascertained in order to stop the disease outbreak and prevent its recurrence. The need to identify pathogens quickly, and to balance patient benefit and cost, complicate the task.

To be effective, the professional clinical laboratory staff must interact with the infectious disease staff. Laboratory scientists should make infectious disease rounds. They should keep abreast of new developments in tests, equipment, and classification and should communicate this information to their medical colleagues. They should interpret, qualify, or explain laboratory reports. If a name is changed or a new species is reported, the laboratory should provide background information, including a reference.

The clinical laboratory must be run efficiently. A concerted effort must be made to eliminate or minimize inappropriate and contaminated specimens, unwarranted tests, and after-hours service in the absence of an emergency. Standards for the collection, submitting, and transport of specimens should be drawn up, put in both laboratory and nursing procedure manuals, and reviewed periodically by a committee composed of medical, nursing, and laboratory staff.

Most laboratories today use either commercially available, miniaturized, biochemical test systems or automated instruments for biochemical tests and for susceptibility testing. The miniaturized kit systems for assessment of *Enterobacteriaceae* are shown in Table 17-1. These kits usually contain 10-21 tests. The test results are converted to numerical biochemical profiles that are looked up in a codebook for identification. Identification is accomplished in 4-16 hours.

Automated instruments can be used to identify all gram-negative fermenters and nonfermenters; most can be used for gram-positive pathogens, but not for anaerobes. Antimicrobial susceptibility can be performed with this equipment by giving approximate minimum inhibitory drug concentrations. Both tasks are accomplished in 3-16 hours. If semiautomated instruments are used, varying amounts of manipulation are done by the technician, and the cultures (in miniature cards or microtiter plates) are incubated outside of the instrument. The test containers are then read rapidly by the instrument and the identification is made automatically. Some other instruments designed to speed laboratory diagnosis of bacteria are those that detect (but do not identify) bacteria in blood cultures in 8-18 hours, and those that remove antimicrobials from blood to facilitate culture of blood from patients who are undergoing antimicrobial therapy. Also available are a large number of rapid screening systems for the detection of one or a series of specific bacteria, including staphylococci, streptococci, salmonellae, and chlamydia. These screening systems are based on fluorescent antibody, agglutination, or rapid biochemical plating procedures.

It is important to try to identify pathogens presumptively before identification is completed, so that appropriate therapy can be initiated as quickly as possible. A Gram stain, spot indole test, rapid oxidase test, and spore and acid-fast stains may allow presumptive identification within minutes. Rapid enzymatic tests can render presumptive identification in 1 hour or less.

Despite recent advances, the armamentarium of the clinical laboratory is far from complete. Few laboratories can or should conduct the animal experiments that are often essential for distinguishing virulent from avirulent strains. Serotyping is done only for a few species; phage typing is done only rarely. Few pathogenicity tests are performed. Not many laboratories can conduct comprehensive biochemical tests on strains that cannot be identified readily by commercially available biochemical systems. Even fewer laboratories are equipped to do plasmid profiles, gene probes, or DNA hybridization. These and other specialized tests for the serologic or biochemical identification of some exotic bacteria, as well as pathogenic yeasts, fungi, protozoans, and viruses, are best done in district, state, or federal reference laboratories. It is not cost effective to keep, and control the quality of, reagents and media for tests that are seldom run or that are quite complex.

Specific genetic probes are now available for the identification directly in tissue or body fluid of many bacteria and viruses including cholera toxin, heat labile and heat stable *E coli* enterotoxins, pathogenicity plasmids in invasive *E coli* and *Yersinia enterocolitica*, salmonellae, legionellae, and *Neisseria gonorrhoeae*. These probes are now available in only a few research laboratories, but should become commercially available soon. Eventually, gene probes will allow identification by species or pathogenicity factors within 48 hours of sampling—without the need to isolate the organism.

Interfacing With Public Health Laboratories

Hospital and local clinical laboratories interact with district, state, and federal health laboratories in several important ways. The clinical laboratories participate in quality control and proficiency testing programs that are conducted by their state health department laboratories or by the CDC. The reference laboratories supply cultures and often reagents for use in quality control, and conduct training programs for clinical laboratory personnel.

All types of laboratories should interact closely to provide diagnostic services and epidemic surveillance. The primary concern of the clinical laboratory is identifying infectious disease agents and studying nosocomial and local outbreaks of disease. The local laboratory may ask the state laboratory for help in identifying an unusual organism, serotyping or phage typing various bacteria, discovering the cause or mode of transmission in a disease outbreak, or performing specialized tests not done routinely in clinical laboratories. The local laboratory's request should be justified. Cultures should be pure, and should be sent on appropriate media with pertinent clinical laboratory information, including: name and address of the submitting laboratory and the person to be contacted if additional information is required; culture or specimen number, and type of specimen; date sent; patient name (or number), birthdate, and sex; clinical diagnosis, associated illness, date of onset, and present condition; laboratory test requested; category of agent, specific agent suspected, and any other organisms isolated; origin, source, and date of isolation of specimen; relevant epidemiologic and clinical data; treatment of patient; and previous laboratory results (biochemical or serologic tests).

These data allow the state laboratory to test the specimen properly and quickly, and also provide information about what is happening within the state. For example, a food-borne outbreak might extend to many parts of the state (or beyond its boundaries). The state laboratory can alert local physicians to the possibility of such outbreaks.

Another necessary interaction between local and state laboratories is the reporting of **notifiable diseases** by the local laboratory. The state laboratory makes available to local laboratories summaries of the incidence of these diseases. The state laboratories also submit the summaries to the CDC weekly (or, for some diseases, yearly), and national summaries are published weekly in the *Morbidity and Mortality Weekly Report* (see Chapter 24).

Interaction between the CDC and state and federal laboratories is very similar to that between local and state laboratories. The CDC provides quality control cultures and reagents to state laboratories, and serves as a national reference laboratory for diagnostic services and epidemiologic surveillance. The CDC participates in disease outbreaks only when invited to do so by a state laboratory. Local laboratories cannot send specimens or cultures directly to the CDC; instead, they must send specimens to the state health laboratory, which, when necessary, forwards them to the CDC. The CDC reports its results back to the state laboratory, which then reports to the local laboratory.

Hazards of Clinical Laboratory Work

Clinical laboratory personnel, including support and clerical people, are subject to the risk of infection, chemical hazards, and, in some laboratories, radioactive contamination. Risks can be prevented or minimized by a laboratory safety program.

Personnel who work with radioactive materials should take a radioactivity safety course, wear radiation monitor badges, and be aware of the methods for decontaminating hands, clothing, work surfaces, and equipment. They should wear gloves when working with radioactive compounds; when they work with high level radiation they should use a hood and stand behind a radiation shield. Preparative radioactive work should be done in a separate room to which only personnel who are involved directly in the work have access.

Chemicals can harm laboratory personnel through inhalation or skin absorption of volatile compounds, bodily contact with acids, bases, and other harmful chemicals, or introduction of poisonous or skin-damaging liquids into the mouth. Good laboratory practices require that volatile compounds be handled only under a hood, no mouth pipetting of hazardous chemicals be done, and gloves and eye guards be worn by those working with skin-damaging chemicals. Workers should be familiar with procedures for chemical decontamination.

Microbiologic contamination is the greatest hazard in clinical microbiology laboratories. Laboratory infections are a danger not only to the clinical laboratory personnel, but also to anyone else who enters the laboratory, including janitors, clerical and maintenance personnel, and visitors. The risk of infection is governed by the frequency and length of contact with the infectious agent, its virulence, the dose and route of administration, and the susceptibility of the host. The inherent hazard of any infectious agent is affected by factors such as the volume of infectious material used, handling of the material, effectiveness of safety containment equipment, and soundness of laboratory methods.

If possible, agents that are treated differently, such as viruses as opposed to bacteria or *Mycobacterium tuberculosis* in contrast to *E coli,* should be handled in different laboratories or in different parts of the same laboratory. When the risk category of an agent is known, it should be handled in an area with appropriate containment. All specimens sent for isolation of infectious agents and all organisms sent to the laboratory for identification should be assumed to be pathogenic. A separate area should be set aside for the receipt of specimens. Personnel should be aware of the handling and potential hazards of improperly packed, broken, or leaking packages and of the proper methods for their handling and decontamination.

To prevent infection, personnel should wear laboratory coats at all times, wash their hands at the conclusion of each exposure to pathogenic agents, be forbidden to use mouth pipetting and not carry food or cigarettes into the laboratory. Immunization may be appropriate for employees who are exposed often to certain infectious agents, including yellow fever, rabies, and polio viruses, *Yersinia pestis, S typhi,* and *Francisella tularensis.*

Infectious agents are assigned to biosafety levels from 1 to 4 on the basis of their virulence. The containment levels for organisms should correlate with the biosafety level assigned. Biosafety level 1 is for well-defined organisms not known to cause disease in healthy humans; it includes certain *E coli* strains (such as K-12) and *Bacillus subtilis.* Containment level 1 involves standard microbiologic practices and safety equipment is not needed.

Biosafety level 2, the minimum level for clinical laboratories, is for moderate risk agents associated with human disease. Containment level 2 includes limited access to the work area, decontamination of all infectious wastes, use of protective gloves, and a biologic safety cabinet for use in procedures that may create aerosols. Examples of biosafety level 2 agents are: nematode, protozoan, trematode, and cestode human parasites; all human fungal pathogens except *Coccidiodes immitis;* all *Enterobacteriaceae* except *Y pestis; Bacillus anthracis;* brucellae; *Clostridium tetani; Corynebacterium diphtheriae; Haemophilus* sp; leptospires; legionellae; mycobacteria other than *M tuberculosis;* pathogenic *Neisseria* sp; staphylococci, streptococci, *Treponema pallidum; V cholerae;* and hepatitis and influenza viruses.

Biosafety level 3 is for agents that are associated with risk of serious or fatal aerosol infection. In containment level 3, laboratory access is controlled, special clothing is worn in the laboratory, and containment equipment is used for all work with the agent. *M tuberculosis, Coccidiodes immitis, Coxiella burnetii,* and many of the arboviruses are biosafety 3 level agents. Containment level 3 usually is recommended for work with rickettsiae, brucellae, *Y pestis,* and a wide variety of viruses.

Biosafety level 4 indicates dangerous and novel agents that cause diseases with high fatality rates. Maximum containment and decontamination procedures are used in containment level 4, which is found in only a few reference and research laboratories. Only some viruses (Lassa, Ebola, and Marburg) are classified in biosafety level 4.

References

Buchanan, R.E., Gibbons, N.E., (editors): *Bergey's manual of determinative bacteriology,* 8th ed. Baltimore: The Williams and Wilkins Co, 1974.

Center for Infectious Diseases: *Reference/diagnostic services.* Atlanta: Centers for Disease Control, 1973.

Gregg, M.B., (editor): *Morbidity and Mortality Weekly Report.* Atlanta: Centers for Disease Control, 1984.

Krieg, N.R., Holt, J.G., (editors): *Bergey's manual of systematic bacteriology.* vol 1. Baltimore: The Williams and Wilkins Co, 1984.

Lapage, S.P., et al: *International code of nomenclature of bacteria.* 1975 revision. Washington, D.C.: American Society for Microbiology, 1975.

Lennette, E.H., et al: *Manual of clinical bacteriology,* 3rd ed. Washington, D.C.: American Society for Microbiology, 1980.

Richardson, J.H., Barkley, W.E., (editors): *Biosafety in microbiological and biomedical laboratories* (Draft). Atlanta and Bethesda: Centers for Disease Control and National Institutes of Health, 1983.

Skerman, V.B.D., McGowan, V., Sneath, P.H.A., (editors): Approved lists of bacterial names. *Int J Syst Bacteriol* 1980; 30:225–420.

18 Cultivation

C. P. Davis, PhD

General Concepts

Bacterial multiplication consists of cell growth and division. Although the term *growth* commonly refers to increasing bacterial cell numbers, growth can also refer to an increase in mass of cellular material brought about by synthesis of proteins, polysaccharides, lipids, and nucleic acids. In bacteriology, however, most investigators consider growth to be restricted to the narrower aspect of bacterial multiplication—bacterial division.

The precise nutritional requirements for growth vary among bacteria, but all bacteria require water, some source of carbon, nitrogen, energy, hydrogen donors and acceptors, and inorganic ions. These basic nutritional requirements often are taken for granted because most growth factors are provided in complex culture media such as meat infusion broths. Key nutritional factors become evident when chemically defined culture media are employed, or when fastidious or nutritionally demanding bacteria are cultured. Some bacteria of medical importance, such as *Treponema pallidum* and *Mycobacterium leprae,* cannot be cultured in vitro because key metabolites remain unknown. This chapter presents essential aspects of bacterial growth, its measurement, and the basic components of culture media.

Measurement of Bacterial Growth

Under optimal conditions, the average bacterium grows and divides about once every half hour. Exceptions include *Mycobacterium tuberculosis,* which divides about once a day (a rate similar to mammalian cells in culture). The half-hourly rate of cell division in *Escherichia coli,* for example, produces a large number of cells in a short time. Rapid bacterial doubling time is responsible, in part, for the speedy onset and progression of disease. Further, *E coli* can be grown to cell densities ranging from 10^8 to 10^{10} cells per milliliter, depending on culture conditions. Higher cell densities (10^{12}/mL) can be achieved if toxic products of growth are removed and fresh nutrients are added continuously.

Bacterial cells can be enumerated by several commonly used methods: viable cell counts, direct particle (microbial) counts, and turbidimetric density determinations. **Viable cell counts** are made by estimating the total number of colony-forming units (CFU) in a bacterial culture. Colony-forming units represent those organisms capable of growing and dividing to form distinct colonies visible on an agar surface. **Direct particle counts** are performed by counting both viable and nonviable cells. These estimates can be derived by direct observation using a bacteria counting chamber on a microscope stage. **Turbidimetric determinations** differ from the previous two methods by indirectly measuring growth. In these determinations, the turbidity of a culture is estimated and then correlated with viable cell or particle counts.

Viable cells are determined routinely with the aid of serial dilutions that decrease the number of bacteria so they can be counted. Usually a series of tenfold or a hundredfold dilutions of the culture are made, because cultures frequently contain large numbers of bacteria. Figure 18-1 shows a typical dilution series. This dilution method may be used to gain a good estimate of viable cells. Viable cell counts may be equal, or nearly equal, to total cell counts. However, if bacterial cells are dying in a culture and are not undergoing lysis, then the viable cell count may be considerably lower than the direct particle counts.

Bacterial Growth Curve

Most bacteria follow a similar pattern of growth involving four phases: lag, logarithmic, stationary, and decline (Figure 18-2). When bacteria are inoculated into a nutritious medium, cell growth and division occur following a short **lag phase.** This phase allows sufficient time for the bacteria to adapt to the culture medium. Progression through the lag phase consists of generation of the proper oxidation-reduction potential, sidero-phore (an iron chelator) production, and protein synthesis. These adaptive metabolic activities occur in cells preparing for division. Also, cell elongation and cell septum formation usually occur before the first daughter cell is formed. During lag phase, these activities increase cell mass but do not increase cell number.

Following lag phase, the cells progress to the **logarithmic phase** of growth, during which the most rapid cell division occurs. In the log phase, bacterial cell number can double in as few as 20 minutes, depending on the individual bacterium's generation,

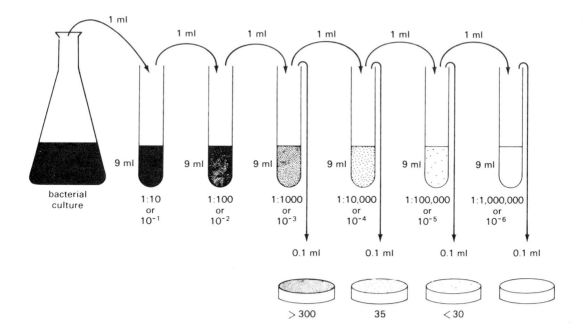

Figure 18-1 Typical tenfold dilution series of a bacterial culture. Serial 1 mL volumes of broth culture are transferred to 9 mL dilution blanks containing saline or other diluent. Usually, 3–4 consecutive dilutions are selected for plating onto solid medium in duplicate. After incubation of plates, the number of bacterial colonies from a given dilution yielding 30–300 colonies is enumerated and multiplied by appropriate dilution to estimate number of viable bacteria per 0.1 mL sample of original culture. Customarily, values are multiplied by 10, and viable cell counts are expressed as colony-forming units/mL (CFU/mL). Here, CFU/mL is 3.5×10^6 (or the CFU/0.1 mL is 3.5×10^5).

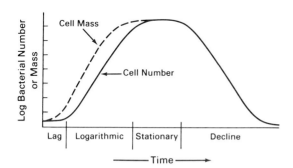

Figure 18-2 Bacterial growth curve with relative location of phases of growth.

or doubling, time. The net result is an exponential increase in cell number. Each cell division is preceded by an increase in cell mass (see Figure 18-2). The log phase lasts only as long as nutrients are available or until toxic waste products inhibit growth.

During the **stationary phase,** the rate of cell division equals the rate of cell death. As a result, the number of viable cells remains constant. During this phase, the cells continue adaptive changes to the environment (for example, sporulation in spore-forming genera and synthesis of inclusion bodies, or granules, in other genera). The stationary phase may last for an extended period (a matter of days) depending on environmental factors.

The **decline phase** varies considerably according to species, temperature, environment (especially pH), and the presence or absence of moisture. Cells die much more rapidly under dry conditions than under moist ones. The half-lives (time required for death of 50% of the population) of certain bacteria during the phase of decline may vary greatly (36 hours for *E coli* compared to 1600 hours for *Mycobacterium* sp). The point to be emphasized is that bacteria survive for prolonged periods under moist conditions. Moist soiled bandages and bedding are therefore potential sources of infection unless properly sterilized.

Calculation of Bacterial Generation Time

During log phase, most organisms undergo division at a constant rate, called the **generation time,** which is defined as the average time needed to double the bacterial number. The generation time can be easily calculated. Plot the growth curve (see Figure 18-2) on semi-log paper and find two points on the linear part of the logarithmic portion of the curve that represents a doubling of viable cell number. Draw a line to the abscissa (x axis) from both points. The length of the line on the abscissa between the two points represents the generation time of the organisms.

Synchronous Growth

The events depicted in the growth curve of Figure 18-2 represent the average of those occurring in the bacterial population as a whole. Sometimes it is desirable to have most cells in the population dividing in synchrony to permit analysis of the sequential events during cell growth and division.

Synchronous growth can be achieved by any of several methods. First, because thymine is needed for DNA synthesis in thymine-starved, thymine-requiring bacteria, cell division can be arrested by withholding thymine. Addition of thymine allows most cells to continue the growth cycle in synchrony. Second, by growing the cells at alternate cycles of low and optimum temperatures, bacteria can be converted to a synchronous mode of growth (for example, growing *E coli* alternately at 25 and 37 C can slow or increase growth rates to aid in synchronizing a bacterial culture). Third, promotion of spore germination in spore-forming bacteria often yields vegetative cells in the same mode of growth. Fourth, separating cells of various ages on the basis of size can be done by selective filtration methods or by density-gradient centrifugation. This method separates younger (small) cells from older or dividing (large) cells. In all cases, however, synchrony persists for only one to four division cycles, after which the cells become more and more out of phase until their division times again become completely random.

Factors Affecting Growth and Division

The essential compounds required for growth (hydrogen donors, hydrogen acceptors, energy source, carbon source, nitrogen source, inorganic salts, and growth factors) are discussed first, followed by the physical factors that limit growth.

Hydrogen Donors

Hydrogen (proton and electron) donors are substances that can be oxidized and usually serve as an energy source for the bacterium. Both organic and inorganic compounds may serve as hydryogen donors; typical organic hydrogen donors include carbohydrates, fatty acids, alcohols, methane, and occasionally amino acids. Sulfur, hydrogen sulfide, nitrites, ammonia, and hydrogen are common inorganic "hydrogen" (actually electron) donors. Some of these substances may serve multiple functions, discussed later in terms of cellular synthesis.

Hydrogen Acceptors

Hydrogen (proton and electron) acceptors, substances that can be reduced, are required for the coupling of oxidation-reduction reactions. Bacteria utilize hydrogen acceptors during respiration or fermentation. The hydrogen acceptor during aerobic respiration is oxygen; however, many bacteria grow where oxygen is not readily available. Under these conditions of reduced oxygen concentration, partially oxidized organic compounds or inorganic compounds can be used as hydrogen acceptors. In bacteria capable of anaerobic fermentation, partially oxidized organic compounds serve as hydrogen acceptors. These organic compounds include pyruvate, lactate, fatty acids, and aldehydes. In contrast, anaerobic respiration utilizes inorganic compounds such as nitrate and sulfate as hydrogen acceptors.

Energy Source

Bacteria may utilize a large variety of compounds as energy sources. Chemosynthetic bacteria derive energy from many of the compounds listed as hydrogen donors. Although most bacteria of medical importance are chemosynthetic, some bacteria in nature are photosynthetic, utilizing light as an energy source. Chapter 19 provides extensive coverage of energy metabolism.

Carbon Source

All bacteria require a source of carbon, if not as an energy source then as a structural component of DNA, RNA, structural proteins, enzymes, carbohydrates, and lipids. Bacteria are broadly classified by their main source of carbon. **Autotrophs** utilize carbon dioxide as the sole source of carbon, whereas **heterotrophs** require, in addition to carbon dioxide, carbohydrates, amino acids, or some additional organic compounds.

Nitrogen Source

Nitrogen sources include amino acids, nitrates, nitrites, hydroxylamine, ammonia, and nitrogen gas. Considerable variation exists among bacteria in their capacities to utilize these sources of nitrogen.

Inorganic Salts (Minerals)

Certain ions (Mg^{++}, K^+, Na^+, and $PO_4^=$) are required in relatively high concentrations for bacterial growth and must be added to chemically defined media. Other ions are required in only trace amounts and are found as contaminants in reagent-grade chemicals and most commercially available culture media.

Growth Factors

Some bacteria require additional growth factors in the form of organic compounds that cannot be synthesized by particular bacteria. Examples are water-soluble vitamins, nucleic acid derivatives, and certain amino acids.

Physical Factors

Bacteria have an optimum temperature for growth; however, they can also grow at a measurable rate within a broad temperature range. **Psychrophiles,** bacteria with an optimum temperature of approximately 10 C, include *Pseudomonas fluorescens* and many marine bacteria. **Mesophiles,** with an optimum temperature of 20-40 C, include most pathogenic types of bacteria. **Thermophiles,** bacteria with an optimum temperature of 50-60 C, include bacteria from hot springs such as *Bacillus stearothermophilus*. The temperature of incubation is critical in determining rate of growth. A reduction of 10 C from the optimum temperature at least doubles the generation time of a bacterium, although the final cell yield will be the same. As would be expected, a reduction in temperature also extends the viability of a culture. In fact, freezing in liquid nitrogen is an excellent way to preserve microorganisms. In contrast, elevation of temperature above the optimum incubation temperature reduces viability. Temperatures exceeding 50 C are usually lethal for most pathogenic bacteria (see Chapter 27).

The pH of the culture medium is another factor affecting bacterial growth. Most bacteria have an optimal pH of 6-7, although some bacteria can tolerate extremes (for example, *Vibrio cholerae*, pH 8; *Thiobacillus*, pH 3). If bacteria are introduced into an environment with a pH beyond their tolerance range, they will not survive.

Osmotic pressure normally presents no problem for the growth of most bacteria because of their rigid cell wall; however, some bacteria lack a cell wall and are particularly sensitive to changes in osmotic pressure. Such cell wall-deficient bacteria include *Mycoplasma* sp and bacterial L forms.

Some bacteria can tolerate and grow slowly in 6% sodium chloride, which has almost twice the tonicity of sea water. Examples of salt-tolerant bacteria are *Micrococcus*, *Staphylococcus* sp, and enteric streptococci.

Culture Media

All culture media for bacteria must contain the necessary nutrients and must provide appropriate physical conditions for bacterial growth. Some bacteria can grow in simple media; others require chemically complex media. Furthermore, pathogenic bacteria frequently are incubated in special media that select for certain genera or contain indicators that aid in rapid identification of certain biochemical characteristics possessed by the pathogen. Selective media frequently are used to identify pathogens in clinical

Table 18-1   Characteristics of Typical Culture Media

Bacteriologic Culture Media		Use	Mechanism
Minimal Medium for Escherichia coli		Assays for utilization of glucose as sole organic carbon source	Only glucose is available for an organic carbon source
Sodium monohydrogen phosphate	7.0 g		
Potassium dihydrogen phosphate	3.0 g		
Ammonium chloride	1.0 g		
Magnesium sulfate	0.1 g		
Glucose (or certain other carbohydrates)	2.0 g		
Distilled water	1000.0 mL		
pH adjusted to 7.0			
Nutrient Broth		Allows growth of many fastidious organisms	Provides many complex substances such as amino acids
Beef extract	3.0 g		
Peptone	5.0 g		
Distilled water	1000.0 mL		
pH, 6.8			
Sugar Fermentation Broth		Determines presence of metabolic pathway to utilize added sugar	Use of sugar results in acid production and change of indicator color
Nutrient broth (no added carbohydrate)	1000.0 mL		
Sugar (e.g., glucose)	10.0 g		
Brom cresol purple pH indicator: yellow at pH 5.2 and lower; violet at pH 6.8 and higher	0.01 g		
pH 7.0			
Selective and Differential Medium		Selects for colonies of *Salmonella* and *Shigella* and suppresses growth of most other bacteria	Bile salts and dyes at this concentration are somewhat toxic for many related gram-negative bacteria but are tolerated by *Salmonella* and *Shigella*
Beef extract	5.0 g		
Proteose peptone	5.0 g		
Lactose	10.0 g		
Bile salts	8.5 g	Also indicates whether H_2S is formed or lactose is fermented	FeS precipitates when H_2S is produced
Sodium citrate	8.5 g		
Sodium thiosulfate	8.5 g		
Ferric citrate	1.0 g		
Agar	13.5 g		Lactose fermentation lowers pH
Dye (brilliant green)	0.33 mg		
Dye (neutral red) pH indicator	25.0 mg		
Distilled water	1000.0 mL		

specimens containing both pathogens and residents of the normal flora. Table 18-1 gives examples of several media types.

References

Davis, B.D.: Energy production. In: *Microbiology*, 3rd ed. Davis, B.D., et al (editors). Hagerstown, Md.: Harper & Row, 1980.

Gale, E.F.: *The chemical activities of bacteria.* New York: Academic Press, 1952.

Harder, W., Dijkhaizen, L.: Physiological responses to nutrient limitation. *Ann Rev Microbiol* 1983; 37:1-23.

Ingledew, W.J., Poole, R.K.: The respiratory chains of *Escherichia coli. Microbiol Rev* 1984; 48:222-271.

Thimann, K.V.: *The life of bacteria*, 2nd ed. New York: Macmillan Pub. Co., 1966.

19 Metabolism

Peter Jurtshuk, Jr., PhD

General Concepts

Metabolism refers to all the biochemical reactions that occur in a cell or organism. The study of bacterial metabolism focuses on the chemical diversity of substrate oxidations and unusual **dissimilation reactions,** which normally occur in bacteria to generate energy. Also within the scope of bacterial metabolism is the study of the uptake and utilization of the inorganic or organic compounds required for growth and maintenance of cellular steady state (**assimilation reactions**). These respective **exergonic** (energy-yielding) and **endergonic** (energy-requiring) **reactions** are catalyzed within the living bacterial cell by integrated enzyme systems, the end result being self-replication of a bacterial cell. The capability of microbial cells to live, function, and self-reproduce in an appropriate chemical milieu (such as bacterial culture media) and the chemical changes that result during this transformation constitute the scope of bacterial metabolism.

The bacterial cell is a highly specialized energy transformer. Chemical energy generated by substrate oxidations is conserved by formation of high-energy compounds

Chapter figures by Ms. Moon Vanko

like adenosine diphosphate (ADP) (AMP~P) and adenosine triphosphate (ATP)

$$\overset{O}{\underset{\|}{}}$$

(AMP~P~P), or compounds containing the thioester bond (R—C~S—R), as ace-tyl~SCoA or succinyl~SCoA. In the presence of proper enzyme systems, these compounds can then be used as energy sources to synthesize the new complex organic compounds needed during growth for a self-replicating cell. All living cells must maintain steady-state biochemical reactions for growth and reproduction.

Kluyver and Donker (1924–1926) recognized that bacterial cells, regardless of species, were in many respects similar chemically to all other living cells. For example, these investigators recognized that hydrogen transfer is a common and fundamental feature of all metabolic processes. Bacteria, just as mammalian and plant cells, require ATP or the high-energy phosphate bond (~P) as the primary chemical energy source. Bacteria also require the B-complex vitamins as functional coenzymes for many oxidation-reduction reactions needed for growth and energy transformation. An organism like *Thiobacillus thiooxidans*, grown in a medium containing only sulfur and inorganic salts, synthesizes large amounts of thiamin, riboflavin, nicotinic acid, pantothenic acid, pyridoxine, and biotin. Thus, Kluyver proposed the **unity theory of biochemistry** (*Die Einheit in der Biochemie*), which stated that all basic enzymatic reactions supporting and maintaining life processes within cells of all organisms had more similarities than differences. This concept of biochemical unity stimulated many investigators to use bacteria as model systems for studying related eukaryotic biochemical reactions that are essentially "identical" at the molecular level. From a nutritional, or metabolic, viewpoint, three major physiologic types of bacteria exist: the heterotrophs (or chemoorganotrophs), the autotrophs (or chemolithotrophs), and photosynthetic bacteria (or phototrophs) (Table 19-1).

Heterotrophic Metabolism

Heterotrophic bacteria, which include all pathogens, obtain energy from oxidation of organic compounds. Carbohydrates (in particular, glucose), lipids, and protein are the most commonly oxidized compounds. Biologic oxidation of these organic compounds by bacteria results in synthesis of ATP as the chemical energy source. This process also permits generation of simpler organic compounds (precursor molecules) needed by the bacteria cell for biosynthetic or assimilatory reactions.

The Krebs cycle intermediate compounds serve as precursor molecules (building blocks) that are needed to synthesize the new complex organic compounds in bacteria through the energy-requiring biosynthetic pathways. Degradation reactions that simulta-neously produce energy and generate precursor molecules for the biosynthesis of new cellular constituents are called **amphibolic.**

All heterotrophic bacteria require preformed organic compounds. These carbon- and nitrogen-containing compounds are growth substrates, which are used aerobically or anaerobically to generate reducing equivalents (for example, reduced nicotinamide adenine dinucleotide; NADH + H$^+$); these reducing equivalents in turn are chemical energy sources for all biologic oxidative and fermentative systems. Heterotrophs are the

Table 19-1 Nutritional Diversity Exhibited by Physiologically Different Bacteria

Physiologic Type	Required Components for Bacterial Growth			
	Carbon Source	Nitrogen Source	Energy Source	Hydrogen Source
Heterotrophic (chemoorganotrophic)	Organic	Organic or inorganic*	Oxidation of organic compounds	—
Autotrophic† (chemolithotrophic)	CO_2	Inorganic*	Oxidation of inorganic compounds	—
Photosynthetic†				
Photolithotrophic				
Bacterial	CO_2	Inorganic*	Sunlight	H_2S or H_2
Cyanobacterial	CO_2	Inorganic*	Sunlight	Photolysis of H_2O‡
Photoorganotrophic	CO_2	Inorganic*	Sunlight	Organic compounds§

*Common inorganic nitrogen sources are NO_3^- or NH_4^+ ions; nitrogen fixers can use N_2.
†Many phototrophs and chemotrophs are nitrogen-fixing organisms.
‡Results in O_2 evolution (or oxygenic photosynthesis) as commonly occurs in plants.
§Organic acids such as formate, acetate, and succinate can serve as hydrogen donors.

most commonly studied bacteria in microbiology; they grow readily in media containing carbohydrates, proteins, or other complex nutrients such as blood. Also, growth media may be enriched by the addition of other naturally occurring compounds such as milk (to study lactic acid bacteria) or hydrocarbons (to study hydrocarbon-oxidizing organisms).

Respiration

Glucose is the most common substrate used for studying heterotrophic metabolism. Most aerobic organisms oxidize glucose completely by the following reaction equation:

$$C_6H_{12}O_6 + 6O_2 \rightarrow 6CO_2 + 6H_2O + Energy$$

This equation expresses the cellular oxidation process called **respiration.** Respiration occurs within the cells of plants and animals, normally generating 38 ATP molecules (as energy) from the oxidation of one molecule of glucose. This yields approximately 380,000 calories (cal) per mole of glucose (1 ATP ≃ 10,000 cal/mole). Thermodynamically, the complete oxidation of one mole of glucose should yield approximately 688,000 cal; the energy that is not conserved biologically as chemical energy (or ATP formation) is liberated as heat (308,000 cal). Thus, the cellular respiratory process is at best about 55% efficient.

Glucose oxidation is the most commonly studied dissimilatory reaction leading to energy production or ATP synthesis. The overall respiration equation for complete oxidation of glucose requires three fundamental biochemical pathways. The first is the glycolytic or the Embden-Meyerhof-Parnas (EMP) pathway (Figure 19-1). Second is the Krebs cycle (also called the citric acid cycle or tricarboxylic acid cycle). Third are the membrane-bound electron transport oxidations coupled to oxidative phosphorylation.

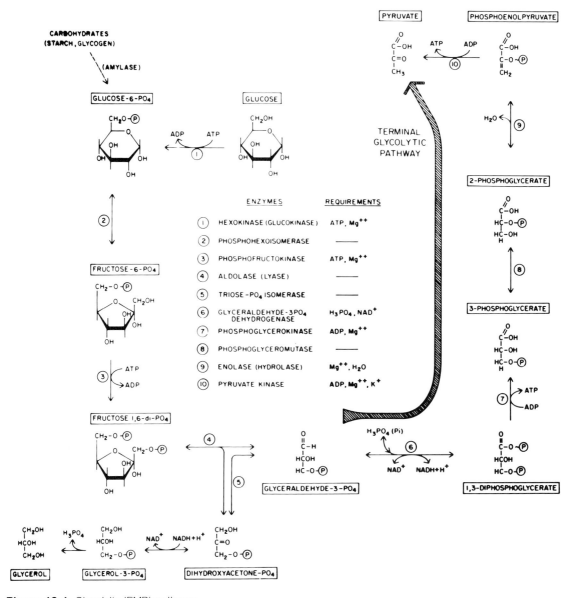

Figure 19-1 Glycolytic (EMP) pathway.

Respiration takes place when any organic compound is oxidized completely to CO_2 and H_2O. In aerobic respiration, molecular O_2 serves as the terminal acceptor of electrons. For anaerobic respiration, NO_3^-, SO_4^-, CO_2, or fumarate can serve as terminal electron acceptors, depending on the bacterium studied. The end result of the respiratory process is the complete oxidation of the organic substrate molecule, and the end products formed are primarily CO_2 and H_2O. Ammonia (NH_3) is formed also if protein (or amino acid) is the substrate oxidized. The biochemical pathways normally involved in oxidation of various naturally occurring organic compounds are summarized in Figure 19-2.

Metabolically, bacteria are unlike cyanobacteria (blue-green algae) and eukaryotes in that glucose oxidation may occur by one or more multiple pathways. In bacteria, glycolysis (EMP) represents one of several pathways by which bacteria can catabolically attack glucose. The glycolytic pathway is most commonly associated with anaerobic or

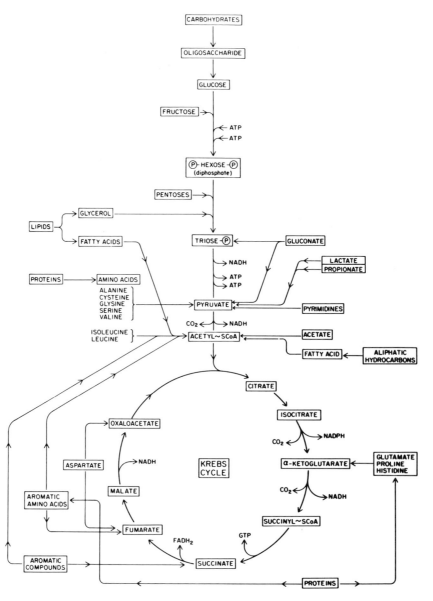

Figure 19-2 Heterotrophic metabolism, general pathway.

fermentative metabolism in bacteria and yeast. In bacteria, other minor heterofermentative pathways also exist, such as the phosphoketolase pathway.

In addition, two other glucose-catabolizing pathways are found in bacteria: the oxidative pentose phosphate pathway (hexose monphosphate shunt, or HMS) shown in Figure 19-3 and the Entner-Doudoroff pathway, which is almost exclusively found in obligate aerobic bacteria (Figure 19-4). The highly oxidative *Azotobacter* and most

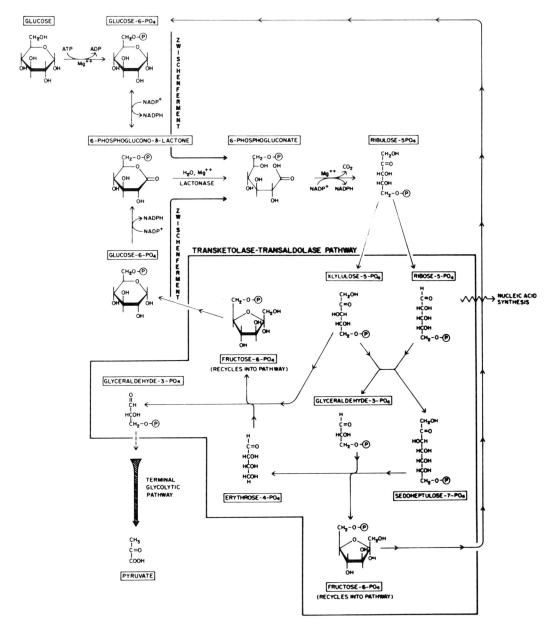

Figure 19-3 Hexose monophosphate (HMS) pathway.

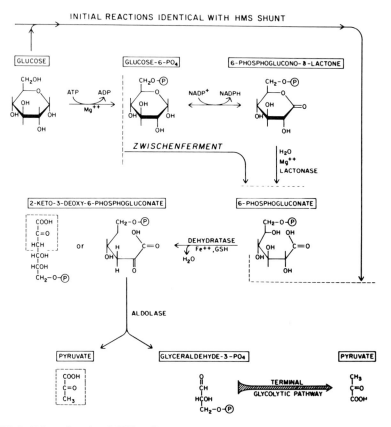

Figure 19-4 Entner–Doudoroff (ED) pathway.

Pseudomonas spp, for example, utilize the Entner-Doudoroff pathway for glucose catabolism, because the organisms of these two genera lack the enzyme phosphofructokinase. Thus, they cannot synthesize fructose 1,6-diphosphate, a key intermediate compound in the glycolytic pathway. (Phosphofructokinase is also sensitive to molecular O_2 and does not function in obligate aerobes.) Other bacteria lacking the enzyme aldolase (which splits fructose 1,6-diphosphate into two triose phosphate compounds) also cannot have a functional glycolytic pathway. Although the Entner-Doudoroff pathway is usually associated with obligate aerobic bacteria, it is present in the facultative anaerobe *Zymomonas mobilis* (formerly *Pseudomonas lindneri*). This organism dissimilates glucose to ethanol, and represents a major alcoholic fermentation reaction in a bacterium.

Hexose dissimilation also occurs by the hexose monophosphate shunt (see Figure 19-3). This oxidative (pentose phosphate) pathway was discovered in tissues that actively metabolized glucose in the presence of two glycolytic pathway inhibitors (iodoacetate and fluoride). Neither inhibitor had an effect on glucose dissimilation, and NADPH + H^+ generation occurred directly from the oxidation of glucose-6-phosphate (to 6-phosphoglucono-δ-lactone) by glucose-6-phosphate dehydrogenase. The pentose phosphate pathway subsequently permits the direct oxidative decarboxylation of glucose to pentoses. The capability of an oxidative metabolic system to bypass glycolysis explains the term shunt.

The biochemical reactions of the Entner-Doudoroff pathway are a modification of the hexose monophosphate shunt, except that pentose sugars are not directly formed. The initial reaction sequences of these two pathways are identical and remain so until formation of 6-phosphogluconate (see Figure 19-4), at which point the two pathways differ. In the Entner-Doudoroff pathway, no oxidative decarboxylation of 6-phosphogluconate occurs, and no pentose compound is formed. For this pathway, a new 6-carbon compound intermediate (2-keto-3-deoxy-6-phosphogluconate) is generated by the action of 6-phosphogluconate dehydratase (an Fe^{++} and glutathione-stimulated enzyme); this intermediate compound is then directly cleaved into the triose (pyruvate) and a triose-phosphate compound (glyceraldehyde-3-phosphate) by the 2-keto-3-deoxy-6-phosphogluconate aldolase. The glyceraldehyde-3-phosphate is further oxidized to another pyruvate molecule by the same enzyme systems that catalyze the terminal glycolytic pathway (see Figure 19-4).

Thus, bacteria have more than one pathway for glucose dissimilation: the glycolytic Embden-Meyerhof-Parnas pathway may be the major one existing concomitantly with the minor oxidative pentose phosphate hexose monophosphate shunt pathway; the Entner-Doudoroff pathway also may function as a major pathway with a minor hexose monophosphate shunt. In a few bacteria only one pathway is found. All cyanobacteria, *Acetobacter suboxydans*, and *A xylinum* possess only the hexose monophosphate shunt pathway; *Pseudomonas saccharophilia* and *Z mobilis* possess solely the Entner-Doudoroff pathway. Thus, the end products of glucose dissimilatory pathways are as follows:

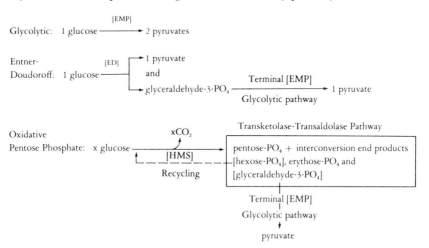

The glucose dissimilation pathways used by specific microorganisms are shown in Table 19-2.

All major pathways of glucose or hexose catabolism have several metabolic features in common. First, there are the preparatory steps by which key intermediate compounds like the triose-PO_4, glyceraldehyde-3-phosphate and/or pyruvate are generated. These two compounds are almost universally required for further assimilatory or dissimilatory

Table 19-2 Glucose Dissimilatory Pathways Utilized By Bacteria, Cyanobacteria and Eucaryotic Yeasts

Bacterium	EMP* (Glycolytic)	HMS† (Oxidative Pentose Phosphate)	Entner-Doudoroff
Acetobacter suboxydans		sole	
Acetobacter xylinum		sole	
Agrobacterium spp			major
Azotobacter‡ vinelandii			major
Bacillus subtilis	major	minor	
Caulobacter spp			major
Escherichia coli	major	minor	
Lactobacillus delbrueckii	major		
Leuconostoc mesenteroides		major	
Neisseria gonorrhoeae		minor	major
Neisseria meningitidis		minor	major
Neisseria perflava		major	
Neisseria sicca		major	
Pseudomonas‡ aeruginosa			major
Pseudomonas saccharophilia			sole
Rhizobium spp			major
Sarcina lutea	major	minor	
Spirillum spp			major
Streptococcus fecalis	major		(major)§
Streptomyces griseus	major	minor	
Zymomonas anaerobia			sole
Zymomonas mobilis			sole
All cyanobacteria		sole	
All yeasts	major	minor	

*Embden-Meyerhof-Parnas (EMP) pathway.
†Hexose monophosphate shunt (HMS).
‡Most species utilize the Enter-Doudoroff as major pathway.
§Induced by growth on gluconate.

reactions within the cell. Second, the major source of phosphate for all reactions involving phosphorylation of glucose or other hexoses is ATP, not inorganic phosphate (Pi). Actually, chemical energy contained in ATP must be initially spent via kinase-type enzymes to generate glucose-6-PO_4, which initiates the reactions involving hexose catabolism. Third, NADH + H^+ or NADPH + H^+ is generated as reducing equivalents (potential energy) directly by one or more of the enzymatic reactions involved in each of these pathways.

Fermentation

Fermentation, another example of heterotrophic metabolism, requires an organic compound as a terminal electron (or hydrogen) acceptor. In fermentations, simpler organic end products are formed from the anaerobic dissimilation of glucose (or some other compound) by microorganisms. Energy (ATP) is generated through the dehydrogenation reactions that occur as glucose is broken down enzymatically. The simpler organic end products formed from this incomplete biologic oxidation process also serve as final electron and hydrogen acceptors. On reduction, these organic end products are secreted into the media as waste metabolites (usually alcohol or acid). In fermentations, the organic substrate compounds are incompletely oxidized by bacteria yet yield sufficient energy for microbial growth. Glucose is the most common hexose used to study fermentation reactions.

In the late 1850s, Pasteur demonstrated that fermentation was a vital process requiring microorganisms. He proved that all fermentative reactions were the end result of microbial growth. Pasteur showed that as fermentation occurred, it was accompanied by the growth of specific types of microorganisms and that each type of fermentation could be defined by the principal organic end product formed (lactic acid, ethanol, acetic acid, or butyric acid).

In his studies on butyric acid fermentation, which led directly to discovery of anaerobic microorganisms, Pasteur observed that the butyric acid bacteria became immobile and lost viability on contact with air; this discovery inspired his classic statement, *"La fermentation est la vie sans l'air."* Pasteur concluded that oxygen had an inhibitory effect on the microorganisms responsible for butyric acid fermentation and that butyric acid formation ceased when air was bubbled into the reaction mixture. Pasteur also first introduced the terms aerobic and anaerobic. Pasteur's views on fermentation are made clear from his microbiologic studies on the production of beer (from *Etudes sur la Biere*, 1876):

> In the experiments which we have described, fermentation by yeast is seen to be the direct consequence of the processes of nutrition, assimilation and life, when these are carried on without the agency of free oxygen. The heat required in the accomplishment of that work must necessarily have been borrowed from the decomposition of the fermentation matter.... Fermentation by yeast appears, therefore, to be essentially connected with the property possessed by this minute cellular plant of performing its respiratory functions, somehow or other, with the oxygen existing combined in sugar.

For most microbial fermentations, glucose dissimilation occurs through the glycolytic pathway (Figure 19-1). The simpler organic compound most commonly generated is pyruvate, or a compound derived enzymatically from pyruvate such as acetaldehyde, α-acetolactate, acetyl~CoA, or lactyl~CoA (see Figure 19-5). Acetaldehyde can then be reduced by $NADH + H^+$ to ethanol, which is then excreted by the cell. In the case of lactic acid fermentation, which occurs in streptococci (*Streptococcus lactis*) and many lactobacilli (*Lactobacillus casei, L pentosus*), the end product can be a single organic acid, lactic acid. Organisms that produce only lactic acid from glucose fermentation are **homofermenters.** Homofermentative lactic acid bacteria dissimilate glucose exclusively through the glycolytic (EMP) pathway. Organisms that ferment glucose with the production of multiple end products, such as acetic acid, ethanol, formic acid, and CO_2, are referred to as **heterofermenters.** Examples of heterofermentative bacteria include *Lactobacillus, Leuconostoc,* and *Microbacterium.* Heterofermentative fermentations are more common among bacteria, as in the mixed-acid fermentations carried out by bacteria of the family *Enterobacteriaceae* (for example, *Escherichia* *coli, Salmonella, Shigella,* and *Proteus* sp). Many of these glucose fermenters usually produce CO_2 and H_2 gas with different combinations of acid end products (formate, acetate, lactate, and succinate). Other bacteria such as *Enterobacter aerogenes, Aeromonas,*

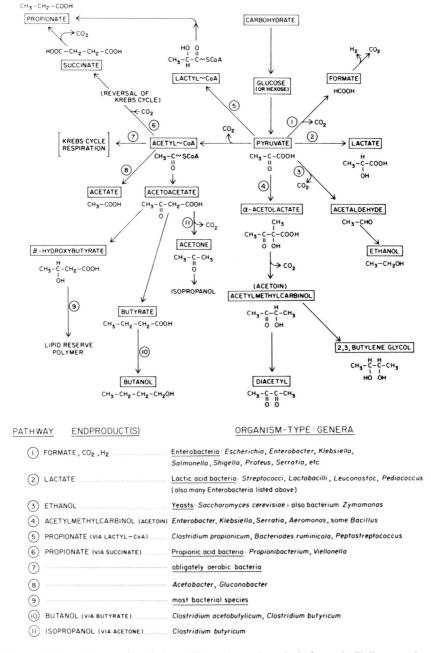

PATHWAY   ENDPRODUCT(S)   ORGANISM-TYPE : GENERA

① FORMATE, CO_2, H_2 .... Enterobacteria: *Escherichia, Enterobacter, Klebsiella, Salmonella, Shigella, Proteus, Serratia, etc.*

② LACTATE .... Lactic acid bacteria: *Streptococci, Lactobacilli, Leuconostoc, Pediococcus* (also many Enterobacteria listed above)

③ ETHANOL .... Yeasts: *Saccharomyces cerevisiae*; also bacterium *Zymomonas*

④ ACETYLMETHYLCARBINOL (ACETOIN) *Enterobacter, Klebsiella, Serratia, Aeromonas,* some *Bacillus*

⑤ PROPIONATE (VIA LACTYL~CoA) .... *Clostridium propionicum, Bacteriodes ruminicola, Peptostreptococcus*

⑥ PROPIONATE (VIA SUCCINATE) .... Propionic acid bacteria: *Propionibacterium, Viellonella*

⑦ .... obligately aerobic bacteria

⑧ .... *Acetobacter, Gluconobacter*

⑨ .... most bacterial species

⑩ BUTANOL (VIA BUTYRATE) .... *Clostridium acetobutylicum, Clostridium butyricum*

⑪ ISOPROPANOL (VIA ACETONE) .... *Clostridium butyricum*

Figure 19-5 Fermentative pathways of bacteria and the major end products formed with the organism type carrying out the fermentation.

Serratia, Erwinia, and *Bacillus* spp also form CO_2 and H_2 as well as other neutral end products (ethanol, acetylmethylcarbinol (acetoin), and 2,3-butylene glycol). Many obligately anaerobic clostridia (*Clostridium saccharobutyricum, C thermosaccharolyticum*) and *Butyribacterium* sp ferment glucose with the production of butyrate, acetate, CO_2, and H_2, whereas other *Clostridium* spp (*C acetobutylicum* and *C butyricum*) also form these same fermentation end products plus others (butanol, acetone, isopropanol, formate, and ethanol). Similarly, the anaerobic propionic acid bacteria (*Propionibacterium* spp) and the related *Veillonella* spp ferment glucose to form CO_2, propionate, acetate, and succinate. In these bacteria, propionate is formed by the partial reversal of the Krebs cycle reactions and involves a CO_2 fixation by pyruvate (the Wood-Werkman reaction) that forms oxaloacetate (a four-carbon intermediate). Oxaloacetate is then reduced to malate, fumarate, and succinate, which is decarboxylated to propionate. Propionate is also formed by another three-carbon pathway in *C propionicum, Bacteroides ruminicola,* and *Peptostreptococcus,* involving a lactyl~CoA intermediate. The obligately aerobic acetic acid bacteria (*Acetobacter* and the related *Gluconobacter* sp) can also ferment glucose, producing acetate and gluconate. Figure 19-5 summarizes the pathways by which the various major fermentation end products form from the dissimilation of glucose by the common intermediate pyruvate.

For thermodynamic reasons, bacteria that rely on fermentative processes for growth cannot generate as much energy as respiring cells. In respiration, 38 ATP (or approximately 380,000 cal/mole) can be generated as biologically useful energy from the complete oxidation of one molecule of glucose (assuming 1 NAD(P)H = 3 ATP and 1 ATP $\rightarrow$ ADP + Pi = 10,000 cal/mole). Table 19-3 shows comparable bioenergetic parameters for the lactate and ethanolic fermentations by the glycolytic pathway:

Table 19-3 Energy Obtained from Bacterial Fermentations by Substrate Phosphorylations

	Energy		
	Actual *(cal/mole)*	*Theory* *(cal/mole)*	*Efficiency* *(%)*
Homolactic (also homofermentative): $$C_6H_{12}O_6 \xrightarrow{[EMP]} 2CH_3-\overset{\overset{\displaystyle H}{\displaystyle |}}{\underset{\underset{\displaystyle OH}{\displaystyle |}}{C}}-COOH +$$ (Glucose) (Lactic acid)	$\simeq 20,000$	57,000	35
Alcoholic (also heterofermentative): $$C_6H_{12}O_6 \xrightarrow{[EMP]} 2CH_3-\overset{\overset{\displaystyle H}{\displaystyle |}}{\underset{\underset{\displaystyle H}{\displaystyle |}}{C}}-OH + 2CO_2 +$$ (Glucose) (Ethanol)	$\simeq 20,000$	58,000	34

Although 2 ATP are generated by the glycolytic (or EMP) pathway, for the lactate or ethanolic fermentation, this is apparently sufficient energy to permit anaerobic growth of lactic acid bacteria and the ethanolic fermenting yeast, *Saccharomyces cerevisiae*. The ATP-synthesizing reactions in the glycolytic pathway (Figure 19-1) specifically involve the substrate phosphorylation reactions catalyzed by phosphoglycerokinase and pyruvic kinase. Although all the ATP molecules available for fermentative growth are believed to be generated by these substrate phosphorylation reactions, some energy equivalents are also generated by proton extrusion reactions (acid liberation), which occur with intact membrane systems and involve the Mitchell hypothesis of energy conservation as it applies to fermentative metabolism.

Krebs Cycle

The Krebs cycle functions oxidatively in respiration and is the metabolic process by which pyruvate or acetyl~CoA is completely decarboxylated to CO_2. In bacteria, this reaction occurs through acetyl~CoA, which is the first reaction product in the oxidative decarboxylation of pyruvate by the pyruvate dehydrogenase. Bioenergetically, the following overall exergonic reaction occurs:

$$CH_3-\overset{\overset{\text{O}}{\|}}{C}-COOH + 5O \xrightarrow[\substack{\text{Electron transport and} \\ \text{oxidative phosphorylation}}]{\text{[Krebs Cycle (via } CH_3-\overset{\overset{\text{O}}{\|}}{C}-O\sim SCoA)]}} 3CO_2 + 2H_2O + 15ATP\ (\approx150,000\ \text{cal/mole})$$

(Pyruvate) $\left(\begin{array}{c}\text{Oxygen}\\\text{atoms}\end{array}\right)$

If two pyruvate molecules are obtained from the dissimilation of one glucose molecule, then 30 ATP are generated totally. The decarboxylation of pyruvate, isocitrate, and α-ketoglutarate accounts for all CO_2 molecules generated during the respiratory process. Figure 19-6 shows the enzymatic reactions in the Krebs cycle. The chemical energy conserved by the Krebs cycle is contained in the reduced compounds generated ($NADH + H^+$, $NADPH + H^+$, and succinate). The potential energy inherent in these reduced compounds is not available as ATP until the final step of respiration (electron transport and oxidative phosphorylation) occurs.

The Krebs cycle is therefore another preparatory stage in the respiratory process. If one molecule of pyruvate is oxidized completely to three molecules of CO_2, generating 15 ATP, the oxidation of one molecule of glucose will yield as many as 38 ATP, provided glucose is dissimilated by glycolysis and the Krebs cycle (further assuming that the electron transport/oxidative phosphorylation reactions are bioenergetically identical to those of eukaryotic mitochondria).

Glyoxylate Cycle

In general, the Krebs cycle functions similiarly in bacteria and eukaryotic systems, but major differences are found among bacteria. One difference is that in obligate aerobes, L-malate may be oxidized directly by molecular O_2 via an electron transport chain. In

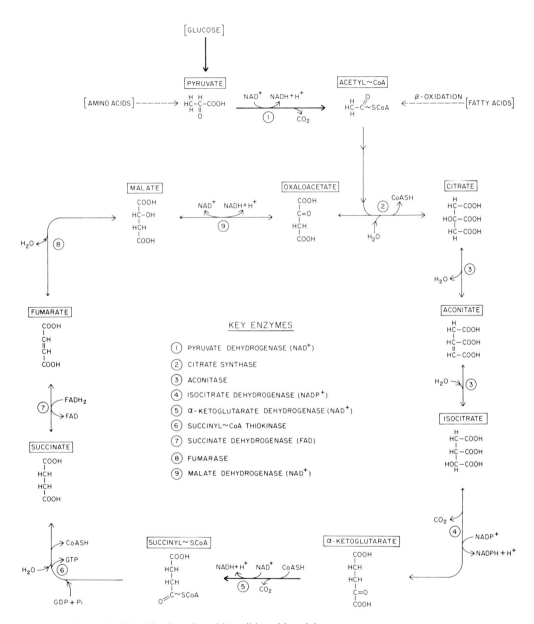

Figure 19-6 Krebs cycle (also tricarboxylic acid or citric acid cycle).

other bacteria, only some Krebs cycle reactions occur because α-ketoglutarate dehydrogenase may be missing.

A modification of the Krebs cycle may exist in other bacteria, commonly called the glyoxylate cycle, or shunt (Figure 19-7). This cycle functions similarly to the Krebs cycle but lacks many of the same enzyme reactions. The glyoxylate cycle is primarily an oxidative pathway in which acetyl~SCoA is generated directly from acetate oxidation,

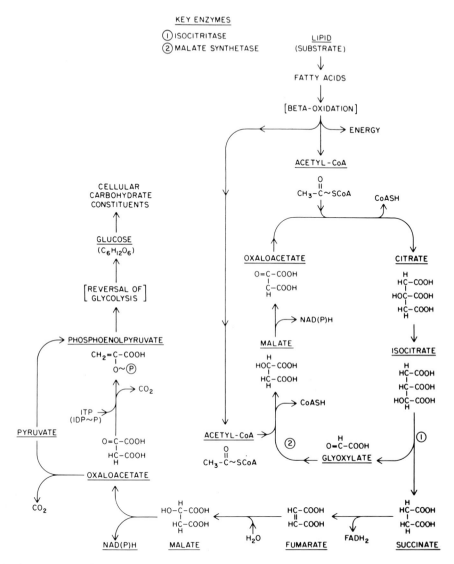

Figure 19-7 Glyoxylate shunt.

or more commonly from the oxidation of fatty acids by the β-oxidation pathway. Pyruvate oxidation is not directly involved in the glyoxylate shunt, yet this cycle yields sufficient succinate and malate, which are required for energy production (see Figure 19-7). The glyoxylate cycle also generates other precursor compounds needed for biosynthesis (see Figure 19-7). The glyoxylate cycle was discovered as an unusual metabolic pathway during an attempt to learn how lipid (or acetate) oxidation in bacteria and plant seeds could lead to the direct biosynthesis of carbohydrates, required by most organisms. The glyoxylate cycle converts oxaloacetate either to pyruvate and CO_2 (catalyzed by pyruvate carboxylase) or to phosphoenolpyruvate and CO_2 (catalyzed by the ITP [inosinetriphosphate]-dependent phosphoenolpyruvate carboxylase kinase). Either triose compound can then be converted to glucose by reversal of the glycolytic [EMP] pathway. Thus a new C_4 oxidative pathway was discovered in bacteria. The glyoxylate cycle is commonly found in many bacteria, like *A vinelandii* and in particular those organisms that can grow well in media in which acetate and other dicarboxylic acid intermediates of the Krebs cycle are used as the sole carbon sources. One primary function of the glyoxylate cycle is to replenish the tricarboxylic and dicarboxylic acid intermediates needed by the cell that are normally provided by the Krebs cycle. A pathway whose primary purpose is to replenish such intermediate compounds is called **anaplerotic.**

Electron Transport and Oxidative Phosphorylation

The final stage of respiration yields energy through sequential electron transfer reactions that occur concomitantly with oxidative phosphorylation. Electron transport enzymes reside on the bacterial inner (cytoplasmic) membrane. Subcellular structural entities called respiratory vesicles, lamellar vesicles, or mesosomes are membrane invaginations of the inner cytoplasmic membrane, the site of electron transport and oxidative phosphorylation. The mesosome may be the premitochondrial equivalent of mitochondria found in eukaryotic cells.

Among bacteria, respiratory electron transport chains vary greatly; in some organisms they are absent. The respiratory mitochondrial electron transport chain oxidizes $NADH + H^+$, $NADPH + H^+$, and succinate (as well as the coacylated fatty acids like acetyl~SCoA). The bacterial electron transport chain also oxidizes these compounds, and it can directly oxidize, via *non*-pyridine nucleotide dependent pathways, a larger variety of reduced substrates such as lactate, malate, formate, α-glycerophosphate, H_2, and glutamate. The respiratory electron carriers in bacterial electron transport systems are more varied and are usually branched at the site(s) reacting with molecular O_2. Some electron carriers are common to both the bacterial and mammalian respiratory electron transport chains (like nonheme iron centers and ubiquinone Q [coenzyme Q]). In other bacteria, the naphthoquinones or vitamin K may be found with ubiquinone Q. In still other microorganisms, bacterial vitamin K serves in the absence of ubiquinone Q; naphthoquinones have no function in eukaryotic respiration. In mitochondrial respiration, only one cytochrome oxidase component is found (cytochrome $a + a_3$ oxidase). In bacteria there are multiple cytochrome oxidases, including cytochromes a_1, d, o, and occasionally cytochrome $a + a_3$ (Figure 19-8).

In bacteria, cytochrome oxidases are diverse entities that usually occur in multiple combinations of a_1:d:o and $a + a_3$:o, respectively. Bacteria also possess mixed-function oxidases like cytochromes P-450 and P-420 and cytochromes c' and $c'c'$-types, which also react with carbon monoxide. These diverse types of oxygen-reactive cytochromes undoubtedly have evolutionary significance. Bacteria were present before O_2 was formed; when O_2 became available as a metabolite, bacteria evolved in different ways, which accounts for the diversity in bacterial oxygen-reactive hemoproteins.

Cytochrome oxidases in many pathogenic bacteria are studied by the bacterial oxidase reaction, which subdivides gram-negative organisms into two major groups, oxidase-positive and oxidase-negative. This oxidase reaction is assayed for by N, N, N',

MITOCHONDRIA (EUKARYOTIC)

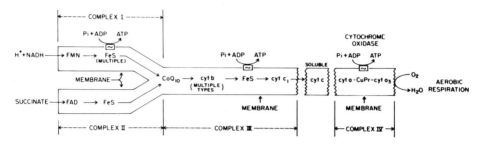

Paracoccus (Micrococcus) denitrificans (FACULTATIVE ANAEROBE)

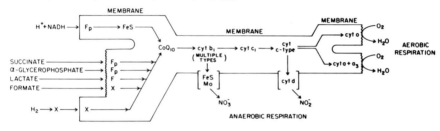

Azotobacter vinelandii (OBLIGATE AEROBE)

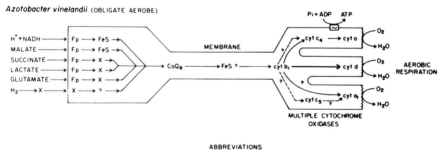

ABBREVIATIONS

FMN = FLAVINMONONUCLEOTIDE	CoQ = COENZYME Q or UBIQUINONE Q
FAD = FLAVINADENINEDINUCLEOTIDE	cyt = CYTOCHROME
FeS = NON-HEME IRON CENTER	Pi = INORGANIC PHOSPHATE (H_3PO_4)
Fp = FLAVOPROTEIN DEHYDROGENASE	~ = HIGH ENERGY INTERMEDIATE COMPOUND
X = UNKNOWN COMPONENT(S)	CuPr = COPPER PROTEIN

Figure 19-8 Respiratory electron transport chains.

N'-tetramethyl-*p*-phenylenediamine oxidation (to Wurster's blue) or by indophenol blue synthesis (with dimethyl-*p*-phenylenediamine and α-naphthol). Oxidase-positive bacteria contain integrated [cytochrome *c*-type:oxidase] complexes; the oxidase component most frequently encountered is cytochrome *o*, and occasionally cytochrome *a* + *a₃*. The cytochrome oxidase responsible for the indophenol oxidase reaction complex was isolated from membranes of *Azotobacter vinelandii,* a bacterium with the highest respiratory rate of any known cell. The cytochrome oxidase was found to be an integrated cytochrome c_4:o *complex*, which most recently was shown to be present in *Bacillus* sp. These *Bacillus* strains were also highly oxidase-positive, and most were found in morphological group II.

What is common to both bacterial and mammalian electron transfer systems is their capacity to carry out electron transfer (oxidation) reactions with $NADH + H^+$, $NADPH + H^+$, and succinate. Energy generated from such membrane oxidations is conserved within the membrane and is then transferred in a coupled manner (linkage) so that concomitant oxidative phosphorylation occurs. This electron transfer sequence is accomplished entirely within membrane-bound enzyme systems. As the electrons are transferred by a specific sequence of electron carriers, ATP is synthesized from ADP + inorganic phosphate (Pi) or phosphoric acid (H_3PO_4) as shown in Figure 19-8.

In respiration, the electron transfer reaction is the primary mode of generating energy; electrons ($2e^-$) from a low-redox-potential compound such as $NADH + H^+$ are sequentially transferred to a specific flavoprotein dehydrogenase or oxidoreductase (flavin mononucleotide [FMN]-type for NADH or a flavin adenine dinucleotide [FAD]-type for succinate); this electron pair is then transferred to a nonheme iron center (FeS) and finally to a specific ubiquinone Q or a naphthoquinone derivative. This transfer of electrons causes a differential chemical redox potential change so that within the membrane enough chemical energy is conserved to be transferred by a coupling mechanism to a high-energy compound (for example, ADP + Pi → ATP). ATP molecules represent the final stable high-energy intermediate compound formed.

A similar series of redox changes also occurs between ubiquinone Q and cytochrome *c* but with a greater differential in the oxidation-reduction potential level, which allows for another ATP synthesis step. The final electron transfer reaction occurs at the cytochrome oxidase level between reduced cytochrome *c* and molecular O_2; this reaction is the terminal ATP synthesis step.

Mitchell Hypothesis

A highly complex but attractive theory to explain energy conservation in biologic systems is the chemiosmotic coupling theory of oxidative and photosynthetic phosphorylations, commonly called the **Mitchell hypothesis.** This theory attempts to explain the conservation of free energy on the basis of an osmotic potential caused by proton concentration differential (or proton gradient) across a proton-impermeable membrane. Energy is generated by the membrane-bound electron transport reactions, which in essence serve as proton pumps; energy conservation and coupling subsequently follow (an obligatory membrane phenomenon). The energy thus conserved (again within a membrane) is coupled to ATP synthesis. This would occur in all biologic cells, even in the lactic acid bacteria that lack a cytochrome-dependent electron transport chain. In this hypothesis, the membrane allows for charge separation, thus forming a proton gradient that drives all bioenergization reactions. By such means, electromotive forces can be generated by oxidation-reduction reactions that can be directly coupled to ion translocations, as in the separation of H^+ and OH^- ions in electrochemical systems. Thus, an enzyme or an electron transfer carrier on a membrane that undergoes an oxidation-reduction reaction serves as a specific conductor for OH^- (or O^-), and "hydrodehydration" provides electromotive power, as it does in electrochemical cells.

The concept underlying Mitchell's hypothesis is complex and many modifications have been proposed, but the theory's most attractive feature is that it unifies all bioenergetic conservation principles into a single concept requiring an intact membrane vesicle to function properly. Figure 19-9 shows how the Mitchell hypothesis might be used to explain energy generation, conservation, and subsequent transfer by a coupling process. The least satisfying aspect of the chemiosmotic hypothesis is the lack of understanding of how chemical energy is actually conserved within the membrane and how it is transmitted by coupling for ATP synthesis.

Bacterial Photosynthesis

Prokaryotes (bacteria as well as cyanobacteria) possess phototrophic modes of metabolism (see Table 19-1). The types of photosynthesis occurring in the two groups of prokaryotes differ mainly with regard to which type of compound serves as the hydrogen donor needed for the reduction of CO_2 to glucose (see Table 19-1). Phototrophic organisms differ from heterotrophic organisms in that they utilize the glucose synthesized intracellularly for biosynthetic purposes (as in starch synthesis) or for energy production, which usually occurs through cellular respiration.

Heterotrophs, unlike phototrophs, require glucose (or some other organic compound) that is directly supplied as a substrate from an exogenous source. Heterotrophs cannot synthesize large concentrations of glucose from CO_2 by specifically using H_2O (or H_2S) as a hydrogen source and sunlight as energy. Plant metabolism is a classical example of photolithotrophic metabolism: plants need CO_2 and sunlight; H_2O must be provided as a hydrogen source and usually NO_3^- is the nitrogen source for protein synthesis. Organic nitrogen, supplied as fertilizer, is converted to NO_3^- in all soils by bacteria via the process of ammonification and nitrification. Although plant cells are

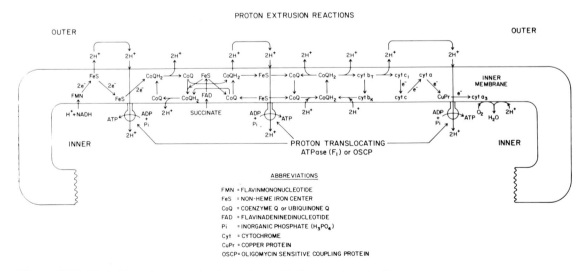

Figure 19-9 Mitchell hypotheses, a chemiosmotic model of energy transduction.

Table 19-4 Characteristics Commonly Exhibited by Phototrophic Bacterial*

Photosynthetic Type	Characteristics	Representative Families (f) and Genera (g)

I. *Purple bacteria*
  A. Sulfur-type
  (formerly *Thiorho-daceae*)
  Photolithotrophic bacteria
	Obligate phototrophes
	Strict anaerobes
	H_2S (or H_2) serve as [H] source
	Possess S granules when H_2S used
	Contain bacteriochlorophyll types a or b
		(f) *Chromatiaceae*
		(g) *Chromatium*
		(g) *Thiospirillum*
		(g) *Thiosarcina*
		(g) *Thiocapsa*

B. Non–sulfur-type (formerly *Athiorhodaceae*) *Photoorganotrophic bacteria*	Facultative phototrophes (have respiratory mechanisms and will grow heterotrophically) Oxygen-tolerant anaerobes Most require one or more B vitamins Simple organic compounds serve as [H] source Contain bacteriochlorophyll type a or b	(f) *Rhodospirillaceae* (g) *Rhodopseudomonas* (g) *Rhodospirillum* (g) *Rhodomicrobium*
II. *Green bacteria* *Photolithotrophic bacteria*	Obligate phototrophes Strict anaerobes Contains chlorobium chlorophyll, which is currently referred to as bacteriochlorophyll type c and d Many require vitamin B_{12} S_2 deposited extracellularly	(f) *Chlorobiaceae* (g) *Chlorobium* (g) *Chloropseudomonas*

*All are gram-negative; if motile, they exhibit polar flagellation. Most species are anaerobic, although some purple nonsulfur bacteria (family *Athiorhodaceae*) are *facultative phototrophes*, and can grow as heterotrophes by using *anaerobic* respiratory mode of metabolism, and thus are oxygen-tolerant. For further information, see Part 1, *Bergey's Manual*, 8th Edition.

phototrophic, they also exhibit a heterotrophic mode of metabolism in that all plants respire. For example, plants catabolize by classical respiration glucose that is generated photosynthetically. Mitochondria as well as the soluble enzymes of the glycolytic pathway are required for glucose dissimilation, and these enzymes are also found in all plant cells. The soluble Calvin cycle enzymes, which are required for glucose synthesis in photosynthesis, are also found in plant cells. A plant cannot be fed by pouring a glucose solution on it, but water supplied to a plant will be "photolysed" by chloroplasts in the presence of light; the hydrogen(s) generated from H_2O is used to reduce $NADP^+$ to $NADPH + H^+$. With these reduced pyridine nucleotides, CO_2 is reduced intracellularly to glucose. This metabolic process is carried out in an integrated manner by the Calvin cycle enzymes. Table 19-4 summarizes the characteristics of known photosynthesis bacteria.

Autotrophy

Bacteria that grow solely at the expense of inorganic compounds (mineral ions), without sunlight as an energy source, are called autotrophs, chemotrophs, chemoautotrophs, or chemolithotrophs. Like photosynthetic organisms, all autotrophs use CO_2 as a carbon source for growth; their nitrogen comes from inorganic compounds like NH_3, NO_3^-, or N_2 (see Table 19-1). Interestingly, the energy source for such organisms is obtained from the oxidation of specific inorganic compounds. Which inorganic compound is oxidized depends on the bacteria in question (see Table 19-5). Many autotrophs will not grow on media that contain organic matter, even agar.

Also found among the autotrophic microorganisms are the sulfur-oxidizing or sulfur-compound–oxidizing bacteria, which seldom exhibit a strictly autotrophic mode of metabolism like the obligate nitrifying bacteria (see discussion of nitrogen cycle on page 234). The representative sulfur compounds oxidized by such bacteria are H_2S, S_2, and S_2O_3. Among the sulfur bacteria are two very interesting organisms: *Thiobacillus ferrooxidans*, which gets its energy for autotrophic growth by oxidizing elemental sulfur or ferrous iron, and *T denitrificans*, which gets its energy by oxidizing S_2O_3 anaerobically, using NO_3^- as a sole terminal electron acceptor. *T denitrificans* reduces NO_3^- to molecular N_2, which is liberated as a gas; this biologic process is called **denitrification.**

All autotrophic bacteria must assimilate CO_2, which is reduced to glucose, from which organic cellular matter is synthesized. The energy for this biosynthetic process is

Table 19-5 Inorganic Oxidation Reactions Used by Autotrophic Bacteria as Energy Sources

Chemosynthetic Type	Inorganic Compounds Oxidized as Energy $(\sim E)$ Source	Representative Bacteria* Families (f), Genera (g), and Species (s)	Nitrogen Cycle Reaction
NH_3 oxidizers (aerobic)	$NH_3 \longrightarrow NO_2$ $(\sim E)$ $(\sim E)$ = chemical energy line ATP produced	(f) *Nitrobacteriaceae* (g) *Nitrosomonas* (g) *Nitrosococcus* (g) *Nitrosospira*	Nitrification Nitrification Nitrification Nitrification
NO_2 oxidizers (aerobic)	$NO_2 \longrightarrow NO_3$ $(\sim E)$	(f) *Nitrobacteriaceae* (g) *Nitrobacter* (g) *Nitrococcus*	Nitrification Nitrification Nitrification
Sulfur oxidizers† (aerobic) Iron oxidizers (aerobic)	$S_2 \longrightarrow SO_4$ $(\sim E)$ $Fe^{++} \longrightarrow Fe^{+++}$ $(\sim E)$ use both reactions	(g,s) *Thiobacillus thiooxidans* (g,s) *Thiobacillus ferrooxidans* (g) *Ferrobacillus* (g) *Leptothrix*	— — — —
Sulfur-compound oxidizers (anaerobic)	S_2O_3 oxidized; NO_3 reduced	(g,s) *Thiobacillus denitrificans*	Denitrification

*All are gram-negative species; see Part 12, *Bergey's Manual.*
†Strict autotrophic modes of metabolism are not present in sulfur and sulfur-compound oxidizing bacteria. For example, heterotrophic sulfur-compound oxidizers are known; the aerobic spp being able to oxidize $H_2S \longrightarrow S_2$, for example, *Beggiatoa* and *Thiothrix* spp.
$(\sim E)$

derived from the oxidation of inorganic compounds discussed in the previous paragraph. Note that all autotrophic and phototrophic bacteria possess essentially the same organic cellular constituents found in heterotrophic bacteria; from a nutritional viewpoint, however, the autotrophic mode of metabolism is unique, occurring only in bacteria.

Anaerobic Respiration

Bacteria may also exhibit a unique mode of respiration called anaerobic respiration. This type of metabolism generally occurs with heterotrophic bacteria that will not grow anaerobically unless a specific chemical component, which serves as a terminal electron acceptor, is added to the medium. Among these electron acceptors are NO_3^-, SO_4^-, the organic compound fumarate, and CO_2. Bacteria requiring one of these compounds for anaerobic growth are said to be obligate anaerobic respirers.

A large group of anaerobic respirers are the nitrate reducers (Table 19-2). The nitrate respirers are predominantly heterotrophic bacteria, which possess a complex electron transport system(s) allowing the NO_3^- ion to serve anaerobically as a terminal acceptor of electrons ($NO_3^- \xrightarrow{2e^-} NO_2^-$; $NO_3^- \xrightarrow{5e^-} N_2$; or $NO_3^- \xrightarrow{8e^-} NH_3$). The organic compounds that serve as specific electron donors for these three known nitrate reduction processes are shown in Table 19-6. The nitrate reductase activity is common in bacteria and is routinely used to identify bacteria by the simple nitrate reductase test (see *Bergey's Manual of Determinative Bacteriology*, 8th ed.).

$$4AH_2 + HNO_3 \xrightarrow{\text{Nitrate reduction}} 4A + NH_3 + 3H_2O + \text{Energy}$$

(AH$_2$ = organic substrate, which serves as electron donor)

A second group of anaerobic respirers, the sulfate reducers, utilizes $SO_4^=$ ion in similar fashion ($SO_4^= \xrightarrow{8e^-} H_2S$):

$$4AH_2 + H_2SO_4 \xrightarrow{\text{Sulfate reduction}} 4A + H_2S + 4H_2O + \text{Energy}$$

The third group, the fumarate respirers, are anaerobic bacteria that require exogenously added fumarate to media (HOOC—CH=CH—COOH) in order to grow. Fumarate is reduced to succinate (HOOC—CH$_2$—CH$_2$—COOH), which is secreted as a by-product.

$$AH_2 + HOOC-\overset{\overset{\displaystyle H}{|}}{C}=\overset{\overset{\displaystyle H}{|}}{C}-COOH \xrightarrow{\text{Fumarate reduction}} A + HOOC-CH_2-CH_2-COOH + \text{Energy}$$

Organisms of still another specialized group of anaerobic respirers, the methanogens, which produce methane gas ($CO_2 \xrightarrow{8e^-} CH_4$) as a metabolic end product of microbial growth. H$_2$ gas is the substrate.

$$4H_2 + CO_2 \xrightarrow{\text{CO}_2 \text{ reduction}} CH_4 + 2H_2O + \text{Energy}$$

Table 19-6   Nitrate Reducers (respirers) Among Bacteria

Physiologic Types of Nitrate Reductases	Electron Donor(s)	Representative Organisms
Respiratory ($NO_3^- \rightarrow NO_2^-$)	Formate NADH	E coli K aerogenes
Denitrifying ($NO_3^- \rightarrow N_2$)	NADH Pyruvate NADH, succinate	P aeroginosa C perfringens Paracoccus denitrificans
Assimilatory ($NO_3^- \rightarrow NH_3$)	Lactate H_2, formate NADH, succinate NADH NADH, lactate, glycerol-phosphate	S aureus V succinogenes B stearothermophilus E aerogenes E coli

The methanogens are among the most anaerobic bacteria known, being very sensitive to small concentrations of molecular O_2. They are also archaebacteria, or organisms that live in unusual and deleterious environments.

All of the above anaerobic respirers obtain chemical energy for growth using these anaerobic energy-yielding oxidation reactions.

The Nitrogen Cycle

Nowhere can the total metabolic potential of bacteria and their diverse chemical-transforming capabilities be more fully appreciated than in the geochemical cycling of the element nitrogen (N). All basic chemical elements (S, O, P, C, and H) required to sustain living organisms have geochemical cycles similar to the nitrogen cycle. The recycling process provides the specific chemical components (both organic and inorganic) needed for growth or energy or both. The actual compound needed depends on the nutritional type of organism in question. To sustain life, these basic constituents must be available in sufficient concentrations and in proper environments so they can be utilized as nutrients.

The nitrogen cycle, in an almost ideal manner, demonstrates how bacteria, plants, and animals function in an interdependent ecologic manner. Nitrogen is recycled when organisms utilize one form of nitrogen for growth and excrete another nitrogenous compound as a waste product. This waste product is in turn utilized by another type of organism as a growth or energy substrate. Figure 19-10 shows the nitrogen cycle diagrammatically, enumerating the specific physiologic steps in the chemical transformation of nitrogen.

Ammonification is an essential step in the nitrogen cycle. When the specific breakdown of organic nitrogenous compounds occurs, that is, when proteins are degraded to amino acids (proteolysis) and then to inorganic NH_3 by heterotrophic bacteria, the process is called **ammonification.** At death, the organic constituents of

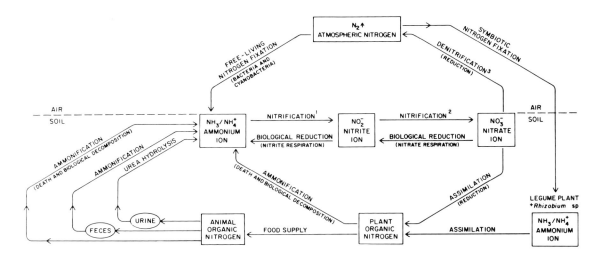

Figure 19-10 The nitrogen cycle.

[1] Carried out primarily by chemoautotrophes of the genus *Nitrosomonas*

[2] Carried out by chemoautotrophes of the genus *Nitrobacter*

[3] Carried out by denitrifying bacteria, a property exhibited by some heterotrophic bacteria

the tissues and cells decompose biologically to inorganic constituents by a process called **mineralization;** these inorganic end products can then serve as nutrients for other life forms. The NH_3 liberated in turn serves as a utilizable nitrogen source for many other bacteria. The breakdown of solid sewage wastes (feces) and soluble wastes (urine) also occurs by ammonification.

The other important biological processes in the nitrogen cycle include: **nitrification** (the conversion of $NH_3 \rightarrow NO_3$ by autotrophes in the soil; **denitrification** (the anaerobic conversion of $NO_3^- \rightarrow N_2$ gas) carried out by many heterotrophes); and finally **nitrogen fixation** ($N_2 \rightarrow NH_3^-$ cell protein). The latter is a very specialized procaryotic process carried out both by free-living bacteria (such as *Azotobacter, Derxia, Beijerinckia* and *Azomonas* spp) as well as by symbionts such as *Rhizobium* spp with legume plants (soybeans, peas, clover, bluebonnets), and *Frankia* spp with angiospermous higher plants, like speckled alder. All plant life relies heavily on the availability of NO_3^- as a nitrogen source; most animals rely on plant life for nutrients.

References

Gibson, T., Gordon, R.E. (editors): *Bergey's Manual of determinative bacteriology,* 8th ed. Baltimore: Williams and Wilkins, 1974.

Green, D.E.: A critique of the chemosmotic model of energy coupling. *Proc Natl Acad Sci USA* 1981; 78:2249–2253.

Haddock, B.A., and Hamilton, W.A. (editors): *Microbial energetics,* 27th Symposium of the Society of General Microbiology. London: Cambridge University Press, 1977.

Hempfling, W.P.: *Microbial respiration.* Benchman Papers in Microbiology No. 13. Stroudsburg, Pa.: Downden, Hutchinson and Ross, 1979.

Hill, R.: The biochemists' green mansions: The photosynthetic electron-transport chain in plants. In *Essays in biochemistry*. Vol 1, Campbell, P.N., Greville, C.D. (editors). New York: Academic Press, 1965.

Jurtshuk, P., Jr., Mueller, T.J., Acord, W.C.: Bacterial terminal oxidases. *CRC Crit Rev Microbiol* 1975; 3:359-368.

Jurtshuk, P., Jr., Liu, J.K.: Cytochrome oxidase and analyses of *Bacillus* strains: Existence of oxidase positive species. *Intern J Syst Bacteria* 1983; 33:887-91.

Jurtshuk, P., Jr., Mueller, T.J., Wong, T.Y.: Isolation and purification of the cytochrome oxidase of *Azotobacter vinelandii*. *Biochim Biophys Acta* 1981; 637:374-382.

Jurtshuk, P., Jr., Yang, T.Y.: Oxygen reactive hemoprotein components in bacterial respiratory systems. In: *Diversity of bacterial respiratory systems*, Vol. 1. Knowles, C.J. (editor). Boca Raton, Fla.: CRC Press, 1980.

Kamp, A.F., La Riviere, J.W.M., Verhoeven, W. (editors): *Jan Albert Kluyver: His life and work*. New York: Interscience, 1959.

Kluyver, J.A., Van Niel, C.B.: *The microbe's contribution to biology*. Cambridge, Mass.: Harvard University Press, 1956.

Kornberg, H.L.: The role and maintenance of the tricarboxylic acid cycle in *Escherichia coli*. In: *British biochemistry past and present*. Goodwin T.W. (editor). Biochemistry Society Symposium No. 30. London: Academic Press, 1970.

Lemberg, R., Barrett, J.: Bacterial cytochromes and cytochrome oxidases. In: *Cytochromes*. New York: Academic Press, 1973.

Mandelstam, J., McQuillen, K., Dawes, I. (editors): *Biochemistry of bacterial growth,* 3rd ed. Oxford: Blackwell Scientific Publications, 1982.

O'Leary, W.M.: *The chemistry and metabolism of microbial lipids*. Cleveland: World Publishing Co., 1967.

Thauer, R.K., Jungermann, K., Decker, K.: Energy conservation in chemotrophic anaerobic bacteria. *Bacteriol Rev* 1977; 41:100-180.

Thimann, K.V.: *The life of bacteria,* 2nd ed. New York: Macmillan, 1966.

20 Genetics

Randall K. Holmes, MD, PhD

General Concepts

Genetics is the biologic science that concerns heredity and variation. When a bacterium is cultivated under defined conditions, its characteristics remain constant from generation to generation. The properties of a bacterium may change if the conditions of cultivation are changed, but the range of possible characteristics is limited and genetically determined. The **genome** is the complete set of genetic determinants of an organism. **Mutations** are heritable changes in the genome that can occur spontaneously or be induced by a variety of chemical or physical agents (mutagenic agents). The specific genetic determinants of a bacterial strain constitute its **genotype;** the observable properties of a bacterium at any particular time are its **phenotype.** Changes in phenotype caused by mutations are called **genotypic variations;** changes that are normal physiologic responses to altered growth conditions are called **phenotypic variations** and result from regulation of gene function.

Most bacteria are haploid and contain one complete set of genetic determinants encoded in their DNA. Plasmids and bacteriophages can provide additional genetic information in bacteria. **Plasmids** are autonomous, self-replicating, extrachromosomal genetic elements that are usually not essential for bacterial survival. **Bacteriophages** (bacterial viruses) are infectious agents that can replicate within bacteria, releasing infectious bacteriophage progeny and usually killing their bacterial hosts. Temperate bacteriophages can also establish **lysogeny,** a state in which the phage genomes are perpetuated as **prophages** in persistently infected bacteria. Bacterial cells can exchange genetic information in several different ways, called **transformation, transduction,** and **conjugation. Transposons** are segments of DNA that behave as mobile genetic elements; they can move from place to place within a genome or between genomes. **Recombination** is the rearrangement of genetic determinants from donor and recipient genomes to form new, hybrid genomes. Mutations are responsible for generating diversity among bacteria; recombination provides a mechanism for reassortment of traits among genetically compatible bacteria.

Hybrid molecules, called **recombinant DNA,** can be made in vitro by joining together fragments of DNA from different sources. Plasmids and viral DNAs can be used as **vectors** into which foreign DNA fragments can be introduced. The insertion of specific genes in such vectors is called **gene cloning.** The structure and function of cloned genes can be analyzed at the molecular level. Recombinant DNA technology and gene cloning are widely used for both basic research and biotechnology, including vaccine development, production of biologics, diagnosis of infectious or genetic diseases, and many other applications.

Nature of Genetic Information in Bacteria

The genetic information of living organisms is encoded in nucleic acids. The genetic material of all bacteria is deoxyribonucleic acid (DNA); bacterial plasmids are also composed of DNA. Bacteriophages have DNA or ribonucleic acid (RNA) as genetic material. The two essential functions of genetic material are replication and expression. Genetic material must replicate accurately so that all progeny of a bacterium inherit the specific genetic determinants (genotype) of the parental organism. When replication is inaccurate, mutations occur. Expression of specific genetic material under a particular set of growth conditions determines the observable characteristics (phenotype) of a microorganism.

Nucleic Acid Structure

Nucleic acids are large polymers consisting of repeating nucleotide units. Figure 20-1 depicts the structure of DNA. Each nucleotide contains one phosphate group, one pentose or deoxypentose sugar, and one purine or pyrimidine base. In DNA, the sugar is

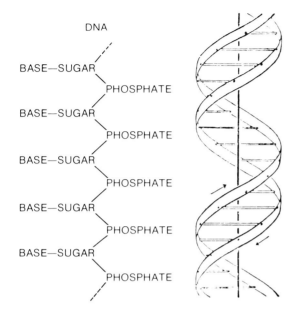

DNA

BASE—SUGAR

PHOSPHATE

BASE—SUGAR

PHOSPHATE

BASE—SUGAR

PHOSPHATE

BASE—SUGAR

PHOSPHATE

BASE—SUGAR

PHOSPHATE

BASE—SUGAR

PHOSPHATE

Figure 20-1 Structure of DNA. Diagram at left illustrates polymeric structure of a single strand of DNA. Backbone is composed of alternating phosphate and D-2-deoxyribose residues joined in phosphodiester linkages; a purine or pyrimidine base is attached to each sugar residue. Diagram on right represents helical structure of double-stranded DNA. The two ribbons symbolize two phosphate-sugar chains with opposite polarities (arrows). Each pair of complementary bases joined by hydrogen bands is represented by a bar extending from one ribbon to the other. The solid vertical line is the axis around which the double helix is oriented. The diameter of the double helix is 2 nm. Each full turn of double helix is 3.4 nm long and corresponds to 10 nucleotide pairs. Reprinted by permission from *Nature*, Vol. 171, p. 964. Copyright © 1953 Macmillan Journals Limited.

D-2-deoxyribose; in ribonucleic acid (RNA), the sugar is D-ribose. In DNA, the purine bases are adenine (A) and guanine (G); the pyrimidine bases are thymine (T) and cytosine (C). In RNA, uracil (U) replaces thymine. Chemically modified purine and pyrimidine bases are found in some bacteria and bacteriophages. The repeating molecular structure of nucleic acids forms a long polymer with alternating sugar and phosphate residues. The 3'-hydroxyl and 5'-hydroxyl groups of adjacent sugar residues are linked by phosphodiester bonds; these chemically asymmetric phosphodiester linkages define a polarity for each single-stranded molecule of nucleic acid. A purine or pyrimidine base is linked at the 1'-carbon atom of each sugar residue and projects from the repeating sugar-phosphate backbone. Double-stranded DNA is arranged in a double helix. The complementary purine and pyrimidine bases on opposite strands are linked by hydrogen bonds and the polarities of the two strands are opposite. Adenine forms hydrogen bonds with thymine; guanine pairs with cytosine. Chemical analyses of double-stranded DNA reveal equimolar amounts of purines and pyrimidines with adenine equal to thymine and guanine equal to cytosine. The amount of guanine plus cytosine (C + G) as a molar fraction of the total purine and pyrimidine bases in double-stranded DNA can vary widely from organism to organism, but the G + C ratio is reproducible and characteristic for each bacterial or viral strain. The extent of nucleotide sequence homology between DNA from different microorganisms is the most stringent criterion for determining how closely they are related.

DNA Replication

Replication of DNA during bacterial growth depends on the structural features previously summarized. Because of the constraints of base pairing in double-stranded DNA, the sequences of purine and pyrimidine bases on the two polynucleotide strands are complementary. Thus, during replication of double-stranded DNA, each polynucleotide strand can serve as the template for enzymatic synthesis of an appropriate complementary strand. Each newly replicated double-stranded DNA molecule thus contains one old polynucleotide strand and one newly synthesized strand. This mechanism for replication of bacterial DNA is called semiconservative. In bacteria, replication of chromosomal DNA occurs at intracellular sites associated with the plasma membrane. When bacteria divide by binary fission after completion of DNA replication, the membrane-associated DNA molecules are partitioned into each of the daughter cells. These characteristics of DNA replication during bacterial growth fulfill the requirements of the genetic material to be reproduced accurately and to be inherited by each daughter cell at the time of cell division.

Transcription and Translation

Genetic information in nucleic acids is encoded in the specific sequences of purine and pyrimidine bases. Genetic information in DNA is expressed by synthesis of specific RNA and protein molecules. Individual strands of DNA can serve not only as templates for synthesis of complementary strands during DNA replication but also as templates for synthesis of complementary single-stranded molecules of RNA. The DNA-directed synthesis of RNA is called transcription. Some RNA molecules, including **ribosomal RNAs (rRNAs)** and **transfer RNAs (tRNAs),** are components of the biosynthetic machinery of bacterial cells. Other RNA molecules, designated **messenger RNAs (mRNAs),** are templates for protein synthesis; their base sequences are translated into the amino acid sequences of specific polypeptides.

How do sequences of the four purine and pyrimidine bases in mRNA molecules determine the sequences of the 20 amino acids in polypeptides? The answer to this question is the essence of the genetic code. In an RNA molecule of random sequence, the base in any single nucleotide is A, G, U, or C. In a random dinucleotide sequence, 16 (4×4) arrangements of the four bases are possible; in a random trinucleotide sequence, 64 $(4 \times 4 \times 4)$ arrangements are possible. Thus, a minimum of three nucleotides is required to provide at least one unique sequence of the bases A, G, U, and C corresponding to each of the 20 amino acids. The genetic code is, in fact, a triplet code in which 61 of the 64 possible triplet sequences (**codons**) correspond to specific amino acids (Table 20-1). Synonyms exist in the code, since more than one codon can specify the same amino acid. The code is described as nonoverlapping because adjacent codons in a mRNA molecule correspond to adjacent trinucleotides, with no overlap in the individual nucleotides of adjacent codons. A region of mRNA that codes for a polypeptide is translated sequentially in the 5' to 3' direction from a specific starting point until a codon is reached that specifies termination of translation. The three chain-terminating codons for polypeptide synthesis are UAA, UAG, and UGA. These chain-terminating codons are also called **nonsense codons.** The nascent polypeptide grows sequentially from its amino-terminal end to its carboxy-terminal end. Thus, the sequence of amino acid residues in a polypeptide is colinear with the sequence of nucleotide residues in the corresponding mRNA and in the DNA molecule from which the mRNA was transcribed. In a double-stranded DNA molecule, only one of the two strands can serve as template for a specific mRNA molecule, because the other strand contains a sequence of bases that is complementary to the template strand and opposite

Table 20-1   The Genetic Code*

First Nucleotide of Codon	Second Nucleotide of Codon				Third Nucleotide of Codon
	U	*C*	*A*	*G*	
U	Phe	Ser	Tyr	Cys	U
	Phe	Ser	Tyr	Cys	C
	Leu	Ser	Termination	Termination	A
	Leu	Ser	Termination	Trp	G
C	Leu	Pro	His	Arg	U
	Leu	Pro	His	Arg	C
	Leu	Pro	His	Arg	A
	Leu	Pro	His	Arg	G
A	Ileu	Thr	Asn	Ser	U
	Ileu	Thr	Asn	Ser	C
	Ileu	Thr	Lys	Arg	A
	Met	Thr	Lys	Arg	G
G	Val	Ala	Asp	Gly	U
	Val	Ala	Asp	Gly	C
	Val	Ala	Glu	Gly	A
	Val	Ala	Glu	Gly	G

*Abbreviations: ala, alanine; arg, arginine; asn, asparagine; asp, aspartic acid; cys, cysteine; gln, glutamine; glu, glutamic acid; gly, glycine; his, histidine; ileu, isoleucine; leu, leucine; lys, lysine; met, methionine; phe, phenylalanine; pro, proline; ser, serine; thr, threonine; tyr, tyrosine; trp, tryptophan; val, valine.

in polarity. Specific enzymatic reactions involved in DNA, RNA, and protein synthesis are beyond the scope of this chapter, and the interested reader is directed to the references.

Expression of genetic determinants in bacteria involves the unidirectional flow of information from DNA to RNA to protein. In bacteriophages, either DNA or RNA can serve as genetic material. During infection of bacteria by RNA bacteriophages, RNA molecules are templates for RNA replication and also carry messages for protein synthesis. Studies with oncogenic (tumor-inducing) RNA animal viruses reveal that DNA molecules can be synthesized from RNA templates by enzymes designated as RNA-dependent DNA polymerases (reverse transcriptases). This reversal of the usual direction for flow of genetic information, from RNA to DNA instead of from DNA to RNA, is an important mechanism for enabling information from RNA tumor viruses to be encoded in DNA and to become incorporated into the genomes of animal cells.

Organization of Genetic Material

Chromosomal DNA

The common intestinal bacterium *Escherichia coli* contains about 2.4×10^9 daltons of DNA per cell—only 0.1% of the DNA in a human cell. The simplest, free-living bacteria (genus *Mycoplasma*) have significantly smaller genomes than *E coli* and contain about

0.5×10^9 daltons of DNA. The DNA content of a cell determines the maximum amount of genetic information that can be present. For example, the DNA of *E coli* is about four million nucleotide pairs, sufficient to code for several thousand different polypeptides of 30,000–60,000 daltons each.

Although prokaryotic cells do not contain chromosomes like those of eukaryotic cells, the DNA corresponding to the bacterial genome is often called the bacterial chromosome. Genetic and biochemical data indicate that the chromosome of *E coli* is a single circular molecule of double-stranded DNA with a contour length of approximately 1.35 mm. The DNA is several hundred times longer than the bacterial cell, and it is present within the bacterium in a tightly packed state. Nevertheless, replication of the chromosomal DNA in *E coli* is a highly coordinated process, as depicted in Figure 20-2. Synthesis of DNA is initiated in a specific region of the chromosome called the origin of replication. DNA synthesis proceeds sequentially from the origin in a bidirectional manner until the entire chromosome has been replicated. The replication of DNA in *E coli* is complex and is known to involve many different proteins.

The chromosome of *E coli* is thus a single molecule of DNA that replicates as a unit within the bacterial cell. DNA molecules coding for functions that permit them to replicate as discrete units in bacteria are called **replicons.** In some *E coli* strains, chromosomal DNA corresponds to the entire complement of DNA within the cell; other bacterial strains may have additional replicons.

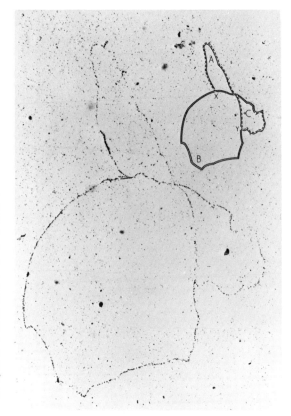

Figure 20-2 Autoradiograph of intact replicating chromosome of *E coli.* Bacteria were radioactively labeled with tritiated thymidine for approximately two generations and were lysed gently. Bacterial DNA was then examined by autoradiography. Insert shows replicating bacterial chromosome in diagrammatic form. The chromosome is circular, and two forks (X and Y) are present in replicating structure. The segments of chromosome represented by double lines had completed two replications in presence of tritiated thymidine, whereas segments represented by a solid line and a dotted line had replicated only once in presence of tritiated thymidine. The density of grains in the autoradiogram was twice as great in the segments of chromosome that had completed two cycles of replication in presence of tritiated thymidine. Bar, 100 μm. From Cairns, J.P.: *Cold Spring Harbor Symposia on Quantitative Biology* 1963; 28:44.

Plasmids

Plasmids are replicons that are maintained as discrete, extrachromosomal genetic elements in bacteria. Usually, the bacterial chromosome codes for all metabolic functions that are essential for bacterial viability, and the functions encoded by plasmids are not essential. Plasmids vary considerably in size, but are usually much smaller than the bacterial chromosome. The average number of copies of a plasmid per copy of the bacterial chromosome is called its copy number. The copy number is characteristic for each plasmid but can vary from plasmid to plasmid. Large plasmids often are present in small numbers (sometimes only one per chromosome), whereas small plasmids often are present in larger numbers (10-20 per chromosome).

Plasmids are classified into two major groups: conjugative and nonconjugative. Conjugative plasmids code for functions that promote transfer of plasmid DNA from one bacterial cell to another. Nonconjugative plasmids do not promote their own transfer from cell to cell. Some plasmids control important phenotypic properties of pathogenic bacteria, such as resistance to multiple antibiotics and production of toxins, colonization (adherence) factors, or other virulence factors. Other plasmids are cryptic and have no recognizable effects on the phenotypes of the bacterial cells that harbor them. Examples of medically important toxins that can be encoded by plasmids include heat-labile and heat-stable enterotoxins of *Escherichia coli,* exfoliative toxin of *Staphylococcus aureus,* and tetanus toxin produced by *Clostridium tetani.* The biologic significance of plasmids in the evolution of resistance to antibiotics and the role of some conjugative plasmids as sex factors in bacteria are discussed further in subsequent sections of this chapter.

Bacteriophages

Bacteriophages (bacterial viruses, phage) are infectious agents that replicate as obligate intracellular parasites in bacteria. The life cycle of phages includes an extracellular phase in which they exist as metabolically inert, infectious particles called virions; these particles can be visualized by electron microscopy.

Several distinct morphologic classes of phage have been described; these include polyhedral, filamentous, and complex virions. Bacteriophages with complex virions have polyhedral heads to which tails and other appendages may be attached, as illustrated in Figure 20-3. Chemical analyses indicate that phages contain protein and DNA or RNA as major components. A few phages contain lipids and are highly susceptible to inactivation by lipid solvents. The nucleic acid of bacteriophages is tightly packaged, and the proteins of the virion are arranged in an organized array to form a protective shell surrounding the nucleic acid. Infection of bacteria is initiated by absorption of virions to specific receptors on the bacterial surface, followed by entry of the phage DNA or RNA into the bacterial cells. During lytic infections, the bacteriophage RNA or DNA is replicated to produce many new copies of the phage genome, and phage-specific proteins are synthesized within the bacterium. Next, progeny are assembled from the phage structural components in the cytoplasm of the infected bacteria. Finally, the newly formed virions are released, usually by cell lysis. For discussions of structure, multiplication, and classification of animal viruses, see Section IV.

Bacteriophages are classified into two major groups: virulent and temperate.

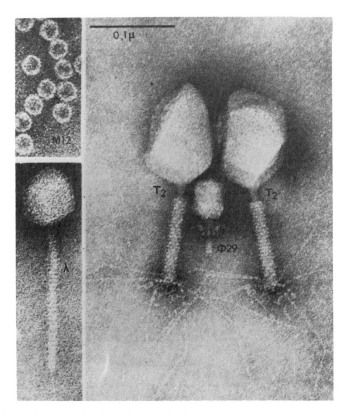

Figure 20-3 Morphology of selected bacteriophages. Electron micrographs of negatively stained virions of phages M12, λ, T2, and ϕ29 at same magnification. M12 is a small polyhedral phage containing an RNA genome and 180 copies of a single structural polypeptide. Phages λ, T2, and ϕ29 are DNA phages with complex structures involving several different kinds of structural polypeptides. Negatively stained preparations of ϕ29 and T2 are by D.L. Anderson, and preparation of λ is by F. Eiserling. From Kellenberger, E., Edgar, S.: In: *The bacteriophage lambda.* Hershey, A.D. (editor). Cold Spring Harbor, N.Y.: Cold Spring Harbor Laboratories, p. 272, 1971.

Growth of virulent phages in susceptible bacteria eventually destroys bacterial cells. The life cycle of temperate phages is more complex. Infection of susceptible bacteria by temperate phages can have either of two different outcomes: lytic growth or lysogeny. Lytic growth of temperate and virulent bacteriophages is similar, leading to production of progeny and death of the host bacteria. In contrast, lysogeny is a specific type of persistent infection in which the phage genome replicates as a genetic determinant (prophage) in the bacterial cell. The physical state of the prophage is not identical for all temperate viruses. For example, the prophage of bacteriophage λ in *E coli* is integrated into the bacterial chromosome at a specific site and replicates as part of the bacterial chromosome, whereas the prophage of bacteriophage P1 in *E coli* replicates as a plasmid.

Although lysogenic bacteria harbor the genomes of temperate phages as prophage, they do not normally contain infectious virions. In cultures of lysogenic bacteria, however, lytic phage development occurs spontaneously in a small fraction of the cells, leading to release of infectious phages. For some temperate phages, the change from the lysogenic state to lytic growth can be induced by treating the bacterial cultures with physical or chemical agents such as ultraviolet light or mitomycin C. Sometimes the genetic information corresponding to the prophage in a lysogenic cell is lost, and the cell becomes nonlysogenic. The loss of a prophage or a plasmid from a bacterial cell is called curing.

Some temperate phages contain genes that determine bacterial properties; these determinants are not essential for lytic bacteriophage growth or maintenance of the prophage. Phenotypic expression of phage genes that determine bacterial properties is called phage conversion. Examples of phage conversion that are important for medical microbiology include production of diphtheria toxin in *Corynebacterium diphtheriae*, production of erythrogenic toxin in *Streptococcus pyogenes*, production of botulinum toxin in some strains of *Clostridium botulinum*, and control of O antigen specificity in many strains of *Salmonella*.

Mutation and Selection

Mutations are heritable changes in the genome. Spontaneous mutations occur randomly and infrequently in individual bacteria. Some mutations cause changes in phenotypic characteristics; the occurrence of such mutations can be inferred from the phenotypic effects they produce. In studies of bacterial genetics, specific reference bacteria are designated as wild-type strains. Descendants of wild-type strains that have mutations in their genomes are called **mutants.** Thus, mutants are characterized by the inherited differences between them and the ancestral wild-type strains. To simplify the description of bacterial genotypes, symbols are used as convenient abbreviations for genetic determinants. Plus signs are used as superscripts with genotypic symbols to designate the specific determinants in a wild-type strain. For example, the genotypic symbol for the ability to ferment lactose is lac^+, and mutants that cannot ferment lactose are designated *lac*. Similar genotypic symbols are used to describe genetic determinants of bacteriophages or plasmids.

Selective and Differential Media

Selective and differential media are helpful for isolating bacterial mutants. Some selective media permit particular mutants to grow but do not allow the wild-type strains to grow. Rare mutants can be isolated by using such selective media. Differential media permit both wild-type and mutant bacteria to grow and form colonies that differ in appearance. Detection of rare mutants on differential media may be limited by constraints on the total number of colonies that can be observed. The examples in the following paragraphs illustrate some general principles concerning the use of selective and differential media for isolating bacterial mutants.

Consider a wild-type strain of *E coli* that is susceptible to the antibiotic streptomycin (genotypic symbol: str^s) and can utilize lactose as the sole source of carbon (genotypic symbol: lac^+). Streptomycin-resistant (str^r) mutants can grow in selective media containing high concentrations of streptomycin, but the wild-type str^s bacteria will be killed. Although spontaneously occurring str^r mutants are rare and are usually found at frequencies of less than one per 10^9 bacteria in cultures of wild-type *E coli*, such str^r mutants can be isolated easily by using selective media.

Isolation of lactose-negative (*lac*) mutants of *E coli* poses a different set of practical problems. On minimal media with lactose as the sole source of carbon, lac^+ wild-type strains can grow, but *lac* mutants will not grow. On differential media such as MacConkey's agar or eosin-methylene blue-lactose agar, *lac*⁺ wild-type and *lac* mutant strains of *E coli* can be distinguished, but spontaneous *lac* mutants may be too rare to be isolated easily. Selective media for *lac* mutants of *E coli* can be made by incorporating chemical analogs of lactose that are converted into toxic metabolites by *lac*⁺ bacteria but not by *lac* mutants. The *lac* mutants can grow on such media, but the *lac*⁺ wild-type bacteria are killed.

Spontaneous Mutations

In analyzing the origin of bacterial mutations, investigators sought to determine whether mutations occurred spontaneously in the absence of selective agents or were induced by exposure to the selective agents. They established that spontaneous mutations in bacteria can occur in the absence of selective agents. This principle was first demonstrated by using a statistical method known as the fluctuation test, represented diagrammatically in Figure 20-4. The frequencies of occurrence of phage-resistant

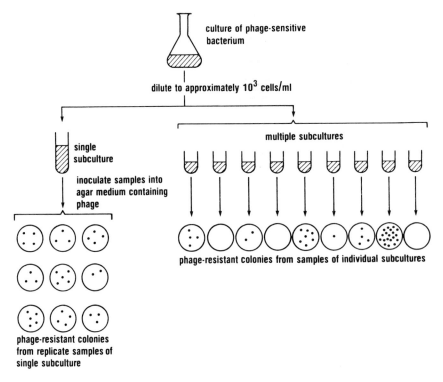

Figure 20-4 The fluctuation test. Differences in numbers of colonies of phage-resistant mutants in replicate samples from single subculture were small and reflected only expected fluctuations due to sampling errors. In contrast, numbers of phage-resistant colonies in samples from individual subcultures were more variable and reflected both sampling errors and the independent origins of mutants in individual subcultures. Sizes of clonal populations of mutants in each culture reflected numbers of generations of growth between times that mutations occurred and time of sampling.

mutants of *E coli* were measured and compared in replicate cultures grown from small inocula, and in replicate samples taken from a single bacterial culture. If the phage-resistant mutants arose only after exposure of the bacteria to the phage, the distribution of mutant frequencies should have been similar under both sets of conditions. In contrast, if the phage-resistant mutants arose during bacterial growth before exposure to the phage, the distribution of mutant frequencies should have been more variable for the replicate cultures grown independently from small inocula. The experimental data supported the second model and proved that mutations conferring resistance to phage T1 in *E coli* occurred spontaneously during growth of the bacteria in the absence of the phage.

Subsequently, the technique called **replica plating** was used to confirm the spontaneous origin of bacterial mutants. For replica plating, a flat, sterile, velveteen surface is used to pick up an inoculum from the surface of an agar plate called the master plate and to transfer samples to other agar plates called the replica plates. In this manner, samples of the bacterial population from the master plate can be transferred to replica plates without distorting their spatial arrangement.

In Figure 20-5, a sample of a bacteriophage-susceptible strain of *E coli* was inoculated onto the master plate and allowed to grow in the absence of phage. Before the bacterial inoculum was transferred from the master plate, the surfaces of the replica plates were inoculated with phage. The susceptible bacteria transferred to the replica plates were killed by infection with the phage, and colonies were formed on the replica plates only by mutant bacteria resistant to phage infection. After the positions on the replica plates at which resistant bacterial colonies developed were noted, bacteria were recovered from corresponding positions on the master plate and tested for resistance to phage. In this manner, phage-resistant mutants of *E coli* that had never been exposed to the selective action of the bacteriophage were isolated. Similar experiments were performed using streptomycin as the selective agent, and str^r mutants were isolated from wild-type *E coli* that never had been exposed to streptomycin. These experiments demonstrated that mutations conferring resistance had occurred spontaneously without exposure of the bacteria to the selective agents.

Structural Genes

Mutations in bacteria can be analyzed in terms of their effects on the function of genetic determinants, the structure of genetic material, or both. Because bacteria have few genetically determined structural or developmental features that can be observed easily, changes in biochemical capabilities are useful for analysis as phenotypic manifestations of mutations. For example, mutants may lose the ability to catabolize particular organic compounds or to synthesize specific amino acids, purines, pyrimidines, sugars, vitamins, or other required molecules. Early studies with the mold *Neurospora crassa* demonstrated that specific biochemical mutants had genetic defects in specific enzymes. These observations provided the basis for the one gene–one enzyme hypothesis. Subsequent investigations established that many sequences of DNA in bacterial genomes are transcribed into mRNA and translated into specific polypeptides. The individual polypeptides function as discrete units in bacterial metabolism, as enzymes, subunits of enzymes, or structural components of bacterial cells. Therefore the one gene–one

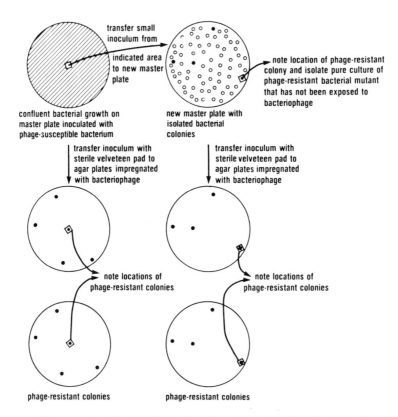

Figure 20-5 Detecting bacterial mutants by replica plating. Master plate was heavily inoculated with sample from pure culture of phage-susceptible bacterium. After incubation, bacteria from master plate were transferred by replica plating to duplicate agar plates impregnated with bacteriophage. Phage-susceptible bacteria were killed by the bacteriophage. Colonies of phage-resistant bacteria appeared at identical positions on duplicate plates, indicating that phage-resistant bacteria had been transferred to each replica plate from the corresponding locations on master plate. Bacterial inocula selected from appropriate locations on master plate contained a higher proportion of phage-resistant mutants than original bacterial culture. By repeating these procedures several times, it was possible to isolate pure cultures of phage-resistant bacterial mutants that had never been exposed to bacteriophage.

enzyme hypothesis was replaced by the one gene–one polypeptide concept. However, other DNA sequences are transcribed into tRNAs or rRNAs that also serve as discrete functional units in bacterial metabolism without being translated into polypeptides. Therefore, it is appropriate to define structural genes as segments of the genome coding for specific macromolecular products that function as discrete units in cellular metabolism. Structural genes are also called **cistrons.**

Complementation Tests

Complementation tests are used to determine if mutations in independently isolated mutant strains with similar phenotypes are located in the same or different structural genes (Figure 20-6). Complementation tests are performed with partially diploid bacterial strains that contain two copies of the region of the bacterial chromosome harboring the mutations, with each copy derived from a different mutant strain. If both mutations inactivate the same gene product, then the partially diploid strain will express the mutant phenotype. In contrast, if the two mutations are in different cistrons, then a wild-type gene corresponding to each mutant structural gene will be present. If the products of the wild-type structural genes can function normally in the partially diploid cell, the wild-type phenotype will be expressed. This phenomenon is called **complementation.** Thus, a positive result in a complementation test indicates that the two mutations being tested are in different cistrons. Complementation tests can be performed and interpreted even if the specific biochemical functions of the gene products are unknown.

As an example, consider using a complementation test to characterize two independently derived *lac* mutants of *E coli*. The biochemical pathway for utilization of lactose requires β-galactoside permease (structural gene: *lacY*) to transport lactose into the bacterial cell and β-galactosidase (structural gene: *lacZ*) to convert lactose into D-glucose and D-galactose. Mutants that lack β-galactoside permease or β-galactosidase cannot utilize lactose for growth. If the mutations in both *lac* mutants inactivated the same gene product, either β-galactoside permease or β-galactosidase, then a partially diploid strain containing the *lac* genes from both mutants would be unable to utilize lactose and complementation would not be observed. In contrast, if the genotypes of the two mutants were *lacZ$^+$ lacY* and *lacZ lacY$^+$*, the partially diploid bacterium would produce active β-galactosidase from the *lacZ$^+$* determinant and active β-galactoside permease from the *lacY$^+$* determinant. Complementation would occur under these circumstances, and the partially diploid strain would be able to utilize lactose.

Molecular Basis of Mutations

Because DNA is the genetic material of bacteria, the molecular basis for mutation is alteration of the nucleotide sequence of DNA. Thus, mutations can be classified on the

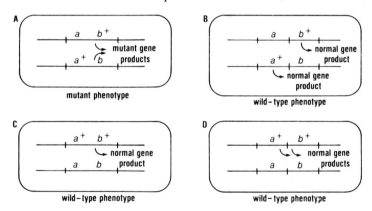

Figure 20-6 Complementation tests. Two mutants with similar phenotypes were isolated. Mutations in these strains were designated *a* and *b*, and the wild-type alleles were *a$^+$* and *b$^+$*. Partially diploid heterozygous strains containing *a*, *a$^+$*, *b*, and *b$^+$* were constructed and tested to determine if the mutations *a* and *b* were in same structural gene (cistron). **A,** If *a* and *b* are in the same structural gene, neither *ab$^+$* nor *a$^+$b* codes for the normal gene product. The mutant phenotype will be expressed (no complementation occurs). **B,** If *a* and *b* are in different cistrons, the *a$^+$* and *b$^+$* determinants code for normal gene products. In the presence of the *a$^+$* and *b$^+$* gene products, the wild-type phenotype is expressed (complementation occurs). **C** and **D,** These strains are tested as positive controls to demonstrate that presence of *a* and *b* mutations in heterozygous cells does not interfere with expression of wild-type *a$^+$b$^+$* chromosomal segment.

Table 20-2 Classification of Mutations

Change in DNA	Effect on Polypeptide Structure	Effect on Function of Polypeptide	Comments
Nucleotide substitution	1. None	1. None	1. Silent mutation (no phenotypic change)
	2. Amino acid substitution	2. Variable	2. Missense mutation (usually CRM$^+$)*
	3. Premature termination	3. Usually lost	3. Nonsense mutations (CRM$^-$ or CRM$^+$); Extragenic suppression common
Microdeletion or microinsertion	Frameshift mutation	Usually lost	Intragenic suppression common
Large insertions	Altered	Usually lost	See section on transposons
Large deletions	Altered	Usually lost	Do not revert

*CRM, cross-reacting material. Mutant polypeptides are CRM$^+$ if they share antigenic determinants with the corresponding wild-type polypeptides.

basis of the kinds of structural changes that occur in DNA, which are summarized in Table 20-2. Some mutations are localized within short segments of DNA (for example, nucleotide substitutions, microdeletions, and microinsertions). Other mutations involve large regions of DNA and include deletions, insertions, or other rearrangements of segments of DNA.

Nucleotide substitutions are called **transitions** when a pyrimidine is substituted for another pyrimidine or a purine is substituted for another purine within a single polynucleotide strand in DNA. Substitution of a purine for a pyrimidine or vice versa is called a **transversion.** If a nucleotide substitution occurs in a region of DNA that codes for a polypeptide, one of the three nucleotides within a single codon of a corresponding mRNA molecule will be changed. Because synonyms exist in the genetic code, some substitutions cause the exchange of one codon in mRNA for another that codes for the same amino acid, and no change in polypeptide structure or function occurs. Other substitutions cause one amino acid to be replaced by another at the specific position within the polypeptide corresponding to the altered codon. Mutations that result in replacement of one amino acid for another within a polypeptide chain are called **missense mutations.** The effects of amino acid replacements on the function of a polypeptide gene product can vary and depend on the location and the identity of the amino acid replacement. Mutant polypeptides containing amino acid replacements usually share antigenic determinants with the wild-type polypeptide and often have some residual biologic activity. Still other nucleotide substitutions in DNA create chain-terminating codons within the mRNA. These are also called **nonsense muta-tions.** Premature chain termination during polypeptide synthesis produces an amino-terminal fragment of the normal polypeptide gene product. Mutations that produce premature chain termination often result in complete loss of biologic activity.

Because of the triplet nature of the genetic code, the consequences of mutations caused by insertions or deletions of small numbers of nucleotides (microinsertions, microdeletions) depend on the number of nucleotides involved and on the specific sequences of those oligonucleotides. Deletion or addition of multiples of three nucleotide pairs decreases or increases the number of codons in mRNA without affecting the reading frame, causing deletion or addition of appropriate numbers of amino acids at one site within the polypeptide gene product. If a new chain-terminating codon is introduced, premature chain termination occurs within the polypeptide gene product. In contrast, addition or deletion of other numbers of nucleotide pairs alters the reading frame for the entire segment of mRNA from the mutation to the distal end of the structural gene. Therefore, frameshift mutations are likely to cause drastic changes in the structure and activity of polypeptide gene products.

Reversion and Suppression

Mutations that convert the phenotype from wild-type to mutant are called **forward mutations.** Other mutations change the phenotype from mutant back to wild-type and are called **reverse mutations** (reversions). Bacterial strains that contain reverse mutations are called **revertants.** Analysis of mutations that cause phenotypic reversion yields useful information. Reverse mutations that restore the exact nucleotide sequence of the wild-type DNA are true reversions. True revertants are identical to wild-type strains genotypically and phenotypically. Reverse mutations that do not restore the exact nucleotide sequence of the wild-type DNA are called **suppressor mutations** (suppressors). Some revertants that harbor suppressor mutations are phenotypically indistinguishable from wild-type strains. Other revertants, called pseudorevertants, can be distinguished phenotypically from wild-type strains, for example, by subtle differences in the characteristics of an enzymatic activity that has been regained (such as specific activity, substrate specificity, kinetic constants, or susceptibility to thermal or chemical inactivation). Recognition of pseudorevertant phenotypes should suggest the presence of suppressor mutations.

Suppressor mutations can be intragenic or extragenetic in location. Intragenic suppressors are located in the same structural genes as the forward mutations that they suppress. Within any given structural gene, the possible locations and nature of intragenic suppressors are variable and are determined by the original forward mutation and by the relationships between the primary structure of the gene product and its biologic activity. Extragenic suppressors are located in different structural genes than are the forward mutations whose phenotypic effects they suppress. The ability of extragenic suppressors to suppress a variety of independent mutations can be tested. Some extragenic suppressors are specific for particular genes, some are specific for particular codons, and some have other specificity patterns. Extragenic suppressor mutations that reverse the phenotypic effects of specific chain-terminating codons have been well characterized and found to alter the structure of specific tRNAs. A particular suppressor tRNA can permit a specific chain-terminating codon to be translated, resulting in incorporation of a specific amino acid into the nascent polypeptide at the position corresponding to the chain-terminating codon. In a bacterium that has a chain-terminating mutation in a structural gene and an appropriate extragenic suppressor, translation of the mRNA for that structural gene can lead to premature chain-termination or to formation of a suppressed full-length polypeptide. Individual suppressor tRNAs that recognize the same chain-terminating codon but specify different amino acids can differ in their efficiency for translating the chain-terminating codon. The biologic activity of the suppressed mutant protein therefore depends on the amount of protein made and on the functional consequences of the specific amino acid replacement determined by the suppressor tRNA.

Conditionally Lethal Mutations

If the function of a particular gene is essential for survival of a haploid bacterium, a mutation that destroys the activity on that gene will be lethal; however, under certain experimental conditions, mutations that inactivate essential genes can be studied. For example, a chain-terminating mutation that inactivates an essential gene is lethal in a wild-type strain of *E coli* but may not be lethal if an appropriate, codon-specific, extragenic suppressor is present simultaneously in the bacterial cell. Similarly, a mutation that increases the thermolability of an essential gene product may prevent growth of an *E coli* strain at 42 C, although the mutant may still grow at 25 C. These examples illustrate the properties of conditionally lethal mutations. Expression of conditionally lethal mutations (bacterial death) occurs only under nonpermissive conditions subject to experimental control. Temperature-sensitive mutations and suppressible, chain-terminating mutations in essential genes are the best-studied classes of conditional lethal mutations and have been extremely useful for experimental studies of genetics in bacteria and bacteriophages.

Mutation Rates

The rate at which mutations occur in bacteria is determined in part by the accuracy of DNA replication and repair of damage to DNA. For a particular bacterial strain under defined growth conditions, the mutation rate for any specific gene is constant and can be expressed as the probability of mutation per cell division. Although the mutation rate remains constant, the proportion of mutants in a bacterial population changes progressively as growth occurs.

Both environmental and genetic factors affect mutation rates. Exposure of bacteria to mutagenic agents causes mutation rates to increase, sometimes by several orders of magnitude. Many chemical and physical agents, including X rays and ultraviolet light, have mutagenic activity. Chemicals that are carcinogenic for animals are often mutagenic for bacteria, or can be converted by animal tissues to metabolites that are mutagenic for bacteria. Standardized tests for mutagenicity in bacteria are useful screening procedures to identify environmental agents that may be carcinogenic in humans. Mutator genes in bacteria are genes that cause an increase in spontaneous mutation rates for a wide variety of other genes. The overall mutation rate, the probability that a mutation will occur somewhere in the bacterial genome per cell division, appears to be a significant factor in determining the fitness of a bacterial strain for survival in nature. The high probability that most mutations will be deleterious for individual bacteria must be balanced against the positive value of mutability as a mechanism for adaptation of bacterial populations to changing environmental conditions.

Exchange of Genetic Information

The interaction of parental bacteria to produce recombinant progeny has two principal requirements. First, all or part of the genome of the donor bacterium must enter the recipient bacterium. Second, a hybrid genome must be formed. The reassortment of genetic determinants from donor and recipient genomes to form new hybrid genomes is called recombination. Generally, recombination does not occur unless the donor and recipient bacteria are from the same or closely related taxonomic groups.

Detection of recombinant bacteria requires two additional criteria. The phenotypes of the parental bacteria must be sufficiently different to distinguish appropriate recombinants from the parental strains. After a recombinant genome is formed, at least one generation of growth may be required before the recombinant bacterium can be detected. This lag may be due to the time required for segregation of the haploid, recombinant genome (segregation lag), or for physiologic expression of the recombinant phenotype (phenotypic lag), or both. Because the mechanisms for exchange of genetic information in bacteria are often inefficient, recombinant bacteria may be rare. Appropriate selective media are useful for detecting rare bacterial recombinants.

Testing for linkage (nonrandom reassortment of parental genes in the recombinant progeny) is possible if the parental bacterial strains differ with respect to several genetic determinants. If two different genes are linked, they are more likely to be coinherited from the donor parent than if they are not linked. Quantitative analysis of linkage permits construction of genetic maps. The genetic map of *E coli* is circular and is illustrated in Figure 20-7. Some genomes have been studied by genetic mapping (linkage analysis) and by physical mapping (determining gene locations on DNA molecules). Colinearity between the arrangements of genes on the genetic maps and the corresponding DNA molecules has been demonstrated. Similar genetic mapping procedures can be used to analyze recombination in bacteriophages and plasmids.

Several mechanisms exist for exchange of genetic information in bacteria. These mechanisms differ in the way DNA is transferred from one bacterial cell into the cytoplasm of another bacterium (Figure 20-8). In transformation, pieces of extracellular DNA released from donor bacteria are taken up directly by recipient bacteria. In transduction, fragments of DNA from donor bacteria are packaged in bacteriophage virions replacing phage DNA; the aberrant virions serve as vectors for transfer of the donor DNA into phage-susceptible, recipient bacteria. In conjugation, donor and recipient bacteria establish cell-to-cell contact and DNA is transferred from donor to recipient bacteria through cytoplasmic bridges. Although the entire bacterial chromosome can be transferred from donor to recipient bacteria by conjugation, transfer of fragments of the bacterial chromosome of varying size is much more likely. Therefore, the zygotes that occur as transient intermediates in the formation of bacterial recombinants by transformation, transduction, or conjugation are usually merozygotes (partial zygotes).

Transformation

Transformation was discovered in *Streptococcus pneumoniae* and has been reported in other bacterial genera including *Haemophilus, Neisseria, Bacillus,* and *Staphylococcus.* One

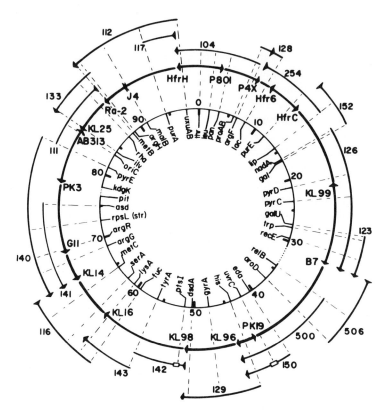

Figure 20-7 Circular genetic map of *E coli*. Positions of representative genes are indicated on inner circle. Distances between genes are calibrated in minutes, based on times required for transfer during conjugation. Position of threonine (*thr*) locus is arbitrarily designated as 0 minutes, and other assignments are relative to *thr*. On next circle, symbols and arrowheads identify specific Hfr donor strains of *E coli* and their characteristics. For each Hfr strain the point of arrowhead is the origin for chromosomal transfer; oriented transfer of chromosome during conjugation proceeds from point of arrowhead, followed immediately by base of the arrowhead, and so on. F′ plasmids are identified by numbers, and the fragment of the *E coli* chromosome present in each F′ plasmid is represented by an arc corresponding to a specific segment of the circular genetic map. See text for definitions of Hfr and F′ donor strains and for description of the conjugal mating system in *E coli*. From Bachman, B.J., Low, K.B. *Microbiol Rev* 1980; 44:31.

of the genetic traits analyzed extensively in early studies of transformation was control of type-specificity of the capsular polysaccharides that are essential virulence factors in *S pneumoniae*. Characterization of the transforming principle from *S pneumoniae* provided the first direct evidence that DNA is the genetic material of bacteria.

To be highly active in transformation, DNA molecules must be quite large (approximately 3×10^5 daltons or larger). Transforming activity is destroyed rapidly by treatment of the DNA with deoxyribonuclease. In transformation, recombination occurs between single molecules of transforming DNA and the chromosomes of individual recipient bacteria. Because large molecules of transforming DNA correspond to small fragments of the bacterial chromosome, simultaneous transformation of two or

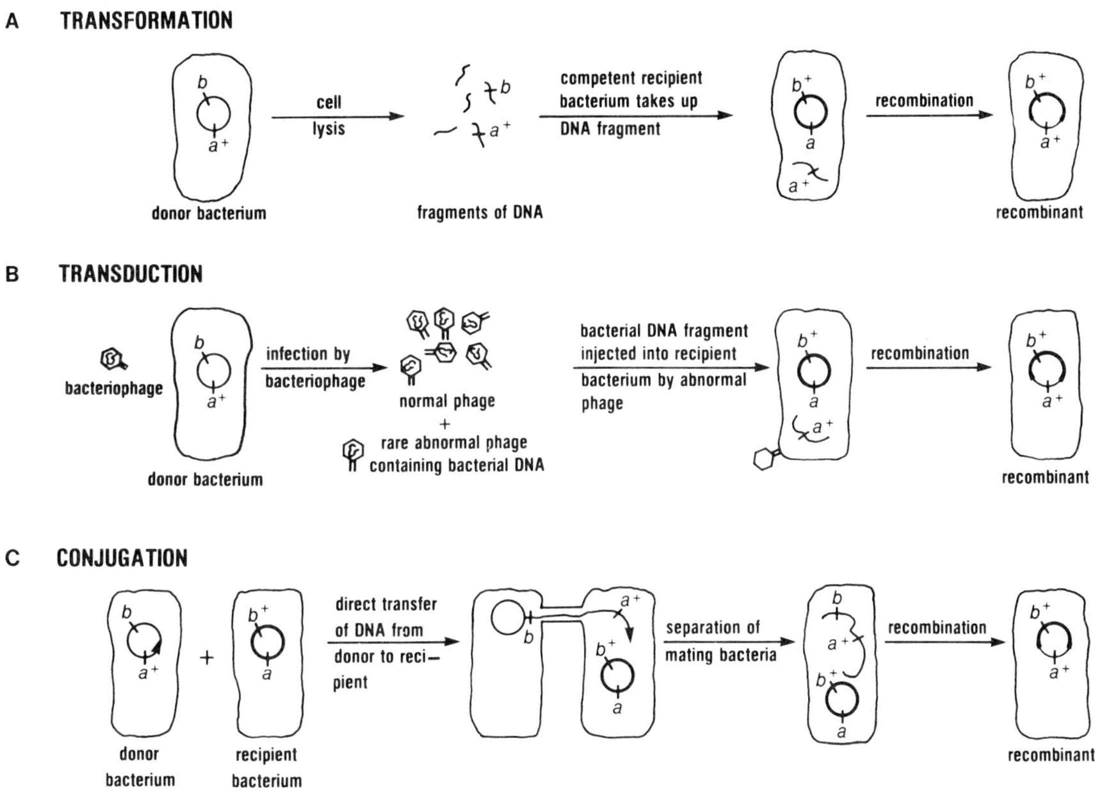

A   TRANSFORMATION

B   TRANSDUCTION

C   CONJUGATION

Figure 20-8 Exchange of genetic information in bacteria. Transformation, transduction, and conjugation differ in means for introducing DNA from donor cell into recipient cell. **A,** In transformation, fragments of DNA released from donor bacteria are taken up by competent recipient bacteria. **B,** In transduction, abnormal bacteriophage particles containing DNA from donor bacteria inject their DNA into recipient bacteria. **C,** Conjugation occurs by formation of cytoplasmic connections between donor and recipient bacteria, with direct transfer of newly synthesized donor DNA into the recipient cells. In all three cases, recombination between donor and recipient DNA molecules is required for formation of stable recombinant genomes. Bacterial genome is represented diagrammatically as a circular element in bacterial cells. Donor and recipient DNA are indicated by fine lines and heavy lines, respectively. In each recombinant genome, the a^+ allele from donor strain has replaced the a allele from recipient strain, and the b^+ allele is derived from recipient strain.

more traits is unlikely unless the appropriate genes are so closely linked that they can be encoded on a single DNA fragment. The ability of bacteria to take up extracellular DNA and to become transformed is called **competence** and varies with the physiologic state of the bacteria. Recent studies of transformation in *Haemophilus* and *Neisseria* have demonstrated that uptake of transforming DNA of these bacteria depends on recognition of specific oligonucleotide sequences. In contrast, uptake of DNA by *S pneumoniae* is not sequence-specific. Competent bacteria can also take up intact bacteriophage DNA or plasmid DNA; this process is called **transfection.** A replicon such as a plasmid can replicate as an extrachromosomal genetic element after it is introduced into a recipient bacterium by transfection. In contrast, a piece of chromosomal DNA from a donor bacterium cannot be maintained permanently in a recipient bacterium unless it becomes part of a hybrid replicon by recombination. Transformation has also been demonstrated with appropriate donor and recipient bacteria when they are cultured together or are used simultaneously to infect experimental animals.

Transduction

During lytic growth of bacteriophages, mature virions are assembled from their structural components in infected bacterial cells. For some DNA-containing bacterio-phages (called generalized transducing phages), the mechanisms responsible for packaging of DNA can permit rare, aberrant virions to form that contain bacterial DNA instead of phage DNA. The pieces of bacterial DNA packaged in this manner are bacterial genome fragments that are comparable in size to the phage genome. When a susceptible bacterium is infected by a transducing phage, the DNA fragment derived from the donor bacterium is injected into the recipient bacterium. Recombination can then occur between the genome of the recipient bacterium and the DNA fragment from the donor bacterium. Because any gene from the donor can be introduced into the recipient and appear in recombinant progeny, this process is called generalized transduction. Major differences between generalized transduction and transformation include the larger size of the donor DNA fragment transferred by transduction and resistance of the donor DNA fragment in a transducing bacteriophage to degradation by extracellular deoxyribonuclease.

After a donor DNA fragment is introduced into a recipient bacterium by a transducing phage, formation of a stable hybrid genome by recombination occurs independently from expression of the structural genes encoded by the donor DNA fragment. If the donor DNA fragment can persist in the cytoplasm of the recipient bacterium without participating in recombination, then abortive transduction may occur. In abortive transduction, the nonreplicating donor DNA fragment in the bacterial cytoplasm segregates into only one of the two daughter cells formed when the bacterium divides. This linear pattern of inheritance of the donor DNA can occur throughout several cycles of cell division. The products encoded by the donor DNA fragment are made only in the bacterial cell that has inherited it. After the donor DNA fragment is lost, the donor gene products are reduced to half of their previous concentrations at each cell division. If a specific donor gene product enables the bacteria to grow on a selective medium, abortively transduced bacteria form minute colonies on the selective medium. Such abortive transductants can be distinguished from recombinant bacteria that have arisen by generalized transduction and that form colonies of normal size on the selective medium. The frequency of abortive transduction is usually greater than the frequency of generalized transduction, demonstrating that formation of a stable recombinant genome occurs in only a fraction of the recipient cells that receive an appropriate fragment of the donor genome.

Another type of transduction is called specialized transduction (or localized transduction) because only a specific set of bacterial genes is transduced. Specialized transduction is observed only with temperate bacteriophages. When lytic phage development occurs in cultures of lysogenic bacteria, rare specialized transducing phages may be formed. The specialized transducing phages have recombinant genomes containing segments of the bacterial chromosome that were adjacent to the sites of prophage integration in the ancestral, lysogenic bacterial strains. Therefore, only a restricted set of bacterial genes can be present in specialized transducing phages; these bacterial genes behave as integral parts of the phage genomes. The formation of specialized transducing phages is discussed further in the subsequent section on recombination. Segments of the normal phage genome are deleted from specialized transducing phages to compensate for the added bacterial DNA. For this reason, specialized transducing phages often lack functions essential for lytic growth. Defective phages can grow, however, in bacteria simultaneously infected with wild-type phages that provide the missing functions by complementation. The bacterial genes in specialized transducing phages can be expressed phenotypically in lysogenic cells and in infected susceptible cells during lytic phage growth.

Conjugation

Conjugation in bacteria was discovered in *E coli* and also occurs in many other bacteria. The ability of bacterial strains to function as genetic donors is determined by specific conjugative plasmids called fertility factors. The special feature of fertility factors is their capacity to promote transfer of both plasmid and chromosomal DNA from donor to recipient bacteria. The F plasmid in *E coli* is considered here as the prototype for fertility plasmids. Bacteria that lack fertility plasmids may function as recipients but not as donors in conjugal matings. Bacteria containing fertility factors may function as donors and under some circumstances as recipients.

The ability to promote transfer of DNA from donor to recipient bacteria is determined by a cluster of 15 transfer (*tra*) genes in the F plasmid. Some of these *tra* genes code for synthesis and assembly of specific F pili on the surface of donor bacteria. Interactions between F pili on the donor bacteria and receptors on the recipient bacteria are essential for cytoplasmic connections to form between the mating bacteria. If the F plasmid is present in the donor cell as an extrachromosomal genetic element, only the F plasmid DNA is transferred through the cytoplasmic bridge from the donor to the recipient bacterium during conjugation. Transfer begins from a unique origin within the F plasmid. Only one specific strand of the F plasmid DNA is transferred, and the transfer proceeds sequentially from the 5' end to the 3' end of that polynucleotide strand. In the recipient bacterium, DNA synthesis converts the single-stranded molecule of F plasmid DNA to the double-stranded form characteristic of the F plasmid. In the donor bacterium, synthesis of a new strand of F plasmid DNA is coordinated with displacement of the original single strand for transfer to the recipient cell. This asymmetric pattern of DNA replication in the donor cell during conjugation, which uses only one of the two polynucleotide strands of the F plasmid DNA as a template, differs from the symmetric, semiconservative pattern of DNA replication described previously for the bacterial chromosome during normal bacterial growth. After conjugative transfer of the F plasmid has occurred, the F plasmid is present in both of the exconjugant bacteria. Thus, the F plasmid, like other conjugative plasmids, can spread in an infectious manner from donor to compatible recipient cells in a mixed population of bacteria.

The F plasmid can exist in *E coli* as an extrachromosomal element or as part of the bacterial chromosome (Figure 20-9). Because the F plasmid and the bacterial chromosome are both circular DNA molecules, reciprocal recombination between them can

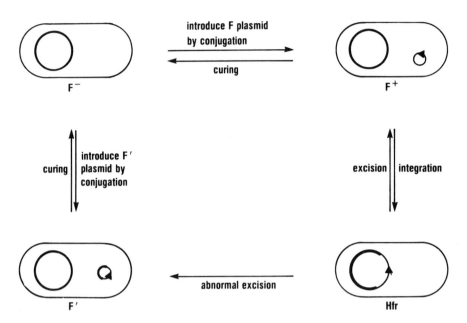

Figure 20-9 Donor and recipient strains of *E coli*. The F plasmid is representative of specific conjugative plasmids that control donor ability in *E coli*. F⁻ strains lack the F plasmid and are genetic recipients. F⁺ donor strains harbor the F plasmid as a cytoplasmic element. F plasmid can become integrated into bacterial chromosome at various locations to produce Hfr (high-frequency recombination) donor strains. Abnormal excision of F plasmid can result in formation of F′ plasmids that contain segments of bacterial chromosome of variable length. The arrowhead in F plasmid defines origin for transfer of DNA during conjugation. F plasmid and chromosomal DNA are indicated by fine lines and heavy lines, respectively. For additional data concerning the genomes of Hfr and F′ strains, see Figure 20-7.

produce larger, circular DNA molecules. Called integration, this process results in the linear insertion of the F plasmid DNA into the bacterial chromosome at the site of recombination. Integration of the F plasmid can occur at many different sites on the chromosome of *E coli*.

An *E coli* strain with an integrated F plasmid retains its ability to function as a donor in conjugal matings. In such matings, transfer of single-stranded DNA begins from the same unique origin within the F plasmid and proceeds in the same sequential manner described. The entire hybrid genome containing the F plasmid and the bacterial chromosome can be transferred from the donor to the recipient bacterium. Thus, for each specific donor strain with an integrated F plasmid, the origin of transfer of chromosomal genes is determined by the site at which the F factor is integrated; the polarity of transfer of chromosomal genes is determined by the relative orientations of the F plasmid DNA and the bacterial chromosome. The circularity of the genetic map for the chromosome of *E coli* was deduced from the overlapping, circularly permuted sequences of specific gene transfer by individual donor strains in which the F factor was integrated at different chromosomal locations (see Figure 20-7).

Transfer of the entire bacterial chromosome from donor to recipient bacteria requires approximately 100 minutes. The mating bacteria usually separate spontaneously at some time during conjugation, resulting in transfer of fragments of the donor chromosomes into the recipient bacteria. Thus, genes transferred early by each specific donor strain are transferred with higher efficiency than those transferred late. The mating cells can also be broken apart by treatment with strong shearing forces such as those generated in a mechanical blender. Thus conjugal matings can be terminated experimentally at defined times after cultures of the donor and recipient bacteria are mixed together. Interrupted mating experiments have been used to demonstrate the specific origins of chromosomal transfer by particular donor strains, the polarity of transfer of donor genes, and the lower probability that genes transferred late will appear in recombinant progeny.

Strains of E $coli$ are designated F^- if they contain no F plasmids, F^+ if they have cytoplasmic F plasmids, or Hfr if they have chromosomally integrated F plasmids. Hfr strains with integrated F plasmids are highly efficient as donors of chromosomal genes in conjugal matings with F^- bacteria (Hfr indicates *high frequency* of *recombination*). In matings between F^+ and F^- strains, the F plasmid is transferred from donor to recipient bacteria with high efficiency, but the bacterial chromosome is transferred with very low efficiency. Rare Hfr cells in populations of F^+ cells are apparently responsible for the transfer of the donor chromosome observed in matings between F^+ and F^- bacteria. In matings between Hfr and F^- strains, the segment of the F plasmid containing the *tra* region is transferred last, after the entire bacterial chromosome has been transferred. Most recombinants from matings between Hfr and F^- cells fail to inherit the entire F plasmid and behave as do genetic recipients. In contrast, in matings between F^+ and F^- strains, the cytoplasmic F plasmid spreads rapidly throughout the bacterial population and most recombinant bacteria are F^+.

The integrated F plasmids in Hfr strains can also become excised from the bacterial chromosome. If the recombination events leading to excision are precise reversals of the integration process, F^+ cells containing cytoplasmic F plasmids are produced. On rare occasions, excision occurs by recombination involving sites on the bacterial chromosome some distance from the original integration sites; segments of the bacterial chromosome become incorporated into the excised, cytoplasmic F plasmids (see Figure 20-9). Recombinant F plasmids that contain segments of the bacterial genome are called F' plasmids. Both F' plasmids and specialized transducing phages have hybrid genomes that contain segments of the bacterial chromosome. Therefore, the partially diploid bacterial strains required for complementation tests and other purposes can be constructed by introducing appropriate F' plasmids or specialized transducing phages into properly selected recipient bacteria.

Recombination

Recombination involves breakage and joining of parental DNA molecules to form hybrid, recombinant molecules. Several distinct kinds of recombination have been identified that depend on different structural features of the participating genomes and require the activities of different gene products. Specific enzymes that act on DNA (for example, exonucleases, endonucleases, polymerases, ligases) participate in recombination. Detailed discussion of the biochemical events in recombination is beyond the scope of this chapter.

Generalized recombination involves donor and recipient genomes that have homologous polynucleotide sequences. Reciprocal exchanges can occur between any homologous sites in the donor and recipient DNA molecules. In *E coli,* the product of the *rec*A gene is essential for generalized recombination, but other gene products also participate.

Site-specific recombination occurs only between specific sites in donor and recipient genomes. The *rec*A gene product is not required for site-specific recombination. Integration of the temperate bacteriophage λ into the chromosome of *E coli* is a well-studied example of site-specific recombination (Figure 20-10). The specific attach-

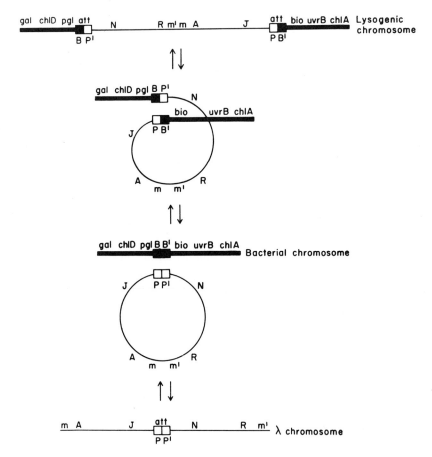

Figure 20-10 Integration of bacteriophage λ into chromosome of *E coli* is an example of site-specific recombination. Arrangement of genes in DNA from phage λ is shown at the bottom. A, J, N, and R are phage genes, m and m' are ends of λ DNA molecule, and *att* PP' is phage attachment site involved in insertional recombination. Bacterial attachment site is designated *att* BB', and *gal, chl*D, *pgl, bio, urv*B, and *chl*A are bacterial genes adjacent to *att* BB'. In infected cell, λ DNA becomes circular by joining m to m', and site-specific recombination between *att* BB' and *att* PP' results in insertion of λ chromosome into bacterial chromosome. Arrangement of prophage genes in lysogenic chromosome is a circular permutation of arrangement of genes in the DNA from λ virions. From Campbell A. In: *The bacteriophage lambda.* Hershey, A.D., (editor). Cold Spring Harbor, N.Y.: Cold Spring Harbor Laboratories, p. 14, 1971.

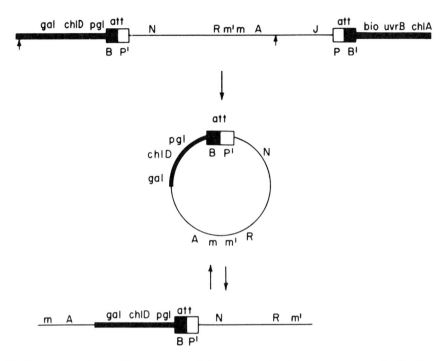

Figure 20-11 Abnormal excision of bacteriophage λ from lysogenic chromosome occurs by illegitimate recombination. When aberrant recombination occurs between the two nonhomologous sites (indicated by arrows), the excised phage (called λ *gal*) contains segment of bacterial genome required for galactose utilization (*gal*) and has lost a segment of λ genome between A and *att*P. Phage λ *gal* can function as a specialized transducing phage, but it lacks functions essential for viral growth and is therefore defective. From Campbell A. In: *The bacteriophage lambda*. Hershey, A.D., (editor). Cold Spring Harbor, N.Y.: Cold Spring Harbor Laboratories, p. 15, 1971.

ment (*att*) sites on the *E coli* and λ phage genomes have a common core sequence, 15 nucleotides long, within which reciprocal recombination occurs, flanked by adjacent sequences that are not homologous in the phage and bacterial genomes. In phage λ the product of the *int* gene (integrase) is required for the site-specific integration event in lysogenization; the products of the *int* and *xis* (excisionase) genes are both needed for the complementary site-specific excision event that occurs during induction of lytic phage development in lysogenic cells.

Illegitimate recombination is the term used to describe nonhomologous, aberrant recombination events such as those involved in formation of specialized transducing phages (Figure 20-11). The mechanisms of illegitimate recombination are unknown.

Transposons

Transposable elements (**transposons**) are segments of double-stranded DNA that can move from place to place within a genome or between genomes. They have been identified both in bacteria and in eukaryotic cells, but the discussion here focuses on bacteria. The insertion of a transposon into a new site in DNA is called **transposition;**

transposons are named for this characteristic function. Such an insertion often will disrupt the integrity of a gene at the target site, inactivate it, and cause a mutation. Transposons also can mediate other rearrangements in the genome, including fusion of replicons and deletion or inversion of segments of DNA. Maintenance of transposons in bacteria depends on their integration into replicons such as the bacterial chromosome or plasmids.

Transposons have characteristic structural features. The simplest transposons are called **insertion sequences (IS)**. The known IS vary in length from approximately 700 to 1500 base pairs, and short inverted complementary nucleotide sequences are present on each DNA strand at the ends of the IS (Figure 20-12). The lengths of these inverted terminal repeats, as well as their base sequences, vary from one IS to another. The DNA between the inverted terminal repeats encodes one or more polypeptides that are essential for transposition. A bacterial chromosome or plasmid can contain multiple copies of several different IS at various locations. Integration of F into the chromosome of *E coli* to produce Hfr strains (see Figures 20-7 and 20-9) is an example of IS-mediated replicon fusion that can occur by either of two mechanisms. First, an IS located in one replicon (the F plasmid or the chromosome) can cause it to fuse with the other replicon during transposition. Second, copies of a single IS located in the F plasmid and the chromosome provide regions of nucleotide-sequence homology at which generalized recombination can occur, and reciprocal recombination between the two circular DNA molecules will join them into a single, cointegrate circular molecule.

The transposons in a second group have composite structures and contain IS or ISlike elements as modules at each end. They are large and vary in length from about

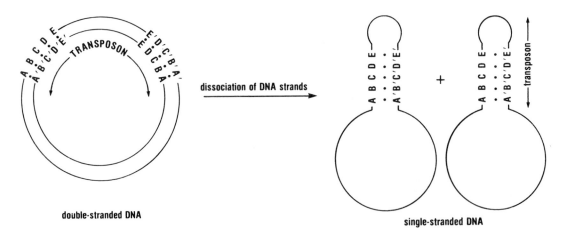

double-stranded DNA   single-stranded DNA

Figure 20-12 Diagrammatic representation of basic transposon in circular DNA molecule. Two strands of DNA are indicated by lines; sequences of letters correspond to inverted, complementary sequences of nucleotides at ends of transposon. A is complementary to A', B is complementary to B', and so on. Dots indicate hydrogen bonds between purine and pyrimidine bases in complementary nucleotides. The DNA between the inverted terminal repeats of the transposon codes for one or more polypeptides that are essential for transposition. When double-stranded DNA molecule is dissociated, the inverted, complementary nucleotide sequences within each single-stranded DNA molecule can associate with each other to form double-stranded segment. Transposon assumes characteristic stem and loop structure that can be visualized by electron microscopy.

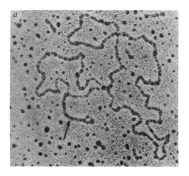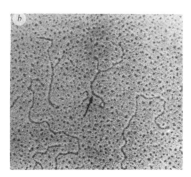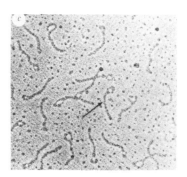

Figure 20-13 Electron micrographs of single-stranded DNA molecules with transposon (Tn1681) that encodes *E coli* heat-stable enterotoxin (ST). Arrows indicate typical stem and loop structures formed by ST transposons. Inverted, complementary sequences forming stems are about 760 nucleotides long and correspond to a known genetic element in *E coli* called insertion sequence 1 (IS1). **A,** Plasmid ESF3001. **B,** A 3.4-kilobase fragment of ESF3001 containing the intact ST transposon. **C,** A 1.4-kilobase fragment of ESF3001 including loop and part of stem of ST transposon. Plasmid ESF3001 is a hybrid plasmid constructed in vitro by recombinant DNA techniques. Reprinted by permission from *Nature,* Vol. 277, p. 454. Copyright © 1979 Macmillan Journals Limited.

2,000 to more than 40,000 base pairs. The terminal IS or ISlike modules of composite transposons usually have inverted orientations. The DNA between the terminal modules is large enough to encode several different functions. In medically important bacteria, genes that determine virulence factors or resistance to antibiotics often are located in such transposons. A composite transposon that encodes heat-stable enterotoxin (ST) in *E coli* is shown in Figure 20-13.

Transposon Tn3, which determines resistance to ampicillin, is representative of another family of transposons, the Tn*A* family. These relatively large transposons have short terminal inverted repeat sequences, but they do not have the ISlike modules of composite transposons. The Tn*A* family has an important place in the history of medical microbiology. The development of high-level resistance to ampicillin in *Haemophilus influenzae* and *Neisseria gonorrhoeae* during the 1970s, which severely limits the usefulness of ampicillin for treatment of gonococcal and *Haemophilus* infections in areas where such strains are prevalent, was caused by the dissemination of Tn*A* resistance determinants from plasmids in the enterobacteriaceae to plasmids in *Haemophilus* and *Neisseria.*

Some bacteriophage are transposons. Bacteriophage mu, a temperate phage capable of integrating at many different sites in the *E coli* chromosome, is one well-studied example. The entire genome of bacteriophage mu functions as a transposon. Bacteriophage mu appears to have evolved such that the process of transposition was utilized as an essential step for replication and integration of the phage genome.

The mechanisms responsible for the genetic rearrangements produced by transposons are not fully defined. Transposition in *E coli* is distinct from generalized recombination and does not require the function of the *rec*A gene product. Transposition does involve specific recognition of the inverted, complementary nucleotide sequences at the ends of the transposon. This feature of transposition resembles site-specific recombination. Transposition differs from site-specific recombination, however, in several important respects. There is relatively little specificity for the DNA sequences into which transposons can be integrated. Furthermore, transposition involves replication of the transposon. After transposition is completed, the transposon is found both at its original site and at its new location. Finally, a short nucleotide sequence at the target site is duplicated during transposition, and the transposon is inserted between the two copies of the directly repeated sequence. Thus, transposition is a unique type of nonhomologous recombination that involves replication of the transposon.

Transposons have an important role in the evolution of bacterial genomes; this has been well studied in the case of antibiotic resistance. Many plasmids that determine resistance to multiple antibiotics contain several different transposons, each of which has genes for resistance to one or more antibiotic. The acquisition of resistance determinants by plasmids, therefore, can proceed through several independent transposition events. Although the initial incorporation of any specific gene into a transposon presumably occurs rarely, the frequency of subsequent transposition can be quite high. Therefore, transposition is an efficient genetic mechanism for moving genes that have been incorporated into a transposon from one place to another in a genome. In the case of antibiotic-resistance genes, environmental factors such as the widespread use of antibiotics in human and veterinary medicine and the incorporation of antibiotics into animal feeds may provide significant selective pressure to maintain plasmids that have acquired resistance to multiple antibiotics. Conjugation, transduction, and transfection provide opportunities for dissemination of newly evolved multiple-resistance plasmids within and between bacterial species. After a plasmid carrying a transposon has been introduced into a new bacterial host, the transposon and the determinants that it carries can jump into the chromosome or indigenous plasmids of the new host. Therefore, stability of the mobilizing plasmid is not essential for persistence of a transposon in a new host. Recently, enterobacteriaceae collected before the antibiotic era were studied to determine the characteristics of their plasmids. They contained many plasmids that are related to the drug-resistance plasmids in current clinical isolates, but the plasmids from the older strains rarely determined resistance to antibiotics. These studies demonstrated the important role of transposons in the evolution from the plasmid pool that existed in the preantibiotic era to the multiple drug resistance plasmids now observed.

Recombinant DNA and Gene Cloning

The scope of molecular genetics has been expanded greatly by the development of methods to isolate and characterize specific genes. The preparation of hybrid or chimeric DNA molecules, called **recombinant DNA,** and the isolation of specific genes in hybrid replicons, known as **gene cloning,** have central roles in the technology of genetic engineering. Some of the highlights of these developments are summarized here.

Analysis of the phenomena of host-controlled restriction and modification in bacteriophage ultimately led to the discovery of **restriction endonucleases.** Many of these enzymes have characteristics that make them extremely valuable as tools for analyzing DNA. They recognize short, oligonucleotide target sequences called **palin-**

dromes that have twofold rotational symmetry, and they cleave both strands of DNA within these symmetric target regions. The targets of individual restriction enzymes differ with respect to length (usually four to six nucleotide pairs) and base sequence. Some restriction enzymes break both DNA strands at coincident sites, whereas others make cuts at staggered positions on the two strands. The specificity of representative restriction endonucleases is illustrated in Table 20-3.

Restriction enzymes can be used to obtain physical maps of DNA. Each restriction enzyme will cleave a specific DNA molecule, such as a bacterial chromosome, a plasmid, or a phage genome, into a characteristic set of fragments. The number of restriction fragments will be determined by the frequency with which the target site for the specific enzyme appears in the DNA molecule, and the lengths of the fragments will be determined by the distances between adjacent target sites. An inverse relationship exists between the length of the target sequence for a restriction enzyme and the probable frequency of its occurrence in a DNA molecule. By analyzing the fragments produced by digestion with several different restriction enzymes, researchers can determine the positions of the target sites for each enzyme within the intact DNA molecule, and thus construct a restriction map. In practice, enzymes that cut at relatively few sites are used to construct preliminary restriction maps, and enzymes that cut at larger numbers of sites are used to create more detailed maps of specific regions of interest. **Restriction maps** are physical maps of DNA molecules; when the locations of individual genes on specific restriction fragments are determined, the physical map can be compared with the corresponding genetic map.

Restriction fragments, which are homogeneous populations of DNA molecules with defined ends, are also used as starting materials for determining nucleotide sequences. Several methods for sequence analysis are available, but they are based on similar principles. Populations of single-stranded molecules are produced that have overlapping sequences extending from a common origin at one end and terminating at each of the positions where a particular nucleotide (A, T, G, or C) occurs. By arranging

Table 20-3   Recognition Sites for Selected Restriction Endonucleases*

Restriction Endonuclease	Microorganism	Recognition Site in Double–Stranded DNA*	
		Length	Sequence (5′ → 3′)
MboI	*Moraxella bovis*	Tetranucleotide	↓GATC
HpaII	*Haemophilus parainfluenzae*	Tetranucleotide	C↓CGG
HaeII	*Haemophilus aegypticus*	Tetranucleotide	GG↓CC
HhaI	*Haemophilus haemolyticus*	Tetranucleotide	GCG↓C
EcoRII	*Escherichia coli* R245	Pentanucleotide	↓CC($_T^A$)GG
EcoRI	*Escherichia coli* RY13	Hexanucleotide	G↓AATTC
HindIII	*Haemophilus influenzae* Rd	Hexanucleotide	A↓AGCTT
BglII	*Bacillus globigii*	Hexanucleotide	A↓GATCT
PstI	*Providentia stuartii* 164	Hexanucleotide	CTGCA↓G

*Modified from Roberts, R.J.: In: *Recombinant molecules: impact on science and society.* Beers, R. F., Jr., Bassett, E. G. (editors). New York: Raven Press, 1977.
†Each sequence is a palindrome. The complementary sequence is an inverted repeat of the sequence given. Arrows designate sites of cleavage.

all such molecules that terminate at each of the four nucleotides in order of increasing length, the sequence of the DNA molecule from which they were derived is established. Sequences up to several hundred nucleotides in length can be obtained by such methods. The accuracy of the data can be checked by determining independently the sequence of the complementary DNA strand. Long sequences can be deduced by assembling data from a set of overlapping short sequences.

Many successful strategies for gene cloning have been developed. All are based on the finding that small replicons, such as plasmids or phages, can serve as carriers, or **cloning vectors,** for foreign DNA. Insertion of foreign DNA into a cloning vector at an appropriate site does not inactivate the vector functions required for replication in bacteria. Hybrid vectors, therefore, can be amplified by replication in bacteria, and the recombinant DNA molecules or the gene products that they encode can be purified and studied. Restriction endonucleases are used frequently to introduce foreign DNA into cloning vectors. Enzymes are chosen that cut the cloning vector at only one site or a few sites. Restriction endonucleases that produce symmetrically staggered cuts in palindromic target sequences are particularly useful because they produce short, single-stranded ends with complementary nucleotide sequences (cohesive ends) that can associate by hydrogen bonding under appropriate conditions. Samples of vector DNA and DNA to be cloned, therefore, can be cut by the same restriction enzyme, mixed together, and permitted to associate randomly to form recombinant DNA molecules. The noncovalently associated hybrid replicons can then be converted into intact DNA molecules by treatment with DNA ligase and introduced into appropriate bacterial strains in which they can replicate and express their genetic determinants. This general strategy (see Figure 20-14) leads to random insertion of restriction fragments into the vector, and is called **shotgun cloning.** A collection of strains with recombinant DNA molecules that contain the various restriction fragments is a **genomic library.** Alternatively, if the restriction fragment containing the gene of interest has previously been identified, the desired fragment can be purified and inserted directly into an appropriate cloning vector. Other general methods for constructing recombinant DNA molecules include attachment of complementary synthetic oligonucleotides to the ends of the linearized vector DNA and the fragments to be cloned, followed by association and ligation, or use of DNA ligase to join blunt-ended fragments of vector and donor DNA previously generated by appropriate restriction enzymes or mechanical shearing. Recombinant DNA can be introduced directly into recipient bacteria by transformation. Recombinant DNA molecules also can be prepared with phage vectors or cosmid vectors (cosmids are plasmids that contain the *cos* site required for packaging of DNA into phage), encapsidated in phage coats in vitro, and introduced into phage-susceptible bacteria by infection.

Many methods are available to identify bacteria that contain recombinant DNA molecules. Most cloning vectors have genes for traits that can be positively selected, such as resistance to antibiotics. Furthermore, it is often possible to introduce foreign DNA into the cloning vector at a site that inactivates a nonessential, but easily recognizable, vector function. If both of these conditions are fulfilled, bacteria that contain recombinant molecules can be selected and distinguished from bacteria that contain only the vector by testing for their failure to express the insertionally inactivated gene. Bacteria in a genomic library that contain a particular cloned gene of interest can be identified by using biochemical or immunologic methods to test for the desired gene product. If specific radioactively labeled DNA or RNA probes are available, it is even possible to identify cloned genes by using DNA-DNA or DNA-RNA hybridization. By using specialized vectors called shuttle vectors that can replicate in two different cell types, such as bacteria and eukaryotic cells, researchers can clone genes from eukaryotes in convenient bacterial systems and subsequently reintroduce them into eukaryotic cells for analysis in their natural environment.

Use of recombinant DNA methods makes it technically feasible to clone specific DNA fragments from any source into vectors that can be studied in well-characterized bacteria, eukaryotic cells, or in vitro (Figure 20-14). During the last decade, recombinant DNA technology has revolutionized the analysis of gene structure and function; the theoretical and practical applications of DNA cloning in biology and medicine are pervasive. Applications of recombinant DNA technology in medicine range from the prenatal diagnosis of human genetic diseases to the characterization of oncogenes and their role in carcinogenesis. Pharmaceutical applications include large-scale production from cloned human genes of biologic products such as interferon, insulin, and growth hormone. In the fields of infectious diseases and public health, genetic engineering has assumed a central role in development of new vaccines, and specific DNA probes are being developed for rapid diagnosis, by DNA-DNA hybridization, of infections caused by specific bacterial, viral, or other pathogens.

Regulation of Gene Expression

The phenotypic properties of bacteria are determined by their genotypes and by the environmental conditions used for their cultivation. For bacteria in pure cultures, physiologic adaptations to defined changes in conditions can occur rapidly, in a predictable manner, and in all members of the population; however, the range of possible adaptations is genetically determined for each bacterial strain.

Physiologic adaptations are often associated with striking changes in metabolic activities. The flow of metabolites through particular biochemical pathways can be regulated by controlling the synthesis of specific enzymes, by altering the activities of existing enzymes, or both. Mechanisms for regulating the activities of existing enzymes are discussed in Chapter 19. Factors that control the production of specific enzymes and other gene products are discussed here.

Formation of enzymes for catabolic pathways is often induced when the initial substrates for those pathways are present in the growth medium; the synthesis of many biosynthetic enzymes is repressed when their specific metabolic end products are present. **Induction** and **repression** are important physiologic mechanisms that enable bacteria to regulate production of specific gene products in response to appropriate environmental stimuli. Enzymes that participate in a single biochemical pathway often are induced or repressed coordinately; their structural genes may occupy adjacent positions on the bacterial chromosome. **Operons** are groups of contiguous genes with coordinately regulated expression. The organization of genes into operons is an important strategy for regulating gene expression in bacteria.

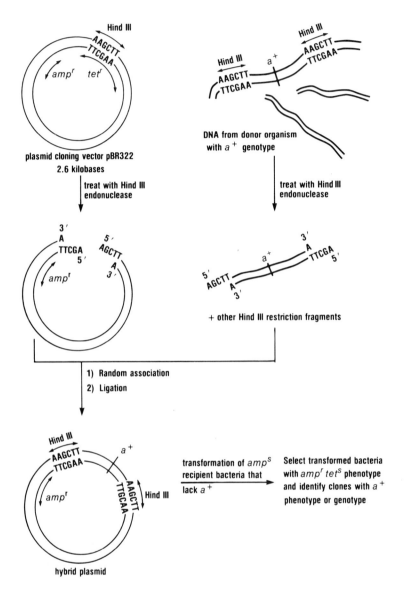

Figure 20-14 Diagrammatic representation of gene cloning experiment. Plasmid cloning vector pBR322 is 4.36 kilobases in size, has genes for resistance to ampicillin (*amp*[r]) and to tetracycline (*tet*[r]), and has only one HindIII restriction site that is located within the *tet*[r] locus. HindIII is used to treat samples of DNA from plasmid pBR322 and from a donor organism with a gene, designated *a*[+], to be cloned. The donor can be a prokaryotic or a eukaryotic organism. If HindIII restriction sites are located adjacent to *a*[+] in donor DNA, but do not occur within *a*[+], a restriction fragment carrying intact *a*[+] marker can be generated from donor DNA. Hybrid plasmids can be formed by random association and ligation of the HindIII-treated donor and vector DNA fragments. Although pBR322 is *tet*[r], hybrid plasmids will be *tet*[s] because the donor DNA fragments are inserted at the HindIII restriction site within the *tet*[r] locus. After transformation of *amp*[s]-recipient bacteria that also lack *a*[+], transconjugants with hybrid plasmids can be selected by their *amp*[r] *tet*[s] phenotypes. Strains in which the *a*[+] gene is present can then be identified by expression of the *a*[+] phenotype or by presence of polynucleotide sequence corresponding to *a*[+]. The pBR322 plasmid contains other unique restriction sites that can also be used for cloning (PstI in *amp*[r] or SalI and BamHI in *amp*[r]). Many other cloning vectors and restriction endonucleases have also been used for gene cloning experiments.

Regulatory genes control the expression of many operons. Some regulatory genes code for cytoplasmic gene products; others are regions in DNA that bind to the cytoplasmic regulatory macromolecules.

mRNAs as Transcriptional Units

DNA-dependent RNA polymerase catalyzes the transcription of mRNAs from DNA templates, using ribonucleoside triphosphates as substrates. Binding of RNA polymerase holoenzyme to DNA occurs at specific sites called **promoters** and is facilitated by a polypeptide component of the holoenzyme that is called **sigma factor.** After synthesis of mRNA is initiated at promoters, sigma factor dissociates from the polymerase. Elongation of mRNA is catalyzed by RNA-polymerase core enzyme, and transcription is completed at specific termination sites. A protein called **rho factor** is essential for termination at some sites.

Individual mRNA molecules may code for one polypeptide or for several. Molecules of mRNA that code for several polypeptides are called **polycistronic mRNAs.** Translation of polycistronic mRNAs leads to coordinate synthesis of the encoded polypeptides; although each polypeptide is synthesized as a separate molecule. Thus, formation and translation of polycistronic mRNAs provide the biochemical basis for the coordinate expression of genes in operons.

Messenger RNAs in bacteria are degraded rapidly with an average half-life of several minutes. In contrast, tRNAs and rRNAs are metabolically stable. Although mRNAs represent about half of the newly synthesized RNA in bacteria, only a small fraction of the total RNA is mRNA. The short half-life of mRNAs has important consequences for gene expression. If the synthesis of a specific mRNA is suddenly prevented, synthesis of the corresponding polypeptides declines rapidly.

The most common mechanism for regulating gene expression in bacteria controls the rate of synthesis of specific mRNAs. Because the rate of chain elongation during synthesis of mRNA is approximately constant, the major factors that control mRNA synthesis are the rate of transcription initiation and the probability that initiation will result in formation of a complete mRNA transcript.

Regulation of Transcription Initiation

Some mRNAs are initiated and synthesized at constant rates in each bacterial cell, resulting in constitutive production of the corresponding polypeptides; the synthesis of other mRNAs is regulated in response to changing environmental conditions. The maximal rate for initiating transcription is determined by the interaction of RNA polymerase with the promoter and can vary greatly from one promoter to another.

Additional regulatory genes participate in the control of transcription initiation of some operons. The oligonucleotide sequences in DNA to which specific regulatory proteins bind are called **operators.** The operator and promoter regions in an operon are close together and may have overlapping DNA sequences. Binding of a specific regulatory protein to an operator can inhibit or stimulate the initiation of transcription by RNA polymerase at the adjacent promoter. Regulatory proteins that stimulate transcription exert positive control on operon function, whereas regulatory proteins that inhibit transcription exert negative control. Proteins that function as negative regulators of transcription initiation are usually called repressors. Because regulatory proteins can diffuse through the cytoplasm to interact with operators, the structural genes for specific regulatory proteins do not have to be linked closely to their target operons.

The recognition of specific substrates or metabolic products and the coupling of their detection to changes in the rates of synthesis of specific gene products are important aspects of induction and repression. Regulatory proteins offer one solution to this problem of metabolic stimulus-response coupling. Regulatory proteins are bifunctional molecules that bind specifically not only to appropriate operators but also to particular ligands such as individual sugars, amino acids, purines, pyrimidines, or vitamins. Furthermore, regulatory proteins are allosteric molecules that can exist in different conformational states. In their alternate conformations, regulatory proteins have different binding affinities for their specific operators and for their specific ligands. A sufficient concentration of ligand stabilizes the regulatory protein in the conformational state that has high affinity for the ligand, and the ligand-binding conformation has either high affinity or low affinity for the corresponding operator. In this manner the binding of specific ligand to a regulatory protein affects directly the ability of the regulatory protein to bind to the appropriate operator.

The lactose (*lac*) operon of *E coli* illustrates these mechanisms for regulating gene expression (Figure 20-15). The *lac* operon is an example of an inducible, negatively regulated operon. The *lac* repressor binds to the *lac* operator and prevents initiation of

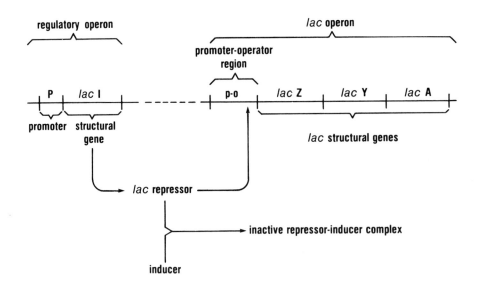

Figure 20-15 Regulation of *lac* operon in *E coli*. Structural genes *lacZ*, *lacY*, and *lacA* code for β-galactosidase, β-galactoside permease, and β-galactoside transacetylase, respectively. The physiologic role of *lacA* is unknown. The *lac* repressor is product of *lacI* gene in separate regulatory operon. Transcription of *lac* mRNA is negatively regulated, and binding of *lac* repressor to operator *lacO* prevents initiation of transcription of *lac* mRNA at promoter *lacP*. Inducer binds to *lac* repressor and inactivates it. Roles of cAMP and cAMP receptor protein (CRP) in positive regulation of expression of *lac* operon are discussed in text.

transcription of polycistronic *lac* mRNA at the *lac* promoter; however, when the specific ligand, called an **inducer,** binds to the *lac* repressor, the repressor undergoes a conformational change, loses its affinity for the *lac* operator, and can no longer prevent transcription of *lac* mRNA. If other conditions are favorable, transcription and translation of *lac* mRNA can proceed, resulting in induced synthesis of β-galactosidase, β-galactoside permease, and β-galactoside transacetylase. The structural gene for the *lac* repressor is separate from the *lac* operon; the *lac* repressor is synthesized constitutively at a slow rate. Synthesis of the enzymes of the *lac* operon can be induced by lactose or by structurally related analogs such as isopropyl-β-D-thiogalactoside (IPTG). Allolactose, formed from lactose by β-galactosidase, is the natural inducer of the *lac* operon. Although IPTG is active as an inducer of the *lac* operon, it cannot be hydrolyzed by β-galactosidase and cannot serve as a carbon or energy soure for *E coli.* Inducers like IPTG that do not serve as substrates for the induced enzyme are called gratuitous inducers.

The mechanisms of repression and induction in negatively regulated operons are similar; however, in repressible operons, the repressor-ligand complex, not the free repressor, binds to the operator and prevents transcription of mRNA. The metabolic products that function as regulatory ligands in repressible systems are often called **corepressors.** Repression occurs in many biosynthetic operons including the tryptophan (*trp*) operon of *E coli.*

The arabinose (*ara*) operon in *E coli* provides an example of enzyme induction in a positively regulated system. Binding of the active form of the regulatory protein to an operator site called the *ara* initiator stimulates transcription of polycistronic mRNA for the *ara* operon.

When *E coli* grows in medium containing lactose and glucose, the glucose is utilized preferentially, and induction of the *lac* operon is delayed until the available supply of glucose has been consumed. This phenomenon is called **diauxic growth.** The action of glucose in preventing induction of the *lac* operon is an example of a more general phenomenon called **catabolite repression.** Catabolite repression is mediated by cyclic-3′,5′-adenosine monophosphate (cAMP) and a specific cAMP receptor protein (CRP). The cAMP-CRP complex interacts with several different promoters in *E coli,* including the *lac* promoter, and stimulates the initiation of transcription by RNA polymerase. Therefore, the cAMP-CRP complex functions as a positive regulator of gene expression. The intracellular concentration of cAMP is low in *E coli* grown in rich medium containing glucose or other substrates that are highly efficient as energy sources. In contrast, high intracellular cAMP concentrations are found during growth in media with poor energy-yielding substrates. Therefore, maximal expression of cAMP-dependent operons cannot occur when highly efficient energy sources are present and intracellular cAMP concentrations are low.

During sporulation, as well as during infection by certain lytic phages in *Bacillus subtilis,* the transcription of many different genes is turned on or off in a coordinated manner. These regulatory phenomena reflect global switches in initiation that are determined by production of new sigma factors. Each sigma factor directs RNA polymerase to initiate transcription at a different set of promoters, and substitution of one σ factor for another in RNA polymerase causes transcription from one group of genes to cease as transcription from another set begins.

Regulation of Transcription Termination

The production of functional mRNAs from operons can be prevented by blocking the initiation of transcription, as described previously, or by aborting transcription after initiation has occurred. **Attenuation** is a mechanism for regulation of operons that is based on premature termination of transcription of mRNAs. Control of transcription initiation and attenuation are independent regulatory mechanisms, although both are present in some operons. Attenuation occurs in several operons involved in biosynthesis of amino acids including the tryptophan (*trp*), histidine (*his*), threonine (*thr*), and isoleucine-valine (*ilv*) operons in *E coli*.

The secondary structure of mRNA has an important role in the mechanism of attenuation. Messenger RNAs have leader sequences of variable length corresponding to the segments between their transcriptional origin and the beginning of the coding region for their first structural gene. In the *trp* operon, the leader sequence for *trp* mRNA is encoded by the *trpL* region (see Figure 20-16). The *trp* mRNA leader contains several complementary oligonucleotide sequences that can participate in hydrogen bonding with each other to form double-stranded RNA segments. The diagram at the left of Figure 20-17 shows that nucleotides 114 through 141 of the *trp* mRNA leader can form a hairpin loop with a G-C–rich, double-stranded stem that is followed by a string of U residues. This structure resembles other rho factor–independent termination signals; when it is recognized by RNA polymerase, transcription terminates at the attenuator and the distal part of the *trp* operon is not transcribed.

In contrast, the diagram at the right of Figure 20-17 shows that the *trp* mRNA leader sequence can assume an alternative double-stranded structure that is incompatible with formation of the termination signal described above. This alternative conformation of the mRNA leader sequence enables RNA polymerase to continue transcription through the attenuator to the end of the operon. The decision to terminate transcripts at the

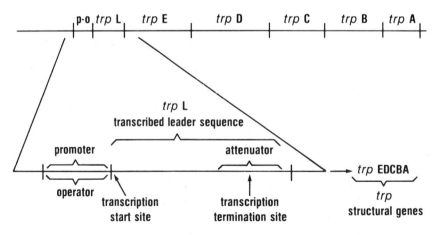

Figure 20-16 Regulatory and structural genes of *trp* operon of *E coli*. Transcription initiation is controlled at promoter-operator. Transcription termination is regulated at attenuator in transcribed 162 base pair leader region *trpL*. The five structural genes *trpE*, *trpD*, *trpC*, *trpB*, and *trpA* encode polypeptides that catalyze terminal sequence of reactions in tryptophan formation. Modified from *Nature,* Vol. 289, pp. 751–758. Copyright © 1981 Macmillan Journals Limited. By permission.

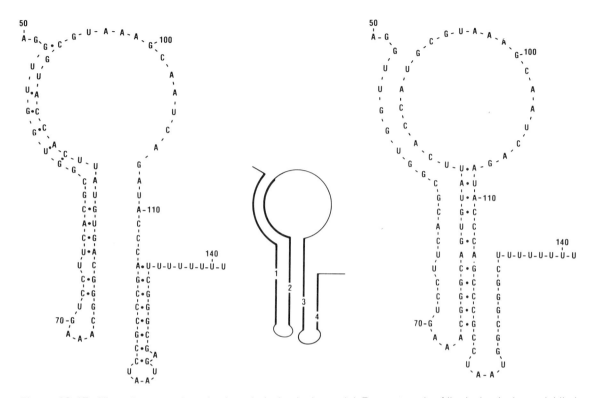

Figure 20-17 Alternative secondary structures in *trp* leader transcript. Four segments of the *trp* leader transcript that can participate in hydrogen-bonding with each other are shown schematically as heavy lines in the center diagram. Secondary structure at left is associated with short transcripts terminated at attenuator, whereas alternative secondary structure at right is thought to prevent transcription termination at attenuator. In secondary structure at left, two hairpin loops are formed by pairing of segment 1 with segment 2 and segment 3 with segment 4. In secondary structure at right, segments 2 and 3 are paired with each other and cannot simultaneously pair with segment 1 or 4. Dots represent hydrogen bonds between complementary purine and pyrimidine bases, and nucleotides are numbered sequentially from origin of *trp* leader transcript. Modified from *Nature,* Vol. 289, pp. 751–758. Copyright © 1981 Macmillan Journals Limited. By permission.

attenuator or extend them to a terminator at the distal end of the operon is the central feature of control of the *trp* operon by attenuation.

In the amino acid biosynthetic operons controlled by attenuation, the machinery of protein synthesis is used to detect depletion of the supply of a specific amino acid and to couple this detected signal with transcription of the appropriate mRNA beyond its attenuator. After transcription is initiated, ribosomes attach to the growing mRNA molecule and begin to translate it; hence, proximal segments of the mRNA are translated at the same time that the distal part of the mRNA is being transcribed. The mRNA leader sequence includes a short region that can be translated to form a peptide; typically, this peptide contains several molecules of the amino acid that correspond to the product of the pathway controlled by the operon. For example, the peptide encoded by the *trp* mRNA leader sequence includes two adjacent tryptophan residues, and the peptide encoded by the *his* mRNA leader sequence has a series of seven consecutive histidine residues. When the supply of a particular amino acid is deficient, the corresponding tRNA is not fully charged, translation of the mRNA leader peptide for the corresponding amino acid biosynthetic operon cannot proceed normally, and ribosomes remain bound at the codons of the mRNA leader sequence that corresponds to the deficient amino acid. The location of these codons is critically important because parking of the ribosomes at these specific sites prevents the mRNA leader sequence from assuming the conformation in which the termination signal is expressed. Consequently, transcription does not terminate at the attenuator, the complete polycistronic mRNA for the operon is made, and the enzymes required for synthesis of the amino acid that was deficient are produced. In contrast, when the supply of the specific amino acid is plentiful, ribosomes do not stop at the critical site within the mRNA leader sequence. Under these conditions, the favored conformation for the mRNA leader sequence is the one that results in premature termination of transcription at the attenuator and prevents full expression of the operon.

A second mechanism that causes premature termination of transcription is **polarity.** Nonsense mutations in structural genes cause termination of polypeptide-chain elongation during protein synthesis. Some nonsense mutations not only affect the functions of the genes in which they are located, but also block expression of other genes located more distally in the operon. This phenomenon, polarity, is often associated with absence of the mRNA that corresponds to the distal genes. Strong polar effects are believed to result from the presence of rho factor–dependent potential termination sites that are located between nonsense codons and the distal ends of the operons. Such potential termination sites are expressed only in the mutants and not in the wild-type strains, because of the way that the rho factor works. Normally, rho factor binds to the 5′ end of a growing mRNA molecule, moves along the mRNA until it encounters RNA polymerase that has paused at a rho factor–dependent termination site, interacts with the polymerase, and causes it to cease transcription and dissociate from its DNA template and its mRNA product. The attachment of rho factor or its movement along mRNAs can be blocked by ribosomes on the mRNAs. In wild-type strains, normal translation prevents rho factor from interacting with RNA polymerase and terminating transcription at sites within the structural genes. During translation of the mutant mRNAs, however, ribosomes are released prematurely when they encounter nonsense codons. This enables rho factor to interact with RNA polymerase that has paused at sites corresponding to locations within the mutant structural genes and thereby cause termination of transcription.

In summary, attenuation and polarity are both examples of premature termination of transcription. Attenuation is a normal physiologic mechanism for regulating operons for amino acid biosynthesis in response to changing availability of specific amino acids; polarity is associated with nonsense mutations and blocks expression of structural genes (in an operon) that are distal to the site of the nonsense mutation.

In some biologic systems, antitermination is used as a positive regulatory mechanism to control gene expression; phage λ provides a particularly well-studied example. Immediately after infection of E coli by λ, the bacterial RNA polymerase binds at two different promoters in λ DNA and initiates transcription of genes that code for immediate early functions. Each of the two immediate early transcripts terminates at a rho factor–dependent termination site. The protein product of gene N, one of the immediate early genes, interacts with RNA polymerase and with specific recognition sites on λ DNA called *nut* (for N *u*tilization) to permit transcription to continue to a second set of termination sites. In this way, the N protein activates expression of the delayed early genes of phage λ. The protein product of λ gene Q, one of the delayed early genes, functions at another location in the λ genome to block termination of transcription of a different mRNA and activate expression of λ late genes. Therefore, antitermination has a key role in controlling the cascade of gene expression that occurs during growth of phage λ.

Control of Translation

Translational control of gene expression in bacteria occurs, but it appears to be significantly less common than transcriptional control. An example of translational control is provided in the case of ribosome biosynthesis. The translation of the mRNAs that code for certain ribosomal proteins is inhibited by the free ribosomal proteins that accumulate when synthesis of rRNA and assembly of complete ribosomes is prevented.

Control of rRNA Synthesis

Normally, a close coupling occurs between the rates of protein synthesis and ribosomal RNA synthesis in *E coli*. When ribosomes participating in protein synthesis encounter uncharged tRNAs corresponding to the codon to be translated, a sequence of events is initiated that results in prompt cessation of rRNA synthesis. This is called the stringent response. A novel nucleotide called guanosine-3′-diphosphate-5′-diphosphate (ppGpp) accumulates during amino acid starvation and appears to be a mediator of the stringent response, but the precise regulatory mechanisms are unknown.

Control of Protein Turnover

Proteins in bacteria are usually stable, and turnover of cellular proteins occurs at a slow rate. During starvation, however, the rate of turnover of cellular proteins increases strikingly. This stimulation during starvation in *E coli* also depends on ppGpp. The breakdown of cellular proteins to generate a pool of amino acids that can be used for synthesis of new proteins may facilitate survival of bacterial cells during adaptation to adverse environments.

Interactions of Regulatory Systems

The various regulatory systems in bacteria work together to maximize metabolic efficiency and growth in a wide variety of environmental conditions. Control of operon expression at the level of transcription initiation (by regulator-operator interactions) or premature termination of transcription (by attenuation) conserves metabolic energy because transcription is the first specific step in the DNA-directed synthesis of proteins. Control of mRNA initiation is formally analogous to feedback inhibition of the first specific enzyme of a metabolic pathway by the product of that pathway. Many of the metabolites that function as effectors in feedback inhibition of enzyme activity or in regulator-operator interactions can be obtained from environmental sources or by biosynthesis. The intracellular concentrations of such compounds may reflect their extracellular concentrations, the activities of specific transport systems, and the rates of their synthesis and utilization. Therefore, these regulatory systems are particularly well suited to respond promptly to changes in the availability of specific compounds in the environment. In contrast, the key metabolic signal for attenuation is the extent to which specific tRNAs are charged. This is determined not only by the availability of the corresponding amino acids but also by the activity of specific aminoacyl-tRNA synthetases, the overall rate of protein synthesis, and other factors. Attenuation appears particularly well suited for adjusting the rates of synthesis of specific amino acids to correspond with the rates of their utilization for protein synthesis.

Several regulatory systems in bacteria control the expression of more than one operon. A broad network of regulatory interactions is illustrated by the role of cAMP and CRP as positive effectors for many different operons. The cAMP-CRP system permits the adequacy of the energy supply to serve as a determinant for the expression of a whole family of bacterial genes. The stringent response involving ppGpp illustrates another regulatory network by which production of additional machinery for protein synthesis (new ribosomes) is coupled closely to an adequate supply of the entire family of charged tRNAs required for protein synthesis.

The metabolic interactions that are required for bacteria to grow and divide under steady-state conditions and to adapt to changing growth conditions are both complex and highly regulated. The examples of regulation of gene expression just described illustrate some of the genetic and physiologic mechanisms that permit relatively simple organisms like bacteria to perform complex metabolic functions and to respond to chemical signals in their environment.

References

Campbell, A.: Evolutionary significance of accessory DNA elements in bacteria. *Ann Rev Microbiol* 1981; 35:55-83.

Datta, N., Hughes, V.M.: Plasmids of the same Inc groups in Enterobacteria before and after the medical use of antibiotics. *Nature* 1983; 306:616-617.

Drake, J.W., Glickman, B.W., Ripley, L.S.: Updating the theory of mutation. *Am Sci* 1983; 71:621-630.

Elwell, L.P., Shipley, P.L.: Plasmid mediated factors associated with virulence of bacteria to animals. *Ann Rev Microbiol* 1980; 34:465-496.

Hendrix, R.W., et al. (editors): Lambda II. Cold Spring Harbor, N.Y.: Cold Spring Harbor Laboratory, 1983.

Holmberg, S.D., et al.: Drug-resistant salmonella from animals fed antimicrobials. *N Engl J Med* 1984; 311:617-622.

Kleckner, N.: Transposable elements in prokaryotes. *Ann Rev Genet* 1981; 15:341-404.

Kolter, R., Yanofsky, C.: Attenuation in amino acid biosynthetic operons. *Ann Rev Genet* 1982; 16:113-134.

Lewin, B.: *Genes.* New York: John Wiley, 1983.

Maas, W.K.: Genetics of bacterial virulence. In: *Genetics as a tool in microbiology,* thirty-first symposium of the Society for General Microbiology. Glover SW, Holwood DA (editors). Cambridge: Cambridge University Press, 1981.

Maniatis, T., Fritsch, E.F., Sambrook, J.: *Molecular cloning: A laboratory manual.* Cold Spring Harbor, N.Y.: Cold Spring Harbor Laboratory, 1982.

Miller, J.H., Reznikoff, W.S. (editors): *The operon.* Cold Spring Harbor, N.Y.: Cold Spring Harbor Laboratory, 1978.

Novick, R.P.: Plasmids. *Sci Am* 1980; 243:103-123.

Shapiro, J.A. (editor): Mobile genetic elements. New York: Academic Press, 1983.

Ward, D.F., Gottesman, M.E.: Suppression of transcription termination by phage lambda. *Science* 1982; 216:946-951.

21 Normal Flora

C. P. Davis, PhD

Raza Aly, PhD

H. I. Maibach, MD

General Concepts

Human beings have diverse microbial flora associated with their skin and mucous membranes from shortly after birth until death. With 10^{13} body cells, human beings routinely also have about 10^{14} bacteria associated with the body. This bacterial population is the **normal microbial flora,** which consists of relatively stable genera of microorganisms that populate certain body regions at particular time spans during an individual's life.

Anaerobic bacterial genera (such as *Bacteroides* and *Streptococcus* sp, both facultative and anaerobic species) comprise the bulk of the microbial flora in the large intestine. The microorganisms that comprise the normal flora may aid the host (by competing for microenvironments more effectively than such pathogens as *Salmonella* or by producing nutrients the host can use), harm the host (by causing dental caries, abscesses, or other infectious diseases), or be commensals (living together for long periods with no harm or benefit to either). Even though the vast majority of the normal microbial flora that inhabit human skin, nails, eyes, oropharynx, genitalia, and gastrointestinal tract usually cause no harm, these organisms frequently cause disease in compromised hosts. Viruses and parasites are not considered members of the normal microbial flora by most investigators because they are not commensals and do not aid the host.

This chapter introduces some of the genera that localize, usually in an identifiable sequence (a bacterial succession), on certain parts of the human body. A few characteristics of individual members of the flora are presented, but the reader should refer to specific chapters for detailed characteristics of the various genera.

Significance of Normal Flora

That normal flora substantially influence the well-being of the host was not well understood until germ-free animals became available. Germ-free animals were obtained by caesarian section and maintained in special isolators, thus allowing the investigator to raise them in an environment free from detectable viruses, bacteria, and other organisms. Two interesting observations were made about animals raised under germ-free conditions. First, the germ-free animals lived almost twice as long as their conventionally maintained counterparts, and second, the major causes of death were different for each group. Infection often caused death in conventional animals, but intestinal atonia frequently killed germ-free animals. Other investigations showed that germ-free animals have anatomic, physiologic, and immunologic features not shared with conventional animals. For example, in germ-free animals, the alimentary lamina propria is underdeveloped, little or no immunoglobulin is present in sera or secretions, intestinal motility is reduced, and the intestinal epithelial cell renewal rate is approximately one-half that of normal animals (4 rather than 2 days).

Although the foregoing suggests that bacterial flora may be undesirable, studies with antibiotic-treated animals suggest that the flora protects individuals from pathogens. Investigators have used streptomycin to reduce the normal flora and have then infected animals with streptomycin-resistant *Salmonella*. Normally, about 10^6 organisms are needed to establish a gastrointestinal infection, but in streptomycin-treated animals whose flora are altered, fewer than ten organisms were needed to cause infectious disease. Further studies suggested that fermentation products (acetic and butyric acids) produced by the normal flora inhibited *Salmonella* growth in the gastrointestinal tract.

Normal flora in humans usually develops in an orderly sequence after birth (**succession**), leading in turn to stable populations of bacteria that comprise the normal flora. The main factor determining the composition of the normal flora in a body region is the nature of the local environment, which is determined by pH, temperature, redox potential, and oxygen, water, and nutrient level. Other factors such as peristalsis, saliva, lysozyme, and secretion of immunoglobulins also play a role in flora control. The local environment is like a concerto in which one principal instrument usually dominates. For example, an infant begins to contact organisms as it moves through the birth canal. A gram-positive population (bifidobacteria and lactobacilli) predominates in the gastrointestinal tract early in life if the infant is breast-fed. This bacterial population is reduced and displaced somewhat by a gram-negative flora (Enterobacteriaceae) when the baby is bottle-fed. The type of liquid diet provided to the infant is the principal instrument of this flora control; immunoglobulins and, perhaps, other elements in breast milk may also play a significant role.

What, then, is the significance of normal flora to humans? Animal and some human studies suggest that the flora influence human anatomy, physiology, lifespan, and, ultimately, cause of death. Although the causal relationship of flora to death and disease in humans is accepted, other roles of the human microflora need further study.

Normal Flora of Skin

Skin provides good examples of various microenvironments. Skin regions have been compared to geographic regions of earth: the desert of the forearm, the cool woods of the scalp, and the tropical forest of the armpit.

Composition of the skin's microbial flora varies according to the environment of its site. Different bacterial flora characterize each of three regions of skin: (a) axilla, perineum, and toe webs; (b) hand, face, and trunk; and (c) upper arms and legs. Skin sites with partial occlusion (axilla, perineum, and toe webs) harbor greater numbers of microorganisms than do less occluded areas (legs, arms, and trunk). These quantitative differences may relate to increased amount of moisture, higher body temperature, and greater concentrations of skin surface lipids. The axilla, perineum, and toe webs are more frequently colonized by gram-negative bacilli than are drier areas of the skin.

The number of bacteria on an individual's skin remains relatively constant; bacterial survival and the extent of colonization probably depends partly on the exposure of skin to a particular environment and partly on the innate and species-specific bactericidal activity in skin. Also, a high degree of specificity is involved in the adherence of bacteria to epithelial surfaces. Not all bacteria attach to skin; staphylococci, which are the major flora of the nose, possess a distinct advantage over viridans streptococci in colonizing the nasal mucosa. Conversely, viridans streptococci are not seen in large numbers on the skin or in the nose but constitute the major flora of the mouth.

The microbiology literature is inconsistent about the density of bacteria on the skin; one reason for this is the variety of methods used to collect skin bacteria (swabs, contact plates, and scrub methods; Table 21-1). The scrub method yields more accurate and higher counts for a given skin area. Most microorganisms live in the superficial layers of the stratum corneum and in the upper parts of the hair follicles. Some bacteria, however, reside in the deeper areas of the hair follicles and are beyond the reach of ordinary disinfection procedures. These bacteria are a reservoir for recolonization after the surface bacteria are removed.

Staphylococcus epidermidis

S epidermidis is a major inhabitant of the skin, and in some areas it comprises more than 90% of the resident aerobic flora. *S epidermidis* is divided into four biotypes on the basis of variable acid production from carbohydrates. *S epidermidis* biotype I is the main type found on the skin and frequently causes infection following the insertion of a ventriculoatrial shunt in the treatment of hydrocephalus.

Table 21-1 Quantitative Aerobic Microbial Flora Recoverable from Adults by Contact and Scrub Techniques

Contact Plate Technique*		Scrub Technique†	
Site	CFU‡/plate	Site	CFU‡/cm²
Forehead	348	Axilla	5.4×10^6
Temple	560	Groin	2.4×10^6
Cheek	548	Toe web	4×10^6
Back of neck	211	Finger web	9.3×10^5
Side of neck	316	Forearm	2.3×10^4
Shoulder	43	Forehead	4×10^5
Subclavicle	83		
Axilla	106		
Upper arm	42		
Forearm	41		
Subscapular	128		
Hip	104		

Adapted from Ulrich J.: In *Skin bacteria and their role in infection.* Maibach, H., Hildick-Smith, G. (editors). New York: McGraw-Hill 1965; and from Aly, R., Maibach, H.I.: *Appl Environ Microbiol* 1977; 33:97.
*Agar pressed to skin.
†Cylinder pressed over skin, nutrient broth (or saline) and Tween 80 added and skin scrubbed with Teflon-tipped rod.
‡Viable bacteria expressed as colony-forming units (CFU).

Staphylococcus aureus

The nose and perineum are the most common sites of *S aureus,* which is present in 10% to more than 40% of normal adults. *S aureus* is prevalent (67%) on vulvar skin. Its occurrence in the nasal passages varies with age and is greater in the newborn, less in adults. *S aureus* is extremely common (80%-100%) on the skin of patients with certain dermatologic diseases such as atopic dermatitis, but the reason for this is unclear.

Micrococci

Micrococci are not as common as staphylococci and diphtheroids; however, they are frequently present on normal skin. *Micrococcus luteus (Sarcina luteus),* the predominant species, usually accounts for 20%-80% of the micrococci isolated from the skin. Micrococci and staphylococci can be separated by several key tests, such as glucose utilization: micrococci utilize glucose oxidatively, whereas staphylococci utilize it both oxidatively and fermentatively.

Diphtheroids (coryneforms)

The term diphtheroids denotes a wide range of bacteria belonging to the genus *Corynebacterium.* Classification of diphtheroids remains unsatisfactory; for convenience, cutaneous diphtheroids have been categorized into four groups composed as follows: lipophilic or nonlipophilic diphtheroids; anaerobic diphtheroids; diphtheroids producing porphyrins (coral red fluorescence when viewed under ultraviolet light); and those that possess some keratinolytic enzyme and are associated with trichomycosis axillaris (infection of axillary hair). Lipophilic diphtheroids are extremely common in the axilla, whereas nonlipophilic strains are found more commonly on glabrous skin.

Anaerobic diphtheroids are most common in rich sebaceous gland areas. Although the term *Corynebacterium acnes* was originally used to describe skin anaerobic diphtheroids, these are now classified as *Propionibacterium acnes (C acnes)* and *P granulosum (C granulosum)*. *P acnes* is seen eight times more frequently than *P granulosum* in acne lesions and is probably involved in acne pathogenesis. Children younger than 10 years of age are rarely colonized with *P acnes*. The appearance of this organism on the skin is probably related to the onset of sebum (a semifluid substance composed of fatty acids and epithelial debris secreted from sebaceous glands) secretion at puberty. *P avidum,* the third species of cutaneous anaerobic diphtheroids, is rare in acne lesions and is more often isolated from the axilla.

Streptococci

Streptococci, especially β-hemolytic streptococci, are rarely seen on normal skin. The paucity of β-hemolytic streptococci on the skin is attributed at least in part to the presence of skin lipids, or fatty acids, as these lipids are lethal to streptococci. Other groups of streptococci, such as α-hemolytic streptococci, exist primarily in the mouth, from where they may, in rare instances, spread to the skin.

Gram-Negative Bacilli

Gram-negative bacteria form a small proportion of the skin flora. In view of their extraordinary numbers in the gut and in the natural environment, their scarcity on skin is striking. Gram-negative bacteria are seen in moist intertriginous areas such as the toe webs and axilla and not on dry skin. Dessication is the major factor preventing the multiplication of gram-negative bacteria on intact skin. *Enterobacter, Klebsiella, Escherichia coli,* and *Proteus* spp are the predominant gram-negative organisms. *Acinetobacter* sp (formerly *Mima-Herellia*) occurs on the skin of normal individuals and, like other gram-negative bacteria, is more commonly found in the moist, intertriginous zones of the skin.

Nail Flora

The microbiology of a normal nail is generally similar to that of the skin. Under the nails, dust particles and other extraneous materials may get trapped, depending upon the nails' contacts. In addition to resident skin flora, these dust particles may carry fungi and bacilli. *Aspergillus, Penicillium, Cladosporium,* and *Mucor* are the major types of fungi encountered in this area.

Oral and Upper Respiratory Tract Flora

The oral flora are involved in causing dental caries and periodontal disease, conditions which affect about 80% of the population in the western world. The oral flora, their interactions with the host, and their alterations by environmental factors are thoroughly discussed in Chapter 116. Anaerobes in the oral flora are responsible for many of the brain, face and lung infections that are frequently manifested by abscess formation.

The pharynx and trachea primarily contain those bacterial genera found in the normal oral cavity (for example, α- and β-hemolytic streptococci); however, anaerobes, staphylococci, neisseriae, diphtheroids, and others are also present. Potentially pathogenic organisms such as *Hemophilus*, mycoplasmas, and pneumococci may also be found in the pharynx. Anaerobic organisms also are found frequently. The upper respiratory tract is so often the site of initial colonization of pathogens (*Neisseria meningitidis, C diphtheriae, Bordetella pertussis,* and many others) that it could be considered the first region of attack for such organisms. In contrast, the lower respiratory tract (small bronchi and alveoli) is usually sterile, because particles the size of bacteria do not readily reach it. If bacteria do reach these regions, they encounter host defense mechanisms, such as alveolar macrophages, that are not present in the pharynx.

Intestinal Tract Flora

The stomach is a relatively hostile environment for bacteria. It contains those bacteria swallowed with the food and those dislodged from the mouth. Acidity lowers the bacterial count, which is highest (approximately 10^3-10^6 organisms per gram of contents) after meals and lowest (frequently undetectable) after digestion. The cultured aspirates of duodenal or jejunal fluid contain approximately 10^3 organisms per milliliter in most individuals. Most bacteria cultured (streptococci, lactobacilli, enterobacteria, bacteroides) are thought to be transients. Levels of 10^5-10^7 bacteria per milliliter in such aspirates usually indicate an abnormality in the individual's digestive system (for example, achlorhydria or malabsorption syndrome). Rapid peristalsis and bile secretions may explain in part the paucity of organisms in the upper gastrointestinal tract. Further along the jejunum and into the ileum, bacterial populations begin to increase, and at the ileocecal junction they reach levels of 10^6-10^8 organisms per milliliter, with streptococci, lactobacilli, enterobacteria, bacteroides, and bifidobacteria accounting for most of the flora.

Concentrations of 10^9-10^{11} bacteria per gram of contents are frequently found in human colon contents and feces. These are composed of a bewildering array of bacteria (more than 400 species have been identified); nonetheless, 95%-99.9% are anaerobic genera such as *Bacteroides, Bifidobacterium, Eubacterium,* anaerobic streptococci (*Peptococcus* and *Peptostreptococcus*), and *Clostridium.*

In this highly anaerobic region of the intestine, these genera proliferate, occupy most available niches, and produce metabolic waste products such as acetic, butyric, and lactic acids. Thus, strict anaerobic conditions, physical exclusion (as occurs in animal studies), and bacterial waste products are factors that inhibit the growth of other bacteria in the large bowel.

Although normal flora can inhibit pathogens, many genera that comprise the normal intestinal flora can produce disease in humans. Anaerobes in the intestinal tract are the primary causative agents of intraabdominal abscesses and peritonitis. Bowel perforations, produced by appendicitis, malignancy, infarction, surgery, or gunshot wounds, almost always seed the peritoneal cavity and adjacent organs with the normal flora. Anaerobes can also cause problems within the gastrointestinal lumen. Treatment with antibiotics may allow certain flora to become predominant and cause disease. For example, *Clostridium difficile*, which can remain viable in a patient undergoing antimicrobial therapy, may produce a pseudomembranous colitis. Other intestinal pathologic conditions or surgery can cause bacterial overgrowth in the upper small intestine. Anaerobic bacteria can then deconjugate bile acids in this region and bind available vitamin B_{12} so that the patient malabsorbs the vitamin and fats. In these situations, the patient usually has been compromised in some way; thus, the infection caused by the normal intestinal flora is secondary to another problem.

There is more information available on animal microflora than on human microflora. Research on animals has revealed that unusual filamentous microbes attach to ileal epithelial cells and modify host membranes with few or no harmful effects. Microbes have been observed in thick layers on gastrointestinal surfaces (Figure 21-1) and in the crypts of Lieberkühn. Other studies indicate the immune response can be modulated by intestinal flora. Intestinal flora studies of vitamin K biosynthesis and other host-utilizable products, conversion of bile acids (perhaps to cocarcinogens), and ammonia production (which can play a role in hepatic coma) show the dual role microbial flora play in influencing the host's health. More basic studies of human bowel flora are necessary to define their effect on humans.

Urogenital Flora

The type of bacterial flora found in the vagina depends on the age, pH, and hormonal levels of the host. *Lactobacillus* sp predominate in female infants (vaginal pH approximately 5) during the first month of life. Glycogen secretion seems to cease from about 1 month of age to puberty. During this time, diphtheroids, *S epidermidis*, streptococci, and *E coli* predominate at a higher pH (approximately 7). At puberty, glycogen secretion occurs, the pH drops, and women acquire an adult flora in which *L acidophilus*, corynebacteria, peptococci, peptostreptococci, staphylococci, streptococci, and bacteroides predominate. After menopause, pH again rises, less glycogen is secreted, and the flora returns to that found in prepubescent girls. Yeasts *(Torulopsis* and *Candida)* are occasionally found in the vagina (10%-30% of women); these sometimes increase and cause vaginitis.

In the anterior urethra of humans, *S epidermidis*, *S faecalis*, and diphtheroids are found frequently; *E coli*, *Proteus*, and *Neisseria* are found occasionly (10%-30%). The normal flora in the urethra are responsible for the care that must be taken in clinically interpreting urine cultures, as they may occur at levels of 10^4 organisms/mL of urine if a midstream (clean-catch) specimen is not obtained.

Conjunctiva

The conjunctival flora are sparse. Approximately 17%-49% of culture samples are negative. Lysozyme, secreted in tears, may play a role in controlling the bacteria by interfering with their cell wall formation. When positive samples show bacteria, corynebacteria, neisseriae, and moraxellae are cultured. Staphylococci and streptococci are also present, and recent reports indicate *Haemophilus parainfluenzae* can be found in 25% of conjunctival samples.

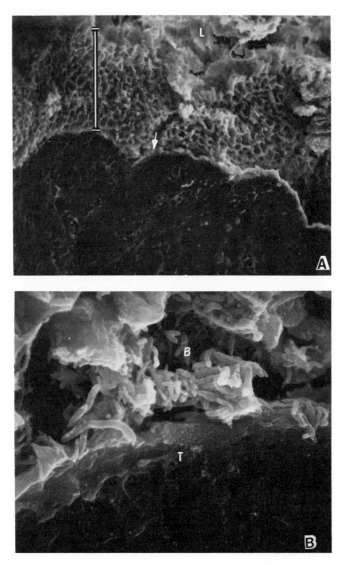

Figure 21-1 Scanning electron microscopy of cross section of rat colon. **A,** Bar indicates extensive layer of bacteria extending toward lumen (L). Arrow indicates where Figure 21-1B was photographed (X262). **B,** Mass of bacteria (B) immediately adjacent to colonized intestinal tissue (T) (X2,624). (**B** From Davis, C.P.: *Appl Environ Microbiol* 1976; 31:310.)

Host Infection by Normal Flora

This chapter has briefly described the normal human flora; however, it has not discussed the pathogenic mechanisms of various genera or the clinical syndromes in which they are involved. Although such material is presented in other chapters, note that breaches in mucosal surfaces often result in the host becoming infected by members of the normal flora. Caries, periodontal disease, abscesses, foul-smelling discharges, and endocarditis are hallmarks of infections with normal human flora. In addition, impaired hosts (for example, those with heart failure or leukemia) or impaired host defenses (due to immunosuppression, chemotherapy, irradiation) may result in failure of the normal flora bacteria to suppress transient pathogens or may cause them to invade the host themselves. In either situation, death of the host often may result.

References

Aly, R., Maibach, H.I.: *Clinical skin microbiology.* Springfield, Ill: Charles C Thomas, 1978.

Bitton, G., Marshall, K.C.: *Adsorption of microorganisms to surfaces.* New York: John Wiley and Sons, 1980.

Draser, B.S., Hill, M.J.: *Human intestinal flora.* London: Academic Press, 1974.

Freter, R., et al: Survival and implantation of *Escherichia coli* in the intestinal tract. *Infect Immun* 1983; 39:686-703.

Hentges, D.J., et al: Protective role of intestinal flora against *Pseudomonas aeruginosa* in mice: Influence of antibiotics on colonization resistance. *Infect Immunol* 1985; 47:118-122.

Marples, M.J.: Life in the skin. *Sci Am* 1969; 220:108-115.

Maibach, H., Aly, R.: *Skin microbiology: relevance to clinical infection.* New York, Heidelberg, Berlin: Springer-Verlag, 1981.

Savage, D.C.: Microbial ecology of the gastrointestinal tract. *Ann Rev Microbiol* 1972; 31:107-133.

22 Pathogenesis and Nonspecific Defenses

L. Joe Berry, PhD

Johnny W. Peterson, PhD

C. P. Davis, PhD

General Concepts
Pathogenic Mechanisms
   Bacterial Infectivity
   Colonization of Host Tissues
   Invasion and Spread of Infection
   Endotoxin
   Exotoxins

Other Virulence Factors
Genetic Mechanisms (R factors)
Nonspecific Host Defenses
   Anatomic Factors
   Physiologic Factors
   Inflammation and Phagocytosis

General Concepts

Equilibrium between the pathogenic potential of the bacterium and the nonspecific defense mechanisms of the host is the critical issue in the initial interaction of bacteria with an animal host. The pathogenic potential of bacteria can involve many factors acting either separately or together, such as ability to colonize body surfaces, increase in number, move on to other sites, penetrate the barriers to invasion, or produce toxic substances. Nonspecific defense mechanisms of the animal host include physical barriers to impair entry of foreign substances, mechanical clearance mechanisms, chemical barriers, competition with organisms comprising the normal microbial flora, and cellular clearance mechanisms. The pathogenic potential of bacteria is not necessarily designed to cause host injury but, in many cases, is probably related to the ability of bacteria to multiply and survive. Likewise, nonspecific defense mechanisms probably evolved as multipurpose mechanisms for host survival (for example, stomach acidity and bile secretions aid in food digestion in addition to serving as microbial barriers). When the equilibrium between bacteria and the host tips to favor the host, potential for disease is reduced or eliminated. Conversely, when bacteria overwhelm the nonspecific defense mechanisms, disease may ensue. Although nonspecific defense mechanisms continue to combat bacterial disease, these defense mechanisms may still function in tandem with specific immune defense mechanisms in an attempt to protect the host (see Chapter 23).

Pathogenic Mechanisms

Bacterial Infectivity

Infection is the invasion of the host by microbes, which then multiply in close association with the host's tissues. Infection is distinguished from disease, a morbid process that does not necessarily involve infection (for example, diabetes is a disease with no known specific causative agent). Bacteria can cause a multitude of different infections, ranging in severity from inapparent to fulminating. Table 22-1 lists these types of infections.

The capacity of a bacterium to cause disease reflects its relative **pathogenicity.** On this basis, bacteria can be organized into three major groups. When isolated from a patient, **frank pathogens** are considered to be probable agents of disease (for example, when the cause of diarrheal disease is identified by the laboratory isolation of *Salmonella* from feces). **Opportunistic pathogens** are those isolated from patients whose host defense mechanisms have been compromised. They may be the agents of disease, for example, in patients who have been predisposed to urinary tract infections with *Eshericia coli* by catheterization. Finally, some bacteria, such as *Lactobacillus acidophilus*, are considered to be **nonpathogens,** because they rarely or never cause human disease. Their categorization as nonpathogens may change, however, because of the adaptability of bacteria and the detrimental effect of modern radiation therapy, chemotherapy, and immunotherapy on resistance mechanisms. In fact, some bacteria previously considered to be nonpathogens are now known to cause disease. *Serratia marcescens,* for example, has been found to cause urinary tract infections and bacteremia in compromised hosts.

Virulence is the measure of an organism's pathogenic potential (pathogenicity). The degree of virulence is related directly to the bacterium's capacity to cause disease despite host resistance mechanisms; it is affected by numerous variables such as the number of infecting bacteria, route of entry into the body, specific and nonspecific host defense mechanisms, and virulence factors of the bacterium. Virulence can be measured experimentally by determining the number of bacteria required to cause animal death, illness, or lesions in a defined period of time, after the bacteria are administered by a designated route. Consequently, calculations of a lethal dose affecting 50% of a population of animals (LD_{50}) or an effective dose causing a disease symptom in 50% of a population of animals (ED_{50}) are useful in comparing the relative virulence of different bacteria.

The widely used method for determining virulence, which was devised by Reed and Muench nearly 50 years ago, is illustrated in Table 22-2. The infectious dose is increased

Table 22-1 Types of Bacterial Infections

Types of Infection	Description	Examples
Inapparent (subclinical)	No detectable clinical symptoms of infection	Asymptomic gonorrhea in women and men
Dormant (latent)	Carrier state	Typhoid carrier
Accidental	Zoonosis and environmental exposures	Anthrax and cryptococcal infection
Opportunistic	Infection caused by normal flora or transient bacteria when normal host defenses compromised	*Serratia* or *Candida* infection of the genitourinary tract
Primary	Clinically apparent invasion and multiplication of microbes in body tissues causing local tissue injury	*Shigella* dysentery
Secondary	Microbial invasion subsequent to primary infection	Bacterial pneumonia following viral lung infection
Mixed	Two or more microbes infecting same tissue	Anaerobic abscess (*E. coli* and *B. fragilis*)
Acute	Rapid onset (hrs or days); brief duration (days/weeks)	Diphtheria
Chronic	Prolonged duration (months, years)	Mycobacterial diseases (tuberculosis and leprosy)
Localized	Confined to a small area or to an organ	Staphylococcal boil
Generalized	Disseminated to many body regions	Gram-negative bacteremia (gonococcemia)
Pyogenic	Pus-forming	Staphylococcal and streptococcal infection
Retrograde	Microbes ascending in a duct or tube against the flow of secretions or excretions	*E coli* urinary tract infection
Fulminant	Infections that occur suddenly and intensely	Airborne *Yersinia pestis* (pneumonic plague)

Table 22-2 Calculation of the LD_{50}

Infectious Dose of Bacteria	Number of Mice Alive	Number of Mice Dead	Cumulative Survivors (Add Up)	Cumulative Deaths (Add Down)	Cumulative Total (Add Across)	Percent Dead (Cumulative)
2×10^4	9	1	32	1	33	3
4×10^4	7	3	23	4	27	15
6×10^4	6	4	16	8	24	33
8×10^4	6	4	10	12	22	55
10×10^4	3	7	4	19	23	83
12×10^4	1	9	1	26	27	97

$$LD_{50} = 60,000 + 20,000 \left(\frac{50 - 33}{55 - 33} \right)$$

$$LD_{50} = 60,000 + 15,455$$

$$LD_{50} = 7.5 \times 10^4$$

by uniform increments to make calculation simpler. Ten animals are infected, by the same route, with each challenge dose. The dead and surviving animals in each group are listed in columns 2 and 3. The number of cumulative survivors is determined by assuming that any animal capable of surviving a large dose of organisms would survive a smaller dose. Therefore, by starting at the bottom of column 4 and adding upward, the researcher can determine the number of animals capable of surviving each challenge. Similarly as an animal that dies from a small dose would probably die if given a larger dose, cumulative deaths are determined by adding downward in column 5. The cumulative total shown in column 6 is the sum, at each dose, of the number of survivors and deaths. These values are used to calculate the percentage of dead animals listed in column 7. The final step is to interpolate between 33% and 55% mortality by using the 6×10^4 bacteria that killed an estimated 33% of the animals and then finding the fraction of 2×10^4 (the increment) that yields the 50% point). Thus, by rounding out fractions, the LD_{50} in this example is found to be 7.5×10^4.

Colonization of Host Tissues

The virulence of a bacterium is increased substantially by structures that permit colonization of the host's surface. Flagella propel the bacterium to areas in which nutritional factors favor its growth and multiplication; they also appear to be important in assisting some bacteria to establish close physical contact with surface epithelial cells of the host. For example, *Vibrio cholerae*, which causes cholera, must migrate through a layer of mucus that covers the small intestinal epithelium before attaching to the surface. In the pathogenesis of a *Vibrio* infection, the flagella of the bacteria may allow them to adhere to the epithelial cells by adhesins and reach the appropriate sites. More frequently, attachment of bacteria is mediated by pili. In gonorrhea, a common genital infection, colonization is achieved by pili-mediated adherence (see Chapter 30). Pili also play an essential role in the virulence of enteropathogenic *E coli* (Chapter 41), in which, in some cases, the attachment sites on cells can be blocked by the addition of a specific sugar, mannose. Regardless of the adherence mechanism, the selective retention of pathogenic bacteria to specific host cells increases the probability that disease will ensue.

Invasion and Spread of Infection

For disease to result following colonization, one of two possible mechanisms must prevail: the bacterium, while close to the host, must release potent toxins detrimental to the host, or it must enter the host's tissues and set up disseminated foci of infection. Although toxin production inside or outside the host often is the immediate cause of disease, the invasive potential of the bacterium may be crucial in the delivery of toxins to the target organ. Some bacteria invade mucosal epithelial surfaces of the respiratory, intestinal, and genitourinary tracts. The precise mechanisms that allow most bacteria to invade host cells are poorly understood; some bacteria seem to enter by pinocytosis, whereas others appear to secrete cytotoxic substances that affect the integrity of the host cell membrane. Many bacteria tend not to invade the host unless damage to the body surface occurs. Thus, trauma in the form of wounds, surgical incisions, or abrasions allows the entrance of bacteria that otherwise would not have access to the host. If these bacteria can survive the normal defense mechanisms of the host, disease will likely result.

Once inside the host, some bacteria may exhibit **organotropisms** (preference for a specific organ or organs), which most likely result from **chemotaxis** (movement toward or away from a chemical stimulus). A classical example of organotropism occurs in cattle infected with *Brucella abortus*. Abortion is a prominent feature of brucellosis in cattle, because the bovine uterus is rich in erythritol, a carbohydrate preferred by this bacterium. Bacterial organotropisms also occur in humans; a good example is the invasion of the central nervous system by *Neisseria meningitidis*. Most mechanisms of organotropism are not well understood.

Several mechanisms allow bacteria to survive and spread throughout the body of the host; those of the staphylococci and streptococci are among the best characterized. Staphylococci, streptococci, and clostridia produce hyaluronidase, an enzyme that hydrolyzes hyaluronic acid, the intercellular ground substance of connective tissue, and thus loosens the integrity of tissue barriers. As a result, the enzyme facilitates the spread of these bacteria through tissues. Many bacteria produce other substances (for example, proteases, neuraminidase, and cytotoxins) that increase the probability of their migration in the host. Spread of bacteria in the host occurs through lymph, blood, tissues, and migrating phagocytes. The routes of entry and spread account for the typical localization of certain pathogens, although some bacteria may be deposited at some sites because of chemotaxis. Regardless of bacterial localization, numerous bacterial substances, discussed in the following sections, are responsible for the pathogenesis of bacterial diseases.

Endotoxin

Endotoxin is a lipopolysaccharide moiety that constitutes part of the outer membrane of all gram-negative bacteria (see Chapter 16). It is considered to be responsible for the pathogenic manifestations of many gram-negative infections, even though proof of this in many cases has not been established. For the following pathogenic bacteria, the only confirmed toxic component of the cell is endotoxin: *N gonorrhoeae*, *N meningitidis*, the nonenterotoxigenic strains of *E coli*, members of the genera *Brucella*, *Haemophilus*, *Francisella*, *Proteus*, *Serratia*, and probably some species of *Salmonella*, *Shigella*, *Klebsiella*, and *Pasteurella*. Only a few produce one or more toxic proteins in addition to endotoxin.

Endotoxin has been known for years to act as a potent pyrogen, and it causes a characteristic biphasic fever response (Table 22-3 shows other biologic effects). The fever causation is mediated through an endogenous pyrogen released in response to endotoxin from macrophages distributed in a variety of organs, such as the liver, spleen, and lymph nodes. The pyrogen has been purified to homogeneity, and antibody against it has been found to neutralize the pyrogenic effect of endotoxin in homologous laboratory animals. Fever is produced when the endogenous pyrogen reaches the thermoregulatory center in the hypothalamus and raises the body's "thermostat" so that body temperature is maintained at a nearly constant elevated level. Because fever is pathognomonic for many infectious diseases, especially those caused by gram-negative

Table 22-3   Biologic Effects of Endotoxin

Type of Response	Preferred Animal for Study	Target Cells or Organ
Fever	Rabbits and primates	Endogenous pyrogen on neurons in hypothalamus
Cardiovascular shock	Dogs and primates	Probably vascular endothelium
Increase in nonspecific resistance	All species	Decrease in serum iron and increase in interferon
Adjuvanticity and immune stimulation	All species	B lymphocytes, macrophages, and probably T lymphocytes
Sanarelli-Shwartzman reaction	Rabbits	Skin and platelets (intravascular fibrin formation)
Protection against X-irradiation	Mice	Stimulation of myelocytic cells
Susceptibility to stress (heat, cold)	Mice	Glucocorticoid antagonist from macrophages
Lethality	All species	Combinations of above

microorganisms, the release of endogenous pyrogen is presumably responsible for fever induction.

Endotoxin causes profound changes in the vascular system. When endotoxin is administered intravenously to dogs, the animals become hypertensive almost immediately, probably in response to the release of biogenic amines such as histamine and 5-hydroxytryptamine. This transitory phase is followed quickly by a prolonged and progressively severe hypotension. Tissue perfusion diminishes, and death usually occurs because of circulatory collapse. Patients who die from gram-negative septic shock have symptoms that are similar to those seen in experimental animals after a lethal dose of endotoxin. The underlying cause of the vascular changes induced by endotoxin has not been established conclusively.

Originally Sanarelli and, later, Shwartzman observed that a second immunizing dose of a vaccine or culture supernatant from a gram-negative bacterium often produced a skin lesion at the site of the first vaccine injection (localized Sanarelli-Shwartzman reaction). This reaction can be duplicated in rabbits, especially if the interval between the two injections is only a few hours. The initial or preparatory dose should be intradermal, and the eliciting dose should be intravenous. The two injections need not contain antigenically related vaccines or the same bacterium derivative. If both injections are given intravenously, bilateral renal cortical necrosis and intravascular coagulation (generalized Sanarelli-Shwartzman reaction) occur and death often results.

Endotoxin has some interesting effects on the immune system. It is a potent adjuvant, it activates the alternate complement pathway, and it leads to the consumption of large amounts of the complement components along this pathway, designated as $C'3-C'9$, thereby diminishing the hemolytic activity of fresh serum incubated with endotoxin. The polysaccharide moiety of lipopolysaccharide is highly antigenic, whereas the lipid A component is only weakly antigenic when used as an isolated product that has been made soluble by complexing with a suitable protein such as albumin. Researchers have suggested, however, that antibodies against lipid A may provide protection against infectious challenge with gram-negative bacteria of unrelated species. Thus, livers and spleens of animals treated with endotoxin undergo hypertrophy as a result of the proliferation of cells of the reticuloendothelial system. Particulate matter, including microorganisms, is cleared more rapidly from the blood of such animals, and phagocytosis is enhanced as a result of the increase in number of cells.

The effects of endotoxin on the elements involved in host defense may explain why an injection of endotoxin increases an animal's nonspecific resistance to a wide array of infectious diseases caused by a variety of pathogens (bacteria, fungi, parasites, viruses). This remarkable effect, which has been confirmed by many investigators, has never been explained fully, but it may result from the decrease in levels of circulating iron that accompanies an injection of endotoxin. The microorganisms must compete with the host for iron needed for growth. When less iron is available, microbial proliferation is suppressed, thereby permitting host defenses to cope with the slow-growing pathogens.

Endotoxin recently has been observed to stimulate the release or production of several mediators (other than endogenous pyrogen) from various cells of the animal host, including colony-stimulating factor, interferon, tumor-necrotizing factor, leukocyte-endogenous mediator, glucocorticoid-antagonizing factor, serotonin, histamine and related compounds, kinin production, and, probably, various lymphokines. The functions of these mediators are discussed in the first section. All actions attributed to endotoxin may be caused by mediators, as the chemical structure and molecular size of lipopolysaccharide make endotoxin an unlikely sole cause of its biologic effects.

Exotoxins

Exotoxins constitute another broad category of toxins that are distinguished from the lipopolysaccharide endotoxin. Virtually all exotoxins are proteins released from viable bacteria. Most exotoxins are heat-labile and constitute a class of poisons that is among the most potent, per unit weight, of all toxic substances. Unlike endotoxin, which is a structural component of all gram-negative cells, exotoxins are produced by only some members of gram-positive and gram-negative genera. In most instances, the functions of these exotoxins for the bacteria are unknown. In contrast to the extensive systemic and immunologic effects of endotoxin on the host, the site of action of most exotoxins is more localized and is confined to particular cell types or cell receptors. Tetanus toxin, for example, affects only internuncial neurons. In general, exotoxins are excellent antigens that elicit specific antibodies, or antitoxins. The resulting antitoxins can react with the exotoxin and neutralize it, whereas antibody to endotoxin reacts with the lipopolysaccharide complex and has little effect on the biologic activity of the complex. Exotoxins can be grouped into several categories (neurotoxins, cytotoxins, and enterotoxins), based on their biologic effect on host cells.

Neurotoxins are best exemplified by the toxins produced by *Clostridium* sp. One example of a neurotoxin is botulinum toxin, produced by *C botulinum*. This potent neurotoxin acts on motor neurons by preventing the release of acetylcholine at the myoneural junction, thereby preventing muscle excitation and producing flaccid paralysis (see Chapter 34). In comparison, cytotoxins constitute a larger, more heterogenous grouping with a wide array of host cell specificities and toxic manifestations. One cytotoxin is diphtheria toxin, which is produced by *Corynebacterium diphtheriae*. This cytotoxin can act on many cell types, but its primary mode of action always is the same. Diphtheria toxin produces ADP-ribosylation of elongation factor II, which blocks elongation of the growing peptide chain and thus terminates protein synthesis.

Enterotoxins are those exotoxins that stimulate the hypersecretion of fluid and electrolytes from the intestinal epithelial surface. Some enterotoxins may also disturb normal smooth muscle contraction, and thereby cause abdominal cramping.

Enterotoxigenic *E coli* and *V cholerae* produce diarrhea if they attach to the intestinal mucosa while elaborating a toxin that causes fluid and electrolyte loss from the blood into the intestinal lumen. Neither pathogen can invade the body in substantial numbers, so penetration of the intestinal mucosa is not an essential aspect of virulence in these organisms. In contrast, organisms responsible for shigellosis (*Shigella dysenteriae, S Boydii, S flexneri,* and *S sonnei*) must penetrate the mucosal surface of the colon and terminal ileum to proliferate and cause ulcerations, which then lead to loss of blood into the stools. This limited invasiveness appears to be an essential requirement for virulence, although the pathogens rarely become blood-borne and systemic. Endotoxin is the bacterial component believed to be responsible for producing the symptoms of shigellosis. It is present in all *Shigella* species capable of producing disease, and host responses are consistent with those known to be caused by endotoxin. On the other hand, the pathogenic role of enterotoxin, detected after in vitro growth of *S dysenteriae*, is problematic because some *Shigella* sp that cause dysentery have not been demonstrated to produce the enterotoxin under the same conditions. Laboratory animals infected with *S flexneri* have been reported to form antitoxic antibodies; however, toxin synthesis may occur under in vivo growth conditions that have not yet been duplicated *in vitro*.

In contrast to shigellosis, typhoid fever and other forms of salmonellosis are characterized by bacterial penetration of the intestinal wall. Bacteremia and systemic infection result. Intestinal ulceration often occurs through rupture of Peyer's patches, placing the patient at risk for more serious complications. The bacteria also may be discharged from the gallbladder into the digestive tract, which may become a chronic condition in patients who are carriers. Whether one or more exotoxins are involved in the pathogenesis of salmonellosis has not been established clearly. *Salmonella* sp have been reported to produce an enterotoxin.

Other Virulence Factors

Numerous structural and metabolic virulence factors have evolved among bacteria, enhancing the survival rate of the bacteria in the host. Capsule formation has long been recognized as a protective mechanism for bacteria. Encapsulated strains of many bacteria (for example, pneumococci) are more virulent and more resistant to phagocytosis and intracellular killing. Many organisms are killed by fresh human serum that contains complement components; organisms that cause bacteremia are less sensitive to killing by fresh human serum and are called serum-resistant. Serum resistance may be related to the amount and structure of capsular antigens, as well as to the structure of the lipopolysaccharide.

The relationship between surface structure and virulence also is important in infections with *Borrelia* sp. As the bacteria encounter increasing resistance to infection in the host, bacterial surface antigens are altered by bacterial mutation and selection.

Salmonella typhi and some of the paratyphoid organisms contain a surface antigen thought to enhance virulence. Accordingly designated the Vi antigen, it is composed of a polymer of galactosamine and uronic acid in 1,4-linkage. Its role in virulence has not been defined, but antibody against it is protective.

Some bacteria and parasites have the ability to survive and multiply inside phagocytic cells. *Mycobacterium tuberculosis,* whose survival seems to depend upon the structure of its cell surface (see Chapter 48), is a classic example. *Toxoplasma gondii* (see Chapter 99) has the remarkable ability to block the fusion of lysosomes with the phagocytic vacuole. The hydrolytic enzymes contained in the lysosomes are unable, therefore, to contribute to the destruction of the parasite. The mechanisms by which other bacteria, such as *Brucella abortus* and *Listeria monocytogenes,* remain unharmed inside phagocytes are not understood.

Some bacteria may survive in the host because of substances called siderophores. Perhaps the most important function of siderophores is chelating iron in competition with the host. Strains of bacteria that do not secrete siderophores have markedly reduced virulence in animal models (for example, the enterochelin in enteric bacteria). Some other virulence factors (teichoic acids, envelopes, and cell walls) have not been mentioned in this section; this chapter covers only the major factors in survival and multiplication of bacteria in the host.

Genetic Mechanisms (R factors)

In 1959, during an outbreak of dysentery, Japanese microbiologists observed that freshly isolated cultures of *S dysenteriae* were simultaneously resistant to four antibiotics: streptomycin, chloramphenicol, tetracycline, and sulfonamide. Subsequent incubation of resistant cells with sensitive cells resulted in frequent transfer of multiple resistance. Because resistance to each drug is determined by a separate gene, it was evident that all four genes must be located on one plasmid, called an R factor. R factors are now known to be widespread in enteric bacteria; exchange can occur between species within one genus or between species of different genera. Genetic exchange is thought to be a regular occurrence within the digestive tract; it may occur more frequently when the selective pressure of antibiotic therapy is involved. Resistance to as many as 11 or 12 antibacterial agents, including antibiotics and heavy metals, is known to be transferred by a single plasmid.

Plasmids do not normally encode for essential enzymes; thus, resistance to each antibiotic probably depends on a nonessential plasmid-encoded enzyme that inactivates the drug. For example, β-lactamase hydrolyzes the β-lactam ring of penicillin. Other specific enzymes adenylate streptomycin, acetylate chloramphenicol, or phosphorylate kanamycin. Chromosomal resistance usually results from modification of the antibiotic receptors on the bacterial cell, which diminishes drug effectiveness.

Antibiotic therapy may increase the incidence of drug resistance and the frequency of R factor transfer. Therefore, administration of antimicrobial agents is indicated only when laboratory and sensitivity tests have established the efficacy of the treatment. Prescribing an antibiotic for a febrile patient without first identifying the causative organism and showing its susceptibility to the drug of choice is unacceptable medical practice.

Other important plasmids can code for pathogenic mechanisms such as colonization factors (for example, antigens), enterotoxin production (for example, *E coli* heat-labile toxin), and siderophore synthesis. Some of these plasmids may become integrated with the bacterial chromosome and thus can be transmitted by conjugation. Bacteriophages also may contribute to the virulence of bacteria. Toxin production by *C diphtheriae* occurs as a result of lysogenic infection of the bacterium by a bacteriophage containing the gene for toxin synthesis. Similarly, several serologic types of botulin toxin are encoded by bacteriophages specific for *Clostridium* species (see Chapters 34 and 48).

Nonspecific Host Defenses

Nonspecific host defenses are a collection of nonimmunologic protective mechanisms in the host that limit access of microorganisms to the body. They are categorized as either anatomic or physiologic factors.

Anatomic Factors

Perhaps the most important barrier to microorganisms is the skin. The outermost layer of squamous cell epithelium is continually being sloughed and replaced, a process that constantly removes a portion of the microbial flora colonizing the skin. Mucosal epithelium of the intestinal, respiratory, and genitourinary tracts is also replaced continuously. In addition, portions of the respiratory tract are lined with cilia, hair, and a layer of mucus to prevent microorganisms from migrating into the lungs. The cilia beat in an upward, rhythmic movement to ensure expulsion of the mucous layer and its microbial flora. When this mechanism functions properly, the lungs are kept free of microorganisms. Similarly, peristalsis, a movement that produces a washing action on the gut wall, constantly removes substances from the gastrointestinal tract. In addition, body orifices are protected from potentially pathogenic organisms by such structures as sphincters, eardrums, and nasal hairs.

Physiologic Factors

One important physiologic factor in nonspecific host defense is the local or systemic fever response that accompanies many infections. The rise in body temperature often suppresses bacterial multiplication, allowing phagocytic cells greater opportunity to remove the microbes. In contrast to temperature rise during acute infection, some regions of the body, such as the skin and upper respiratory tract, have temperatures lower than 37 C, which limits the multiplication of some pathogens. These body regions are normally colonized by microorganisms with lower temperature optima. Normal skin has a low pH and high fatty acid content, both of which are toxic for some bacteria.

Likewise, gastric acidity (pH 2) kills many bacteria so quickly and effectively that the duodenum is almost devoid of organisms. In addition, the body produces several enzymes that inhibit bacterial growth and colonization. Proteases are found in the gastrointestinal tract, as are bile acids, which can lyse bacteria such as pneumococci. Another enzyme, lysozyme, which is found in saliva and tears, effectively disrupts the peptidoglycan in bacterial cell walls, allowing osmotic lysis of the microorganisms.

The blood contains many substances that contribute nonspecifically to host defense. Transferrin is a substance that binds iron, thereby making it unavailable to bacteria. Properdin, a basic globulin that interacts with certain bacteria and the complement cascade, is found in all normal blood. Two other components found in varying concentrations in normal blood are the so-called natural antibodies and interferon. Although both of these substances probably result from heteroantigenic stimulation, they are so commonplace that they are considered to be nonspecific host defense mechanisms.

Inflammation and Phagocytosis

An inherent nonspecific host defense of all normal mammals from birth is the ability of certain cell types (polymorphonuclear leukocytes, macrophages, and Küpffer cells) to phagocytize and digest certain substances. These cells phagocytize any substance recognized as either foreign material or as altered host cells. When a pathogen disrupts the host cells or enters the body, inflammation and phagocytosis usually occur simultaneously.

Inflammation is a cellular response to injury or abnormal stimulation by physical, chemical, or biologic agents. Its features include local or systemic temperature increase, increased vascular permeability, and migration of certain cell types (polymorphonuclear leukocytes, macrophages, and lymphocytes). This cellular infiltration and vasodilation is caused by release of a small number of mediators, including histamine, 5-hydroxytryptamine, and kinins from various cell types such as lymphocytes and histiocytes.

Phagocytosis can occur in many cell types, but nonspecific host defense relies mainly on polymorphonuclear leukocytes and macrophages. Phagocytosis has two main steps: engulfment, which requires firm attachment, and subsequent chemical dissolution, or killing, of bacteria. This latter phenomenon is facilitated by opsonins directed against specific bacteria. Chemical dissolution of bacteria and other substances occurs inside phagolysosomes bound by membranes. In polymorphonuclear leukocytes, myeloperoxidase, in combination with H_2O_2, halide ions, and a low pH value is particularly important in killing bacteria. Also generated is a toxic superoxide radical. In addition, because the pH is low (3–4), lysozyme is present. In macrophages, large amounts of lysosomal enzymes and proteases are formed, although the myeloperoxidase system is absent. This nonspecific armamentarium usually can confine and eliminate most microbes.

References

Berry, L.J.: Bacterial toxin. *CRC Crit Rev Toxicol* 1977; 5:239–318.
Eisenstein, T.K., Actor, P., Friedman, H.: *Host defenses to intracellular pathogens.* New York: Plenum Press, 1983.

Foster, T.J.: Plasmid-determined resistance to antimicrobial drugs and toxic metal ions in bacteria. *Microbiol Rev* 1983; 47:361–409.

Mims, C.A.: *The pathogenesis of infectious disease.* London: Academic Press, 1976.

Sack, R.B.: Human diarrheal disease caused by enterotoxigenic *Escherichia coli. Ann Rev Microbiol* 1975; 29:333–351.

Schlessinger, D. (editor): *Microbiology 1980.* Washington, D.C.: American Society for Microbiology, 1980.

Smith, H.: Microbial surfaces in relation to pathogenicity. *Bacterial Rev* 1977; 41:475–500.

Smith, H., Skehel, J.J., Turner, M.J. (editors): *The molecular basis of microbial pathogenicity.* Deerfield Beach, FL: Verlag Chemie, 1980.

23 Specific Acquired Immunity

John P. Craig, MD

General Concepts
Biologic Basis of Acquired Resistance
Antibody-Mediated Resistance Mechanisms
Cell-Mediated Resistance Mechanisms
Acquired Resistance to Infectious Disease
Artificial Immunization

General Concepts

Bacterial infections, like all infections, are usually followed by a state of specific acquired resistance to reinfection by the same microorganism. This specific acquired resistance is one facet of the host's immune response to the intrusion of the foreign antigens present in the infecting microbe.

In bacterial infections, both humoral (antibody-mediated) and cellular immune responses may play important roles in acquired resistance. Bacteria vary greatly in their rates of growth, mechanisms of pathogenesis, and preferred sites of multiplication within the host. Some produce acute diseases, whereas others cause chronic infections associated with prolonged survival and multiplication of organisms within phagocytic cells. Therefore, the nature and effectiveness of the immune response in bacterial infections vary greatly, depending on the properties of the infecting bacterium and its location within the host.

Biologic Basis of Acquired Resistance

Acquired specific resistance is initiated by the stimulation and expansion of lymphocyte clones that can respond to specific antigens in the infecting microbe (see Section I on immunology). Expansion of specific populations of B lymphocytes or T lymphocytes mediates resistance. B lymphocytes mature into plasma cells that synthesize and release immunoglobulins, the mediators of humoral immunity. T lymphocytes play a major role in cell-mediated immune mechanisms and as helper cells in some B-cell-mediated responses. Either one or both of these immune responses may be involved in the increased resistance that an animal exhibits following natural infection or artificial exposure to microbial antigens (vaccination).

The common features of antibody-mediated and cell-mediated immunity are specificity and memory. Memory results from the persistence of increased populations of specifically primed, antigen-reactive lymphocytes following exposure to antigen. These cells respond quickly to subsequent exposure to the same antigen by vigorous differentiation and population expansion. This cellular response leads to more rapid and greater production of antibody or cell-mediated reactivity or both.

Determining the change in specific immune resistance and distinguishing specific resistance from preexisting innate and nonspecific resistance require a method for measuring resistance. This can be achieved only by observing the differences in morbidity and mortality between immune and nonimmune animals following live microbial challenge. Although in vitro measurement of antibody and cell-mediated immunity may sometimes correlate with resistance, such measurements can never subsitute fully for in vivo challenge of the whole animal. In vitro measurements do not necessarily correlate with protection against disease because some in vitro assays measure activities of antibodies or lymphocytes that may not be protective in vivo.

Antibody-Mediated Resistance Mechanisms

Antibody-mediated immunity in bacterial infections may be directed against antigenic toxic products (**antitoxic immunity**) or against antigens on the bacterial surface (**antibacterial immunity**). Antitoxic immunity resembles antibody-mediated antiviral immunity in that the combination of antibody with the toxin antigen prevents attachment or entry of the toxin into the target cells. This process is called **toxin neutralization.**

Antitoxin may be circulating IgG or secretory IgA, but only circulating IgG antitoxins have been clearly shown to protect against bacterial toxins in human disease. Bacterial infections in which the major manifestations of disease are caused by highly potent, secreted toxic proteins (exotoxins) are called **toxinoses;** diphtheria, tetanus, botulism, scarlet fever, and cholera are examples. Specific antitoxins can be effective in conferring resistance if they can combine with exotoxin and neutralize it before the toxin combines with specific receptors on target cell membranes. Once exotoxins have attached to susceptible cells and entered them, antitoxin is ineffective. Therefore, in diseases in which the exotoxin must be distributed by the blood from the site of synthesis to the target cell (diphtheria, tetanus, botulism, and scarlet fever) humoral antitoxic immunity is relatively effective because antitoxin can neutralize the toxin before it binds to target cell membranes. In cholera, on the other hand, exotoxin is produced by bacteria adhering to the luminal surface of small intestinal epithelial cells, which are also the target cells for the toxin. Passage of the toxin through the bloodstream does not occur and, in humans, serum antitoxin has not been shown to be protective. It is not clear whether IgA antitoxin effectively protects against cholera in humans, but because the distance from the toxin source to its target is so short, successful neutralization even by local secretory antitoxin may prove difficult.

Antibody directed against bacterial surface antigens may enhance phagocytosis by combining with surface or capsular antigens, inhibit attachment of bacteria to cell surfaces by combining with bacterial surface structures (for example, fimbriae), inhibit motility by combining with flagellar antigens, or promote complement-mediated bacteriolysis. Precipitation of bacterial macromolecules and agglutination of whole bacterial cells probably play little or no role in increasing resistance in vivo, even though serum from a resistant host may readily exhibit these reactions in vitro.

In infections with organisms that possess polysaccharide capsules such as *Neisseria meningitidis*, *Streptococcus pneumoniae*, and *Haemophilus influenzae*, specific acquired resistance can be attributed mainly to anticapsular antibody, which alters the bacterial surface and thereby renders the microbe more susceptible to phagocytosis and intracellular killing by granulocytes. This process is called **opsonization**, and the antibodies are called **opsonins**. Figure 23-1 shows the reciprocal relationship between the incidence of meningococcal infection and antibody titers specific for the three most common types of capsular polysaccharide in the general population. A vaccine composed of type-specific capsular polysaccharide has been tested and proved highly effective in preventing disease caused by meningococci of the same capsular type.

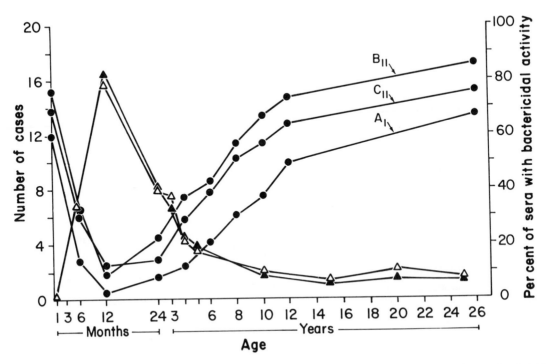

Figure 23-1 Age-related incidence of meningococcal disease in United States and prevalence of serum bactericidal activity against three pathogenic strains of *N meningitidis*. Number of cases/100,000 age-specific population, 1965, ▲——▲; 1966, △——△. Percent sera having bactericidal titer of 1:4 or greater against meningococcal strains A_1, B_{11} and C_{11}, ●——●. From Goldschneider, I., Gotschlich, E.C., Artenstein, M.S. *J Exp Med* 1969; 129:1307.

Secretory antibody directed against surface structures may inhibit adherence of bacteria to mucosal surfaces and prevent colonization, which is a necessary step in the pathogenesis of several bacterial infections. For example, antibodies against fimbriae appear to confer resistance against infections with enterotoxinogenic strains of *Escherichia coli* that cause diarrhea; they may also function in resistance against gonococcal infections of the genitourinary tract mucosa.

Antibody-mediated immunity can be judged to play a decisive role in resistance only if passive transfer of serum from an immune animal specifically protects a nonimmune animal against live bacterial challenge. Studies of passive transfer usually are done in animals; a few studies in human volunteers have assessed the value of passive immunoprophylaxis against naturally occurring disease. For certain virus infections, for example, poliomyelitis and hepatitis A, controlled studies have shown that injection of serum containing specific antibody does indeed afford protection, but similar studies in humans have not been done for bacterial infections. The successful use of tetanus antitoxin as a routine immunoprophylactic measure for patients with wounds strongly suggests that antitoxin alone is sufficient to prevent tetanus in humans, but, for ethical reasons, adequately controlled studies have not been performed in humans.

Cell-Mediated Resistance Mechanisms

In some bacterial infections, particularly those characterized by intracellular survival and multiplication of the microbe in mononuclear phagocytes, cell-mediated immunity may be the major factor in resistance. As noted previously, this immunity arises by stimulation and expansion of specific clones of T cells following exposure to those specific microbial antigens for which they possess preexisting receptors. Sensitized T lymphocytes respond to a second exposure of the original antigen by producing lymphokines. One of these lymphokines, **macrophage-activating factor** (MAF), increases the capacity of macrophages to destroy ingested bacteria. This enhanced capacity for intraphagocytic killing is independent of antibody and is the major mechanism of acquired specific resistance in infections with pathogens such as brucellae, tubercle bacilli, listeriae, *Francisella tularensis,* and *Salmonella typhi*. These intracellular bacteria, as well as certain bacterial components such as endotoxin (lipopolysaccharide) can also induce T cells to produce interferons that can nonspecifically enhance intracellular killing of bacteria, protozoa, and viruses by macrophages.

The *cell* in the term *cell-mediated immunity* refers to the immunologically committed T lymphocyte and not to the macrophage, which is the ultimate executor in the cell-mediated immune response. In cell-mediated immunity, although the lymphocyte response is antigen-specific, the increase in bactericidal activity of macrophages is nonspecific; it acts effectively against a variety of unrelated organisms. Cell-mediated resistance declines after recovery from infection, but it can be recalled by reexposure of the residual population of immunologically committed lymphocytes to the antigens of the originally infecting microbe. Cell-mediated immunity of this type may be conferred on normal animals by the transfer of lymphocytes from actively immunized animals. Bactericidal activity of the macrophages of the recipient increases following reexposure of the recipient to the specific antigen.

Infections that elicit cell-mediated immunity usually also elicit a state of delayed hypersensitivity, which can be demonstrated by either intracutaneous injection or topical application of antigen. Delayed hypersensitivity is manifested as an area of redness and firm swelling that is characterized by a localized infiltration of mononuclear cells at the site of antigen deposition, which reaches a peak 24–48 hours after the sensitized host is exposed. A positive tuberculin skin test (Mantoux test) is an example of this kind of response. Like cell-mediated immunity, delayed hypersensitivity can be transferred by lymphocytes. Delayed hypersensitivity is mediated by a lymphokine, **migration inhibition factor** (MIF), which is produced with other lymphokines such as MAF when microbial antigens interact with immunologically committed lymphocytes. By inhibiting macrophage migration, MIF promotes accumulation of macrophages in areas of higher antigen concentration. This series of events is the basis for skin reactions of delayed hypersensitivity as in the positive tuberculin test. The precise relationship between delayed hypersensitivity and enhanced cellular immunity is not known. Both are phenomena mediated by immunologically committed T lymphocytes, but they do not always increase and decrease together.

In many infections, delayed hypersensitivity may be associated with tissue destruction. Intense accumulation of mononuclear cells at sites of high antigen concentration in tissues may lead to marked disturbance of function and even tissue death. The classic example of the harmful effect of delayed hypersensitivity is seen in tuberculosis. Sensitivity to the antigens of *Mycobacterium tuberculosis* may be followed by caseation necrosis (death of host tissue that produces a homogeneous mass with cheeselike consistency and appearance). Therefore, although cell-mediated immunity and delayed hypersensitivity may be associated with increased resistance to exogenous challenge with living bacteria, they may also be associated with tissue destruction during the natural course of disease.

Acquired Resistance to Infectious Disease

In different bacterial diseases, humoral and cell-mediated immunity contribute to specific acquired resistance in varying proportions. Antibody tends to be a decisive factor in infections in which the bacteria remain chiefly extracellular and in those in which exotoxins are major pathogenetic factors. Cell-mediated immunity appears to be more important in those infections in which multiplication occurs chiefly in mononuclear phagocytes, which interfere with antibody access. In these infections, resistance ultimately depends on heightened intraphagocytic killing, which results from the interaction of specific antigen with immunologically committed lymphocytes and is independent of antibody.

Figure 23-2 illustrates the synergistic activity of humoral and cell-mediated immunity. Antibody-coated *Salmonella typhimurium* undergoes moderate intracellular killing when engulfed by normal macrophages. In comparison, when phagocytized by activated macrophages (activated by the product [MAF] of the interaction between *S typhimurium* antigen and immunologically committed lymphocytes), intracellular killing is accelerated and enhanced.

In most infections, more than one mechanism of acquired immunity develops during the course of disease, and it is the synergistic effect of this mosaic of mechanisms

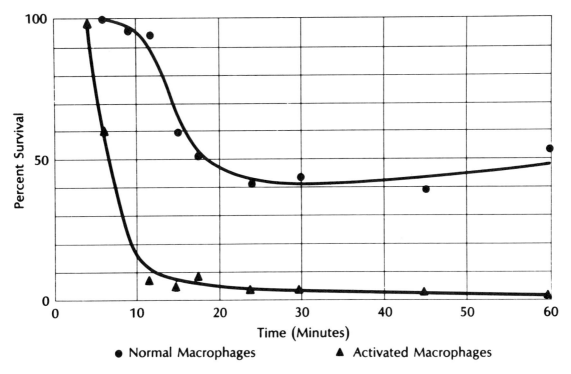

Figure 23-2 Faster onset of killing and greater bactericidal capability of activated vs. normal macrophages was demonstrated in this experiment with opsonized *Salmonella typhimurium*. From Mackaness, G.B.: *Hosp Practice* 1970; 5:73. Reproduced with permission.

that constitutes the specific acquired resistance displayed by the host when rechallenged with a given microbe. The relative influence of each mechanism involved probably varies from individual to individual, depending upon the host's unique immunologic response to the microbe's antigens. Therefore, although the above generalizations usually are valid, it must be emphasized that each kind of infection, in each host species, and even in each individual of a species, must be evaluated separately.

Artificial Immunization

Having observed the natural acquisition of resistance after recovery from smallpox (a virus disease), the ancient Chinese became the first to attempt artificial immunization by inoculation of scab material from patients with mild smallpox (variolation). The danger of inducing severe disease was recognized, and the price paid was often high. Many centuries later, Edward Jenner's recognition that inoculation (vaccination) with material taken from a mild disease related to smallpox (cowpox) could protect humans against smallpox led to artificial immunization with attenuated or killed microbial vaccines.

Jenner's vaccine has so far proved to be the most successful artificial immunizing agent that has been developed. As a result of a concerted worldwide vaccination campaign, the last reported case of smallpox occurred in 1978, and the World Health

Organization has declared the disease eradicated. Whether the smallpox virus has indeed disappeared as a natural human parasite remains to be seen, but the achievement is unique. Eradication of smallpox by vaccination has been possible because the disease is limited to humans, only one antigenic type of virus exists, and persistent infection following recovery does not occur.

The term vaccine (derived from *vaccinia,* the Latin name for cowpox) originally referred only to smallpox vaccine. Today, however, the term vaccine can be properly applied to any **active immunizing agent,** including those composed of whole bacteria or viruses, living or killed, as well as bacterial components or products or their detoxified toxins (toxoids).

In a few bacterial and viral infections, **passive immunization** is attempted by injecting antibody-containing serum or purified immunoglobulins from animals or human volunteers who have previously been actively immunized. Such passive immunizing agents are called antisera or antitoxins.

Table 23-1 lists the major immunizing agents in current use against human bacterial infections. Antisera may be used as immunoprophylactic agents if they are given before exposure to prevent disease or as immunotherapeutic agents if used in the treatment of disease. The active immunizing agents (vaccines) are, of course, always used as prophylactic agents.

Although no bacterial diseases are likely to be eradicated by vaccination in the near future, a few of the vaccines listed in Table 23-1 have contributed significantly to the reduction in morbidity and mortality from these diseases. Bacterial infections will be difficult to eradicate by vaccination because many bacteria persist in animal reservoirs or in the environment, many can colonize the immunized human host and are a source of infection for others, and many have multiple antigenic types. It has been difficult to develop bacterial vaccines because some organisms cannot be cultivated *in vitro* (for example, *Treponema pallidum,* the spirochete of syphilis) or, when grown *in vitro,* they may not produce the appropriate antigenic components that evoke protective immunity (for example, *B pertussis*). Moreover, in many bacterial infections, it is not clear which antigens are responsible for the resistance that follows recovery from natural disease and which route of administration would be most successful in stimulating this resistance.

Infections in which bacteria multiply exclusively on mucosal surfaces of the respiratory, intestinal, or genitourinary tracts pose a particularly difficult problem in vaccine development. In such infections, adherence to the host cell luminal membrane is essential to pathogenesis. Adherent organisms can deliver toxic products to cell surface receptor molecules more efficiently, and thus can make microbial antigens more available to the initiators of the secretory immune system than can organisms free in the lumen. Adherence may be mediated by specialized fimbriae (pili), as in enterotoxinogenic *E coli* and gonococci, or by less structured macromolecular adhesins, as in *Vibrio cholerae.*

Secretory IgA directed against adherence factors has been shown to protect the host by preventing the chain of events initiated by adhesion. Because attachment is the first step in invasion of mucosal cells, sIgA that inhibits attachment can be the major antiinvasive immune mechanism in infections in which pathogenesis is mainly associated with intracytoplasmic multiplication, such as shigellosis and diarrhea caused by enteroinvasive *E coli.*

Table 23-1   Major Immunizing Agents Used Against Bacterial Infections of Humans

General Category	Disease	Agent	Comments
Passive immunization (anti-sera)	Diphtheria	Antitoxin (usually horse serum)	Used chiefly in treatment of diphtheria, effectiveness uncertain.
	Tetanus	Antitoxin (horse serum or human tetanus immune globulin)	Used both for immunoprophylaxis (effective) and for treatment of tetanus (effectiveness uncertain)
	Botulism	Polyvalent antitoxin against several serotypes of *Clostridium botulinum* toxin	Used chiefly for treatment of botulism; probably effective if given early
Active immunization (vaccines)	Diphtheria	Toxoid (formalin-detoxified toxin of *Corynebacterium diphtheriae*)	Widely used, effective, long-lasting
	Tetanus	Toxoid (formalin-detoxified toxin of *Clostridium tetani*)	Widely used, effective, long-lasting
	Pertussis	Killed *Bordetella pertussis* whole cell vaccine	Widely used in children under 6 years of age; effective
	Typhoid fever	Killed *Salmonella typhi* whole cell vaccine	Moderately effective against low challenge doses
		Living attenuated oral vaccine (galactose epimerase deficient mutant of *S. typhi*)	New; more effective than killed vaccine
	Cholera	Killed *Vibrio cholerae* whole cell vaccine	Moderate, short-lived effectiveness
	Plague	Killed *Yersinia pestis* whole cell vaccine	Moderate, short-lived effectiveness
	Tuberculosis	Living attenuated strain of *Mycobacterium bovis* (BCG)	Moderate, long-lasting effectiveness but used only in high-risk groups
	Pneumococcal pneumonia	Polyvalent capsular polysaccharide vaccine prepared from 14 serotypes of *Streptococcus pneumoniae*	Effective in high-risk groups
	Meningococcal infections	Types A and C capsular polysaccharides from *Neisseria meningitidis*	Effective in high-risk groups
	Typhus fever	Killed *Rickettsia prowazekii* whole cell vaccine	Moderately effective
	Rocky Mountain spotted fever	Killed *Rickettsia rickettsii* whole cell vaccine	Moderately effective; used only for special high-risk groups

Circulating IgA, IgG, and IgM are of little value in protecting against surface infections. As an example, cholera toxoid, which evoked impressive levels of circulating IgG antitoxin, failed to protect against cholera in controlled field trials. The available evidence now suggests that sIgA directed against adherence factors or toxins, and present in the appropriate mucosal secretions, is probably necessary to provide specific acquired resistance against these surface pathogens. This kind of immunoglobulin probably can be raised to protective levels only by exposing the appropriate mucosal surface to the relevant antigen *in the proper molecular form*. Thus, antigen forms that may be capable of evoking protective antibody when introduced to macrophages in the tissues (as by injection) may not be recognized by the M (membrane) cells of the Peyer's patches of the ileum when the same antigen is applied to the mucosa. Homing of sIgA-producing cells to the site of antigen exposure has also been shown to occur. These findings emphasize the importance of selecting the proper antigen form and site of delivery in the development of vaccines against surface infections.

Systemic infections, in which the microbe or its toxins must pass through tissues containing antibody or sensitized lymphocytes to reach their sites of multiplication or toxic activity, do not present the same obstacles to vaccine development.

A living, enzyme-deficient mutant of *Salmonella typhi* recently has been introduced as an oral vaccine against typhoid fever. The vaccine strain probably undergoes one or two divisions in the recipient's intestine, but the exact site of this limited multiplication and the other prerequisites for conferring immunity are not known. Nevertheless, this vaccine has afforded a high level of protection against typhoid fever in controlled field trials. It evokes both cell-mediated immunity and specific antibodies that could serve as opsonins. The relative contributions of these two mechanisms to the acquisition of resistance is not yet clear, but animal studies suggest that both are necessary to achieve maximal protection.

Smallpox vaccine was developed before the biologic mechanisms of specific immunity were known, which emphasizes the fact that the methods needed for measuring resistance are completely independent of an understanding of the mechanism by which that resistance is acquired and expressed. There is no doubt, however, that a better understanding of these immune mechanisms will greatly improve our future chances of developing vaccines that can provide protection more nearly approaching that conferred by natural disease.

References

Collins, F.M.: Vaccines and cell-mediated immunity. *Bacteriol Rev* 1974; 38:371-402.

Goldschneider, I., Gotschlich, E.C., Artenstein, M.S.: Human immunity to the meningococcus. I. The role of humoral antibodies. *J Exp Med* 1969; 129:1307-1326.

Lurie, M.B.: *Resistance to tuberculosis.* Boston: Harvard University Press, 1964.

McNabb, P.C., Tomasi, T.B.: Host defense mechanisms at mucosal surfaces. *Ann Rev Microbiol* 1983; 35:477-96.

Wahdan, M.H., et al: A controlled field trial of live *Salmonella typhi* strain Ty21a oral vaccine against typhoid: three year results. *J Infect Dis* 1982; 145:292-295.

Wilson, G.S., Miles, A.A., Parker, M.T. (editors): *Topley and Wilson's principles of bacteriology, virology, and immunity,* Vol. 1, 7th ed. Baltimore: Williams and Wilkins, 1983.

24 Epidemiology

Philip S. Brachman, MD

General Concepts

This chapter reviews the general concepts of *epidemiology*, which is the study of the determinants, occurrence, distribution, and control of health and disease in a defined population. Epidemiology is a descriptive science and includes the determination of rates, that is, the quantification of disease occurrence within a specific population. The most commonly studied rate is the attack rate, or the number of cases of the disease divided by the population among whom the cases have occurred. Epidemiology can accurately describe the occurrence of a disease before its cause is identified. For example, Snow described many aspects of the epidemiology of cholera in the late 1840s, fully 30 years before Koch described the bacillus. One goal of epidemiologic studies is to define the parameters of a disease, including risk factors, in order to develop the most effective and efficient measures for control and prevention of future cases. This chapter includes a discussion of the chain of infection, the three main epidemiologic methods, and how to investigate an epidemic.

Proper interpretation of disease-specific epidemiologic data requires information concerning past as well as present occurrence of the disease. The collection, collation, analysis, and reporting of these data is called **surveillance,** and an active, sensitive, and specific surveillance program is necessary to develop adequate information about the occurrence of a disease. For example, the United States abides by an international agreement to report four diseases (cholera, plague, smallpox [now declared eradicated], and yellow fever). In addition health departments of individual states also report to the Centers for Disease Control (CDC) the occurrence of 33 diseases weekly and of another 7 diseases either annually or as they occur.

Diseases Recommended to be Reported to the United States Centers for Disease Control

Acquired immunodeficiency syndrome
(AIDS) (W, A, CR)
Amebiasis (A)
Anthrax (W, A)
Arboviral infections
(CR)
Aseptic meningitis
(W, A, CR)
Bacterial meningitis
(CR)
Botulism (W, A)
Brucellosis
(W, A, CR)
Chickenpox (W, A)
Cholera (W, A)
Diphtheria (W, A, CR)
Encephalitis
Primary (W, A, CR)
Postinfectious
(W, A, CR)
Enterovirus (CR)
Foodborne disease
(CR)
Hepatitis
A (infectious)
(W, A, CR)
B (serum)
(W, A, CR)
Non-A, Non-B
(W, A, CR)
Unspecified
(W, A, CR)
Influenza (CR)
Intestinal parasites
(CR)

Legionellosis
(W, A, CR)
Leprosy (W, A, CR)
Leptospirosis
(W, A, CR)
Malaria (W, A, CR)
Measles (rubeola)
(W, A)
Meningococcal infections
Total (W, A)
Civilian (W, A)
Military (W, A)
Mumps (W, A)
Pertussis (whooping
cough) (W, A, CR)
Plague (W, A)
Poliomyelitis (CR)
Total (A)
Paralytic (W, A)
Nonparalytic (W)
Unspecified (W)
Psittacosis (W, A, CR)
Rabies
In animals
(W, A, CR)
In humans (W, A)
Rheumatic fever
(acute) (A)
Rubella (German measles) (W, A)
Congenital
(W, A, CR)
Salmonellosis (excluding typhoid fever;
A, CR)

Shigellosis (A, CR)
Smallpox (W, A)
Tetanus (W, A, CR)
Toxic shock syndrome
(W, A, CR)
Trichinosis (W, A, CR)
Tuberculosis (W, A,
CR)
Tularemia (W, A)
Typhoid fever (W, A,
CR)
Typhus fever
Murine (flea-borne)
(W, A)
Rocky Mountin
spotted fever
(tick-borne) (W,
A, CR)
Venereal diseases
Gonorrhea (W, A,
CR)
Civilian (W, A)
Military (W, A)
Syphilis (W, A, CR)
Civilian (W, A)
Military (W, A)
Chancroid (A, CR)
Granuloma inguinale (A, CR)
Lymphogranuloma
venereum (A,
CR)
Waterborne disease
(CR)
Yellow Fever (W, A)

W, Notifiable weekly through *Morbidity and Mortality Weekly Report* (MMWR).
A, Notifiable annually through *MMWR Annual Summary*.
CR, Notifiable by case report form.

Infection, Infectiousness, and Occurrence

Infection is the replication of organisms in the tissue of a host; **disease** is the overt clinical manifestation of infection. In inapparent, or subclinical, infection, an immune response can occur without overt clinical disease. A **carrier** (or colonized individual) is a person in whom organisms are present and may be multiplying, but who shows no clinical response to their presence. The carrier state may be permanent, with the organism always present; intermittent, with the organisms present for varying periods; or temporary, with carriage for only a brief period. **Dissemination** is the movement of an infectious agent from a source individual directly into the enviroment; when infection results from dissemination, the source individual is referred to as a dangerous disseminator.

Infectiousness is the transmission of organisms from a source, or reservoir (see page 310), to a susceptible individual. A human may be infective during the preclinical, clinical, postclinical, or recovery phase of an illness. The **incubation period** is the interval in the preclinical period between the time at which the causative agent first infects the host and the onset of clinical symptoms, during which time the agent is replicating. The greatest period of infectiousness may be during the incubation period for some diseases such as measles; in other diseases such as shigellosis, transmission occurs during the clinical period. The individual may be infective during the convalescent phase or become an asymptomatic carrier and remain infective for prolonged periods, as do approximately 5% of persons with typhoid fever.

The spectrum of occurrence of disease in a defined population includes **sporadic** (occasional occurrence); **endemic** (regular, ongoing occurrence); **epidemic** (significantly increased occurrence); and **pandemic** (epidemic occurrence in multiple countries).

Chain of Infection

The chain of infection describes the interaction of three factors that lead to infection: the etiologic agent, the method of transmission, and the host. For the most effective and efficient utilization of resources, the characterization of these links in the chain should precede implementation of control and prevention measures. Environmental factors may influence any of the links; thus their effect also must be evaluated.

Etiologic Agent

The **etiologic agent** may be any microorganism that can cause infection. The **pathogenicity** of an agent is its ability to cause disease; pathogenicity is further characterized by describing the organism's virulence and invasiveness. **Virulence** refers to the severity of infection. Some organisms are highly virulent, for example, *Yersinia pestis* (the causative agent of plague, which almost always causes severe disease in the susceptible host). An organism with low virulence is *Staphyloccoccus epidermidis* (a frequent skin contaminant that only rarely causes significant disease).

Invasiveness of an organism refers to its ability to invade tissue. *Vibrio cholerae* organisms are noninvasive, causing symptoms by releasing into the intestinal canal an exotoxin that acts on the tissues. In contrast, *Shigella* organisms in the intestinal canal are invasive and migrate into the tissue.

No microorganism is completely avirulent. An organism may have very low virulence, but if the host is highly susceptible, as when therapeutically immunosuppressed, infection with that organism may cause disease. The poliomyelitis virus in the oral vaccine is highly attenuated and thus has low virulence, but in some highly susceptible individuals it can cause paralytic disease.

Other factors should be considered in describing the agent. The **infecting dose** (the number of organisms necessary to cause disease) varies according to the organism, method of transmission, site of entrance of the organism into the host, host defenses, and host species. Another agent factor is specificity; some agents (for example, *Salmonella typhimurium*) can infect a broad range of hosts; others have a narrow range of hosts. *S typhi*, for example, infects only humans. Other agent factors include antigenic composition, which can vary within a species (as in influenza virus or *Streptococcus*); antibiotic sensitivity; resistance transfer plasmids; and enzyme production.

The **reservoir** of an organism is the site where it resides, metabolizes, and multiplies. The **source** of the organism is the site from which it is transmitted to a susceptible host, either directly or indirectly through an intermediary object. The reservoir and source can be different; for example, the reservoir for *S typhi* could be the gallbladder of an infected individual, but the source for transmission might be food contaminated by the carrier. The reservoir and source can also be the same, as in an individual who is a permanent nasal carrier of *S aureus* and who disseminates organisms from this site. The distinction can be important when considering where to apply control measures.

Method of Transmission

The method of transmission is the means by which the agent goes from the source to the host. The four major methods of transmission are contact, common vehicle, airborne, and vector borne.

In **contact transmission** the agent may be spread directly, indirectly, or by droplet. Direct contact transmission takes place when organisms are transmitted directly from the source to the susceptible host without involving an intermediate object; this is also referred to as person-to-person transmission. An example is the transmission of hepatitis A virus from one individual to a susceptible host by hand contact. Indirect transmission occurs when the organisms are transmitted from a source, either animate or inanimate, to a host by means of an inanimate object. An example is *Pseudomonas* organisms transmitted from one individual to another by means of a shaving brush contaminated from the first individual. Droplet spread refers to organisms that travel through the air very short distances, that is, less than 3 feet from a source to a host. Thus, the organisms are not airborne in the true sense. An example of a droplet-spread disease is measles.

Common vehicle transmission refers to agents transmitted by a common inanimate vehicle with multiple cases resulting from such exposure. This category includes diseases in which food or water as well as drugs and parenteral fluids are the vehicles of infection. Examples include food-borne salmonellosis, waterborne shigellosis, or bacteremia resulting from use of intravenous fluids contaminated with a gram-negative organism.

The third method of transmission, **airborne**, refers to infection spread by droplet nuclei or dust. To be truly airborne, the particles should travel more than 3 feet through the air from the source to the host. Droplet nuclei are the residue from the evaporation of fluid from droplets, are light enough to be transmitted more than 3 feet from the source, and may remain airborne for prolonged periods. Tuberculosis is primarily an airborne disease; the source may be an infected patient who, when coughing, creates aerosols of droplet nuclei that contain tubercle bacilli. Infectious agents may be contained in dust particles, which may become resuspended and transmitted to hosts. An example occurred in an outbreak of salmonellosis in a newborn nursery in which *Salmonella*-contaminated dust in a vacuum cleaner bag was resuspended when the equipment was used repeatedly, resulting in infections among newborns.

The fourth method of transmission is **vector borne** disease, in which insects are the vectors. Vector transmission may be external or internal. External, or mechanical, transmission occurs when organisms are carried mechanically on the vector (for example, *Salmonella* that contaminate the legs of flies). Internal transmission occurs when the organisms are carried *within* the vector. If the organism is not changed by its carriage within the vector, the form of internal transmission is called **harborage** (as when a flea ingests plague bacilli from an infected individual or animal and contaminates a susceptible host when it feeds again; the organism is not changed while in the flea). The other form of internal transmission is called **biologic.** In this form, the organism is changed biologically during its passage through the vector (for example, malaria parasites in the mosquito vector).

Infectious agents may be transmitted by more than one route of transmission. For example, *Salmonella* may be transmitted by a common vehicle (food) or by contact spread (human carrier). *Francisella tularensis* may be transmitted by any of the four routes.

Host

The third link in the chain of infection is the host. The organism may enter the host through the skin, mucous membranes, lungs, gastrointestinal tract, genitourinary tract, or into fetuses through the placenta. Frequently, the resulting disease reflects the point of entrance, but this may not always be the case; meningococci may enter the host through the mucous membranes, but they nonetheless cause meningitis. Development of disease in a host reflects agent characteristics (see previous discussion) and is influenced by host defense mechanisms, which may be nonspecific or specfic.

Nonspecific defense mechanisms refer to the skin, mucous membranes, secretions, excretions, enzymes, inflammatory response, genetic factors, hormones, nutrition, behavioral patterns, and presence of other diseases. Specific defense mechanisms or immunity may be natural, resulting from exposure to the infectious agent, or artificial, resulting from active or passive immunization (see Chapter 23).

The environment can affect any link in the chain of infection. Temperature can assist or inhibit multiplication of organisms at their reservoir, air velocity can assist the airborne movement of droplet nuclei, low humidity can damage mucous membranes, and ultraviolet radiation can kill the microorganisms. In any investigation of disease, it is important to evaluate critically the effect of environmental factors and to react accordingly. At times, environmental control measures are instituted more on emotional grounds than on epidemiologic fact. It should be apparent that the occurrence of disease results from the interaction of many factors; some of these factors are outlined here.

Epidemiologic Methods

The three major epidemiologic techniques are descriptive, analytic, and experimental. Although all three can be used in investigating the occurrence of disease, the method used most is descriptive epidemiology. Once the basic epidemiology of a disease has been described, specific analytic methods can be used to study the disease further, and a specific experimental approach can be developed to test a hypothesis.

Descriptive Epidemiology

In descriptive epidemiology, data that describe the occurrence of the disease are collected by various methods from all relevant sources. The data are then collated by time, place, and person. Four time trends are considered in describing the epidemiologic data. The **secular** trend describes the occurrence of disease over a prolonged period of time, such as years; it is influenced by the degree of immunity in the population and possibly nonspecific measures such as improved socioeconomic and nutritional levels among the population. For example, the secular trend of tetanus in the United States since 1920 shows a gradual and steady decline.

Agent, Host, and Environmental Factors That Influence Disease Occurrence

Agent Factors
  Direct
    Pathogenicity
      Virulence
      Invasiveness
    Dose
    Specificity
    Stability
    Antigenic composition
    Antibiotic susceptibility
    Resistance transfer plasmids
    Enzyme production
  Indirect
    Reservoir
    Source
    Duration of dissemination

Host Factors
  Site of Deposition
  Defense Mechanisms
    Genetic
    Nonspecific
      Primary
        Skin, mucous membranes, respiratory tract
      Secondary
        Physiologic (cough, tears)
        Other (age, sex, diet)
      Environmental factors
        Temperature
        Humidity
        Radiation
  Specific Immunity
    Active
      Natural (following clinical or subclinical disease)
      Acquired (vaccination)
    Passive
      Natural (transplacental)
      Acquired (tetanus antiserum)

The second time trend is the **periodic trend.** A temporary modification in the overall secular trend, the periodic trend usually indicates a change in the antigenic characteristics of the disease agent. For example, the change in antigenic structure of the prevalent influenza A virus every 2–3 years results in periodic increases in the occurrence of clinical influenza caused by lack of natural immunity among the population. Additionally, a lowering of the overall immunity of a population or segment thereof can result in an increase in the occurrence of the disease. This can be seen with some immunizable diseases when periodic decreases occur in the level of immunization in a defined population.

The third time trend is the **seasonal trend.** This trend reflects seasonal changes in disease occurrence following changes in environmental conditions that enhance the agent's ability to replicate or be transmitted. For example, food-borne disease outbreaks occur more frequently in the summer, when temperatures are more favorable for multiplication of bacteria to infective dose levels. Examining the occurrence of salmonellosis on a monthly basis makes this trend evident (Figure 24-1).

The fourth time trend is the **epidemic occurrence** of disease. This trend reflects the sudden increased occurrence of cases of the disease due to prevalent factors that support disease transmission.

A description of epidemiologic data by place indicates the site where the susceptible host came in contact with the infectious agent. The location of the host when disease becomes clinically apparent can differ from the place where the infection occurred. This difference is important to consider in attempting to prevent additional

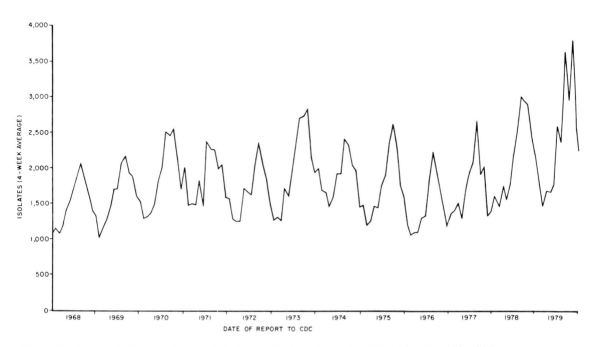

Figure 24-1 Reported human *Salmonella* isolations, by 4-week average, United States, 1968–1982.

cases. For example, an individual who develops gastroenteritis in one city may have been infected in another city; this distinction must be made to prevent additional cases.

The third descriptive factor is person; it requires identifying all the pertinent characteristics that describe an individual: age, sex, occupation, personal habits, socioeconomic status, immunization history, presence of underlying disease, and other data.

Once the descriptive epidemiologic data have been analyzed, the features of the epidemic should be clarified so that additional areas for investigation become apparent.

Analytic Epidemiology

The second epidemiologic method is analytic epidemiology, which analyzes disease determinants for possible causal relations. The two main analytic methods are the case-control (or case-comparison) method and the cohort method. The case-control method starts with the effect (disease) and retrospectively investigates the cause that led to the effect. The case group consists of those individuals with the disease; a comparison group is selected whose members are similar to the case group except for absence of the disease. These two groups are then compared to determine differences that would explain the occurrence of the disease. An example of a case-control study is selecting individuals with meningococcal meningitis and a comparison group matched for age, sex, socioeconomic status, and residence, but who do not have meningococcal meningitis, to see what factors may have influenced the occurrence in the group who developed disease.

The second analytic approach is the cohort method, which prospectively studies two populations: one that has had contact with the suspected causal factor under study and a similar group that has had no contact with the factor. When both groups are observed, the effect of the factor should become apparent. An example of a cohort approach is to observe two similar groups of people, one composed of individuals who received blood transfusions and the other group who did not. Noting the occurrence of hepatitis in both groups permits an association between blood transfusions and hepatitis to be made; that is, if the transfused blood was contaminated with hepatitis B virus, the recipient cohort should have a higher incidence of hepatitis than the nontransfused cohort.

The case-control approach is relatively easy to conduct and is inexpensive and reproducible; however, bias may be introduced in selecting the two groups, it may be difficult to exclude subclinical cases from the comparison group, and a patient's recall of the past events may be faulty. The advantages of a cohort study are the accuracy of collected data and the ability to make a direct estimate of the disease risk resulting from factor contact; however, cohort studies take longer and are more expensive to conduct.

Experimental Epidemiology

The third epidemiologic method is the experimental approach. A hypothesis is developed and an experimental model is constructed in which one or more selected factors are manipulated. The effect of the manipulation will either confirm or disprove the hypothesis. An example is the evaluation of the effect of a new drug on a disease. A group of people with the disease is identified, and some members are randomly selected to receive the drug. If the only difference between the two groups is use of the drug, the clinical differences between the two groups should reflect the effectiveness of the drug.

Epidemic Investigation

An epidemic investigation describes the factors relevant to an outbreak of disease; once the circumstances related to the occurrence of disease are defined, appropriate control and prevention measures can be identified. In an epidemic investigation, data are collected, collated according to time, place, and person, and analyzed, and inferences are drawn.

In the investigation, the first action should be to confirm the existence of the epidemic by discussing the occurrence of the disease with physicians or others who have seen or reported cases by examining patients and reviewing laboratory and hospital records. These diagnoses should then be verified. A case definition should be developed so that some specificity exists as to which patients are actual cases, which are suspected or presumptive cases, and which should be omitted from further study. Additional cases may be sought or additional patient data obtained, and a rough case count made.

This initial phase consists basically of collecting data, which then must be organized according to time, place, and person. The population at risk should be identified and a hypothesis developed concerning the occurrence of the disease. If appropriate, specimens should be collected and transported to the laboratory. More specific studies may be indicated. Additional data from these studies should be analyzed and the hypothesis confirmed or altered. After analysis, control and prevention measures should be developed and, insofar as possible, implemented. A report containing this information should be prepared and distributed to those involved in investigating the outbreak and in implementing control and/or prevention measures. Continued surveillance activities may be appropriate to evaluate the effectiveness of the control and prevention measures.

In the United States, the CDC assists state health departments by providing epidemiologic and laboratory support services on request. Its assistance supports disease investigations and diagnostic laboratory activities and includes various training programs conducted in the states and at the CDC. A close working relationship exists between the CDC and state health departments. Additionally, physicians frequently consult with CDC personnel on a variety of health-related problems and attend public health training programs.

The use of epidemiology to characterize a disease before its etiology has been identified is exemplified by the initial studies of acquired immunodeficiency syndrome (AIDS). The first cases came to the attention of the CDC when an increase was observed in requests for pentamidine for treatment of *Pneumocystis carinii* pneumonia. This initiated specific surveillance activities and epidemiologic studies that provided important information about this newly diagnosed disease.

Initial symptoms include fever, loss of appetite, weight loss, extreme fatigue, and enlargement of lymph nodes. A severe immunodeficiency then develops, which appears to be associated with opportunistic infections. These infections include *P carinii* pneumonia, diagnosed in 52% of cases; Kaposi's sarcoma in 26% of cases; and both *P carinii* pneumonia and Kaposi's sarcoma in 7% of cases. The remaining 15% of AIDS patients have other parasitic, fungal, bacterial, or viral infections associated with immunodeficiencies. Among the first 2640 cases reported to the CDC, there were 1092 deaths, a case-fatality rate of 41%. Approximately 95% of the cases were male; 70% were 20-49 years of age at the time of diagnosis. Approximately 40% of the cases were reported from New York City, 12% from San Francisco, 8% from Los Angeles, and the remainder from 32 other states. Cases were reported from at least 16 other countries. Among the 90% of patients who were categorized according to possible risk factors, those at highest risk included were homosexuals or bisexuals (70%), intravenous drug abusers (17%), Haitian entrants into the United States (95%), and persons with hemophilia (1%).

Analysis of these initial data, collected before the etiologic agent of AIDS was identified, supported the hypothesis that transmission occurred primarily by sexual contact, receipt of contaminated blood or blood products, or contact with contaminated intravenous needles. Spread through casual contact did not seem likely. The epidemiologic data indicated that AIDS was an infectious disease. It has now been determined that AIDS results from infection with a retrovirus of the human T cell leukemia/lymphoma virus (HTLV) family, which has been designated HTLV-III.

References

Benenson, A.: *Control of communicable disease in man*. Washington, D.C.: American Public Health Assn, 1980.

Bennett, J.V., Brachman, P.S.: *Hospital infections*, 2nd ed. Boston: Little, Brown & Co 1985.

Fox, J.P., Hall, C.E., Elveback, L.R.: *Epidemiology, man and disease*. New York, MacMillan Publ. Co., 1970.

Langmuir, A.D.: The surveillance of communicable diseases of national importance. *N Engl J Med* 1963; 268:182-192.

Lilienfeld, A.M.: *Foundations of epidemiology*. New York, Oxford University Press, 1980.

MacMahon, B., Pugh, T.F.: 1970. *Epidemiology principles and methods*. Boston: Little, Brown & Co., 1970.

Smith, D.M., Haupt, B.J.: Hospital discharge data used as feedback in planning research and education for primary care. *Public Health Rept* 1983; 98:457-66.

World Health Organization. The surveillance of communicable diseases. *WHO Chronical* 1968; 22:439-444.

25 Principles of Diagnosis

Martin Goldfield, MD

General Concepts

Some infectious diseases may be associated with distinctive features that permit their recognition solely by clinical means. Most pathogenic microbial agents, however, may each be responsible for a wide spectrum of clinical syndromes in humans and, conversely, a single clinical syndrome may result from infection with any one of many microbial agents. Influenza virus infection, for example, may result in so wide a variety of respiratory syndromes in humans as to be indistinguishable from those caused by streptococci, mycoplasmas, or more than a hundred different viruses.

Most often, therefore, it is necessary to apply microbiologic methods in the study of infectious diseases to identify a specific etiologic agent. Diagnostic medical microbiology is the discipline that recognizes and identifies etiologic microbial agents of disease. Inevitably, its setting tends to be the clinical laboratory. The job of the clinical microbiology laboratory is to identify in specimens from patients microorganisms that are, or may be, a cause of the patient's illness, and to provide information, when appropriate, about the in vitro activity of antimicrobial drugs against the microorganisms identified.

Some common contentions may be misleading: that the clinician caring directly for a patient decides what laboratory procedures will be helpful in making a diagnosis; that the responsibility of the laboratory is to perform those, and only those, procedures requested by the clinician; and that the laboratory does not help in making a diagnosis but merely reports results to the clinician who is alone expected to interpret them. Thus, it is widely and erroneously believed that only the clinician providing direct patient care can utilize laboratory results to make a diagnosis.

The clinical microbiology laboratory unfortunately cannot provide optimum diagnostic services by strict attention to these dicta. No procedures have ever been devised that would permit recognition of all known potentially pathogenic microbial agents from any type of clinical specimen, so that rote processing of specimens by some arbitrarily established routine techniques never can be fully satisfactory. Generally speaking, many clinicians cannot keep pace with the rapid advances in knowledge of microbial agents that may be related to a given clinical syndrome. They cannot be expected to know which laboratory procedures would be most useful in a given case, and are often even unequipped to make appropriate decisions as to the type of specimens to be collected, the optimum timing of collection during the course of a patient's illness, and the proper method of collection. They may not be thoroughly informed regarding optimum conditions for storage and transportation of clinical microbiologic specimens. Finally, it is unrealistic to expect clinicians to keep fully abreast of knowledge concerning the time of appearance, peaking, and persistence of antibodies measured by various techniques for a multitude of microbiologic agents; therefore, they are in no position to interpret certain laboratory results.

A diagnostic medical microbiology laboratory ideally should be staffed with personnel competent to serve in a consultative capacity rather than as passive recipients of specimens. They should be given salient information on a patient, such as age and sex, details of the clinical syndrome presented, date of onset, possibly significant exposures, prior antibiotic therapy, immunologic status, and underlying conditions. They should play a role in decisions regarding the microbiologic diagnostic studies to be performed on a patient, the type and timing of specimens to be collected, and the techniques to be employed for their transportation and storage. Above all, the medical microbiology laboratory, whenever appropriate, should not hesitate to provide an interpretation of laboratory results.

One important limitation in applying microbiologic techniques is that isolation of a microorganism does not necessarily establish the etiology of a disease. Strictly speaking, the laboratory usually provides evidence that a patient is, or has been, infected or colonized by one or more microbial agents that are potentially pathogenic. Identification of infection, the process of lodgement and multiplication of a microorganism in tissues of the host, does not necessarily provide adequate proof that the agent is causally related to the host's illness. In those instances when study of a normally sterile tissue or body cavity reveals clinical and/or pathologic evidence of an inflammatory process and of the presence of a potentially pathogenic microbial agent, it is highly likely that the two are causally associated. For example, organisms found to be multiplying in a patient's abdominal cavity are likely to be causally related to the peritonitis with which he or she presents, and those isolated from cerebrospinal fluid are probably a cause of a patient's meningitis. But the interpretation of results of bacteriologic studies of anatomic sites that are normally colonized by bacteria (for example, the upper respiratory tract, the skin, and the gastrointestinal tract) can be far more difficult. In such instances, the clinician must play a major role in decisions regarding the causal association of microbiologic findings.

The major goal of the diagnostic microbiologic process is to provide information for selection of appropriate therapeutic procedures for a patient. However, diagnostic microbiology does have other goals. For example, identification of a pathogenic microorganism infecting a patient may not help in the selection of appropriate antimicrobial therapy for that patient, but may be of critical importance in detecting nosocomial disease and determining the appropriate isolation procedures to minimize the role of spreading the infection to medical personnel and other patients. Identification of a salmonella isolate from a number of patients may provide the first clue in an epidemiologic study to detect a common source in water or food and prevent widespread disease in the community.

Similarly, viral studies of an encephalitis patient may not aid clinicians to select therapy for that patient if an arbovirus infection is identified, but may lead them to recognize an arthropod-borne disease and prevent an epidemic by permitting the institution of appropriate control measures in the community. Most serologic studies provide information too late to be useful in the treatment of patients, but identification of measles, rubella, and influenza infections may provide valuable information on the advisability of instituting emergency immunization programs to prevent additional spread in a hospital or community.

It is understandable that clinical medical personnel are concerned chiefly with individual patients. The aims of diagnostic microbiology should not be so narrowly construed, however, as to limit potential benefits to a patient's family and associates, and other patients in the local community.

The diagnostic microbiologic process is presented schematically in Figure 25-1. Four basic approaches are useful in establishing a diagnosis of an infectious disease: direct examination of specimens, cultivation and identification of microbial agents, detection of microbial products or components in host tissue, and documentation of immunologic responses.

Direct Examination of Clinical Specimens

Microscopic Examinations

Microbial agents in certain clinical specimens can be recognized most quickly by direct examination. Microscopic examination of wet mounts or stained smears may provide valuable information for the selection of immediate therapeutic intervention strategies. A simple hanging drop preparation of untreated vaginal fluids, for example, may serve to detect *Trichomonas vaginalis* infections, and dark-field examination of fluids collected from lesions may reveal the characteristic spirochetes of syphilis.

**A. Collection of Appropriate Specimens
Potentially Harboring Pathogenic
Microbial Agents or Their Products**

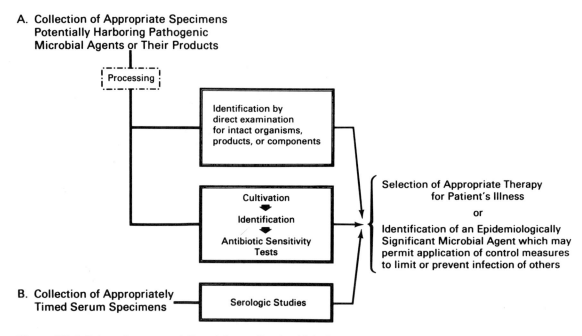

Figure 25-1 Schematic representation of diagnostic microbiologic process.

More often, however, smears are stained in some fashion before microscopic examination. Stained blood smears are useful in detecting malaria and certain other parasites; stained preparations of spinal fluid may reveal organisms resembling pneumococci, *Haemophilus influenzae*, or meningococci. Gonorrhea in men is most expeditiously diagnosed by the finding of intracellular diplococci of typical morphology in urethral exudates; inclusion bodies of cytomegalovirus can be recognized by microscopic study of stained urine sediment. Stained smears of conjunctival scrapings are useful in the diagnosis of trachoma; corneal impression smears may be of value in the recognition of rabies. Occasionally, negative staining of specimen material is useful, as in India ink preparations of spinal fluid specimens that provide contrast for the visualization of unstained *Filobasidiella (Cryptococcus) neoformans*. Specific antisera acting on pneumococci or *H influenzae* cause a swelling of the bacterial capsule; this swelling is discernible when the preparation is negatively stained with methylene blue. This technique permits specific identification of these organisms in spinal fluid.

In some instances, the clinical specimen should be treated prior to microscopic examinations. Sputum specimens to be studied for the presence of mycobacteria are routinely treated with a sodium hydroxide (or substitute) preparation to liquefy mucus and exudate and to achieve maximal destruction of other microorganisms. The increased concentration of relatively resistant *Mycobacterium tuberculosis* permits more ready visualization with the help of differential ("acid-fast") stains. Concentration by centrifugation is also routinely employed before direct microscopic examination of fecal extracts for the presence of helminth ova and larvae and protozoan cysts.

Electron Microscopy

Despite early enthusiasm for its potential value, direct examination of clinical specimens by electron microscopy has had only limited application. High equipment cost, need for highly trained operators, and high concentration of microorganisms required for visualization (usually $>10^6$ per mL) have thus far outweighed the advantages of speed and simplicity. Electron microscopy has been used for rapid differentiation of herpesviruses from vaccinia or variola viruses in vesicle fluid samples and for study of fecal extracts for the presence of rotaviruses among patients with gastroenteritis.

Electron-dense materials such as ferritin or peroxidase can be coupled to antibody and used to stain infected cells and tissues, which are then studied in thin sections under the electron microscope. This technique is termed immune electron microscopy. With a technique called immune aggregate electron microscopy, untreated antibody preparations can be mixed with suspensions containing a virus to promote aggregation, and the immune aggregates can be identified by electron microscopy. These methods have been most commonly applied to study agents that cannot as yet be recognized by other immunologic or cultivation techniques. Agents of acute infectious nonbacterial gastroenteritis and hepatitis A virus are identifiable in fecal extracts by immune electron microscopic techniques.

Fluorescence Microscopy

Some substances have the capacity to absorb light energy of one wavelength and to emit visible light of a longer wavelength, a process known as fluorescence. *Mycobacterium tuberculosis* can be selectively stained with auramine in smears of concentrated sputum; when viewed under a specially equipped microscope illuminated with ultraviolet light, the bacterium appears brightly fluorescent on a relatively dark background. The procedure, referred to as **fluorochrome staining**, can be exceedingly useful in enhancing the efficiency of a microscopic search for organisms.

Fluorescein can be coupled to antibody preparations without loss of their specific reactivity with antigens. They can then be used to stain microorganisms, and the antigen-antibody-fluorescein complex can be visualized under the microscope by excitation with ultraviolet light, a procedure called direct fluorescent antibody or direct immunofluorescent staining.

Fluorescent antibody staining of clinical laboratory specimens has been used routinely to detect *T pallidum* in syphilis; rabies antigens in impression smears of brain and cornea; viruses such as herpes simplex and eastern, western, and St. Louis encephalitis in human and animal brains; and herpes simplex, varicella-zoster, and vaccinia virus in fluids from vesicular lesions. Recently, fluorescent antibody staining has been used to identify *Toxoplasma* cysts and trophozoites in sections of a cervical lymph node. In some instances, it is advantageous to incubate a clinical specimen for a brief time in a cultivating medium before performing fluorescent antibody staining. Group A streptococci can be identified routinely in throat swabs with a sensitivity equaling or exceeding conventional 48-hour culture techniques by fluorescent antibody staining following a 4-hour incubation in Todd Hewitt broth; various viruses can be identified by fluorescent antibody after a brief, overnight incubation in selected cell cultures.

Unfortunately, the direct demonstration of microbial organisms by fluorescent antibody staining of clinical specimens is limited in application by the need for very large numbers of organisms in the specimen, for relative freedom from contaminating materials that contribute nonspecific fluorescence, and for highly specific antiserum.

Immunoenzymatic Staining

It is possible to couple an enzyme to antibody molecules and to use the labeled antibody in a manner similar to fluorescent antibody staining. Horseradish peroxidase-labeled antibody preparations are coming into more widespread use because an ordinary light microscope is more practical than the cumbersome and expensive apparatus required for fluorescence microscopy. The labeled antibody on a slide is visualized by providing a substrate (H_2O_2) containing an indicator compound, such as 3,3'-diaminobenzidine, that deposits a colored precipitate at the molecular sites of peroxidase activity.

Cultivation and Identification of Microbiologic Agents

The process of cultivating, isolating in pure culture, and identifying microorganisms associated with disease states remains the most definitive method of medical microbiology, despite the expenditure of time and effort it entails, and the consequent delays in providing information that might permit effective therapeutic intervention. It is still the most commonly used method for studying bacterial, mycotic, and chlamydial agents of disease, and is second only to immunologic studies for viral, rickettsial, and mycoplasma agents. Only among the parasitic diseases are cultivation, isolation, and identification rarely attempted; however, even if sensitive and specific rapid techniques to identify virtually all microbiologic agents of disease were devised, cultivation methods would still be required because of the need for pure cultures in antimicrobial drug sensitivity testing.

Pretreatment of Contaminated Specimens

Clinical specimens collected from such sites as skin, throat, upper respiratory tract, and gastrointestinal tract are almost invariably heavily contaminated with bacteria and fungi. It is often advantageous to pretreat heavily contaminated specimens before attempting to cultivate an agent of interest. Specimens for viral culture are almost always pretreated by the addition of antibacterial and antimycotic antibiotics, and bacterial populations may be reduced further by high-speed centrifugation, or eliminated by passage through filters of appropriate pore size. The use of sodium hydroxide for the pretreatment of sputum specimens, as cited previously, was introduced by Koch for the study of tuberculosis a century ago, and is still used today.

Use of Appropriate Host Systems

Bacteria, fungi, and mycoplasmas usually are cultivated in artificial media, whereas chlamydiae, viruses, and rickettsiae require living host systems. Artificial culture media are either of liquid or solid consistency. Liquid media generally offer the advantage of greater sensitivity to smaller inocula of organisms and the disadvantage of overgrowth by contaminating organisms. Cultures of blood are usually performed in liquid media. Use of a solid medium promotes discrete growth in isolated colonies and permits individual microorganisms to be chosen for study from a mixed sample.

Selective media contain substances that stimulate the growth of a desired microorganism or inhibit the growth of others. Selective media are consequently often referred to as enrichment media. In bacteriology, certain aniline dyes, phenol, telluric acid, bile salts, and many other substances are used to inhibit the growth of saprophytes in specimens from normally contaminated sites. Brilliant green may be used to inhibit common lactose-fermenting enteric bacteria. Conversely, blood, serum, ascitic fluid and special mixtures of growth factors may be used to stimulate the growth of organisms being sought.

Indicator media contain a substance that changes color or appearance in certain circumstances. *Corynebacterium diphtheriae* reduces sodium tellurite and, when culti-vated in medium containing tellurite, produces black colonies that are readily discernible. Selective and indicator media may be combined, as in MacConkey's agar, in which neutral red and lactose are used as indicators of lactose utilization and bile salts are added to inhibit growth of a variety of contaminating bacteria. In other instances, an indicator may be added after growth has occurred, as in use of reagents to detect catalase production among mycobacteria and oxidase activity in colonies of *Neisseria gonorrheae*.

Viruses are most often propagated in a variety of cell culture systems, but animal hosts such as suckling mice, chick embryos, guinea pigs, rabbits, hamsters and primates may be required as well. One of the most sensitive methods of propagating a virus from tissue specimens consists of preparing a culture of host cells from the tissue specimen itself or by promoting fusion of the dispersed viable host cells from the tissue specimen with an established cell culture system.

Identification of Cultivated Microorganisms

When a culture system has shown evidence of growth, it is the microbiologist's responsibility to identify the organisms present. Isolated varieties may be examined for the appearance of colonies on solid media and for the morphology and staining characteristics of individual organisms. Their shape, size, motility, internal structure, number and distribution of flagella, shape and location of spores and other structures, and presence of capsules may be studied. Their biochemical properties are often defined according to oxidative or fermentative activity on selected carbohydrate and alcohol substrates, their ability to utilize salts such as citrate and tartrate, their proteolytic and lipolytic activity, and their production of substances such as catalase, indole, ammonia, or hydrogen sulfide. Often, cultural appearance, staining characteristics, morphology, and biochemical properties provide enough information to identify the isolated microorganism. When more definitive identification is required, its antigenic structure must be studied by a variety of immunologic techniques. This is virtually always the case with viruses and rickettsiae.

Detection of Microbial Products or Components

To identify the etiologic agent as rapidly as possible by highly sensitive and specific techniques so that appropriate therapy can be applied promptly is vitally important in managing patients with infectious diseases. Unfortunately, until recently, medical microbiology has been armed with relatively few rapid diagnostic methods. The direct examination of clinical specimens by conventional staining techniques is often too insensitive to permit visualization of an infecting organism when its population density is inadequate, and frequently fails to provide identification. Immune electron microscopy, immunofluorescent staining, and immunoenzymatic methods may provide enhanced specificity but fail to provide adequate sensitivity. Cultivation generally requires too much time to serve as a rapid diagnostic tool. Therefore, the significant advances that have been made in the development of rapid diagnostic microbiologic techniques during the past decade are exciting. These newer techniques are based on detection of microbial components by sensitive and specific immunologic methods or on chemical identification of metabolites.

Immunodiffusion and Counterimmunoelectrophoresis

When an antigen is placed in a well cut in a matrix such as agar or agarose, it diffuses through the medium in all directions. If an antiserum is placed in another well separated from the first by a short distance, an antigen-antibody reaction will form an immunoprecipitate in a line between the wells where optimal proportions of diffusing antigen and antibody are attained. This technique, called double immunodiffusion, can be highly specific but generally requires high antigen concentrations and long time periods for visualization of a precipitin band. In counterimmunoelectrophoresis, a current is applied to impel the negatively charged antigen to migrate toward the anode. The resulting concentration of antigen results in rapid development of an immunoprecipitin band (30-60 minutes), and provides several magnitudes of increased sensitivity over double immunodiffusion.

Counterimmunoelectrophoresis has been applied to the diagnosis of bacterial meningitis. Pneumococcus, meningococcus, and *H influenzae* organisms can be detected in spinal fluid in more than 90% of bacteriologically proved cases with few or no nonspecific reactions. The technique provides the added advantage of permitting identification of the etiologic agent in spinal fluid as long as 1 or 2 days after antibiotic administration has precluded their cultivation. Counterimmunoelectrophoresis also permits identification of the pneumococcus by detection of antigen in serum, pleural fluids, and urine of patients with pneumonia, and has received wide application as a test of intermediate sensitivity for detecting hepatitis B surface antigen in serum. It has also been used to detect soluble polysaccharide from *Filobasidiella (Cryptococcus) neoformans* in spinal fluid, serum, and urine of patients with meningitis, and to detect antigenic components of several other bacterial, viral, and protozoal agents.

Radioimmunoassay

Antigens and antibodies can be labeled with a radioisotope (most commonly ^{125}I), and the tagged reagents may be used in a variety of ways to provide the most sensitive and specific procedures now available for the diagnosis of infectious diseases. Radioimmunoassay procedures to detect various microbial agents of disease have developed rapidly, and new applications will be discovered in the future.

Radiolabeled antigen can be added to a biologic specimen, followed by the addition of a limiting concentration of an unlabeled antibody preparation. Antigen in the specimen competes for antibody sites and decreases the amount of labeled antigen that will be bound by antibody. Free radiolabeled antigen can be separated from that bound by antibody by various techniques, and the distribution of radioactivity in the two fractions provides a sensitive test system. This technique is known as **competitive binding radioimmunoassay.**

In **solid-phase radioimmunoassay** techniques, antigen or antibody is fixed to a glass or plastic surface. One variant, for example, has been widely used to detect hepatitis B surface antigen in serum. A serum to be tested is incubated with a polystyrene bead to which antibody has been affixed. The bead is then washed and treated with a labeled antibody preparation that reacts with antigen adhering to the antibody-coated surface. After washing again, the amount of radiolabeled antibody left on the bead is, within limits, proportional to the amount of antigen that was present in the serum specimen.

Radioimmunoassays have been developed to detect antigenic components of a wide variety of viruses, (for example, hepatitis A, herpes simplex, influenza, and measles) and, to a lesser extent, have been applied to identification of bacterial antigens and exotoxins. They provide the advantages of high sensitivity and specificity but require the use of radioactive materials and expensive radiation-counting equipment.

Enzyme Immunoassay

Antigens or antibodies can be linked to an enzyme rather than an isotope and the labeled products can be used in a manner analogous to the radioimmunoassay technique. Tagged reagent is detected by adding a substrate that will result in a color change when acted on by enzyme, and the reaction can be quantified with an ordinary spectrophotometer. This technique is simple, sensitive, and potentially specific, and, unlike radioimmunoassay, may be performed using inexpensive equipment with stable reagents. It has already been used to detect viruses (hepatitis A and B, herpes simplex, rotavirus), bacteria, protozoa, and fungi. It appears likely that immunoenzymatic techniques will play an increasingly important role in the diagnosis of infectious disease over the next few years.

Particle-Agglutination Techniques

Latex particles coated with antibody agglutinate in the presence of antigen and have been used for the detection of microbial antigens in body fluids. Cryptococcal polysaccharide, for example, can be detected in serum and spinal fluid by this simple and rapid technique. Unfortunately, however, as much as 1%–2% of human sera contains antibodies that nonspecifically agglutinate the coated latex particles. Thus, specificity generally does not approach levels attainable by radioimmunoassay and immunoenzymatic methods.

Erythrocytes may be coated with an antigen and suspended in a clinical specimen to which antibody has been added. In the absence of antigen in the clinical specimen, the erythrocytes will be agglutinated. Antigen in the specimen inhibits agglutination. This hemagglutination inhibition technique has been used for the detection of *Candida* cell wall polysaccharide antigen in the serum of infected patients, but thus far has received little additional attention.

Immune adherence agglutination is an even more promising technique. It is based on the principle that antigen-antibody interactions can activate complement, which results in the binding of antigen-antibody complexes to human and other primate erythrocytes. Adherence of complexes is measured by hemagglutination.

Immune adherence hemagglutination can be highly sensitive and has been used to detect hepatitis A, hepatitis B, and cytomegalovirus antigens.

Gas Chromatography

Gas chromatography has received wide application in the identification of anaerobic bacteria that have been isolated by conventional techniques. For example, volatile, short-chain organic acids that are products of bacterial metabolism are identifiable by this technique. Recently, however, gas chromatographic techniques have been used to study body fluids, and chromatographic patterns in serum have permitted detection of pneumococcal, streptococcal, and pseudomonal infections. Tuberculous, cryptococcal, and viral meningitis have been differentiated by examining spinal fluid; streptococci, staphylococci, and gonococci have been identified in joint fluid of patients with septic arthritis. Gas chromatography requires expensive equipment and highly trained personnel to yield results; however, it is potentially high in sensitivity and specificity and may provide rapid results.

Other Promising Techniques

Spectrophotometric measurement of turbidity can be used to provide early evidence of bacterial multiplication in liquid media. Similarly, bacterial growth in a medium containing ^{14}C-labeled glucose may be detected rapidly by measurement of the radioactivity associated with the CO_2 that is released. Sensitive microcalorimetric techniques can detect changes in heat output resulting from the growth of bacteria. Bacterial ATP can be measured by the luminescence emitted in a medium when a luciferin-luciferase reagent is added. Minute quantities of endotoxin produced by gram-negative bacteria have been detected by endotoxin's ability to cause gelation of a lysate of amebocytes from the horseshoe crab, *Limulus polyphemus*. The *Limulus* lysate assay for endotoxin has varied in sensitivity and specificity in the hands of different investigators. Additional experience may prove the value of this assay as a rapid technique for detecting gram-negative bacterial sepsis.

Documentation of Serologic Responses

Some infectious diseases are accompanied by serologic responses that are not directed specifically against the invading microorganism. Heterophile antibodies that develop in the serum of infectious mononucleosis patients may be detected by their ability to agglutinate sheep erythrocytes. Cold agglutinins develop early in the course of primary atypical pneumonia and are assayed by their ability to agglutinate adult human type O erythocytes at 4 C. Similarly, rickettsial infections may stimulate the early appearance of antibodies that can agglutinate certain strains of *Proteus*.

Most serologic diagnostic tests, however, are based on the demonstration of a significant increase in antibody levels specifically directed to a given microorganism or one of its component structures. Generally, this requires testing an acute phase serum specimen collected early after the onset of illness and a convalescent serum specimen obtained 1-6 weeks later. Thus, most serologic diagnoses are retrospective, although detection of transient antibody in a single serum specimen may be of value in indicating a recent viral infection. Another disadvantage is the need to suspect a particular infectious agent in order to detect it. Furthermore, an antibody response may not develop, or may be delayed, if an antigenic stimulus is aborted by antibiotic therapy. In some instances, as in respiratory syncytial virus infection of infants, an immunologic response is detected by the techniques currently employed in only a proportion of those infected.

On the other hand, serologic diagnostic methods present distinct advantages. Some infectious agents cannot be found at any available portal or in any accessible body fluid. In nonfatal cases of St. Louis, eastern, and western encephalitis, virus is not shed from the respiratory or gastrointestinal tract, is not found in blood after onset of clinical disease, and is rarely detectable in spinal fluid. Moreover, cultivation of many agents may be difficult, time consuming, expensive, and beyond the capabilities of available laboratory resources. In such instances, serologic studies may provide results more rapidly, and certainly more cheaply, than conventional cultural techniques. Also, the sensitivity of cultivation methods currently employed rarely approaches 100% and may be as low at 50%. Failure to cultivate and identify a particular agent from a patient does not, therefore, rule out the possibility that the patient was nevertheless infected. It is not uncommon, for example, to document influenza virus infections among patients whose respiratory secretions fail to yield virus.

Immunologic responses to the infectious diseases are measured by a wide variety of techniques. Antibodies may be titrated by precipitin, particle agglutination, neutralization, complement-fixation, immunodiffusion, counterimmunoelectrophoresis, hemagglutination inhibition, indirect fluorescent antibody staining, radioimmunoassay, immunoenzymatic, or other methods too numerous to be detailed here. Complement-fixation, one of the most widely applied serologic procedures, appears to measure IgG antibodies only, whereas neutralization and hemagglutination inhibition tests reflect concentrations of antibodies of both IgG and IgM. As a consequence, complement-fixation antibodies tend to appear and peak later, a distinct advantage for diagnostic studies of some diseases where peak neutralization and hemagglutination inhibition titers may develop within days after onset. Complement-fixation antibodies, on the other hand, tend to be more short-lived, disappearing in many instances in a few years after onset of illness. They are not, therefore, a reliable measure of lifetime experience. Radioimmunoassay and immunoenzymatic methods for detection of antibody are relatively new but are presently receiving wider application and use. They appear to provide highly specific results and a higher level of sensitivity than has been attainable previously.

References

Chernesky, M.A., Ray, C.G., Smith, T.F.: Laboratory diagnosis of viral infections. In: *Cumulative techniques and procedures in clinical microbiology.* Drew, W.L., (editor). Washington, D.C.: American Society for Microbiology, 1982.

Halsted, C.H., Halsted, J.A., (editors) In: *The laboratory in clinical medicine, Infectious diseases* (section 12). Philadelphia: W.B. Saunders Co., 1981.

Howard, C.R., (editor): *New developments in practical virology.* New York: Alan R. Liss, 1982.

Lorian, V., (editor): *Significance of medical microbiology in the care of patients.* Baltimore: Williams & Wilkins, 1982.

Rytel, M.W., (editor): *Rapid diagnosis in infectious disease.* Boca Raton, Fla.: CRC Press, 1979.

Sommers, H.M.: Laboratory diagnosis of bacterial and fungal infections. In: *The biological and clinical basis of infectious disease.* Youmans, G.P., Paterson, P.Y., Sommers, H.M., (editors). Philadelphia: W.B. Saunders Co., 1975.

26 Antimicrobial Chemotherapy

Harold C. Neu, MD

General Concepts

In the past 50 years, the development of new natural, semisynthetic, and synthetic antimicrobial agents has been continuous. Moreover, the biochemical bases for the actions of such agents have been described. The basic mechanisms of antimicrobial activity have been shown to be inhibition of cell walls, production of damage to cytoplasmic membranes, inhibition of ribosome function, and inhibition of nucleic-acid synthesis. A great number of antimicrobial agents are now available but, unfortunately, bacteria have developed several mechanisms to overcome the action of many of them. Such mechanisms involve the modification or duplication of target enzyme, prevention of access of antimicrobial agents to the targets, and synthesis of enzymes that modify or destroy the antimicrobial agents. Bacterial resistance has become a serious problem in many parts of the world, since the resistance genes exist on plasmids and transposons that can be disseminated widely. The techniques that have been used to overcome this resistance include the molecular modification of antimicrobial agents and the administration of combinations of antimicrobial agents. Understanding how antimicrobial agents affect bacteria and how resistance develops is extremely important in the prevention of human bacterial diseases.

Historical Overview

As noted in other chapters, humans and microorganisms coexist in a very tenuous relationship, just as nations exist in delicate balance. Some organisms are naturally pathogenic, some produce disease only when host defenses are disrupted, and some microorganisms protect us from the deleterious effects of other bacteria or fungi. In considering the role of chemotherapy in our evolving society it is important to remember that chemotherapeutic agents not only can affect the intended pathogens, but they may also have profound effects on the microecology of individuals and the macroecology around them.

The earliest successes of chemotherapy occurred in ancient Peru where the Indians used bark from the cinchona tree to treat malaria. Other substances were used in ancient China, and many of the poultices used by primitive peoples probably contained antibacterial and antifungal substances. Modern chemotherapy dates back to the work of Paul Ehrlich in Germany who systematically sought to discover effective agents to treat trypanosomiasis and syphilis. He discovered p-rosaniline, which had antitrypanosomal effects, and arsphenamine, which could be used against syphilis. Ehrlich postulated that it would be possible to find chemicals that were selectively toxic for parasites but not toxic to humans. Success with this "magic bullet" was minimal until the 1930s when Gerhard Domagk discovered the protective effects of prontosil, the forerunner of sulfonamide. Ironically, Fleming discovered penicillin G fortuitously in 1929, and his original papers indicate that he did not initially appreciate the magnitude of his discovery. Fortunately, in 1939, Florey, Chain and their colleagues at Oxford University found a way to develop methods of isolating penicillin. In 1944, Waksman, working at the Rutgers Institute, isolated streptomycin and later antibiotics such as chloramphenicol, tetracyclines, and erythromycin were found in organisms from soil samples. By the 1960s, improvements in fermentation techniques and advances in medicinal chemistry paved the way for the development of novel molecular modifications of existing compounds that also could be used therapeutically. Much less progress has been made in developing effective but nontoxic antifungal and antiviral agents. Amphotericin B, isolated in the 1950s, remains the most effective antifungal agent. Recently nucleoside analogues such as adenosine arabinoside or acyclovir have offered hope for the treatment of selected viral infections.

Biochemical Basis of Antimicrobial Action

Bacterial cells repeatedly grow and divide to reach the large numbers present in infection or on the body surfaces. As organisms multiply and divide, they make new molecules of DNA, RNA, and protein, and also make or obtain from their environment the smaller units such as amino acids or sugars they need for their walls and membranes. Antimicrobial agents act by interfering with one or more areas of the organisms's functioning (Figure 26-1). For example, they can inhibit (1) bacterial and fungal cell wall synthesis; (2) the organization or formation of cytoplasmic membranes; (3) nucleic acid synthesis; and (4) ribosomal functioning (Table 26-1). Antimicrobial agents that inhibit bacteria and fungi may do so in either a bactericidal or bacteriostatic manner. Ideally bacteria should be killed, but even agents that only inhibit growth of bacteria can be beneficial, since the normal defenses of the host can then destroy the weakened microorganisms.

Inhibition of Bacterial Cell Wall Synthesis

Bacteria, as noted in earlier chapters, are divided into gram-positive and gram-negative organisms on the basis of staining characteristics. Gram-positive bacterial cell walls contain peptidoglycan and teichoic or teichuronic acid, and the bacteria may be surrounded by a protein or polysaccharide envelope. Gram-negative bacteria contain

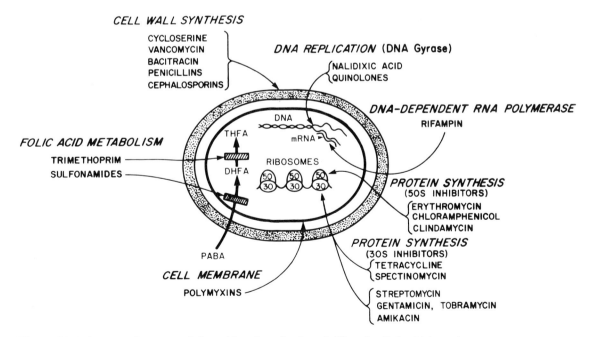

Figure 26-1 Diagramatic representation of the sites of action of different antimicrobial agents.

Table 26-1 Mechanisms of Action of Antimicrobial Agents

Inhibition of Bacterial Cell Wall Synthesis
Inhibition of biosynthetic enzymes
—fosfomycin
—cycloserine
Antibiotics that combine with carrier molecules
—bacitracin
Inhibition of polymerization and attachment of new peptidoglycan to cell wall
—penicillins
—cephalosporins
—thienamycins
—monobactams
Antibiotics that combine with substrates of wall
—vancomycin

Inhibition of Cytoplasmic Membranes
Drugs disorganizing cytoplasmic membrane
—polymyxins
Drugs producing pores in membranes
—gramicidins
Drugs altering sterol structure of fungi
—polyenes (amphotericin)

Inhibition of Nucleic Acid Synthesis
Inhibitors of nucleotide metabolism
—5-fluorocytosine (fungi)
—adenosine arabinoside (viruses)
—acyclovir (viruses)
Agents that impair DNA template function: intercalating agents
—chloroquin (parasites)
Inhibitors of RNA polymerase
—rifampin
Inhibitors of DNA replication
—nalidixic acid agents
—nitroimidazoles

Inhibition of Ribosomal Function
Inhibitors of 30S units
—streptomycin
—kanamycin, gentamicin, etc.
—spectinomycin
—tetracyclines
Inhibitors of 50S unit
—chloramphenicol
—clindamycin
—erythromycin
Inhibition of folate metabolism
Inhibition of pteroic acid synthetase
—sulfonamides
Inhibition of dihydrofolate reductase
—trimethoprim

Inhibitors of Mycobacteria
Isoniazid
Ethambutol
Rifampin
Streptomycin

peptidoglycan, lipopolysaccharide lipoprotein, phospholipid, and protein (Figure 26-2). The critical attack site of antimicrobial agents is the peptidoglycan layer, which is essential for the bacteria's survival in hypotonic environments; its damage or removal results in loss of rigidity of the bacterial cell wall and death of the organism.

Peptidoglycan synthesis occurs in three stages, and certain antimicrobials can affect each stage. The first stage occurs within the cytoplasm where low-molecular-weight precursors UDP-GlcAc and UDP-MurNAc-L-ala-D-glu-meso-Dap-D-ala-D-ala are synthesized. UTP and GluNAcl-P are converted to UDP-GluNAc, which is subsequently converted to UDP-MurNAc by the enzyme phosphoenolpyruvate: UDP-GlcNAc-

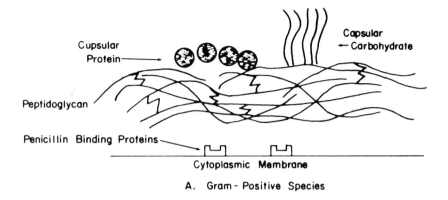

A. Gram - Positive Species

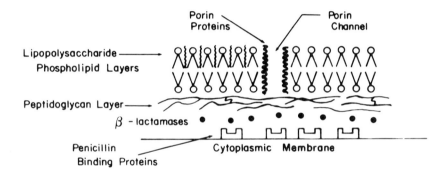

B. Gram-Negative Species

Figure 26-2 Diagrammatic representation of cell walls of gram-positive species (**A**), and gram-negative species (**B**). This illustrates that there is a difference in complexity of the cell walls and that antimicrobial agents must pass through porin channels to reach their sites of action.

3-enol-pyruvyl transferase. *Fosfomycin* and related analogues block this transfer by a direct nucleophilic attack on the enzyme. Fortunately, enzymes such as enolase, pyruvate kinase and carboxykinases and shikimate enoloases, which are important components of mammalian metabolic pathways, are not inhibited by these compounds. Three amino acids are added to the muramyl peptide to yield a tripeptide.

The dipeptide D-alanyl-D-alanine is synthesized from two molecules of D-alanine by the enzyme D-alanyl-D-alanine synthetase. D-alanine is produced from L-alanine by an alanine racemase. *Cycloserine* inhibits both alanine racemase and D-alanine-D-alanine synthetase, because it is structurally so similar to D-alanine; cycloserine actually binds to the enzymes better than the D-alanine.

The second stage of cell wall synthesis is catalyzed by membrane-bound enzymes. The nonnucleotide portion of the precursor molecules previously made are transferred sequentially to a carrier in the cytoplasmic membrane. This carrier is a phosphorylated undecaprenyl alcohol. The lipid carrier functions as a point of attachment to the membrane for the precursors and allows for transport of the subunits across the hydrophobic interior of the cytoplasmic membrane to the outside surface.

Bacitracin is a peptide antibiotic that specifically interacts with the pyrophosphate derivate of the undecaprenyl alcohol, hence preventing further transfer of the muramyl-pentapeptide from the precursor nucleotide to the nascent peptidoglycan.

The third stage of cell wall synthesis involves polymerization of the subunits and the attachment of nascent peptidoglycan to the cell wall. Polymerization occurs by transfer of the new peptidoglycan chain from its carrier in the membrane to the nonreducing N-acetyl glucosamine of the new saccharide-peptide attached to the membrane. The new peptidoglycan is attached to preexisting cell wall peptidoglycan by a transpeptidase reaction that involves peptide chains in both polymers, one of which must possess a D-alanyl-D-alanine terminus. It is believed that the transpeptidase enzyme leaves the peptide bond between two D-alanyl residues in the pentapeptide and becomes acetylated via the carbonyl group of the penultimate D-alanine residue. Beta-lactam antibiotics inhibit this final reaction.

Beta-lactam antibiotics include penicillins (penams), cephalosporins such as oxa-cephems, cephamycins, penems, thienamycins (carbapenems), and aztreonam (mono-bactams) (Figure 26-3). These drugs bind to the enzymes involved in this final process of cell wall formation, preventing them from functioning properly. Called *penicillin-binding proteins (PBPs),* these enzymes differ in gram-positive and gram-negative bacteria and in anaerobic species. These differences in the PBPs explain to some extent differences in antibacterial activity of the β-lactam antibiotics. The PBP to which a particular β-lactam antibiotic binds also affects the morphological response of the bacterium to the agent. Some antibiotics bind to a PBP that is involved in septum formation, and the bacteria continue to grow into long filaments, which eventually die. Binding to another PBP results in rapid lysis of a bacterium because the wall bulges and the bacterium bursts. Some penicillins, such as mecillinam, an amdino penicillin, do not bind to the PBPs of gram-positive bacteria and do not kill gram-positive bacteria. Aztreonam, a monobactam, binds only to gram-negative PBPs and does not inhibit gram-positive or anaerobic species.

Another important antibiotic is *vancomycin,* which interferes with cell wall synthesis by combining with substrates essential for cell wall formation. A complex polypeptide of large molecular weight, vancomycin cannot enter the cytoplasmic membrane and cannot pass through the complex outer wall of gram-negative bacteria. Instead, it binds to the D-ala-D-ala termini of growing peptidoglycan attached to the undecaprenyl pyrophosphate and prevents interaction of muramidases with the glycan chain. The specificity of vancomycin and other antibiotics of the teichoplanin class for the acyl-D-ala-D-ala site, and their inability to enter the cell may explain the lack of resistance to these antibiotics.

Inhibition of Cytoplasmic Membrane Functioning

Bacterial Cytoplasmic Membranes

The cytoplasmic membrane acts as a diffusion barrier for water, ions, and nutrients, and aids in the transport of molecules into and out of the cell. Most workers now believe

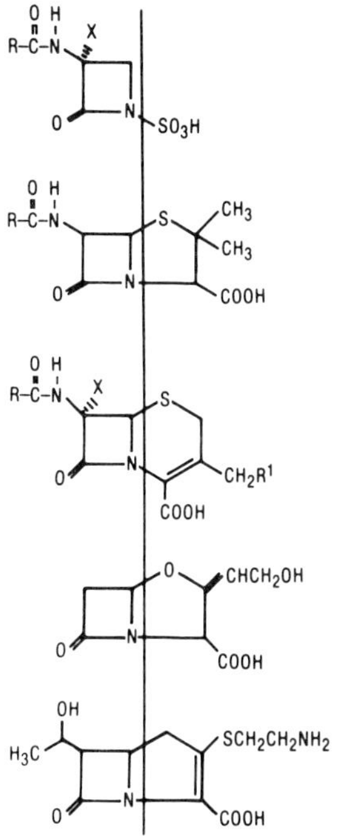

Figure 26-3 Basic structures of β-lactam antibiotics. Penicillins and cephalosporins/cephamycins are the agents most widely used inhibiting both gram-positive and gram-negative bacilli. Monobactams inhibit only aerobic gram-negative bacilli, clavulanic acid acts as a β-lactamase inhibitor, and thienamycin inhibits a wide range of aerobic and anaerobic species.

membranes to be a lipid matrix with globular proteins randomly distributed throughout the lipid bilayer and, to a lesser extent, the aqueous component of the membrane. A number of cationic, anionic, and neutral agents can cause disorganization of the membrane. The best known of these are the polymyxins, polymyxin B and colistimethate (polymyxin E). These compounds are octapeptides characterized by high molecular weight. They inhibit gram-negative bacteria, which have negatively charged lipids at the surface. Since the activity of the agents can be antagonized by cations Mg^{++} and Ca^{++}, the polymyxins probably competitively displace Mg^{++} or Ca^{++} from the negatively charged phosphate groups present on membrane lipids. Basically, polymyxins disorganize membrane permeability and nucleic acid, allowing cations to leak out of the bacterial cell.

Polymyxins cannot be used systemically, since they bind to various ligands in body tissues and are toxic to the kidney and nervous system. Gramicidins are also membrane-active antibiotics, but these agents appear to produce aqueous pores in the membranes.

Fungal Membrane-Active Agents

Fungal membranes contain sterols, whereas bacterial membranes do not. The polyene antibiotics contain a rigid hydrophobic center and a flexible hydrophilic section.

Structurally, these agents are tightly packed rods held in rigid extension by the polyene portion. They interact with fungal cells to produce a membrane-polyene complex that alters the membrane permeability, resulting in internal acidification of the fungus with exchange of K^+ and sugars, loss of phosphate esters, organic acids, and nucleotides, and eventual leakage of cell protein. In effect the polyene makes a pore in the fungal membrane and the contents of the fungus leaks out. Prokaryotic cells neither bind nor are inhibited by polyenes. Although numerous polyene antibiotics have been isolated, only amphotericin B is used systemically. Nystatin is used as a topical agent and primaricin as an ophthalmic preparation.

Another class of compounds referred to as imidazoles interfere with the synthesis of fungal lipid membranes. Such agents are micronazole, ketoconazole, and clotrimazole. They inhibit the incorporation of subunits into ergosterol and also may damage the membranes directly.

Inhibition of Nucleic Acid Synthesis

Antimicrobial agents can interfere with nucleic acid synthesis at several different levels. They can inhibit nucleotide synthesis or cause an interconversion of nucleotides. They can also prevent DNA from functioning as a proper template, and can interfere with polymerases involved in the replication and transcription of DNA.

Interference with Purine or Pyrimidine Synthesis

A large number of agents interfere with purine and pyrimidine synthesis, causing interconversion of nucleotides or acting as nucleotide analogues which are incorporated into polynucleotides.

5-fluorocytosine, an antifungal agent, inhibits yeast species. It is converted within the fungal cell to 5-fluoruracil, which inhibits thymidylate synthetase, resulting in deprivation of thymine nucleotides and consequent impairment of DNA synthesis.

Adenosine arabinoside inhibits viruses. This agent is phosphorylated in the virus and acts as a competitive analogue of dATP, thus inhibiting the incorporation of dATP into DNA. Acyclovir is a nucleoside analogue, which inhibits thymidine kinase and DNA polymerase of herpes viruses.

Agents That Impair the Template Function of DNA

A number of substances bind to DNA by intercalation. Although neither is used as an antibacterial, chloroquine and miracil D (lucanthone) inhibit plasmodia and schistoma, respectively. These agents are thought to intercalate into the DNA, thereby inhibiting further nucleic acid synthesis. Acridine dyes such as proflavine also act by this intercalation mechanism, but they cannot be used as antibacterial agents due to their effects on mammalian systems and the danger that they may promote oncogenic changes with photoactivation.

Inhibition of DNA-Directed RNA Polymerase

Rifamycins inhibit DNA-directed RNA polymerase activity. Rifampin binds to RNA polymerase noncovalently but very strongly. RNA polymerase is an enzyme of four α and four β subunits. Its polypeptide chains attach to a σ factor, which confers specificity for the recognition of the correct promoter sites required to initiate transcription of the DNA. Rifampin binds to a β subunit and interferes specifically with the initiation process, but it has no effect after polymerization has begun.

Inhibition of DNA Replication

DNA gyrase is an enzyme that changes negative supercoiled strands of DNA into closed circular duplex DNA; it is essential for replication of circular chromosomes. It also is involved in breakage and reunion of DNA strands. The gyrase consists of two components, A and B, with the A subunit more abundant. Nalidixic acid, a quinolone, binds to the A component of DNA gyrase and inhibits its action. Nalidixic acid inhibits only gram-negative species, whereas recently synthesized fluorinated carboxyl derivatives in this class, such as ciprofloxacin and enoxacin, inhibit gram-positive species as well as anaerobic bacteria.

The DNA gyrase B subunit can be inhibited by agents such as novobicin and coumermycin. Novobicin is no longer used and coumermycin is still investigational; the latter may become an important agent, since it inhibits methicillin-resistant staphylococci.

Nitroimidazoles such as metronidazole inhibit DNA replication in anaerobic bacteria and protozoa. The nitro group of the nitrosohydroxyl amino part of the compound is reduced by anaerobic bacteria. The drug then diffuses into the organisms, where it is concentrated and reduced by an electron transport protein. The reduced drug causes strand breaks in the DNA, leaving mammalian cells unharmed because they lack the enzymes to reduce the nitro group.

Inhibition of Ribosomal Function

The structure and function of ribosomes are discussed elsewhere in this text. Basically bacterial ribosomes contain 65% protein and 35% RNA. They can be dissociated into subunits, referred to as 50S and 30S ribosomal subunits. Since it is possible to dissociate ribosomes into subunits, it is possible to localize the action of antibiotics to one or both units (Figure 26-4). It is also possible to isolate specific proteins in the ribosome units to which the agent binds and to isolate mutants of bacteria, which can be shown to lack a specific ribosomal protein and thereby be resistant to a particular agent.

Aminoglycosides are complex sugars derived from various species of *Streptomyces* that interfere with the function of bacterial ribosomes. These antibiotics can differ by virtue of their nuclei, which can be streptidine or 2-deoxystreptidine, and by the aminohexoses linked to the nuclei. Essential to the activity of these agents are free NH_4 and $-OH$ groups by which aminoglycosides bind to specific ribosomal proteins.

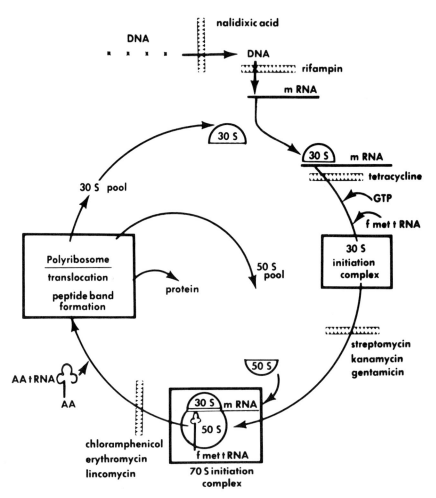

Figure 26-4 Diagramatic representation of protein biosynthesis cycle with examples of inhibition by agents that affect 30S and 50S ribosomes.

Streptomycin was the first aminoglycoside studied, and in the course of learning about its mode of action, many facets of protein synthesis were elucidated. However, streptomycin is rarely used clinically today because of toxicity, and its mode of action differs from the other clinically useful aminoglycosides, which are 2-deoxystreptidine derivatives such as gentamicin, tobramycin, and amikacin.

Streptomycin binds to a specific S12 protein in the 30S ribosome. The outcome of the in vitro binding is achieved at much higher concentrations than are possible in vivo. Many textbooks continue to discuss the misreading of the genetic code caused by aminoglycosides. Although this occurs in vitro, it is unlikely to occur in vivo.

Other aminoglycosides bind to the S12 protein of the 30S ribosome, but they also bind to some extent to the L6 protein of the 50S ribosome. This latter binding is quite important in the resistance of bacteria to aminoglycosides. Indeed, the aminoglycoside-type drugs have multiple binding sites on 30S ribosomes, and they ultimately cause death of bacteria by forming aberrant initiation complexes, sequestering the ribosomes from the ribosome pool (Figure 26-4 and 26-5).

Aminoglycosides bind tightly to 30S ribosomes and act as bactericidal agents. Spectinomycin is an aminocylitol antibiotic closely related to the aminoglycosides. It binds to a different protein in the ribosome and is not bactericidal. It is used to treat gonorrhea.

Tetracyclines also bind to 30S ribosomes (Figure 26-6). These agents appear to inhibit the binding of aminoacyl tRNA into the A site of the bacterial ribosome. Binding is a transient affair; hence the tetracyclines are bacteriostatic. Nonetheless, tetracyclines inhibit a wide variety of bacteria chlamydia and mycoplasma and are useful antibiotics.

Three important classes of drugs inhibit the larger 50S ribosomal subunit: chloramphenicol, macrolide, and lincinoid antibiotics. Chloramphenicol is a bacteriostatic agent that inhibits gram-positive and gram-negative bacteria. It inhibits peptide bond formation by binding to a peptidyl transferase enzyme on the 50S ribosome.

Inhibition of 30s ribosome-RNA complex formation

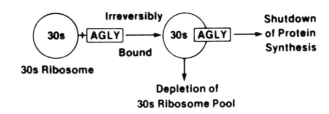

Misreading of code on mRNA

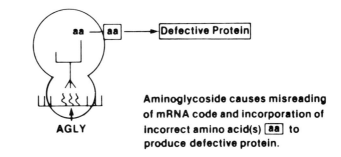

AGLY: Aminoglycoside antibiotic

Figure 26-5 Inhibition of protein biosynthesis by aminoglycosides.

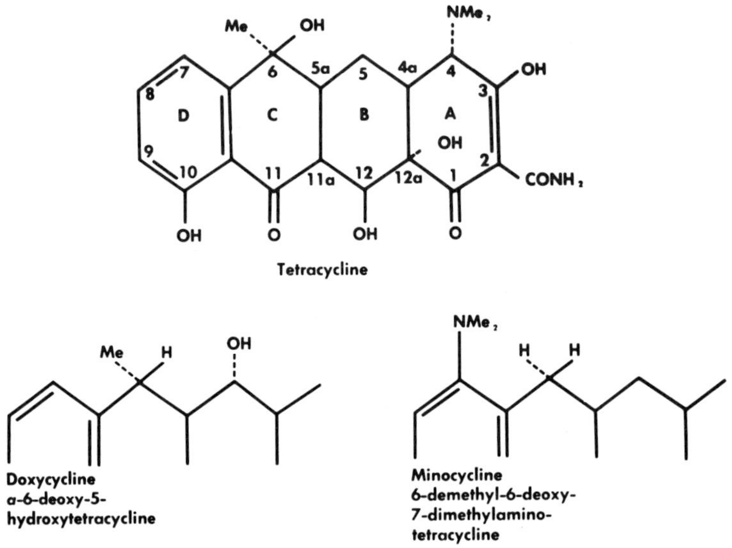

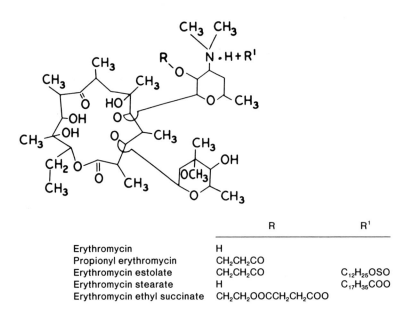

Figure 26-6 Structure of tetracycline and the two major tetracycline derivatives that have slightly different antimicrobial properties from the parent compound.

	R	R'
Erythromycin	H	
Propionyl erythromycin	CH_2CH_2CO	
Erythromycin estolate	CH_2CH_2CO	$C_{12}H_{25}OSO$
Erythromycin stearate	H	$C_{17}H_{35}COO$
Erythromycin ethyl succinate	$CH_2CH_2OOCCH_2CH_2COO$	

Figure 26-7 Structure of erythromycin, prototype of macrolide antibiotics that bind to 50S ribosomes and inhibit protein biosynthesis.

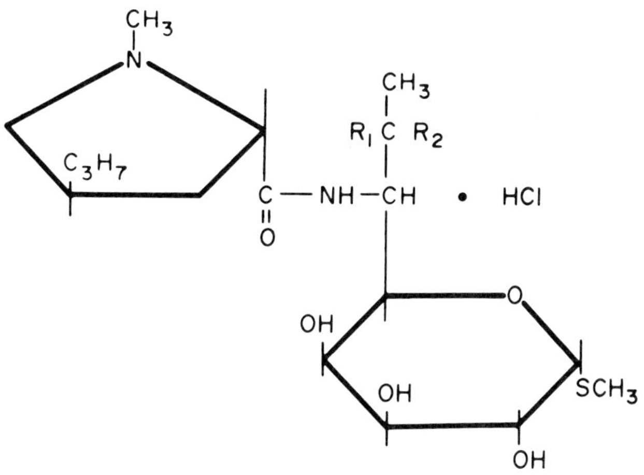

LINCOMYCIN R_1 = OH ; R_2 = H

CLINDAMYCIN R_1 = H ; R_2 = Cl

Figure 26-8 Structure of lincomycin and clindamycin that bind to 50S ribosomes.

Macrolides are large lactone ring compounds that bind to 50S ribosomes and appear to impair a peptidyl transferase reaction, translocation, or both reactions (Figure 26-7). The most important macrolide is erythromycin, which inhibits gram-positive species and a few gram-negative species such as *Haemophilus*, mycoplasma, chlamydia and *Legionella*. Lincinoids (Figure 26-8), of which the most important is clindamycin, have a similar site of activity as the macrolides. Both macrolides and lincinoids are bacteriostatic and only inhibit the formation of new peptide chains.

Inhibition of Folate Metabolism

Both trimethoprim and sulfanomides interfere with folate metabolism of the bacterial cell by competitively blocking the biosynthesis of tetrahydrofolate—a precursor of folinic acid (Figure 26-9). Unlike mammals, bacteria and protozoan parasites usually lack a transport system that would enable them to use preformed folic acid, which is abundant in their environment. Most organisms must synthesize folates, although some are capable of using exogenous thymidine and circumventing the need for folate metabolism.

Sulfonamides competitively block the conversion of pteridine and para-aminobenzoic acid (PABA) to dihydrofolic acid. Sulfonamides have a greater affinity for the enzyme that performs the conversion than does PABA. Trimethoprim has a tremendous affinity for the enzyme dihydrofolate reductase (10,000 to 100,000 times more for the bacterial enzyme than for the mammalian enzyme). It binds to this enzyme and inhibits synthesis of tetrahydrofolate, which acts as a cofactor for carriers of 1-carbon fragments and is necessary for the ultimate synthesis of DNA, RNA, and bacterial cell wall proteins.

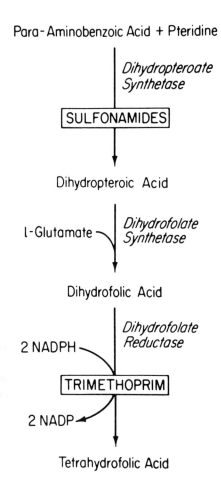

Figure 26-9 Sites of inhibition of folic acid cycle by sulfonamides and trimethoprim.

Inhibition of Mycobacteria

Isoniazid is a nicotinamide derivative that inhibits mycobacteria. Its precise mode of action is not known, but it affects synthesis of lipid, nucleic acid, and the mycolic acid of the cell walls of these species. Ethambutol also is an antimycobacterial agent whose mechanism of action is unknown. It is mycostatic whereas isoniazid is mycocidal. The other antituberculosis drugs, rifampin and streptomycin, affect mycobacteria in the same manner that they inhibit other bacterial species.

Bacterial Resistance

Over the past four decades, bacteria have proved themselves to be adept at becoming resistant to each new antimicrobial agent that is discovered in nature or synthesized by the medicinal chemist. Just as it has been possible to develop antibacterial agents to interfere with each critical step in the growth mechanism or in production of the protective walls of bacteria, bacteria have evolved novel mechanisms of resistance to thwart our attack.

Most of the early studies of bacterial resistance focused on single-step mutational events of chromosomal origin. Resistance to the early sulfonamides resulted from a change in a single amino acid in the enzyme dihydropeteroic synthetase, so that sulfonamides bound less well than paraaminobenzoic acid. Similarly a single-step mutation altered a ribosomal protein, and bacteria were able to resist the action of streptomycin. However, in the late 1950s, Japanese workers found that enteric bacteria such as *Shigella dysenteriae* had become resistant not only to sulfonamides but also to the tetracyclines and chloramphenicol. This resistance was shown to be due not to a chromosomal change, but rather to the presence of transmissible extrachromosomal DNA. This resistance, now referred to as *plasmid resistance,* was formerly called R-factor; that is, resistance-factor resistance.

Resistance-conferring plasmids have been shown to be present in virtually all bacteria (Table 26-2), and they have been widely dispersed in nature, appearing in *Haemophilus influenzae* in 1974 and in *Neisseria gonorrhoeae* in 1976.

In the past decade we have realized that, in addition to plasmids, bacteria can contain transposons, so-called jumping genes. Transposons can enter plasmids and also the chromosome (Figure 20-12). Transposon-mediated resistance to most of the major antibiotics has been found in the past few years. Of greater concern is the possibility that plasmids will pick up chromosomal genes of resistance and transfer these genetic elements via plasmids, which are highly transferable by conjugation.

Antimicrobial agents exert a strong selective pressure on the development of both chromosomal and plasmid-mediated resistance. The use of antibiotics in any environment, whether in a hospital or within an individual patient, destroys antibiotic-

Table 26-2 Bacteria Found to Contain R-Plasmids

Gram-Negative	*Gram-Positive*
Escherichia coli	*Staphylococcus aureus*
Shigella sp	*Staphylococcus epidermidis*
Salmonella sp	*Streptococcus faecalis*
Proteus spp	*Bacillus* spp
Klebsiella spp	*Streptococcus pyogenes*
Serratia marcescens	*Streptococcus pneumoniae*
Enterobacter sp	*Clostridium* spp
Pseudomonas aeruginosa	
Aeromonas sp	
Vibrio sp	
Yersinia sp	
Haemophilus influenzae	
Neisseria gonorrhoeae	
Bacteroides sp	
Providencia spp	
Proteus-Morganella spp	
Citrobacter spp	

susceptible bacteria and permits the proliferation of bacteria that are intrinsically resistant or have acquired extrachromosomal resistance. From an epidemiological viewpoint, plasmid resistance is the most threatening, since it is transmissible, is usually highly stable, confers resistance to many different classes of antibiotics simultaneously, and often is associated with other characteristics that enable a microorganism to colonize and invade a susceptible host.

Microorganisms develop resistance to antimicrobials by (1) developing altered receptors for a drug, (2) decreasing the amount of a drug that reaches the receptor by altering the means of entry or removal of a drug, (3) destroying or inactivating a drug, or (4) by synthesizing resistant metabolic pathways.

Bacteria may make use of one or all of these mechanisms simultaneously. Table 26-3 summarizes a number of mechanisms used by organisms that result in increased or complete resistance to antimicrobials.

Resistance Based on Altered Receptors for a Drug

β-lactams

Analyses of changes in receptors for β-lactams in competition experiments in which ^{14}C penicillin was inhibited from binding to PBPs has explained a number of cases of resistance of bacteria to penicillins and cephalosporins. In 1977, *Streptococcus pneumoniae* resistant to penicillin G was encountered in patients in Johannesberg and Durban, South Africa. Numerous studies have not shown plasmids that confer resistance, and β-lactamases are not present in these isolates of *S pneumoniae*. The Tomasz laboratory at Rockefeller University has shown that the penicillin-resistant *S pneumoniae* have altered PBPs. Other workers have confirmed these observations for isolates of *S pneumoniae* from South Africa and from other parts of the world. Resistance of *S pneumoniae* to penicillin has been increasing and there are relatively resistant isolates (MIC 0.1–1.0 μg/mL) in many parts of the world.

The presence of altered receptors also seems to explain why some *Staphylococcus aureus* are resistant to β-lactamase-stable penicillins. The precise mechanism of this methicillin resistance in *S epidermidis* has not been worked out, but it seems probable that the β-lactam resistance of *S epidermidis* is also the result of altered PBPs. Staphylococcal organisms resistant to methicillin are resistant to all penicillins and cephalosporins.

Table 26-3   Resistance Mechanisms

1. Modification of a target enzyme so that it is insensitive to an inhibitor but still functions
2. Reduction in physiological importance of a target
3. Duplication of a target enzyme
4. Prevention of access to the target
5. Depression of metabolic activity that normally converts an inert agent into an active agent
6. Synthesis of enzymes that:
   - inactivate an antimicrobial agent
   - modify the agent to alter energy or binding to a receptor

The resistance of enterococci of the group D streptococci to β-lactam antibiotics appears to be the result of lower affinity of the PBPs for the penicillins and particularly for cephalosporins, which do not inhibit these species.

One gram-negative species for which resistance to β-lactam antibiotics can be correlated with diminished affinity of the target enzymes is *Neisseria gonorrhoeae*. There are no well established examples of altered PBPs in *Enterobacteriaceae*, but some *Pseudomonas aeruginosa* may owe part of their resistance to altered PBPs.

Macrolide-Lincomycin Resistance

The occurrence of macrolide-lincomycin resistance in clinical isolates of staphylococci and streptococci has been recognized for the past several decades. The mechanism of resistance is the methylation of two adenine nucleotides in the 23S component of 50S RNA; the genetic basis of the resistance is plasmid, and the resistance is present on transposons. An enzyme that is normally repressed in nonresistant bacteria is induced, and the methylated RNA binds macrolide-lincomycin-type drugs less well than unmethylated RNA. Induction of resistance varies by species; erythromycin is a more effective inducer of resistance in most gram-positive species than are lincomycin or clindamycin. Plasmids in streptococci and staphylococci that mediate macrolide-lincomycin resistance are very similar structurally, indicating that these plasmids readily pass between these species.

Rifampin Resistance

Resistance of bacteria to rifampin develops because of altered DNA-directed RNA polymerase. A change of one amino acid in the beta subunit of DNA-directed RNA polymerase alters binding of rifampin. The degree of resistance is related to the degree that the enzyme is changed but does not correlate strictly with enzyme inhibition. This form of resistance exists at a low level in any population of bacteria and develops during therapy. Appearance of such resistance is not due to a new mutational event, but rather to selection of a subset of the bacterial population that possesses an RNA polymerase with poor affinity for rifampin. Such organisms are more common among the *Enterobacteriaceae*, which explains why organisms that cause urinary tract infections rapidly become resistant to rifampin. Resistance of *Neisseria meningitidis* to rifampin appeared in closed military settings in which rifampin had been used for prophylaxis.

Sulfonamide-Trimethoprim Resistance

The presence of an altered or new dihydropeteroic synthetase that has poor affinity for sulfonamides will preferentially bind PABA and preclude a block of the folic acid synthesis cycle. Sulfonamide resistance of this type can be the result of a point mutation or the presence of a plasmid that causes synthesis of a new enzyme. A serious problem is an increase in resistance to trimethoprim, which is plasmid- and transposon-mediated and due to production of an altered dihydrofolate reductase. Distinct dihydrofolate reductases have been characterized that differ by molecular weight and serologically. The new enzymes have markedly reduced affinity for trimethoprim. Since the genetic information for synthesis of the enzymes resides on transposons, we can anticipate even greater resistance to trimethoprim in the future.

Quinolone Resistance

Resistance of bacteria to older quinolone antibiotics such as nalidixic acid, cinoxacin, and oxalinic acid appears to be due either to altered DNA gyrase or, in some bacteria, to failure of entry of the agent. This is not a plasmid-mediated form of resistance, but rather is a mutational event or selection of such strains from the bacterial population. The mechanism of the resistance of bacteria to the new fluorinated carboxy quinolones such as norfloxacin, enoxacin, and ciprofloxacin has not yet been elucidated. These agents are active against DNA gyrase A and B mutants that are resistant to nalidixic acid.

Decreased Entry of a Drug

Tetracycline uptake by *Enterobacteriaceae* is a biphasic process with an initial energy-independent rapid phase that is believed to represent binding of the drug to cell-surface layers and passage by diffusion through the outer layers of the cell. The second phase of uptake is energy-dependent as the tetracycline crosses the cytoplasmic membrane, probably by means of a proton motive force.

Tetracycline resistance is common in both gram-positive and gram-negative bacteria. In most cases it is plasmid-encoded and inducible, but chromosomal, constitutive resistance is present in some species such as *Proteus*. Thus far, five plasmid-specified tetracycline-resistance determinants have been found in enteric bacteria. The most common of these determinants, Tet B, is also present in *H influenzae*. Most tetracycline resistance in *S aureus* is due to small plasmids that exist in multiple copies; chromosomal resistance is rare. Tetracycline resistance is found in *S faecalis* on nonconjugative plasmids, and in the chromosomes of *S pneumoniae*, *S agalactiae* (group B streptococci), and oral streptococci such as *S mutans*. *Clostridia* such as *C difficile* harbor chromosomal genes for tetracycline resistance.

Basically, tetracycline resistance is due to a decrease in drug accumulation. A drug efflux mechanism in which decreased uptake and efflux occur simultaneously probably influences its development as well. Resistant bacteria clearly bind less tetracycline, and the tetracycline they do accumulate is lost by an energy-dependent process when they are in a drug-free milieu.

Plasmid resistance to tetracyclines can be partially overcome in gram-positive species by molecular modification of the tetracycline nucleus. Thus, minocycline and doxycycline will inhibit some streptococci such as *S pneumoniae* and some *S aureus* at acceptable doses. Molecular modification has not been successful in overcoming tetracycline resistance of *Enterobacteriaceae* amd *Pseudomonas* nor of most *Bacteroides*.

Tetracycline resistance is a major concern. Tetracycline resistance is located on plasmids near insertion sites, and it appears that tetracycline plasmids can readily acquire other genetic information to enlarge the spectrum of resistance. The widespread use of tetracycline in animal feeds has been thought to be a factor in the extensive, worldwide resistance of *Enterobacteriaceae,* particularly enteric species such as *Salmonella,* to tetracyclines and subsequently to many other drugs. Not only tetracycline resistance can move among the *Enterobacteriaceae* on plasmids, but plasmids mediating tetracycline resistance have moved between *S aureus, S epidermidis, S pyogenes, S pneumoniae,* and *S faecalis.*

Fosfomycin Resistance

Fosfomycin and fosmidomycin, which inhibit cell wall synthesis, enter bacteria by means of a glycerol-phosphate or glucose-6-phosphate transport system. Gram-positive bacteria that have a poorly developed glucose 6-phosphate transport system will not take up the drugs in adequate concentrations to inhibit the cell wall synthesis. This resistance usually is chromosomally mediated. Resistance of gram-negative bacteria to this class of agents is related primarily to the presence of some bacteria in any population of cells that can function without the transport system. This resistance appears as a single step at a high level. Recently, plasmids and transposons that transfer resistance to fosfomycin have been found in the bacteria *Serratia.*

Aminoglycoside Resistance

Formerly, we would have classified the cause of the resistance of bacteria to aminoglycosides as inactivation of the drugs. Strictly speaking, this is inaccurate, since aminoglycosides are highly stable and resist most attempts at denaturation. All aminoglycosides contain free amino and hydroxyl groups, which are essential for their binding to ribosomal proteins in the 30S ribosome and to both 30S and 50S ribosomes in selected situations. Amino groups can be acetylated and hydroxyl groups can be phosphorylated or adenylated by the enzymes shown in Figure 26-10.

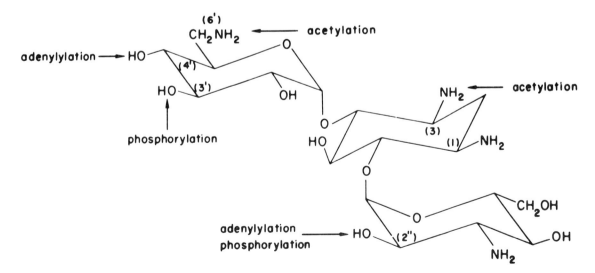

Figure 26-10 Prototype structure of an aminoglycoside, which consists of aminohexoses linked to glycosidic linkage to a central 2-deoxystreptamine nucleus common to these antibiotics. Hydroxyl and amino groups are sites at which these compounds can be inactivated by phosphorylation, adenylation, or acetylation.

The most important aminoglycoside resistance is due to poor uptake of the compounds by bacteria, which results from the structural modification of the compounds when they are phosphorylated, adenylated, or acetylated. Other forms of resistance, such as altered binding sites on 30S ribosomes, occur much less frequently. In *Enterobacteriaceae* and *Pseudomonas*, the aminoglycosides pass through the cell wall by going through channels through which charged molecules enter the periplasmic spore. These channels are *porin channels* (porin proteins line the channel and the channels are, so to speak, pores). Aminoglycosides that reach the cell membrane are moved across the membrane by a proton motive force and enter the cytoplasm where they bind to ribosomes just below the membrane. The initial uptake of aminoglycoside into the membrane is energy dependent. Aminoglycosides that enter the cell will bind only to ribosomes actively engaged in protein synthesis. Binding to the ribosomes induces a protein involved in the uptake of the aminoglycosides.

Unfortunately, bacteria may contain in the periplasmic space enzymes that will acetylate, phosphorylate, or adenylate aminoglycosides to varying degrees depending on the molecular configuration of the molecule. Whether the enzymes are free in the periplasmic space or bound to the cytoplasmic membrane is not clear. Aminoglycosides that are acetylated, phosphorylated, or adenylated do not bind well to ribosomes, and hence uptake is poor or does not occur.

Aminoglycoside-modifying enzymes have been found in gram-positive species such as *S aureus*, *S faecalis* and *S pyogenes,* and *S pneumoniae*. These enzymes are particularly prevalent in *Enterobacteriaceae* and *P aeruginosa*. Many of the aminoglycoside modifying enzymes are present on transposons.

Anaerobic species such as *Bacteroides* are resistant to aminoglycosides because they lack an oxygen-dependent transport system for getting the drug into and across the cytoplasmic membrane. Although most resistance of *S aureus* to aminoglycosides is due to modifying enzymes, small colony variants of staphylococci are resistant because they have a defect in adenyl cyclase or in cyclic AMP binding proteins; the cells with reduced growth rates do not transport aminoglycosides into the cytoplasm. Finally, some *Enterobacteriaceae* and *P aeruginosa* appear to be resistant because of altered porin channels, which means that these bacteria do not take up any drug or possess aminoglycoside-inactivating enzymes.

Destruction or Inactivation of a Drug

Chloramphenicol Resistance

Many gram-positive and gram-negative bacteria, including recently some *Haemophilus influenzae*, are resistant to chloramphenicol because they possess the enzyme chloramphenicol transacetylase, which acetylates hydroxyl groups on the chloramphenicol structure. Acetylated chloramphenicol binds less well to the 50S ribosome, allowing the bacteria to continue their protein synthesis. This enzyme, unlike the aminoglycoside inactivating enzymes and β-lactamases, is an intracellular enzyme of larger molecular weight and subunit structure. It is in most instances plasmid mediated.

β-Lactam Resistance

The best known mechanism of bacterial resistance is that of the penicillinase. Resistance of *E coli* to penicillin was recognized in 1940, before penicillin was clinically useful. Subsequently in the 1940s, resistance of staphylococci was shown to be due to a penicillinase. With the advent of other β-lactam compounds such as cephalosporins, carbapenems, and monobactams, it became more appropriate to designate these enzymes as β-lactamases, since their attack on the β-lactam nucleus is the most important aspect of their activity (Figure 26-11). β-lactamases are widely distributed in nature and can be classified in various ways, but usually they are referred to on the basis of the principle compounds they destroy; hence, they are penicillinases or cephalosporinases. β-lactamases can be chromosomally or plasmid-mediated, constitutive, or inducible enzymes.

In gram-positive species, β-lactamases are primarily exoenzymes; that is, they are excreted into the milieu around the bacteria. Virtually all hospital isolates of staphylococci, both *S aureus* and *S epidermidis,* possess β-lactamases and 50% to 80% of community staphylococcal isolates produce β-lactamases. In gram-negative species,

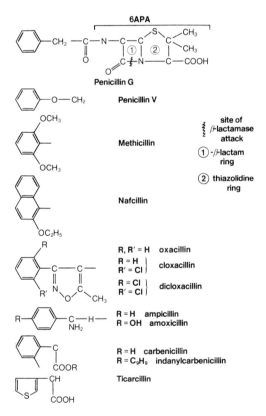

Figure 26-11 Structural modification of basic penicillin nucleus, which consists of β-lactam ring fused to thiazolidine ring. Penicillin V, ampicillin, and carbenicillin are hydrolyzed by β-lactamases. Oxacillin, cloxacillin, and other agents containing bulky side chains are not.

aerobic and anaerobic β-lactamases are contained in the periplasmic space, protecting the PBPs.

Resistance of staphylococci to β-lactams was overcome with the development of the antistaphylococcal penicillins and the cephalosporins. Some strains of *S aureus*, however, do produce larger amounts of β-lactamase constitutively, and can be resistant to some of the cephalosporins.

In 1974, *H influenzae* was shown to possess a plasmid-mediated β-lactamase. At present, 10% to 35% of *H influenzae* in the United States are β-lactamase–positive. The TnA transposon has become more widespread and the resistance of *Haemophilus* to penicillin G and ampicillin seems to be increasing yearly. The β-lactamase of *Haemophilus* is the same structurally as the enzyme found in *E coli, Salmonella, Shigella,* and *N gonorrhoeae*. The enzyme has generally been called the TEM enzyme, named after the first three initials of the Greek girl from whom an *E coli* that contained a plasmid beta-lactamase was isolated by Datta and Kontomichalou in 1964. These enzymes are also called Richmond-Sykes class IIIa enzymes according to a classification proposed by Richmond and Sykes in 1973. This β-lactamase also is present in *N gonorrhoeae*. By far the most common plasmid β-lactamase found in nature is the TEM-1 enzyme, which has been reported to account for 75% to 80% of plasmid-mediated β-lactamase resistance worldwide.

Chromosomally mediated β-lactamases are present in many *Enterobacter, Citrobacter, Proteus-Providencia* and *Pseudomonas*. All *Klebsiella* possess a β-lactamase that acts primarily as a penicillinase and is chromosomally mediated. Constitutively produced β-lactamase also are present in many anaerobic species.

Table 26-4 illustrates the major β-lactamases of clinical importance. β-lactamases vary in their ability to destroy penicillins and cephalosporins. β-lactamase activity studied with isolated or purified β-lactamases may not reflect the activity of a compound against gram-negative bacteria, since resistance of gram-negative bacteria to β-lactams is a combination of decreased entry, β-lactamase stability, and affinity of the compound for PBPs.

Synthesis of Resistant Metabolic Pathway

No bacteria have yet been able to synthesize a cell wall resistant to β-lactams, although some, particularly streptococci, lack hydrolytic enzymes necessary for forming a new cell wall and thus β-lactams do not cause lysis of these bacteria. An altered hydrolytic system thus converts a bactericidal antibiotic into a bacteriostatic agent. Whether such resistance occurs in gram-negative species is not clear.

Some thymidine-requiring streptococci fail to be inhibited by trimethoprim and sulfonamides. These organisms cause some urinary tract infections, albeit rarely, but fail to undergo the thymineless death that occurs normally with bacteria exposed to these agents. Other bacteria produce adequate dTMP by alternate methods, and as a result survive exposure to these folate inhibitors.

Certain yeasts of the *Candida* or *Cryptococcus* species are resistant to the compound 5-fluorocytosine, because they fail to convert 5-fluorocytosine to its active component 5-fluorouracil. Other fungi are resistant to the polyenes and imidazoles because their

Table 26-4   R-Plasmid–Mediated Resistance

Antibiotic	Mechanism	Organisms
Penicillin, ampicillin, carbenicillin, etc.	β-lactamase hydrolysis	Gram (+), (−)
Oxacillin, methicillin, etc.	β-lactamase hydrolysis	Gram (−)
Cephalosporins	β-lactamase	Gram (+), (−)
Chloramphenicol	Acetylation	Gram (+), (−)
Tetracyclines	Permeability block	Gram (+), (−)
Aminoglycosides		
Streptomycin	Acetylation	
Neomycin	Phosphorylation	Gram (+), (−)
Kanamycin	Adenylation; alters binding to ribosomes and uptake of drug	
Gentamicin		
Tobramycin		
Amikacin		
Macrolides-Lincinoids		
Erythromycin	Altered 23S RNA	Gram (+), (−)
Clindamycin		
Trimethoprim	Altered dihydrofolate reductase	Gram (−)
Sulfonamides	Altered tetrahydropteroic synthetase	Gram (−)
Nitrofurans	Unknown	Gram (−)
Fosfomycin	Altered glucose transport system	Gram (+), (−)

membranes are not disrupted by the agents, since different metabolic mechanisms are used to synthesize the membranes.

Combinations of Antimicrobial Agents

Antibiotics are frequently used in combination (1) to combat a life-threatening infection, (2) to prevent emergence of bacterial resistance, (3) to treat mixed infections (aerobic and anaerobic bacteria), (4) to enhance antibacterial activity, and (5) to allow the use of a lower dose of a toxic drug. Of these reasons, combined treatment is reasonable when the precise etiologic agents causing a serious infection are unknown. Use of two or more drugs to prevent emergence of resistance has been shown to be effective for tuberculosis and for therapy of some chronic infections. The use of combinations to achieve synergy is more complicated. **Synergy** has been defined as the correlated action of two drugs that causes inhibition or killing of a microorganism at a fourfold lower concentration of both component drugs. **Indifference** of drugs means that the combined action is the same as either component. Finally, **antagonism** refers to a reduction in the activity of one or both components in the presence of the other.

Some important examples of bacterial synergy include (1) use of agents that inhibit cell walls along with aminoglycoside antibiotics, (2) use of β-lactamase inhibitors with β-lactam antibiotics, and (3) administration of agents that act on sequential steps in bacterial metabolic or synthetic pathways. Combining penicillin and streptomycin to treat *Streptococcus faecalis* endocarditis and carbenicillin and gentamicin to treat *Pseudomonas aeruginosa* infections have been particularly useful. Recently, β-lactamase inhibitors, such as clavulanic acid, have been combined with amoxicillin (an amino penicillin) to inhibit *Staphylococcus aureaus, Klebsiella pneumoniae,* and *Haemophilus influenzae,* all of which are resistant to amoxicillin when they contain β-lactamases. The combination of sulfamethoxazole and trimethoprim attacks two parts of the folic acid cycle and synergistically inhibits many bacteria. Finally, combining two penicillins that affect different stages of cell wall synthesis in gram-negative bacteria is synergistic. This is true for the combination of mecillinam (amdinocillin), which binds to PBP2 of bacteria, and other penicillins or cephalosporins, which bind to PBPs 1 and 3.

Antagonism, by which one agent reduces the effectiveness of another can occur when a bacteriostatic agent is combined with a bactericidal agent. The most common example is the combination of chlortetracycline and penicillin used to treat pneumococcal meningitis. This effect has not been explained from a molecular standpoint, however, and tetracyclines and penicillins or cephalosporins are used to treat mixed infections such as pelvic inflammatory disease due to *Neisseria gonorrhoeae* and *Chlamydia.* Some β-lactam antibiotics can induce β-lactamases that inactivate other β-lactams, and antagonism can be shown in the test tube—but the relevance for clinical infections is not established.

Toxicology of Antimicrobial Agents

Antimicrobial agents can cause toxicity directly, they can interact with other drugs to influence the toxicity of another agent, or they can, by altering microbial flora, result in infection with organisms that are normally saprophytic. Allergic reactions can be caused by any agent, but penicillins can produce either immediate, IgE-mediated, or delayed hypersensitivity reactions. Cutaneous reactions have been reported with every class of antimicrobial. Hematological reactions can range from the life-threatening events that occur in 1 in 60,000 individuals who receive chloramphenicol to the development of hemolytic anemia in individuals who take sulfonamides and lack the enzyme glucose-6-phosphate dihydrogenase. Many antimicrobials depress blood platelet activity, and almost all antibiotics, by altering the gastrointestinal flora, can cause an overgrowth of a *Clostridium difficile,* which produces a toxin that causes serious colon reactions. Alteration of intestinal flora by antibiotics also can result in overgrowth of *Candida* in the mouth, vagina, or gastrointestinal tract. Since a number of antibiotics are metabolized in the liver, damage to the liver can occur; this has been of particular concern when isoniazid is used to treat tuberculosis. Damage to the kidneys can follow use of aminoglycosides, but other drugs may damage renal tubular cells. Neurologic toxicity is fairly uncommon, but the aminoglycosides can damage the auditory or vestibular apparatus if the clinician does not pay close attention to the amount given to the patient.

Implications of Resistance

Bacteria continue to evolve new mechanisms of resistance to old and new antimicrobial agents. Some bacteria, such as *P aeruginosa,* are particularly adept at utilizing a number

Table 26-5 Mechanisms to Reduce Antibiotic Resistance

1. Control, reduce, or cycle antibiotic usage
2. Improve hygiene in hospitals and among hospital personnel and reduce movement of patients to eliminate the dissemination of resistant organisms within hospitals
3. Discover new antibiotics from nature or develop synthetic antimicrobial agents
4. Modify existing antibiotics chemically to produce compounds inert to known resistance mechanisms
5. Develop inhibitors of antibiotic-modifying enzymes
6. Find agents that can "cure" resistance plasmids

of different mechanisms simultaneously to become resistant to agents in virtually every class, and to agents that have such diverse sites of action as cell walls, protein biosynthesis, or DNA and RNA synthesis. It is probable that developments in other areas of medicine will keep alive patients who become nosocomially infected with resistant pathogens.

Mechanisms to Reduce Bacterial Resistance

Proper selection of new antibiotics should be a major force in slowing the development of antimicrobial resistance. Proper hygienic practices should reduce plasmid transfer and the establishment of bacteria that can resist many drugs in the hospital, and delay the appearance of such species in the community. Table 26-5 lists a number of mechanisms to prevent bacterial resistance. The health care providers must be continually alert to the appearance of antibiotic resistance within their hospital and community.

References

Bryan, L.E.: *Bacterial resistance and susceptibility to chemotherapeutic agents*. London: Cambridge University Press, 1982.

Davies, J., Smith, D.: Plasmid-determined resistance to antimicrobial agents. *Ann Rev Microbiol* 1978; 32:469-518.

Gale, E.F., et al: *The molecular basis of antibiotic action*, 2nd ed. New York: John Wiley and Sons, 1981.

Garrod, L.P., Lambert, H.P., O'Grady, F.: *Antibiotic and chemotherapy*, 5th ed. New York: Churchill Livingstone, 1981.

Moellering, R.C., Jr., Krogstad, D.J.: Combinations of antimicrobial agents—mechanisms of interaction against bacteria. In: *Antibiotics in laboratory medicine*. Lorian, V. (editor). Baltimore, MD: Williams & Wilkins, 1980.

Neu, H.C.: The pharmacology and toxicology of antimicrobial agents. In: *Medical microbiology and infectious diseases*. Braude, H. (editor). Philadelphia: Saunders, 1981.

Neu, H.C.: The emergence of bacterial resistance and its influence on empiric therapy. *Rev Infect Dis* 1983; 5 (Suppl): 9-20.

Sykes, R.B., Mathew, M.: The beta-lactamases of gram-negative bacteria and their role in resistance to beta-lactam antibiotics. *J Antimicrob Chemother* 1976;2:115-157.

Waxman, D.J., Strominger, J.L.: Beta-lactam antibiotics: biochemical modes of action. In: *Chemistry and biology of beta-lactam antibiotics*. Morin, R.B., Gorman, M. (editors). New York: Academic Press, 1982.

27 Sterilization and Disinfection

James G. Shaffer, ScD†
C. P. Davis, PhD

General Concepts
Sterilization
Disinfection

General Concepts

Disinfection and sterilization are fundamental processes in microbiology. Without sterile substrates, the pure culture of microorganisms would be impossible; without sterile materials, major surgery would be impossible. Disinfection is crucial in disease prevention and in food preparation and preservation. Both processes have been used for centuries, but only within the past 150 years has a relatively sophisticated understanding of their nature developed. In the late 1820s, Collins in Dublin and, some years later, Semmelweis in Vienna demonstrated that puerperal sepsis could be controlled using chemical disinfection, sterilization by heat, and isolation of mothers who had fever.

Disinfection and sterilization are terms with which many are familiar, but too few understand. Simply defined, sterilization is an act or process that frees an item of all viable agents, thus making it sterile. Substances cannot be partially sterile; if they are not sterile, they are contaminated. Disinfection is an act or process by which microorganisms are removed or destroyed, or both, to render an item incapable of transmitting infection. Disinfection can result in complete destruction of organisms, but this may not be necessary to accomplish the purpose. In either process, contaminating organisms are removed or killed by chemical or physical means.

---

†Deceased.

Certain basic principles apply to all methods of reducing the microbial content of an item. First, the antimicrobial process, whether physical or chemical, must be able to affect the microorganism directly. Second, the item must be cleaned in a manner that removes all extraneous soil that might interfere with access to chemical or physical action or the penetration of heat. Third, effective action of chemicals or gas requires moisture, either in the air or on the item itself. Finally, the time required to kill microorganisms depends on four factors: nature of the organism, nature of the agent being used, number of organisms present on the object, and temperature of the process.

Sterilization

Sterilization is routinely accomplished with heat, a toxic gas, radiation, or filtration. The heat used may be dry or moist, depending on the nature of the material to be sterilized. Moist heat in the form of superheated steam (steam under pressure) works most rapidly and should be used whenever possible.

The autoclave is commonly used for steam sterilization. Modern autoclaves are complex machines that operate automatically. To attain a sterile condition the steam, which denatures the vital proteins of microorganisms, must penetrate to each item. The autoclave is similar to a large, automatic pressure cooker. Temperatures sufficient to kill all organisms, including the most resistant spores, are easily reached in a short time.

To obtain the best results from autoclaving, certain criteria must be fulfilled. Air must be completely eliminated. Most autoclaves now can be evacuated before steam is introduced; remaining air is released through an automatic valve. It is critical that the sterilization temperature be reached and held for the appropriate time (see Table 27-1). Items also must be packaged so that air will be removed and replaced by steam. In addition, the autoclave must be loaded to provide for free circulation of steam, which should reach a pressure of at least 15 psi at 121 C to prevent fluids from boiling in the chamber.

Table 27-1   Sterilization

Method	Temp. (C)	Time* (min.)	Pressure	Mode of Action	Controls
Moist heat (autoclave)	121†	15	15 psi	Protein denaturation	Chemical indicator‡
	126	10			
	134	3			Spore strip
Dry heat (oven)	160	45§	Atmospheric	Protein denaturation and oxidation	May use spore strip
	170	18			
	180	7.5			
	190	1.5			

*Time should be extended when large packs of items are being sterilized.
†Temperatures above the boiling point of water are attained by raising steam pressure.
‡Chemical indicators used in each sterilization cycle; spore strips once a week.
§These times assume the organism has been at that temperature.

To ensure that an autoclave is functioning properly, one can monitor the temperature on a tape with a chemical heat indicator placed in each package. Effective autoclaving will also eradicate the inhabitants of a bacterial spore strip (containing 1×10^6 spores of *Bacillus stearothermophilus* or *B subtilis* var *niger*) placed in the center of the largest package.

Sterilization with dry heat is slower than with moist heat. Table 27-1 shows the minimal times needed for killing spores. In practice, sterilization often requires longer times than those shown in Table 27-1 to allow for uniform heating. Ovens for dry-heat sterilization have fans to distribute the heated air uniformly and a thermostat to regulate temperature. Dry-heat sterilization is useful for glassware and instruments that cannot be damaged by heat. Items wrapped in paper or gauze or plugged with cotton may char if the temperature is too high or if the procedure is prolonged. Packing the oven to allow for adequate circulation of air is essential. Packaged items are commonly heated at 160 C for 2 hours.

Gas sterilization is an important process because it can sterilize items, particularly plastics, that would be damaged by heat. Ethylene oxide (ETO) is used most extensively, and special gas sterilizers are available. Certain interdependent factors are crucial in gas sterilization: temperature, relative humidity, gas concentration, and time. A temperature of 72 C, relative humidity above 40%, and an ETO concentration of 400 mg/L of space are particularly effective. Because different materials absorb varying amounts of gas, sterilization times range from 2 to 30 hours. Chemical indicators can be used to assure adequate sterilization, but spore strips are the most dependable controls. The chamber should be evacuated after sterilization is complete. To eliminate gas residue, all items must be exposed to free air for 48 hours before use.

ETO kills microorganisms by alkylation of essential cell components. Other gases (propylene oxide, betapropiolactone, methyl bromide, and formaldehyde) have been used for sterilizing or disinfecting, but each has one or more serious drawback. ETO itself is a strong irritant for skin and mucous membranes and is explosive under some circumstances. Recently ETO was designated as a potential carcinogen, which may limit its use in the future.

When using gas sterilization, the operator should use proper equipment and follow the manufacturer's directions to prevent harm to him- or herself and to those who use the sterilized items.

Radiation with cobalt gamma rays and laser beta rays has been used for sterilization in large commercial installations but is not suitable for ordinary laboratory use. Sterilization of fluids or gases may be accomplished by filtration through appropriate filters which remove particles the size of bacteria (0.2 μm pore size is routinely used for most bacteria); however, viruses and flexible organisms such as mycoplasma will pass through these filters.

Disinfection

Before the advent of antibiotics, disinfection meant removing mainly pathogenic microorganisms, mostly bacteria and fungi, from the item in question. In recent years, the number of potential pathogens has greatly increased because of the population's changing susceptibility and the discovery of new bacterial and viral agents. As a result, the goal is now to reduce microbial contents rather than to kill specific organisms.

The first step in disinfection is thorough cleaning. On hard, smooth surfaces, such cleaning may remove 60%–90% of the offending microorganisms. Studies of carpeting found that vacuuming a dry carpet could remove as much as 90% of the surface bacteria.

Numerous chemical substances have been used as disinfectants. The most important groups are presented in Table 27-2 with their ranges of activity and other pertinent information.

Many formulations using these agents are available. A company can devise a formula and market it under a trade name, with a label listing the ingredients. The exception is alcohol, which according to federal law must be called by its generic name.

All federally registered disinfectants are tested for effectiveness by methods devised by the Association of Official Analytical Chemists (AOAC). These methods are complex and exacting procedures and should never be attempted by inexperienced personnel. The choice of a disinfectant depends on the nature of the material to be disinfected, the type of contamination, and the results desired. It is always best to use products of reputable manufacturers and to follow their directions.

Many products have been developed and marketed as disinfectants in spray cans or other kinds of dispensers or fogging devices. Most are expensive and the results obtained may not meet advertising claims. Although fogging has been suggested as a means of disinfecting rooms and elevators in hospitals, its effectiveness is questionable. Claims that fogging effectively penetrates remote areas have not been substantiated; thus caution is recommended.

The effectiveness of ultraviolet light as a physical method of disinfecting has been somewhat controversial for many years. Effectiveness depends on time, intensity, humidity, and direct access to the organism. Microorganisms must be exposed directly to the rays for a sufficient period. The more intense the radiation, the shorter the time required; intensity decreases as the square of the distance from the source. When the relative humidity is above 55%, effectiveness declines rapidly. In addition, ultraviolet rays do not penetrate dust particles and soil.

These rays have been used with success in entries to sterile rooms and as barriers between infectious areas in hospitals. Intensity sufficient to kill microorganisms will also damage living tissue and eyesight. The extensive literature on ultraviolet light should be consulted before its use, since some of the failures reported may have been the result of improper use.

Antisepsis and sanitization are often used to destroy or inhibit microorganisms. **Antiseptics,** which are substances used on tissues to reduce chances of infection, are generally milder than disinfectants, and their effects are bacteriostatic rather than bactericidal. Most disinfectants, such as the iodophors or phenolics, can be used as antiseptics when adequately diluted. Often disinfectants are contained in 70% alcohol, which also has strong antimicrobial effects. Silver nitrate is a common antiseptic and is instilled in the eyes of newborn infants. Antisepsis thus may be viewed as a mild form of disinfecting.

Sanitization, a process used extensively in the food and dairy industries, implies removing and destroying microorganisms to prevent spoilage of food and/or transmission of infection by a food product such as milk. Heat, hot water, cleansing agents, and easily removed disinfectants are used.

Table 27-2 Disinfectants

Group	Range (vegetative)*‡	Effect on Spores	Speed	Nature of Activity	Remarks
Alcohols (ethyl, isopropyl)	Gram +, gram −, and acid fast	Poor (bacteriostatic)	Rapid	Bactericidal Fungistatic	Effective range 50%-85% by volume; not effective below 50% by volume; denatures protein.
Phenolics†	Gram +, gram −, and acid fast	Moderate	Good	Bactericidal	Many modifications of phenol; denatures protein; stable to drying & mild heat.
Quaternary ammonia‡	Gram +, gram −	Negative	Moderate	Bactericidal or bacteriostatic	Many quaternary compounds have detergent effects; some are absorbed by fabrics and neutralized by soap; good when used properly; acts on cell walls.
Amphoteric surfactants§	Gram +, gram −	Questionable	Rapid	Bactericidal	Activity probably depends on surface or membrane alternations.
Halogens: chlorine, iodine	Gram +, gram −, and acid fast	Moderate	Rapid	Bactericidal	Activity depends on release of halogen from some complex such as hypochlorite; inactivates enzymes.
Iodophor‖	Gram +, gram −, and acid fast	Moderate	Rapid	Bactericidal	Produced as a complex by combining iodine with detergent; iodine affects enzyme systems.
Glutaraldehyde	Gram +, gram −, and acid fast	Excellent	Rapid	Bactericidal	Effective in 2% aqueous alkaline concentration; cross-links proteins.
Formaldehyde	Gram +, gram −, and acid fast	Excellent	Moderate	Bactericidal	Used as formaline (8% formaldehyde in water = 20% formaline); acts on proteins.
Metallic ions: mercury, silver, copper	Gram +, gram −	Poor	Moderate	Bactericidal Fungicidal	Direct toxicity or removal, by competition, of an essential trace metal; inactivates enzymes by forming mercaptides.

*In general, the agents listed here have effects on viruses similar to those on bacteria.
†Corrosive; irritates skin.
‡Bland; may be bacteriostatic at lower concentrations.
§Trade name TEGO; produced and used extensively in Europe.
‖Effectiveness due to release of iodine.

References

Block, S.S.: *Disinfection, sterilization and preservation,* 3rd ed. Philadelphia: Lea and Febiger, 1983.

Borick, P.M.: *Chemical sterilization.* Stroudsburg, Pa.: Dowden, Hutchinson and Ross, 1973.

Howard, J.M., et al.: Postoperative wound infections: the influence of ultraviolet irradiation of the operating room and of various other factors. *Ann Surg* 1964; 160 (suppl.):1-92.

National Institute for Occupational Safety and Health (NIOSH): *Ethylene oxide (ETO).* Current Intelligence Bulletin 35. Washington, D.C.: DHHS (NIOSH) Publication No. 81-130, 1981.

Shaffer, J.G.: The role of laboratory in infection control in the hospital. In: *Control of infections in hospitals, proceedings of an institute.* Ann Arbor, Mich.: University of Michigan, School of Public Health, 1965.

Spaulding, E.H.: Chemical disinfection and antisepsis in the hospital. *J Hosp Res* 1972; 9:5-31.

Vesley, D., et al.: A cooperative microbiological evaluation of floor-cleaning procedures in hospital patient rooms: a committee report. *Health Lab Sci* 1970; 1:256-264.

28 *Staphylococcus*

Jay O. Cohen, PhD

General Concepts

Traditionally, the staphylococci have been divided into two groups according to their ability to clot blood plasma (the coagulase reaction). Coagulase-positive staphylococci are in the species *Staphylococcus aureus*. They are considered to be opportunistic pathogens in humans and some other mammals. The coagulase-negative staphylococci are considered to be saprophytes, even though they are occasionally responsible for infections. Recently, the coagulase-positive strains have been subdivided according to the animal host, kind of plasma coagulated, serotype, and phage type. In general, new species names have not been proposed for the subspecies of coagulase-positive staphylococci.

By contrast, the coagulase-negative staphylococci, once referred to as *Staphylococcus epidermidis,* have been further differentiated according to biochemical characteristics and cell wall chemistry. New names also have been proposed. The new terminology differentiates the urinary tract pathogen *Staphylococcus saprophyticus* from *S epidermidis* and other "nonpathogenic" staphylococci.

Over the years the coagulase-positive staphylococci have been isolated from deep-seated human infections, such as pneumonia, osteomyelitis, septicemia, abscesses, and wound infections. These serious infections, however, have been the exception. Usually, staphylococci are isolated from superficial skin infections, such as boils, styes, and the lesions of infantile impetigo. The introduction of antibiotics in the treatment of human diseases and the long hospitalization of chronically ill persons resulted in a dramatic change in the host-parasite relationship. Chronically ill, debilitated patients such as burn or cancer victims often suffer severe infections caused by *S aureus* strains that are resistant to many frequently used antibiotics.

The staphylococci form a variety of extracellular substances (Table 28-1), some of which have been correlated with virulence. Overall virulence probably results from the cumulative effect of several of these substances during infection. Antibodies are effective in neutralizing the toxic effects of the staphylococcal toxins and enzymes, but both antibiotics and surgical drainage are often necessary to cure abcesses, large boils, and wound infections.

Distinctive Properties

Structure

Staphylococci are gram-positive cocci, about 0.5–1.0 μm in diameter; they are arranged in clusters, pairs, and occasionally in short chains. The clusters arise because staphylococci divide in two planes. The configuration of the cocci helps distinguish micrococci and staphylococci from streptococci, which usually grow in chains. Observations must

Table 28-1   Extracellular Substances Formed by Staphylococci

Toxins and Enzymes	Action
Hemolysins	Causes lysis of erythrocytes
α-toxin	Most active against rabbit RBC
β-hemolysin	Most active against sheep RBC
δ-hemolysin	Weak hemolysin
ϵ-hemolysin	Weak hemolysin
Leukocidin	Lethal toxicity for leukocytes and macrophages
Enterotoxins (serologically distinct types, A–E)	Intestinal fluid secretion
Exfoliative (epidermolytic) toxins	Dermonecrosis
Toxic shock syndrome toxin	Pyrogenic toxin perhaps leading to death
Coagulase	Clot formation
Fibrinolysin (staphylokinase)	Dissolves fibrin clots
DNAse (nuclease)	Hydrolyzes the 5′ phosphodiester bond of DNA
Lipases (lipase, esterase, and phosphatidase)	Lipid hydrolysis
Hyaluronidase	Hydrolyzes hyaluronic acid in tissues

be made on cultures grown in broth, because streptococci grown on solid medium may appear in clumps. Several fields should be examined before concluding there is a prevalence of clumps or chains.

The catalase test is also important, as it distinguishes the streptococci, which are catalase-negative, from other gram-positive cocci. The test can be performed by flooding an agar slant or broth culture with several drops of 3% hydrogen peroxide. If a culture is catalase-positive, bubbles evolve at once. The test should be done on a duplicate culture because peroxide is bactericidal, but it should not be done on blood agar plates because the blood itself may produce bubbles.

Antigens

S aureus strains have group-specific and type-specific antigens. Over 90% of *S aureus* strains have protein A at the surface. This antigen is not found on coagulase-negative staphylococci and has not been reported in any other microbial species. Protein A reacts with the IgG immunoglobulins of humans, mice, rabbits, and other mammals. The reaction occurs through the Fc fragment of the IgG molecule and is thus different from the usual antibody reaction. The ability to react does not appear to require antigenic stimulation. Protein A reactions have been observed by serum gel precipitation, fluorescent antibody, and slide agglutination tests. The amounts of reactive immunoglobulin and the intensities of the reactions differ from animal to animal.

The ability of *S aureus* to attract IgG antibodies that attach at the Fc portion, or back end, is the basis for various serologic tests for both soluble and dispersed insoluble antigens, as this characteristic makes possible a process called **coagglutination.** The IgG in these tests is from specific antisera against the antigen being measured. A quantitative measurement of antigen can be obtained by preparing serial dilutions. The specific antibody-combining sites are free to react with antigen even though the other end of the molecule is attached to the staphylococcal cell. Combination with the antigen causes the staphylococci to agglutinate, thus providing a useful test to detect numerous antigens.

Another surface antigen that is group-specific for *S aureus* is a specific ribitol teichoic acid, also known as polysaccharide A. An α-linked glucosyl glycerol teichoic acid has been identified in coagulase-negative staphylococci and named polysaccharide B. The teichoic acids can be identified and distinguished by serum-gel diffusion tests.

In addition to the group-specific antigens of staphylococci, type-specific antigens have been used for serotyping *S aureus*. Staphylococci have usually been further differentiated by **bacteriophage (phage) typing,** that is, distinguishing strains by the pattern of susceptibility to lysis by specific bacterial viruses (bacteriophages).

Toxins

S aureus strains have been shown to release several toxins into the environment. No one strain produces all of the toxins. Most of these toxins are specifically identified by serum-gel precipitation. They also can be identified by a neutralization test, that is, by counteracting the toxic effects with specific antiserum.

Hemolysins.   Hemolysins cause red blood cells to lyse, and they act against cell membranes with some degree of specificity. α-Toxin is most active against rabbit erythrocytes. It is found in almost all human strains of staphylococci and in most animal strains. β-Hemolysin (a sphingomyelinase) is much more active against sheep erythrocytes than against human or rabbit erythrocytes. This toxin is found in 88% of *S aureus* animal strains, but in only 10% of human *S aureus* strains. Two other hemolysins, δ and ϵ, have been identified. These weaker hemolysins are found in human and animal strains.

Leukocidin.   Many strains of *S aureus* produce leukocidins, which are toxins that kill leukocytes and macrophages. The Panton–Valentine leukocidin (P–V) is the only toxin that attacks leukocytes but no other cells. Woodin has shown that P–V is composed of two separate proteins, both of which are required for a strong antileukocytic effect. The two components have been separated on carboxymethylcellulose and are recognized as nonidentical antigens in serum-gel precipitations when diffused against rabbit immune serum.

Enterotoxins.   Some *S aureus* strains release enterotoxins into foods. When the food is eaten, enterotoxins cause a form of food poisoning. Usually the food is contaminated with large numbers of staphylococci. Symptoms of staphylococcal food poisoning, which occur within a few hours after ingestion of food, are vomiting, and sometimes diarrhea. Most people recover after 24 hours. The several serologically distinct staphylococcal enterotoxins (A, B, C, C_1, C_2, D, and E) are resistant to the proteolytic enzymes of the digestive tract, although they are simple, single-chain, globular proteins. The known enterotoxins, A–E, can be identified by serologic tests such as serum-gel diffusion and radioimmunoassay. At present, only a few laboratories have the capability to identify these toxins routinely. When the toxin in a food cannot be identified, epidemiologic evidence of staphylococcal food poisoning usually shows large numbers of staphylococci in samples of the food eaten by most of the sick persons.

Scalded Skin Syndrome (Exfoliative or Epidermolytic) Toxins.   *S aureus* strains, particularly some of those of bacteriophage group II, cause a type of impetigo in children called the scalded skin syndrome, in which the outer layers of the epidermis peel off, revealing "scalded" skin. Recently, two of these toxins were demonstrated in bacteriophage group II strains, one plasmid coded and the other inherited chromosomally. The two toxins are distinct immunologically.

A case of toxic epidermal necrolysis due to *S aureus* has been described in an infant who developed toxic shock syndrome and died. It is important that this syndrome be distinguished from staphylococcal scalded skin syndrome, which usually is self-limiting.

Toxic Shock Syndrome Toxin.   In 1980, a new disease was observed that affects young women when they are menstruating. The symptoms of the disease resemble those reported by Todd et al. (1978), who isolated a new toxin from cultures of the staphylococci from skin infections. The new disease was called toxic shock syndrome (TSS). Shortly thereafter, reports of TSS in women were made in which there were severe symptoms and some deaths. Unlike earlier cases, these women did not have skin infections or any other overt sign of infection. Almost invariably, the women were menstruating at onset of TSS, and almost all had been using tampons. TSS is an important disease because of the severity of symptoms in affected individuals. Seventy-three deaths were reported to the CDC in 941 cases. The disease, however, is relatively rare when one considers the millions of women at risk and the small percentage who show symptoms of disease. A few cases of TSS have been reported in men and nonmenstruating women. More of these patients had overt staphylococcal infections.

Recent work, done independently in two different laboratories, has resulted in the isolation and identification of an exotoxin (exotoxin C) or an enterotoxin that was present in all strains of staphylococci from TSS. The toxin is pyrogenic in rabbits but does not lead to the rash seen in humans. The capacity to identify the toxin enhances the ability to study the epidemiology and toxicology of this new disease. At a recent symposium, researchers agreed to call the toxin TSS toxin 1 (TSST 1).

Extracellular Enzymes

In addition to known toxins of *S aureus*, enzymes are produced by staphylococci that diffuse from the cells and are active on extracellular substrates. Some of these have been considered to be pathogenicity factors primarily because they are often found in the more virulent strains of staphylococci.

Coagulase. Aside from its taxonomic importance in delineating potentially pathogenic strains, coagulase has been assigned a pathogenic role in infections by some investigators. This role in infections is debatable because of the frequency with which humans and animals carry coagulase-positive staphylococci without apparent harm. If coagulase is a factor in infections, it does not appear to be involved in the early stages of disease. Some authors have distinguished between two different molecular forms of coagulase, as the substrate of one is human plasma and that of the other, bovine plasma. Some strains produce both forms of coagulase simultaneously, and each is active on its substrate in the presence or absence of the other.

Fibrinolysin (Staphylokinase). About 95% of coagulase-positive staphylococci from humans produce fibrinolysin, an enzyme that dissolves fibrin clots. Only 9% of 115 animal strains made fibrinolysin. This difference is important in distinguishing animal and human strains. Fibrinolysin has not been shown to be an important pathogenicity factor. An enzyme similar to fibrinolysin from group A streptococci has been purified and used in human medicine to help debride wounds in which fibrin is part of the lesion.

DNAse (Nuclease). *S aureus* strains produce a thermostable, calcium-activated enzyme called deoxyribonuclease (DNAse). The enzyme hydrolyzes the 5' phosphodiester bond and thereby differs in action from pancreatic DNAse and some other phosphodiesterases. The ability to produce this DNAse is a property of virulent staphylococci, but the contribution of DNAse to virulence in microorganisms is not well understood.

Lipases. Staphylococci produce several lipid-hydrolyzing enzymes. Lipolysis probably depends on three enzymes—lipase, esterase, and phosphatidase. About 99.5% of human strains of *S aureus* are lipolytic as well as 30% of coagulase-negative strains. One of the tests used to demonstrate lipases involves the ability of some strains of staphylococci to break down egg yolk, usually in an agar medium. The relationship between egg yolk positivity and potential pathogenicity has been a subject of much controversy; some reports indicate that possession of egg yolk lysing factor delineates more pathogenic strains, and other reports make the opposite inference, that it is the egg-yolk–negative strains that are more capable of spreading and setting up systemic infections. These contrary opinions still exist, and the argument has not been resolved.

Hyaluronidase. Hyaluronidase hydrolyzes hyaluronic acid of human and animal tissues. Duran-Reynolds in 1929 described this activity as the spreading factor and showed that such enzymes could enhance the spread of viral or microbial infections in animals. Modern researchers use the term hyaluronic lyases for these factors. Abramson and Friedman in 1964 demonstrated the presence of four multiple molecular forms of this enzyme. The pathogenicity of the enzyme is not well known, but it does tend to be found in strains that are coagulase-positive and that produce pathogenicity factors such as fibrinolysin, DNAse, lipases, and protease.

Pathogenesis

The staphylococci are often viewed as microorganisms on their way toward a commensal, nonpathogenic relationship with humans. All coagulase-negative staphylococci, except perhaps *S saprophyticus,* are considered noninvasive and only occasionally pathogenic. *S epidermidis* is found on normal human skin, but coagulase-positive staphylococci, the *S aureus* strains, appear to be carried naturally in the anterior nares and in the axillary areas of the body, although they are occasionally isolated from skin. The use of antibiotics in hospitals has allowed populations of antibiotic-resistant bacteria to develop; these bacteria are often carried by hospital personnel and patients. Hospital epidemics caused by specific strains of *S aureus* in nurseries and in surgical and burn wards have been detected by phage typing and serotyping and by determining antibiotic resistance patterns (antibiograms).

Pigeons, dogs, and other animals carry coagulase-positive staphylococci peculiar to the host animal. Because these animals seldom become infected with staphylococci, the relationship appears to be commensal. Dairy animals suffer udder infections, a disease called mastitis. Streptococci of groups B and C were responsible for most cases of bovine mastitis before the introduction of penicillin for treatment of mastitis. Today coagulase-positive staphylococci resistant to penicillin account for most cases of bovine mastitis.

Coagulase-positive staphylococci are notorious for causing boils, furuncles, styes, and other skin infections in humans (Figure 28-1). They cause more serious infections in persons debilitated by chronic illness, traumatic injury, burns, or immunosuppressant therapy. These infections include staphylococcal pneumonia, deep abscesses (Figure 28-2), osteomyelitis, acute endocarditis, phlebitis, mastitis, and meningitis. *S aureus* has been isolated from infections of all organs of the body; however, the disease

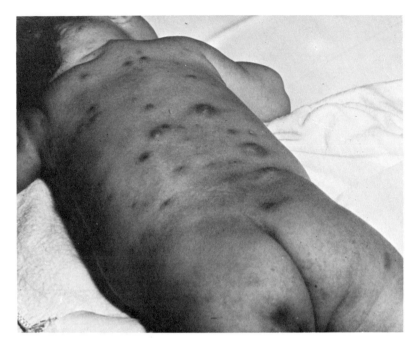

Figure 28-1 Widespread staphylococcal furunculosis in an infant. Photograph by Centers for Disease Control. From Shulman, J.A., Nahmias, A. J. In: *The staphylococci.* Cohen, J. O. (editor). New York: John Wiley & Sons, 1972, p. 461.

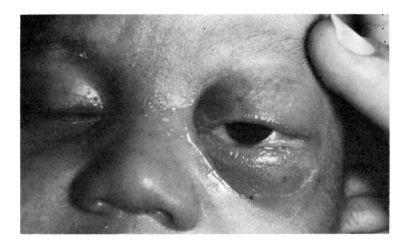

Figure 28-2 Child with thrombosis of the cavernous sinus (venous space in dura mater), a serious complication of staphylococcal skin infection. Photograph by Centers for Disease Control. From Shulman, J.A., Nahmias, A.J. In: *The staphylococci.* Cohen, J.O. (editor). New York: John Wiley & Sons, 1972, p. 462.

mechanisms are not well understood. Many factors found in *S aureus* strains, but not in coagulase-negative strains, are considered virulence factors, such as heat-resistant DNAse, coagulase, α-hemolysin, leukocidin, and protein A. Strains from serious infections have been shown to have more of these factors than strains from carriers, but little is known about the role these factors play in initiating infections or about the interactions that may allow staphylococci to invade the host. All strains capable of producing enterotoxin do not necessarily cause food poisoning. The strain must also be capable of growing well in a specific food, and it must produce significant amounts of toxin.

Thus, the staphylococci are enigmatic. They can be isolated from human flora, but their presence may not be significant; however, isolation from a deep abscess, pleural fluid, bone, spinal fluid, superficial abscess, or blood indicates serious infection. Large numbers of staphylococci should be isolated and identified except in blood specimens, in which any bacteria isolated are significant.

Host Defenses

S aureus appears to have been associated with humans for a long time. Both parasite and host have developed factors against each other and even against the defense factors. Human serum contains a heat-labile opsonin that facilitates the phagocytosis of staphylococci. Some *S aureus* strains can live inside the leukocyte and eventually kill it. Some strains produce a specific capsule, making them refractory to phagocytosis. Humans can make antibody to these capsules and thereby promote opsonization of these virulent strains for phagocytosis.

Several examples of interaction between *S aureus* and its hosts have been reported. Protein A of staphylococci can attract IgG antibodies to the staphylococcal surfaces without regard to the specificity of the antibodies. This attraction apparently does not lead to opsonization of, or injury to, the staphylococci. This reaction may also block complement-mediated bactericidal mechanisms by binding the Fc portion of IgG and masking complement receptor sites on the staphylococcus-specific immunoglobulin.

For each of the staphylococcal protein pathogenicity factors, such as toxins and enzymes, specific antibodies can be evoked in humans to inactivate the factor. Even before antibiotic therapy is introduced into the struggle, the host and bacterium engage in a complex tug-of-war.

Antibody defenses against *S aureus* can be arbitrarily divided into four categories: first, naturally occurring antibodies and antibodylike activities; second, group antibodies, found in adult humans, against a common staphylococcal antigen (teichoic acid or peptidoglycan); third, specific antibodies evoked in response to vaccines or infections, perhaps against only a few strains; and fourth, antibodies against staphylococcal toxins. The interplay between these factors and cell-mediated immunity leading to recovery from infections is not understood. Despite the development of significant immunologic responses, antibiotics and surgical drainage usually are necessary to cure abcesses, large boils, and wound infections.

Epidemiology

Although serious infections have been observed since the beginning of modern bacteriology, the epidemiology of *S aureus* infections has changed dramatically since penicillin and other antibiotics were introduced. Almost all *S aureus* strains were at first sensitive to penicillin. By the mid-1950s, however, hospital strains of staphylococci were invariably resistant to penicillin and often to several other antibiotics as well. By the 1970s, the majority of community-acquired staphylococcal infections were due to penicillinase-producing staphylococci. Penicillin resistance was shown to be caused by production by *S aureus* of a β-lactamase (penicillinase) enzyme that inactivates penicillin. Epidemics caused by certain virulent strains of *S aureus* occurred in hospital nurseries, burn wards, and surgical wards; severe illnesses and some deaths resulted. Antibiotic resistance, especially penicillin resistance, can be transferred genetically from one *S aureus* cell to another by a plasmid introduced into the new strain by a bacteriophage in a process called **transduction.**

The staphylococci are still responsible for serious infections, but hospital epidemics have decreased, probably because synthetic penicillins have been introduced that are resistant to penicillinase and are therefore effective against penicillin-resistant bacteria. New procedures to prevent cross-infection in hospital nurseries are credited with the decline of serious outbreaks in these areas. Strains of staphylococci resistant to methicillin have been reported in hospitals in Europe and the United States. The mechanism of resistance is not enzymatic. The strains have not been epidemic, but the possibility of serious hospital infections remains. Changes in staphyloccocal disease have been caused by the introduction of new antibiotics and by the placement of most debilitated patients in hospitals.

Diagnosis

Isolation and Identification

The presence of staphylococci in a lesion might first be suspected after examination of a direct Gram stain of a specimen. (Because of the small numbers of staphylococci present in blood, they are more likely to be detected by culture than by Gram stain.) With the Gram stain, only the presence of gram-positive cocci can be detected. Specific early identification can be achieved by direct fluorescent antibody staining with antistaphylo-coccal serum.

The organism usually is isolated by streaking material from a swab onto solid media such as blood agar, trypticase soy agar, or heart infusion agar. Specimens likely to be highly contaminated with other microorganisms can be plated on selective media, such as mannitol salt agar, which contains 7.5% sodium chloride, or potassium tellurite agar. A Gram stain should be made of the isolated organism and tests run for catalase and coagulase production. Other tests are useful in confirming a diagnosis of *S aureus*, specifically one that demonstrates heat-stable DNAse and another that tests lysostaphin sensitivity. *S aureus* is readily lysed by 50 μg/mL of lysostaphin (an extracellular peptidase made by a coagulase-negative staphylococcus); most coagulase-negative staphylococci are resistant to this level of lysostaphin, but higher levels lyse these staphylococci. Micrococci are completely refractory to lysostaphin. A test that demonstrates protein A on the cells or in the broth supernatants or both confirms identification of *S aureus*.

Isolation of coagulase-negative staphylococci from the skin is not considered medically significant because they are part of the normal microbial flora. However, these organisms, especially *S epidermidis,* have been implicated as the cause of subacute endocarditis. Therefore, isolation of coagulase-negative staphylococci from blood is important. A test should be set up to observe the ability of the isolate to ferment glucose anaerobically.

All staphylococci are capable of anaerobic growth with fermentation of glucose, but micrococci are not. Organisms belonging to the genus *Micrococcus* seldom have been shown to be the primary pathogen in specimens from infections. In a blood sample, the micrococci are considered chance contaminants unless they have been isolated repeatedly. All members of the genus *Micrococcus* are coagulase-negative and exhibit a guanine and cytosine mole percent of 57-75, whereas staphylococci exhibit one between 30 and 40. This is an important taxonomic difference, but only research laboratories have the capability to perform the test.

A single isolation of coagulase-negative cocci from a blood culture may result from chance contamination; repeated isolation usually indicates an infection. If several consecutive isolates have the same biotype, phage type, or antibiogram, or are identical by some other valid marker system, infection rather than chance contamination is probable.

Bacteriophage Typing and Serotyping

S aureus organisms are ubiquitous on humans and in their environment. In epidemics, a single virulent strain is often at fault; other staphylococci in the environment are not involved. Determination of the source of the epidemic and its extent requires knowledge of the type as well as the species. This knowledge is usually gained by bacteriophage typing, which is based on different lytic patterns obtained when different strains of bacteriophage are dropped on agar plates previously seeded with the test cultures of *S aureus*. After a period of incubation, usually at 30 C, the plate is examined for areas of lysis. In the international basic set of 24 bacteriophages, each bacteriophage has been assigned an Arabic numeral. Thus, if a culture is lysed by bacteriophages 80 and 81, its bacteriophage type is 80/81. The bacteriophages used have been carefully selected for this purpose, that is, for specificity coupled with the ability to lyse a reasonable percent of strains. Bacteriophage typing is usually done in a reference laboratory such as that of a state public health department.

Serotyping

Methods for serotyping staphylococci were developed before bacteriophage typing. At first, the staphylococci could not be divided into enough different types by the antisera available. Recent research has resulted in successful systems of typing to identify multiple factors. The validity of serotyping and bacteriophage typing has been demonstrated by comparative studies. Despite these successes, bacteriophage typing is usually preferred because it is more readily available, easier to do, and can be performed under international standards. The use of both methods for the same group of isolates results in better differentiation of the strains.

Control

Infections

Because staphylococci are part of the normal flora, with *S aureus* frequently found in the nose and *S epidermidis* found normally on the skin, they cannot be eliminated from humans. It is probable that in past generations most staphylococcal infections were superficial or limited to the skin. More serious infections probably occurred in people debilitated by burns, injury, or by failure of their immune system. These people were primarily infected by their own staphylococci. Today, however, many staphylococcal infections are produced by hospital strains of staphylococci, which have caused epidemics in nurseries, burn wards, and surgical wards.

The circumstances that resulted in the development of reservoirs of antibiotic-resistant *S aureus* in hospitals have been complex; often, the procedures to limit spread of hospital staphylococci and to combat epidemics also have been complex. When development of new antibiotics did not offer security against epidemics in the nursery, innovative measures were taken to prevent colonization with epidemic strains. One such measure was to implant penicillin-sensitive *S aureus,* strain 502A, in the nose and on the umbilical cord of each newborn. Though this technique was successful, other procedures for preventing cross-infections between babies and the introduction of synthetic penicillins were primarily responsible for reducing the threat of epidemics in nurseries. Isolation equipment, designed like the isolators used in germ-free animal research, has limited opportunities for staphylococci and other pathogens to contaminate burn patients.

Food poisoning

Enterotoxin production by *S aureus* remains the most common cause of food poisoning. Recent research has led to development of better diagnostic procedures for identifying the staphylococcal enterotoxins. Today, when an outbreak occurs because a commercially produced food is contaminated by a food handler, it is possible to determine which lots of food contain enterotoxin. In addition, recently developed procedures for preparing food for large groups of people reduce opportunities for bacterial contamination.

Treatment

Patients with staphylococcal infections are usually treated with antibiotics and by surgical drainage. In emergencies, when antibiotic sensitivity information is not yet available, a synthetic penicillin that is resistant to penicillinase (methicillin, nafcillin, or oxacillin) is chosen. When penicillin allergy precludes the use of penicillin derivatives, appropriate second-line antibiotics are cephalosporins, vancomycin, or clindamycin. When time permits, therapy of patients with staphylococcal infections should be based on the results of antibiotic sensitivity testing. Some *S aureus* strains from the community are penicillin-sensitive, in which case maintaining an adequate level of penicillin in the patient for 7 days or more is the treatment of choice.

Future Trends

The future course of a disease is unpredictable when the causative organisms are so intimately associated with humans and their environment. In other animals, a true commensal relationship frequently exists between *S aureus* and the host. Factors that enhance immunity in chronically ill and immune-deficient persons reinforce the possibility of commensal relationship, but the continued introduction of new antibiotics tends to prolong the existing situation, in which antibiotic-resistant staphylococci predominate in hospitals. But whether the staphylococci exist as commensals, as serious pathogens, or both, they no doubt will be intimately associated with humankind.

References

Chesney, P.J., et al.: Exfoliative dermatitis in an infant. Association with enterotoxin F-producing staphylococci. *Am J Dis Child* 1983; 137:899–901.

Christensen, P., et al.: New method for the serological grouping of streptococci with specific antibodies adsorbed to protein A-containing staphylococci. *Infect Immunol* 1973; 7: 881–885.

Cohen, J.O., (editor): *The staphylococci.* New York: John Wiley and Sons, 1972.

Cohen, J.O.: Serological typing of staphylococci for epidemiological studies. In: *Recent advances in staphylococcal research.* Yotis WW (editor), *Ann NY Acad Sci* 1974; 236: 485–494.

Cohen, J.O., Smith, P.B.: Serological typing of *Staphylococcus aureus.* II. Typing by slide agglutination and comparison with phage typing. *J Bacteriol* 1964; 88:1364–1371.

Kloos, W.E.: Natural populations of the genus *Staphylococcus. Ann Rev Microbiol* 1980; 34: 559–592.

Kloos, W.E., Schleifer, K.H.: Simplified scheme for routine identification of human *Staphylococcus* species. *J Clin Microbiol* 1975; 1: 82–88.

Oeding, P., Digranes, A.: Classification of coagulase-negative staphylococci in the diagnostic laboratory. *Acta Pathol Microbiol Scand* 1977; B 85: 136–142.

Shinefield, H.R., et al.: Bacterial interference between strains of *S aureus.* In: *Recent advances in staphylococcal research.* Yotis WW (editor). *Ann NY Acad Sci* 1974; 236: 444–455.

Todd, J., et al.: Toxic-shock syndrome associated with phage-group-1 staphylococci. *Lancet* 1978; 2:1116–1118.

Woodin, A.M.: Assay of the two components of staphylococcal leukocidin and their antibodies. *J Pathol Bacteriol* 1961; 81:63–68.

29 *Streptococcus*

M. Jevitz Patterson, MD, PhD

General Concepts

The genus *Streptococcus* consists of a heterogeneous group of gram-positive bacteria with broad significance in medicine and industry. Member organisms are important ecologically as part of the normal microbial flora of animals or humans; they can also cause diseases that range from subacute to acute or even chronic. Among the significant human diseases attributable to streptococci are scarlet fever, rheumatic heart disease, glomerulonephritis, and pneumococcal pneumonia. Streptococci are essential in industrial and dairy processes and as indicators of pollution.

Nomenclature for streptococci, especially in medical use, has been based largely on serogroup identification of cell wall components rather than on species names. For several decades, interest has focused on two major species that cause severe infections: *S pyogenes* (group A streptococci) and *Diplococcus pneumoniae* (pneumococci). The similarity of pneumococci to the other streptococci has long been recognized; therefore, a recent classification resulted in a change in nomenclature from *Diplococcus pneumoniae* to *Streptococcus pneumoniae*.

In recent years, increasing attention has been given to other streptococcal species, partly because of innovations in serogrouping methods. Advances in understanding the significance of these other species in pathogenesis and epidemiology have been made. A variety of cell-associated and extracellular products are produced by streptococci, but no clear scheme of pathogenesis has been defined. Some of the other medically important streptococci are *S agalactiae* (group B), etiologic agents of neonatal disease; *S faecalis* (group D), a major cause of endocarditis; and *S mutans* and *S sanguis* (viridans group), which are involved in dental caries. These and other streptococci of medical importance are listed in Table 29-1 by serogroup designation, normal ecologic niche, and associated disease.

In humans, diseases associated with the streptococci occur chiefly in the respiratory tract, bloodstream, or as skin infections. Group A streptococci are the most commonly isolated bacteria linked to human disease. Acute group A streptococcal disease occurs principally as respiratory infection (pharyngitis or tonsillitis) or skin infection (pyoderma). Also medically significant are the late immunologic sequelae of group A infections (rheumatic fever following respiratory infection and glomerulonephritis following respiratory or skin infection), which are becoming more prevalent in tropical countries. Much effort is being directed toward clarifying the risk and mechanisms of these sequelae and identifying rheumatogenic and nephritogenic strains. Of major biologic importance is a renewed interest in safe and effective streptococcal vaccines.

Table 29-1   Medically Important Streptococci

Type Species	Lancefield Serogroup	Normal Habitat	Significant Human Disease
S pyogenes	A	Humans	Acute pharyngitis and others
S agalactiae	B	Cattle, humans	Neonatal meningitis and sepsis and other infections in adults
S equisimilis	C	Wide human and animal distribution	Endocarditis, bacteremia, pneumonia, meningitis, mild upper respiratory infection
S faecalis (enterococcus) *S bovis* (nonenterococcus)	D	Human and animal intestinal tracts, dairy products	Urinary tract infection, endocarditis, bacteremia
S milleri	F*	Humans	Subcutaneous or organ abscesses, endocarditis
S anginosus	G	Humans, dogs	Endocarditis, mild upper respiratory infection
S sanguis	H	Humans	Endocarditis, caries
S salivarius	K	Humans	Endocarditis, caries
None	O	Humans	Endocarditis
S suis	R	Swine	Meningitis
"Viridans"†: *S mitis, S mutans*	None identified	Humans	Caries, endocarditis
Anaerobic or microaerophilic	None identified	Wide human and animal distribution	Brain and pulmonary abscesses, gynecologic infections
S pneumoniae	None identified	Humans	Lobar pneumonia and others

*Strains of *S milleri* may possess antigens of group A, C, F, G or no identifiable Lancefield group antigen.
†Other viridans streptococci (*S sanguis, S salivarius, S milleri, S bovis, S faecalis*) have identified group antigen(s).

Distinctive Properties

Both *S pyogenes* and *S pneumoniae* are gram-positive cocci, nonmotile, and nonsporulating; they usually require complex culture media. *S pyogenes* characteristically are round-to-ovoid, 0.6–1.0 μm cocci. They divide in one plane and thus occur in pairs or, especially in liquid media or from clinical material, in chains of varying lengths. *S pneumoniae* appear as 0.5–1.25 μm diplococci, typically described as lancet-shaped but sometimes difficult to distinguish morphologically from other streptococci. Streptococcal cultures older than logarithmic phase may lose their gram-positive staining characteristics.

All streptococci lack the enzyme catalase, unlike the staphylococci described in Chapter 28. Most are facultative anaerobes, but some are obligate anaerobes. Streptococci often have a mucoid or smooth colonial morphology, with *S pneumoniae* colonies exhibiting a central depression caused by rapid partial autolysis. As *S pneumoniae* colonies age, viability is lost during fermentative growth in the absence of catalase and peroxidase because of the accumulation of peroxide. Some group B and D streptococci produce pigment. Recently, streptococcal nutritional variants, which form satellite thiol- or pyridoxal-dependent colonies adjacent to staphylococcal colonies, have been reported. These variants do not grow on routine subculture but have gained increasing attention as important agents of endocarditis.

The type of hemolytic reaction displayed on blood agar has long been used to classify the streptococci. β-Hemolysis is associated with complete lysis of red cells surrounding the colony, whereas α-hemolysis is a partial or greening hemolysis associated with reduction of red cell hemoglobin. Nonhemolytic colonies have been termed γ-hemolytic. Hemolysis is affected by species and age of red cells, as well as by other properties of the base medium. Use of hemolytic reaction in classification is not completely satisfactory. Some group A streptococci appear nonhemolytic; group B can manifest α-, β-, or even γ-hemolysis; most *S pneumoniae* are α-hemolytic but can produce β-hemolysis during anaerobic incubation. The viridans group, although linked by the property of α-hemolysis, is actually an extremely diverse group of organisms, whose taxonomy is particularly confused (Table 29-1).

Structural Antigens

The cell wall structure of group A streptococci is among the most studied of any bacteria. The cell wall is composed of repeating units of N-acetylglucosamine and N-acetylmuramic acid, the standard peptidoglycan. For decades definitive identification of streptococci has rested on serologic reactivity of cell wall polysaccharide antigen, originally delineated by Rebecca Lancefield. Eighteen group-specific antigens were established. The group A polysaccharide is a polymer of N-acetylglucosamine and rhamnose. Some group antigens are shared by more than one species; no Lancefield group antigen has been identified for *S pneumoniae* or for some other α- or γ-streptococci. With advances in serologic methods, other streptococci have been shown to possess several established group antigens.

The cell wall consists, in addition, of several structural proteins (Table 29-2). In group A streptococci, the R and T proteins may serve as epidemiologic markers, but the

Table 29-2   Structural and Metabolic Growth Products of Group A Streptococci

Cell-associated	*Extracellular*
Cytoplasmic membrane	Streptolysins (O and S)
Cell wall	
Peptidoglycan	NADase
N-acetylglucosamine	
N-acetylmuramic acid	Hyaluronidase
Alanine, glutamic acid	
Lysine, glycine	Streptokinases (A and B)
Group carbohydrate	
N-acetylglucosamine	Streptodornases (A, B, C, D)
Rhamnose	
Protein	
Fimbriae (M protein and	
lipoteichoic acid)	Erythrogenic toxins
Other (R and T proteins)	(A, B, C)
Capsule	
Hyaluronic acid	

M proteins are clearly virulence factors associated with resistance to phagocytosis. More than 50 types of *S pyogenes* M proteins have been identified, based on antigenic specificity. Both the M proteins and lipoteichoic acid are external to the cell wall on fimbriae and particularly the lipoteichoic acid appears to mediate bacterial attachment to host epithelial cells. M protein, N-acetylglucosamine of the peptidoglycan, and group-specific carbohydrate portions of the cell wall have antigenic moieties similar in size and charge to those of mammalian muscle and connective tissue.

The capsule of *S pyogenes* is composed of hyaluronic acid, which is chemically similar to that of host connective tissue and is therefore nonantigenic. In contrast, the antigenically reactive and chemically distinct capsular polysaccharide of *S pneumoniae* allows the single species to be separated into more than 80 serotypes. The antiphagocytic *S pneumoniae* capsule is the sole virulence factor of these organisms; type 3 *S pneumoniae*, which produces copious quantities of capsular material, are the most virulent. Unencapsulated *S pneumoniae* are avirulent.

Finally, the cytoplasmic membrane of *S pyogenes* has antigens similar to those of human cardiac, skeletal, and smooth muscle, heart valve fibroblasts, and neuronal tissues.

Extracellular Growth Products

The importance of the interaction of streptococcal products with mammalian blood and tissue components is receiving increasing recognition. The soluble extracellular growth products or toxins of the streptococci, especially *S pyogenes* (see Table 29-2), have been studied intensely. Streptolysin S is an oxygen-stable cytolysin; streptolysin O is a reversibly oxygen-labile cytolysin. Both, in addition to NADase, are leukotoxic. Hyaluronidase (spreading factor) can digest host connective tissue hyaluronic acid as well as the organism's own capsule. Streptokinases participate in fibrin lysis. Streptodornases A-D possess deoxyribonuclease activity; B and D possess, in addition, ribonuclease activity. When *S pyogenes* is lysogenized by certain bacteriophages, the erythrogenic toxin is produced that is associated with damage to small blood vessels and the rash in scarlet fever. Nonlysogenized strains are atoxic.

This large repertoire of products may be important in the pathogenesis of *S pyogenes* by enhancing virulence; however, antibodies to these products appear not to protect the host even though they have diagnostic importance.

Virulence factors in the other streptococcal species are less well identified. In group B, carbohydrate surface antigens associated with antiphagocytosis have been identified, as well as neuraminidase, which may also play a role in pathogenesis.

Pathogenesis

Streptococcus pyogenes and *Streptococcus pneumoniae*

Streptococci vary widely in pathogenic potential. Despite the remarkable array of cell-associated and extracellular products previously described (see Table 29-2), no clear scheme of pathogenesis has been defined. *S pneumoniae* and, to a lesser extent, *S pyogenes* are part of the normal human nasopharyngeal flora. Their numbers are usually limited by competition from the nasopharyngeal microbial ecosystem and by nonspecific host defense mechanisms, but failure of these mechanisms can result in disease. More commonly, disease can result from acquisition of a new strain, following alteration of the normal flora. *S pyogenes* causes inflammatory purulent lesions with resulting tissue damage directly at the portal of entry, often the upper respiratory tract or the skin. Some strains of streptococci show a predilection for the respiratory tract; others, for the skin. Generally, streptococcal isolates from the pharynx and respiratory tract do not cause skin infections.

Invasion of other portions of the upper or lower respiratory tracts results in infections of the middle ear (otitis media), sinuses (sinusitis), or lungs (pneumonia). In addition, meningitis can occur by direct extension of infection from the middle ear or sinuses to the meninges or by way of bloodstream invasion from a pulmonary focus. Bacteremia can also result in infection in bones (osteomyelitis) or joints (arthritis).

S pyogenes (a group A streptococcus) is the leading cause of bacterial pharyngitis and tonsillitis. Indeed, only group A streptococci are sought routinely in pharyngitis, although groups B, C, and G are sometimes identified. *S pyogenes* infections can also result in sinusitis, otitis, mastoiditis, pneumonia, arthritis, or bone infections, and, more infrequently, meningitis or endocarditis. *S pyogenes* infections of the skin can be superficial (impetigo) or deep (cellulitis). Although scalet fever was formerly a severe complication of streptococcal infection, it is now little more than streptococcal pharyngitis accompanied by rash. Similarly, erysipelas, a form of cellulitis accompanied by fever and systemic toxicity, is less common today (Figure 29-1).

The capsule of *S pneumoniae* renders it resistant to phagocytosis. Evading this important host defense mechanism, *S pneumoniae* can survive, multiply, and spread to

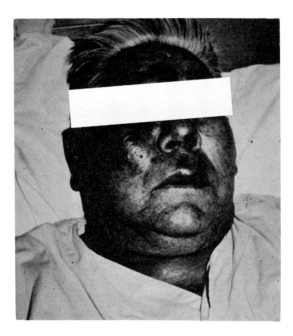

Figure 29-1 Patient with streptococcal erysipelas. Photograph courtesy of C. G. Ray, MD, University of Arizona.

various organs. *S pneumoniae* is the leading cause of bacterial pneumonia in adults. This organism is also the most common cause of sinusitis, acute bacterial otitis media, and conjunctivitis beyond early childhood. Dissemination from the respiratory focus results in serious disease: outpatient bacteremia in children, meningitis, occasionally acute septic arthritis and bone infections in patients with sickle cell disease and, more rarely, peritonitis or endocarditis.

The postinfection sequelae of *S pyogenes* (but not *S pneumoniae*) are acute rheumatic fever and acute glomerulonephritis, which occur 1–3 weeks after the acute illness. Whether all *S pyogenes* strains are rheumatogenic is still controversial, but clearly not all are nephritogenic; however, these differences in pathogenic potential are not yet understood.

Acute rheumatic fever follows only pharyngeal infections, but acute glomerulonephritis follows infections of the pharynx or the skin. Although there is no adequate explanation for the precise pathogenesis of acute rheumatic fever or for its failure to occur after streptococcal pyoderma, an abnormal or enhanced immune response seems essential. Also persistence of the organism, due perhaps in part to greater avidity of organism adherence to host pharyngeal cells, is associated with increased likelihood of the rheumatic fever sequel. Acute glomerulonephritis results from deposition of antigen-antibody-complement complexes on the basement membrane of kidney glomeruli. The antigen may originate in streptococci or in host tissue with antigenic determinants similar to those of the streptococci. In the United States, incidence of acute rheumatic fever has decreased dramatically. Less than 1% of sporadic streptococcal pharyngitis infections result in acute rheumatic fever; however, recurrences are common, and life-long antibiotic prophylaxis is recommended following a single case. Incidence of acute glomerulonephritis in the Unites States is more variable perhaps due to cycling of nephritogenic strains, but also appears to be decreasing; recurrences are uncommon and prophylaxis following an initial attack is unnecessary. Reversal of the decreasing trends of these sequelae remains possible.

Other Streptococcal Species

Streptococcal groups B, C, and G initially were recognized as animal pathogens (see Table 29-1) and as part of the normal human flora. Recently, the pathogenic potential for humans of some of these non–group-A streptococci has been clarified. Group B streptococci, a major cause of bovine mastitis, are a leading cause of neonatal septicemia and meningitis and, thus, account for significant mortality. Recently, they also have been associated with pneumonia in elderly patients. Group B streptococci are part of the normal oral and vaginal flora and have also been isolated from adult urogenital infections, meningitis, bacteremia, and endocarditis. They have not been implicated in acute rheumatic fever or acute glomerulonephritis. Streptococci of groups C and G are associated with mild as well as severe human disease. Group D streptococci are important etiologic agents in urinary tract infections as well as in cases of disseminated infection, bacteremia, and endocarditis. In particular, *Streptococcus bovis* bacteremia has been recognized more often in cases of bowel disease. Group F streptococci are associated with abscess formation and purulent disease. Group R streptococci, well-documented causes of meningitis and septicemia in pigs, also pose a serious health hazard to workers in the pork industry.

The diverse group of organisms classified as viridans streptococci and other nongroupable streptococci of the oral cavity includes important etiologic agents of subacute bacterial endocarditis. Dental manipulation and dental disease are the most common predisposing factors in subacute bacterial endocarditis. *S mutans* and *S sanguis* are responsible for the formation of dental plaque, the dense adhesive microbial mass that colonizes teeth and is linked to caries and other human oral disease (see Chapter 116). *S mutans* is the most cariogenic of the two species, and its virulence is directly related to its ability to synthesize glucan from fermentable carbohydrates as well as to modify glucan in promoting increased adhesiveness.

Like their aerobic counterparts, anaerobic streptococci are part of the normal flora, particularly of the mouth and intestinal tract; they are also part of the normal flora of the upper respiratory and genital tracts and the skin. These anaerobic organisms are linked to a wide variety of serious infections of the female genital tract as well as brain, pulmonary, and abdominal abscesses.

Host Defenses

The streptococci are part of the endogenous microbial flora of the nasopharynx; disease results from circumvention of normal specific or nonspecific host defense mechanisms. More commonly, both *S pyogenes* and *S pneumoniae* may be exogenous secondary invaders following viral disease or disturbances in the normal bacterial flora.

In the normal host, nonspecific defense mechanisms prevent organisms from penetrating beyond the superficial epithelium of the upper respiratory tract. These mechanisms include mucociliary movement and the cough, sneeze, and epiglottal reflexes. The host phagocytic system is a second line of defense against pathogens. Opsonization of organisms can be facilitated by activation of the classical or alternate complement pathways or by specific immunoglobulin binding.

The capsules of both *S pyogenes* and *S pneumoniae* allow escape from effective opsonization. The hyaluronic acid outer surface of *S pyogenes* is only weakly antigenic; however, protective immunity results from the development of type-specific antibody to the M protein of the fimbriae, which protrude from the cell wall through the capsular structure. This antibody, which follows respiratory and skin infections, is persistent. Presumably, IgA in the respiratory secretions and serum IgG are the important protective antibody classes. *S pyogenes* is rapidly killed following opsonization enhanced by specific antibody. Rapid effective antibiotic treatment of streptococcal infections may preclude development of this persistent antibody. Evidence has shown that antibody to the erythrogenic toxin involved in scarlet fever is also long lasting. This remains the basis of the Dick test, an in vivo skin test rarely used today, which measures host antitoxin.

The capsular polysaccharides of *S pneumoniae* are highly antigenic and type-specific. Type-specific anticapsular antibodies result in effective opsonization and host recovery. In untreated *S pneumoniae* infections, recovery clearly is due to opsonizing antibody. Even in the face of adequate and appropriate antibiotic therapy, the contribution of opsonizing antibody to recovery from pneumococcal disease is probably significant. The normal host is somewhat resistant to *S pneumoniae* disease, but compromised hosts of several types are highly susceptible to serious infections: alcoholics, the semicomatose, the very young and the very old, those who have undergone splenectomy, and patients with underlying diseases (specifically sickle cell anemia, leukopenia, multiple myeloma, and diabetes).

Cross-reactive antigens, especially of *S pyogenes* and various mammalian tissues, help explain the autoimmune mechanisms following some infections. The level of humoral response to infection with *S pyogenes* is more elevated in patients with rheumatic fever than in patients with uncomplicated pharyngitis.

Neonatal susceptibility to group B streptococci may result from impaired neonatal phagocytic function, humoral immunity, or cell-mediated immunity, or from lack of passively acquired maternal antibody. Complete polymorphonuclear neutrophil function encompasses mobility, chemotaxis, ingestion, and the subsequent metabolic processes involved in bactericidal activity (generation of a group of toxic oxygen products including hydrogen peroxide, hydroxyl radicals, superoxide, or singlet oxygen).

Recent evidence from the rhesus monkey animal model in dental research shows that IgG may be a more important antibody class than IgA or IgM in protection against caries. This may be ascribed partly to IgG being the most efficient antibody class to enhance phagocytosis of *S mutans*. Cell-mediated immunity appears also to be part of the protective host response against caries.

Epidemiology

The streptococci are widely distributed in nature and frequently are part of normal flora in humans (see Table 29-1). Approximately 5%-15% of humans carry *S pyogenes* or *S agalactiae* in the nasopharynx. *S pneumoniae* infects humans exclusively, and no reservoir is found in nature. The carrier rate of *S pneumoniae* in the normal human nasopharynx is 20%–40%.

All ages, races, and sexes are susceptible to streptococcal disease. *S pneumoniae* is a particularly labile organism, sensitive to heat, cold, and drying. Acquisition requires close person-to-person contact, factors that lower host resistance, as described in the preceding section, or the introduction of more virulent strains. In the United States, pneumococcal disease is most prevalent during winter, coinciding with increased rates of acquisition but not necessarily of carriage. Respiratory disease attributed to *S pyogenes* shows a peak at about 6 years of age, a second rise at 13 years of age, and is most common during the late winter and early spring in temperate climates. Skin infections are most common among preschool-age children and prevalent in late summer and early fall in temperate climates, when hot, humid weather prevails, or at all times in tropical climates. *S pyogenes* is spread by respiratory droplets or by contact with fomites used by the index individual, either patient or carrier. Skin infections often follow minor skin irritation, such as insect bites. Occasional outbreaks traced to rectal carriers, as well as food-borne and vector-borne outbreaks of streptococcal disease, have been reported.

The world prevalence of the serious late sequelae of *S pyogenes* infections, acute rheumatic fever and acute glomerular nephritis, has shifted from temperate to tropic climates. These diseases particularly affect persons with a low standard of living and limited access to medical care. Whether ethnic or racially determined factors affect this shift is not known.

Other streptococcal groups show striking epidemiologic features. An increasing prevalence of non–group-A as compared to group A streptococci in throats has been reported. Studies of the vaginal flora among women of child-bearing age show a *S agalactiae* carrier rate of 2%–30%. Transmission of the organisms to neonates of vaginally infected mothers ranges from 1%–25%, but the incidence of neonates with disease in contrast to colonized, healthy neonates is low. *S suis* has been linked to meningitis among meat handlers. Isolation of *S milleri* or *S bovis* from the bloodstream should raise suspicion of visceral abscess formation and bowel disease (including carcinoma), respectively.

Diagnosis

Diagnosis of streptococcal pharyngitis or tonsillitis on clinical grounds alone usually is not possible. Accurate differentiation from viral pharyngitis is difficult even for the experienced clinician, and therefore the use of bacteriologic methods is essential. When documented streptococcal pharyngitis is accompanied by an erythematous punctiform rash, the diagnosis of scarlet fever can be made. Rheumatic fever is a late sequel to pharyngitis and is marked by fever, polyarthritis, and carditis. The other late sequel, acute glomerulonephritis, is preceded by pharyngitis or pyoderma and is characterized by fever, blood in the urine (hematuria), and edema, and it is sometimes accompanied by hypertension and elevated blood urea nitrogen (azotemia). Pneumococcal pneumonia is a life-threatening disease, often characterized by edema and rapid lobar consolidation.

S pyogenes is usually isolated from throat cultures; *S pneumoniae* is usually isolated from sputum or blood. Precise streptococcal identification is based on the Gram stain and on biochemical properties as well as serologic characteristics when group antigens are present. Table 29-3 shows biochemical tests that provide sensitive group-specific

Table 29-3   Characteristics for the Presumptive Identification of Streptococci of Human Clinical Importance

Procedure	A	B	D (entero-coccus)	D (nonentero-coccus)	Non A, B, D	S pneumoniae	"Viridans"
Hemolysis*	β	β, α, γ	α, β, γ	α, γ, β	β, α, γ	α	α
Bacitracin sensitivity	+	−(+)†	−	−	−(+)	±	−
Growth at 45 C	−	−	+	+	−	−	+
Optochin sensitivity	−(+)	−(+)	−	−	−(+)	+	−
Hydrolysis of sodium hippurate	−	+	−(+)	−	−	−	−(+)
Tolerance to 6.5% NaCl	−	±	+	−	−	−	−
Hydrolysis of esculin in presence of 40% bile	−	−	+	+	−	−	−(+)

*In general order of frequency.
†Signs in parentheses indicate occasional.

Table 29-4   Methods for Serogrouping Streptococci

Nature of Streptococcal Antigen	Techniques
Whole cells	Fluorescent antibody Direct bacterial agglutination Coagglutination with staphylococcal protein A Carrier agglutination (antibody-coated latex particles) Quellung reaction (for S pneumoniae)
Soluble extract	Precipitation (classical capillary or counterimmunoelectrophoresis) Coagglutination with staphylococcal protein A Carrier agglutination (antibody-coated latex particles)

characteristics permitting presumptive identification of gram-positive catalase-negative cocci.

Hemolysis should not be used as a stringent identification criterion. Bacitracin susceptibility is a widely used screening method for presumptive identification of *S pyogenes*; however, some *S pyogenes* are resistant to bacitracin (up to 10%) and some group C and G streptococci (about 3%–5%) are susceptible to bacitracin. *S pneumoniae* can be separated from other α-hemolytic streptococci on the basis of sensitivity to surfactants such as bile or optochin (ethylhydrocupreine hydrochloride). These agents activate autolytic enzymes in the organisms that hydrolyze peptidoglycan.

In many instances, presumptive identification is not carried further. Serologic grouping has not been performed as often as it might be because of the lack of available methods and the practical constraints of time and cost; however only serologic methods, as listed in Table 29-4, provide definitive identification of the streptococci. The Lancefield capillary precipitation test is the classical serologic method. *S pneumoniae*, lacking a demonstrable group antigen by the Lancefield test, is conventionally identified by the quellung or capsular swelling test that employs type-specific anticapsular antibody.

New methods for serogrouping that show sensitivity and specificity now are being explored. Organisms from throat swabs, incubated for only a few hours in broth, can be examined for the presence of *S pyogenes* using the direct fluorescent antibody technique. *S pneumoniae* can be identified rapidly by counterimmunoelectrophoresis (see Chapter 25), a modification of the gel precipitin method. The coagglutination test, described in Chapter 28, is a more sensitive modification of the conventional direct bacterial agglutination test. The Fc portion of group-specific antibody binds to the protein A of dead staphylococci, leaving the Fab portion free to react with specific streptococcal antigen. The attachment of antibody to other carrier particles in suspension (for example, latex) also is being explored. The ability to use whole streptococcal cells in recently developed methods circumvents the difficulties involved with extraction of components that retain appropriate antigenic reactivity. With increased use of these newer serogrouping methods, it should become more practical to identify not only β-hemolytic isolates from the blood or normally sterile sites, but also α- and nonhemolytic strains. Such information will expand understanding of the importance of non-group-A streptococci.

Antibodies to some of the extracellular growth factors of the streptococci are not protective but can be used in diagnosis. The antistreptolysin O (ASO) and anti-NADase titers are more commonly elevated after pharyngeal infections than after skin infections. In contrast, antihyaluronidase is elevated after skin infections; anti-DNase B rises after both pharyngeal and skin infections. Titers observed during late sequelae, acute rheumatic fever and acute glomerulonephritis, reflect the site of primary infection. Although it is not as well known as the ASO test, the anti-DNase B test appears superior because high titered antibody is detected following skin and pharyngeal infections and during the late sequelae.

Although not used in diagnosis, bacteriocin production and phage typing of streptococci are employed in research and epidemiologic studies.

Control

Penicillin remains the drug of choice for *S pyogenes* and *S pneumoniae* infections. Unlike the other streptococci, group D enterococci are resistant to penicillins, including penicillinase-resistant penicillins such as methicillin, nafcillin, dicloxacillin, and oxacillin and are becoming increasingly resistant to many other antibiotics. Group B streptococci are often resistant to tetracycline and kanamycin but remain sensitive to the clinically achievable blood levels of penicillin, even though they have penicillin minimal inhibitory concentrations (MIC) considerably higher than *S pyogenes*. Although duration of penicillin therapy varies with degree of invasiveness, streptococcal pharyngitis is generally adequately treated with 10 days of antibiotic therapy, and pneumococcal pneumonia with 7–14 days. If penicillin allergy occurs, an alternative drug for treating pharyngitis is erythromycin, although sporadic erythromycin and tetracycline resistance has been reported recently. Life-long prophylaxis against recurrences of rheumatic fever is achieved with low-dose penicillin or erythromycin. Sulfonamides are no longer used because *S pyogenes* is often resistant to sulfa drugs. Although streptococcal pharyngitis is usually a benign self-limited disease, therapy is important to prevent rheumatic fever and probably glomerulonephritis.

Treating the asymptomatic pharyngeal carrier of *S pyogenes* remains controversial, although recent evidence suggests that there may be no risk to the carrier or to others and that the carrier state is frequently difficult to eradicate despite exquisite sensitivity of the organism to penicillin in vitro. Similar failure of antibiotic therapy to eradicate nasopharyngeal carriage or to prevent reinfection with *S pneumoniae* also occurs. Treating pregnant women who are carriers of group B streptococci or their colonized neonates in an effort to avoid risk of serious neonatal disease remains controversial for several reasons: the high carrier rate documented in several parts of the country, the associated high risk of penicillin hypersensitivity, the potential increase in infections with penicillin-resistant organisms, the difficulty in effecting eradication, and the low risk of neonatal disease.

Clearly, penicillin has reduced the severe morbidity and mortality associated with *S pneumoniae*. Serious infections with group D enterococci often require the synergistic combination of penicillin and an aminoglycoside, although complicated urinary tract infection with enterococci can be treated with ampicillin alone.

Antibiotic resistance among the streptococci is an increasing problem. Genetic studies show that in vitro resistance can be plasmid-mediated. Mechanisms involved in the in vivo genetic exchange are not clearly defined. Evidence is accumulating that oral streptococci may be the important donors of resistance plasmids. The first penicillin-resistant *S pneumoniae* were reported in 1967 in Australia and in 1974 in North America. In New Guinea, where the first penicillin-resistant strains were reported in 1971, one-third of *S pneumoniae* isolates from patients with severe pneumococcal disease were resistant by 1978. Some strains resistant to erythromycin or tetracycline also have been reported, as well as some multiply resistant strains. In South Africa, outbreaks of infection with strains of *S pneumoniae* resistant to β lactam antibiotics (penicillin and cephalosporins) as well as tetracycline, chloramphenicol, erythromycin, streptomycin, clindamycin, sulfonamides, and rifampin have been reported. Although antibiotic resistance among *S pneumoniae* is presently infrequent in the United States, it should be monitored, especially in serious pneumococcal disease, or in settings with particularly susceptible patients, such as debilitated young children or immunocompromised individuals. No penicillin-resistant *S pyogenes* have been described, although rare erythromycin-resistant strains, reported as early as 1959 and increasing in prevalence, have recently been reported to be a significant problem in Japan.

With the introduction of antibiotics, previously successful pneumococcal vaccines fell into disuse; however, although antibiotics have reduced the serious consequences of *S pneumonniae* infections, the disease incidence remains unchanged and attention has recently been redirected to vaccines for *S pneumoniae* as well as for other streptococci. Pneumococcal vaccines (containing the pneumococcal polysaccharides of the most prevalent serotypes) have been licensed in several countries, including the United States. Initial use shows them to be useful and safe and ongoing efficacy studies are in progress. In 1983, the United States Food and Drug Administration licensed a vaccine containing 23 serotypes representing coverage against 87% of the pneumococcal isolates submitted to the CDC. The population target of pneumococcal vaccines includes those at high risk for serious pneumococcal disease: elderly individuals and patients with sickle cell anemia, asplenia, nephrotic syndrome, or chronic cardiopulmonary disease. Vaccines for the other streptococci remain experimental.

Vaccine production for the streptococci presents several formidable problems. For both *S pyogenes* and *S pneumoniae,* a large number of serotypes must be included in effective vaccines. Continuing surveillance to determine prevalent serotypes is necessary to insure that the vaccine formulations remain appropriate. For *S pyogenes,* it is critical to determine rheumatogenic and nephritogenic strains to limit the required multivalency of the vaccines. Toxicity has been associated with M protein preparations, but lack of immunogenicity in highly purified preparations of antigens is still a problem. Studies of mild extraction of M proteins have increased in frequency. With streptococcal vaccines, the potential risk of antigenic cross-reactivity with cardiac tissue and an associated increased risk of acute rheumatic fever must be appreciated. Passive immunity in group B streptococcal neonatal infection appears protective; artificial induction of this immunity with undegraded sialic acid containing polysaccharide group B antigens is being explored.

The streptococci are ubiquitous, and their significance in medicine is remarkable. Exciting advances are being made in diagnosis, in the understanding of the mechanisms of pathogenesis, as well as in control of these well-known organisms. Problems with antibiotic resistance must preclude complacency in dealing with these common pathogens.

References

Breese, B.B., Hall, C.B.: *Beta hemolytic streptococcal diseases.* Boston: Houghton Mifflin, 1978.

Dillon, H.C.: Post-streptococcal glomerulonephritis following pyoderma. *Rev Infect Dis* 1979; 1:935-943.

Facklam, R.R., et al: Presumptive identification of group A, B, and D streptococci. *Appl Microbiol* 1974; 27:107-113.

Gray, B.M., Converse, G.M., Dillon, H.C.: Epidemiologic studies of *Streptococcus pneumoniae* in infants: Acquisition, carriage, and infection during the first 24 months of life. *J Infect Dis* 1980; 142:923-933.

McCarty, M.: An adventure in the pathogenetic maze of rheumatic fever. *J Infect Dis* 1981; 143:375-385.

McGhee, J.R., Michalek, S.M.: Immunobiology of dental caries: microbial aspects and local immunity. *Ann Rev Microbiol* 1981; 35:595-638.

Parker, M.T. (editor): *Pathogenic streptococci: proceedings of the VIIth international symposium on streptococci and streptococcal diseases.* Surrey, England: Reedbooks, 1979.

Patterson, M.J., Hafeez, A.E.B.: Group B streptococci in human disease. *Bacteriol Rev* 1976; 40:774-792.

Skinner, F.A., Quesnel, L.B. (editors): *Streptococci.* New York: Academic Press, 1978.

Stollerman, G.H.: Global changes in group A streptococcal disease and strategies for their prevention. *Adv Intern Med* 1982; 27:373-406.

Thore, M., et al: Anaerobic phagocytosis, killing and degradation of *Streptococcus pneumoniae* by human peripheral blood leukocytes. *Infect Immunol* 1985; 47:277-281.

Wannamaker, L.W.: Changes and changing concepts in the biology of group A streptococci and the epidemiology of streptococcal infections. *Rev Infect Dis* 1979; 1:967-973.

Ward, J.: Antibiotic resistant *Streptococcus pneumoniae:* Clinical and epidemiologic aspects. *Rev Infec Dis* 1981; 3:254-266.

30 *Neisseria, Branhamella, Moraxella,* and *Acinetobacter*

Stephen A. Morse, PhD

General Concepts

The family Neisseriaceae is comprised of the genera *Neisseria, Branhamella, Moraxella,* and *Acinetobacter.* The only pathogens among these genera that cause significant human disease are *N gonorrhoeae*, the causative agent of gonorrhea, and *N meningitidis*, a causative agent of acute bacterial meningitis. Infections caused by *N gonorrhoeae* have a high frequency and a low mortality, whereas infections caused by *N meningitidis* have a low frequency and a high mortality.

Gonococcal infections are acquired by sexual contact and usually affect the urethra in men and the cervix in women, although dissemination of the infection to a variety of tissues may occur. The pathogenic mechanism involves the attachment of the gonococci to ciliated epithelial cells via pili (fimbriae) and the production of cytotoxic factors (endotoxin). Similarly, lipopolysaccharide of meningococci is highly toxic, but an additional virulence factor is the antiphagocytic capsule. Both pathogens produce proteases that cleave human IgA, and evidence suggests that the enzymes are involved in circumventing the local host defense. Meningococci inhabit the nasopharynx of many normal individuals, whereas gonococci are present only if sexual contact with an infected person has occurred. Epidemics of meningococcal meningitis occur sporadically. Epidemics of gonococcal infections occur frequently and affect large numbers of sexually active people. Other species of this family are primarily parasites on mucosal surfaces of humans and other animals. Human disease caused by these organisms usually is associated with opportunistic infections in compromised patients.

NEISSERIA

Members of the genus *Neisseria* inhabit the mucosal surfaces of warm-blooded animals. The genus includes two species that are pathogenic for humans: *N gonorrhoeae* (the gonococcus), the causative agent of gonorrhea, and *N meningitidis* (the meningococcus), a causative agent of acute bacterial meningitis. It also includes several nonpathogenic species (Table 30-1), which may be part of the normal flora and, therefore, can be confused with gonococci and meningococci.

Neisseria are gram-negative cocci, 0.6-1.0 μm in diameter. The organisms are usually seen in pairs with their adjacent sides flattened. *Neisseria* are nonflagellated; however, twitching motility may sometimes be observed with piliated organisms. Gonococci and meningococci have an optimum growth temperature ranging from 36-39 C.

Neisseria are aerobic microorganisms that contain high levels of cytochrome *c* oxidase. This enzyme, an important taxonomic characteristic of this genus, can be measured by reduction of *N,N*-dimethyl-*p*-phenylenediamine (or tetramethyl-*p*-phenylenediamine). The principal species of *Neisseria* and their differential characteristics are listed in Table 30-1.

Carbohydrates are utilized by oxidative pathways resulting primarily in accumulation of acetic acid. *N gonorrhoeae* and *N meningitidis* metabolize glucose by a combination of the Entner–Doudoroff and pentose phosphate pathways. Each species exhibits a characteristic pattern of acid production from specific carbohydrates that can be used to aid speciation. Testing for acid production is generally accomplished by inoculating the surface of a semisolid cystine trypicase agar (CTA) deep. The initial pH (7.3) of the medium is important, as only small amounts of acid are generated in positive reactions. Rapid methods (under 4 hours) employing heavy suspensions of organisms are also used.

The pathogenic species are fastidious microorganisms (the gonococcus more so than the meningococcus) with complex growth requirements. Both organisms are sensitive to growth inhibition by free fatty acids present in various peptones or in agar. The toxic effect of the free fatty acids can be eliminated by adding a binding agent such as soluble starch, serum, or charcoal to the medium.

Table 30-1 Differential Characteristics of Organisms in the Genera *Neisseria* and *Branhamella**

Characteristic†	N gonorrhoeae	N meningitidis	N lactamica	N sicca	N subflava‡	N flavescens	N cinerea	N mucosa	B catarrhalis
Acid from									
Glucose	+	+	+	+	+	–	–	+	–
Maltose	–	+	+	+	+	–	–	+	–
Lactose	–	–	+	–	–	–	–	–	–
Fructose	–	–	–	+	V	–	–	+	–
Sucrose	–	–	–	+	V	–	–	+	–
Growth on									
TM, or MTM, or NYC medium^π	+	+	+	–	–	–	–	–	d
Chocolate or blood agar at 22 C	–	–	V	V	V	+	–	+	+
Nutrient agar at 35 C	–	–	+	+	V	+	+	+	+
Polysaccharide synthesis from									
5% sucrose	φ	φ	?	+§	d	+	–	+	–
Production of H₂S	–	–	–	+	+	+	?	+	–
Presence of capsule	V	d	?	V	+	–	?	+	+
Reduction of nitrate	–	d	–	–	–	–	–	+	+
Reduction of nitrite§	+	d	+	+	+	+	+	+	+
Deoxyribonuclease	–	–	–	–	–	–	+	–	+
IgA₁ protease	+	+	–	–	–	–	?	–	–
Utilization of									
transferrin-bound iron	+	+	–	–	–	–	d	–	+
lactoferrin-bound iron	d	+	–	–	–	–	d	–	?

*All species contain catalase and cytochrome oxidase.

†+, most strains positive (≥90%); –, most strains negative (≥90%); d, some strains positive; V, character inconstant within single strain; φ, no growth on medium with 5% sucrose; ?, not known.

‡New species consisting of *N subflava*, *N flava*, and *N perflava*.

§*N sicca* forms an iodine-positive product when grown on trypticase soy agar without 5% sucrose. This reaction, which does not occur with *N subflava*, may be used as a differentiating characteristic.

^π T.M., Thayer–Martin medium; MTM, modified Thayer–Martin medium; NYC, New York City medium.

§0.001% (w/v) nitrite. Higher concentrations of nitrite (≥0.1%) are toxic for many species.

Neisseria gonorrhoeae

Distinctive Properties

The gonococcus is susceptible to drying and dies within 1-2 hours outside the body. Older cultures of gonococci typically undergo autolysis. Many strains of gonococci require increased atmospheric CO_2 concentrations (4%-8%) for initial isolation, but this requirement is often lost after repeated subculture. Colonies of freshly isolated strains consist of fimbriated organisms (type 1 and type 2 colonies). Fimbriated cells are virulent when inoculated experimentally into the urethra of the human or chimpanzee male or intravenously into chicken embryos. During nonselective transfer, fimbriated colonial types are often replaced by less virulent, nonfimbriated organisms (type 3 and type 4 colonies).

Recently, each of these colony types has been found to represent a combination of several phenotypic characteristics. In addition to fimbriation, colony coloration and opacity characteristics are important. Gonococci isolated from the urethras of males are characteristically fimbriated, form colonies of intermediate or marked opacity, and are killed in vitro by trypsin. Gonococci isolated from cervices vary in their colonial characteristics, depending on the point in the menstrual cycle at which the culture is obtained. Near ovulation or midcycle, gonococci have characteristics similar to those from male urethras; gonococci cultured from menstruating women are fimbriated, trypsin-resistant, and nearly all produce transparent colonies. These colonial characteristics can be maintained by selective subculture at daily intervals. The opacity or transparency of the colonies has been correlated to the presence or absence of one or more of a group of heat-modifiable outer membrane proteins (protein II).

Pathogenesis

The gonococcus usually enters the body during sexual activity, when one sex partner is already infected. The primary sites of infection are the urethra in men and the cervix in women. Other common sites are the pharynx and the anorectal region of both sexes. The gonococcus may spread by direct local invasion or by the bloodstream to produce major complications. Local spread results in infection of the fallopian tubes (salpingitis) or of Bartholin's glands (bartholinitis) in women, and occasionally in epididymitis and periurethral abscess in men. Disseminated gonococcal infection is usually manifested by arthritis and cutaneous lesions and occasionally by endocarditis, hepatitis, myocarditis, or meningitis.

The presence of fimbriae on *N gonorrhoeae* is not unique, as nonpathogenic species and *N meningitidis* also possess fimbriae. Gonococcal fimbriae are primarily protein and exhibit marked antigenic heterogeneity between strains. Fimbriae are important in attachment to host cells and in overcoming the long-range electrostatic repulsion between the negatively charged gonococci and the host cell surfaces. In fallopian tube organ cultures, gonococci attach almost exclusively to nonciliated mucosal cells (Figure 30-1). This attachment is mediated in part by fimbriae. Once attached, gonococci elaborate cytotoxic substances that damage the ciliated epithelial cells of the fallopian tube mucosa. Pilus-specific antibody is known to be opsonic and to prevent attachment

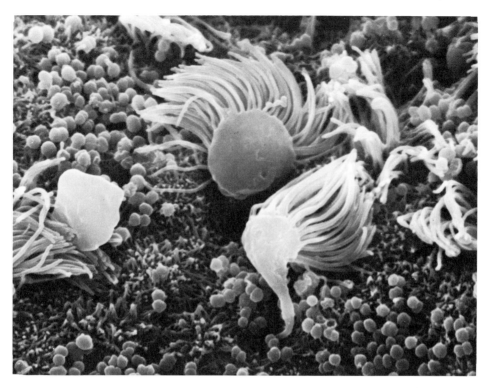

Figure 30-1 A scanning electron micrograph of an organ culture of human fallopian tubes after 20 hours of infection with piliated cells of a laboratory strain of *N gonorrhoeae*. The micrograph shows morphologically intact ciliated cells (far right and top), two sloughing ciliated cells with an apparently full complement of cilia (center), and gonococci attached almost exclusively to the microvilli of nonciliated cells but not attached to sloughing ciliated cells (×3,126). From McGee, Z., et al: *J Infect Dis* 1981; 143:413.

of gonococci to epithelial cells. Whether fimbriae play an antiphagocytic role is controversial.

Freshly isolated gonococci appear to be encapsulated. The capsule is antiphagocytic and can be removed easily from the gonococcal cell surface. Environmental and nutritional factors are important in capsule synthesis. The chemical nature and heterogeneity of capsular types are unknown.

The gonococcal outer membrane contains relatively few proteins, with one protein accounting for as much as 66% of total outer membrane protein. This protein (protein I) exhibits antigenic heterogeneity and has been used as both a serogroup and serotype antigen. Antibodies against this protein are bactericidal. Gonococcal lipopolysaccharide is a relatively small molecule devoid of O-antigen repeat units. Serological analysis indicates that three distinct antigenic determinants exist: common, variable, and serotype antigens. The common antigen is found on all gonococcal lipopolysaccharides, whereas the variable antigen may not be present. At least six different serotype antigens have been found. Gonococcal lipopolysaccharide contains a site(s) that is important in killing by normal human serum. The gonococcus produces an enzyme that degrades the polysaccharide portion of the lipopolysaccharide. Gonococcal endotoxin is one of the cytotoxic factors that damages ciliated epithelial cells in fallopian tube cultures (Figure 30-1).

Pathogenic species of *Neisseria* produce an extracellular protease that cleaves a prolyl-threonyl peptide bond on the heavy chain of the IgA_1 subclass of IgA, thus causing a loss of antibody activity. This enzyme may play a role in pathogenesis.

Gonococci must obtain iron from the host to grow. All gonococcal strains can use transferrin-bound iron; about one-half can use lactoferrin-bound iron. Considerable controversy exists concerning whether gonococci produce an extracellular sidero-phore.

The survival and multiplication of the gonococcus in an intracellular environment also is controversial. Fimbriated cells tend to remain extracellular, whereas nonfim-briated cells are ingested readily. Although most of the ingested cells are killed, some may survive and multiply within phagocytes.

Gonococci in urethral exudates usually are resistant to the bactericidal activity of the patient's serum, but they lose this resistance after subculture on laboratory medium. The molecular basis of gonococcal serum resistance has not been fully defined. It has been suggested that changes in the lipopolysaccharide, protein I, and protein II species contribute to the sensitivity of gonococci to normal human sera. Genetic loci have been described that govern the level of serum resistance of *N gonorrhoeae*. Environmental factors can also affect the phenotypic expression of serum resistance of *N gonorrhoeae*.

Host Defenses

Gonococcal infection stimulates local immunity; however, whether the secretory immune response that occurs is protective is not known. Acquired IgA and IgG serum antibody enhances the association of gonococci with the polymorphonuclear leuko-cytes in vitro. Protection against disseminated infections requires a functional comple-ment pathway. Individuals who are genetically deficient in the late complement components often have repeated bacteremic infections caused by serum-sensitive or serum-resistant strains of pathogenic *Neisseria* sp. In contrast, disseminated infections in individuals with a functional complement pathway are usually caused by strains that resist the bactericidal activity of normal human serum and complement. This form of serum resistance may be mediated by a blocking antibody in the serum.

Gonococci isolated from uncomplicated infections generally activate complement by the classical pathway, whereas gonococci isolated from disseminated infections activate complement by the alternate pathway. The release of chemotactic factors is slower during the activation of complement by the alternate pathway than during activation by the classical pathway. Thus, the activation of complement by the alternate pathway by disseminated strains may explain the paradoxical situation that strains capable of causing disseminated disease also produce asymptomatic local infections.

Epidemiology

Gonococci can colonize various mucosal surfaces lined by transitional or columnar epithelial cells such as the cervix, anal canal, urethra, throat, and conjunctiva. The gonococcus is almost always venereally transmitted. The only natural host for the gonococcus is the human; primary reservoirs of infection are asymptomatic women and men.

Gonorrhea is a worldwide problem. An estimated 3 million cases of gonorrhea were treated in the United States alone during 1982. The highest attack rate for gonorrhea in both men and women occurs among those 15-29 years old. Host-related factors such as number of sexual partners, contraceptive practices (for example, use of birth control pills and failure to use a condom), homosexuality, and population mobility contribute to the incidence of uncomplicated gonorrhea.

Not everyone exposed to gonorrhea acquires the disease. Whether this is due to varations in virulence, the size of the inoculum, nonspecific resistance, or to specific immunity is uncertain.

Diagnosis

Definitive diagnosis cannot be made solely on clinical grounds. In men, a gram-stained smear of urethral exudate showing the presence of intracellular gram-negative diplococci is sufficient to diagnose gonorrhea. When a direct smear is not definitive, a culture specimen from the anterior urethra should be inoculated onto a selective medium (modified Thayer-Martin, Martin-Lewis, or New York City medium); plates must be incubated in a candle jar or CO_2 incubator. The combination of oxidase-positive colonies and gram-negative diplococci provides a presumptive identification of *N gonorrhoeae*. Fluorescent antibody staining, coagglutination, or the production of acid from glucose (but not from maltose, sucrose or fructose; see Table 30-1) may be used for confirmation. In homosexual men, additional specimens should be obtained from the anal canal and pharynx and processed in the manner described above.

Gram-stained smears of exudate are not recommended for diagnosis of gonorrhea in women. Culture specimens should be obtained from the cervix and the anal canal and treated as described above. Pharyngeal cultures also should be taken from persons who engage in oral-genital sex. Serologic tests for gonorrhea have not proved satisfactory in men or women.

Control

Sulfonamides were used to treat gonorrhea until the end of World War II, when the organism's resistance to these drugs became so extensive that therapy was no longer effective. Penicillin was introduced at about this time. Initially, gonococci were extremely sensitive, with minimum inhibitory concentration values ranging from 0.003-0.03 units/mL. Treatment with a single injection of 150,000 units of penicillin gave cure rates of 90% or more. Since the mid-1950s, however, gonococci have shown reduced sensitivity to penicillin as well as to other antibiotics. This low-level penicillin resistance was not caused by the presence of β-lactamase and has required an increase in the recommended dosage to 4.8 million units.

Since 1976, penicillin-resistant strains of gonococci, originating in the Far East and Africa, have been isolated; they contain an R factor that codes for the synthesis of β-lactamase. Infections with these strains can be treated successfully with spectinomycin.

At present, no effective vaccine against gonorrhea exists, but experimental vaccines composed of gonococcal pili and the principal outer membrane protein (protein I) are being evaluated. Condoms are effective in preventing gonorrhea. As with other sexually transmitted diseases, the sex partner or partners of the patient should be treated to control effectively the spread of disease.

Neisseria meningitidis

Distinctive Properties

Meningococcal capsular polysaccharides provide the basis for grouping these organisms. The serogroups and the chemical composition of their capsular polysaccharide, where known, are listed in Table 30-2. Meningococcal capsular polysaccharides are immunogenic when the intact bacterium is presented to humans and rabbits. Highly specific anticapsular antibodies produced by rabbits are utilized in an agglutination test to divide meningococcal isolates into serogroups.

Serogroups B and C meningococci have been further subdivided according to the presence of outer membrane protein serotype antigens. Most disease by both groups B and C meningococci is caused by a single serotype, type 2. The type 2 antigens from groups B and C meningococci are chemically and serologically identical. All known group A strains have the same protein sterotype antigens in the outer membrane. Antibodies against the serotype antigens are bactericidal.

Pathogenesis and Host Defenses

Purified meningococcal lipopolysaccharide is highly toxic and is as lethal for mice as the lipopolysaccharide from *Escherichia coli* or *Salmonella typhimurium;* however, meningococcal lipopolysaccharide is 5–10 times more effective than enteric lipopolysaccharide in eliciting a dermal Shwartzman reaction in rabbits. Meningococcal lipopolysaccharides suppress leukotriene B_4 synthesis in human polymorphonuclear leukocytes. The loss of leukotriene B_4 deprives the leukocytes of a strong chemokinetic and chemotactic factor. Humans develop antibodies against meningococcal lipopolysaccharide during systemic disease; however, a role for these antibodies in immunity to meningococcal infection remains to be demonstrated.

Untreated meningococcal meningitis in humans has a mortality rate of approximately 85%. Meningococci can establish systemic infections in only individuals that lack serum bactericidal antibodies directed against capsular or noncapsular antigens of the invading strain, or in patients deficient in the late-acting complement components (C_5-C_9). In addition, IgM-deficient individuals are at greater risk from meningococcal infections than are normal hosts. The virulence of *N meningitidis* depends partly on the antiphagocytic properties of its capsule. Antibodies directed against the capsular polysaccharide are bactericidal. In the animal host, meningococci behave as extracellular parasites. Although they are often visible within polymorphonuclear leukocytes, no evidence suggests that they can multiply intracellularly.

Strains of *N meningitidis* produce two distinct IgA proteases that cleave the heavy chain of human IgA$_1$ at different points within the hinge region. Type 1 protease cleaves a prolyl-seryl peptide bond and type 2 protease cleaves a prolyl-threonyl peptide bond

Table 30-2 Chemical Composition of the Capsular Polysaccharides of *N meningitidis*

Serogroup	Components*	Structural Repeating Unit
A[+] (homopolymer)	ManNAc, phosphate, NAc and OAc	ManNAc—(1—P $\xrightarrow{\alpha}$ 6)——— 3 | | | OAc
B (homopolymer)	NeuNAc	NeuNAc—(2 $\xrightarrow{\alpha}$ 8)———
C‡ (homopolymer)	NeuNAc, OAc	NeuNAc—(2 $\xrightarrow{\alpha}$ 9)——— 7 8 | \\ | \\ | \\ | \\ OAc OAc
W-135 (disaccharide repeating unit)	Gal, NeuNAc	6-D-Gal(1 $\xrightarrow{\alpha}$ 4)—NeuNAc(2 $\xrightarrow{\alpha}$ 6)———
X	GlcNAc, phosphate	DOG1cNAc(1—P $\xrightarrow{\alpha}$ 4)———
Y (BO)§ (disaccharide repeating unit)	Glc, NeuNAc, OAc	6-D-Glc(1 $\xrightarrow{\alpha}$ 4)-NeuNAc(2 $\xrightarrow{\alpha}$ 6) | | | O-Ac
Z (monosaccharide-glycerol repeating unit)	GalNAc, glycerol phosphate	D-GalNAc, (1 $\xrightarrow{\alpha}$ 1′)-glycerol-(3′-P $\xrightarrow{\alpha}$ 4)———
29-e (disaccharide repeating unit)	GalNAc, KDO, OAc	D-GalNAc(1 $\xrightarrow{\beta}$ 7)-KDO(2 $\xrightarrow{\alpha}$ 3)——— 4,5 | | | O-Ac
L (trisaccharide repeating unit)	GlcNAc, phosphate	3-D-GlcNAc(1→3)-D-GlcNAc(1-3)-D-GlcNAc(1-P-)

Adapted from DeVoe, I.W. 1982. The meningococcus and mechanisms of pathogenicity. *Microbiol Rev* 46:180.
*Gal, galactose; Glc, glucose; GlcNAc, N-acetylglucosamine (2-acetamido-2-deoxy-D-glucose); KDO, 3-deoxy-D-manno-octulosonic acid; ManNAc, N-acetyl-mannosamine (2-acetamido-2-deoxy-D-mannose); NeuNAc, N-acetyl neuraminic acid (sialic acid); OAc, O-acetylated; NAc, N-acetylated; phosphate, phosphodiester linkage.
†Group A is substituted with O-acetyl at C_3 on about 70% of the ManNac-P residues.
‡Group C is substituted on C 7 or C 8 with 1 mol of O-acetyl per mol of sialic acid. One-quarter of the sialyl residues are not acetylated. Some di-O-acetylated (C 7 and C 8) may exist.
§The Y polysaccharide contains 1.3 mol of O-acetyl per NeuNAc residue. The most probable site for acetylation is C 3, C 4, or C 7. [13]C nuclear magnetic resonance studies have shown that the serogroup B0 polysaccharide is identical to serogroup Y, although B0 contains 1.8 mol of O-acetyl per mol of NeuNAC.

(similar to the gonococcal enzyme) in the unique IgA_1 subclass duplicated octapeptide sequence Thr-Pro-Pro-Thr-Pro-Ser-Pro-Ser. Each meningococcal isolate elaborates only one of these two enzymes. Circumstantial evidence suggests that these enzymes may have a role in the infectious process.

Epidemiology

The meningococcus usually inhabits the human nasopharynx without causing detectable disease. This carrier state may last for a few days to months and is important because it not only provides a reservoir for meningococcal infections but also enhances host immunity. From 3%-30% of normal individuals are carriers at any given time, yet few develop meningococcal disease. Even during epidemics of meningococcal meningitis in military recruits, when the carrier rate may reach 95%, the incidence of systemic disease is less than 1%. Carriers are usually over 20 years of age, but the attack rates are highest in children: with group B, 5 years of age; with group C, 4-14 years of age. The low incidence of disseminated disease following colonization suggests that host rather than bacterial factors play an important determining role.

Meningococcal meningitis occurs sporadically and in epidemics, with highest incidence during late winter and early spring. Most epidemics are caused by group A strains, but small outbreaks have occurred with group B and group C strains. Sporadic cases generally are caused by group B, group C, and group Y strains. Whenever group A strains become prevalent in the population, the incidence of meningitis increases markedly.

Diagnosis

Specimens of blood, cerebrospinal fluid, and nasopharyngeal secretions should be examined for presence of *N meningitidis* in cases of suspected meningococcal disease. Specimens should be collected before administration of any antimicrobial agents. Success in isolation is reduced by prior therapy; however, the microscopic diagnosis is not significantly affected. The cerebrospinal fluid should be concentrated by centrifugation and a portion of the sediment cultured on chocolate or blood agar. The plates should be incubated in a candle jar or CO_2 incubator. The presence of oxidase-positive colonies and gram-negative diplococci provides a presumptive identification of *N meningitidis*. Production of acid from glucose and maltose, but not sucrose, lactose, or fructose, may be used for confirmation. The serologic group may be determined by a slide agglutination test, using first polyvalent then monovalent antisera.

Nasopharyngeal specimens must be obtained from the posterior nasopharyngeal wall behind the soft palate and then should be inoculated onto selective medium (modified Thayer-Martin, Martin-Lewis, or New York City) and processed in the manner described previously.

Gram-stained smears of cerebrospinal fluid may be diagnostic; however, organisms in these smears are often more difficult to find than in those examined for pneumococcal meningitis. Quellung tests may be of value.

Control

Meningococcal disease arises from association with infected individuals, as evidenced by the 500-800 times greater attack rate among household contacts than among the general population. Because such household members are at high risk, they require chemoprophylaxis. Sulfonamides were the chemoprophylactic agent of choice until the emergence of sulfonamide-resistant meningococci. At present, approximately 25% of clinical isolates of *N meningitidis* in the United States are resistant to sulfonamides; rifampin is therefore the chemoprophylactic agent of choice.

Penicillin is the drug of choice to treat meningococcal meningitis. Although penicillin does not penetrate the normal blood-brain barrier, it does so readily when the meninges are acutely inflamed.

Group A and group C capsular polysaccharide vaccines are available. These vaccines provide a highly protective immunity against strains of these serogroups. Protection is provided through complement-mediated bactericidal antibodies that persist for at least 5 years following a single parenteral injection of vaccine. The capsular polysaccharide from serogroup B organisms is not immunogenic for young children.

BRANHAMELLA

Members of the species *B catarrhalis* (formerly *N catarrhalis*) are cocci that morphologically resemble *Neisseria*. Other relevant characteristics are presented in Table 30-1. *B catarrhalis* is a parasite of the mucous membranes of mammals. It was formerly placed in the genus *Neisseria;* however, studies of DNA base content, fatty acid composition, and genetic transformation showed that this organism did not belong in that genus. *B catarrhalis* should be considered more than a harmless commensal of the mucous membranes of humans. It is an infrequent, yet significant, cause of severe systemic infections such as pneumonia, meningitis, and endocarditis. It has been implicated in acute pulmonary infections in coal miners and in infections of compromised patients. It has also been implicated as a pathogen in otitis media and acute axillary sinusitis in children. *B catarrhalis* may cause clinical syndromes indistinguishable from those caused by gonococci. Thus, care must be taken to distinguish these organisms from one another. Many strains produce β-lactamase.

MORAXELLA

The genus *Moraxella* is comprised of organisms that are morphologically similar to *Acinetobacter;* however, *Moraxella* is oxidase-positive and shows no serologic cross-reactivity with *Acinetobacter*. Fimbriated strains may exhibit "twitching" motility on solid surfaces. Other relevant characteristics are presented in Table 30-3.

Members of *Moraxella* are parasites of the mucous membranes of humans and other warm-blooded animals. Many species are nonpathogenic. *M lacunata* can be isolated from the eye and may cause conjunctivitis in humans living under poor hygienic conditions. *M nonliquefaciens* is found in the upper respiratory tract, especially the nose, and may be a secondary invader in respiratory infections. *M urethralis* can be isolated from urine and the female genital tract. Some strains formerly designated as *Mima polymorpha* var. *oxidans* belong in this species. These organisms can be mistaken for *N gonorrhoeae* unless appropriate biochemical characteristics (for example, acid production from glucose) are determined (see Tables 30-1 and 30-3). Unlike *Acinetobacter*, *Moraxella* is sensitive to penicillin.

Table 30-3 Differential Characteristics of Organisms in the Genera *Moraxella* and *Acinetobacter*

Characteristics*	M lacunata	M bovis	M nonliquefaciens	M phenylpyruvica	M osloensis	M kingii†	M urethralis†	A calcoaceticus
Catalase	+	+	+	+	+	−	+	+
Cytochrome oxidase	+	+	+	+	+	+	+	−
Oxidation of:								
Glucose	−	−	−	−	−	+	−	d
Galactose	−	−	−	−	−	−	−	d
Mannose	−	−	−	−	−	−	−	d
Xylose	−	−	−	−	−	−	−	d
10% lactose	−	−	−	−	−	−	−	d
Gelatin or serum liquefaction	+	+	−	−	−	−	−	d
Hemolysis on:								
Blood agar	−	+	−	−	−	+	−	d
Chocolate agar	+	+	−	−	−	−	−	?
Phenylalanine deaminase	−	−	−	+	−	−	−	−
Reduction of nitrate	+	−	+	+	d	d	−	−
Reduction of nitrite	−	−	−	−	−	−	−	−
Presence of capsule	v	v	v	?	?	?	−	d
Production of H₂S	−	−	−	−	−	−	−	−

*+, most strains positive (≥90%); −, most strains negative (≥90%); d, some strains positive, some negative; v, character inconstant within single strain; ?, not known.
†Tentatively placed in the genus *Moraxella*.

ACINETOBACTER

Organisms of the genus *Acinetobacter* are typically short rods about 1.0-1.5 by 1.5-2.5 μm in the logarithmic phase; they are coccoid in the stationary phase. Cells occur predominantly in pairs and short chains. No spores are formed and flagella are not present. Fimbriated strains may exhibit twitching motility on solid surfaces. Other relevant characteristics are presented in Table 30-3.

Acinetobacter sp have been somewhat difficult to classify in the past because they do not process a sufficient number of unique phenotypic properties to differentiate them with certainty from other similar-looking organisms. All strains of *Acinetobacter* studied are strict aerobes. They resemble saprophytic *Pseudomonas* sp in their ability to use any one of a large number of organic compounds as a carbon and energy source for growth in a mineral medium. Strains capable of utilizing glucose as a carbon and energy source for growth degrade this compound exclusively by the Entner-Doudoroff pathway (see Chapter 19). Some strains produce an extracellular lipase and gelatinase. Many strains isolated from humans show hemolysis on blood agar plates. The hemolysin has phospholipase C activity and is excreted during growth. Strains of *Acinetobacter* grow almost as well at 40 C as at 30 C, although the optimum temperature is 34-35 C. Aquatic strains appear to be psychrotropic and grow at from 2-30 C.

Acinetobacter is usually associated with opportunistic infections in compromised patients. Some infections may be serious, but most are minor. Usually, isolation of these organisms is of slight clinical significance, representing only contamination or secondary invasion of damaged tissues. Strains of *Acinetobacter* are usually resistant to 5 units of penicillin; many strains are highly resistant due to production of β-lactamase. Organisms are usually sensitive to gentamicin, tobramycin, kanamycin, polymyxin B, colistin, or the tetracyclines.

References

Brooks, G.F., et al., (editors): *Immunobiology of Neisseria gonorrhoeae.* Washington, D.C.: American Society for Microbiology, 1978.

Danielsson, D., Normark, S.: *Genetics and immunobiology of pathogenic Neisseria.* EMBO Workshop, Hemavan, Sweden, 1980.

DeVoe, I.W.: The meningococcus and mechanisms of pathogenicity. *Microbiol Rev* 1982; 46:162-190.

Doern, G.V., Miller, M.J., Winn, R.E.: *Branhamella (Neisseria) catarrhalis* systemic disease in humans. *Arch Int Med* 1982; 141:1690-1692.

Juni, E.: Genetics and physiology of *Acinetobacter.* In: *Annual review of microbiology.* Star, M.P., Ingraham, J.L., Raffel, S., (editors). Palo Alto, Calif: Annual Review, Inc., 1978.

Morse, S.A.: The biology of the gonococcus. *CRC Crit Rev Microbiol* 1978; 7:92-189.

Sippel, J.E.: Meningococci. *CRC Crit Rev Microbiol* 1981; 8:267-302.

Watt, P.J., Ward, M.E.: Adherence of *Neisseria gonorrhoeae* and other *Neisseria* species to mammalian cells. In: *Bacterial adherence.* Beachey, E.H., (editor) New York: Chapman and Hall, 1980.

31 *Bacillus*

James C. Feeley, PhD
George C. Klein, MA

General Concepts
Distinctive Properties
Pathogenesis
Host Defenses
Epidemiology
Diagnosis
Control

General Concepts

Forty-eight *Bacillus* species are listed in the eighth edition of *Bergey's Manual of Determinative Bacteriology*. Most are saprophytes or insect pathogens, except for *B anthracis* and *B cereus*. Although *B anthracis* primarily infects animals, it rarely infects humans, and it does so usually through contact with contaminated animal tissues or materials such as wool, hide, or hair. The fatality rate for animals is high, but it varies for humans according to type of illness. Approximately 85% of pulmonary and 50% of gastrointestinal illnesses are fatal, whereas untreated cutaneous infections have a 5%–20% fatality rate. Recovery from anthrax requires early diagnosis and prompt effective therapy. No cases of person-to-person spread have been reported. The pathogenesis of *B anthracis* has been linked to its production of three toxic factors.

Although *Bacillus* sp generally do not cause human illness, reports of various species causing clinical infections are increasing. *B cereus* causes food poisoning and has been isolated and recognized as the actual pathogen in a wide variety of clinical specimens. Other species are isolated, usually as opportunistic pathogens, from

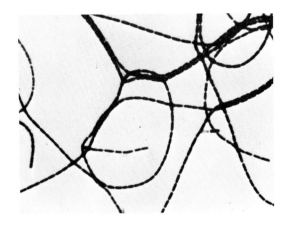

Figure 31-1 Gram stain of *B anthracis.*

individuals who are debilitated, have neoplastic disease, or are compromised immunologically. In this chapter, the *Bacillus* sp are considered as three groups: *B anthracis*, *B cereus*, and other *Bacillus* sp.

Distinctive Properties

The *Bacillus* sp are characteristically gram-positive, rod-shaped bacteria that produce endospores and require oxygen for growth (Figure 31-1). Some species and strains are exceptions; these are gram-negative or have the capability of growing as facultative anaerobes. The *Bacillus* sp resemble bacteria of the genus *Clostridium* in structure and production of endospores and Gram stain reaction; however, the clostridia are distinctly different from bacilli by characteristically growing only under anaerobic conditions.

Bacillus sp are distinguished from each other by a combination of morphologic and biochemical characteristics. The size and shape of the spore and its location within the vegetative cell allow tentative identification of a bacterium as one of several species in a group having similar characteristics. Definitive identification is accomplished with specific biochemical tests designated to separate species within each group (Table 31-1).

Bacillus sp share common antigens in the cell walls of their vegetative cells and, to a lesser degree, in their spores. Although other species produce capsules composed of polysaccharides, *B anthracis* produces a capsule composed of D-glutamic acid (glutamyl polypeptide) only when grown in vivo or on bicarbonate agar that is incubated in air supplemented with 10% CO_2. *B anthracis* and *B cereus* produce exotoxins that differ from each other in structure, antigenicity, and physiologic action.

Pathogenesis

Anthrax infections result only when animals or individuals are infected with *B anthracis* bacteria that produce both capsules and exotoxin. The capsule enables the anthrax

Table 31-1 Characteristics of 17 *Bacillus* Species*

	Percentage of Positive Tests†			Spore		Anaerobic Growth	Differential Test	
	Arabinose	Mannitol	Xylose	Centrally Located	Swells Rods		Result	Test
B anthracis	−	−	−	+	−	+	+	Phage‡
B cereus	−	−	−	+	−	+	−	Phage
B thuringiensis	−	−	−	+	−	+	−	Phage§
B alvei	−	−	−	d	+	+	−	Phage
B sphaericus	−	+	−	−	+	−	−	Phage
B pumilus	+	+	+	+	−	−	−	Nitrate
B licheniformis	+	+	+	+	−	+	+	Nitrate
B subtilis	+	+	+	+	−	−	+	Nitrate
B megaterium	d	d	+	+	−	−	d	Nitrate
B polymyxa	+	+	+	d	+	+	+	Dihydroxy acetone
B macerans	+	+	+	−	+	+	−	Dihydroxy acetone
B circulans	+	+	+	d	+	d	−	Dihydroxy acetone
B stearothermophilis	d	d	d	−	d	−	−	Indol
B coagulans	d	−	d	d	d	+	−	Indol
B firmus	−	+	−	+	−	−	+	Starch
B laterosporus	−	+	−	+	−	+	−	Starch‖
B brevis	−	d	−	d	+	−	−	Starch

*Compiled from *Bergey's Manual of determinative bacteriology*, 8th ed.
†+, positive for ≥90% of strains; −, negative for ≥90% of strains; d, reactions differ; positive for 11%–89% of strains.
‡Other special tests positive for *B. anthracis* are encapsulation on bicarbonate agar, susceptibility to penicillin in which cells round-up like a "string of pearls," and direct fluorescent antibody straining.
§*B. thuringiensis* contains crystalline protein bodies toxic for larvae of Lepidoptera.
‖*B. laterosporus* spores have laterally attached spindle-shaped bodies.

bacillus to survive phagocytosis, multiply, and release exotoxin that is composed of three components. Although British investigators have called these components factors I, II and III, American workers have named them, respectively, edema factor, protective antigen, and lethal factor. When pure preparations of each are injected separately into animals, each is not toxic; however, when combined, they are toxic. A mixture of protective antigen and lethal factor is lethal when injected intravenously into mice; a mixture of protective antigen and edema factor produces gross local edema when injected into the skin of guinea pigs or rabbits.

The exact mode of action of these factors has not been determined. It has been shown that the edema factor is an adenylate cyclase that increases cyclic AMP concentrations in eukaryotic cells, thus eliciting an edematous response in the skin. Recent evidence suggests that toxin production in *B anthracis* is mediated by large-molecular-weight plasmids. *B anthracis* strains that were cured of their resident extrachromosomal gene pools by sequential passage at 42.5 C also lost the ability to produce detectable amounts of lethal toxin and edema-producing activities. The involvement of these plasmids in the production of toxin was established by the transformation of nontoxigenic, heat-passaged strains into toxigenic strains by means of plasmid DNA obtained from the toxigenic parent strain. The exact role that these plasmids play in the production of exotoxin, however, remains to be demonstrated.

Human clinical anthrax is classified according to route of entry: cutaneous, inhalation, or gastrointestinal. Cutaneous illness develops when *B anthracis* spores are deposited beneath the skin through abrasion, insect bite, or other means. Spores germinate, and the resulting vegetative cells multiply and produce toxin. A small pruritic pimple appears within 1–7 days and enlarges into a vesicle or, occasionally, a ring of vesicles with an overall diameter of 0.5–1.0 cm.

The vesicle may be circumscribed by a small ring of erythema and nonpitting edema, which is usually minimal unless the lesion is located on the face, neck, or upper thorax. The vesicle at first contains clear serous fluid that later becomes hemorrhagic and blue-black. It ruptures within a few days, leaving a round sharp-edged ulcer crater that contains a hemorrhagic necrotic coagulum or developing "black eschar." This lesion usually is not painful in itself but may be if extensive edema or secondary infection is present. Gradually the black eschar dries, its edges separate from the surrounding skin, and it sloughs off. It should be noted that even when appropriate therapy is started early and is effective, the lesion still develops fully and results in an ulcerative black eschar lesion. Only 5% of patients have been reported to develop septicemia and generalized infection.

Inhalation anthrax results when dust particles contaminated with *B anthracis* spores are inhaled and deposited in the terminal alveoli. These particles, usually ≤ 5 μm in diameter, are engulfed by macrophages and transported to the regional lymph nodes in the mediastinum. The spores germinate, and the resulting vegetative cells multiply and produce toxin. Death usually results. Autopsy usually reveals extensive necrotic hemorrhage in the mediastinum. Multiple organs are involved.

Gastrointestinal anthrax results usually from ingestion of meat contaminated with *B anthracis*. The exact pathogenesis of this illness is not known. Organisms somehow penetrate either the oropharynx or the intestinal mucosa and are deposited in the submucosal tissue, where they multiply and produce toxin. The infection usually extends to the regional lymph nodes, and systemic symptoms finally develop. The fatality rate is approximately 50%.

B cereus has been associated with food poisonings and several clinical infections. The food poisonings are intoxications rather than infections. Illness results from ingestion of bacterial exotoxins produced by bacteria, which multiply rapidly and release exotoxins in food that has been stored improperly. The exotoxin (enterotoxin) associated with diarrheal illness is believed to activate adenylate cyclase and cause fluid loss through the intestinal mucosa. The mechanism of action of the exotoxin associated with the vomiting type of illness is not understood.

In addition to food poisoning, *B cereus* has been associated with several clinical conditions such as abscess formation, eye and ear infections, meningitis, osteomyelitis, and endocarditis. Exotoxins are also believed to play a major role in these infections. The pathogenic mechanisms of other *Bacillus* spp have not been delineated.

Host Defenses

Anthrax has been documented in a wide variety of warm-blooded animals. Species such as the rat, chicken, and dog are less susceptible to infection than other species such as cattle, sheep, and horses. Anthracidal substances found in the sera of these animals were once thought to account for this resistance, but detection of these substances in highly susceptible animals such as the guinea pig and rabbit has discredited this belief. Although the specific mechanisms for resistance are unknown, animal species that have a high level of phagocytic activity for *B anthracis* are more resistant than animals that do not.

Specific immunity occurs with development of antibodies to components of the exotoxin released by *B anthracis*. The antigen component of the toxin in the noncellular vaccine elicits protective antibody in the host. The same mechanism is at work in the avirulent spore vaccine administered to animals. The polyglutamic acid capsule of *B anthracis* is poorly immunogenic, and antibodies to the polysaccharide and other components contained in the cell walls of the organism are not protective.

To date, there is no evidence that *B cereus* food poisoning and infections with *B cereus* and other *Bacillus* species elicit immunity. A vaccine against the toxins of *B cereus* has not been developed.

Epidemiology

Most *Bacillus* sp are present worldwide in soil as saprophytes and alternate between vegetative and spore states. When soil and climate conditions facilitate growth, these bacteria actively grow and multiply in the vegetative state. When environmental conditions deteriorate, they sporulate and persist as spores. It is postulated that *B anthracis* alternates between these two states but is present only in soils contaminated by animals dying of anthrax. *B anthracis* bacteria persist in areas where animal anthrax has occurred; such areas in the United States are the Gulf Coast regions of Louisiana and Texas, the eastern parts of South Dakota and Nebraska, and some central parts of California. Nonvaccinated animals foraging on soils in these areas periodically become infected with the disease.

Humans are infected through association with infected animals or contaminated animal products such as goat hair and wool. Spores apparently can survive in soil for as long as 60 years. Woolsorters (woolsorters' disease) and hide handlers are the most frequently infected individuals. The worldwide incidence of human anthrax is estimated to be between 2,000 and 5,000 cases yearly. Most cases (95%) are cutaneous lesions, which are associated with agricultural or industrial occupations. The remaining 5% are the inhalation type. Only a few cases occur in the United States. No well-documented gastrointestinal anthrax ever has been reported in the United States.

The incidence of *B cereus* diarrheal illness varies from country to country and depends on local customs of preparing, cooking, and storing foods. Although only a few outbreaks have occurred in the United States, numerous outbreaks have occurred worldwide. *B cereus* was the third most common cause of bacterial food poisoning between 1960 and 1968 in Hungary. The outbreak was attributed to the seasoning of meat dishes with spices that contained spores of *B cereus* and other *Bacillus* sp, which were not killed during cooking. These spores germinated during unsatisfactory postcooking storage, and the resulting vegetative cells multiplied.

Outbreaks of *B cereus* vomiting-type illness have been reported from numerous countries where Chinese restaurants are popular. In England, nearly all of the more than 100 outbreaks that have occurred since 1971 have been associated with fried rice. The practice of bulk cooking of rice, storing portions of it at room temperature, and only rapidly frying the rice before serving allows surviving spores to germinate.

Increasing numbers of reports of *B cereus* and other *Bacillus* sp are associated with infections. Isolates of *B cereus* have been made from wounds, blood, cerebrospinal fluids, lung abscesses, and numerous other clinical specimens.

These isolates of *Bacillus* sp must not be dismissed simply as contaminants, especially when they are isolated from wounds resulting from trauma, insect bite, or surgical incision; from individuals who have predisposing factors (such as debilitation, neoplastic disease, and compromised immunity); or repeatedly from the same patient.

Diagnosis

Only cutaneous anthrax and *B cereus* food poisonings cause clinical symptoms that are sufficiently characteristic to permit early diagnosis. The first stages of inhalation and gastrointestinal anthrax cannot be distinguished from early stages of other diseases. Diagnosis is generally made too late for the patient's benefit. Most cases of inhalation anthrax have been discovered on autopsy. Infections with other *Bacillus* sp are usually determined from laboratory results.

Cutaneous lesions and other clinical specimens suspected of containing *B anthracis* bacteria should be examined microscopically and culturally. Smears should be prepared and stained with Gram stain and direct immunofluorescent reagents. They also should be inoculated onto a sheep blood agar plate and incubated aerobically at 36 C. *B anthracis* colonies are off-white, flat, and nonhemolytic; they have irregular margins, which may have comma-shaped outgrowths (Figure 31-2). When a portion of a *B anthracis* colony is lifted with a bacteriologic needle, it remains standing—an indication of the colony's tenacity. *B anthracis* is further distinguished from *B cereus* by other special tests (Table 31-1). Serologic diagnosis of anthrax can be made by means of a

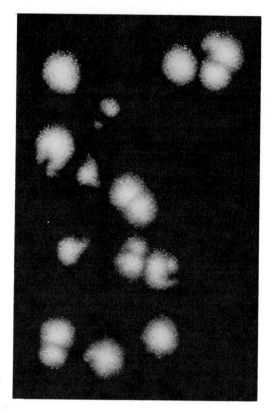

Figure 31-2 Colonies of *B anthracis* (×3).

microhemagglutination test specific for antibodies to the protective antigen component of the exotoxin of *B anthracis*.

B cereus food poisoning has two distinct clinical forms: the vomiting type and the diarrheal type. The vomiting type has a short incubation period of 1-6 hours, consists predominantly of vomiting with or without diarrhea, and is associated with eating contaminated fried rice. The diarrheal form has a longer incubation period, 10-12 hours, and consists predominantly of abdominal pain with profuse, watery diarrhea, which usually lasts no longer than 12-24 hours.

Because *B cereus* can be found in stools of healthy individuals, control specimens from healthy individuals should be collected along with stool specimens from infected individuals. Isolates should be sent to a special reference laboratory for serologic typing. Plate counts of *B cereus* should be done on feces and on any epidemiologically incriminated food using blood agar plates. Counts of *B cereus* greater than 10^5/g are considered diagnostic. Identification of *B cereus* isolates is made according to tests listed in Table 31-1.

Control

Ultimate prevention of infection with *Bacillus* sp is possible only by eradicating these organisms from the environment, an impractical and improbable solution. These bacteria are ubiquitous. Their spores have enabled them, and will continue to enable them, to persist in soil and dust for years.

Limited decontamination, on the other hand, is feasible and effective. Goat hair contaminated with *B anthracis* bacteria has been decontaminated by scouring in 2% formaldehyde or by cobalt radiation, but this no longer is done routinely. Contaminated buildings have been decontaminated with formaldehyde vapor having a final concentration of 18-21 mg/L. Also, anthrax infections have been prevented in animals by periodic immunization with an avirulent spore vaccine and, in humans working in mills contaminated with infected goat hair, with a cell-free vaccine. To prevent further anthrax infections, animals that are suspected of dying of anthrax must be examined by a qualified veterinarian. Carcasses should be disposed of by burial in a 6-foot-deep pit with 5% lye spread around the burial site, or by burning.

No vaccines are available against other *Bacillus* sp. Consequently, prevention of infection consists primarily of good housecleaning. *B cereus* food poisoning can be prevented by preparing and storing foods properly.

For treatment of anthrax, penicillin is currently recommended in countries such as the United States, where no penicillin-resistant strains have been detected. In other countries, such as England, where resistant strains have been encountered, tetracycline should be used. Only broad-spectrum antibiotics should be used to treat infections with the other *Bacillus* sp, because most of them, especially *B cereus*, are resistant to penicillin. Most are still sensitive to tetracycline, chloramphenicol, and gentamicin, although final selection of the antibiotic should be based on results of antibiotic sensitivity testing of the isolate.

References

Brachman, P.S.: Anthrax. In: *Clinical medicine,* Vol. II. Spittel, J.A. Jr., (editor). Hagerstown, Md.: Harper & Row, 1980.

Farrar, W.E.: Serious infections due to "non-pathogenic" organisms of the genus *Bacillus. Am J Med* 1963; 34:134-137.

Gibson, T., Gordon, R.E., (editors): *Bergey's manual of determinative bacteriology,* 8th ed. Baltimore: Williams and Wilkins, 1974.

Lennette, E.H., et al. (editors): *Manual of clinical microbiology,* 3rd ed. Washington, D.C.: American Society for Microbiology, 1980.

Leppla, S.H.: Anthrax toxin edema factor: A bacterial adenylate cyclase that increases cyclic AMP concentrations in eukaryotic cells. *Proc Natl Acad Sci USA* 1982; 79:3162-3166.

Mikesell, P., et al.: Evidence for plasmid-mediated toxin productions in *Bacillus anthracis. Infect Immun* 1983; 39:371-376.

Parry, J.M., Turnbull, P.C.B., Gibson, J.R., (editors): *A colour atlas of Bacillus species.* London: Wolfe Medical Publications Ltd, 1983.

Poretz, D.M.: In: *Principles and practise of infectious diseases,* Mandell, G.L., Douglas, R.G., Bennett, J.E., (editors). New York: John Wiley & Sons, 1979.

Riemann, H., Bryan, F.L., (editors): *Food-borne infections and intoxications,* 2nd ed. New York: Academic Press, 1979.

Turnbull, P.C.B., et al.: Severe clinical conditions associated with *Bacillus cereus* and the apparent involvement of exotoxins. *J Clin Pathol* 1979; 32:289-293.

Von Gravenitz, A.: The role of opportunistic bacteria in human disease. *Ann Rev Microbiol* 1977; 31:447-471.

32 Miscellaneous Pathogenic Bacteria

Robert M. Pike, PhD

General Concepts

The microorganisms discussed in this chapter are taxonomically unrelated but share the tendency to cause human infection less frequently than most medically important bacteria. Some of these infections can be fatal; others tend to be self-limited. Recognition of them depends largely on proper use of bacteriologic methods, which is important not only to insure appropriate therapy, but also to exclude other possible causative agents.

Listeria monocytogenes is a common animal pathogen that occasionally causes meningitis and septicemia in chronically debilitated adults, as well as in prenatal or neonatal infants. *Streptobacillus moniliformis* may infect individuals who have been bitten by an infected rodent. Septicemia frequently occurs upon ulceration of the skin at the site of the bite. *Erysipelothrix rhusiopathiae* may cause a painful inflammatory infection at the site of abraded skin, but septicemia is rare. *Propionibacterium acne* often is isolated from the skin lesions of patients with acne, but whether it causes acne is still controversial. *Calymmatobacterium (Donovania) granulomatis* causes granuloma inguinale, a venereal disease that should not be confused with lymphogranuloma venereum.

LISTERIA

Distinctive Properties

Listeria monocytogenes is a small, gram-positive bacillus. In smooth colonies, coccobacilli in pairs and short chains predominate and may be mistaken for streptococci. The organisms tend to be arranged in palisades suggestive of diphtheroids (corynebacteria other than *Corynebacterium diphtheriae*). Long filaments appear as the change from smooth to rough occurs. Spores are not formed and capsules, although usually not seen, have been described. The organism is motile, but flagella develop better at room temperature than at 37 C. Consequently, cultures may at first be thought to be nonmotile. Four main serologic types have been recognized; types 1 and 4 predominate in the United States.

The organism will grow in an unenriched medium, but grows more readily on blood agar, which also permits detection of a narrow zone of β-hemolysis around colonies of most strains. The colonies are small (0.5–1.5 mm) and translucent.

Pathogenesis

L monocytogenes is naturally pathogenic for a wide variety of animals. Meningoencephalitis is the predominant disease caused by it in cattle and other ruminants. Systemic infections have also been observed in rabbits, guinea pigs, swine, and other animals, often with focal necrosis in various organs. The organism sometimes causes abortion.

In recent years, listeriosis in humans has been recognized with increased frequency. Although the infection can result in a variety of clinical manifestations, the infections commonly seen are meningitis in adults or prenatal or postnatal disease. The meningitis may or may not be accompanied by septicemia. Disseminated infection occurs most often in persons with other chronic debilitating disease. Infection in utero results in death of the fetus or in death of the infant shortly after birth. In such cases, the mother shows no symptoms at all or has a mild febrile illness during the third trimester of pregnancy.

Host Defenses

The relative infrequency of human listeriosis, despite wide distribution of *L monocytogenes* and existence of asymptomatic infection, suggests that humans are fairly resistant. In infected tissues, the organisms are largely intracellular; immunologically activated macrophages appear to be the body's main defense.

Epidemiology

Many potential sources of *L monocytogenes* exist. In addition to infections in animals, the organism has been isolated from plants and soil. Except in the case of transmission from mother to infant, no evidence suggests person-to-person transmission. The epidemiology is not completely understood, but the pattern is that of a saprophyte that humans acquire from the environment.

Diagnosis

Listeriosis can be diagnosed definitively only by isolating and identifying the organism. Blood and cerebrospinal fluid should be cultured in cases of suspected meningitis. Direct smears of the spinal fluid sediment may show gram-positive bacilli, which may be confused with *Haemophilus influenzae* if not properly stained. Specimens from the genital tract of the mother should be cultured when in utero infection is suspected, and various tissues should be cultured at autopsy. Primary isolation is often facilitated by storing the specimen or a suspension of the material to be cultured at 4 C and making cultures periodically up to 6 months if growth is not obtained before that time. All cultures should be incubated in 10% CO_2.

Blood agar plates are examined for colonies that have the macroscopic and microscopic characteristics previously described. Catalase production and motility at room temperature distinguish *L monocytogenes* from *Erysipelothrix rhusiopathiae* and from streptococci. *L monocytogenes* is pathogenic for mice on intraperitoneal injection, and a drop of culture instilled into the eye of a rabbit or guinea pig characteristically produces purulent conjunctivitis. Intravenous injection in the rabbit causes a marked monocytosis. Final identification and typing are accomplished by agglutination with specific antisera prepared against flagellar and somatic antigens.

Control

No specific means of preventing listeriosis exist. If infection in the mother can be recognized early, infection of the infant can be prevented by adequate treatment, but the maternal infection is often not apparent. The organism is susceptible to penicillin, erythromycin, and tetracyclines; antibiotic therapy has reduced the fatality rate appreciably except in neonatal infections, which usually are fatal regardless of therapy.

STREPTOBACILLUS

Distinctive Properties

Streptobacillus moniliformis is a gram-negative, nonmotile rod with microscopic and cultural properties so distinctive that recognition usually presents no problem. In young cultures, the bacilli are about 1 μm in width and up to 5 μm in length. As growth progresses, an extreme pleomorphism develops, resulting in the appearance of long convoluted filaments that stain unevenly. These filaments may show swellings, either elongated or spherical (moniliform), as much as 5 μm in diameter.

Growth in an artificial medium depends on the presence of blood, serum, or ascitic fluid and is enhanced by an atmosphere containing increased CO_2. In a fluid medium, the organisms form macroscopic clumps that settle out, leaving a clear supernatant fluid. Colonies are 1-2 mm in diameter on blood agar. Spontaneous variation takes place, resulting in the production of L-phase colonies (cell wall-deficient bacteria) that are barely visible to the naked eye. Under a low-power lens, these tiny colonies often outnumber the parent colonies. Because L-phase colonies are embedded in the agar, no organisms are visualized in smears made in the usual way. They are indistinguishable from other L-phase organisms and from *Mycoplasma* (see Chapter 52).

Pathogenesis

Humans usually are infected with *S moniliformis* through the bite of a wild or laboratory rat; the resulting disease is called rat-bite fever. (A similar clinical entity, also known as rat-bite fever, is caused by another organism, *Spirillum minor;* see Chapter 50). An ulcer that heals spontaneously may or may not develop at the site of the bite, and within a few days the organisms spread to the regional lymphatics and lymph nodes and to the bloodstream, causing abrupt onset of fever and general malaise. Other characteristics of the disseminated infection include a rash and painful, swollen joints, which may persist in the chronic form of the disease. Endocarditis is a possible serious complication. Up to 10% of untreated cases are fatal.

Although sporadic cases following the bite of a rat are the most frequently observed form of infection, outbreaks and isolated cases caused by ingestion of contaminated milk have occasionally been reported and are referred to as Haverhill fever.

Mice are susceptible to artificial inoculation, but rats are usually resistant.

Epidemiology

S moniliformis inhabits the upper respiratory tract of healthy rats. Its infectivity for humans depends on its introduction into a wound or, less frequently, on ingestion with food or drink. Because of its inability to resist acid, the organism probably cannot survive the gastric environment.

Diagnosis

The acute onset of chills and fever several days following a rat bite suggests the possibility of *S moniliformis* infection. In most instances, the only way to isolate the organism is by culturing the blood. The culture should be incubated in 10% CO_2 and examined periodically (without disturbing the sedimented blood cells) for small fluffy balls of growth lying on the layer of sedimented cells. These balls can be removed with a capillary pipette, smeared on slides for microscopic examination, and spread on a blood agar plate to be incubated in increased CO_2. Plates should be examined with the aid of a hand lens or low-power microscope to detect the characteristic L-phase colonies in addition to colonies visible with the naked eye. Visual colonies can be smeared and stained in the usual way, but, to examine the L-phase colonies or to subculture them, a small block of agar containing the colonies must be removed. Isolation of an extremely pleomorphic, gram-negative bacillus plus the spontaneous production of L-phase colonies strongly suggest the presence of *S moniliformis*. Occasionally exudate is obtainable on a swab at the site of the bite or fluid can be aspirated from a swollen joint; these materials should be cultured in broth and streaked on blood agar plates to be incubated and examined as described previously.

Control

Rat-bite fever is a potential hazard of wild rat infestation. Also, laboratory workers should take precautions against bites by experimental rats. Penicillin and streptomycin have been reported effective in treatment, but since the L-phase organisms, which lack cell walls, are not susceptible to penicillin, broad-spectrum antibiotics should be used in patients who do not respond to penicillin.

ERYSIPELOTHRIX

Distinctive Properties

Erysipelothrix rhusiopathiae is a small, nonmotile bacillus that forms neither spores nor capsules. Although gram-positive, it is easily decolorized. Organisms in smooth colonies are fairly uniform in appearance, but long filaments tend to occur in rough colonies. Growth is slow in the absence of blood, serum, or glucose. Smooth colonies are small (1 mm or less); rough colonies are somewhat flatter and larger. Growth occurs aerobically but may be enhanced by the presence of increased CO_2, particularly on primary isolation.

Lack of motility, failure to produce β-hemolysis on blood agar, and the absence of catalase help to distinguish *E rhusiopathiae* from *Listeria*, with which it may initially be confused. These organisms are also antigenically distinct.

Pathogenesis

Naturally acquired erysipeloid infections (skin or tissue) have been seen in various domestic animals and fowl. Among the more frequent are swine erysipelas and an infection of the long bones of turkeys and chickens. Mice are susceptible to experimental inoculation; guinea pigs are not. In humans, erysipeloid infections usually take place after a slight skin abrasion. Although the painful inflammation at the site of inoculation spreads peripherally, swelling in the central portion of the lesions subsides. No pus is formed. Most infections are self-limited and disappear in a few weeks. On rare occasions, septicemia develops and can be fatal if not properly treated.

Host Defenses

The characteristic limited erysipeloid infection in humans, a contrast to the more extensive infection that often occurs in animals, suggests that humans have a fair degree of natural resistance to *E rhusiopathiae*. Because reinfection may occur, immunity to natural infection evidently is not permanent.

Epidemiology

E rhusiopathiae has a wide and varied distribution. In addition to its presence in infections of animals and fowls, it has been found in fresh and saltwater fish. Human infection most often occurs in individuals such as veterinarians, slaughterhouse workers, and fish handlers, whose occupations bring them in contact with these sources. Men are more often infected than women because of their prevalence in these occupations. The organism is not unusually resistant to heat or to drying, but it can survive for several months in salted or pickled meat and in decaying carcasses.

Diagnosis

History of possible occupational exposure and the presence of a typical nonsuppurating lesion on the hand might lead to suspicion of erysipeloid. Isolation and identification of the organism are required for confirmation. As collecting a suitable specimen with a swab is not possible, a biopsy should be taken near the margin of the lesion or a small amount of saline should be injected into the skin and aspirated. Direct smears of these materials are of little value. The specimen should be obtained aseptically, placed in glucose broth, incubated for 24 hours, and then plated on blood agar. More than 24 hours incubation of the broth is sometimes required before growth can be obtained on subculture. Besides the characteristics already described, the ability of *E rhusiopathiae* to produce H_2S in triple sugar iron agar is said to be an aid in distinguishing it from other gram-positive non-spore-forming bacilli.

Control

Although most cases of erysipeloid are self-limited, chemotherapy is essential for the occasional disseminated infection and may prevent complications in localized infections. Penicillin is the drug of choice; erythromycin is also effective.

PROPIONIBACTERIUM

The genus *Propionibacterium* includes several species formerly classified as *Corynebacterium*. They are gram-positive, non-spore-forming, nonmotile rods with a tendency to pleomorphism exemplified by uneven staining and by forms that vary from coccoid to elongate. Some cells are club-shaped. Strains of *Propionibacterium* are at least microaerophilic; some strains prefer strictly anaerobic conditions. Propionic and acetic acids are important products of fermentation.

Members of this genus are frequently found in dairy products, the intestinal tracts of humans and animals, and on human skin. The species most often suspected of contributing to human infection is *P acnes*. The common occurrence of *P acnes* on the skin of patients explains why this is the most common contaminant in anaerobic cultures and why it is difficult to establish its causal role in disease. Instances have occurred, however, in which *P acnes* has been isolated repeatedly from the blood, spinal fluid, bone marrow, and abcesses, alone or in combination with other organisms. Its frequent presence in acne lesions has led to the suspicion that it may be involved in the etiology of this disease, a view that is not universally held and is difficult to prove.

CALYMMATOBACTERIUM

Distinctive Properties

Calymmatobacterium (Donovania) granulomatis is a gram-negative, nonmotile, encapsulated bacillus. This morphology and cross-complement fixation with *Klebsiella* suggest it is related to this genus. Although growth was originally obtained only in the yolk sac of the developing chick embryo and this is still the most reliable means of cultivation, the organism also grows in a medium containing egg yolk if cultures are incubated in a microaerophilic atmosphere.

Pathogenesis

C granulomatis is not pathogenic for laboratory animals. In humans, the disease typically caused by this organism is granuloma inguinale (not to be confused with lymphogranuloma venereum, a chlamydial infection). It consists of chronic granulomatous lesions that tend to ulcerate and that may be confined to the external genitalia; they may also appear anywhere in the genital region, including the cervix and vagina. Other parts of the body may be infected with or without genital involvement.

The infection tends to spread from the initial site, destroying the skin and subcutaneous tissue as it spreads. The regional lymphatics may be infected, but lymphadenopathy is not a characteristic feature of the disease. Systemic infection is rare. Large numbers of phagocytes invade the infected area, and the mononuclear cells filled with the encapsulated bacteria are found in material obtained from the lesions. Superinfection is the most frequent complication.

Epidemiology

Granuloma inguinale has been considered a venereal disease, partly because of the principal location of the lesions and partly because of the presence of the disease in marital partners; however, infection in the marital partners of infected individuals varies, suggesting a low degree of transmissibility. The presence of the organisms in feces and the low incidence of the disease in marital partners reported by some observers suggest that sexual transmission may not be the only means of disseminating the infection. It has been argued that *C granulomatis* is a normal inhabitant of the intestinal tract, where it causes no pathologic change, and that it is transmitted to the skin by autoinoculation or by heterosexual or homosexual venereal contact.

Granuloma inguinale occurs most frequently in the tropics and in the lower socioeconomic stratum. In the United States, it is seen seven times more often in blacks than in whites and twice as often in men as in women.

Diagnosis

The early lesions of granuloma inguinale are not sufficiently characteristic to establish a clinical diagnosis and must be distinguished from those caused by *Treponema pallidum* and *Haemophilus ducreyi*. Many patients with granuloma inguinale also have syphilis. Although antibodies to *C granulomatis* have been demonstrated in patients' serum by complement fixation, serologic procedures have not been developed to provide the sensitivity and specificity required for a reliable diagnostic test. Diagnosis is therefore confirmed by demonstrating the organisms in the lesions. This is done most conveniently by direct microscopic examination. To obtain material suitable for examination, the investigator should first wash the lesion with a sterile sponge wet with saline to remove many of the contaminating organisms usually present. Tissue is then removed with a biopsy punch, and smears or tissue spreads are made from this material. When stained with Wright's stain, large mononuclear cells containing dumbbell-shaped encapsulated rods are characteristic of *C granulomatis*. These are the Donovan bodies originally associated with this disease. Extracellular organisms may also be present, but they only suggest a positive diagnosis. Microscopic examination, properly done, is so reliable that cultivation of the organisms is usually not attempted. Cultivation has been accomplished, however, by inoculating the specimen into the yolk sac of 5-day-old chick embryos and by inoculating slants made from coagulated egg yolk.

Control

The only means of preventing granuloma inguinale are cleanliness and the avoidance of close contact with infected persons. Tetracycline and erythromycin are effective in treatment.

References

French, R.S., et al.: Chronic meningitis caused by *Propionibacterium acnes*. *Neurology* 1974; 24:624-28.

Gray, M.L., Killinger, A.H.: *Listeria monocytogenes* and listeric infections. *Bacteriol Rev* 1966; 30:309-82.

Grieco, M.H., Sheldon, C.: *Erysipelothrix rhusiopathiae*. *Ann NY Acad Sci* 1970; 174:523-32.

Lal, S., Nicholas, C.: Epidemiological and clinical features in 165 cases of granuloma inguinale. *Br J Vener Dis* 1970; 46:461-63.

Proceedings of the Third International Symposium on listeriosis. Utrecht: Rijks Institut voor de Volksgesond-heid, 1966.

Rogosa, M.: *Streptobacillus moniliformis* and *Spirillum minor*. In: *Manual of clinical microbiology*, 2nd ed., Lennette, E.H., Spaulding, E.H., Traunt, J.B., (editors). Washington, D.C.; American Society for Microbiology, 1974.

Whiteside, J.A., Voss, J.G.: Incidence and lipolytic activity of *Propionibacterium acnes* (*Cornyebacterium acnes* group I) and *P. granulosum* (*C. acnes* group II) in acne and normal skin. *J Invest Dermatol* 1973; 60:94-97.

Wing, E.J.: Effect of acute nutritional deprivation on host defenses against *Listeria monocytogenes*. *Adv Exp Med Biol* 1983; 162:245-50.

33 Anaerobes: General Characteristics

David J. Hentges, PhD

General Concepts
Oxygen Toxicity
Pathogenic Anaerobes
Processing Clinical Specimens

General Concepts

The broad classification of bacteria as **anaerobes, aerobes,** or **facultative microorganisms** depends on the types of reactions they employ to generate energy for growth and other activities. In their metabolism of energy-containing compounds, aerobes require molecular oxygen as a terminal electron acceptor and cannot grow in its absence. Anaerobes, on the other hand, cannot grow in the presence of oxygen. Oxygen is toxic for them, and they must therefore depend on other substances as electron acceptors. Their metabolism frequently is a fermentative type in which they reduce available organic compounds to various end products such as organic acids and alcohols. The facultative organisms are the most versatile. They preferentially utilize oxygen as a terminal electron acceptor, but also can metabolize in the absence of oxygen by reducing other compounds. Much more usable energy, in the form of high-energy phosphate, is obtained when a molecule of glucose is completely catabolized to carbon dioxide and water in the presence of oxygen (38 ATP) than when it is only partially catabolized by a fermentative process in the absence of oxygen (2 ATP). The ability to utilize oxygen as a terminal electron acceptor provides organisms with an extremely efficient mechanism for generating energy. Understanding these general characteristics of anaerobic bacteria provides insight into how these organisms can proliferate in damaged tissue, and why special care is needed in processing clinical specimens that may contain anaerobes.

Oxygen Toxicity

Several studies indicate that aerobic microorganisms can survive in the presence of oxygen only by virtue of an elaborate system of defenses. Without these defenses, key enzyme systems in the organisms fail to function and the organisms die. Obligate anaerobic bacteria, which live only in the absence of oxygen, do not possess effective defenses that make aerobic life possible and therefore cannot survive in air.

During growth and metabolism, oxygen reduction products are generated within microorganisms and secreted into the surrounding medium. The superoxide anion, one oxygen reduction product, is produced by univalent reduction of oxygen:

$$O_2 \xrightarrow{e^-} O_2^-$$

It is generated during the interaction of molecular oxygen with various cellular constituents, including reduced flavins, flavoproteins, quinones, thiols, and iron-sulfur proteins. The exact process by which the superoxide anion causes intracellular damage is not known; the anion, however, is capable of participating in a number of destructive reactions potentially lethal to the cell. Moreover, products of secondary reactions may amplify toxicity. For example, one hypothesis holds that the superoxide anion reacts with hydrogen peroxide in the cell:

$$O_2^- + H_2O_2 \longrightarrow OH^- + OH^{\cdot} + O_2$$

This reaction, known as the Haber–Weiss reaction, generates a free hydroxyl radical (OH$^{\cdot}$), which is the most potent biologic oxidant known. It can attack virtually any organic substance in the cell. A subsequent reaction between the superoxide anion and the hydroxyl radical produces singlet oxygen (O_2^*), which is also damaging to the cell:

$$O_2^- + OH^{\cdot} \longrightarrow OH^- + O_2^*$$

The excited singlet oxygen molecule is very reactive. Therefore, superoxide must be removed for the cells to survive in the presence of oxygen.

Most facultative and aerobic organisms contain a high concentration of an enzyme called superoxide dismutase (SOD). This enzyme converts the superoxide anion into ground-state oxygen and hydrogen peroxide, thus ridding the cell of destructive superoxide anions:

$$2O_2^- + 2H^+ \xrightarrow{\text{SOD}} O_2 + H_2O_2$$

The hydrogen peroxide generated in this reaction is an oxidizing agent, but it does not damage the cell as much as the superoxide anion and tends to diffuse out of the cell. Many organisms possess the enzymes catalase or peroxidase or both to eliminate the H_2O_2. Catalase uses H_2O_2 as an oxidant (electron acceptor) and a reductant (electron donor) to convert peroxide into water and ground-state oxygen:

$$H_2O_2 + H_2O_2 \xrightarrow{\text{Catalase}} 2H_2O + O_2$$

Peroxidase uses a reductant other than H_2O_2:

$$H_2O_2 + H_2R \xrightarrow{\text{Peroxidase}} 2H_2O + R$$

One study showed that facultative and aerobic organisms that lack superoxide dismutase possess high levels of catalase or peroxidase. The presence of these enzymes at high levels may alleviate the need for superoxide dismutase, because they effectively scavenge H_2O_2 before it can react with the superoxide anion to form the more active hydroxyl radical. However, most organisms show a positive correlation between the activity of superoxide dismutase and resistance to the toxic effects of oxygen.

In another study, facultative and aerobic organisms demonstrated high levels of superoxide dismutase. The enzyme was present, generally at lower levels, in some of the anaerobes studied, but was totally absent in others. The most oxygen-sensitive anaerobes as a rule contained little or no superoxide dismutase. In addition to the activity of superoxide dismutase, the rate at which an organism takes up and reduces oxygen was determined to be a factor in oxygen tolerance. Very sensitive anaerobes, which reduced relatively large quantities of oxygen and exhibited no superoxide dismutase activity, were killed after short exposure to oxygen. More tolerant organisms reduced very little oxygen or else demonstrated high levels of superoxide dismutase activity.

The continuous spectrum of oxygen tolerance among bacteria appears to be due partly to the activities of superoxide dismutase, catalase, and peroxidase in the cell, and partly to the rate at which the cell takes up oxygen. Clearly, other factors influence tolerance: the location of protective enzymes in the cell (surface versus cytoplasm); the rate at which cells form toxic oxygen products (for example, the hydroxyl radical or singlet oxygen); and the sensitivities of key cellular components to the toxic oxygen products.

Pathogenic Anaerobes

Anaerobic bacteria are widely distributed in nature in oxygen-free habitats. Many indigenous human flora are anaerobic bacteria, including spirochetes and gram-positive and gram-negative cocci and rods. For example, the human colon, where oxygen tension is low, contains large populations of anaerobic bacteria, exceeding 10^{11} organisms per gram of colon content. Anaerobes in this region frequently outnumber facultative organisms by a factor of at least 100 to 1. Oxygen-sensitive organisms also are numerous in other areas of the body, such as the gingival crevices, tonsillar crypts, nasal folds, hair follicles, the urethra and vagina, and on tooth surfaces.

Anaerobic indigenous flora components are potentially pathogenic if displaced from their normal habitat. Most anaerobic infections are endogenously acquired from the microflora, although *Clostridium,* found principally in the soil, also produce infections in humans. Proliferation of anaerobic bacteria in tissue depends on the absence of oxygen. Oxygen is excluded from the tissue by impairment of local blood supply by trauma, obstruction, or surgical manipulation. Anaerobes multiply well in dead tissue. Multiplication of aerobic or facultative organisms in association with anaerobes in infected tissue also diminishes oxygen concentration and develops a habitat that supports growth of anaerobic bacteria.

Infections produced by anaerobic bacteria occur in all parts of the human body. The infected tissues usually contain a mixture of several kinds of anaerobes, and frequently also contain aerobic and facultative bacteria. The types of infections commonly produced by anaerobic bacteria are:

1. Intraabdominal infections. Abscesses, postoperative wound infections, and generalized peritonitis produced by anaerobes occur as a consequence of bowel perforation during surgery or injury.

2. Pulmonary infections. Anaerobic lung infections may originate in the bronchi or the blood. Aspirations from the upper respiratory tract, which contain large numbers of anaerobic bacteria, are responsible for initiating infection in the bronchi.

3. Pelvic infections. Anaerobic infections of the vagina and uterus sometimes occur after gynecologic surgery or in association with malignancy of pelvic organs.

4. Brain abscesses. Anaerobes infrequently produce meningitis, but are a common cause of brain abscesses. The infecting organisms usually originate in the upper respiratory tract.

5. Skin and soft tissue infections. Combinations of anaerobes, aerobes, and facultative organisms often act synergistically to produce these infections.

6. Oral and dental infections. These local infections frequently extend to the face and neck, and sometimes to other areas of the body such as the brain.

7. Bacteremia and endocarditis. Anaerobic bacteremia may occur following disturbance in an area of the body where an established flora or an infection exists. Endocarditis, an inflammation of the endothelial lining of the heart cavities, is occasionally caused by anaerobic bacteria, especially anaerobic streptococci.

With the exception of the clostridia, which have been studied extensively, the mechanisms by which anaerobes cause infections in humans are not well understood. *Clostridium* sp are known to produce various toxins that destroy tissue cells, and two species, *C botulinum* and *C tetani,* release the neurotoxins responsible for botulism and tetanus. Enzymes excreted by other anaerobic bacteria, including proteases, lipases, hyaluronidase, chondroitin sulfatase, and neuraminidase, may play a role in infection by causing tissue cell destruction, and β-lactamase may act as a virulence factor by inactivating antibiotics that possess a β-lactam ring, such as the penicillins and cephalosporins. In addition, the capsules surrounding some anaerobic bacteria probably interfere with phagocytosis and act as a barrier against penetration of antimicrobial agents.

Processing Clinical Specimens

When collecting specimens from patients for isolation and identification of anaerobic bacteria associated with infections, precautions must be taken to exclude air. Materials for anaerobic culture are best obtained with a needle and syringe. Unless the specimen can be sent to the laboratory immediately, it is placed in an anaerobic transport tube containing oxygen-free carbon dioxide or nitrogen. The specimen is injected through the rubber stopper in the transport tube and remains in the anaerobic environment of the tube until processed in the bacteriology laboratory. If the specimen is collected with a swab, only a special commercially available anaerobic swab transport system is used.

Specimens should be free of contaminating bacteria. Material from sites that are normally sterile, such as blood, spinal fluid, or pleural fluid, poses no problem provided the usual precautions are taken to decontaminate the skin properly before puncturing it to obtain the specimen. Fecal specimens, sputum specimens, or vaginal secretions cannot be cultured routinely for pathogenic anaerobes, because they normally contain other anaerobic organisms. Aspirates from abscesses or the specific sites of infections must be obtained in these cases to avoid undue contamination with indigenous flora components.

Although several techniques are available for maintaining an oxygen-free environment during the processing of specimens for anaerobic culture, the anaerobic jar is used most commonly. It consists of a medium-sized glass or plastic jar with a tightly fitting lid containing palladium-coated alumina particles, which serve as a catalyst. The anaerobic jar can be set up by two methods. The easiest uses a commercially available hydrogen and carbon dioxide generator envelope (Gas Pak) that is placed in the jar along with the culture plates. The generator is activated with water. Oxygen within the jar and the hydrogen that is generated are converted to water in the presence of the catalyst, thus producing anaerobic conditions. Carbon dioxide, which is also generated, is required for growth by some anaerobes and stimulates the growth of others. An alternative method for achieving anaerobiosis in the jar consists of evacuation and replacement. Air is evacuated from the sealed jar containing the culture plates and is replaced with an oxygen-free mixture of 80% nitrogen, 10% hydrogen, and 10% carbon dioxide.

More sophisticated procedures are used to isolate extremely oxygen-sensitive microorganisms that cannot be recovered by the anaerobic jar technique. One called the roll tube method consists of a stoppered test tube containing oxygen-free gas and a thin layer of prereduced agar medium on its inside surface. The medium in the tube is inoculated with a loop while the tube is rotated. This produces a spiral track on the agar surface. The tube is flushed with a stream of carbon dioxide to prevent entry of air while it is open during innoculation.

The anaerobic glove box isolator is another innovation developed for isolating anaerobic bacteria. It is essentially a large clear vinyl chamber, with attached gloves, containing a mixture of 80% nitrogen, 10% hydrogen, and 10% carbon dioxide. A lock at one end of the chamber is fitted with two hatches, one leading to the outside and the other to the inside of the chamber. Specimens are placed in the lock, the outside hatch is closed, and the air in the lock is evacuated and replaced with the gas mixture. The inside hatch is then opened to introduce the specimen into the chamber. Conventional bacteriologic procedures are employed to process the specimen in the oxygen-free atmosphere.

Although these complex systems are needed to isolate anaerobic flora components, studies have shown that the anaerobic jar is adequate to recover clinically significant anaerobes. The extremely oxygen-sensitive bacteria of the microflora apparently are not associated with infectious processes.

Procedures for cultivation and identification of anaerobic bacteria are well established (Figure 33-1). A variety of selective and nonselective media is available for cultivation of anaerobes. A reliable, nonselective medium consists of *Brucella* agar

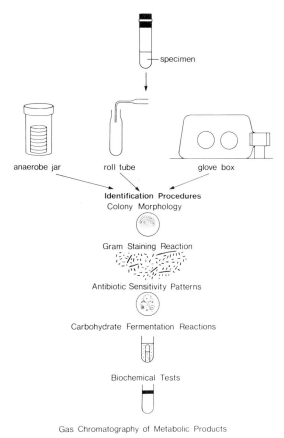

specimen

anaerobe jar

roll tube

glove box

Identification Procedures

Colony Morphology

Gram Staining Reaction

Antibiotic Sensitivity Patterns

Carbohydrate Fermentation Reactions

Biochemical Tests

Gas Chromatography of Metabolic Products

Figure 33-1 Isolation and identification of anaerobes.

supplemented with sheep blood, hemin, cysteine, sodium carbonate, and menadione. Usual bacteriologic procedures are used to identify anaerobes. These are based on gram-staining reactions, cellular and colony morphology, antibiotic sensitivity patterns, carbohydrate fermentation reactions, and other biochemical tests. Analysis of metabolic end products, especially organic acids, provides additional information useful in classifying these organisms.

References

Balows, A., et al., (editors): *Anaerobic bacteria*. Springfield, Ill.: Charles C Thomas, 1974.

Finegold, S.M.: *Anaerobic bacteria in human disease*. New York: Academic Press, 1977.

Holdeman, L.V., Cato, E.P., Moore, W.E.C., (editors): *Anaerobe laboratory manual*, 4th ed. Blacksburg, Va.: The Virginia Polytechnic Institute and State University Anaerobe Laboratory, 1974.

Lennette, E.H., Spaulding, E.H., Truant, J.P., (editors): *Manual of clinical microbiology*, 2nd ed. Washington, D.C.: American Society for Microbiology, 1974.

Morris, J.G.: The physiology of obligate anaerobiosis. In: *Advances in microbial physiology*, Vol. 12. Rose, A.H., Tempest, D.W., (editors). London: Academic Press, 1975.

Sutter, V.L., Citron, D.M., Finegold, S.M.: *Wadsworth anaerobic bacteriology manual*, 3rd ed. St. Louis: The C.V. Mosby Co., 1980.

34 Clostridia

Carol L. Wells, PhD
Tracy D. Wilkins, PhD

General Concepts

Of the anaerobes that infect humans, the clostridia are the most widely studied. They are involved in a variety of human diseases, the most important of which are gas gangrene, tetanus, botulism, pseudomembranous colitis, and food poisoning (Table 34-1). In most cases, clostridia are opportunistic pathogens, that is, one or more species establishes a nidus of infection in a particular site in a compromised host. Each clostridial species produces protein exotoxins (such as botulinum and tetanus toxins) that play an important role in the pathogenesis of each clostridial disease.

Many generalizations can be made about the clostridia as a genus, although nearly every generalization has an exception. The clostridia are classically anaerobic rods, but some species can become aerotolerant on subculture; a few species (*Clostridium carnis, C histolyticum,* and *C tertium*) can grow under aerobic conditions. Most species are gram-positive, but a few are gram-negative. Also, with many gram-positive species, the gram reaction may be easily lost, resulting in gram-negative cultures.

The clostridia form characteristic spores, and the position of the spore is useful in species identification; however, some species do not sporulate unless exposed to exacting cultural conditions. Many clostridia are transient or permanent members of the normal flora of the human skin and the gastrointestinal tracts of humans and animals. The clostridia are somewhat unusual members of the human bacterial flora, as most of these organisms can also be found worldwide in the soil.

Thus, the clostridia are ubiquitous saprophytes, and the clinician should be aware that most clostridia isolated from clinical specimens are accidental contaminants and are not involved in a disease process. Because these organisms are normally found on the

Table 34-1   Diseases Caused by the Clostridia

Disease	Etiologic Agent	Pathogenesis
Gas gangrene	*C perfringens* and/or other clostridial species	Organisms grow in traumatized tissue with low redox potential; exotoxins cause necrosis and toxemia
Tetanus	*C tetani*	Organisms grow in traumatized tissue with low redox potential; neurotoxin fixes to gangliosides and blocks glycine release.
Botulism (adult)	*C botulinum*	Ingestion of neurotoxin or release of neurotoxin from organisms growing in traumatized tissue with low redox potential; neurotoxin interferes with acetylcholine release.
Botulism (infant)	*C botulinum*	Organisms replicate and produce neurotoxin in intestinal tract of infants.
Pseudomembraneous colitis (antibiotic-induced)	*C difficile*	Antibiotic therapy gives organism a competitive advantage in the intestinal tract; exotoxin causes colonic pathology.
Food poisoning (relatively mild form)	*C perfringens*	Ingestion of live organisms results in sporulation and concomitant enterotoxin production.

skin, even a pure culture of clostridia isolated from the blood may have no clinical significance. In determining the importance of a clinical isolate of clostridia, the clinician should consider the frequency of isolation of the species, the presence of other microbes of pathogenic potential, and the clinical symptoms of the patient. All clostridial infections can be controlled by antibiotic therapy (penicillin, chloramphenicol, vancomycin) and, in some cases, tissue debridement. Antitoxin therapy and toxoid immunization are clearly useful in some clostridial infections, such as tetanus.

GAS GANGRENE AND RELATED CLOSTRIDIAL WOUND INFECTIONS

Distinctive Properties

Clostridial wound infections may be divided into three categories: gas gangrene or clostridial myonecrosis, anaerobic cellulitis, and superficial contamination. These infections usually are polymicrobic because the source of wound contamination (feces, soil) is polymicrobic. In gas gangrene and anaerobic cellulitis, the primary pathogen can be any one of various clostridial species including *C perfringens* (80%), *C novyi* (40%), *C septicum* (20%) and, occasionally, *C bifermentans*, *C histolyticium*, or *C fallax*. Other bacterial isolates may be any of a wide number and variety of organisms (for example, *Proteus, Bacillus, Escherichia, Bacteroides, Staphylococcus*).

The distinctive or unique properties of the causative agents of gas gangrene are difficult to list; morphologic characteristics and biochemical reactions vary among these species, and a reliable laboratory manual should be consulted for their proper identification. Isolation of 10^7 or more clostridia per mL of wound exudate is strong evidence for a clostridial wound infection.

Gas gangrene can have a rapidly fatal outcome and requires prompt, often severe, treatment. The more common clostridial wound infections are much less acute and require much less radical treatment; however, they may share some characteristics with gas gangrene and must be included in the differential diagnosis. Superficial wound contamination caused by clostridia usually involves *C perfringens,* with staphylococci or streptococci or both as frequent coisolates.

Pathogenesis

All clostridial wound infections occur in an anaerobic tissue environment caused by an impaired blood supply secondary to trauma, surgery, foreign bodies, or malignancy. Contamination of the wound by clostridia from the external environment or from the host's normal flora produces the infection.

Gas gangrene is an acute disease with a poor prognosis and often fatal outcome. Initial trauma to host tissue damages muscle and impairs blood supply. This lack of oxygenation causes the oxidation-reduction potential to decrease and allows the growth of anaerobic clostridia. Initial symptoms are generalized fever and pain in the infected tissue. As the clostridia multiply, various exotoxins (including hemolysins, collagenases, proteases, and lipases) are liberated into the surrounding tissue, causing more local tissue necrosis and systemic toxemia. Infected muscle is discolored and edematous and produces a foul-smelling exudate; gas bubbles form from the products of anaerobic fermentation. As capillary permeability increases, the accumulation of fluid increases, and venous return eventually is curtailed. As more tissue becomes involved, the clostridia multiply within the increasing area of dead tissue, releasing more toxins into the local tissue and into the systemic circulation. Because ischemia plays a significant role in the pathogenesis of gas gangrene, the muscle groups most frequently involved are those in the extremities that are served by one or two major blood vessels.

Clostridial septicemia, although rare, may occur in the late stages of the disease. Severe shock with massive hemolysis and renal failure is usually the ultimate cause of death. The incubation period, from the time of wounding until the establishing of gas gangrene, varies with the infecting clostridial species from 1-6 days, but it may be as long as 6 weeks. Average incubation times for the three most prevalent infecting organisms are as follows: *C perfringens*, 10-48 hours; *C septicum*, 2-3 days; and *C novyi*, 5-6 days. Because the organisms need time to establish a nidus of infection, the time lag between wounding and appropriate medical treatment is a significant factor in the initiation of gas gangrene.

Like gas gangrene, clostridial cellulitis is an infection of muscle tissue, but here the infecting organisms invade only tissue that is already dead; the infection does not spread to healthy, undamaged tissue. Clostridial cellulitis has a more gradual onset than gas gangrene and does not include the systemic toxemia associated with gas gangrene. Pain is minimal, and although only dead tissue is infected, the disease can spread along the planes between muscle groups, causing the surrounding tissue to appear more affected than it actually is. Anaerobic cellulitis may cause formation of many gas bubbles, producing infected tissue that looks similar to the gaseous tissue of gas gangrene. Some tissue necrosis does occur, but it is caused by decreased blood supply and not invasion by the infecting organism. With adequate treatment, anaerobic cellulitis has a good prognosis.

Superficial contamination, the least serious of the clostridial wound infections, involves infection of only necrotic tissue. Usually, the patient experiences little pain, and the process of wound healing proceeds normally; however, occasionally an exudate may form and the infection may interfere with wound healing.

Discussion of the differential diagnosis of clostridial wound infections appropriately includes streptococcal myositis, as this disease can be characterized by an edematous, necrotizing, often gaseous lesion. Like anaerobic cellulitis and superficial contamination with clostridia, streptococcal myositis is a relatively localized disease, but its later stages may include some systemic toxicity that mimics the toxemia of gas gangrene.

Host Defenses

Host defenses against gas gangrene and other clostridial wound infections are essentially absent. Even repeated episodes of clostridial wound infection do not seem to produce effective immunity.

Epidemiology

The clostridia are ubiquitous microorganisms in the soil, on human skin, and in the gastrointestinal tracts of humans and animals. Thus, the causative agents of clostridial wound infections are not environmentally restricted. Even operating theaters can be habitats for infecting clostridial organisms and spores. The incidence of clostridial wound infections has declined with the advance of prompt, adequate medical treatment. Historically, war casualties have had the greatest incidence of gas gangrene; however, the prompt evacuation and medical attention given United States casualties in the Vietnam war greatly decreased the incidence of gas gangrene in these soldiers, emphasizing the importance of undelayed medical treatment.

Diagnosis

Diagnosis of clostridial wound infections is based on clinical symptoms coupled with Gram stains and bacterial culture of clinical specimens. Characteristic lesions and the presence of large numbers of gram-positive bacilli (with or without spores) in a wound exudate provide strong presumptive evidence. Spores are rare in cultures of *C perfringens*, the most common etiologic agent of these diseases. Gas gangrene, once initiated, may spread and cause death within hours. By the time the typical lesions of gas gangrene are evident, the disease usually is firmly established and the physician must treat the patient on a clinical basis without waiting for laboratory confirmation.

Control

Correction of the anaerobic conditions combined with antibiotic treatment forms the basis for therapy. Penicillin is the drug of choice for all clostridial wound infections; chloramphenicol is a second-choice antibiotic. Successful treatment of the less severe forms of clostridial wound infections include local debridement and antibiotic therapy; patient recovery usually proceeds along a steady, positive course. Treatment of gas gangrene includes radical surgical debridement coupled with high doses of antibiotics. Blood transfusions and supportive therapy for shock and renal failure also may be indicated.

The usefulness of gas gangrene antitoxin is currently a disputed matter. Some physicians maintain that the efficacy of this polyvalent antitoxin has been proved in the past, but better medical care now may have eliminated the need for its use. Others believe that because of insufficient data, antitoxin should be administered systemically as early as possible after diagnosis, and that the antitoxin should be injected locally into tissue that cannot be excised.

Disagreements also exist concerning the efficacy of hyperbaric oxygen therapy. Certain chelating agents such as ethylenediamine tetracetic acid (EDTA) and diethylene-triamine pentacetic acid (DTPA) may aid in treatment of gas gangrene caused by *C perfringens*, as these agents have been found to inhibit the activity of α-toxin (the most damaging toxin released by this organism).

Obviously, prevention of wound contamination is the single most important factor in controlling clostridial wound infections. In the past, immunization has been considered as a possible preventive measure for gas gangrene; however, several factors have discouraged the use of active immunization, including difficulty in preparing a suitable antigenic toxoid, availability of prompt wound treatment, and accessibility of effective therapeutic agents.

TETANUS AND *CLOSTRIDIUM TETANI*

Distinctive Properties

C tetani is an anaerobic gram-positive rod that forms terminal spores, giving it a characteristic squash racquet appearance. Some strains do not sporulate readily, and spores may not appear until the third or fourth day of culture. Most strains are motile with peritrichous flagella; colonies often swarm on agar plates, but some strains are nonflagellated and nonmotile. The presence of *C tetani* should be suspected on isolation of a swarming rod that produces indole and has terminal spherical spores, but does not produce acid from glucose. This organism usually produces three toxins, but nontoxigenic strains also exist. These three toxins are responsible for the infamous toxemia called tetanus. The two animal species most susceptible to this toxemia are horses and humans.

Pathogenesis

As with all clostridial wound infections, the initial event in tetanus is trauma to host tissue, followed by accidental contamination of the wound with *C tetani*. Tissue damage is needed to lower the oxidation-reduction potential and provide an environment suitable for growth. Once growth is initiated, the organism itself is not invasive and remains confined to the necrotic tissue, where the vegetative cells of *C tetani* elaborate the lethal toxins. The incubation period from the time of wounding to the appearance of symptoms varies from a few days to several weeks, depending on the infectious dose and the site of the wound (the more peripheral the wound, the longer the incubation time).

Tetanus can be initiated in two different ways, resulting in either ascending or descending tetanus. In the ascending form, toxins travel along the neural route (peripheral nerves), causing a disease confined to the extremities and seen most often in inadequately immunized persons. In descending tetanus, all of the toxin cannot be absorbed by local nerve endings; therefore, it passes into the blood and lymph with subsequent absorption by all the motor nerves. The most susceptible centers are the head and neck; the first symptom is usually trismus (lockjaw), with muscle spasms descending from the neck to the trunk and limbs. As the disease progresses, the spasms increase in severity, becoming very painful and exhausting. Spasms often are initiated by environmental stimuli that may be as insignificant as the flash of a light or the sound of a footstep. Portions of the body may become extremely rigid, and opisthotonos (a spasm in which the head and heels are bent backward and the body bowed forward) is common. Complications include fractures, bowel impaction, intramuscular hematoma, muscle ruptures, and pulmonary, renal, and cardiac problems.

The three toxins of *C tetani* are a spasmogenic toxin (tetanospasmin) responsible for the classical symptoms of the disease; a nonspasmogenic toxin that acts peripherally and may have paralytic effects; and tetanolysin, a hemolysin that is inactivated by cholesterol and thus may not be important in humans.

The spasmogenic toxin fixes to gangliosides in neural tissue and blocks the release of glycine, a transmitter substance that normally prevents contraction of antagonistic muscles. Muscle spasms and convulsions result. Tetanospasmin also may act on the sympathetic nervous system, the neurocirculatory system, and the neuroendocrine system. Tetanospasmin may be as potent as the toxin of *C botulinum;* as little as 130 μg constitutes a lethal dose for humans. The mortality rate in tetanus is 55%-65%, and the ultimate cause of death is usually pulmonary or cardiac failure.

Host Defenses

Apparently, innate immunity to tetanus toxin does not exist. Also, one or more episodes of tetanus do not produce immunity to future attacks. The reason for the lack of immune response may be twofold: the toxin is potent, and the amount released may be too small to trigger immune mechanisms but still be enough to cause symptoms and, because the toxin binds firmly to neural tissue, it may not interact effectively with the immune system.

Epidemiology

C tetani can be isolated from the soil in almost every environment throughout the world. Occasionally, the organism can be found among the gastrointestinal flora of humans and horses. Isolation of *C tetani* from the intestinal flora of horses, coupled with the high frequency of equine tetanus, led to the erroneous assumption that the horse was the animal reservoir of *C tetani*.

Generalized outbreaks of tetanus do not occur, but certain populations can be considered at risk. Historically, wounded soldiers have had a high incidence of tetanus, but this phenomenon has declined with widespread use of immunizations. Umbilical tetanus (tetanus neonatorum) usually is a generalized, fulminating, fatal disease that occurs with the neonates of unimmunized mothers who have given birth under unsanitary conditions. In the United States, heroin addicts using septic injection techniques have become another population with an increasing incidence of clinical tetanus. Tetanus is rare in most developed countries (the United States has about one case per million per year); however, in some underdeveloped tropical countries, tetanus is still one of the ten leading causes of death.

Diagnosis

Diagnosis of tetanus is obvious in advanced cases; however, successful treatment depends on early diagnosis before a lethal amount of toxin becomes fixed to neural tissue. The initial symptom is cramping and twitching of muscles around a wound. The patient usually has no fever but sweats profusely and begins to experience pain, especially in the area of the wound and around the neck and jaw muscles. The patient should be treated on a clinical basis without waiting for laboratory data. *C tetani* can be recovered from the wound in only about one-third of the cases, and a wound is not even evident in 10%-20% of cases. Note that toxigenic strains of *C tetani* can grow actively in the wound of an immunized person, but the presence of antitoxin antibodies prevents initiation of tetanus.

Numerous syndromes have symptoms similar to those of tetanus and must be considered in the differential diagnosis. Ingestion of strychnine (found in rat poison) can cause symptoms that closely resemble those of tetanus. Trismus can occur in encephalitis, phenothiazine reactions, and diseases involving the jaw.

Control

Injections of tetanus toxoid are prophylactic. Currently, booster doses are recommended only every 10 years by the CDC. More frequent boosters are unnecessary and may cause local reactions resembling the Arthus phenomenon, or a delayed hypersensitivity reaction (see Chapter 9).

Treatment of diagnosed tetanus has a number of aspects. The source of the offending organism must be removed by local debridement. Pencillin or chloramphenicol is administered to kill the offending organisms, but may not be a necessary adjunct in therapy. Human tetanus immunoglobulin is given in an attempt to neutralize unbound systemic toxin; the recommended dose is at least 3000 units intramuscularly into three different sites, including the involved extremity. Supportive measures, such as respiratory assistance and intravenous fluids, are often critical to patient survival. Recommended tranquilizers and sedatives to relieve muscle spasms include meprobamate and diazepam.

In cases of clean, minor wounds, tetanus toxoid should be administered only if the patient has not had a booster dose within the past 10 years. For more serious wounds, toxoid should be administered if the patient has not had a booster dose within the past 5 years. All patients who have a reasonable potential for contracting tetanus should receive injections of 250 units of human tetanus immunoglobulin.

BOTULISM AND *CLOSTRIDIUM BOTULINUM*

Distinctive Properties

Most species of bacteria consist of strains that have a close genetic relationship and similar cultural characteristics. This is not true of *C botulinum*. This species consists of several distinct groups of organisms that have a common name solely because they produce similar toxins. The name *C botulinum* is only a convenience that reflects the medical importance of the species. A strain of *C botulinum* usually produces only one of eight toxin types designated A, B, C_1, C_2, D, E, F, and G. The toxins produced by *C botulinum* types C and D have been shown to be coded by the genetic material contained in bacteriophages that infect the bacteria. *C botulinum* types C and D can be interconverted by use of specific bacteriophage. Also, types C and D even can be transformed into *C novyi* by curing bacteria of the botulinum phage and substituting a phage that codes for a *C novyi* toxin. Thus, the production of a pharmacologically similar neurotoxin is the single distinctive property of a clostridium that places it in the botulinum species. All the organisms that produce these toxins are anaerobic rods, gram-positive, and motile by peritrichous flagella. Oval, subterminal spores are produced in extremely variable numbers, depending on the particular isolate and on the culture medium. Cultural reactions vary greatly, and the species includes highly proteolytic and nonproteolytic strains as well as saccharolytic and nonsaccharolytic strains.

Pathogenesis

The pathogenesis of *C botulinum* depends entirely on neurotoxin production. In humans, these toxins cause the well-known form of food poisoning resulting from ingestion of toxin in improperly preserved food; wound botulism, a rare disease that results from *C botulinum* growing in the necrotic tissue of a wound; and infant botulism, in which the organism grows and produces toxin in the intestines of infants.

The Toxins

The neurotoxins of *C botulinum* are differentiated serologically into eight types (A, B, C_1, C_2, D, E, F, and G); humans are most susceptible to toxin types A, B, E, and F. Types C and D are most toxic for animals, and type G is so rare that its specificity has not yet been determined. The toxins often are released from the bacteria as inactive proteins that must be cleaved by a protease to expose the active site. These proteases may be produced by the cell itself or may be in the body fluids of the infected host.

Type A toxin is the most potent poison known. Ingestion of only 10^{-8} g of this toxin can kill a human or, put another way, the amount of toxin that could be held on the tip of a dissecting probe could kill 40 medical students.

From its site of entry into the body, the toxin travels through the blood and lymphatic systems (and possibly the nervous system). It then becomes fixed to cranial and peripheral nerves, but exerts almost all its action on the peripheral nervous system. The toxin appears to bind to receptor sites at the neuromuscular junctions of parasympathetic nerves, and prevents impulses from passing from motor nerves to muscle fibers by interfering with the release of acetylcholine, the transmitter substance. The result is muscle paralysis. The cranial nerves are affected first, followed by a descending symmetric paralysis of motor nerves. The early involvement of cranial nerves causes problems with eyesight, hearing, and speech. Double or blurred vision, dilated pupils, and slurred speech are common symptoms. Decreased saliva production causes a dryness of the mouth and throat, and swallowing may be painful. An overall weakness ensues, followed by descending paralysis with critical involvement of the respiratory tree. Death usually is caused by respiratory failure, but cardiac failure also can be the primary cause. Mortality from botulism is decreasing and it now occurs in less than 20% of cases. Individuals over 20 years of age have a higher mortality than those who are younger. Mortality is highest for type A, followed by type E and then type B, possibly reflecting the affinities of the toxins for neural tissue: type A binds most firmly, followed by type E, then type B. Fatality rates are directly proportional to the infectious dose and inversely proportional to the incubation time of the disease.

Food Poisoning

In food poisoning, the toxin is produced by the vegetative cells of *C botulinum* in contaminated food, and preformed toxin then is ingested with the contaminated food.

The incubation time for botulism food poisoning can vary from a few hours to 8 days, but most commonly is 18–36 hours. Only a small, but effective, percentage of the ingested toxin is absorbed through the intestinal mucosa; the remainder is eliminated in the feces.

Gastrointestinal disturbances are early symptoms of the disease in about one-third of the patients with toxin types A or B, and in almost all of the cases involving type E toxin. These symptoms include nausea, vomiting, and abdominal pain. Diarrhea often is present, but constipation also may occur. Symptoms of toxemia then become apparent. No fever occurs in the absence of complicating infections.

Wound Botulism

Wound botulism is a rare disease. The initial event is contamination of a wound by *C botulinum*. The organisms are not invasive and are confined to the necrotic tissue, where they replicate and elaborate the lethal neurotoxin. The incubation time varies from a few days to as long as 2 weeks. The only differences in the symptoms of wound botulism and food poisoning (in addition to a possibly longer incubation time) are that wound botulism lacks gastrointestinal symptoms, and a wound exudate or a fever or both may be present. *C botulinum* may rarely be present in a wound and create no botulism symptoms.

Infant Botulism

In contrast to food poisoning with toxemia caused by ingestion of preformed toxin, infant botulism results from germination of spores in the gastrointestinal tract. Here vegetative cells replicate and release the botulinum toxin. The reasons for spore germination and bacterial replication in the intestine of infants are unclear, but they appear to be related to the composition of the intestinal flora of infants. Almost all reported cases have occurred in infants between 2 weeks and 6 months of age. This is not a new disease, but has been recognized only recently. As of January 1, 1983, there had been over 300 reported hospitalized cases, but many, and perhaps most, cases have not been properly diagnosed or reported. The usual first indication of illness, constipation, is often overlooked. The infant then becomes lethargic and sleeps more than normally. Suck and gag reflexes diminish, and dysphagia often becomes evident as drooling. Later, head control may be lost, and the infant becomes flaccid. In the most severely affected babies, respiratory arrest can occur.

Host Defenses

Host defenses against *C botulinum* are undefined. Some people can tolerate ingestion of botulinum toxin better than others. The reason for this phenomenon is obscure, but could be due to differences in the efficiency of transporting toxin to neural tissue. An attack of botulism does not produce effective immunity. The small amount of toxin in the circulation and its affinity for neural tissue probably prevent adequate amounts of toxin from interacting with the immune system.

Epidemiology

C botulinum is found worldwide in the soil (including sea sediments) and in low numbers in the gastrointestinal tracts of some birds, fish, and mammals. In the United States, the most frequent isolate is type A, followed by B and E, with an occasional isolate of type F. In Europe, B is the most frequent isolate, whereas A is comparatively rare. Despite the worldwide occurrence of *C botulinum* in the environment, wound botulism is a comparatively rare disease.

Originally, botulism food poisoning was thought to be associated only with contaminated meat, especially sausage; however, it is now known that *C botulinum* can grow equally well in most types of food, including vegetables, fish, fruits, and condiments. Home canning using inadequate sterilization techniques has been responsible for most cases of botulism during this century. The toxin is usually produced at pH 4.8-8.5. Acid foods such as canned tomatoes were once thought incapable of containing preformed toxin; however, canned tomatoes have been responsible for several recent cases of botulism food poisoning. In addition, certain culture conditions have been shown to cause toxin production at pH values lower than 4.6. In general, germination of botulinum spores is favored in food kept at warm temperatures under anaerobic conditions for a long period of time at a pH less than 6.

Diagnosis

Although all forms of botulism are difficult to diagnose, prompt diagnosis and treatment are crucial to patient survival. The symptoms of botulism occur in the alimentary tract and the nervous system of the patient and, as a result, many diseases enter into the differential diagnosis, including pharyngitis, gastroenteritis, intestinal obstruction, myasthenia gravis, encephalitis, muscular dystrophy, meningitis, poliomyelitis, cerebrovascular accident, Guillain-Barré's syndrome, chemical food poisoning, and tick paralysis. For infant botulism, additional syndromes enter into the differential diagnosis: failure to thrive, acute infantile polyneuropathy, dehydration, and various hereditary and metabolic disorders. Infant botulism often is missed by physicians, but it always should be considered if any of these symptoms are present.

Although laboratory tests offer little in establishing an initial diagnosis of botulism, the finding of a normal cerebrospinal fluid can help eliminate many of the diseases concerned with central nervous system disorders. In infant botulism, but not in adult botulism, an electromyogram pattern of brief, small-amplitude overabundant motor reaction potentials often is seen.

Confirmation of the initial diagnosis rests on demonstrating toxin in the patient's feces, serum, or vomitus. In adult botulism, serum samples rarely yield type A toxin because of the strong affinity of this toxin for neural tissue. In infant botulism, no toxin of any type has been detected in serum samples. Fecal samples are the best specimens for detecting toxin in infants because only a small percentage of ingested toxin is absorbed through the intestinal mucosa and toxin may be excreted for days or even weeks following botulism food poisoning. Toxin is usually detected by its lethal effect in mice coupled with neutralization of this effect with specific antisera. In infants, the organism can be cultured from the stool.

C botulinum spores exist throughout the environment; all adults have likely ingested these spores with no ill effects. For some infants, the ingestion of such spores can cause poisoning, so obvious sources of such spores should be eliminated from the infant's environment and especially the infant's diet. Honey is the only dietary ingredient that has been implicated, and honey is no longer recommended for infants under 1 year of age. The majority of cases are not caused by ingesting honey, however, so this will not eliminate the disease. The other more common environmental sources of spores, such as soil and dust, are not so easily controlled. There is no evidence for infant-to-infant transmission of *C botulinum*.

Control

The best way to control botulism food poisoning is to use adequate food preservation methods and to heat all canned food before eating. Because botulinum toxin is heat-labile, boiling food for a few minutes will eliminate toxin contamination; however, the spores themselves are not destroyed by boiling and proper canning procedures must be followed to kill clostridial spores.

Once a case of wound botulism or food poisoning has been diagnosed, therapy has four objectives: to eliminate the source of the toxin, to eliminate any unabsorbed toxin, to neutralize any unbound toxin with specific antitoxin, and to provide general supportive care.

Food Poisoning in Adults and Wound Botulism

In food poisoning, the unabsorbed toxin may be eliminated by stomach lavage and high enemas. In wound botulism, debridement and antibiotic therapy with penicillin are used to eliminate the offending organism. Antibiotic therapy is of questionable value in food poisoning, but it is advocated by those who believe the organism can replicate in the intestinal tract of adults.

For both food poisoning and wound botulism, antitoxin therapy is most effective if administered early; however, clear-cut evidence for the efficacy of antitoxin therapy exists for only type E toxin. Antitoxin is available from the CDC in various forms of monovalent, bivalent, and multivalent preparations. Unfortunately, all antitoxins are equine preparations, and a significant percentage of patients experience reactions typical of anaphylaxis and serum sickness. Thus, before they receive antitoxin, all patients should be tested for sensitivity to horse serum. The most important aspect of treatment in botulism is close observation of the patient and availability of adequate facilities for immediate respiratory support. Respiratory failure may occur within minutes, and immediate respiratory assistance often saves the lives of patients with botulism toxemia.

All cases of botulism food poisoning should be reported immediately to local, state, or federal authorities, who will then take steps to minimize the chance of an outbreak. All persons suspected of ingesting contaminated food should be closely observed. Antitoxin should be administered to those with overt symptoms and those who have definitely ingested contaminated food.

Infant Botulism

Treatment for infant botulism is similar to that for adult botulism food poisoning with a few exceptions. Oral antibiotic therapy is not indicated, because it may unpredictably alter the intestinal microecology and allow accidental overgrowth of *C botulinum*. The value of antitoxin therapy in infants still is disputed for the following reasons: antitoxin therapy has not been shown to have a definite therapeutic effect; toxin never has been demonstrated in the serum of infants. The most significant aspect of therapy for infant botulism is supportive care. The infant should be kept under close supervision, with facilities for respiratory support immediately available.

PSEUDOMEMBRANOUS COLITIS AND *CLOSTRIDIUM DIFFICILE*

Distinctive Properties

Diarrhea has come to be accepted as a natural accompaniment of treatment with many antibiotics. Although this diarrhea usually causes only minor concern, it can evolve into a life-threatening enterocolitis. Many antibiotics have been associated with pseudomembranous colitis, including ampicillin, cephalosporins, clindamycin, tetracyclines, and chloramphenicol. Patients treated with clindamycin have a higher incidence of the disease, but most cases are found in patients treated with other antibiotics because of the more widespread use of these agents.

Pseudomembranous colitis is caused by the growth of *C difficile* in the colon. The organism appears unable to compete successfully in the normal colon ecosytem, but can compete when the normal flora are disturbed by antibiotics. During growth, *C difficile* produces two potent toxins. Toxin A is an enterotoxin that causes fluid accumulation in the bowel; toxin B is primarily a cytopathic agent. Both toxins kill experimental animals, and both probably are involved in the pathology of the disease. Cytotoxicity tests on fecal filtrates depend on the neutralization of toxin B activity with antitoxin. Toxin A never has been found in the absence of toxin B, or vice versa.

C difficile is a slender, gram-positive bacillus that produces large, oval, subterminal spores. It is an anaerobe, and some strains are extremely sensitive to oxygen. It is nonhemolytic and does not produce lecithinase or lipase reactions on egg yolk agar. Its proteolytic ability is weak and limited to digestion of gelatin. The products of fermentation are many and complex; they include acetic, butyric, isovaleric, valeric, isobutyric, and isocaproic acids, but only small amounts of each are produced.

Pathogenesis

In pseudomembranous colitis, many of the anaerobic microflora are eliminated by antibiotic therapy, allowing overgrowth of *C difficile*. This organism then replicates and secretes toxins; the resulting pathology is largely limited to the colon. The first symptoms are severe abdominal pain with a watery, nonbloody diarrhea. Leukocytosis is a common laboratory finding, and complications may include intractable colitis, intestinal perforation, and toxic megacolon. Histologically, the colon responds to the toxin by a leukocytic infiltrate into the lamina propria and by elaboration of a mixture of fibrin, mucus, and leukocytes, which form gray, white, or yellow patches on the mucosa. These areas are called pseudomembranes; hence the common term pseudomembranous colitis. Pseudomenbranes usually develop after 4-10 days of treatment, but they may appear 1-2 weeks after all antibiotic therapy has stopped. Mortality is high: 27%–44% of untreated patients with pseudomembranous colitis die. The ultimate cause of death often is difficult to determine, as most patients show a nonspecific deterioration over a period of weeks.

Host Defenses

The toxin of *C difficile* can be neutralized by antitoxin preparations. A formalin-treated toxoid is a good antigen, and high-titered antisera has been raised in rabbits and goats. Host defenses for pseudomembranous colitis are unknown. The role of protective antibody has not been elucidated.

Epidemiology

The incidence of pseudomembranous colitis varies greatly from hospital to hospital. This seems to be due in part to contamination of hospital environments with the spores of *C difficile* and in part to different types of patient populations in various hospitals. Patients with pseudomembranous colitis excrete large numbers of *C difficile* spores; care should be taken not to expose other patients receiving antibiotics. Healthy adults do not carry significant numbers of the organism, but healthy infants may have large numbers of these organisms in their feces. The toxins also are present in these infants' stools, but for unknown reasons appear to have no effect on the infants. The same amounts of toxins are associated with disease in adults.

Diagnosis

Diagnosis of pseudomembranous colitis has required demonstration of the pseudo-membrane by colonoscopy. Most cases of severe diarrhea are not caused by *C difficile* and pseudomembranes are not present in these patients.

C difficile can be isolated from the stools of almost all patients with this disease, and a good selective medium has been developed for this purpose. The isolates should be checked for the production of a cytopathic toxin (toxin B), which can be neutralized with specific antitoxin. Some strains do not produce toxins. The cytotoxicity test also can be done directly on fecal filtrates and yields information on the amount of toxin present. The presence of toxin is not sufficient for diagnosis of pseudomembranous colitis; some patients have toxin present but no colonic involvement.

Control

In most cases, symptoms resolve 1-14 days after antibiotic therapy is discontinued. Vancomycin or metronidazole are the antibiotics of choice. *C difficile* is susceptible to all these agents, but symptoms can reappear when therapy is discontinued. Some patients have had many repeated relapses; fecal enemas can help such patients establish a normal flora. Supportive therapy is needed to compensate for the often severe fluid and electrolyte loss.

OTHER PATHOGENIC CLOSTRIDIA

Food Poisoning and *Clostridium perfringens*

C perfringens is a major cause of food poisoning in the United States. The disease results from ingestion of a large number of organisms in contaminated food, usually meat or meat products. Food poisoning usually does not occur unless the food contains at least 10^6–10^7 organisms per gram. The spores are ubiquitous and, if present in food, can be triggered to germinate when the food is heated. For some heat-sensitive strains, heating is not necessary for germination. After germination, the number of organisms quickly increases in warm food because the generation time can be extremely short (12 minutes) and can encompass a wide temperature range. After the organisms in contaminated food are ingested, they sporulate in the intestine and produce enterotoxin.

C perfringens type A is the usual causative agent, and serotyping is necessary and available for epidemiologic studies. Incubation time is 8–22 hours after ingestion of contaminated food, with a mean of 14 hours. Symptoms include diarrhea, cramps, and abdominal pain. Fever, nausea, and vomiting are rare, and the disease lasts only about 24 hours. The mortality rate is essentially zero, but elderly and immunologically compromised patients should be closely supervised.

Necrotizing Enteritis and *Clostridium perfringens*

Necrotic enteritis in humans has not been well documented. The disease appears to result from ingesting large amounts of food contaminated with *C perfringens*, usually type C. It usually follows ingestion of a large meal, implicating bowel distention and bacterial stasis as contributing factors. The intestinal pathology varies considerably, and may include sloughing of intestinal mucosa, marked inflammation, and hemorrhagic necrosis with gas bubbles in the mucosa, submucosa, and mesenteric lymph nodes. Intestinal perforations occur frequently. The best-documented cases of this disease involve the natives of New Guinea, who develop necrotic enteritis ("pig-bel") after eating large quantities of improperly cooked pork that has been contaminated with the bowel contents of the animal. The course of the disease is fulminant, and the mortality rate is high. Scattered cases of necrotizing enteritis with *C perfringens* as the prominent bacterial isolate have been reported in Western countries. In these cases, controversy exists concerning whether *C perfringens* is a primary invader, an accidental contaminant, or an opportunistic pathogen.

Some evidence suggests that acute necrotizing enterocolitis of infants may be caused by a clostridium, but definitive reports are lacking. This theory is supported by the fact that penumatosis cystoides intestinalis, a syndrome that can be caused by *C perfringens*, often is present in cases of acute necrotizing enterocolitis of infants.

Malignancy and *Clostridium septicum*

C septicum is a spindle-shaped rod that is motile in young cultures. The organism produces toxins designated alpha, beta, gamma, and delta; the alpha toxin is necrotizing and lethal for mice. Whether *C septicum* is a member of the host's normal flora or whether it takes advantage of a compromised host is uncertain. The organism is not strongly invasive, but has been associated with gas gangrene. Interestingly, recent studies correlate *C septicum* bacteremia with the presence of malignancy somewhere in the body. The most frequent association is with colorectal cancer, but other types of malignancies have been noted, including leukemia, lymphoma, and sarcoma. In a survey of *C septicum* bacteremia, 49 of 59 (83%) cases had an underlying malignancy and, in 28 of these cases, the portal of entry appeared to be the distal ileum or the colon. Thus, in the absence of an overt infection, isolation of *C septicum* should alert the physician to the possible presence of a malignancy, most likely in the ileum or the colon. Immediate antibiotic therapy is indicated because most patients die quickly of the infection if not treated. Penicillin is the antibiotic of choice, but chloramphenicol, carbenicillin, and cephalothin also have been used successfully.

Clostridum ramosum

Little, if anything, is known about the pathogenesis of *C ramosum*, but it usually is listed with the ten anaerobic species most frequently isolated from clinical specimens. This frequency suggests that *C ramosum* may have an as yet unrecognized pathogenic significance. *C ramosum* frequently is misidentified, as the Gram reaction is lost easily, and spores are difficult to detect.

References

Arnon, S.S.: Infant botulism, *Ann Rev Med* 1980; 3:541-60.

Finegold, S.M.: *Anaerobic bacteria in human disease.* New York: Academic Press, 1977.

Finegold, S.M., et al.: *Scope monograph on anaerobic infections.* Kalamazoo, Mich.: Upjohn Co., 1972.

George, W.L., et al.: Diarrhea and colitis associated with antimicrobial therapy in man and animals. *Am J Clin Nutr* 1979; 32:251-257.

George, W.L., et al.: Selective and differential medium for isolation of *Clostridium difficile. J Clin Microbiol* 1979; 9:214-219.

Gorbach, S.L., Bartlett, J.G.: Colitis associated with clindamycin therapy. Pseudomembranous enterocolitis: a review of its diverse forms. *J Infect Dis* 1977; 135:S89-S94.

Holdeman, L.V., Cato, E.P., Moore, W.E.C., (editors): *Anaerobic laboratory manual,* 4th ed. Blacksburg: V.P.I. Anaerobic Laboratory, Virginia Polytechnic Institute and State University, 1977.

Koransky, J.R., Stargel, M.D., Dowell, V.R.: *Clostridium septicum* bacteremia, its clinical significance. *Am J Med* 1979; 66:63-66.

Lyerly, D.M., et al.: Effects of *Clostridium difficile* toxins given intragastrically to animals. *Infect Immunol* 1985; 47:349-352.

Richardson, S.A., Alcock, P.A., Gray, G.: *Clostridium difficile* and its toxin in healthy neonates. *Br Med Q* 1983; 287:878-879.

Schwan, A.: Relapsing *Clostridium difficile* enterocolitis cured by rectal infusion of homologous feces. *Lancet* 1983; 2:845.

Smith, I.D.S.: *Botulism. The organism, its toxins, the disease.* Springfield, Ill.: Charles C Thomas, Publisher, 1977.

Sullivan, N.M., Pellet, S., Wilkins, T.D.: Purification and characterization of toxins A and B of *Clostridium difficile. Infect Immun* 1982; 35:1032-1040.

35 Anaerobic Cocci

Susan E.H. West, MS
Tracy D. Wilkins, PhD

General Concepts
Distinctive Properties
Pathogenesis
Host Defenses
Epidemiology
Diagnosis
Control

General Concepts

Anaerobic cocci are opportunistic pathogens that cause a multitude of infections. They are part of the normal microbial flora of a healthy individual, but they can and do cause infections involving traumatized tissue or infections in the compromised host. They are isolated most often from a wide variety of polymicrobic infections (usually along with *Bacteroides* sp or with facultative organisms or both), indicating a synergistic role in these infections. Approximately 10%-15% of all isolates of anaerobic cocci come from pure culture infections, thus indicating that these organisms can be significant pathogens rather than innocuous commensals. The anaerobic cocci represent 25%-30% of all anaerobic clinical isolates; among anaerobes, they are second only to the gram-negative anaerobic bacilli in frequency of isolation from clinical specimens. Anaerobic cocci are part of the normal flora of the skin, the mouth, and the intestinal and genitourinary tracts of healthy individuals.

Distinctive Properties

Pathogenic anaerobic cocci belong to the genera *Peptococcus, Peptostreptococcus, Streptococcus,* and *Veillonella*. In the past, these organisms received little attention and usually were referred to only as anaerobic streptococci, anaerobic staphylococci, or microaerophilic streptococci. Today, because of an increased awareness of their pathogenic potential and of improved methods for culturing and identifying anaerobic bacteria, microbiologists often identify the anaerobic cocci according to species. The pathogenic anaerobic cocci and their incidence of isolation from clinical specimens are listed in Table 35-1.

The anaerobic cocci are a physiologically diverse group. Both gram-negative and gram-positive species exist. Not all anaerobic cocci require stringent anaerobic conditions; for example, strains of *Streptococcus intermedius* are quite aerotolerant and may grow under reduced oxygen tension. Anaerobic cocci may be proteolytic or saccharolytic or both. They produce a variety of short-chain volatile fatty acids (for example, acetic, propionic, butyric, caproic, and lactic acids) from the fermentation of simple sugars and amino acids. Both *Peptococcus magnus* and *Peptostreptococcus anaerobius* possess species-specific cell wall antigens; in other anaerobic cocci, species-specific antigens have not yet been identified.

The anaerobic cocci have received little attention from microbiologists and clinicians; consequently, it is not known if these organisms produce toxins, capsules, or have other pathogenic attributes.

Pathogenesis

Anaerobic cocci are not involved in any single specific disease process; rather, they may be present in a great variety of infections involving all areas of the human body. These infections may range in severity from mild skin abscesses, which disappear sponta-

Table 35-1   Species of Anaerobic Cocci Isolated from Clinical Specimens

Species	Incidence* (% of anaerobic isolates)
Peptococcus asaccharolyticus	2–6
P magnus	6–12
P prevotii	2–5
P saccharolyticus	0.3
Peptostreptococcus anaerobius	3–4
P micros	2
P parvulus	0.5
P productus	1
Streptococcus constellatus	1.5
S intermedius	3–4
S morbillorum	2
Veillonella parvula	0.5–2

*Data compiled from Holland, J.W., Hill, E.O., Altemeier, W.A.: *J Clin Microbiol* 1977; 5:20; Wren, M.W., et al.: *J Med Microbiol* 10:49; and Applebaum, P.C., Holloway, Y., Hallett, A.F.: *S Afr Med J* 1976; 50:1435.

neously after incision and drainage, to more serious and life-threatening infections such as brain abscess, bacteremia, necrotizing pneumonia, and septic abortion. Infection by anaerobic cocci (and by anaerobes in general) usually involves invasion of devitalized tissue by organisms that are part of the normal flora of the affected tissue or of the surrounding areas.

Brain abscess, with a mortality rate of 40%, is one of the more serious infections involving anaerobic cocci. Anaerobes, rather than facultative or aerobic organisms, are a major cause; anaerobic cocci, *Bacteroides* and *Fusobacterium,* respectively, are the predominant groups isolated. Anaerobic cocci often have been isolated in pure culture from brain abscesses. Chronic otitis media or mastoiditis frequently is the primary source of the organisms and results as a direct extension of the infection into the brain. Pleuropulmonary infection, sinusitis, congenital heart defects, and bacterial endocarditis are other conditions predisposing to brain abscess by blood-borne metastases.

Pleuropulmonary infections in which anaerobic cocci may be etiologic agents are lung abscesses, necrotizing pneumonia, aspiration pneumonitis, and empyema. The incidence of anaerobes in these infections is 50%–90%; anaerobic cocci account for about 40% of the anaerobic isolates. *F nucleatum* and *B melaninogenicus* are often isolated concomitantly. These organisms are part of the normal microbial flora of the mouth and enter the lower respiratory tract as the result of aspiration, usually in association with altered consciousness. Anaerobic pleuropulmonary infections frequently develop slowly and often are chronic. The mortality rate is about 15%.

Anaerobic cocci are involved in several skin and soft tissue infections that may be confused with clostridial myonecrosis (gas gangrene). These infections are anaerobic streptococcal myonecrosis, progressive bacterial synergistic gangrene, necrotizing fasciitis, crepitant cellulitis, chronic burrowing ulcer, and synergistic necrotizing cellulitis. These are severe infections, and the mortality rates may be as high as 75%. These conditions may be characterized by a purulent exudate, by varying degrees of tissue necrosis involving the skin, fascia, and/or underlying muscles, and sometimes by systemic toxicity. The infecting organisms often produce gas. Anaerobic cocci often are isolated with other organisms in these infections. They are characteristically found with *Staphyloccoccus aureus* and *Streptococcus pyogenes* in progressive bacterial synergistic gangrene, and also are found with gram-negative aerobic or facultative bacilli or *Bacteroides* or both in synergistic nonclostridial myonecrosis and synergistic necrotizing cellulitis. Diabetes mellitus and vascular insufficiency (often associated with trauma) are predisposing factors. Decubitus ulcers and postoperative wound infections are other soft-tissue infections from which anaerobic cocci have been isolated.

Anaerobic cocci have been recognized as significant pathogens in puerperal fever and septic abortion since the early 1900s. Other infections of the female genital tract in which anaerobic cocci have been implicated are pyometra, tuboovarian abscesses, postoperative wound infections following gynecologic surgery, and pelvic inflammatory disease, often in association with gonococci. Anaerobic cocci (notably *P prevotii, P anaerobius and S intermedius*) and *B fragilis* are the most frequently isolated anaerobes from these infections. Like the anaerobic cocci in other infections, these organisms are part of the normal flora of the affected area or of the surrounding tissues—in this case, the vagina.

Peritonitis, intraabdominal abscesses, and abscesses of the liver, spleen, and pancreas are types of intraabdominal infections from which anaerobic cocci have been isolated. *P prevotii and P anaerobius* are the species isolated most frequently. Again, these are polymicrobic infections; concomitant isolates may be *Bacteroides* sp, *E coli* and *Streptococcus* sp.

Recently, with increasing study of the anaerobic cocci as pathogens, certain species are being associated with specific types of infection. As noted above, *P prevotii* and *P anaerobius* are associated with female genital tract and intraabdominal infections. *P magnus*, the most frequently isolated anaerobic coccus, is associated most often with chronic bone and joint infections and ankle ulcers. Pure cultures of this organism are not rare; they account for 15% of all *P magnus* isolates. The presence of foreign bodies, such as prosthetic joints, seems to be particularly significant in *P magnus* infections.

Veillonella and the anaerobic *Streptococcus* are the anaerobic cocci isolated most frequently from infected human bites. These organisms are part of the normal oral flora.

Host Defenses

P magnus infection (in pure culture) of hip prostheses has produced serum antibody response; however, in most cases, specific immune responses to anaerobic cocci have not been investigated.

Epidemiology

Anaerobic infections generally occur in the compromised host; that is, in patients who have impaired host defense mechanisms. The primary host defense deficiency in these infections is the disruption of natural barriers (such as the skin and mucous membranes). Diabetes mellitus, connective tissue disorders, atherosclerotic disease, cancer (especially of the colon, uterus, and lung), irradiation damage, immunosuppressive treatment, and alcoholism are conditions that may disrupt these natural barriers.

Diagnosis

To establish a definite role for anaerobic cocci in infections, the causative organism must be isolated from the affected tissue or the bloodstream. Because anaerobic cocci are a significant part of the normal flora, the proper choice of specimen is critical. For example, coughed sputum, feces, and vaginal swabs, all of which could be contaminated with normal microbial flora, are unacceptable.

Sodium polyanethol sulfonate, a common anticoagulant in blood culture media, inhibits the growth of *P anaerobius;* however, this inhibitory effect can be reversed by including 1.2% gelatin in the medium. Therefore, an appropriate choice of blood culture system is essential when specimens are obtained for anaerobic blood cultures.

Procedures for isolating and identifying the anaerobic cocci are outlined in the Virginia Polytechnic Institute *Anaerobe Laboratory Manual* and the *Wadsworth Anaerobic Bacteriology Manual*. Definitive species identification requires determination of the metabolic end products by gas-liquid chromatography; however, inhibition of *P anaerobius* by sodium polyanethol sulfonate can be used for a presumptive identification of this organism. *Veillonella* can be presumptively identified by the red fluorescence of colonies under ultraviolet light. This fluorescence is lost rapidly on exposure to oxygen.

Control

Treatment of infections caused by anaerobic cocci consists of antibiotic therapy and drainage, debridement, or both of necrotic tissue. In general, penicillin is the drug of choice, and clindamycin is used for the patient allergic to penicillin; however, the clinician should be aware that in vitro antimicrobial susceptibility tests have shown that some strains of anaerobic cocci are resistant to penicillin or to clindamycin. In a study by Sutter and Finegold, 3% of the peptostreptococci tested were resistant to 8 units/mL or greater of penicillin; 14% of the peptococci tested were resistant to 8 μg/mL of clindamycin. Brain abscesses must be treated with an antimicrobial agent such as chloramphenicol or penicillin or both, sufficient doses of which can cross the blood barrier. Frequently *B fragilis*, an anaerobic gram-negative rod, is present in infections containing anaerobic cocci; this organism produces a β-lactamase that can protect other organisms in the infection from the action of penicillin.

References

Bourgault, A.M., Rosenblatt, J.E., Fitzgerald, R.H.: Peptococcus magnus: A significant human pathogen. *Ann Intern Med* 1980; 93:244-248.

Brook, I., Walker, R.I.: Pathogenicity of anaerobic gram-positive cocci. *Infect Immunol* 1984; 320-324.

Finegold, S.M.: *Anaerobic bacteria in human disease.* New York: Academic Press, 1977.

Finegold, S.M. et al.: Management of anaerobic infections. *Ann Intern Med* 1975; 83:375-389.

Holdeman, L.V., Cato, E.P., Moore, W.E.C.: *Anaerobe laboratory manual,* 4th ed. Blacksburg, Va.: Anaerobe Laboratory, Virginia Polytechnic Institute and State University, 1977.

Lambe, D.W., Jr., Vroon, D.H., Rietz, C.W.: Infections due to anaerobic cocci. In: *Anaerobic bacteria; role in disease.* Balows, A. (editor). Springfield, Ill.: Charles C Thomas, 1974.

Sutter, V.L., Citron, D.M., Finegold, S.M.: *Wadsworth anaerobic bacteriology manual,* 3rd ed. St. Louis: The C.V. Mosby Co., 1980.

Tabaqchali, S.: Rapid techinques for the identification of anaerobic bacteria and presumptive diagnosis. *Scand J Infect Dis* [Suppl] 1982; 35:23-30.

Taylor, A.G., et al.: Infection of total hip prostheses by *Peptococcus magnus,* an immuno-fluorescence and ELISA study of two cases. *J Clin Pathol* 1979; 32:61-65.

36 *Bacteroides* and *Fusobacterium*

Sydney M. Finegold, MD

General Concepts
Distinctive Properties
Pathogenesis
Host Defenses
Epidemiology
Diagnosis
Control

General Concepts

Bacteroides and *Fusobacterium* are genera of gram-negative anaerobic bacilli prevalent in the body as normal flora and involved in various infections throughout the body. These organisms constitute one-third of the total anaerobic isolates from clinical specimens. Within the *Bacteroides* group, *B fragilis* is the most commonly encountered pathogen, followed by *B thetaiotaomicron*. Among the bile-sensitive *Bacteroides* sp, those most commonly encountered clinically are *B melaninogenicus*, *B asaccharolyticus*, and *B ruminicola*. *Fusobacterium nucleatum* is the most commonly encountered member of the genus *Fusobacterium*, but *F necrophorum*, although encountered much less commonly, may produce serious disease. Numerous other species exist in both genera, but these cause infection in humans less frequently or never.

Gram-negative anaerobic bacilli may cause any type of infection throughout the body: those most commonly encountered are pleuropulmonary, intraabdominal, and female genital tract infections (Table 36-1). In addition, gram-negative anaerobic bacilli may play a role in such diverse pathologic processes as periodontal disease and colon cancer. *Bacteroides* and *Fusobacterium* produce enzymes (collagenase, neuraminidase, DNase, heparinase, and proteinases) that may play a role in pathogenesis in that they

Table 36-1 Common Syndromes of Anaerobic Infections

Bite infections	Septicemia with
Oral infection	Malignancy
Aspiration pneumonia	Diabetes
Postabortal and puerperal infections	Corticosteroids
Infections following	"Negative" blood cultures
Bowel and gallbladder surgery	Septic thrombophlebitis
Gynecologic surgery	Gas-forming infections
	Putrid infections

may allow the organisms to penetrate tissues and to set up infection after surgery or other trauma. The incidence of infection by these organisms can best be reduced or eliminated by avoiding conditions that decrease the redox potential of tissues and by preventing introduction of the anaerobes into compromised host tissues.

Distinctive Properties

B fragilis (Figure 36-1), the most important of all anaerobes because of its frequency of occurrence in clinical infection and its resistance to antimicrobial agents, is a gram-negative bacillus with rounded ends 0.5–0.8 μm in diameter and 1.5–4.5 μm long. Most strains are encapsulated. Vacuolization or irregular staining is common, particularly in broth media. A certain degree of pleomorphism also may be seen, particularly in broth media. By electron microscopy, the ultrastructure of *B fragilis* is similar to that of other gram-negative bacteria. The guanine plus cytosine content is 42%. *B melaninogenicus* and *B asaccharolyticus* are short-to-coccoid gram-negative rods; they produce a distinctive pigment (brown to black), which is a heme derivative that colors the colony (Figures 36-2 and 36-3). *B asaccharolyticus* is encapsulated. Many strains of *B melaninogenicus* require Vitamin K, or similar compounds, as well as heme. Other *Bacteroides* are encountered much less commonly.

Numerous studies of the endotoxin of gram-negative anaerobic bacilli have determined that in the case of *B fragilis*, the endotoxin contains no lipid A,

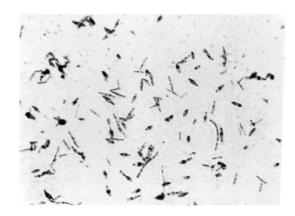

Figure 36-1 Microscopic morphology of *B fragilis* from broth culture. Note irregular staining, rounded ends of bacilli, and some pleomorphism. From Finegold, S.M., and Miller, L.C. Susceptibility to antibiotics as an aid in classification of gramnegative anaerobic bacilli. In *Les Bactéries Anaérobies,* Fredette, V. (ed.). Montreal: Institut Armand-Frappier, 1967.

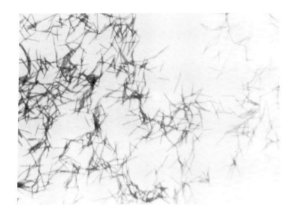

Figure 36-2 Microscopic morphology of *F nucleatum* from broth culture. Note regular staining, and thin, delicate bacilli with tapered ends. Organisms are sometimes found end to end.

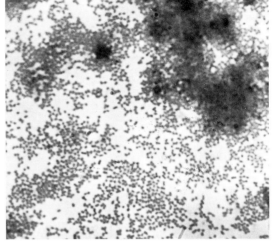

Figure 36-3 Microscopic morphology of *B melaninogenicus*. Organisms are tiny coccobacilli that stain regularly.

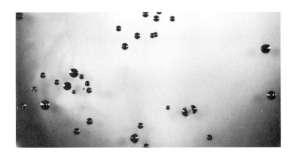

Figure 36-4 Colonial morphology of *B melaninogenicus*. Note jet black pigmented colonies.

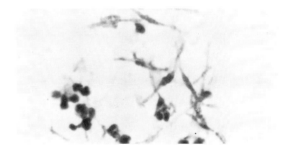

Figure 36-5 Microscopic morphology of *F mortiferum* from broth culture. Note filaments with swollen central portions, large round bodies, and irregular staining. From Finegold, S.M., and Miller, L.C. Susceptibility to antibiotics as an aid in classification of gramnegative anaerobic bacilli. In *Les Bactéries Anaérobies*, Fredette, V. (ed.). Montreal: Institut Armand-Frappier, 1967.

2-ketodeoxyoctanate, or heptose. It also lacks β-hydroxymyristic acid. This endotoxin exhibits little biologic activity in various test systems and little chemotactic activity; what is shown is complement-dependent, using the alternate pathway. Poor biologic activity of endotoxin also has been demonstrated for the closely related species *B thetaiotaomicron*, *B ovatus*, *B vulgatus*, and *B distasonis*. *B asaccharolyticus* also does not have any β-hydroxymyristic acid, and its endotoxin is impotent biologically. *B melaninogenicus* endotoxin contains no heptose or 2-ketodeoxyoctanate, and it and the endotoxin of *B oralis* both show weak biologic activity. Serologic methods have not been reliable for characterizing strains of *Bacteroides*.

Members of the genus *Fusobacterium* (Figures 36-4 and 36-5) may be spindle-shaped or may have parallel sides and rounded ends. Guanine plus cytosine ratios range from

26%-34%. Cells of *F necrophorum* often are elongated or filamentous, curved, and possess spherical enlargements and large, free, round bodies. *F nucleatum*, although not producing infections as serious as those caused by *F necrophorum*, is encountered much more commonly clinically. The cells of this species are usually spindle-shaped, are 5-10 μm long, and are often seen in pairs, end to end.

The lipopolysaccharide of *F necrophorum* is located in a multilayered external coat in the organism. The endotoxin varies from strain to strain in content of 2-ketodeoxyoctanate and sugars. Although biologic activity varies also, many or most strains do show strong biologic activity, comparable to that of *Salmonella enteritidis*. The endotoxin of *F nucleatum* also is variable in its biologic activity, but often exhibits strong activity, comparable to that of *S enteritidis*.

Bacteriophages active against *B fragilis* are not uncommon. They are species-specific and active against most strains. Bacteriocins also are produced by strains of *B fragilis* and *B thetaiotaomicron*. Plasmids have been found in about half of *Bacteroides* strains studied. For the most part, the biologic and clinical significance of these plasmids is not known; however, some have been found to code for resistance to such antimicrobial agents as clindamycin, erythromycin, tetracycline, chloramphenicol, ampicillin, and cephalothin. Antibiotic resistance that is plasmid-mediated has been transferred from strains of *B fragilis* to other strains of this species, to *B thetaiotaomicron*, and to *E coli*. Such resistance also has been transferred from *B distasonis* to *B fragilis*.

Most strains of the *B fragilis* group can deconjugate bile acids and are equally active whether the bile acid is conjugated with glycine or with taurine. Rarely, *B melaninogenicus* may deconjugate bile acids, but in general this species, *B oralis*, and *F nucleatum* are inhibited by bile acids and do not deconjugate them. *F necrophorum* also is active in deconjugating bile acids but is active primarily on taurine conjugates. A few nonspeciated strains of *Bacteroides* can convert primary bile acids to secondary bile acids. *B thetaiotaomicron* can convert some lithocholic acid to its ethyl ester. Because lithocholic acid is toxic in humans and has been shown to exert tumor-promoting activity in animals, this reaction may be important. *B fragilis* has been demonstrated to hydrolyze the conjugated metabolites of benzopyrene. Glucuronidase produced by anaerobic gram-negative bacilli may be of special significance in deconjugating compounds that had previously been detoxified in the liver by combination with glucuronide. There is speculation that this enzyme may be important in promoting bowel cancer. The activity of *B thetaiotaomicron*, *B distasonis*, and other members of the *B fragilis* groups against plant polysaccharides, chondroitin and mucin may be a factor in colon cancer and other disorders. Dietary fiber consists primarily of plant cell wall polysaccharides that are not digested in the stomach or small bowel.

Certain *Bacteroides* sp possess distinguishing enzymes. Superoxide dismutase has been found in *B fragilis*, *B thetaiotaomicron*, *B vulgatus*, and *B ovatus*. In general, a good correlation exists between superoxide dismutase activity and oxygen tolerance. No relationship has been found between catalase activity and oxygen tolerance, however. β-lactamase activity has been demonstrated in several species of *Bacteroides;* it accounts for their resistance to various β-lactam antibiotics such as penicillins and cephalosporins. Urease is produced by *B ureolyticus (B corrodens)*. This organism also produces an agarase, which accounts for pitting of the agar by the colonies. A related pitting organism, *B gracilis*, is much pathogenic and is relatively resistant to antimicrobial agents.

Pathogenesis

Bacteroides and *Fusobacterium* are prevalent as indigenous flora on all mucosal surfaces. They may have an opportunity to penetrate tissues and then to set up infection under certain circumstances such as surgical or other trauma, or when tumors arise at the mucosal surface. In certain cases, such as aspiration pneumonia, anaerobic bacteria from a site of normal carriage may move into another area that is normally free of organisms and infect that site. Tissue necrosis and poor blood supply lower the oxidation-reduction potential, thus favoring the growth of anaerobes. Accordingly, vascular disease, cold, shock, trauma, surgery, foreign bodies, malignancy, edema, and gas production by bacteria may significantly predispose to infection with anaerobes, as may prior infection with aerobic or facultative bacteria. Antimicrobial agents such as aminoglycosides, to which anaerobes are notably resistant, may facilitate anaerobic infection. Conditions predisposing to anaerobic infection are summarized in Table 36-2. The more aerotolerant anaerobes are more likely to survive after the normally protective mucosal barrier is broken and until conditions are satisfactory for their multiplication and invasion. Once anaerobes begin to multiply, they can maintain their own reduced environment by excreting end products of fermentative metabolism. Infections involving *Bacteroides* and *Fusobacterium* often are characterized by abscess formation and tissue destruction, as are most anaerobic infections.

Bacteroides and *Fusobacterium* produce enzymes that may play a role in pathogenesis. *B melaninogenicus* is one of the few bacteria that produce collagenase, an enzyme of considerable importance. Strains of *B melaninogenicus* with high collagenolytic activity produced more acute infection when combined with an anaerobic vibrio than did strains with weak collagenolytic activity. Cell-free extracts of strains of *B melaninogenicus* with collagenolytic activity, when given with a live *Fusobacterium* species, produced more

Table 36-2   Conditions Predisposing to Anaerobic Infection

General	Malignancy
Diabetes	Colon, uterus, lung
Corticosteroids	Leukemia
Leukopenia	Gastrointestinal and female pelvic surgery
Hypogammaglobulinemia	Gastrointestinal trauma
Immunosuppression	Human and animal bites
Cytotoxic drugs	Aminoglycoside therapy
Splenectomy	
Collagen disease	
Decreased redox potential	
Tissue anoxia	
Tissue destruction	
Aerobic infection	
Foreign body	
Calcium salts	
Burns	
Peripheral vascular insufficiency	

severe lesions in rabbits than the organism or the extract given alone. Neuraminidase may be important in the pathogenesis of infection caused by *Bacteroides*. This enzyme alters neuraminic acid-containing glycoproteins of human plasma; strains of *Bacteroides* isolated from clinical specimens have higher neuraminidase activity than those isolated from stools, and strains of *B fragilis* groups have greater activity of this type than do other species of *Bacteroides*. Hyaluronidase is produced by many strains of the *B fragilis* and *B melaninogenicus* groups. Deoxyribonuclease is also produced by *B fragilis* and may be an important factor in infection. Many *Bacteroides* produce phosphatase. A heparinase produced by *B fragilis* strains may contribute to intravascular clotting and increases the dosage requirement for heparin in treating septic thrombophlebitis in infections caused by this organism. The lipopolysaccharides of *B fragilis*, *B vulgatus*, and *F mortiferum* activate Hageman factor and thereby initiate the intrinsic pathway of coagulation. Fibrinolysin is produced by many *B melaninogenicus* group strains and by a few *B fragilis* group strains. *B asaccharolyticus* produces proteinases that render it capable of hydrolyzing gelatin, casein, coagulated protein, plasma protein, azacol, and collagen. A strain of *B melaninogenicus* has been shown to produce phospholipase A.

F necrophorum produces a leukocidin and hemolyses red blood cells of humans, horses, rabbits, and, much less extensively, sheep and cattle. Certain *F necrophorum* cells hemagglutinate the red blood cells of humans, chickens, and pigeons. A bovine isolate of *F necrophorum* demonstrated phospholipase A and lysophospholipase activity. *F gonidiaformans* produces an appreciable inflammatory reaction when inoculated into the skin of rabbits; when injected intraperitoneally into mice, it leads to liver abscesses and occasionally death. A specific toxin has not yet been isolated.

Other factors may be involved in the continued growth and potential pathogenicity of certain anaerobes. For example, *B melaninogenicus* can inhibit the growth of certain other organisms. Also, anaerobes such as *B melaninogenicus* sometimes may inhibit phagocytosis and killing of other organisms during mixed infection. The capsule of organisms such as *B fragilis* may be an important virulence factor. The mechanism by which the capsule may enhance virulence remains to be determined, but it is interesting to note that *B fragilis* strains adhere to rat peritoneal mesothelium better than do unencapsulated species of *Bacteroides*.

Host Defenses

Polymorphonuclear leukocytes have oxygen-dependent and oxygen-independent microbicidal systems. Components of both systems might be important in phagocytic killing of anaerobes under conditions of varying oxygen tension. Specifically, polymorphonuclear leukocytes normally kill *B fragilis* under anaerobic and aerobic conditions. Random migration of polymorphonuclear leukocytes does not differ significantly under aerobic and anaerobic conditions. The same holds true for chemotaxis in response to factors generated by immune complexes in plasma; however, chemotaxis in response to factors generated by bacteria in plasma is markedly depressed under anaerobic conditions.

Studies of host defenses indicate various other interactions may occur between the bacteria and the host's cells. *B fragilis*, one organism utilized in the chemotaxis study described above, is more resistant to the normal bactericidal activity of serum than are other members of the *B fragilis* group. *F mortiferum* is killed by serum alone or by serum plus white blood cells under aerobic and anaerobic conditions. Under anaerobic conditions, *B thetaiotaomicron* and *B fragilis* are phagocytosed and killed intracellularly by human polymorphonuclear leukocytes only in the presence of normal human serum. Similar results are obtained in an aerobic environment, except that *B fragilis* is phagocytosed and killed intracellularly to some extent in the absence of serum. There is evidence that the capsule of certain *Bacteroides* interferes with their phagocytosis.

Immunoglobulin and components of the classical and alternate complement pathways participate in chemotaxis, bacteriolysis, and opsonophagocytic killing of various gram-negative anaerobic bacilli. Antibody to the capsular polysaccharide of *B fragilis* can be induced in animals by infection with encapsulated strains or by implantation of the capsular material itself along with outer membrane components that stimulate antibody response. Such immunization of animals confers significant protection against subsequent abscess development from *B fragilis* strains. Furthermore, a study of women with acute pelvic inflammatory disease demonstrated antibody to the capsular antigen of *B fragilis* in those women whose infecting flora contained *B fragilis;* antibody was quantified by precipitin analysis. Immunodiffusion techniques have also been used on trichloroacetic acid extracts from *B fragilis* in detecting precipitating antibodies against this organism in sera of immune rabbits. Data indicate that more than one serotype exists.

F necrophorum has been demonstrated to persist for an extended period in the liver, where its proliferation in Küpffer cells impairs macrophage function.

There is also evidence that T cells may be involved in immunity to *B fragilis* in humans.

Epidemiology

All infections involving anaerobic gram-negative bacilli arise endogenously when mucosal damage related to surgery, other trauma, or disease permits tissue penetration by indigenous flora. Knowledge of the indigenous flora at various sites under different circumstances permits the clinician to anticipate the likely infecting flora in acute infections in different locations. Pathogenicity of various species also must be taken into account. Ecologic determinants include oxygen sensitivity of various organisms, ability of organisms to adhere (discussed on page 289), and microbial interrelationships. These interrelationships permit one organism to supply growth factor needed by another, to provide assistance with adherence or motility to another organism, and to facilitate production of inhibitory substances.

At birth, an infant's oral cavity usually is sterile; but by 12 months of age, *Fusobacterium* sp can be cultured from 50% of infants and *Bacteroides* from a smaller percentage. In the human gingival crevice area, gram-negative anaerobic rods account for 16%-20% of the total cultivable flora. *B melaninogenicus* is seldom isolated before the age of 6 years, but by the early teens this organism can be isolated from the gingival crevice area of most individuals. In the presence of acute ulcerative gingivitis or advanced chronic periodontal disease, counts of *Fusobacterium* in saliva are higher than the usual 10^4-10^6/mL. Gram-negative anaerobic rods usually constitute from 8%-17% of the cultivable flora of human dental plaque. Selective localization is illustrated by the fact that *B melaninogenicus* is found routinely in the gingival crevice but is not found, or is only rarely found, on the tongue, cheek, or coronal tooth suface.

The stomach normally has few organisms and, as a rule, no anaerobic bacteria; however, in the presence of pathologic conditions such as duodenal ulcer with bleeding or obstruction, abnormal colonization with *B fragilis* may occur in the stomach. In the terminal ileum, approximately equal numbers of facultative aerobes and anaerobes are present, with *Bacteroides* being one of the major anaerobes. *Bacteroides* are almost invariably found in the feces of adult subjects; the mean count is 10^{11}/g. *Fusobacterium* is found in 18% of adults; the mean count is 10^8/g. *B thetaiotaomicron* and *B vulgatus* are the dominant species of *Bacteroides* encountered, followed by *B distasonis*, *B ovatus*, and *B fragilis*. Note that in animal studies, *Bacteroides* protects against infection with *Salmonella* or *Shigella*.

Bacteroides and *Fusobacterium* commonly have been found in the vaginal flora. In one quantitative study of vaginal and cervical flora, *Bacteroides* sp were recovered from one-half of the patients, with mean concentrations of 10^6/g of material. Species of *Bacteroides* recovered from the normal cervical flora of healthy women include *B oralis*, *B fragilis*, *B capillosus*, *B bivius*, *B disiens*, *B ruminicola*, and *B ureolyticus*.

Studies of normal urethral flora are relatively limited, but various *Fusobacterium* and *Bacteroides* sp have been isolated. Fusiform bacilli and *B melaninogenicus* have been found regularly on the external genitalia.

Bacteroides placed on the forearms of human volunteers may persist for a few hours; strains placed on laboratory benches may survive even 10 hours after exposure to air, and *Bacteroides* has been recovered from the hospital environment on occasion. Clearly, however, the source of infection with these organisms is the indigenous flora of the body, particularly of mucosal surfaces.

Diagnosis

The clinical characteristics of infection with *Bacteroides* or *Fusobacterium* are primarily those seen with anaerobes in general. These characteristics include foul odor of the discharge, location of infection in proximity to mucosal surfaces, tissue necrosis, gas in tissues or discharges, association of infection with malignancy, infection related to the use of aminoglycosides, septic thrombophlebitis, infection following human or animal bites, and certain distinctive clinical features. The clinical presentation of *F necrophorum* sepsis may be distinctive in that onset is characterized by sore throat and fever often accompanied by chills. A membranous tonsillitis with foul odor to the breath may be noted, and in the absence of effective therapy, bacteremia and widespread metastatic infection will occur. Black discoloration of blood-containing exudates or red fluorescence under ultraviolet light of such exudates indicates infection with *B melaninogenicus* or *B asaccharolyticus*.

Definitive diagnosis requires demonstrating or isolating the organisms responsible for the infection. Even direct Gram stain may be helpful because of the frequently unique morphology of gram-negative anaerobic bacilli. In general, these organisms are pale staining, and they may stain erratically. *Fusobacterium* may exhibit classical tapered ends and filamentous forms, with or without swollen areas and large round bodies. Direct gas-liquid chromatography of clinical specimens occasionally provides important clues to the presence of certain gram-negative anaerobic bacilli. Large amounts of butyric acid in the absence of isobutyric or isovaleric acid indicate the presence of *Fusobacterium* sp. The presence of succinic acid and only gram-negative rods seen on Gram stain indicates *Bacteroides*. Both succinic and isobutyric acid in the specimen indicates that *Bacteroides* is present. Several studies indicate that both direct and indirect fluorescent antibody techniques may be useful for rapid detection of *Bacteroides* and *Fusobacterium* in clinical material. False-positive reactions may be a problem on occasion. Reagents are available commercially; they will undoubtedly be improved. Use of selective and differential media may facilitate isolation and identification of different members of *Bacteroides* and *Fusobacterium*. Tests for antibody development in response to the infection are not practical.

Control

There are two primary guidelines in preventing anaerobic infections: avoiding conditions that reduce the redox potential of the tissues and preventing introduction of anaerobes of the normal flora to wounds, closed cavities, or other sites prone to infection. Prophylactic antimicrobial therapy is effective in selected situations. Patients with acute leukemia who are to be treated intensively with antitumor chemotherapy may be managed with a diet low in bacterial count and administration of an antimicrobial regimen designed to reduce significantly the total body flora, including anaerobes. Some workers have advocated using antibacterial regimens that are relatively inactive against anaerobes; as a result, anaerobes persist in the bowel and provide colonization resistance against potential aerobic or facultative pathogens.

Anaerobic bacteremia following dental manipulation may be managed effectively by administering an agent such as penicillin 1 hour before the manipulation and continuing for a limited period (12-24 hours) afterward. The effectiveness of prophylactic antimicrobial therapy before bowel surgery is now well established. The physician may use oral neomycin plus erythromycin or oral neomycin plus tetracycline, giving the regimen for a limited time just before surgery to prevent overgrowth of other organisms. Prophylaxis also is effective before certain types of gynecologic surgery. When infection already is established but surgery is indicated (appendectomy, cholecystectomy), antimicrobial therapy just before surgery again may be helpful. Appropriate therapy of established infections such as chronic otitis media and sinusitis may prevent subsequent spread of infection that could lead to intracranial abscess. Precautions to minimize aspiration are helpful in preventing anaerobic pulmonary infection. Care must be observed in feeding feeble or confused patients and patients who have difficulty swallowing. Good surgical technique minimizes the risk of postoperative infection. Minimizing injury and devitalization of tissue during the course of surgery protects against infection. The use of closed methods of bowel resection, when feasible, decreases the likelihood of infection with bowel flora.

Table 36-3 indicates the relative effectiveness of a number of drugs against *Bacteroides* and *Fusobacterium*. Aminoglycosides such as gentamicin and amikacin are generally inactive against most anaerobes. The activity of erythromycin varies significantly according to the testing procedure. Erythromycin and vancomycin are not currently approved by the Food and Drug Administration for anaerobic infections.

Table 36-3 Antimicrobial Susceptibility of *Bacteroides* and *Fusobacterium†*

	Antimicrobial Agent*						
	Peni-cillin	Chloram-phenicol	Clinda-mycin	Erythro-mycin	Tetra-cycline	Metroni-dazole	Vanco-mycin
B fragilis group	1	3	2–3	1–2	1–2	3	1
B melaninogenicus-asaccharolyticus group	2–3	3	3‡	2–3	2	3	1
F varium	2–3	3	1–2	1	2	3	1
Other Fusobacterium sp	4	3	3	1	3	3	1

*4, drug of choice; 3, good activity; 2, moderate activity; 1, poor or inconsistent activity.
†Only drugs that might be used therapeutically are included; not all these agents are routinely used clinically for anaerobic infections and not all are FDA approved.
‡A few strains are resistant.

Most penicillins and cephalosporins are less active than penicillin G; unfortunately, increasing numbers of anaerobes are showing resistance to penicillin, usually on the basis of β-lactamase production. Ampicillin, carbenicillin, and penicillin V are roughly comparable to penicillin G on a weight basis, but the high blood levels safely achieved with carbenicillin and similar penicillins make them effective against 95% of the strains of *B fragilis*. Cefoxitin, a compound resistant to penicillinase and cephalosporinase, is active against 95% of *B fragilis* group strains. Cefamandole is active against most anaerobes other than those in the *B fragilis* group. The third generation cephalosporins are all less active than cefoxitin against the *B fragilis* group. Doxycycline and minocycline are more active than other tetracyclines, but susceptibility testing is indicated to ensure activity.

In addition to antimicrobial therapy, surgical therapy is important in treating anaerobic infection. Surgical therapy includes drainage of abscesses, excision of necrotic tissue, relief of obstruction, ligation or resection of infected veins, and, occasionally, other forms of surgery. Percutaneous nonsurgical drainage may be effective in certain patients. Lung abscess, which responds well to medical therapy, is the primary exception to the rule that abscesses require surgical drainage.

Hyperbaric oxygen therapy is not of value in infections due to *Bacteroides* or *Fusobacterium*. General supportive measures are, of course, important in managing any type of serious infection. Anticoagulation may be useful in patients with septic thrombophlebitis, along with appropriate antimicrobial therapy.

As noted previously, *B fragilis* is the most resistant of all anaerobes to antimicrobial agents. In part, this is related to β-lactamase production by *B fragilis* and related strains, but other mechanisms of resistance exist as well. *B gracilis* is often resistant to penicillins and cephalosporins (including piperacillin and cefoxitin) and to clindamycin. Plasmid-mediated transferable resistance to several antimicrobial agents has been demonstrated with *B fragilis* and related *Bacteroides*. Numerous other species of *Bacteroides* also produce β-lactamases. Chloramphenicol acetyltransferase has been demonstrated in a strain of *B fragilis*, but the clinical significance of this finding has not been evaluated yet. Among the fusobacteria, the primary organism manifesting resistance is *F varium*. Many strains of this species are resistant to clindamycin, and a number are resistant to penicillins and cephalosporins; however, chloramphenicol and metronidazole are active against this organism.

References

Finegold, S.M.: *Anaerobic bacteria in human disease.* New York: Academic Press, 1977.

Finegold, S.M., George, W.L., Rolfe, R.D., (editors): International symposium on anaerobic bacteria and their role in disease. *Rev Infect Dis* 1984; 6(Supp. 1): March–April.

Holdeman, L.V., Cato, E.P., Moore, W.E.C.: *Anaerobe laboratory manual,* 4th ed. Blacksburg, Va.: Virginia Polytechnic Institute and State University, 1977.

Kasper, D.L., Finegold, S.M., (editors): Virulence factors of anaerobic bacteria (Symposium). *Rev Infect Dis* 1979; 1:March–April.

Rosebury, T.: *Microorganisms indigenous to man.* New York: McGraw-Hill Book Co., 1962.

Smith, L., DS.: *The pathogenic anaerobic bacteria,* 2nd ed. Springfield, Ill.: Charles C Thomas, 1975.

Sutter, V.L., Citron, D.M., Finegold, S.M.: *Wadsworth anaerobic bacteriology manual,* 3rd ed. St. Louis: The C.V. Mosby Co., 1980.

37 *Salmonella*

Ralph A. Giannella, MD

General Concepts
Distinctive Properties
Pathogenesis
Host Defenses
Epidemiology
Diagnosis
Control

General Concepts

Salmonellae are ubiquitous human and animal pathogens, and salmonellosis, a disease that infects an estimated 2 million Americans each year, is common throughout the world. Salmonellosis usually occurs in humans as a self-limiting form of food poisoning (gastroenteritis), but may also produce serious systemic infections requiring prompt antibiotic treatment. In addition, salmonellosis causes substantial losses in livestock, poultry, dairy, and food-processing industries.

The pathogenesis of salmonellosis involves both invasion of the intestinal mucosa and production of toxin. Some evidence indicates that inflammatory bowel disease involves both an adenylate-cyclase–activating enterotoxin and a protein-synthesis-inhibiting cytotoxin.

The genus *Salmonella*, one of six major divisions of the family Enterobacteriaceae, is composed of approximately 1800 serotypes. Because of the large number of serotypes, the genus has been classified in various ways. Table 37-1 presents a simple classification of salmonellae that emphasizes ecologic features. In this scheme, all salmonellae are divided into three "species." Salmonellosis is a major public health problem because of

Table 37-1   Ecologic Classification of Salmonellae*

Species	Representative Serotype	Host Preferences
S *choleraesuis*	One only	Animals (swine)
S *typhi*	One only	Humans
S *enteritidis*	Paratyphi-A	Humans
	Schottmuelleri	
	Pullorum	Animals (fowl)
	Dublin	Animals (cattle)
	Typhimurium	
	Derby	
	Enteritidis	Humans and
	Heidelberg and	many animals
	hundreds of	
	related sero-	
	types	

*Adapted from Grady GF, Keusch GT. *N Engl J Med* 1971; 285:831-842.

its large and varied animal reservoir, the existence of human and animal carrier states, and the lack of a concerted nationwide program to control salmonellae.

Distinctive Properties

Salmonellae are gram-negative, flagellated, facultatively anaerobic bacilli possessing three major antigens: H, or flagellar antigen; O, or somatic antigen; and V antigen (possessed by only a few serotypes). H antigen may occur in either or both of two forms called phase 1 and phase 2. The organisms tend to change from one phase to the other. O antigens occur on the surface of the outer membrane and are determined by specific sugar sequences on the cell surface. Vi antigen is a superficial antigen overlying the O antigen; it is present in a few serotypes, the most important being *S typhi*.

Antigenic analysis of salmonellae using specific antisera offers clinical advantages. Determination of antigenic structure is used to identify clinically the organisms and assign them to one of nine serogroups (A-I). H also provides a useful epidemiologic tool to investigate outbreaks of salmonellosis and to determine the infection's source and mode of spread.

As with other gram-negative bacilli, the cell envelope of salmonellae contains a complex lipopolysaccharide structure that is liberated on lysis of the cell and, to some extent, during culture. The lipopolysaccharide moiety may function as an endotoxin, and may be important in determining virulence of the organisms. This micromolecular endotoxin complex consists of three components, an outer O-polysaccharide coat, a middle portion, or R core, and an inner lipid A coat. Lipopolysaccharide structure is important for several reasons. First, the nature of the repeating sugar units in the outer O-polysaccharide chains is responsible for O antigen specificity; it may be a determining factor of the organism's virulence, as well. Salmonellae lacking the complete sequence of O-sugar repeat units are called **rough** because of their rough appearance; they are usually avirulent or less virulent than the **smooth** strains that possess a full complement of O-sugar repeat units. Second, antibodies directed against the R core (common enterobacterial antigen) may protect against infection with a wide variety of gram-negative bacteria sharing a common core structure, or may moderate their lethal effects. Third, the endotoxin component of the cell wall may play an important role in the pathogenesis of many clinical manifestations of gram-negative infections. Endotoxins evoke fever, activate the serum complement, kinin, and clotting systems, depress myocardial function, and alter lymphocyte function, among other functions. Circulating endotoxin may be in part responsible for many of the manifestations of septic shock that can occur in systemic infections (see Chapter 22).

Pathogenesis

Salmonellosis is manifested in several syndromes (gastroenteritis, enteric fever, septicemia, focal infections, and carrier state). Particular serotypes show a strong propensity to produce one or the other of these syndromes (*S typhi, S paratyphi-A,* and *S schottmuelleri* produce enteric fever; *S choleraesuis,* septicemia or focal infections; *S typhimurium* and *S enteritidis,* gastroenteritis); however, on occasion, any serotype can produce any of various syndromes. In general, more serious infections occur in infants, in adults over the age of 50, and in subjects with debilitating illnesses.

Most nontyphoidal salmonellae enter the body when contaminated food is ingested. In addition, person-to-person spread of salmonellae may occur. After ingestion, the organisms colonize the ileum and colon, invade the intestinal epithelium, and then proliferate within the epithelium and lymphoid follicles. The mechanism by which salmonellae invade the epithelium is not understood, but may involve the process of endocytosis or pinocytosis (Figure 37-1). The ability of salmonellae to invade cells may be determined by a 60-megadalton plasmid; loss of this plasmid results in loss of virulence. The organisms then spread to mesenteric lymph nodes and throughout the body via the systemic circulation, and are taken up by the reticuloendothelial cells. The reticuloendothelial system confines and controls spread of the organism; however, depending on the serotype and the effectiveness of the host defenses against that serotype, some organisms may infect the liver, spleen, gallbladder, bones, meninges, and other organs. Fortunately, most serotypes of salmonellae are killed promptly in extraintestinal sites, and the most common human *Salmonella* infection, gastroenteritis, is an infection confined to the intestine.

After invading the intestine, most salmonellae induce an acute inflammatory response, which occasionally can cause ulceration. Salmonellae may elaborate cytotoxins that can inhibit protein synthesis. Whether these cytotoxins contribute to the development of the inflammatory response or to ulceration is not known. Because of the intestinal inflammatory reaction, symptoms of inflammation such as fever, chills, abdominal pain, leukocytosis, and diarrheal stools, which may contain polymorphonuclear leukocytes, blood, and mucus, are seen frequently.

Much is now known about the mechanisms of salmonellae-caused gastroenteritis and diarrhea. Figure 37-2 summarizes the pathogenesis of *Salmonella* enteritis and diarrhea. Only strains of salmonellae that penetrate the intestinal mucosa are associated

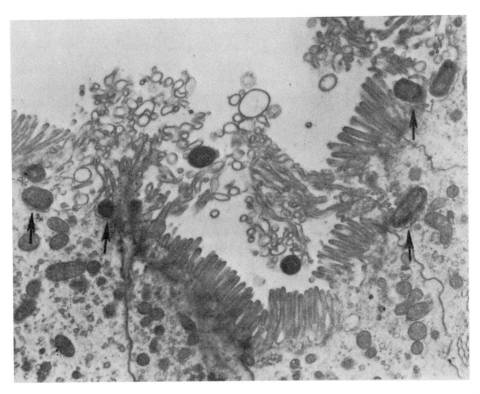

Figure 37-1 Electron photomicrograph demonstrating invasion of guinea pig ileal epithelial cells by *Salmonella typhimurium.* Arrows point to invading *Salmonella* organisms. (Courtesy Akio Takeuchi, Walter Reed Army Institute of Research, Washington, D.C.)

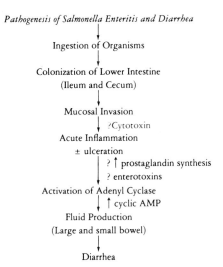

Figure 37-2 Pathogenesis of *Salmonella* enteritis and diarrhea.

with the appearance of an acute inflammatory reaction and diarrhea. After invasion, the small and large intestines secrete fluid and electrolytes, resulting in diarrhea. The mechanisms involved in secretion of salt and water are unclear, but this secretion is not merely a manifestation of tissue destruction and ulceration. Invasion of the intestinal mucosa is followed by activation of mucosal adenylate cyclase; the resultant increase in cyclic AMP induces secretion. The mechanism by which adenylate cyclase is stimulated is not understood; it may involve local production of prostaglandins by the inflammatory reaction. In addition, strains of salmonellae have been reported to elaborate a choleralike toxin that may function as an enterotoxin. However, the precise role of this exotoxin in the pathogenesis of *Salmonella* enterocolitis and diarrhea has not been established.

Host Defenses

Various host defenses are important in resisting intestinal colonization and invasion by *Salmonella*. Normal gastric acidity (pH < 3.5) is lethal to salmonellae. In healthy individuals, the number of ingested salmonellae are reduced in the stomach, so that fewer organisms enter the intestine than are ingested. Normal small intestinal motility also protects the bowel by "sweeping" ingested salmonellae through quickly. Normal intestinal microflora protect against salmonellae, probably through anaerobes, which liberate short-chain fatty acids that are thought to be toxic to salmonellae. Alterations of intestinal anaerobes by antibiotics render the host more susceptible to salmonellosis. Secretory or mucosal antibodies also are thought to protect the intestine against salmonellae. Animal strains genetically resistant to intestinal invasion by salmonellae have been described. These and other factors thought to be involved in host defense against salmonellosis are listed in Table 37-2. When these host defenses are absent or blunted, the host becomes more susceptible to salmonellosis; factors or conditions that render the host more susceptible to salmonellosis are listed in Table 37-3. The role of host defenses in salmonellosis is extremely important, and much remains to be learned.

Table 37-2 Host Defenses Against Salmonellae

Gastric Factors
Gastric acidity
Rate of gastric emptying
Intestinal Factors
Intestinal motility
Normal intestinal flora
Mucus
Secretory antibodies
Genetic resistance to invasion
Nonspecific and Other Possible Factors
Nutritional state
Lactoferrin
Gut reticuloentothelial cells
Lysozyme

Table 37-3 Factors Increasing Susceptibility to Salmonellosis

Stomach
Achlorhydria
Gastric Surgery
Intestine
After antibiotics
After gastrointestinal surgery
? Idiopathic inflammatory
   bowel disease
Hemolytic Anemias
Especially sickle cell anemia and
   other hemoglobinopathies
Impaired Systemic Immunity
Carcinomatosis, leukemias, lymphomas
Immunosuppressive drugs and others

Epidemiology

Contaminated food is the major mode of transmission for nontyphoidal salmonellae because salmonellosis is a zoonosis and has an enormous animal reservoir. The most common animal reservoirs are chickens, turkeys, pigs, and cows; dozens of other domestic and wild animals also harbor these organisms. Because of the ability of salmonellae to survive in meats and animal products that are not thoroughly cooked, animal products are the main vehicle for salmonellosis. The magnitude of the problem is demonstrated by the following recent examples: 41% of turkeys examined in California, 50% of chickens cultured in Massachusetts, and 21% of commercial frozen egg whites examined in Spokane, Washington, yielded salmonellae.

The epidemiology of typhoid fever and the other *Salmonella*-caused enteric fevers primarily involves person-to-person spread because these organisms lack a significant animal reservoir. Contamination with human feces is the major mode of spread, and the usual vehicle is contaminated water. Occasionally, contaminated food (usually handled by an individual who harbors *S typhi*) may be the vehicle of infection. Plasmid fingerprinting and phage lysotyping of *Salmonella* isolates have proved to be powerful epidemiologic tools for studying outbreaks of salmonellosis and tracing the spread of the organisms in the environment.

In typhoid fever and nontyphoidal salmonellosis, two other factors have epidemiologic significance. First, an asymptomatic human carrier state exists for the agents of either form of the disease. Approximately 3% of persons infected with *S typhi* and 0.1% of those infected with nontyphoidal salmonellae become chronic carriers. The duration of the carrier state may vary from many weeks to years. Thus, human as well as animal reservoirs exist. Interestingly, children rarely become chronic typhoid carriers. Second, use of antibiotics in animal feeds, and indiscriminant use of antibiotics in humans, increase antibiotic resistance in salmonellae by promoting transfer of R factors.

Diagnosis

Diagnosis of salmonellosis requires bacteriologic isolation of the organisms from the appropriate clinical specimen. Laboratory identification of the genus *Salmonella* is done by biochemical tests; the serologic type is confirmed by serologic testing. Feces, blood, or other specimens should be plated on several nonselective and selective agar media (blood, MacConkey, eosinmethylene blue, bismuth sulfite, *Salmonella-Shigella*, and brilliant green agars) as well as into enrichment broth such as selenite or tetrathionate. Any growth occurring in enrichment broth is subsequently subcultured onto the various agars. Biochemical reactions on triple sugar iron agar (TSI) and lysine-iron agar (LIA) of suspicious colonies is then determined, and a presumptive identification is made. Recently, biochemical identification of salmonellae has been simplified by systems that permit the rapid testing of 10-20 different biochemical parameters simultaneously. The presumptive biochemical identification of *Salmonella* then can be confirmed by antigenic analysis of O and H antigens using polyvalent and specific antisera. Fortunately, approximately 95% of all clinical isolates can be identified with the available group A-E typing antisera. *Salmonella* isolates then should be sent to a central or reference laboratory for more comprehensive serologic testing and confirmation.

Control

Salmonellae are difficult to eradicate from the environment; however, because the major reservoir is poultry and livestock, reducing the number of organisms harbored in these animals would significantly reduce human exposure. In Denmark, for example, all animal feeds are treated to kill salmonellae before distribution, resulting in a marked reduction in salmonellosis. Other helpful measures include altered and improved animal slaughtering practices to reduce cross-contamination of animal carcasses; more attention to protection of processed foods; training and education in hygienic practices of all food-handling personnel in slaughterhouses, food processing plants, and restaurants; adequate cooking and refrigeration of foods in food processing plants, restaurants, and homes; and continuation and expansion of governmental enteric disease surveillance programs.

Vaccines are available for typhoid fever and are partially effective, especially in children. No vaccines are available for nontyphoidal salmonellosis. Continued research in this area as well as increased understanding of the mechanisms of immunity to enteric infections is of great importance.

General salmonellosis treatment measures include replacing fluid loss by oral and intravenous routes, and controlling pain, nausea, and vomiting. Specific therapy consists of antibiotic administration. Typhoid fever and enteric fevers should be treated with antibiotics; chloramphenicol is the drug of choice. In nontyphoidal salmonellosis, antibiotic therapy should be reserved for the septicemic, enteric fever, and focal infection syndromes. In uncomplicated *Salmonella* gastroenteritis, antibiotics are not recommended, because they do not shorten the illness, and they do significantly prolong the fecal excretion of the organisms and increase the number of antibiotic-resistant strains.

References

Aserkoff, B., Schroeder, S.A., Brachman, P.S.: Salmonellosis in the United States—A five year review. *Am J Epidemiol* 1970; 92:13-24.

Black, P.H., Kunz, L.J., Swartz, M.N.: Salmonellosis—a review of some unusual aspects. *N Engl J Med* 1960; 262:811-817, 864-870, 921-927.

Brunner, F., et al.: The plasmid pattern as an epidemiologic tool for *Salmonella typhimurium* epidemics: Comparison with the lysotype. *J Infect Dis* 1983; 148:7-11.

Committee on Salmonella: *An evaluation of the salmonella problem.* Washington, D.C.: Division of Biology and Agriculture of the National Research Council, 1969.

Ewing, W.H., Martin, W.J.: Enterobacteriaceae. In: *Manual of clinical microbiology,* 2nd ed. Lennette, E.H., Spaulding, E.H., Truant, J.P., (editors). Washington, D.C.: American Society of Microbiology, 1974.

Finkelstein, R.A., et al.: Isolation and characterization of a cholera-related enterotoxin from *Salmonella typhimurium. FEMS Microbiol Lett* 1983; 17:239-241.

Giannella, R.A., Broitman, S.A., Zamcheck, N.: Influence of gastric acidity on bacterial and parasitic enteric infections: A perspective. *Ann Intern Med* 1973; 78:271-276.

Jones, G.W., et al.: Association of adhesive, invasive, and virulent phenotypes of *Salmonella typhimurium* with autonomous 60-megadalton plasmids. *Infect Immun* 1982; 38:476-486.

Koo, F.C.W., Peterson, J.W.: Cell-free extracts of salmonella inhibit protein synthesis and cause cytotoxicity in eukaryotic cells. *Toxicon* 1983; 21:309-320.

Rubin, R.H., Weinstein, L.: *Salmonellosis: microbiologic, pathologic and clinical features.* New York: Stratton Intercontinental Medical Book Corp, 1977.

38 *Shigella*

Samuel B. Formal, PhD
Gerald T. Keusch, MD

General Concepts
Distinctive Properties
Pathogenesis
Host Defenses
Epidemiology
Diagnosis
Control

General Concepts

Bacillary dysentery and the other clinically recognizable enteric diseases (cholera and typhoid) have taken their greatest toll among humans living in crowded, unsanitary conditions. Most vulnerable are those unable to practice good personal hygiene, children under 10 years of age, the malnourished, and those taking part in military campaigns. Gram-negative, facultative anaerobes of the genus *Shigella* are the principal causative agents of bacillary dysentery. Dysentery differs from diarrheal diseases with profuse watery stool, such as cholera, in that the dysenteric stool is scant and contains blood, mucus, and many inflammatory cells. Many individuals suffering from infections with shigellae, however, experience only diarrhea instead of dysentery. The broad designation shigellosis is used to describe the disease that occurs in patients infected with dysentery bacilli.

Recent concepts of shigellosis pathogenesis may explain these two distinct clinical syndromes (diarrhea and dysentery). The shigella organisms produce a toxin in vitro that induces secretion of fluid in the small intestine of experimental animals. This enterotoxin may be responsible for the watery diarrheal syndrome of the naturally occurring disease. In contrast, dysentery is a large intestine manifestation and is associated with bacterial invasion of colonic epithelial cells. The dual clinical presentation of shigellosis thus correlates with distinctive organ abnormalities caused by different pathogenic properties of the dysentery bacillus. Host defenses against shigellosis include gastric acidity and completion of the shigellae with normal intestinal bacteria; however, the susceptibility of these bacteria to killing by phagocytes in intestinal tissue is important in limiting the spread of the bacteria. Shigellosis should be suspected in any patient with dysentery or diarrheal disease. The diagnosis can be confirmed by culture. The best method of controlling shigellosis is to develop safe water supplies and an effective system of feces disposal.

Distinctive Properties

Organisms of the genus *Shigella* belong to the tribe Eshericheae in the family Enterobacteriaceae. They are gram-negative, nonmotile, nonspore-forming rods and are able to grow with or without oxygen. All shigellae ferment glucose and, except for some isolates of *S flexneri* type 6, are anaerogenic; that is, they do not produce gas. None ferment lactose, except for *S sonnei* strains, which do so slowly.

As with other gram-negative organisms, shigellae have a heat-stable toxin (endotoxin) in their cell walls. Polysaccharide side chains, a constituent part of the endotoxin in smooth shigellae, confer immunologic specificity on the organisms and are the basis for serologic typing. For many years, *S dysenteriae* type 1 (Shiga's bacillus) has been known to produce a heat-labile exotoxin in addition to its heat-stable endotoxin. Peripheral paralysis and death occur when this heat-labile toxin is injected into mice or rabbits; for this reason, the toxin has been called a neurotoxin. *Shigella* toxin differs from other classical neurotoxins such as tetanus and botulinum toxins in that its primary site of action appears to be not on nerve cells but on the vasculature of the gray matter of the central nervous system. Preparations with neurotoxin activity inhibit protein synthesis and are highly toxic for some cultured human cell lines; these preparations also are enterotoxic, inducing intestinal fluid secretion in suitable laboratory models. Serotypes of shigellae other than *S dysenteriae* type 1, as well as other members of the family Enterobacteriaceae, have been shown to elaborate a shigalike toxin, but these strains produce the toxin in much smaller amounts than does *S dysenteriae* type 1.

Pathogenesis

Individuals are infected orally with shigellae. The incubation period usually is less than 4 days. Individuals exhibiting signs of illness show histologic changes in the colon that may include a range of lesions varying from a mild acute inflammatory reaction to microulcers or gross ulceration and generalized sloughing of the epithelium. Damage to the terminal ileum has been reported, but these observations have been made at autopsy and undoubtedly represent extreme cases. Lesions of the stomach also have been noted on occasion in humans and monkeys, but their significance is not known.

The lesion, which occurs with varying severity in the colon, is initiated by penetration of the pathogen into the mucosal epithelial cells and causes cell death

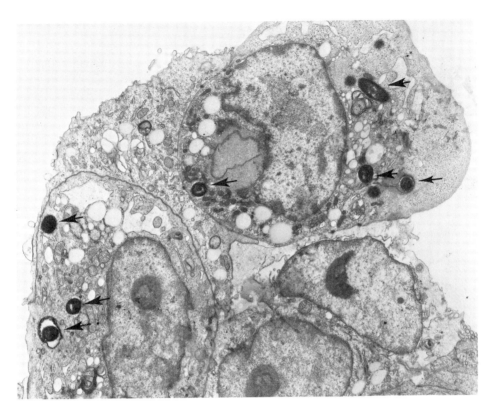

Figure 38-1 Surface colonic epithelium of rhesus monkey 48 hours after oral infection with *S flexneri*. Epithelial cells are being shed into the intestinal lumen. Intraepithelial bacteria (arrows) are enclosed by host membranes or lie free in the cytoplasm. Changes in epithelial cells include loss of microvilli, vacuolization of endoplasmic reticulum, and accumulation of liquid droplets. (×5400.) (Courtesy A. Takeuchi.)

(Figure 38-1). Organisms then spread to adjacent epithelial cells, killing these cells, eroding the epithelium, and ultimately forming ulcers. The role of shigalike toxin in cell death is presently being investigated. Shigellae that enter the lamina propria are rapidly phagocytized and killed. Organisms rarely reach the submucosa or the mesenteric lymph nodes and although bacteremia occurs, it too is infrequent. The ability of dysentery bacilli to penetrate the intestinal epithelial cell is essential to the organism's capacity to cause disease. *Shigella* enteritis may be differentiated from *Salmonella* enteritis by distribution of the lesions they produce: *Shigella* lesions occur in the colon and rarely in the ileum; *Salmonella* lesions commonly occur in the small intestine as well as in the colon.

Physiologic as well as histologic changes occur in the *Shigella*-infected colon. Disruption of the normal motor function of the intestine causes cramps and tenesmus. Fever is thought to be evoked by the action of pyrogens released into the blood from the inflammatory reaction, and endotoxin may be responsible for triggering various combinations of vascular collapse, shock, microangiopathic hemolytic anemia, renal cortical necrosis and, finally, death. Watery diarrhea may be observed in many patients, usually early in the infectious process, and indeed may be the only enteric manifestation of the disease. Studies in rhesus monkeys show that the diarrhea fluid is secreted from the proximal small intestine. This secretion takes place in the absence of any evidence of invasion or histologic change in the jejunum, suggesting that the *S dysenteriae* type 1-like toxin may play a role in the diarrheal phase of the disease; however, more work is required to confirm this hypothesis. The fact that this toxin is elaborated in large amounts by strains of *Escherichia coli* associated with hemorrhagic colitis gives further support to the concept that the toxin is involved in the disease process.

Host Defenses

Gastric acid is considered a first line of defense against enteric pathogens. Although this has been shown to be the case with *Vibrio cholerae* (see Chapter 40), gastric acidity does little to defend against *Shigella* infections. Intestinal secretions, especially bile, also inhibit growth of many microorganisms, but these secretions have little effect on shigellae. A third host defense mechanism is the inhibitory effect of the normal colonic flora on the growth of organisms entering the large intestine. Evidence for this comes from studies that demonstrate an exogenous organism's difficulty in colonizing the intestine of a normal host and its comparative ease of colonization of a gnotobiotic host or of one whose bowel flora is altered by pretreatment with antibiotics.

Type-specific antibody, locally produced and secreted on the mucosal surface, is considered a fourth level of protection against infection. The evidence for such protection in shigellosis is only suggestive, based on the observation that oral vaccines protect against invasion and disease, whereas parenterally administered products are ineffective. A final line of defense, readily apparent following penetration of the mucosa by the pathogen, consists of phagocytic cells in the lamina propria. Shigellae entering the lamina propria are rapidly phagocytized and killed by inflammatory cells; viable organisms rarely spread to the submucosa, the mesenteric lymph nodes, or to the bloodstream. This contrasts with *Salmonella* infections, in which spread to peripheral lymphoid tissue is commonly observed (see Chapter 37). An important role for humoral antibody, other than its possible function in phagocytosis in the lamina propria, has not been demonstrated.

Epidemiology

Shigellosis is distributed worldwide, but its hosts are limited to human beings and subhuman primates. In contrast to many other enteric pathogens, relatively few shigellae are required to initiate clinical disease in healthy human adults. Ten organisms have caused disease in 10% of challenged volunteers, and fewer than 200 shigellae produced illness in 40% of individuals receiving this dose. Although food and water contaminated with organisms from an infected host are common vehicles for the spread of shigellosis, direct person-to-person contact always must be considered as a means of transmission because of the low infectious dose.

All age groups are susceptible to infection with dysentery bacilli; however, 60% of the reported cases in the United States occur in children between the ages of 1 and 10 years. The disease tends to be more severe in children below 4 years of age, and to be highly prevalent in childrens' institutions, mental hospitals, prisons, Native American populations, and among economically disadvantaged or malnourished people. Although there are over 30 serotypes of shigellae, usually only two or three prevail in any given region. Interestingly, *S sonnei* is the most prevalent serotype in developed regions of the world such as northwestern Europe, Japan, and the United States, having replaced *S flexneri* in the past two decades.

Diagnosis

Any person with diarrhea and fever should be suspected of having shigellosis. Mild forms of the disease cannot be distinguished clinically from watery diarrheal disease caused by other microorganisms. In more severe forms of the disease, in which blood is present in the stool, suspicions may be stronger that the cause is *Shigella*. Loose stools containing mucus tinged with bright red blood are uncommon in salmonellosis and do not occur in diarrheal disease caused by enterotoxigenic bacteria. Although blood is common in the stools of patients with amebiasis, it is frequently dark brown rather than bright red as in *Shigella* infections. Furthermore, although ulcers are observed on sigmoidoscopic examination in shigellosis and amebiasis, the generalized inflammation of the mucosa in shigellosis is not common in amebiasis. Nausea and vomiting, uncommon features of shigellosis, often are observed when nontyphoidal salmonellae and enterotoxigenic organisms are the etiologic agents.

Although clinical signs of illness may offer significant information, diagnosis of shigellosis must be made by isolating and identifying the causative agent from feces. Best results are obtained when fecal specimens are taken during the acute phase of the disease. Although rectal swabs passed beyond the anal sphincter may secure adequate samples, freshly passed stool specimens are superior because they can be examined for blood-tinged plugs of mucus, which provide the best source for isolating shigellae.

Note that once a fecal specimen is collected, it must be processed rapidly by the laboratory. If any delay is anticipated, the sample should be deposited into a holding medium. Although processing stools for the purpose of isolating and identifying enteric pathogens differs in detail from laboratory to laboratory, the same general procedure is followed. The specimen is streaked onto Petri dishes containing inhibitory, differential media that inhibit growth of gram-positive organisms and distinguish lactose-fermenting from non–lactose-fermenting organisms. Two kinds of media usually are employed: (a) MacConkey agar or eosin methylene blue agar, which permit the growth of most enterobacteriaceae, (b) *Salmonella-Shigella* (SS) agar, xylose-lysine-desoxycholate (XLD) agar, or Hektoen enteric (HE) agar, which inhibit the growth of most coliforms but allow the propagation of shigellae and salmonellae. A tube of Hajna's gram-negative (GN) broth also is inoculated with a portion of the stool and, following incubation for 6-8 hours, is streaked onto the same media used for the direct plating of the fecal specimen. The gram-negative broth is an enrichment medium for many shigellae. Following overnight incubation at 37 C, lactose-negative colonies are transplanted from the primary plating media to slants containing a medium such as triple sugar iron (TSI) agar.

Next, isolates that give a typical *Shigella* reaction (alkaline slant/acid butt with no bubbles of gas for TSI agar) may be tested in shigellae grouping and typing sera. Positive serologic tests and characteristic reactions on media such as TSI agar slants may be considered as presumptive identification of *Shigella*, but additional biochemical tests are required for definitive identification of an unknown isolate. Usually, correct identification of *Shigella* poses no difficulty. In some instances, however, *E coli* isolates closely resemble *Shigella*. This is especially so with *E coli* strains that cause a dysenterylike disease (see Chapter 42). These *E coli* organisms may be nonmotile and anaerogenic (producing little or no gas); they may fail to ferment lactose or do so slowly; and they may even have cross-reacting or identical somatic antigens with *Shigella*. Nevertheless, they may be differentiated from *Shigella* on the basis of their ability to ferment mucate, to decarboxylate lysine, and to grow on sodium acetate agar (Table 38-1).

Control

The most effective method of controlling shigellosis and many other intestinal infections is to develop a safe water supply and an effective means of feces disposal. When a clinical case is detected, rigorous precautions must be taken to prevent cross-contamination. Because of the low numbers of organisms needed to initiate an infection, asymptomatic carriers also constitute a major source of infection. Parenterally administered vaccines are not effective in preventing the disease, and although the value of live attenuated oral vaccines has been shown, further development is necessary before these vaccines can be used routinely. The prophylactic use of antibiotics has no demonstrated benefit.

The first consideration in treating shigellosis or other diarrheal diseases is correction of the patient's hydration abnormalities. The rapidly rising fever that often results in convulsions in the young must be treated symptomatically. The advantage of employing antibiotics to treat shigellosis has been debated. Because the disease is generally self-limiting, concern has existed that the use of these drugs might alter the intestinal flora to the detriment of the patient. However, appropriate antibiotics reduce the duration of illness from an average of 5 days in untreated patients to an average of 3 days in treated individuals. Treatment also has the added beneficial effect of reducing the

Table 38-1   Differentiation of Shigellae from *E coli*

	S dysenteriae	*S flexneri*	*S boydii*	*S sonnei*	*E coli*
Gas from glucose	−	−*	−	−	+
Glucose	+	+	+	+	+
Lactose	−	−	−	−†	+
Mannitol	−	+	+	+	+
Lysine decarboxylase	−	−	−	−	+
Ornithine decarboxylase	−	−	−	+	+
Mucate	.−	−	−	−	+
Sodium acetate	−	−	−	−	+
Motility	−	−	−	−	+
Serogroup	A	B	C	D	N.A.
Serotypes	1–10	1–6	1–15	2‡	N.A.

*Some strains of *S flexneri*-6 produce gas from glucose.
†*S sonnei* usually ferment lactose slowly.
‡*S sonnei* form I (virulent) dissociates to *S. sonnei* form II (avirulent).

number of days a patient excretes the pathogen after signs of illness subside, and this may reduce the secondary cases within families that commonly occur in shigellosis. This is in contrast to salmonellosis, in which treatment may prolong carriage. Shedding of dysentery bacilli for a period of weeks is not uncommon in untreated individuals, and occasionally an individual may excrete shigellae for more than one year. Life-long carriers of shigellae, however, have not been observed. Excreters of the organism obviously may endanger their close contacts.

The choice of antibiotics for treatment must be made carefully. Absorbable drugs such as ampicillin or tetracycline are effective, but oral nonabsorbable products such as neomycin are not. Because tetracycline is now contraindicated in children of the age group most susceptible to shigellosis, and because the organisms are often resistant in vitro, trimethoprim-sulfamethoxazole is most often used as an alternative to ampicillin. Effective treatment has been complicated by the emergence of single and multiple drug-resistant strains, usually a consequence of plasmid acquisition. Thus, knowledge of patterns of resistance in a community is invaluable as an aid in determining therapeutic choices, and constant surveillance to monitor changes in resistance profiles is necessary.

Drugs that inhibit intestinal peristalsis are commonly prescribed in the treatment of shigellosis; however, in addition to their effect on bowel motility, they may prolong fever and diarrhea and may extend the time the patients shed shigellae. Moreover, megacolon is a recognized complication of the use of these motility-altering drugs. These agents should thus be used only in such selected cases as threatened rectal prolapse.

References

Barada, F.A., Jr., Guerrant, R.L.: Sulfamethoxazole-trimethoprim versus ampicillin in treatment of acute invasive diarrhea. *Antimicrob Agents Chemother* 1980; 17:961-964.

Black, R.E., Gram, G.F., Blake, P.E.: Epidemiology of common source outbreaks of shigellosis in the United States, 1961-1975. *Am J Epidemiol* 1978; 108:47-52.

Edwards, P.R., Ewing, W.H.: *Identification of Enterobacteriaceae*, 3rd ed. Minneapolis: Burgess Publishing Co, 1972.

Keusch, G.T.: Shigella infections. *Clin Gastroenterol* 1979; 8:645-662.

Keusch, G.T., Donohue-Rolfe, A., Jacewicz, M.: Shigella toxin(s): Description and role in diarrhea and dysentery. *J Pharmacol Therapeut* 1982; 15:403-438.

Keusch, G.T., Jacewicz, M.: The pathogenesis of shigella diarrhea. VI. Toxin and anti-toxin in *Shigella flexneri* and *Shigella sonnei* infections in humans. *J Infect Dis* 1977; 135:552-556.

Korzeniowski, D.M., et al.: Value of examination for fecal leukocytes in the early diagnosis of Shigellosis. *Am J Trop Med Hyg* 1979; 28:1031-1035.

Koster, F., et al.: Hemolytic-uremic syndrome after shigellosis. Relation to endotoxemia and circulating immune complexes. *N Engl J Med* 1978; 298:927-933.

LaBrec, E.H., et al.: Epithelial cell penetration as an essential step in the pathogenesis of bacillary dysentery. *J Bacteriol* 1964; 88:1503-1518.

O'Brien, A.D., et al.: Production of *Shigella dysenteriae* type 1-like cytotoxin by *Escherichia coli*. *J Infect Dis* 1982; 146:763-769.

O'Brien, A.D., et al.: *Escherichia coli* 0157:47 strains associated with haemorrhagic colitis in the United States produce a *Shigella dysenteriae* 1 (Shiga)-like cytotoxin. *Lancet* 1983; 2:763.

Rout, W.R., et al.: Pathophysiology of shigella diarrhea in the rhesus monkey: Intestinal transport, morphological, and bacteriological studies. *Gastroenterology* 1975; 68:270-278.

39 *Campylobacter jejuni*

Martin J. Blaser, MD

General Concepts	**Pathogenesis**
Distinctive Properties	**Host Defenses**
Structure	**Epidemiology**
Antigens	**Diagnosis**
Physiology	**Control**

General Concepts

Campylobacters, some of which cause diarrheal illnesses in humans, are gram-negative bacteria widely distributed in the animal kingdom. Although bacteria of this genus have been known to microbiologists as veterinary pathogens for 75 years, their role as enteric pathogens for humans has been realized only recently. Because campylobacters are microaerophilic, neither aerobic nor anaerobic incubation of clinical specimens is appropriate for their isolation. Because they grow more slowly than do the usual enteric flora, selective media and microaerobic incubation are needed to isolate them. Until these methods were used, the significance of campylobacters as enteric pathogens of humans was not recognized.

Only three members of the genus (*C jejuni*, *C coli*, and *C fetus* ssp *fetus*) are known to be pathogenic for humans. *C jejuni* and, less commonly, *C coli* are the agents causing diarrheal disease. Because these two organisms are nearly identical in their characteristics, the name *C jejuni* is commonly used to describe both. Recently, other *C jejuni*-like organisms also have been implicated as pathogens of humans. *C fetus* ssp *fetus* causes systemic illnesses in debilitated hosts but is an uncommon pathogen. Thus, most interest has focused on *C jejuni* because, as a cause of diarrheal illness in previously healthy persons, it is as common as *Salmonella* or *Shigella*.

Distinctive Properties

Structure

C jejuni, like the other campylobacters, is a microaerophilic, gram-negative vibriolike organism. The name *Campylobacter* is a Greek term meaning "curved rod," which describes the appearance of the organisms in light microscopy (Figure 39-1). In young cultures, organisms are comma shaped, spiral, S-shaped, or seagull shaped; as cultures age or are subjected to atmospheric or temperature stresses, round, or coccoid, forms appear. Whether the coccoid forms are viable is not known at present.

Structurally similar to other gram-negative bacilli, *C jejuni* is motile, with a single flagellum at one or both poles of the cell. The cell envelope, typical of gram-negative organisms, has an inner bipolar lipoprotein cell membrane, a thin peptidoglycan layer, an outer bipolar lipoprotein layer with the lipid moiety of a lipopolysaccharide layer embedded in it, and the carbohydrate portion extended to the surface of the cell. Interspersed in the outer layer are membrane proteins, some of which are exposed to the surface and antigenic for infected hosts, and some of which are not. *Campylobacter* lipopolysaccharide has biologic activity like endotoxin from other gram-negative cells.

All campylobacters appear to have similar structures and appearance by light microscopy, although the spiral forms of *C jejuni* are the most tightly coiled. The *Campylobacter* sp and ssp may be differentiated by biochemical reactions (Table 39-1). In

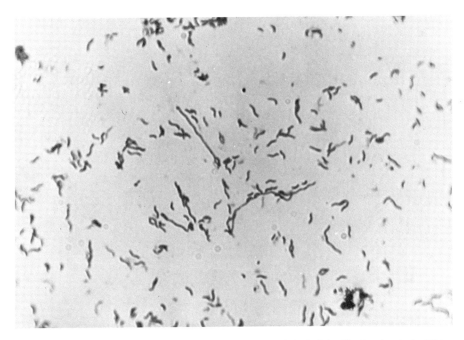

Figure 39-. Forty-eight-hour culture of *C jejuni* (originally King's "related vibrios"), showing typical thin, comma-, S-, or seagull-shaped forms. In broth cultures, chained organisms may appear as elongated forms. All forms are gram-negative and motile (× 1000). (Courtesy Robert Weaver.)

Table 39-1 Differentiation of Several of the Campylobacters

	C jejuni	C fetus ssp fetus	C fetus ssp venerealis	C sputorum ssp sputorum
Catalase	+	+	+	−
Multiplies in				
1% glycine	+	+	−	+
Susceptible to				
naladixic acid	−	+	+	−
Grows at 42 C	+	−*	−	+/−
Grows at 25 C	−	+	+	+
Hydrolyzes hippurate	+†	−	−	−

*Occasionally strains grow at 42 C.
†The biochemical characteristics of C coli strains are nearly identical to those of C jejuni; however, hippurate hydrolysis is nearly always negative.

addition, examining the fatty acids of the cell wall using gas-liquid chromatography has shown the C jejuni usually contains a 19-cyclopropane fatty acid not present in any other member of the genus.

Antigens

At least 50 heat-labile antigens and 60 different heat-stable somatic (O) antigens have been found among isolates of C jejuni; however, 5 of the O group antigens are found in about 50% of the isolates from humans, and similarly several heat–labile antigens account for most isolates from humans. The major outer membrane protein and flagellar proteins also are important antigens.

Physiology

C jejuni utilizes amino acids and tricarboxylic acid (Krebs) cycle intermediates as energy sources for growth; however, carbohydrates such as glucose are neither oxidized nor fermented. Optimal growth occurs when cultures are incubated at 42 C; however, stationary phase cultures may remain viable for several weeks when kept at 4 C in appropriate media. This dichotomy between optimal growth and resting-phase temperatures commonly is observed with other microorganisms.

C jejuni is a microaerophile; for growth, it requires oxygen as the terminal proton acceptor, yet it is unable to grow in air (21% oxygen). The optimum oxygen concentration for growth is 5%. The mechanism of this oxygen toxicity is not well understood, but perhaps C jejuni has a greater sensitivity to exogenous superoxide anions and hydrogen peroxide than do aerotolerant bacteria.

Pathogenesis

The minimal infection-causing dose of C jejuni is not known, although volunteers who ingested as few as 800 organisms became ill. As happens with other enteric pathogens, the attack rate may vary with the ingested dose. In outbreaks of Campylobacter enteritis, the incubation period has ranged from 1-7 days, with the majority ranging between 2-4 days.

Infection leads to multiplication of organisms in the intestines. Ill persons shed 10^6-10^9 *Campylobacter* per gram of feces, concentrations similar to those shed in *Salmonella* and *Shigella* infections. The sites of tissue injury include the small and large bowels, although which is more commonly affected is not known. In both organs, the pathologic lesion is that of acute exudative and hemorrhagic inflammation. Severely ill patients frequently have colonic involvement with infiltration of the lamina propria with neutrophils, eosinophils, and mononuclear cells, and destruction of epithelial glands with crypt abscess formation (Figure 39-2). The pathologic lesions seen in *Campylobacter* colitis may be identical to those in ulcerative colitis; thus, before ulcerative colitis can be diagnosed, *C jejuni* infection must be ruled out.

The mechanisms by which *C jejuni* causes illness are not known. The presence in some patients of bacteremia and the finding of cellular infiltration in biopsy specimens of patients with *Campylobacter* colitis suggest that tissue invasion is a pathogenic mechanism. *C jejuni* has been found to be invasive in vitro to chick embryo cells and causes bacteremia in experimentally infected mice, rabbits, calves, and chicks. Many isolates elaborate both a cytotoxin and an enterotoxin, but the clinical significance of the toxigenicity of these organisms is unknown.

In developed countries, excretion of *C jejuni* by convalescent patients is brief. Several studies of excretion have shown a median duration of 2-3 weeks, with all patients becoming culture-negative by 3 months. There appears to be little variation in

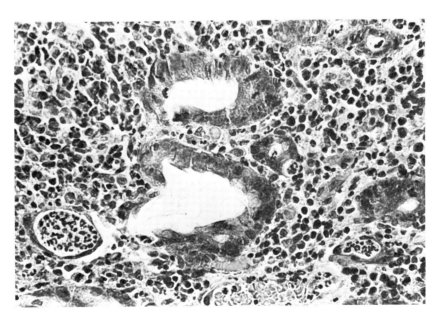

Figure 39-2 Rectal biopsy from patient with *Campylobacter* colitis. There is increased cellularity of the lamina propria with neutrophils, plasma cells, and eosinophils. Glandular epithelial cells are degenerated and thinned, with loss of goblet cells. A crypt abscess is present (lower left). (H & E stain, ×250.)

the duration of excretion by age of the patient. In developing countries, the duration of excretion usually is even shorter, perhaps as a result of acquired immunity.

C jejuni infections may be asymptomatic but often appear to produce symptoms of an acute gastroenteritis. The major symptoms are fever, diarrhea (which may be liquid or bloody or both), and abdominal pain, which may be so severe as to mimic acute appendicitis. Nausea and vomiting are less common complaints. A prodrome with constitutional symptoms may precede the gastroenteritis. The illness may last from 1 day to several weeks; however, illness is frequently self-limited within 7 days. At the more severe end of the spectrum, *Campylobacter* enteritis may resemble inflammatory bowel disease; occasionally, deaths have been reported. *C jejuni* may be isolated from the bloodstream and other sites distant from the intestinal tact, especially in malnourished or immunodeficient persons.

Host Defenses

C jejuni is a pathogen capable of infecting previously healthy persons. In contrast, *C fetus* ssp *fetus* must be considered an opportunistic organism, predominantly affecting persons debilitated by previous disease or at the extremes of age. However, *C fetus* also may cause an acute enteritis in normal hosts.

C jejuni is susceptible to killing by hydrochloric acid, suggesting that normal gastric acidity is an important barrier against infection. The relation of *C jejuni* to the components of the host's immune function have not been studied completely. Neutrophils often are observed in the feces of patients infected with *C jejuni*. Biopsy specimens from patients with *Campylobacter* colitis have shown marked infiltrations with neutrophils, suggesting that these cells may be important in host defense. In mice, macrophages are important for clearance of bacteremia, and in vitro, *C jejuni* antigens stimulate T-cell responses.

Infected persons frequently develop elevated specific serum IgA, IgG, and IgM titers, which may persist for several months. Experimentally infected animals manifest specific intestinal IgA production. Whether this antibody response eliminates the infection or protects against reinfection is not known; however, persons with hypogammaglobulinemia are at increased risk for recurrent or bloodstream infections. *C jejuni* isolates are usually susceptible to complement-mediated killing by normal serum whereas *C fetus* isolates usually are resistant. Regardless of the exact host defense mechanisms involved, most *C jejuni* infections resolve spontaneously.

Epidemiology

Most members of the genus *Campylobacter* normally reside in the intestinal and reproductive tracts of various mammalian and avian species. In particular, *C jejuni* may be part of the intestinal flora of healthy cattle, sheep, swine, chickens, turkeys, dogs, and cats. *C jejuni* may be pathogenic to the animal hosts most often during the primary infection of neonates, and lifelong colonization and immunity usually develop. Because humans frequently contact these animals or their products, the potential for transmission is great. Excreta from these or undomesticated animals also may contaminate soil and water, providing further opportunities for transmission to humans.

In developed countries, 3%-14% of patients with diarrhea seeking medical attention have been shown to be infected with *C jejuni*. Carriage and excretion of the organism by healthy persons are rare. In contrast, in developing countries, up to 40% of healthy children may be carrying the organism at any time. This is an age-related phenomenon, with the highest excretion rates in very young children. The reasons are not known for this marked difference in the epidemiologic pattern in the developed and developing countries. Children in developing countries occasionally may become long-term carriers of the organism without any adverse sequelae after infection. Alternatively, many strains commonly present in developing countries could be nonpathogenic, although disease induction in experimental animals and in travellers argues against this. Another possibility is that reinfection with unrelated strains is common in that environment. Case-to-infection ratios decline with age.

In the developed countries, where infection clearly is associated with illness, the highest isolation rates occur during summer months, as with other enteric pathogens, and in persons 10–29 years old. Infection may be acquired by drinking untreated stream water, drinking unpasteurized milk, eating undercooked foods such as chicken, beef liver, and processed turkey meat, or eating raw clams. Other foods, especially those of animal origin, undoubtedly are sources of infection. Direct contacts with infected puppies and kittens, cattle, sheep, chickens, and wild birds also have been implicated in the transmission of infection. Person-to-person transmission appears to be uncommon except when the index case occurs in someone who is incontinent of feces.

Diagnosis

Campylobacter enteritis cannot be easily distinguished by clinical signs from illness due to other enteric pathogens. Neutrophils or blood in the feces of patients with acute diarrheal illnesses provide important diagnostic clues that suggest *Campylobacter* infection. Examination of a fresh fecal specimen for darting motility or Gram staining to show the characteristic vibrio forms may permit a presumptive diagnosis. Definitive diagnosis of infection is made by isolating the organism from a fecal culture or, rarely, from a blood culture. Because of *C jejuni*'s fastidious growth and requirement for a microaerobic atmosphere, special laboratory methods are needed to isolate it. Plating media must be selective to inhibit the growth of the competing microorganisms in the fecal flora. Most such media developed for isolating *C jejuni* contain antibiotics to which *C jejuni* is resistant but to which most of the usual flora are susceptible. Cultures must be incubated in an environment with reduced oxygen, optimally about 5%, because campylobacters are microaerophilic. For isolating *C jejuni* specifically, incubation at 42 C is helpful, but 37 C is better for isolation of *Campylobacter*-like organisms and *C fetus*. With these methods, any suspicious colonies can be readily identified by their spreading character, mucoid appearance, and grayish color. The series of biochemical reactions outlined in Table 39-1 can differentiate the campylobacters. Serologic methods for diagnosis of infections in humans are only research tools at present and are not generally available.

Control

Control of *Campylobacter* infection depends largely on interruption of transmission of the organism to humans from farm and domestic animals, from foods of animal origin, or from contaminated water. Proper cooking and storing of foods of animal origin, avoiding drinking untreated water and unpasteurized milk, and handwashing after contact with animals or animal products are specific measures by which individuals can reduce the risk of *Campylobacter* infection. The presence of several surface-exposed, broadly specific proteins may permit vaccine development.

Infected persons with severe or prolonged symptoms who have been treated with antimicrobial agents have recovered completely; however, for mild infections, the efficacy of treatment with antimicrobial agents has not yet been demonstrated. When treatment is indicated, erythromycin and tetracycline appear to be the agents of choice.

References

Blaser, M.J., et al.: Campylobacter enteritis: Clinical and epidemiologic features. *Ann Intern Med* 1979; 91:179–185.

Blaser, M.J., et al.: *Campylobacter* enteritis in the United States. A multicenter study. *Ann Intern Med* 1983; 98:360–365.

Butzler, J.P., Skirrow, M.B.: Campylobacter enteritis. *Clin Gastroenterol* 1979; 8:737–765.

Kaplan, R.L.: *Campylobacter.* In: *Manual of clinical microbiology,* 3rd ed. Lennette E (editor). Washington, D.C.: American Society for Microbiology, 1980.

King, E.O.: The laboratory recognition of *Vibrio fetus* and a closely related vibrio isolated from cases of human vibriosis. *Ann NY Acad Sci* 1962; 98:700–711.

Lambert, M.E., et al.: Campylobacter colitis. *Br Med J* 1979; 1:857–859.

Penner, J.L., Hennessey, J.N.: 1980. Serotyping *Campylobacter fetus* subsp. *jejuni* on the basis of somatic (O) antigens. *J Clin Microbiol* 1980; 12:732–737.

Smibert, R.M.: The genus *Campylobacter. Ann Rev Microbiol* 1978; 32:700–773.

Vanhoof, R., et al.: Susceptibility of *Campylobacter fetus* subsp. *jejuni* to twenty-nine antimicrobial agents. *Antimicrob Agents Chemother* 1978; 14:553–556.

Wang, L., et al.: Comparison of antimicrobial susceptibility patterns of *Campylobacter jejuni* and *Campylobacter coli. Antimicrob Agents Chemother* 1984; 26:351–353.

40 *Vibrio cholerae* (and Other Pathogenic Vibrios)

Richard A. Finkelstein, PhD

General Concepts
Distinctive Properties
Pathogenesis
Host Defenses
Epidemiology
Diagnosis
Control

General Concepts

Based upon its Latin derivation (*vibro*, to vibrate), the term vibrio implies a highly motile microorganism, but usage has added the connotation of a curved, or comma-shaped, rod. Of the vibrios that are clinically significant to humans, *Vibrio cholerae*, the causative agent of cholera, is most important. *V cholerae* was first isolated in pure culture by Robert Koch in 1883, although it had been seen earlier by other investigators, including Pacini, who is credited with describing it first in Florence in 1854.

Cholera may be defined as a metabolic disturbance of the epithelial cells of the small bowel of humans caused by a potent, specialized form of exotoxin, the cholera enterotoxin. Also known as choleragen, this enterotoxin produces a copious, life-threatening secretory diarrhea via transfer of ADP-ribose to a substrate within epithelial cells and subsequent increase in cyclic AMP. Treatment consists of fluid and electrolyte replacement; antibiotics alone are not sufficient. Cholera and the cholera enterotoxin are prototypes for an increasingly recognized variety of diarrheal diseases, collectively known as enterotoxic enteropathies; of these, diarrhea due to enterotoxinogenic strains of *Escherichia coli* (discussed in Chapter 42) may be regarded as the most important example.

Humans apparently are the only natural host for the cholera vibrios. Cholera is acquired by the ingestion of water or food contaminated with the feces of an individual who is infected with cholera vibrios. Previously, the disease swept the world in six great pandemics and later receded into its ancestral home in the Indo-Pakistani subcontinent. In 1961, the El Tor biotype (a subset distinguished by physiologic characteristics) of *V cholerae*, not previously implicated in widespread epidemics, emerged from the Celebes (now Sulawesi), causing the seventh great cholera pandemic. In the course of their migration, the El Tor biotype cholera vibrios virtually replaced *V chol⌐ ae* of the classic biotype that formerly were responsible for the annual cholera epidemics of India and East Pakistan (now Bangladesh). The pandemic that began in 1961 is now heavily seeded in Southeast Asia and in Africa. It has also invaded Europe, North America, and Japan, where the outbreaks have been relatively restricted and self-limited because of more highly developed sanitation. Several new cases were reported in Texas in 1981. Interestingly, after nearly 20 years of relative quiescence, *V cholerae* of the classic biotype again are being isolated with increasing frequency in India and Bangladesh.

Other vibrios may be clinically significant also. These include members of a poorly defined and relatively heterogeneous group of nonagglutinable or noncholera vibrios (called NAG vibrios or NCV or non-O group 1 *V cholerae*): *V parahaemolyticus*, a halophilic (salt-loving) vibrio associated with enteritis acquired by ingestion of raw or improperly cooked seafoods. Another halophilic vibrio, which ferments lactose and for this reason was called the L+ vibrio, has recently been identified as *V vulnificus*. It has been associated with wound infections as well as fatal septicemias. Other groups of vibrios, previously referred to as "group F" and EF-6, have recently been classified into species: *V fluvialis*, *V hollisae*, *V furnissi*, and *V damsela*. *V mimicus* is a recently described sucrose-negative species. *V fetus*, a group of anaerobic-to-microaerophilic spirally curved rods associated with venereally transmitted infertility and abortion in domestic animals, is now called *Campylobacter jejuni* and is considered to belong in the family Spirillaceae rather than in the family Vibrionaceae. *C jejuni* has been associated with dysenterylike gastroenteritis as well as with other types of infection, including bacteremic and central nervous system infections in humans (see Chapter 39). Although some similarities in habitat and other properties occur, the Vibrionaceae are separated taxonomically from the Enterobacteriaceae: the oxidase test (vibrios are usually oxidase-positive) is particularly useful. Other vibrios exist, and some of these may be responsible for diseases in fish and other lower animals. As vibrios are widely distributed in the environment, particularly in estuarine waters and in seafoods, reports of their isolation from patients with diarrheal disease do not necessarily always imply an etiologic relationship; vibrios could be merely "passing through."

Distinctive Properties

The cholera vibrios (*V cholerae* OI) are gram-negative, slightly curved rods whose motility depends on a single polar flagellum. Their nutritional requirements are simple. Fresh isolates are prototrophic; that is, they grow in media containing an inorganic nitrogen source, a utilizable carbohydrate, and appropriate minerals. In adequate media, they grow rapidly with a generation time of less than 30 minutes. Although they reach higher population densities when grown with vigorous aeration, they can also grow anaerobically. Vibrios are sensitive to acid pH and succumb rapidly in solutions below pH 6; however, they are quite tolerant of alkaline conditions. This tolerance has been exploited in media used for their isolation and diagnosis.

The vibrios that cause epidemic cholera have been subdivided into two biotypes: classic and El Tor. *V cholerae* of the classic biotype was first isolated by Koch. Subsequently, in the early 1900s, some vibrios resembling *V cholerae* were isolated from Mecca-bound pilgrims at the quarantine station at El Tor that had been established to try to control cholera in the Sinai peninsula. These vibrios resembled classic *V cholerae* in many ways, but were found to cause lysis of goat or sheep erythrocytes in a test known as the Greig test. Because the pilgrims from whom they were isolated did not have cholera, these hemolytic El Tor vibrios were regarded as relatively insignificant except for the possibility of confusing them with true cholera vibrios. In the 1930s, similar hemolytic vibrios were associated with relatively restricted outbreaks of diarrheal disease, called paracholera, in the Celebes. In 1961, cholera caused by El Tor vibrios erupted in Hong Kong and, subsequently, spread virtually worldwide. Although in the course of this pandemic most *V cholerae* biotype El Tor strains have lost their hemolytic activity, a number of ancillary tests differentiate them from vibrios of the classic biotype.

The operational serology of the cholera vibrios, which belong in O antigen group I, is relatively simple. Both biotypes (El Tor and classic) contain two major serotypes, Inaba and Ogawa (Figure 40-1). These serotypes are differentiated in agglutination and vibriocidal antibody tests on the basis of their dominant heat-stable lipopolysaccharide somatic antigens. The cholera group has a common antigen, A, and the serotypes are differentiated by the type-specific antigens, B (Ogawa) and C (Inaba). An additional serotype, Hikojima, which has both specific antigens, has been reported rarely.

Other antigenic components of the vibrios, such as outer membrane protein antigens, have not been extensively studied. The cholera vibrios also have common flagellar antigens. Cross-reactions with *Brucella* and with *Citrobacter* sp have been reported. Because of DNA-relatedness and other similarities, the nonagglutinable vibrios (NAG or NCV) are now classified in the genus and species, *V cholerae*. The term nonagglutinable is a misnomer because it implies that these vibrios are not agglutinable; in fact, they are not agglutinable in antisera against the O antigen group I cholera vibrios, but they are agglutinable in their own specific antisera. More than 50 serotypes are now recognized. Some nonagglutinable vibrio (or non-O group I *V cholerae*) strains cause diarrheal disease by means of an enterotoxin related to the cholera enterotoxin and, perhaps, by other mechanisms, but these strains have not been associated with devastating outbreaks like those caused by the true cholera vibrios. Recently, vibrio

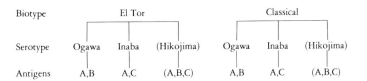

Figure 40-1 *Vibrio cholerae* (O antigen Group I).

strains that agglutinate in some O group I cholera diagnostic antisera but not in others have been isolated from environmental sources. Volunteer feeding experiments have shown that these atypical O group I vibrios are not enteropathogenic in humans. Recent studies using specific toxin gene probes indicate that the environmental isolates are not only nontoxigenic, but they do not possess any of the genetic information encoding cholera toxin, although some isolates from diarrheal stools do.

The cholera vibrios cause many distinctive reactions. They are as a group oxidase-positive. The O group I cholera vibrios almost always fall into the Heiberg I fermentation pattern; that is, they ferment sucrose and mannose but not arabinose, and produce acid but not gas. *V cholerae* also possess lysine and ornithine decarboxylase, but not arginine dihydrolase. Freshly isolated agar-grown vibrios of the El Tor biotype, in contrast to classic *V cholerae*, produce a cell-associated mannose-sensitive hemagglutinin active on chicken erythrocytes. This activity is readily detected in a rapid slide test. In addition to hemagglutination, numerous tests have been proposed to differentiate the classic and El Tor biotypes, including production of a hemolysin, sensitivity to selected bacteriophages, sensitivity to polymyxin, and the Voges–Proskauer (V-P) test for acetoin. El Tor vibrios originally were defined as hemolytic. They differed in this characteristic from classic cholera vibrios; however, during the most recent pandemic, most El Tor vibrios (except for the recent isolates from Texas and Louisiana) have lost the capacity to express the hemolysin. Most El Tor vibrios are V-P positive and resistant to polymyxin and to phage IV, whereas classic vibrios are sensitive to them. As both biotypes cause the same disease, these characteristics have only epidemiologic significance. Strains of the El Tor biotype, however, produce less cholera enterotoxin, but appear to colonize intestinal epithelium better than vibrios of the classic variety; also, they seem somewhat more resistant to environmental factors. Thus, El Tor strains have a higher tendency to become endemic and exhibit a higher infection-to-case ratio than the classic biotype.

Pathogenesis

Recent studies employing laboratory animal models and human volunteers have provided a detailed understanding of the pathogenesis of cholera. Initial attempts to infect healthy American volunteers with cholera vibrios revealed that the oral administration of up to 10^{11} living cholera vibrios rarely had an effect; in fact, the cholera organisms usually could not be recovered from stools of the volunteers. After the administration of bicarbonate to neutralize gastric acidity, however, cholera diarrhea developed in most volunteers given 10^4 cholera vibrios. Thus, gastric acidity itself is a powerful natural resistance mechanism. It also has been demonstrated that vibrios administered with food are much more likely to cause infection.

Cholera is exclusively a disease of the small bowel. To establish residence and multiply in the human small bowel (normally relatively free of bacteria because of the effective clearance mechanisms of peristalsis and mucus secretion), the cholera vibrios have one or more adherence factors that enable them to adhere to the microvilli (Figure 40-2). The motility of the vibrios may also affect virulence by enabling them to penetrate the mucus layer. They also produce mucinolytic enzymes, neuraminidase, and proteases. The growing cholera vibrios elaborate the cholera enterotoxin, choleragen, a polymeric protein (84,000 mol. wt.) consisting of two major domains or regions. The A region

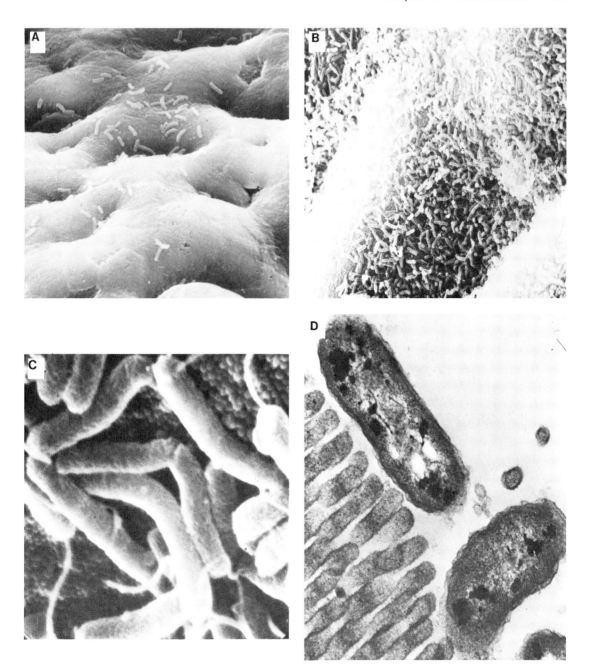

Figure 40-2 *Vibrio cholerae* attachment and colonization in experimental rabbit ileal loops. The events are assumed to be similar in human cholera. **A,** Scanning electron microscopy during early infection. Curved vibrios adhering to epithelial surface. (Approximately 4000×). **B,** Later, vibrios are densely packed, exhibiting a shag rug appearance. **C,** At higher magnification, vibrios can be seen close to tips of microvilli. Single polar flagellum is clearly visible on some of vibrios, but no pili or other surface organelles can be seen. **D,** Transmission electron microscopy of vibrios in both end-on and horizontal modes close to tips of microvilli. From Nelson, E.T., Clements, J.D., Finkelstein, R.A.: *Infect Immunol* 1976;14:527.

(28,000 mol. wt.), responsible for biologic activity of the enterotoxin, is linked by noncovalent interactions with the B region (56,000 mol. wt.), which is composed of five noncovalently associated peptide chains of 11,500 mol. wt. The B region, also known as choleragenoid, binds the toxin to its receptors on host cell membranes. It is also the immunologically dominant portion of the holotoxin. The structural genes that encode the synthesis of cholera enterotoxin reside on the *V cholerae* chromosome, in contrast to those for the heat-labile enterotoxins (LTs) of *E coli* (Chapter 41), which are encoded by plasmids. The amino acid sequences of these structurally, functionally, and immunologically related enterotoxins are very similar: their differences account for the differences in physiochemical behavior and the antigenic distinctions that have been noted. It should also be noted that *V cholerae* exports its enterotoxin whereas the *E coli* LTs occur primarily in the periplasmic space. This may account for the reported differences in severity of the diarrheas these organisms cause.

The molecular events in these diarrheal diseases involve an interaction between the enterotoxins and intestinal epithelial cell membranes. The toxins bind through region B to a glycolipid, the G_{M1} ganglioside, which is practically ubiquitous in eukaryotic cell membranes. Following this binding, the A region, or a major portion of it known as the A_1 peptide (21,000 mol. wt.), penetrates the host cell and enzymatically transfers ADP-ribose from nicotinamide adenine dinucleotide (NAD) to a target protein, the guanosine 5′-triphosphate (GTP)-binding regulatory protein associated with membrane-bound adenylate cyclase. Thus, cholera toxin (and LT) resembles diphtheria toxin in causing transfer of ADP-ribose to a substrate. With diphtheria toxin, however, the substrate is elongation factor 2, and the result is cessation of host-cell protein synthesis. In cholera, the ADP-ribosylation reaction essentially locks adenylate cyclase in its "on mode" and leads to excessive production of cyclic AMP (cAMP). The subsequent cAMP-mediated cascade of events has not yet been delineated, but the final effect is hypersecretion of chloride and bicarbonate, followed by water, resulting in the characteristic isotonic voluminous cholera stool. In hospitalized patients, this can result in losses of 20 L or more of fluid per day. The stool of an actively purging, severely ill cholera patient can resemble rice water—the supernate of boiled rice. Because the stool can contain 10^8 viable vibrios per milliliter, such a patient could shed 2×10^{12} cholera vibrios per day into the environment. Perhaps by production of cholera enterotoxin, the cholera vibrios thus assure their survival by increasing the likelihood of finding another human host.

Various animal models have been used to investigate pathogenic mechanisms, virulence, and immunity. Among these, 10-day-old suckling rabbits develop a fulminating diarrheal disease after intraintestinal inoculation with virulent *V cholerae* or choleragen. Adult rabbits are relatively resistant to colonization by cholera vibrios; however, they do respond, with characteristic outpouring of fluid, to the intraluminal inoculation of live vibrios or enterotoxin in surgically isolated ileal loops. Suckling mice are susceptible to intragastric inoculation of vibrios and to perorally administered toxin. Adult conventional mice are also susceptible to perorally administered toxin, but resist colonization except in isolated intestinal loops. Interestingly, however, germ-free mice can be colonized for months with cholera vibrios. They rarely show adverse effects, although they are susceptible to cholera enterotoxin. Dogs also have been used experimentally, although they are relatively refractory and require enormous inocula to elicit choleraic manifestations. Chinchillas also are susceptible to diarrhea following intraintestinal inoculation with moderate numbers of cholera vibrios. Infections initiated by extraintestinal routes of inoculation (for example, intraperitoneal) largely reflect the toxicity of the lipopolysaccharide endotoxin. The intraperitoneal infection in mice is used to assay the protective effect of conventional killed vibrio vaccines.

Various animals, including humans, rabbits, and guinea pigs, also respond to intradermal inoculation of relatively minute amounts of cholera enterotoxin with a characteristic delayed (maximum response at 24 hours), sustained (visible up to one week or more), erythematous, endematous induration associated with a localized alteration of vascular permeability. In laboratory animals, this response can be measured after injecting a protein-binding dye, such as trypan blue, that extravasates producing a zone of bluing at the site of intracutaneous inoculation of toxin. This observation has been exploited in the assay of cholera enterotoxin and its antibody, and also in the detection of other enterotoxins.

In addition, because of choleragen's broad spectrum of activity on cells and tissues that it never contacts in nature, various in vitro systems can be used to assay the enterotoxin and its antibody. In each, the toxin causes a characteristically delayed, but sustained, activation of adenylate cyclase and increased production of cAMP, and it may cause additional, readily recognizable, morphologic alterations of certain cultured cell lines. The cells most widely used for this purpose are Chinese hamster ovary (CHO) cells, which elongate in response to picogram doses of the toxin, and mouse Y-1 adrenal tumor cells, which round up. Cholera toxin has become an extremely valuable experimental probe to identify other cAMP-mediated responses. It also activates adenylate cyclase in pigeon erythrocytes, a procedure that was used by D. Michael Gill to define the toxin's mode of action.

These assays and models also have been applied in the study of an expanding number of cholera-related and unrelated enterotoxins. These include the heat-labile enterotoxins (LTs) of *E coli*, which are structurally and immunologically similar to it and are effective in any model that is responsive to cholera enterotoxin; the heat-stable enterotoxin (ST) of *E coli*, which activates guanylate cyclase, is rapidly active in the infant mouse and certain other intestinal models, and is clearly unrelated to choleragen: a choleragen-related enterotoxin from certain nonagglutinable (non-O group I) *Vibrio* strains; *Salmonella* enterotoxin, shown to be related immunologically to choleragen; and choleragenlike factors from *Shigella* and *V parahaemolyticus* (thus far only demonstrated in sensitive cell culture systems). Other enterotoxins and enterocytotoxins, which elicit cytotoxic effects on intestinal epithelial cells, also have been described but not clearly defined, from *Klebsiella, Enterobacter, Citrobacter, Aeromonas, Pseudomonas, Shigella, V parahaemolyticus, Campylobacter, Yersinia enterocolitica, B cereus, C perfringens, C difficile*, and staphylococci. The classic staphylococcal enterotoxins perhaps should more properly be called neurotoxins, as they affect the central nervous system rather than the gut directly to cause fluid secretion or histopathologic effects.

Host Defenses

Infection with cholera vibrios results in a spectrum of responses. These range from no observed manifestations except perhaps a serologic response, the most common, to the acutely purging patient, regarded as classic, who requires hospitalization and fluid replacement therapy. The reasons for these differences are not entirely clear, although it is known that individuals differ in gastric acidity and that those individuals who are hypochlorohydric are most prone to cholera. The inoculum size and volume, and whether it is ingested with food, also are significant. Whether individuals differ in the availability of intestinal receptors for cholera vibrios or for their toxin has not been established. Prior immunologic experience of subjects at risk is certainly a major factor. For example, in heavily endemic regions such as Bangladesh, the attack rate is relatively low among adults in comparison with children; in neoepidemic areas, cholera is more frequent among the working adult population. Resistance is related to the presence of circulating antibody and, perhaps more importantly, local IgA antibody against the cholera bacteria or the cholera enterotoxin or both. Intestinal IgA antibody can prevent attachment of the vibrios to the mucosal surface and neutralize, or prevent binding, of the cholera enterotoxin. For reasons that are not clear, individuals of blood group O are slightly more susceptible to cholera.

Recovery from cholera probably depends on two factors: elimination of the vibrios by antibiotics or the patient's own immune response, and regeneration of the poisoned intestinal epithelial cells. As studies in volunteers demonstrated conclusively, the disease is an immunizing process; patients who have recovered from cholera are solidly immune for a period of at least 3 years.

Cholera vaccines consisting of killed cholera bacteria administered parenterally have been used since the turn of the century; however, recent controlled field studies indicate that little, if any, effective immunity is induced in immunologically virgin populations by such vaccines, although they do stimulate preexisting immunity in the adult population of heavily endemic regions. Controlled studies have likewise shown that a cholera toxoid administered parenterally was also ineffective in preventing cholera. Probably the natural disease should be simulated to induce truly effective immunity. Studies in volunteers have shown that a hypotoxinogenic mutant of *V cholerae*, administered perorally, did stimulate effective immunity. Recently, a mutant strain (called Texas Star—SR) has been isolated that produces the B region of the cholera enterotoxin but no A region and is thus avirulent. This mutant has been shown to produce effective active immunity in laboratory animal models and in volunteers. Despite its inability to produce complete cholera toxin, the mutant produced slight diarrhea in some of the volunteers. The results suggest that cholera vibrios may have additional mechanisms of causing intestinal malfunction in addition to the cholera enterotoxin. Perhaps the act of colonization itself is involved or other toxic factors are present. Recent studies in volunteers with genetically engineered tox^- or A^-B^+ strains have indicated that they caused more severe diarrhea (although not cholera) in a more dose-related fashion than the Texas Star strain. If a mutant, lacking undesirable side effects, could stimulate local production of anti-B-subunit antibodies in humans, it might also be effective against the enterotoxic enteropathies that depend on choleragen-related enterotoxins. Studies have established, for example, that the plasmid-mediated, heat-labile enterotoxin of *E coli* is structurally, immunologically, and functionally related to the cholera enterotoxin, and that immunity against cholera toxin is protective against *Salmonella* in an experimental model. Laboratory studies also have shown that perorally administered killed bacteria and inactivated cholera toxin or choleragenoid stimulate effective immunity. Combined preparations of bacterial somatic antigen and toxin antigen act synergistically in stimulating immunity in laboratory animals; that is, the combined protective effort is closer to the product than to the sum of the individual protective effects. Field studies on such orally administered preparations are currently being considered. However, even if they are effective, the requirement for large and repeated doses is likely to make them too expensive for use in the developing areas that are usually afflicted with epidemic cholera.

Epidemiology

Cholera appears to exhibit three major epidemiologic patterns: heavily endemic, neoepidemic (newly invaded, cholera-receptive areas), and occasional limited outbreaks in sanitarily developed countries. These patterns probably depend in large measure on environmental factors (including sanitary and cultural aspects), the prior immune status, or antigenic experience, of the population at risk, and the inherent properties of the vibrios themselves, such as their resistance to gastric acidity, ability to colonize, and toxigenicity. In the heavily endemic region of the India-Pakistan-Bangladesh subcontinent, cholera exhibits some periodicity; this may vary from year to year and seasonally, depending partly on the amount of rain and degree of flooding. Because no extrahuman reservoirs have been incriminated, survival of the cholera vibrios during interepidemic periods probably depends on a relatively constant availability of low-level undiagnosed cases and transiently infected, asymptomatic individuals. Long-term carriers have been reported but are extremely rare. The classic case occurred in the Philippines: "cholera Dolores" harbored cholera vibrios in her gallbladder for 12 years after her initial attack in 1962. Her carrier state resolved spontaneously in 1973; no secondary cases had been associated with her well-marked strain. Recent studies, however, have suggested that cholera vibrios can persist for some time in shellfish in coastal regions of infected areas.

In epidemic periods, the incidence of infection in the sanitarily underdeveloped community is high enough to frustrate the most vigorous epidemiologic control efforts. Although transmission occurs primarily through water contaminated with human feces, infection also may be spread within households and by contaminated foods. Thus, in heavily endemic regions, adequate supplies of pure running water may reduce but not eliminate the threat of cholera.

In neoepidemic cholera-receptive areas, vigorous epidemiologic measures, including rapid identification and treatment of symptomatic cases and asymptomatically infected individuals, education in sanitary practices, and interruption of vehicles of transmission (for example, by water chlorination), may be most effective in containing the disease. In such situations, spread of cholera usually depends on traffic of infected human beings, although spread between adjacent communities can occur through bodies of water contaminated by human feces. Recall that John Snow was credited with stopping an epidemic in London, England, by the simple expedient of removing the handle of the "Broad Street pump" (a contaminated water supply) in 1854, before acceptance of the "germ theory," and before the first isolation of the "Kommabacillus" by Robert Koch.

In such sanitarily developed areas as Japan, Northern Europe, and North America, cholera has been introduced repeatedly in recent years, but has not caused devastating outbreaks; however, Japan has reported secondary cases and, in 1978, the United States experienced an outbreak of about one dozen cases in Louisiana. In that outbreak, sewage was infected, and infected shellfish apparently were involved. Interestingly, the hemolytic vibrio strain implicated was identical to one that caused an unexplained isolated case in Texas in 1973. Several new cases of cholera were reported in Texas in 1981.

Reports of isolation of choleralike vibrios in Maryland's Chesapeake Bay have not been associated with any human cases despite extensive surveillance. These vibrios are probably nonpathogenic nonagglutinable (non-O group I) vibrios, or the atypical O group I vibrios mentioned previously, which do not contain the genes for toxin production, do not colonize, and are avirulent.

Relatively little is known about the epidemiology of nonagglutinable (non-O group I) vibrios. When sought, these vibrios have been found widely in brackish surface waters (sewers, marshes, bogs, and coastal areas), and are generally more numerous in warmer months. They appear to be free-living aquatic organisms; whether particular subsets are potential pathogens is not yet clear. Strains isolated from humans with diarrheal disease more frequently give positive responses in assays for enterotoxins or enteropathogenicity, but the pathogenic mechanism of other isolates associated with shellfish remains undefined.

An epidemiologic pattern is more evident with *V parahaemolyticus*, which is clearly part of the normal flora of coastal and estuarian waters throughout the world. Although originally recognized in Japan, *V parahaemolyticus* enteritis has been reported virtually worldwide within the last decade. Its reported frequency varies widely, partly because of inherent differences in distribution and partly because many laboratories do not use the appropriate culture medium (TCBS, or thiosulfate-citrate-bile salts-sucrose agar) to isolate these organisms.

Two types of clinical syndromes, both usually self-limited, have been observed. The most common is a watery diarrhea, perhaps with associated abdominal cramps, nausea, vomiting, and fever, with a modal incubation period of 15 hours. A dysenteric syndrome with a short incubation period of 2½ hours also has been described. In Japan, about 24% of reported cases of "food poisoning" are attributed to *V parahaemolyticus*. This disease occurs primarily during summer, possibly reflecting the increased presence of the organism in the marine environment during those months, as well as the enhanced opportunity for it to multiply in unrefrigerated foods. It appears to be transmitted exclusively by food and primarily by raw or improperly prepared seafood. As growth of this organism is inhibited at temperatures below 15 C, rapid cooling and refrigeration of seafoods that are eaten raw would vastly reduce the incidence of disease. The organisms are killed by heating to 65 C for 10 minutes; thus, properly handled cooked seafood should present no problem. The role of the thermostable direct hemolysin, which is responsible for the positive Kanagawa phenomenon (a hemolytic reaction around colonies growing on a particular blood agar medium), in virulence and pathogenesis is not yet fully defined. This hemolysin is clearly associated with pathogenicity, but whether it is merely an associated marker or intimately involved in the disease process awaits further research. Be this as it may, only strains that possess the Kanagawa hemolysin are considered pathogenic. In laboratory studies, the isolated hemolysin has been reported to be cytotoxic, cardiotoxic, and lethal.

Diagnosis

Rapid bacteriologic diagnosis offers relatively little clinical advantage to the patient with secretory diarrhea, because essentially the same treatment (fluid and electrolyte replacement) is employed regardless of etiology; nevertheless, rapid identification of the agent can profoundly affect the subsequent course of a potential epidemic outbreak.

Because of their rapid growth and characteristic colonial morphology, *V cholerae* can be easily isolated and identified in the bacteriology laboratory, provided, first, that the presence of cholera is suspected and, second, that suitable specific diagnostic antisera are available. The vibrios are completely inhibited or grow somewhat poorly on usual enteric diagnostic media (MacConkey's agar or eosin methylene blue agar), but they can be isolated from stool samples or rectal swabs from cholera cases on simple meat extract (nutrient) agar or bile salts agar at slightly alkaline pH values. Following observation of characteristic colonial morphology with a stereoscopic microscope using transmitted oblique illumination, they can be confirmed as cholera vibrios by a rapid slide agglutination test with specific antiserum. Classic and El Tor biotypes can be differentiated at the same time by performing a direct slide hemagglutination test with chicken erythrocytes: all freshly isolated El Tor vibrios exhibit hemagglutination; all freshly isolated classic vibrios will not. In practice, this can be accomplished with material from patients as early as 6 hours after streaking the specimen in which the cholera vibrios usually predominate; however, to detect carriers (asymptomatically infected individuals) and to isolate cholera vibrios from food and water, enrichment procedures and selective media are recommended. Enrichment can be accomplished by inoculating alkaline (pH 8.5) peptone broth with the specimen and then streaking for isolation after an approximate 6-hour incubation period; this process enables the rapidly growing vibrios to multiply, and suppresses much of the commensal microflora at the same time. An effective selective medium is TCBS agar, on which the sucrose-fermenting cholera vibrios produce a distinctive yellow colony. However, its usefulness is limited because serologic testing of colonies grown on it occasionally proves difficult, and different lots vary in their productivity. This medium is also useful in isolating *V parahaemolyticus*.

The classic case of cholera, which includes profound secretory diarrhea and should evoke clinical suspicion, can be diagnosed within a few minutes in the prepared laboratory by direct, bright, or dark-field microscopic examination of the liquid stool for the presence of rapidly motile bacteria. Finding such bacteria, the technician can then make a second preparation to which a droplet of specific anti-*V cholerae* O group I antiserum is added. This quickly stops vibrio motility. Another rapid technique is the use of fluorescein isothiocyanate-labeled specific antiserum (fluorescent antibody technique) directly on the stool or rectal swab smear on the culture after enrichment in alkaline peptone broth. For cultural diagnosis, both nonselective and selective (TCBS) media may be used. Although demonstration of typical agglutinating colonies essentially confirms the diagnosis, additional conventional tests such as oxidase reaction, indole reaction, sugar fermentation reactions, gelatinase, lysine, arginine, and ornithine decarboxylase reactions may be helpful. Tests for chicken cell hemagglutination, hemolysis, polymyxin sensitivity, and susceptibility to phage IV are useful in differentiating the El Tor biotype from classic *V cholerae*. Tests for toxinogenesis may be indicated.

Diagnosis can be made retrospectively by confirming significant rises in specific antibody titers. For this purpose, conventional agglutination tests, tests for rises in complement-dependent vibriocidal antibody, or tests for rises in antitoxic antibody can be employed. Convenient microversions of these tests have been developed. Passive hemagglutination tests and enzyme-linked immunosorption assays (ELISA) have also been proposed.

Cultures that resemble *V cholerae* but fail to agglutinate in diagnostic antisera (nonagglutinable or non-O group I vibrios) present more of a problem and require additional tests such as oxidase, decarboxylases, inhibition by the vibriostatic pteridine compound 0/129, and the "string test." The string test demonstrates the property, shared by most vibrios and relatively few other genera, of forming a mucuslike string when colonial material is emulsified in 0.5% aqueous sodium desoxycholate solution. Additional tests for enteropathogenicity and toxigenesis may be useful.

Control

Treatment of cholera consists essentially of replacing fluid and electrolytes in amounts equivalent to those lost. Formerly, this was accomplished intravenously, using costly sterile pyrogen-free intravenous solutions. The patient's fluid losses were conveniently measured by the use of buckets, graduated in half-liter volumes, kept underneath an appropriate hole in an army-type cot on which the patient was resting. Antibiotics such as tetracycline, to which the vibrios are sensitive, are useful adjuncts in treatment. They shorten the period of infection with the cholera vibrios, thus reducing the continuous source of cholera enterotoxin; this results in a substantial saving of replacement fluids and a markedly briefer hospitalization. Note, however, that fluid and electrolyte replacement is all-important; patients who are adequately rehydrated and maintained will virtually always survive, and antibiotic treatment alone is not sufficient.

Recently it has been recognized that almost all cholera patients and others with similar severe secretory diarrheal disease can be maintained by fluids given perorally if the solutions contain a usable energy source such as glucose. Because of this discovery, packets containing appropriate salts are distributed by such organizations as WHO or UNICEF to cholera-afflicted areas, where they are dissolved in water as needed. One such formulation, called ORS for oral rehydration salts, contains NaCl, 3.5 g; KCl, 1.5 g; $NaHCO_3$, 2.5 g; and glucose, 20.0 g. This mixture is dissolved in 1 L of water and taken orally in increments. Flavoring may be added. Unfortunately, this technique, which will save countless millions of lives in countries of the "Third World," has not yet been widely accepted by practicing physicians in developed countries.

The possibility of pharmacologic intervention, for example, a pill that will stop choleraic diarrhea after it has started, has been considered. Two drugs, chlorpromazine and nicotinic acid, have been effective in experimental animals, although the precise mechanism of action has yet to be defined.

Like smallpox and typhoid, cholera under natural circumstances appears to affect only humans; therefore, *V cholerae,* as an etiologic entity, could conceivably disappear with the last human infection. Nevertheless, the spectrum of choleralike diarrheal diseases probably will persist for some time.

Cholera is essentially a disease associated with poor sanitation. The simple application of sanitary principles—that is, protecting drinking water and food from contamination with human feces—would go a long way toward controlling the disease; however, at present, this is not feasible in the underdeveloped areas that are afflicted with epidemic cholera or are considered to be cholera-receptive. Meanwhile, development of a vaccine that would effectively prevent colonization and manifestations of cholera would be extremely helpful. As indicated previously, such vaccines are presently being tested. Antibiotic or chemotherapeutic prophylaxis is feasible and may be indicated under certain circumstances. It also should be mentioned that the incidence of cholera is significantly higher in formula-fed than in breast-fed babies.

Present information indicates that *V parahaemolyticus* enteritis could be almost completely prevented by applying appropriate procedures to prevent multiplication of the organisms in contaminated seafood.

References

Blake, P.A., Weaver, R.E., Hollis, D.G.: Diseases of humans (other than cholera) caused by vibrios. *Ann Rev Microbiol* 1980; 34: 341-367.

Finkelstein, R.A.: Cholera. *CRC Crit Rev Microbiol* 1973; 2: 553-623.

Finkelstein, R.A.: Progress in the study of cholera and related enterotoxins. In: *Mechanisms in bacterial toxinology*. Bernheimer, A.W., (editor). New York: John Wiley & Sons, 1976.

Finkelstein, R.A.: Cholera. In: *Bacterial vaccines*. Germanier, R. (editor). New York: Academic Press, 1984.

Gill, D.M.: Seven toxic peptides that cross cell membranes. In: *Bacterial toxins and cell membranes*. Jeljaszewicz, J., Wadström, T., (editors). New York: Academic Press, 1978.

Kaper, J.B., Moseley, S.L., and Falkow, S.: Molecular characterization of environmental and nontoxigenic strains of *Vibrio cholerae*. *Infect Immunol* 1981; 32: 661-667.

Lai, C-Y.: The chemistry and biology of cholera toxin. *CRC Crit Rev Biochem* 1980; 9: 171-206.

Levine, M.M., Kaper, J.B., Black, R.E., and Clements, M.L.: New knowledge on pathogenesis of bacterial enteric infections as applied to vaccine development. *Microbiol Rev* 1983; 47:510-550.

Levine, M.M., et al.: Evaluation in humans of attenuated *Vibrio cholerae* El Tor Ogawa Strain Texas Star-SR as a live oral vaccine. *Infec Immun* 1984; 43: 515-522.

Marshlewicz, B.A., Finkelstein, R.A.: Immunologic differences among the cholera/coli family of enterotoxins. *Diag Microbiol Infect Dis* 1983; 1: 129-138.

Mekalanos, J.J., et al.: Cholera toxin genes: nucleotide sequence, deletion analysis and vaccine development. *Nature* 1983; 306: 551-557.

Morris, J.G. Jr., Black, R.E.: Cholera and other vibrioses in the United States. *N Engl J Med* 1985; 312:343-350.

Moss, J., and Vaughn, M.: Activation of adenylate cyclase by choleragen. *Ann Rev Biochem* 1979; 48: 581-600.

Ouchterlony, Ö., Holmgren, J., (editors): *Cholera and related diarrheas; molecular aspects of a global health problem*. 43rd Nobel Symposium, co-sponsored by the World Health Organization. Basel: S. Karger, 1980.

van Heyningen, W.E., Seal, J.R.: *Cholera: the American scientific experience, 1947-1980*. Boulder, Colorado: Westview Press, 1983.

41 *Escherichia coli* in Diarrheal Disease

Doyle J. Evans, Jr., PhD

Dolores G. Evans, PhD

General Concepts
Distinctive Properties
Pathogenesis
Host Defenses
Epidemiology
Diagnosis
Control

General Concepts

Escherichia coli is a common bacterial species that colonizes the human large intestine; most strains are nonpathogenic commensals. Members of the species *E coli* are extremely heterogeneous in genetic composition. To date, the only generally accepted subspecies classification scheme devised is based on somatic and surface-associated antigens. *E coli* are transmitted person-to-person with no known animal vectors, and the incidence of *E coli* diarrhea is related to hygiene, food processing, and general sanitation. *E coli* that cause diarrheal diseases generally fit into one of three categories composed of serogroups (somatic O groups) or serotypes (O:H combinations). The organisms of these categories share one of three modes of pathogenesis (Table 41-1). Note that this classification is presumptive, as not every isolate having a particular O:H combination behaves as an enteropathogen. Also, the lists of *E coli* in Table 41-1 are incomplete, as O and H antigens are not virulence factors per se, and other serotypes of *E coli* associated with diarrheal disease have not been adequately researched or detected with sufficient frequency to justify classification. Table 41-1 presents the genetic diversity of *E coli:*

Table 41-1   Major Serogroups and Serotypes of *Escherichia coli* That Cause Diarrheal Disease

Enteropathogenic E coli (EPEC) (Epidemic Infantile Diarrhea)	Shigellalike E coli Serogroups (Dysenterylike Disease)	Entertoxigenic E coli (ETEC) Serotypes (Watery Diarrhea)
020, 026	028, 0112,	06:H16, 06:H⁻,
044, 055,*	0124, 0136,	08:H9, 08:H⁻,
086, 0111,	0143, 0144,	015:H11, 015:H⁻,
0114, 0119,	0152	025:H42, 025:H⁻,
0125, 0126,		063:H12, 063:H⁻,
0127, 0128,†		078:H11, 078:H12,
0142, 0158,		078:H⁻
0159†		

*Serogroups underlined are cross-reactive with 0 groups of *Salmonella*.
†Also frequently found to be enterotoxigenic.

some *E coli* closely resemble *Shigella* species in producing diseases resembling dysentery, others share antigenicity with *Salmonella* species, and others are unique. Production of virulence factors (enterotoxins and colonization factors) of enterotoxigenic *E coli* is determined by extrachromosomal elements (plasmids), which are transmissible between *E coli* strains belonging to different serotypes and which are also susceptible to spontaneous deletion, thus adding to the genetic diversity of such strains. Important host defenses against *E coli* diarrheal disease include gastric acidity, intestinal motility, and the normal intestinal flora.

Distinctive Properties

E coli somatic O-specific antigen (lipopolysaccharide) consists of polysaccharide chains linked to a core oligosaccharide anchored to a lipid A-KDO (2-keto-3-deoxy-mannulosoctonic acid) complex, which is common to all gram-negative bacteria. O-specificity is determined by sugar or amino-sugar composition and the sequence of outer polysaccharide chains. More than 169 different O-specific antigens have been described since Kauffmann began this method of grouping *E coli* in 1943. In normal smooth strains, which possess O-specific antigens, the core lipopolysaccharide complex is buried beneath the O antigen. O-minus mutants also occur, in which the core lipopolysaccharide is exposed; these are called rough strains. Considerable cross-reactivity exists between *E coli* O antigens; many O groups of *E coli* are cross-reactive or identical with specific O groups of *Shigella*, *Salmonella*, or *Klebsiella*.

Many smooth isolates of *E coli* do not react with antisomatic antibody unless the cells are boiled or autoclaved before testing. This was thought to be due to the presence of capsular, or K (after German *Kapsel*), antigens. An elaborate scheme based on indirectly identified K antigens of various types was devised to explain these results. After many years, most inagglutinability has been shown to be attributable to interference by flagellar or fimbrial antigens and not to the presence of capsular antigens; however, inagglutinability with antibody can be caused by the presence of K antigens that are acidic polysaccharides. The only K (A type or heat-stable) antigens now recognized as valid are K1–K57, K62, K74, K82–K84, K87, K92–K98, and K100; others reported in the literature are no longer valid. Two of the heat-labile K antigens (K88 and K99) are now known to be fimbriae.

The H antigens of *E coli* are the flagellar antigens, of which more than 42 have been identified. *E coli* isolates may be nonmotile and nonflagellated and thus H-negative (H⁻). O groups of *E coli* that are more cross-reactive with O groups of *Shigella* are commonly H-negative.

H-typing is important in *E coli* associated with diarrheal disease for two reasons: first, a strain causing an outbreak or epidemic can be differentiated from the normal stool flora by its unique O:H antigenic makeup. Second, most enterotoxigenic *E coli* belong to specific serotypes; this relationship facilitates their identification, even in isolated cases (see Table 41-1). Why specific serotypes are so closely associated with the production of plasmid-determined virulence factors remains a mystery.

Most *E coli* isolates also produce heat-labile surface-associated proteins antigenically unrelated to O and H. These antigens can be seen in electron micrographs as filamentous structures called fimbriae or pili, which are much thinner and usually more rigid than flagella. No serotyping scheme has been devised to classify *E coli* fimbriae, because for years these structures were not considered medically important and preliminary work indicated these proteins were antigenically homogeneous in *E coli*. However, the discovery that the so-called K antigens K88 and K99 are fimbriae, and the more recent discovery of fimbrial colonization factors (CFA/I and CFA/II antigens) on *E coli* that are enterotoxigenic for humans has stimulated renewed interest in *E coli* fimbriae (Figure 41-1). In fact, a preliminary classification scheme exists, as K88, K99, CFA/I, CFA/II, and common fimbriae are each known to be antigenically unique.

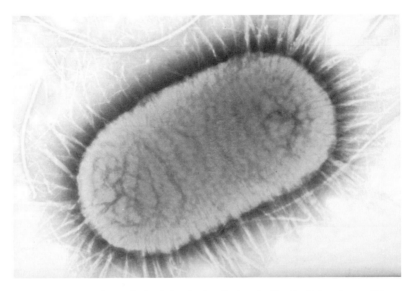

Figure 41-1 Electron micrograph of negatively stained enterotoxigenic *E coli* cell showing peritrichous CFA/I fimbriae. The thicker curved structures are flagella disattached from the cell (original magnification 40,000×; enlarged to 100,000× and reduced for publication).

Pathogenesis

E coli diarrheal disease is contracted orally by ingesting food or water contaminated with a pathogenic strain shed by an infected person. A discussion of the pathogenesis of *E coli* diarrhea requires separate consideration of the three most common types of enteropathogenic *E coli*.

Enterotoxigenic *E coli* diarrhea occurs in all age groups, but mortality is most common in infants in all countries, particularly in the most undernourished or malnourished in developing nations; however, single-source outbreaks of enterotoxigenic *E coli* diarrhea involving contaminated water supplies or food have been reported in adults in the United States and Japan. Adults traveling from temperate climates to more tropical areas, which are usually less sanitized, typically experience travelers' diarrhea caused by enterotoxigenic *E coli*. The high incidence of this diarrhea in travelers is not readily explained, but contributing factors are low levels of immunity and an increased opportunity for infection.

The pathogenesis of enterotoxigenic *E coli* diarrhea is a two-step process: intestinal colonization followed by elaboration of enterotoxin(s). Colonization, or adherence to the mucosal epithelium and subsequent multiplication on the gut surface, is achieved by the fimbriae. Two major colonization factor antigens (CFA/I and CFA/II) exist; which antigen is produced is determined by the enterotoxigenic *E coli* serotype. For example, enterotoxigenic *E coli* serotypes 078:H11 and 025:H42 produce CFA/I, whereas enterotoxigenic *E coli* of serotypes 06:H16 and 08:H9 produce CFA/II. The search for other antigenically unique CFAs continues; two prime candidates (E8775 and CFA/III) have been described, but have not yet been fully evaluated in terms of their geographic distribution, incidence relative to CFA/I and CFA/II, and genetic interrelationships with enterotoxin production. Fatal enterotoxigenic diarrhea of newborn domestic animals is caused by *E coli* organisms of different serotypes that produce different colonization factor antigens. K88 and 987P antigens are the CFAs of enterotoxigenic *E coli* specific for swine, and K99 is the CFA specific for calves and lambs.

Enterotoxigenic *E coli* diarrhea results from hypersecretion of water and electrolytes caused by heat-stable enterotoxin (ST), a heat-labile enterotoxin (LT), or both. The heat-stable enterotoxin is actually a family of toxic peptides ranging from 18 to approximately 50 amino acid residues in length, all having the ability to stimulate intestinal guanylate cyclase, the enzyme that converts guanosine 5'-triphosphate (GTP) to cyclic guanosine 5'-monophosphate (cGMP). Increased intracellular cGMP inhibits intestinal fluid uptake and has a net secretory effect. Both human- and animal-associated enterotoxigenic *E coli* produce one variety of heat-stable enterotoxin (STa or ST-H), which is detectable by the infant mouse assay (see Table 41-2); some animal-associated enterotoxigenic *E coli* produce another variety (STb or ST-P), which is not associated with human diarrhea and not detectable by the mouse assay.

The heat-labile enterotoxin is an antigenic protein whose mechanism of action is similar to that of *V cholerae* enterotoxin. Interestingly, the *E coli* heat-labile enterotoxin shares antigenic determinants with cholera toxin, and their primary amino acid sequences are similar. Heat-labile enterotoxin is composed of two species of subunits. One type of subunit (the B subunit) binds the toxin to the target cells via a specific receptor that has been identified as G_{m1} ganglioside. The other type of subunit (the A subunit) is then activated by cleavage of a peptide bond and internalized. It then catalyzes the ADP-ribosylation (transfer of ADP-ribose from nicotinamide adenine dinucleotide, or NAD) of a regulatory subunit of membrane-bound adenylate cyclase, the enzyme that converts ATP to cAMP. This activates the adenylate cyclase, which produces excess intracellular cAMP and, by some unknown mechanism, hypersecretion of water and electrolytes into the bowel lumen.

Diarrheal disease of infants and young children caused by *E coli* belonging to shigellalike serogroups is bacillary dysentery; that is, bloody diarrhea with mucus. Epithelial tissue destruction is evident, as in shigellosis. The infection centers in the large intestine, and invasive *E coli* strains do not produce either heat-stable or heat-labile enterotoxins. This type of *E coli* disease is limited mostly to impoverished populations living under crowded, unsanitary conditions, and thus is relatively rare in the United States.

Diarrheal disease of infants and young children caused by *E coli* belonging to the enteropathogenic *E coli* serogroups (EEC or EPEC; see Table 41-1) was originally described as epidemic infantile diarrhea. Diarrhea outbreaks associated with entero-pathogenic *E coli* serogroups still occur sporadically, although much less frequently than in the past. Controversy regarding this type of diarrhea has several sources. First, enteropathogenic *E coli* often can be isolated from healthy contacts and healthy individuals; second, *E coli* serotyping is a complex process susceptible to errors in identification, particularly becasue of cross-reactions between different O groups; and third, the mode of pathogenesis of enteropathogenic diarrhea has not been elucidated. Evidence suggests that EPEC infection resembles *Salmonella* infection, and that the bacteria exhibit the limited invasiveness characteristic of enteritis (bacteria invading as far as the lamina propria of the intestinal villi, but not causing massive tissue destruction). Studies of intestinal biopsy specimens from patients with enteropathogenic *E coli* and of EPEC-infected laboratory animals show that the *E coli* attach intimately to the intestinal microvilli and cause a localized degeneration of the epithelial cells, which is characterized by loss of microvilli, and the distortion and disruption of the plasma membranes. Some evidence suggests that these effects are caused by a cytotoxin. Several instances have been noted in which enteropathogenic *E coli* serogroups have gained *ent* plasmids from enterotoxigenic *E coli* serotypes in vivo and thus produce enterotoxins, but most EPEC do not produce enterotoxins according to the standard assays for heat-stable and heat-labile enterotoxins.

Host Defenses

As in any orally transmitted disease, the first line of defense against *E coli* diarrheal disease is gastric acidity. Other nonspecific defenses are small intestine motility and a large population of normal flora in the large intestine. In the case of enterotoxigenic *E coli*, which adhere to mucosal surfaces by fimbriae, the host cells must have specific receptors that recognize these bacterial adhesins. This may easily explain the host specificity of the enterotoxigenic *E coli* because animal species lacking appropriate receptors are naturally resistant.

Information about intestinal immunity against diarrheal disease is somewhat superficial. Circulating antibody responses to *E coli* are erratic and unpredictable; however, immune responses to O antigens, fimbrial antigens, and heat-labile enterotoxins do occur in animals and humans. Passive immune protection of infants and suckling animals by colostral antibody is important. Human breast milk also contains nonimmunoglobulin factors (receptor-type molecules) that can neutralize *E coli* toxins and CFAs. Research on vaccine development indicates that antifimbrial antibody is more efficient than antitoxin antibody in preventing enterotoxigenic *E coli* diarrhea in animals and humans.

Epidemiology

E coli diarrheal disease, of all types, is transmitted person-to-person with no known important animal vectors. The incidence of *E coli* diarrhea is clearly related to hygiene, food processing, general sanitation, and the opportunity for contact. Diagnostic and epidemiologic evidence is based on isolating *E coli* of particular serotypes from diarrheal stool cultures and, where possible, virulence testing of serotyped or randomly chosen isolates. Titration of anti-O, antitoxin, and anti-colonization factor antibody levels in acute and convalescent paired sera is a helpful but not reliable index in naturally acquired diarrhea because circulating antibody responses are erratic.

Besides cases in travelers and common source outbreaks involving adults, *E coli* diarrheal disease occurs most commonly as a nosocomial, hospital-acquired infection in infants. *E coli* is transmitted rapidly in hospital nurseries. Pathogenic strains stay in nurseries for a long time because of fast patient turnover; extreme measure of isolation and quarantine are necessary to stem an outbreak. Deaths are most likely to occur in babies in intensive care units and in premature infants.

Diagnosis

Enterotoxigenic *E coli* diarrhea is characterized by watery stool, with or without associated symptoms such as nausea, malaise, vomiting, fever, or abdominal pain; onset is rapid and duration is short. Shigellalike *E coli* diarrhea is characterized by a dysentery-type stool (blood, mucus, or both and shedding of epithelial cells and polymorphonuclear leukocytes) accompanied by abdominal pain and fever. Enteropathogenic *E coli* diarrhea may be accompanied by a variety of symptoms, and the duration is variable. Neither condition can be diagnosed solely on symptomatolgy, especially as other enteropathogens can produce the same clinical picture and mixed infections are common.

Enteropathogenic *E coli* in general are difficult to identify without specialized facilities for serotyping and virulence testing. *E coli* is usually suspected in cases that appear to be infectious diarrhea but are found to be negative for well-defined enteropathogens such as *Shigella, Samonella,* or intestinal parasites. Serotypic identification (O and H antigens) is presumptive, at best, in isolated cases, but is helpful in institutional or community outbreaks. Representative isolates should be sent to a reference laboratory for confirmation of serotype and, if possible, for testing of virulence and virulence factors.

Virulence testing is impractical for the enteropathogenic *E coli* serogroups because the specific virulence-associated antigens or toxins remain unknown. Virulence of the Shigellalike *E coli* isolates can be confirmed by tests for tissue invasiveness using the

Sereny guinea pig eye test or the HeLa cell tissue culture test. In the Sereny test a drop of broth culture is placed in the conjunctiva, or eye sac, of the guinea pig. Invasive *E coli* cause an eye infection, keratoconjunctivitis, usually within 48 hours. A positive HeLa cell test consists of finding *E coli* within the tissue culture cells. Tests for invasiveness are rarely performed in clinical laboratories because the incidence of Shigellalike *E coli* disease is low.

Tests for virulence factors of suspect enterotoxigenic *E coli* isolates are available at specialized research and reference laboratories. This discussion concerns only the organisms isolated from humans, although the same principles apply to those isolated from animals. Enterotoxigenic *E coli* may produce only heat-stable or heat-labile enterotoxin, or both. Both enterotoxins are released from bacteria during growth in liquid media, so cell-free culture fluids are suitable for testing. Table 41-2 lists the major assays used to detect and quantify these enterotoxins. The permeability factor assay and the tissue culture assays also are suitable for titration of anti–heat-labile enterotoxin antibody in serum. Although the ST peptides are nonantigenic because of their small size, they have been coupled covalently to carrier proteins to produce anti-ST antibody for detecting ST by the enzyme-linked immunosorbent assay, or ELISA. Heat-labile enterotoxin and anti–heat-labile enterotoxin antibody can be quantified in vitro by radioimmunoassay, ELISA, or passive immune hemolysis assay, all of which are extremely sensitive.

Table 41-2   Major Assays Used for the Enterotoxins Produced by Enterotoxigenic *E coli*

Assay	Brief description		Enterotoxin Detected*
	Dose	*Measure*	
Infant rabbit	Peroral or intraluminal injection	Fluid accumulation in intestines	Heat-stable (ST), Heat-labile (LT)
Adult rabbit	Injection into ligated loops of small intestine	Fluid accumulation in loops	ST, LT
Infant mouse†	Direct injection into stomach	Fluid accumulation in intestines	ST only
Permeability factor assay	Intradermal injection into young rabbits or guinea pigs, followed by IV injection of blue dye after 24 hours	Induration and zones of intense blue	LT only
Tissue culture assays† Cultured Y-1 adrenal tumor cells Chinese hamster ovary (CHO) cells		Morphologic changes	LT only
ELISA		Toxin antigens	ST, LT
Gene-probe hybridization		Toxin genes (DNA)	ST, LT

*Heat-labile, but not heat-stable, activity can be further identified by neutralization with anti-LT serum and by observing for heat-inactivation of LT.
†Methods of choice for routine diagnosis.

In human-associated enterotoxigenic *E coli*, the production of ST and LT enterotoxins, and of the CFA/I and CFA/II fimbriae, is determined by genes residing on plasmids. The plasmid encoding for CFA/I also encodes for ST; the plasmid encoding for CFA/II also encodes for both ST and LT. ST-only and LT-only plasmids also occur. Recently, the genes encoding for ST (both STa and STb) and for LT have been isolated and cloned. These specific DNA sequences provide the basis for in vitro assays for ST and LT in clinical isolates. In these gene probe hybridization assays, the toxin genes are radioactively labelled and individually tested for hybridization with DNA obtained from the *E coli* isolates; a positive result is indicated by a spot produced on a radioautograph. Gene probes for the various colonization factor antigens also are under development.

E coli of all varieties, including enterotoxigenic organisms, produce the common form of fimbriae, but only the enterotoxigenic organisms are known to possess fimbriae that play a role in virulence. Also, CFA fimbriae (CFA/I and CFA/II) usually are produced by strains that produce both enterotoxins, rather than those that produce only one. Thus, a positive test for CFA/I or CFA/II tentatively identifies an *E coli* isolate as enterotoxigenic *E coli*. These antigens can be detected by bacterial agglutination using specific anti-CFA serum. CFA fimbriae can be distinguished from common fimbriae because although all fimbriae cause red blood cells to agglutinate, the carbohydrate mannose inhibits only the hemagglutination reaction of common fimbriae; also, only certain species of erythrocytes have the appropriate receptors for CFA fimbriae. Thus *E coli* cells with common fimbriae produce hemagglutination with guinea pig and human erythrocytes that is mannose-sensitive; cells with CFA/I produce hemagglutination with human erythrocytes that is mannose-resistant (not inhibited by mannose); and cells with CFA/I or CFA/II produce hemagglutination with bovine erythrocytes that is mannose-resistant. However, positive hemagglutination tests obtained in screening *E coli* isolates must be confirmed using specific antisera, because other mannose-resistant hemagglutinins may occur on *E coli* isolates and many of these other hemagglutinins have not yet been identified and classified.

Control

Control of *E coli* diarrheal disease is best achieved by preventing transmission by sanitation and sometimes by passive immunization (milk antibodies). The widespread introduction of infant milk formula products into developing countries has created controversy because of the importance of breast-feeding in the passive immune protection of infants against intestinal pathogens, including *E coli*. Attempts at artificial active immunization with vaccines have been unsuccessful, but newer vaccine preparations based on the fimbrial antigens of *E coli* (enterotoxigenic only) offer promise for the future.

Application of antibiotics, or chemotherapeutic agents, for the treatment of *E coli* diarrheal disease usually is reserved for long-term, or chronic, cases, and for the very young in life-threatening situations. Because in most cases death is caused by dehydration, intravenous rehydration is important in severe cases. Oral rehydration therapy is recommended and is gaining popularity, particularly because it is a relatively safe, convenient, and simple procedure to perform.

References

Bäck, E., et al.: Enterotoxigenic *Escherichia coli* and other gram-negative bacteria of infantile diarrhea: Surface antigens, hemagglutinins, colonization factor antigen, and loss of enterotoxigenicity. *J Infect Dis* 1980; 142:318-327.

Darfeuille, A., et al.: A new colonization factor antigen (CFA/III) produced by enteropathogenic *Escherichia coli* 0128:B12. *Ann Microbiol (Inst Pasteur)* 1983; 134A:53-64.

Evans, D.G., Evans, D.J., Jr., Clegg, S.: Detection of enterotoxigenic *Escherichia coli* colonization factor antigen I in stool specimens by an enzyme-linked immunosorbent assay. *J Clin Microbiol* 1980; 12:738-743.

Evans, D.J. Jr., et al.: Hemagglutination typing of *Escherichia coli:* Definition of seven hemagglutination types. *J Clin Microbiol* 1980; 12:235-242.

Klipstein, F.A., et al.: Vaccine for enterotoxigenic *Escherichia coli* based on synthetic heat-stable toxin cross-linked to the B subunit of heat-labile toxin. *J Infect Dis* 1983; 147:318-326.

Moon, H.W., et al.: Attaching and effacing activities of rabbit and human enteropathogenic *Escherichia coli* in pig and rabbit intestine. *Infect Immun* 1983; 41:1340-1351.

Moseley, S.L., et al.: Identification of enterotoxigenic *Escherichia coli* by colony hybridization using three enterotoxin gene probes. *J Infect Dis* 1982; 145:863-869.

Moss, J., et al.: NAD-dependent ADP-ribosylation of arginine and proteins by *Escherichia coli* heat-labile enterotoxin. *J Biol Chem* 1979; 245:6270-6272.

Newsome, P.M., Coney, K.A.: Synergistic rotavirus and *Escherichia coli* diarrheal infection of mice. *Infect Immunol* 1985; 47:573-574.

Rao, M.C., et al.: Mode of action of heat-stable *Escherichia coli* enterotoxin. Tissue and subcellular specificities and role of cyclic GMP. *Biochem Biophys Acta* 1980; 632:35-46.

42 Escherichia, Klebsiella, Enterobacter, Serratia, Citrobacter, and Proteus

M. Neal Guentzel, PhD

General Concepts
   Nosocomial Infections
   Community-Acquired Infections
Distinctive Properties of Organisms
   Structure and Antigens
   Toxins

Pathogenesis
Host Defenses
Epidemiology
Diagnosis
Control

General Concepts

The gram-negative bacilli that constitute members of the genera *Escherichia, Klebsiella, Enterobacter, Serratia, Citrobacter,* and *Proteus* (Table 42-1) are components of the normal flora of the human and animal intestinal tract and may be isolated from a variety of environmental sources. With the exception of *Proteus,* they are sometimes collectively referred to as the coliform bacilli because of shared biochemical properties, particularly the ability of most to ferment the sugar lactose.

At one time, many of these microorganisms were dismissed as harmless commensals. Today, they are known to be responsible for major health problems throughout the world. The increasing incidence of the coliforms, *Proteus,* and other gram-negative organisms in disease reflects in part a better understanding of their pathogenic potential but, more importantly, it reflects the changing ecology of bacterial disease. The widespread and often indiscriminant use of antibiotics has created drug-resistant gram-negative bacilli that readily acquire multiple resistance through transmission of drug-resistance plasmids (R factors). Conjugative resistance plasmids allow transfer of resistance genes among species and genera that normally do not exchange chromosomal

Table 42-1 Taxonomy of the Coliform Bacilli and *Proteus*

Genus	Species	Other Designations
Escherichia	*E coli* *	
Klebsiella	*K pneumoniae* *	Friedländer's bacillus
	K ozaenae	
	K rhinoscleromatis	
	K oxytoca	*K pneumoniae* (indol +, gelatin +)
Enterobacter	*E aerogenes* *	
	E agglomerans	*Erwinia herbicola*
	E cloacae *	
	E sakazakii†	*E cloacae* (yellow pigmented)
	E gergoviae†	
Citrobacter	*C freundii*	
	C diversus	*C intermedius* biotype b
	C amalonaticus†	*C intermedius* biotype a
Serratia	*S marcescens* *	
	S rubidaea	
	S liquefaciens	*Enterobacter liquefaciens*
	S fonticola†	
	S odorifera†	
	S plymuthica	
Proteus‡	*P mirabilis* *	
	P vulgaris	

*Major coliforms in nosocomial and/or community-acquired human disease (prevalent in published reports).
†Relatively new species designations. The quantitative importance of these organisms is not currently well documented.
‡Organisms previously designated as *Proteus morganii* and *Proteus rettgeri* are now classified in the genera *Morganella* and *Providencia*, respectively.

DNA. Resistance genes may move as transposons (see Chapter 20) from a plasmid to the bacterial chromosome or to a bacterial virus. The process of transposition may lead to accumulation of other virulence determinants, such as genes for toxin production and colonization, on the same plasmid.

Development of new surgical procedures, health support technology, and therapeutic regimens has provided new portals of entry and compromised many host defenses. As opportunistic pathogens, the coliforms and *Proteus* take advantage of weakened host defenses to colonize and elicit a variety of disease states.

Nosocomial Infections

Collectively, coliform bacilli and *Proteus* are responsible for approximately 40% of all nosocomial, or hospital-acquired, infections (Table 42-2). The mean nosocomial infection rate for 1979 was 3.3% of patients discharged from hospitals participating in the National Nosocomial Infections Survey. Another recent estimate of nosocomial infections in adult, general medical, and surgical patients in the mainstream of United States hospitals found that 5.2% of the patients had one or more nosocomial infections. Considering that an estimated 37 million acute-care patients are discharged from

Table 42-2   Frequency of Selected Pathogens Causing Nosocomial Infections*

Pathogen	*Percentage of Infections at Site*						
	Primary bacteremia	*Surgical wound*	*Lower respiratory*	*Urinary tract*	*Cutaneous*	*Other*	*All sites*
E coli	14.4	13.4	6.8	31.9	7.1	8.1	18.3
Klebsiella	13.7	5.2	11.2	9.4	4.5	4.5	7.9
Enterobacter	6.3	4.3	6.4	4.0	3.3	2.2	4.3
Serratia	3.9	1.6	3.7	2.1	1.8	1.2	2.2
Proteus-Providencia	2.3	6.1	5.1	9.3	4.9	3.8	6.6
Pseudomonas aeruginosa	4.8	5.9	9.5	11.4	6.0	5.6	8.4
Staphylococcus aureus	13.7	14.8	9.9	1.9	30.1	12.4	9.9
Group D Streptococci	6.8	9.2	1.5	14.2	6.3	5.7	9.2
Other pathogens	33.4	25.0	21.4	14.4	23.2	31.8	21.6
No culture or no pathogen	0.7	14.5	24.5	1.4	12.8	24.7	11.6
Isolates/10,000 discharges	18.5	103.5	64.3	154.6	26.5	48.6	416.0

*Data from the Centers for Disease Control. 1982. *National nosocomial infections study report, annual summary 1979.* Atlanta, Georgia.

hospitals in the United States annually, the coliforms and *Proteus* probably are responsible for hospital-acquired infections in more than 500,000 patients each year.

The highest rates of nosocomial infections routinely are observed on surgical and medical services. Primary sites of infection (in order of decreasing frequency) are: urinary tract, surgical wound, lower respiratory, cutaneous, and primary bacteremia. *E coli,* the predominant nosocomial pathogen, has been the major cause of infection in the urinary tract and in primary bacteremias. *Klebsiella* has been predominant in lower respiratory infections, whereas *Staphylococcus aureus* has been first in cutaneous infections. The major causes of surgical wound infections have been *S aureus* and *E coli.* Data for *Citrobacter* are not shown, but one study suggests this organism is responsible for approximately 1.5% of nosocomial infections.

Other coliform organisms and *Proteus* have been incriminated in various hospital-acquired infections. Members of the *Klebsiella, Enterobacter,* and *Serratia* are frequent causes of bacteremia at some medical centers. They are also involved frequently in infections associated with respiratory tract manipulations, such as tracheotomy and procedures involving use of contaminated inhalation therapy equipment. *Klebsiella* and *Serratia* are commonly involved in infections following intravenous and urinary catheterization and in infections complicating burns. *Proteus* is a frequent cause of nosocomial infections of the urinary tract, surgical wounds, and lower respiratory tract. Less frequently, *Proteus* is a significant cause of bacteremia, most often in elderly patients. A series of nationwide outbreaks of bacteremia (1970–1971 and 1973) caused by contaminated commercial fluids for intravenous injections involved *E cloacae, E agglomerans,* and *C freundii.*

The role of *Citrobacter* in human disease is not well defined. Both *C freundii* and *C diversus* have been isolated, predominantly as superinfecting agents from urinary and respiratory tract infections. *Citrobacter* septicemia may occur in patients with multiple predisposing factors and also has been reported to be a causative agent in meningitis, septicemia, and pulmonary infections of neonates and young children.

Compromised patients often develop infections with coliforms that are not necessarily hospital-acquired. For example, *E coli* is responsible for about 40% of cases of neonatal bacterial meningitis. Infections seen in cancer patients with solid tumors or malignant blood diseases frequently are caused by *E coli, Klebsiella, Serratia,* and *Enterobacter.* Such infections often have a grave and lethal course. Individuals who are immunosuppressed by therapy (for example, cancer patients or transplant recipients) or by congenital defects of host immune systems may develop infections caused by *Klebsiella, Enterobacter,* and *Serratia.* Many additional factors such as diabetes, trauma, and chronic lung disease may predispose to infection by coliforms and other microbes.

Community-Acquired Infections

The coliform organisms and *Proteus* are major causes of diseases acquired outside the hospital; many of these diseases eventually require hospitalization. *E coli* is the causative agent in approximately 85% of cases of urethocystitis (infection of the urethra and bladder), in about 80% of cases of chronic bacterial prostatitis, and in up to 90% of cases of acute pyelonephritis (inflammation of the pelvis and parenchyma of the kidney). *Proteus, Klebsiella,* and *Enterobacter* are among the other organisms most frequently involved in urinary tract infections. *Proteus,* particularly *P mirabilis,* is believed to be the most common cause of renal infection stones, one of the most serious complications of unresolved or recurrent bacteriuria.

Klebsiella was first recognized clinically as a causative agent of pneumonia. *K pneumoniae* accounts for approximately 3% of pneumonia cases; however, extensive damage produced by the organism results in high (up to 90% in untreated patients) case fatality rates. *K rhinoscleromatis* is the causative agent of rhinoscleroma, a chronic destructive granulomatous disease of the respiratory tract that is endemic to Eastern Europe and Central America. *K ozaenae* is an infrequent cause of serious infection. It classically is associated only with ozena, an atrophy of nasal mucosal membranes with a mucopurulent discharge that tends to dry into crusts; however, recent studies indicate that the organism may cause various other disease syndromes involving, on occasion, infections of the urinary tract, soft tissue, middle ear, and blood.

Acute diarrheal diseases, particularly of infants and young children, are a major global health problem. *E coli* is an important cause of diarrhea, and *Klebsiella, Enterobacter, Serratia, Citrobacter,* and *Proteus* occasionally are implicated. *E coli* pathogenic for the intestinal tract may be subdivided into three groups (see Chapter 41). The first are specific serotypes of *E coli,* the classic enteropathogenic *E coli,* which in the past have been implicated in serious outbreaks of disease in newborn nuseries. Today, the classical enteropathogenic serotypes are implicated much less frequently in outbreaks of infantile diarrhea. The second are toxin-producing, or enterotoxigenic, *E coli.* These are major causative agents of traveler's diarrhea, a common disease of tourists from the United States who travel to Mexico or developing countries. The third group are enteroinvasive *E coli* that produce symptoms resembling shigellosis. Invasive *E coli* do not appear to be important agents of diarrhea in the United States.

Distinctive Properties

Structure and Antigens

The generalized structure and antigenic composition of the coliform bacilli, as well as *Proteus* and other members of the family *Enterobacteriaceae,* are depicted schematically in Figure 42-1. Major antigens of coliforms are referred to as H, K, and O antigens. Coliforms and *Proteus* of specific serotypes (based on combinations of these antigens) may be associated with greater virulence or with preferential colonization and production of disease in particular body habitats. The first of these, H antigen determinants, consists of the proteins that make up the flagellar structure. *E coli, Enterobacter, Serratia, Citrobacter,* and *Proteus* are motile by peritrichous flagella; that is, flagella that grow from many places on the cell surface. *Klebsiella* are nonmotile, and nonflagellated, and thus have no H antigens.

Representative strains of all the coliforms and *Proteus* may possess nonflagellar appendages called fimbriae or pili. Fimbriae are associated with adhesive properties that in some cases, have been correlated with virulence. Different fimbrial colonization factors generally are detectable as hemagglutinins that can be distinguished by the type of erythrocyte agglutinated and by the susceptibility of the hemagglutination to inhibition by the sugar mannose. Sex pili are morphologically distinct from fimbriae, are

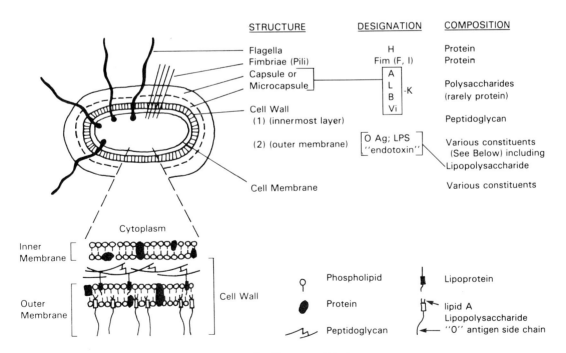

Figure 42-1 Structure and antigenic composition of coliforms and *Proteus.*

less numerous, have receptors for specific bacterial viruses, and are genetically determined by extrachromosomal plasmids. They are important in coliform ecology and in the epidemiology of diseases produced by coliforms and *Proteus* in that types F and I pili are involved in genetic transfer by conjugation (for example, chromosomal- and plasmid-mediated drug resistance or virulence factors).

K antigens (capsule antigens) are additional surface structures, usually in the form of compact polysaccharide capsules. Certain K antigens (K88 and K99 of *E coli*) are fimbriaelike proteins. The K antigens often block agglutination by specific O antisera. In the past, K antigens routinely were differentiated into A, L, and B groups based on differences in their lability to heat; however, the criteria are subject to difficulties that make the distinction tenuous. Some *Citrobacter* serotypes produce Vi (virulence) antigen, a K antigen also found in *Salmonella typhi*. Species of *Proteus, Enterobacter,* and *Serratia* apparently have no regular K antigens. However, the K antigens are important in the pathogenesis of some coliforms. A diffuse slime layer of variable thickness (the M antigen) also may be produced, but unlike the K antigens, it is nonspecific and is serologically cross-reactive among different organisms.

A rigid layer of peptidoglycan is external to the inner cell or plasma membrane and is linked covalently through lipoproteins to the outer membrane of the cell wall. The outer membrane contains receptors for bacterial viruses and bacteriocins (plasmid-mediated, antibioticlike bacteriocidal proteins called colicins in *E coli* that are active against the same or closely related species). It is also an effective barrier to penetration of many chemicals (for example, certain dyes) and antibiotics such as penicillin G and bacitracin. Certain transmembrane proteins, called porins, form water-filled pores through the hydrophobic core of the outer membrane and appear to be responsible for its molecular sieving properties.

The outer membranes of all the organisms contain lipopolysaccharide. Functionally, lipopolysaccharide is divisible into three regions: a heteropolysaccharide chain of repeating oligosaccharide units linked to a central acidic heterooligosaccharide core which, in turn, is linked to a lipoid region called lipid A. The activity of lipopolysaccharide as endotoxin resides in the lipid A portion of the molecule; the repeating sequence of carbohydrates external to the core polysaccharide constitutes the O antigen. Serologic specificity associated with O antigens is based on differences in sugar components, their linkages, and the presence or absence of substituted acetyl groups. Loss of the O antigen by mutation results in a smooth-to-rough transformation, often involving changes in colony type, saline agglutination, and loss of virulence. Certain strains of *P vulgaris* (OX-19, OX-2, and OX-K) produce O antigens that are shared by some rickettsiae. These *Proteus* strains are used in an agglutination test (Weil–Felix test) for antibodies in serum produced against rickettsiae of the typhus and spotted fever groups (see Chapter 53).

Toxins

Aside from endotoxin, which is present in all of the organisms, a number of exotoxins may be produced. Enterotoxigenic *E coli* strains (see Chapter 41) produce a plasmid-coded, heat-labile exotoxin (LT) and a plasmid-coded, heat-stable exotoxin (ST), either in combination or alone. Other enterotoxigenic *E coli* may produce a shigellalike toxin.

Recently, enterotoxigenic strains of *Klebsiella, Enterobacter, Serratia, Citrobacter,* and *Proteus* have been isolated from infants and children with acute gastroenteritis. The enterotoxins of at least some of these organisms are the heat-labile and heat-stable types and have other properties in common with the *E coli* toxins. Some *E coli* strains may produce soluble or cell-bound hemolysins, which are manifested by the production of α-(greening) or β-(clear) hemolysis on blood agar plates.

Pathogenesis

The importance of the coliforms and *Proteus* in hospital- and community-acquired disease states and of factors predisposing to opportunistic infections have been emphasized. Nevertheless, the process of disease production by the coliforms is, in many cases, poorly understood.

Enterotoxigenic *E coli* have been perhaps the best studied coliforms with respect to pathogenesis (see Chapter 41). Briefly, establishment of the causative organisms in the intestinal tract may be promoted by specific plasmid-mediated fimbrial colonization factor antigens (for example, CFA/I and CFA/II), as has been suggested for *E coli* strains enteropathic for porcine (K88 antigen) and bovine (K99 antigen) hosts. The toxins bind to specific membrane receptors and through cyclic AMP (heat-labile toxin) or cyclic GMP (heat-stable toxin) elicit changes in electrolyte flux associated with loss of fluid to the intestinal lumen.

Disease produced by coliforms or *Proteus* in extraintestinal sites often involves specific serotypes of the organisms. For example, respiratory tract infections by *K pneumoniae* predominantly involve capsular types 1 and 2, whereas urinary tract infections often involve types 8, 9, 10, and 24. Similarly, only a few polysaccharide K antigens (types 1, 2, 3, 5, 12, and 13) of *E coli* are found with high frequency in urinary tract and other extraintestinal infections. These observations suggest that some serotypes of coliforms may be more frequent in extraintestinal infections because of special pathogenicity of the strains. An alternative explanation is that such strains may be simply the most prevalent types in the normal gut flora.

Evidence for special pathogenicity of coliform strains involved in extraintestinal infections has been obtained and well documented for *E coli*. The K1 antigen is a virulence factor found in approximately 80% of *E coli* involved in neonatal meningitis, an effect attributable at least in part to increased resistance to phagocytosis of K1 versus non-K1 strains. Certain O antigens (O7 and O18) are found in combination with K1, usually in strains isolated from cases of neonatal bacteremia and meningitis. These findings have been correlated with the increased resistance of the strains to the bactericidal effects of serum complement. Interestingly, the *E coli* K1 antigen, composed of neuraminic acid, is immunologically cross-reactive with the group B meningococcal polysaccharide capsule.

E coli strains isolated from extraintestinal infections are more likely to possess a number of properties not usually found in random fecal isolates. These include production of hemolysin, biosynthesis of colicin V (mediated by the colicin V plasmid), and adherence to target cells.

The enzyme urease, produced by *Proteus* and, to a lesser extent, by *Klebsiella,* is thought to play a major role in the production of infection-induced urinary stones.

Urease hydrolyzes urea to ammonia and carbon dioxide. Alkalinization of the urine by the ammonia can cause supersaturation. The decreasing solubility of magnesium and calcium phosphates leads to the formation of stones composed of struvite and apatite, respectively. Bacteria trapped within the stones may be refractory to antimicrobial therapy. The persisting organisms cause recurrent bacteriuria following discontinuation of therapy. Production of large stones may lead to a decrease in renal function. Ammonia produced by urease also may damage the epithelium of the urinary tract.

Evidence implicating endotoxin as a disease mechanism in most coliform and *Proteus* infections, except for bacteremia, is lacking. Many of the effects produced experimentally by injection of endotoxin into animals are observed in humans with coliform bacteremia, including fever, depletion of complement, release of inflammatory mediators, lactic acidosis, hypotension, vital organ hypoperfusion, irreversible shock, and death.

Host Defenses

The importance of failure of local or generalized host defense mechanisms in disease produced by the coliform organisms and *Proteus* cannot be overemphasized. The normal gastrointestinal flora, which include *E coli* and frequently other coliforms and *Proteus* in smaller numbers, play an important role in preventing disease through bacterial antagonism. Prolonged or indiscriminant antibiotic therapy compromises this defense mechanism by reducing susceptible components of the normal flora, facilitating colonization with nosocomial coliform strains or other bacteria.

The organisms may breach anatomic barriers through third-degree burns, ulceration associated with solid tumors of the skin and mucous membranes, intravenous blood or fluid administration, and surgical or instrumental procedures on the biliary, gastrointestinal, and genitourinary tracts. The lungs may be violated by instrumentation, as in tracheal intubation, or even by contaminated aerosols produced by contaminated nebulizers or humidifiers carrying organisms to the terminal alveoli.

Corticosteroid and radiographic therapy, or the increased steroid levels associated with pregnancy, tend to decrease host control over infections, for example, by depressing the immune response. Cytotoxic drugs also are immunosuppressive. Cancer- or drug-induced neutropenia is an important predisposing factor in bacteremia. Devitalized tissue or foreign bodies may be a source of organisms and provide physical protection from phagocytosis and other antimicrobial factors.

The interaction of multiple predisposing factors often determines the clinical course as well as the eventual outcome of coliform or *Proteus* infection. For example, death rates in bacteremia increase progressively when the underlying disease (for example, cancer or diabetes) is rated as nonfatal, ultimately fatal (death within 5 years), or rapidly fatal (survival less than 1 year). Similarly, coliform and *Proteus* infections commonly are more severe in the very old and very young.

Epidemiology

The epidemiology of coliform and *Proteus* infections is complex and involves multiple reservoirs and modes of transmission. Members of *Klebsiella, Enterobacter, Serratia,*

Citrobacter, and *Proteus* normally are found in water, soil, occasionally in food, and, to a varying degree, in the intestinal tracts of humans and animals. *E coli* presumably is not free-living, and its presence in environmental samples is accepted as proof of recent fecal contamination.

The source of coliform and *Proteus* infections may be exogenous or endogenous. Studies of hospitalized adults and infants have shown that progressive colonization of the intestinal tract by nosocomial coliforms occurs with increasing length of hospitalization. Patients on antibiotics, severely ill patients, and probably infants are more likely to be colonized, and other sites of colonization such as the nose and throat may be important in such patients. A higher risk of nosocomial infections occurs in colonized than in noncolonized patients.

Modes of transfer may be indirect, involving various vehicles, or transfer may occur through direct contact. A variety of contaminated vehicles have been implicated in the spread of nosocomial pathogens. For example, *Klebsiella, Enterobacter,* and *Serratia* have been recovered in high numbers from hospital food, particularly salads, with the hospital kitchen being a primary source. An outbreak of urinary tract infections due to multiply drug-resistant *S marcescens* was associated with exposure of contaminated urine-measuring containers and urinometers. Serious outbreaks or individual cases of bacteremia due to coliforms have been associated with intrinsic contamination of intravenous fluids or caps during manufacture, and with extrinsic contamination of intravenous fluids and administration sets in the hospital environment. Other medical devices and medications have served as vehicles for the spread of nosocomial pathogens. Occasionally, transmission may be through members of the hospital staff who are colonized with nosocomial pathogens in the rectum, vagina, or on the hands; however, passive carriage on the hands of medical personnel constitutes the major mode of transmission.

Certain properties of the coliforms may be important in the epidemiology of hospital-acquired infections. Coliform bacteria other than *E coli* frequently are found in tap or even distilled or deionized water. They may persist or actively multiply in water associated with respiratory therapy or hemodialysis equipment. *Klebsiella, Enterobacter,* and *Serratia,* like *Pseudomonas,* may exhibit increased resistance to antiseptics and disinfectants. The same group of coliforms has been found to have a selective ability over other common nosocomial pathogens (including *E coli, Proteus, P aeruginosa,* and staphylococci) to proliferate rapidly at room temperature in commercial parenteral fluids containing glucose.

The epidemiology of *S marcescens* infections generated public interest because of the United States Army's previous use of it in simulated biologic warfare experiments in United States cities. Red-pigmented strains, like those used by the Army, have an interesting history that dates to antiquity in the form of historical references to the miraculous appearance of blood in food. Because of its assumed innocuous nature, pigmented *S marcescens* has been widely used by scientists as biologic markers. The organisms were used without apparent ill effects to demonstrate a wide range of phenomena such as bacteremia following dental extraction, migration of organisms through urinary catheters, bacterial drifts, and settling of aerosols in hospitals. Pigmented varieties (as shown by 25 C incubation) are rarely isolated from humans and the causative role of *S marcescens* as a nosocomial pathogen has involved specific types of nonpigmented strains.

Diagnosis

Because the coliforms and *Proteus* have been isolated as causative agents from almost all types of infections, a differential diagnosis based on distinctive clinical characteristics rarely can be made. The clinical symptoms depend entirely on the site of infection.

Laboratory identification of coliform and *Proteus* infections demands competent laboratory personnel and properly collected specimens. The organisms have simple nutritional requirements and grow well on mildly selective differential media commonly used for the *Enterobacteriaceae*, but not on some moderately and highly selective enteric-plating media (*Salmonella-Shigella*, bismuth sulfite, and brilliant green agar). Extraintestinal specimens such as urine, purulent material from wounds or abcesses, sputa, and sediment from cerebrospinal fluid should be plated for isolation on blood agar and a differential medium such as MacConkey or eosin-methylene blue agar. Isolation from fecal specimens may be facilitated by adding a moderately selective medium such as xylose-lysine-desoxycholate (XLD) or Hektoen enteric agar. Use of tetrathionate or selenite broths for enrichment of enterotoxigenic strains from feces is not recommended because both inhibit various genera of coliforms. The strong, and occasionally the slow or weak, lactose-fermenting coliforms produce characteristic pigmented colonies on the enteric plating media. A striking characteristic of *Proteus* is its propensity to swarm over the surface of most plating media, making the isolation of other organisms in mixed cultures difficult. The swarming growth appears as a rapidly spreading thin film, sometimes with changing patterns of whirls and bands.

In cases of suspect bacteremia, replicate bottles (one for aerobic, the other for anaerobic cultures) containing 50–100 mL of appropriate medium with anticoagulant are inoculated with 10 mL portions of blood. Multiple specimens usually are required, both before and after initiation of antibiotic therapy. Specimens taken after antibiotic administration permit recognition of therapeutic failure at a time when the bacteremia still may be amenable to medical or surgical treatment.

All the coliforms and *Proteus* are gram-negative, facultative anaerobic, non-spore-forming rods that are typically motile, except for *Klebsiella*, which is nonmotile. The oxidase test is negative, and nitrates are reduced to nitrites (except in certain *Enterobacter*). *Proteus* and all coliforms ferment glucose, but fermentation of other carbohydrates varies. Lactose usually is fermented rapidly by *Escherichia*, *Klebsiella*, and more slowly by *Citrobacter* and some *Serratia*. *Proteus*, unlike the coliforms, deaminates phenylalanine to phenylpyruvic acid, and it does not ferment lactose. Typically, *Proteus* is rapidly urease-positive. Some species of *Klebsiella*, *Enterobacter*, and *Serratia* produce a positive urease reaction, but they do so more slowly. A battery of tests for biochemical properties is required to identify the coliforms and *Proteus* to the species level.

The coliforms are characterized by great antigenic diversity caused by various combinations of specific H, K, and O antigens. For example, approximately 50 H, 90 K, and 160 O antigens have been identified among various strains of *E coli*. In contrast, *Klebsiella*, with no H antigens, has 10 O antigens and approximately 80 K antigens. Serologic identification of the coliforms and *Proteus*, commonly by reference laboratories and sometimes in combination with phage (bacterial virus) or bacteriocin typing, is an extremely important epidemiologic tool. Similarly, antibiograms (patterns of resistance to antimicrobials) and plasmid profiles (determined by agarose gel electrophoresis) have proven to be useful in epidemiologic studies, particularly of multiresistant isolates of coliforms and *Proteus*. In hospital-acquired infections, for example, the same or a small number of serologic or plasmid types suggests single sources of infection. The finding of multiple serotypes or plasmid profiles suggests multiple sources of infection or endogenous infections.

Control

Prevention of coliform and *Proteus* infections, particularly those that are hospital-acquired, is a difficult and perhaps impossible task. An active and aggressive infection control committee can do much to reduce nosocomial infections through a program of recognition and control of predisposing factors, education and training of hospital personnel, and limited microbial surveillance. Except for investigations of potential outbreaks, routine cultures of personnel, patients, and the environment are not warranted. Meticulous hand washing after each patient contact is a highly effective means of reducing the transmission of nosocomial pathogens; however, this practice may be infrequently or poorly performed by some hospital personnel.

Active or passive immunization for coliform and *Proteus* infections presently is not practiced; however, a report from the CDC on an epidemiologic study of gram-negative nosocomial infections concluded that a vaccine or hyperimmune serum for the six common pathogens (*E coli, Klebsiella, Enterobacter, Serratia, P aeruginosa,* and *Proteus*) probably would have a major impact on morbidity and mortality from nosocomial infections. In one trial, the mortality rate was reduced markedly in a group of patients with gram-negative bacteremia who had been given antiserum against a mutant *E coli* with an exposed lipopolysaccharide core.

Ampicillin, sulfonamides, cephalosporins, tetracycline, trimethoprim/sulfamethoxazole, and nitrofurantoin have been useful in treating urinary tract infections from *E coli*. Gentamicin, amikacin, or tobramycin may be useful in treating systemic infections; however, laboratory tests for drug susceptibility are essential for effective antibiotic therapy against coliform and *Proteus* infections. The organisms often have multiple resistance due to presence of R plasmids transmissible by conjugation. In some cases, resolution of the infection may require drainage of abscesses or other surgical intervention.

References

Cooke, E.M., et al.: *Klebsiella* species in hospital food and kitchens: A source of organisms in the bowel of patients. *J Hyg Camb* 1980; 84:97–101.

Chow, A.W., et al.: A nosocomial outbreak of infections due to multiply resistant *Proteus mirabilis:* Role of intestinal colonization as a major reservoir. *J Infect Dis* 1979; 139:621–627.

Dixon, R.E., (editor): Symposium on nosocomial infections. *Am J Med* 1981; 70:379–473 (Part I); 631–744 (Part II); 899–986 (Part III).

Evans, D.J., Jr., Evans, D.G.: Classification of pathogenic *Escherichia coli* according to serotype and the production of virulence factors, with special reference to colonization factor antigens. *Rev Infect Dis* 1983; 5(Suppl):S692–S701.

John, J.F., Jr., Sharbaugh, R.J., Bannister, E.R.: *Enterobacter cloacae:* Bacteremia, epidemiology, and antibiotic resistance. *Rev Infect Dis* 1982; 4:13-28.

Saravolatz, L.D., et al.: An outbreak of gentamicin-resistant *Klebsiella pneumoniae:* Analysis of control measures. *Infect Control* 1984; 5:79-84.

Yu, V.L.: *Serratia marcescens:* Historical perspective and clinical review. *N Engl J Med* 1979; 300:887-893.

Van Furth, R., (editor): Evaluation and management of hospital infections. *New perspectives in clinical microbiology,* Vol 5. The Hague: Martinus Nijhoff Publishers, 1982.

43 *Pseudomonas*

Barbara H. Iglewski, PhD

General Concepts

The genus *Pseudomonas* contains more than 140 species, most of which are saprophytic. More than 25 species of pseudomonads have been associated with humans. Most pseudomonads known to cause disease in humans are associated with opportunistic infections. These include *P aeruginosa, P fluorescens, P putida, P cepacia, P stutzeri, P maltophilia,* and *P putrefaciens.* Only two species, *P mallei* and *P pseudomallei,* have been found to produce specific human diseases: glanders and melioidosis. *P aeruginosa* and *P maltophilia* account for approximately 80% of pseudomonads recovered from clinical specimens. Because of the frequency with which it is involved in human disease, *P aeruginosa* has received the most attention. *P aeruginosa* is a ubiquitous free-living bacterium that can be found in most moist environments. Although this organism seldom causes disease in healthy individuals, *P aeruginosa* is a major threat to hospitalized patients, particularly those with serious underlying diseases such as cancer or cystic fibrosis. The high mortality rate associated with these infections is due to a combination of weakened host defenses, bacterial resistance to antibiotics, and the production of extracellular bacterial enzymes and toxins.

Distinctive Properties

Structure

P aeruginosa is a gram-negative rod measuring 0.5–0.8 μm by 1.5–3.0 μm. Almost all strains are motile by means of a single polar flagellum, and some strains have two or three flagella. The flagella yield heat-labile antigens (H antigen). The significance of antibody directed against these antigens, aside from its value in serologic classification, is unknown. Clinical isolates usually have pili, which may be antiphagocytic and probably aid in bacterial attachment, thereby promoting colonization. In addition to these structures, the cell wall is often surrounded by an antiphagocytic polysaccharide slime layer, which may function as a capsule, although it lacks definite morphology.

The cell envelope of *P aeruginosa,* which is similar to that of other gram-negative bacteria, consists of three layers: the inner or cytoplasmic membrane, the peptidoglycan, and the outer membrane. The outer membrane is composed of phospholipid, protein, and lipopolysaccharide (LPS). The LPS from *P aeruginosa* is less toxic than that of other gram-negative rods. The LPS of most strains of *P aeruginosa* contains heptose, 2-keto-3-deoxyoctonic acid, and hydroxy fatty acids, in addition to side-chain and core polysaccharides. Recent evidence suggests that the LPS of a large percentage of strains isolated from patients with cystic fibrosis may have little or no polysaccharide side chain (O antigen), and that this finding correlates to their being polyagglutinable with typing sera.

Studies of isolated outer membranes suggest strong conservation of many of the outer membrane proteins of *P aeruginosa.* Although numerous serologic types exist (based on evaluations of O-specific antigens), many of the outer membrane proteins from these strains are antigenically cross-reactive.

Physiology

P aeruginosa is a nonfermentative aerobe that derives its energy from oxidation rather than fermentation of carbohydrates. Although able to use over 75 different organic compounds, it can depend on only acetate for carbon and ammonium sulfate for nitrogen. Furthermore, although an aerobe, it can grow anaerobically, using nitrate as an electron acceptor. This organism grows well at 25–37 C, but can grow slowly or at least survive at higher and lower temperatures. Indeed, the ability to grow at 42 C distinguishes it from many other *Pseudomonas* species. In addition to its nutritional versatility, *P aeruginosa* resists high concentrations of salt, dyes, weak antiseptics, and most commonly used antibiotics. These properties help explain its ubiquitous nature and contribute to its preeminence as a cause of nosocomial infections.

Exoenzymes

P aeruginosa produces many factors that may contribute to its virulence. Table 43-1 lists some of them. Almost all strains of *P aeruginosa* are hemolytic on blood agar plates, and several different hemolysins have been described. A heat-stable hemolytic glycolipid consisting of two molecules each of L-rhamnose and 1-β-hydroxy-decenoic acid has

Table 43-1   Products Produced by *Pseudomonas aeruginosa* Strains

Product	Incidence of Production (%)	LD$_{50}$ in Mice	Proposed Role
Endotoxin	100	300 μg/IV	Terminal shock
Heat-stable hemolysin	95	5 mg/IP	Toxic to alveolar macrophages
Leukocidin	4	0.4 μg/IP	Depresses host defenses
Phospholipase C	70	?	Hydrolyses lecithin
Pigments (pyocyanin and fluorescein)	90	?	Antibacterial
Proteases	90	200 μg/IP	Local tissue necrosis and spreading factor
Slime polysaccharide	100	~1 mg/IP	Antiphagocytic
Toxin A	90	0.2 μg/IP	Lethality and inhibition of host defenses
Exoenzyme S	38	?	Local and systemic toxicity

been purified. Although this hemolytic glycolipid is not very toxic to animals (5 mg injected intraperitoneally is required to kill a mouse), it is toxic to alveolar macrophages. Furthermore, *P aeruginosa* strains isolated from respiratory tract infections produce more hemolysin than do environmental strains, suggesting that this glycolipid hemolysin may play a role in *P aeruginosa* pulmonary infections. Correlation of hemolysin production with infections of other sites has not been reported.

Several heat-labile protein hemolysins also have been described. One of these hemolysins may be identical to phospholipase C, which is produced by approximately 70% of all clinical strains of *P aeruginosa*. Phospholipase C, which hydrolyzes lecithin, is of unknown toxicity, and its role in *P aeruginosa* infections also remains unknown. A few strains of *P aeruginosa* produce a thermolabile protein (leukocidin), which lyses leukocytes from many species including humans but is nonhemolytic. This leukocidin damages lymphocytes and various tissue culture cells and is very toxic to mice (minimum lethal dose is 1 μg). Despite its toxicity, leukocidin may be of minor importance as a virulence factor, as only 4% of the *P aeruginosa* strains tested produce it.

In contrast, small amounts of extracellular slime polysaccharide are produced by all strains of *P aeruginosa* tested. Purified slime, although relatively low in toxicity (LD$_{50}$ = 5 mg/mouse), is antiphagocytic and may be important to bacterial survival in humans and animals. Antibodies against slime are type-specific and protect against infection only by serologically identical strains of *P aeruginosa*.

Some strains of *P aeruginosa* produce large amounts of extracellular polysaccharide. These mucoid strains usually are isolated only from patients with cystic fibrosis. The role of these polysaccharides in the pathogenesis of *P aeruginosa* chronic lung infections is unknown, but they may impede phagocytosis and impair diffusion of antibiotics and thus facilitate colonization and persistence.

Most strains of *P aeruginosa* also produce one or more pigments, the most common being pyocyanin (a phenazine pigment) and fluorescein. These pigments are nontoxic in animals. Pyocyanin, however, retards the growth of some other bacteria and thus may facilitate colonization by *P aeruginosa*. One or more of these pigments appears to function in iron acquisition by *P aeruginosa*. Additional work is needed to clarify the role of these pigments in *P aeruginosa* infections.

Approximately 90% of *P aeruginosa* strains produce extracellular protease. Three separate proteases have been purified that differ in pH optimum, isoelectric point, and substrate specificity. Although all are capable of digesting casein, one of them, protease II, also digests elastin. When injected into the skin of animals, purified *P aeruginosa* proteases induce formation of hemorrhagic lesions, which become necrotic within 24 hours. These proteases also cause rapid tissue destruction when injected into the cornea of animal eyes or into rabbit lungs; they also probably contribute to the tissue destruction that accompanies *P aeruginosa* eye or lung infections, and may aid bacteria in tissue invasion. Their effects, however, appear to be localized, and they are not highly toxic (LD_{50} = approximately 200 μg/mouse) to animals (Table 43-1).

Toxin A

Toxin A, the most toxic known product of *P aeruginosa*, is produced by 90% of all strains. The median lethal dose of pure toxin A is about 0.2 μg/mouse. Its toxicity has been attributed to its ability to inhibit protein synthesis in susceptible cells. It achieves this by catalyzing the transfer of the ADP-ribosyl moiety of nicotinamide adenine dinucleotide (NAD) onto elongation factor 2 (EF-2) according to the following reaction:

$$\text{NAD} + \text{EF-2} \overset{\text{toxin}}{\rightleftharpoons} \text{ADP ribosyl-EF-2} + \text{nicotinamide} + \text{H}^+$$

The resultant ADP-ribosyl-EF-2 complex is inactive in protein synthesis. This intracellular mechanism of action of toxin A is identical to that of diphtheria toxin fragment A (see Chapter 48). Also like diphtheria toxin, *Pseudomanas* toxin A is released by *P aeruginosa* as a proenzyme. Toxin A is toxic to animals and cultured cells, but the proenzyme is devoid of enzymatic activity or very low in it. Table 43-2 shows the relationship between the various forms of toxin A and their enzymatic activity and mouse toxicity. Evidence suggesting that toxin A may be a major virulence factor of *P aeruginosa* includes observations that toxin-A–deficient mutants are less virulent in several animal models than their toxin-A–producing parental strains, as well as the observation that most patients surviving *P aeruginosa* sepsis have elevated levels of antitoxin A antibody or are infected with strains that produce little or no detectable

Table 43-2   Comparison of the Structure and Function of Toxin A and Its Fragments

	Daltons	*Mouse LD_{50}*	*Maximum ADP-ribosyl-transferase Activity per μg protein (%)*
Native toxin	70,000	0.2 μg	1–10
Reduced and denatured toxin*	70,000	>5.0 μg	35
Fragment A	27,000	>5.0 μg	100
Fragment B	43,000	Not tested	<1

*Toxin A was preincubated in 4 M urea and 1% dithiothreitol for 15 min.

toxin A in vitro. These studies need to be expanded before firm conclusions can be reached.

Exoenzyme S

A second ADP-ribosyltransferase, exoenzyme S, has been described. Exoenzyme S catalyzes the transfer of ADP-ribose onto a number of unidentified eukaryotic proteins, but it does not modify EF-2. Exoenzyme S is produced by at least 38% of clinical isolates of *P aeruginosa*. Its toxicity in animals is unknown, partly because it has been purified only in small quantities and then only in the presence of detergents. A transposon-induced S-deficient mutant, however, is less virulent in several animal models than its S-producing parental strain; thus, exoenzyme S may be involved in the pathogenesis of some *P aeruginosa* infections.

Pathogenesis

P aeruginosa can cause various diseases. Localized infection following surgery or burns commonly results in a generalized and frequently fatal bacteremia. Urinary tract infections following introduction of *P aeruginosa* on catheters or in irrigating solutions are not uncommon. Furthermore, most cystic fibrosis patients are chronically colonized with *P aeruginosa*. Interestingly, cystic fibrosis patients rarely have *P aeruginosa* bacteremia, probably because of high levels of circulating *P aeruginosa* antibodies; however, many cystic fibrosis patients ultimately die of localized *P aeruginosa* pneumonia. Necrotizing pneumonia also may occur in other patients following the use of contaminated respirators. *P aeruginosa* can cause severe corneal infections following eye surgery or injury. It is found in pure culture, especially in children with middle ear infections. Although rarely, *P aeruginosa* may cause meningitis following lumbar puncture and endocarditis following cardiac surgery. It also has been associated with some diarrheal disease episodes. Since the first reported case of *P aeruginosa* infection in 1890, the organism has been increasingly associated with bacteremia and currently accounts for 15% of all cases of gram-negative bacteremia. The overall mortality rate associated with *P aeruginosa* bacteremia is about 50%. Some infections (for example, eye and ear) remain localized; others, such as wound and burn infections and infections in leukemic and lymphoma patients, result in sepsis. The difference is most likely due to altered host defenses.

P maltophilia is the second most frequently isolated pseudomonad species in clinical laboratories. In nature, *P maltophilia* is found in water and in both raw and pasteurized milk. It has been associated with a variety of opportunistic infections in humans, including pneumonia, endocarditis, urinary tract infections, wound infections, septicemia, and meningitis. *P cepacia*, although primarily a plant pathogen (onion bulb rot), also is an opportunist. Most human infections caused by *P cepacia* are nosocomial in origin and include endocarditis, necrotizing vasculitis, pneumonia, wound infections, and urinary tract infections. Recently, *P cepacia* has been found increasingly to cause chronic lung infections in cystic fibrosis patients. These infections differ from those caused by *P aeruginosa* in that *P cepacia* has become systemic in a number of cystic fibrosis patients, whereas *P aeruginosa* infections remain confined to the lungs in these patients. *P cepacia* is highly resistant to aminoglycosides and other antibiotics, making it very difficult to control.

Unlike most pseudomonads, *P mallei* and *P pseudomallei* can cause disease in otherwise healthy individuals. *P mallei* is the etiologic agent of glanders, which is primarily a disease of equines. Humans generally become infected by inhalation or by direct contract through abraded skin. These infections are frequently fatal within 2 weeks of onset, although chronic infections also have been reported. Today, *P mallei* infections of equines are controlled and are rarely encountered in the western world. Similarly, melioidosis, an endemic glanderslike disease of animals and a pulmonary infection in humans that is caused by *P pseudomallei,* is rare in the western hemisphere. Melioidosis is still found in Southeast Asia and travelers returning from that area are sometimes infected.

Host Defenses

Although 85% of all *P aeruginosa* isolates are serum-resistant, the addition to them of polymorphonuclear leukocytes results in bacterial killing. Killing is most efficient in the presence of type-specific opsonizing antibodies, directed primarily at the antigenic determinants of lipopolysaccharide. This suggests that phagocytosis is an important defense and that opsonizing antibody is the principal functioning antibody in protecting from *P aeruginosa* infections; however, once a *P aeruginosa* infection is established, other antibodies, such as antitoxin, may be important in preventing death. Although evidence suggests interaction between *P aeruginosa* and the cellular immune system, patients with diseases characterized by impaired cellular immune responses (for example, Hodgkin's disease) do not tend to have an increased incidence of severe *P aeruginosa* infections; however, patients with diminished antibody responses caused by underlying disease or its associated therapy have more serious *P aeruginosa* infections. This underscores the importance of the humoral response in controling *P aeruginosa* infections. The exception occurs in cystic fibrosis; most cystic fibrosis patients have high levels of circulating antibodies but are unable to clear *P aeruginosa* efficiently from their lungs.

Epidemiology

P aeruginosa commonly inhabits soil, water, and vegetation. It is found in the skin of some healthy persons and has been isolated from 5% of throats and 3% of stools of nonhospitalized patients. Gastrointestinal carriage rates increase in hospitalized patients to 20% within 72 hours of admission. Within the hospital, *P aeruginosa* finds multiple reservoirs: disinfectants, respiratory equipment, food, sinks, taps, and mops. Furthermore, this organism is constantly reintroduced into the hospital environment on fruits, plants, vegetables, and patients tranferred from other facilities. Spread occurs from patient to patient on the hands of hospital personnel, from direct patient contact with contaminated reservoirs, and from the ingestion of contaminated foods and water.

Several different typing systems are available for epidemiologic studies: serologic, phage, and pyocin. In the pyocin system, pyocins (bacteriocins or aeruginocins) produced by the test strain are assayed for bactericidal activity against a series of indicator strains. A number of different serologic typing systems are used. Some employ combinations of heat-stable and heat-labile antigens, whereas others use only heat-stable antigens. No system is universally accepted.

Diagnosis

Diagnosis of *P aeruginosa* depends on its isolation and laboratory identification. The organism grows well on most laboratory media and commonly is isolated on blood agar plates or eosin-methylthionine blue agar. It is identified on the basis of its Gram morphology, inability to ferment lactose, a positive oxidase reaction, its fruitlike odor, and its ability to grow at 42 C. Fluorescence under ultraviolet radiation helps in early identification of *P aeruginosa* colonies and also is useful in suggesting its presence in wounds. Other pseudomonads are identified by specific laboratory tests.

Control

The spread of *P aeruginosa* can best be controlled by observing proper isolation procedures, aseptic technique, and careful cleaning and monitoring of respirators, catheters, and other instruments. Topical therapy of burn wounds with antibacterial agents such as mafenide or silver sulfadiazine coupled with surgical debridement have dramatically reduced the incidence of *P aeruginosa* sepsis in burn patients.

P aeruginosa is frequently resistant to many commonly used antibiotics. Although many strains are sensitive to gentamicin, tobramycin, colistin, and amikacin, resistant forms have developed, making susceptibility testing essential. The combination of gentamicin and carbenicillin is frequently used to treat severe *Pseudomonas* infections, especially in patients with leukopenia. Several types of vaccines are being tested, but none is currently available for general use.

References

Brown, M.R.W., (editor): *Resistance of* Pseudomonas aeruginosa. New York: John Wiley and Sons, 1975.

Clarke, P.H., Richman, M.N., (editors) *Genetics and biochemistry of* Pseudomonas. New York: John Wiley and Sons, 1975.

Cross, A.S., et al.: Evidence for the role of toxin A in the pathogenesis of infections with *Pseudomonas aeruginosa* in humans. *J Infect Dis* 1980; 142:538-546.

Hancock, R.E.W., et al.: *Pseudomonas aeruginosa* isolates from patients with cystic fibrosis: a class of serum-sensitive, nontypable strains deficient in lipopolysaccharide O side chain. *Infect Immun* 1983; 42:170-177.

Iglewski, B.H., Sadoff, J.C.: Toxin inhibitors of protein synthesis: production, purification and assay of *Pseudomonas aeruginosa* toxin A. In: *Methods in Enzymology*, Vol LX. Grossman L., Moldave K., (editors). New York: Academic Press, 1979.

Liu, P.V.: Extracellular toxins of *Pseudomonas aeruginosa*. *J Infect Dis* 1974; 130(Suppl):S95-S99.

Mutharia, L.M., Nicas, T.I., Hancock, R.E.W.: Outer membrane proteins of *Pseudomonas aeruginosa* serotyping strains. *J Infect Dis* 1982; 146:770-779.

Woods, D.E., Iglewski, B.H.: Toxins of *Pseudomonas aeruginosa*: new perspectives. *Rev Infect Dis* 1983; 5 (Suppl):S715-S722.

Young, L.S., Pollack, M.: Immunological approaches to prophylaxis and treatment of *Pseudomonas aeruginosa* infections. In: *Pseudomonas aeruginosa*. Sabath L.D., (editor). Bern: Hans Huber Publishers, 1980.

44 *Brucella*

G. G. Alton, DVM & S, MRCVS
J. R. L. Forsyth, MD

General Concepts
Distinctive Properties
Pathogenesis
Host Defenses
Epidemiology
Diagnosis
Control

General Concepts

Bacteria of the genus *Brucella* cause disease primarily in domestic animals and in some wild species, but most are also pathogenic for humans. In animals, brucellae typically cause disease of the reproductive organs, and abortion is usually the only sign of the disorder. Human brucellosis is an acute febrile disease, or a chronic disease with a wide variety of symptoms. It is a true zoonosis in that virtually all human infections are acquired from animals. The disease is controlled by the routine practice of pasteurization of milk and milk products, as well as by widespread campaigns to eradicate the disease in domesticated animals exhibiting positive serologic reactions to the organisms. Vaccines are available for protecting cattle, sheep, and goats.

The genus *Brucella* contains six species of bacteria. The three main species (*B abortus* of cattle; *B melitensis* of goats and sheep; and *B suis* of pigs, European hares, and reindeer) are important causes of human disease. Of the others, *B ovis* causes disease only in sheep, mainly rams; *B canis* affects both male and female dogs and causes a mild type of brucellosis in humans; and *B neotomae* has been found only in the American wood rat. Each of the three main species contains a number of biotypes that are distinguished by various metabolic and antigenic properties. Strains of brucellae with characteristics that differ from those just mentioned have been isolated from rodents in Africa, Australia, and the Soviet Union, but their taxonomic position has not yet been determined. The three main species can infect animals other than their preferred hosts; however, such infections are usually mild and seldom transmissible. The pathogenic mechanism is unknown, but the intracellular nature of this bacterium appears to contribute to the chronicity of the infection. Endotoxin probably plays a role in the inflammatory response to this infection.

B melitensis was identified as early as 1886 as the cause of Malta or Mediterranean fever (as human brucellosis was then called). A few years later, on the island of Malta, goats were found to be the source of the human disease. The fact that *B ovis* and *B canis* were not discovered until 1953 and 1967, respectively, has led to speculation that the genus *Brucella* may be in a phase of rapid evolution and that new species may be emerging.

Distinctive Properties

Brucellae are aerobic, but most strains of *B abortus* and *B ovis* require an atmosphere that contains 5%-10% CO_2 for growth in culture. Brucellae are gram-negative coccobacilli or short rods that measure about 0.6-1.5 μm by 0.5-0.7 μm. They are nonmotile and nonsporing, and they possess neither capsules nor flagellae. Their metabolism is mainly oxidative and they show little fermentative action on carbohydrates in conventional media. The guanine + cytosine content of the DNA is 55-58 moles/cm, and hybridization tests indicate a homology of greater than 90%. Antigenic relationships, as determined by serologic tests described later, are important for identification. A collection of phages effective in distinguishing the three main *Brucella* species is available, as is a phage that is lysogenic for rough brucellae. The cell wall of smooth brucellae appears typical of that of gram-negative bacteria, with a lipopolysaccharide possessing both endotoxic activity and determinants of serologic specificity; major outer member proteins are active in stimulating immunity.

Media recommended for growth of *Brucella* include serum-dextrose, trypticase-soy, and tryptose agars. *B abortus* biotype 2 and *B ovis* require 5% serum, blood, or hemoglobin in the medium for growth. Optimum temperature for growth is 37 C. On solid medium, *Brucella* colonies become visible after 2-3 days. Morphologic studies are best made on the fourth day, when typical smooth colonies are 2-4 mm in diameter and are a pale, clear, honey color when viewed from below with the medium held up toward indirect light.

Smooth brucellae readily dissociate to produce rough or mucoid colonies. These changes, which usually occur after prolonged culture in the laboratory, especially in static liquid medium, are accompanied by a reduction in virulence. The three main species of *Brucella* occur in nature in the smooth form, except for *B melitensis*, which is often found in goat's milk in dissociated forms that are mixed with smooth colony types. Colony changes are not obvious to the naked eye; they are best observed under low-power magnification with oblique lighting. Rough and mucoid colonies are more opaque than smooth colonies and can be distinguished by simple tests such as agglutination in acriflavine solution. The two types of colonies are similar, but when touched with a loop, mucoid colonies adhere and stretch. *B ovis* and *B canis* occur only as rough and mucoid colonies respectively. L forms also occur.

Sera from animals infected with any smooth *Brucella* species react (for example, by agglutinating) more or less equally with antigens of other smooth species. The different species and biotypes can be separated, however, into two serotypes, A and M, by agglutination tests with monospecific (absorbed) sera (Table 44-1). The only major serologic cross-reaction with bacteria of other genera is that in which sera from humans or animals infected with *Yersinia enterocolitica* serotype 09 cross-react with smooth *Brucella* antigens, or vice versa. Sera from animals that are infected with rough or mucoid types (for example, *B ovis* or *B canis*) do not react with the smooth antigens used in diagnosing brucellosis caused by the main species. Instead, reaction requires a rough antigen.

The characteristics of the six *Brucella* sp and their biotypes are shown in Table 44-1. The following procedures are used to differentiate the species and biotypes. The need for added CO_2 is determined by incubating duplicate slant cultures with and without CO_2 added to the atmosphere. Tests for H_2S production are performed by using slant cultures with strips of lead acetate paper inserted into the tube; the tip of the paper turns black when H_2S is produced. Dye sensitivity is determined by streaking a suspension of the culture over the surface of agar that contains the appropriate concentration of dye. Agglutination tests with monospecific sera may be done on slides or in tubes. Tests for phage sensitivity require appropriate concentrations of the various phages to be dropped onto a newly sown suspension of the culture on solid medium. Oxidative metabolic tests that measure the oxygen uptake of *Brucella* suspensions in solutions of various amino acids and carbohydrates are also useful in differentiating *Brucella* sp.

Pathogenesis

B melitensis and *B suis* transmit more easily to humans than *B abortus*. The usual portal of entry in humans is by the mouth, either directly by the consumption of untreated dairy products, or indirectly through contact with hands contaminated during work. Infection may also occur by inhaling contaminated dust or by splashing contaminated liquids into the eye. Brucellae can penetrate the skin.

Brucellae are intracellular parasites of the reticuloendothelial system. Upon arrival at the lymph node nearest to the point of entry, the bacteria are phagocytized by polymorphonuclear leukocytes or macrophages and may be destroyed. Some may survive and multiply in these cells and produce a bacteremia, which is followed by localization in certain target organs such as lymph nodes, spleen, liver, and bone marrow (all rich in reticuloendothelial cells). In humans, the lesions produced by *Brucella* consist of minute granulomas that are composed of epithelioid cells, polymorphonuclear leukocytes, lymphocytes, and some giant cells. Necrosis is not common and abscess formation does not occur except in the case of *B suis* infection. The evidence suggests that many of the symptoms of human brucellosis result from the reaction of the host

Table 44-1 Characteristics Used in Differentiating *Brucella* Sp and Biotypes

	Biotype	CO₂ Required	H₂S Production	Growth on Media Thionin*	Growth on Media Basic Fuchsin*	Agglutination with Monospecific Antisera† A	Agglutination with Monospecific Antisera† M	Agglutination with Monospecific Antisera† R	Lysis by Bacteriophage at RTD‡§ Tb	Lysis by Bacteriophage at RTD‡§ Wb	Lysis by Bacteriophage at RTD‡§ Bk
B abortus‖	1	(+)¶	+	−	+	+	−	−	L	L	L
	2	+	+	−	−	+	−	−	L	L	L
	3#	(+)	+	+	+	+	−	−	L	L	L
	4	(+)	+	−	+**	−	+	−	L	L	L
	5	−	−	+	+	−	+	−	L	L	L
	6#	−	(−)¶	+	+	+	−	−	L	L	L
	7	−	(+)	+	+	+	−	−	L	L	L
	9	(−)	+	+	+	−	+	−	L	L	L
B suis	1	−	+	+	−	+	−	−	NL	L	L
	2	−	−	+	−	+	−	−	NL	L	L
	3	−	−	+	+	+	−	−	NL	L	L
	4	−	−	+	(+)	+	+	−	NL	L	L
B melitensis	1	−	−	+	+	−	+	−	NL	NL	L
	2	−	−	+	+	+	−	−	NL	NL	L
	3	−	−	+	+	+	+	−	NL	NL	L
B ovis	/	+	−	+	(+)	−	−	+	NL	NL	NL
B canis	/	−	−	+	−	−	−	+	NL	NL	NL
B neotomae	/	−	+	−††	−	+	−	−	NL or PL	L	L

*Concentration, 1/50,000.
†Monospecific antisera include anti-*B abortis* (A), anti-*B melitensis* (M), and antirough R serum.
‡Bacteriophages Tb (Tblisi), Wb (Weybridge), and Bk (Berkeley) are used at routine test dilution (RTD) in the least concentration giving confluent lysis on host strain.
§L, Confluent lysis; PL, partial lysis; NL, no lysis.
‖*B abortus* biotype 8 is no longer recognized.
¶(+), most strains positive; (−), most strains negative.
#For more certain differentiation of *B abortus* types 3 and 6, thionin at 1/25,000 w/v is used in addition; type 3, +; type 6, −.
**Some strains of this biotype are inhibited by basic fuchsin.
††Not inhibited by thionin at 1/150,000 w/v.

defenses, because hypersensitivity develops rapidly. Many occupationally exposed persons become sensitized without showing symptoms; thus, when a veterinarian accidentally vaccinates himself instead of a calf, he or she usually suffers a hypersensitivity reaction instead of a brucellosis syndrome.

In the more susceptible species of domestic animal (cows, goats, some breeds of sheep, and pigs), enormous multiplication of brucellae occurs in the uterus in the latter part of pregnancy and, to a lesser extent, in the mammary glands during lactation. In the uterus of a pregnant animal, the growth of brucellae is stimulated by the sugar mesoerythritol, which is produced in the fetus and its membranes. Abortion, and sometimes parturition at the normal time, leads to massive contamination of the environment, but excretion does not continue because the uterus is not attractive to brucellae unless the animal is pregnant. On the other hand, excretion of brucellae in the milk, usually in much smaller numbers, may continue for years and, especially in the case of *B melitensis,* this provides a dangerous source of human infection. Orchitis and epididymitis due to *Brucella* occur occasionally in bulls and in male goats, and more frequently in dogs and swine. They are the main manifestations of brucellosis in rams.

Host Defenses

The nonspecific defense mechanism depends largely on cells of the reticuloendothelial system. Specific resistance is mainly cell-mediated, with T lymphocytes playing a major role both directly and in association with phagocytic cells, especially macrophages. Infection also stimulates the production of specific antibody, but antibody plays only a minor role in resistance to brucellosis. Evidence suggests that, in humans, natural infection and complete recovery produce some resistance to reinfection.

Epidemiology

Eradication programs have resulted in the complete or almost complete elimination of bovine brucellosis (*B abortus*) from many developed countries, although it persists in some southern areas of the United States. The disease is moderately prevalent in most other parts of the world.

B melitensis affects goats and some breeds of sheep that are used mainly for milk and cheese production; most other breeds of sheep are almost totally resistant. *B melitensis* infection is prevalent in the Mediterranean area, central Asia, and some parts of Latin America, especially Mexico and Peru; it does not occur in northern Europe, the United States, Canada, Southeast Asia, or Australia.

B suis causes chronic infertility in pig herds. It occurs only rarely in Europe, and an eradication program has decreased its incidence in the United States greatly; however, *B suis* infection is still fairly widespread in Latin America, Southeast Asia, and the Pacific region. *B suis* biotype 2 is unusual in that it does not affect humans. Canine brucellosis due to *B canis* occurs in many countries (including the United States), but poses only a minimal threat to human health.

In countries in which *B abortus* infection still occurs and milk is pasteurized, the human disease is mainly occupational and affects chiefly veterinarians, meat workers, and farm operatives. *B melitensis,* in addition to being a danger to people who handle infected animals, sometimes causes epidemics in persons who consume untreated milk and dairy products, often at a distance from the point of origin of those products. *B suis* is a hazard to pig keepers and meat workers in infected areas, but apparently not to people who eat the meat. Pig farmers have been known to transfer *B suis* infection to the udders of cows, thus giving rise to epidemics among persons who drink the milk.

It must be remembered that in countries in which brucellosis has been eradicated, individuals can acquire the disease by consuming imported dairy products or by visiting countries in which the disease is endemic.

Diagnosis

Brucellosis in humans provides serious diagnostic problems, partly because the clinical presentation is so variable and often so ill-defined and the complications can affect so many systems. In the simple case, the onset is influenza-like with fever reaching 38–40 C but the limb and back pains are unusually severe. However, the fever and malaise persist without treatment for 2 to 4 weeks. Many patients may recover completely at this stage, but others tend to have a series of relapses giving rise to the "undulant fever" picture. Patients tend to have a low or normal leukocyte count with a relative lymphocytosis but few signs bar possible splenomegaly, although malaise and fatigue are severe. Most of these cases will recover within 3 to 12 months, but some will develop complications marked by involvement of various organs, and a few will enter an ill-defined chronic syndrome.

Complications include arthritis and spondylitis, meningitis, uveitis and, occasionally, epididymoorchitis. In women, abortion is not a feature of the disease, unless as a rare concomitant of the acute febrile onset only. Subclinical infections commonly occur, particularly with *B abortus*, and some overt cases have an insidious, rather than an abrupt, onset.

Unequivocal diagnosis depends on the isolation of the organism, usually by blood culture but occasionally from bone marrow or liver biopsy or from sites of localization. Blood cultures need to be performed early in the disease, particularly with infections with *B abortus*. Incubation of the culture bottles for 3 weeks with added CO_2 often is necessary.

Serologic tests are important in diagnosis, but interpretation frequently is difficult. Standard agglutination tests that may involve 2-mercaptoethanol or antiglobulin techniques have been augmented by complement-fixation and ELISA tests. Rising titers of antibody are diagnostic in association with a clinical syndrome. However, patients often present late for investigation and the frequency of subclinical infections complicates the interpretation of stable titers. Standard agglutination titers, especially the 2-mercaptoethanol–resistant IgG, decline fairly rapidly, whereas, with the antiglobulin test, titers persist longer. Persistently positive results with the complement-fixation test may indicate continued active disease, even in a localized site.

The diagnosis of the chronic brucellosis syndrome, without specific localization, is often very unsatisfactory. Cultures are usually negative and results of serologic tests are equivocal. When the question of possible compensation for an occupationally acquired disease also arises, a confident diagnosis is often impossible. Thus, it may be advisable to test occupationally exposed people periodically to establish baseline titers that will facilitate interpretation of serologic results should such people develop symptoms suggestive of brucellosis.

Skin tests are used in some countries. A positive result, however, does not necessarily indicate active infection, although a negative result may be useful in eliminating brucellosis.

Control

Elimination of the animal reservoir of infection eliminates the human disease. Pasteurization of dairy products destroys *Brucella*. Occupationally exposed workers can be protected by wearing impermeable clothing, rubber boots, gloves, and face masks, and by practicing good personal hygiene. Vaccination of humans is practiced in the Soviet Union, but can be recommended only for persons exposed to *B melitensis* or *B suis* infection, and only those who have demonstrated no allergic reaction to the vaccine on a skin test should be vaccinated. Fairly effective, living, attenuated vaccines are available for animals (for example, *B abortus* strain 19 for cattle, and *B melitensis* strain Rev. 1, for goats and sheep). Unfortunately, these vaccines produce antibodies that interfere with subsequent serologic tests. The interference can be minimized, however, by limiting vaccination to immature animals, by reducing the vaccinal dose, and by using more specific serologic tests. Inactivated and sub-unit vaccines are under development.

Diagnosis of brucellosis in animals, especially during eradication campaigns, depends almost entirely on serologic assessment. The tests used are those mentioned earlier for the diagnosis of human brucellosis, along with the buffered brucella antigen tests (card or rose bengal tests) and the simple rapid agglutination tests, which are used often as screen tests. The milk-ring test, an agglutination test that uses a stained antigen, is effective in detecting brucellosis-infected herds of cattle when applied to bulk milk samples. Epidemiologic investigations may be facilitated by isolating and identifying brucellae from dairy products and animal tissues. Selective media that allow the growth of brucellae while inhibiting many extraneous organisms are available.

Tetracycline, or a combination of tetracycline and streptomycin, provides effective treatment of acute brucellosis in humans; regimens of 2-week-long courses of drug therapy with intervals of 2 weeks between treatments have been successful. Patients with chronic brucellosis frequently need symptomatic treatment in addition to antibiotics, and their response to antibiotic treatment is often disappointing.

References

Alton, G. G., Jones, L. M., Pietz, D.E.: *Laboratory techniques in brucellosis,* 2nd ed. WHO Monograph Series No. 55. Geneva: World Health Organization, 1975.

Corbel, M.J., Gill, K.P.W., Thomas, E.L.: *Methods for the identification of Brucella.* Weybridge, England: Central Veterinary Laboratory, 1978.

Spink, W.W.: 1956. *The nature of brucellosis.* Minneapolis: University of Minnesota Press, 1956.

Wise, R.J.: Brucellosis in the United States; past, present and future. *JAMA* 1980; 244:2318-22.

World Health Organization: *A guide to the diagnosis, treatment and prevention of human brucellosis,* rev. ed. Geneva: World Health Organization, 1983.

Young, E.J.: Human brucellosis. *Rev Infect Dis* 1983; 5:821-841.

45 *Yersinia, Francisella,* and *Pasteurella**

Frank M. Collins, PhD, DSc

General Concepts

The small, nonmotile gram-negative coccobacilli, originally grouped in the genus *Pasteurella,* now have been separated into three genera. These organisms cause plague (*Yersinia pestis*), tularemia (*Francisella tularensis*), and local abscesses, usually from animal bites (*Pasteurella* sp). Food-borne intestinal infections may be caused by *Y enterocolitica*. Only two species now remain in the genus *Pasteurella: P multocida* (formerly *P septica*) and *P haemolytica*. *Y pestis,* the plague bacillus, has been placed in a new genus, *Yersinia,* along with *Y enterocolitica* and *Y pseudotuberculosis*. Finally, the causative agent of tularemia has been placed in a new genus, *Francisella,* because *F*

*Studies of *Y enterocolitica* and *P multocida* infections in mice were supported by Grant HL-19774 from the Heart, Lung and Blood Institute of the National Institutes of Health, Bethesda, Md., and Grant RR05705-09 was awarded by the Biomedical Research Support Grant Program, Division of Research Resources, National Institutes of Health.

Table 45-1   Disease and Vector Comparisons Among *Yersinia, Pasteurella,* and *Francisella*

Organisms	Vectors	Human Diseases
Yersinia		
Y pestis	Fleas and aerosols	Bubonic and pneumonic plague
Y enterocolitica	—	Acute enterocolitis
Y pseudotuberculosis	—	Acute enterocolitis
Pasteurella		
P multocida	Cat or dog bites	Localized abcesses
P hemolytica	—	—
Francisella tularensis	(Ticks and deerflies transmit the agent among rabbits and ground squirrels, the reservoir hosts)	Tularemia

tularensis is a facultative intracellular parasite more closely related to *Brucella* than to *Pasteurella.* The diseases and vectors associated with these bacteria are summarized in Table 45-1.

Metabolically, these microorganisms are facultative anaerobes with relatively restricted fermentative capabilities in vitro. They are parasitic for a wide variety of host species and can cause severe systemic infections (bubonic plague, pneumonic pasteurellosis, and intestinal disease). Humans are usually the accidental victims of bites by infected insect vectors. Tetracycline and other antibiotics are generally effective in treating infections caused by these three genera.

YERSINIA

Three organisms of major medical importance occur in the genus *Yersinia: Y pestis* (the causative agent of bubonic and pneumonic plague in humans), *Y enterocolitica,* and *Y pseudotuberculosis.* The second two can cause severe gastrointestinal infections in humans and animals.

Distinctive Properties

Morphologically, these gram-negative coccobacilli exhibit a characteristic bipolar staining (Figure 45-1). Pleomorphic and club-shaped forms can sometimes occur. Freshly isolated strains of *Y pestis* produce a thick slime layer that has been described as a capsule. All yersiniae grow well on enriched nutrient media, but in the presence of blood, *Y pestis* colonies absorb hemin and appear dark brown. Most strains ferment glucose, maltose, and mannitol but not lactose; they produce acid but no gas. Fermentation reactions are not constant enough to reliably distinguish the different species; however, *Y pestis* does not produce urease, whereas the other two species do. Rough colonies often develop after cultivation of *Y pestis* on laboratory media for some

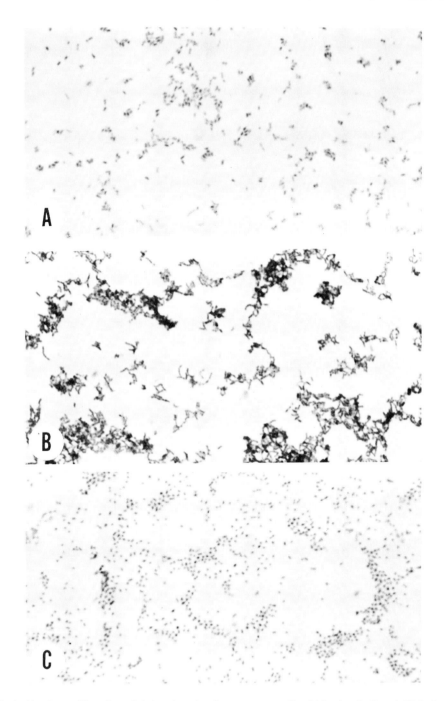

Figure 45-1 A, *Y enterocolitica.* Growth taken from tryptose soy agar after 24 hrs incubation at 37 C. Gram-negative coccoid rods show some bipolar staining (× 1200). **B,** *F tularensis.* Growth taken from chocolate blood agar after 48 hrs incubation at 37 C, showing small pleomorphic rods (× 1200). **C,** *P multocida.* Growth taken from brain-heart infusion agar after 24 hrs incubation at 37 C, showing coccobacillary rods and some bipolar staining (× 1200).

Table 45-2   Antigens of *Yersinia pestis*

Antigen	Composition		Function
Envelope (Fraction 1)			
A	Polysaccharide-protein ⎫		Envelope antigen
B	Polysaccharide ⎬ Water soluble		Low toxicity
C	Insoluble polysaccharide ⎭		Mouse toxic
Somatic			
1	—		Virulence antigen
3	Corresponds to Fl envelope antigen		Immunogenic
4	Heat-stable protein		Nonimmunogenic
5	—		Formed only at 37 C
8	Heat-labile polypeptide		Toxin
V ⎫			Associated with virulence; produced at
W ⎭	Heat-labile; destroyed by trypsin		37 C, not 28 C
Rough	Polysaccharide; heat-stable.		Unknown

time, and such organisms are nonencapsulated and avirulent. *Y pestis* can multiply at 28 C but fails to synthesize a number of virulence antigens at this temperature (see Table 45-2). *Y enterocolitica* is motile when cultured at 28 C, and the bacilli are more virulent for mice than are those grown at 37 C.

Pathogenesis

Y pestis produces an envelope antigen (F1) that is heat-labile, and a number of somatic antigens that are heat-stable (see Table 45-2). Two of the most important somatic antigens are referred to as the V and W antigens; however, they can also occur in some avirulent strains. At least ten somatic antigens have been isolated; some are protective for rats and mice, whereas others are shared with other *Yersinia* strains. The relationship between the somatic antigens and virulence is variable and seems to depend on the host species. Virulent strains of *Y pestis* are toxic for mice and guinea pigs; the toxin being released by autolysis of the cells is antigenically distinct from the smooth somatic endotoxin. Highly virulent strains of *Y pestis* produce F1, the V and W somatic antigens, and potent toxins. Killed vaccines prepared from such strains are highly immunogenic, whereas similar preparations from avirulent organisms are not, unless suspended in a Freund-type adjuvant; however, live attenuated or even avirulent vaccine strains may be protective for experimental mice (Figure 45-2).

Host Defenses

The major defense mechanism against *Yersinia* infection is the production of specific F1 antibodies, which act in vivo as specific opsonins, allowing the polymorphonuclear leukocytes to phagocytose and kill the virulent organisms. Interestingly, *Y pestis,* when recovered from the intestinal tract of the rat flea, does not contain detectable amounts of capsular F1 or VW antigens. As a result, most of the intradermal inoculum is

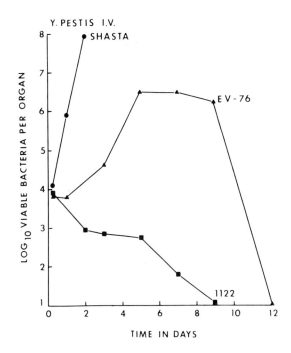

Figure 45-2 Growth of *Y pestis* in intravenously infected mice showing viable counts for combined liver and spleen homogenates. The highly virulent Shasta strain multiplied without an initial lag and resulted in 100% mortality within 3 days. Strain EV-76 was mouse-attenuated, but induced an excellent immune response. Strain 1122 was avirulent for mice. Data from Walker, D.L., et al. *J Immunol* 1953; 70:245.

phagocytosed and killed by polymorphonuclear leukocytes that quickly enter the lesion; however, a few bacilli are taken up by tissue macrophages that are unable to kill the organisms. These phagocytosed bacilli rapidly multiply and produce envelope and VW antigens before killing the macrophage. The virulent bacilli are released into the tissues where they are able to resist uptake by the polymorphonuclear leukocytes. Convalescent patients have high acquired resistance to reinfection; however, some second attacks of plague have been reported, despite the presence of high titers of antibodies to envelope and VW antigen. This observation suggests that activated cellular defense mechanisms may also be involved.

Epidemiology

Plague normally occurs in wild rat populations and seems to occur worldwide. It is carried to humans by the rat flea, and human epidemics of bubonic plague (black death) normally follow an extensive earlier outbreak of rat plague. Bubonic plague is one of the ancient scourges of mankind repeated waves of bubonic and pneumonic plague swept across Europe in the Middle Ages. For unknown reasons, human epidemics have not recurred in Europe in recent times, although endemic plague still occurs throughout Asia, Europe, and the United States. Ecologic studies reveal that *Y pestis* causes recurrent epizootics among pack rats, squirrels, and prairie dogs in the western United States. These continuing outbreaks of sylvatic plague are thought to be responsible for the sporadic cases of human disease reported in this country. For unknown reasons, the sporadic outbreaks do not develop into widespread epidemics, even though the causative organism is highly virulent for humans.

The rat infection is transmitted from a septicemic host to other normal animals by the rat flea. The flea ingests the blood-borne *Y pestis,* which multiply within the flea's intestinal tract until the proventriculus is blocked. After biting another rat, the infected flea regurgitates blood and *Yersinia* into the bite wound. The second rat develops active disease, with death usually occurring within 6-8 days. The infected flea transfers to a new host, which in turn becomes infected and dies. Eventually, fleas are forced to parasitize human beings living in the area, which leads to an outbreak of bubonic plague. Highly virulent strains of *Y pestis* multiply in intravenously infected Swiss mice with a doubling time of about 4 hours, resulting in death of the animal within 2-3 days (see Figure 45-2). In some cases, however, attenuated strains may be unable to establish persistent infections in the liver and spleen even in heavily infected animals.

The primary *Y pestis* infection in the naturally acquired human disease forms a minor intradermal lesion at the site of the flea bite. The plague bacilli multiply freely within the subcutaneous tissues and are carried to the draining lymph node (usually the axillary or the inguinal node). The lymph node becomes enlarged and tender, giving the characteristic inflamed bubo responsible for the name of the disease. Organisms reach the bloodstream after about 1 day, and the developing bacteremia quickly involves the lungs, the spleen, and other reticuloendothelial organs of the host. Many patients develop a severe pneumonia with large numbers of bacilli in the alveolar spaces and sputum. These bacilli are expelled into the air during coughing and can result in direct person-to-person spread (pneumonic plague), especially under conditions of overcrowding and poor sanitation. Pneumonic plague is highly contagious, having mortality rates of 100%. Experimental studies performed with aerogenically challenged rats, guinea pigs, and monkeys have confirmed the extraordinary infectivity and virulence of the plague bacillus by airborne transmission. In addition, infection can enter through the conjunctiva, and probably many laboratory-derived infections occur in this way. (*Y pestis* is a notoriously dangerous pathogen in the laboratory.) Protective glasses and a face mask must always be worn when working with freshly isolated *Yersinia* strains, and the staff should be prevaccinated, preferably with a live attenuated vaccine.

Y enterocolitica is an intestinal parasite found in cows, pigs, rabbits, dogs and birds. It causes diarrhea, lymphadenopathy, necrosis of the Peyer's patches, and severe abscesses in the liver and spleen. Following recovery from the disease, many animals remain healthy carriers, actively excreting organisms in the feces. Increased numbers of human outbreaks of enterocolitis caused by this organism have been reported in recent years, but this probably reflects the increased interest and improved diagnostic procedures now available, rather than a change in overall incidence rates.

Most isolates of *Y enterocolitica* are avirulent for mice. Recently, a mouse-virulent strain (*Y enterocolitica* WA) was isolated from human pathologic material. Orally infected mice develop progressive systemic disease involving the ileal Peyer's patches, the mesenteric lymph nodes, liver, and spleen; most of the animals eventually die. Animals dying late in the infectious period usually suffer from intestinal perforation and peritonitis. The immune response involves polymorphonuclear phagocytes rather than mononuclear defenses, which probably explains the persistent abscess formation in many of these infections.

Y pseudotuberculosis is a relatively large coccobacillus that causes acute enterocolitis in humans. It is also highly infectious for guinea pigs and can lead to devastating outbreaks of pseudotuberculosis, with high mortality rates, in breeding colonies. *Y pseudotuberculosis* can be readily distinguished from the other two *Yersinia* species because it alone is motile when incubated at 22 C.

Diagnosis

Diagnosis must be completed rapidly because of the extraordinary virulence of many strains of *Y pestis*. The mortality rate for untreated bubonic plague is about 50%; the rate for the pneumonic form is 100%, and death may occur within 24 hours of clinical presentation. Sputum and lymph node biopsy material contains large numbers of gram-negative bacilli that exhibit an intense bipolar staining reaction. *Y pestis* isolates can be distinguished by fluorescent antibody staining and by bacteriophage typing. Cultures of *Y pestis* pose a considerable infection hazard for laboratory personnel. Virulence can be checked by mouse inoculation, but only under carefully controlled conditions using ectoparasite-free animals housed under level P-3 containment conditions.

Control

Y pestis is susceptible to streptomycin, chloramphenicol, and tetracycline; so far, few drug-resistant strains have been isolated. Attempts to eliminate the rat plague reservoir have been unsuccessful, but considerable success has been achieved by use of insecticides against the insect vectors. Widespread use of DDT after World War II has been credited with preventing widespread epidemics of this disease in Europe in 1945. Immunization with formalin-killed or with live attenuated vaccines can provide short-term protection for laboratory personnel and other individuals likely to be exposed to endemic plague.

Y enterocolitica is spread to humans by contaminated food or water, and usually can be controlled by adequate water and milk purification methods. The infection's tendency to induce local intestinal abscesses, which often mimic acute appendicitis, may explain why the established infection is so intractable to anything but the most aggressive chemotherapy. The organism is sensitive to ampicillin, chloramphenicol, and polymyxin. Early diagnosis usually prevents severe complications. No vaccine is available for this infection.

Y pseudotuberculosis can cause severe intestinal infections in humans and rodents. The organism is sensitive to ampicillin and to tetracycline; however, the occurrence of large systemic abscesses makes management of this disease relatively difficult. No effective vaccine is available.

FRANCISELLA

One species of the genus *Francisella*, *F tularensis*, has medical importance. The organism causes tularemia in rabbits, and can infect humans, usually when they handle infected rabbit carcasses.

Distinctive Properties

Morphologically, *Francisella* is a nonmotile bacillus that may have a capsule when examined immediately after removal from pathologic material. Many strains exhibit pleomorphism and even filament production after growth on laboratory media (see Figure 45-1). The density of growth is often relatively poor during primary isolation. Growth is usually seen only when the bacillus is cultured on chocolate blood agar or Dorset's egg medium. Large inocula may be required before growth occurs. The organism has an absolute requirement for cysteine or sulfhydril groups in the growth medium. Excellent growth occurs on the chorioallantoic membrane of the developing chick, with death of the embryo 3-4 days later.

Pathogenesis

Tularemia occurs mostly in rabbits and ground squirrels, but it can occur in humans following bites from infected ticks and deer flies (Table 45-1). Mice, rats, and guinea pigs can be infected experimentally by parenteral, nasal, or conjunctival inoculation. *F tularensis* is a facultative, intracellular parasite, and acquired resistance to tularemia is cell-mediated (Figure 45-3). The sharp decline in the viability of the bacterial population in the liver and spleen on the fourth day coincides with development of delayed-type hypersensitivity. These changes are characteristic of a cell-mediated response, as confirmed by an ability to transfer immunity adoptively with immune spleen cells but not with hyperimmune serum. Subcutaneously infected guinea pigs develop enlarged lymph nodes and a spreading systemic infection, resulting in death 5-8 days later. Laboratory-adapted strains may lose virulence and cause chronic infections.

Most rabbit isolates are highly infectious for humans. (The parenteral human infectious dose is fewer than ten viable organisms for many strains.) Laboratory infections are frequent, and vaccination of all high-risk staff is strongly recommended. Infection probably occurs through the conjunctiva. Naturally acquired infections

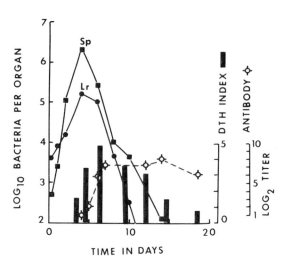

Figure 45-3 Growth of *F tularensis* LVS in the livers (Lr) and spleens (Sp) of intravenously infected Lewis × DA F1 hybrid rats. Histograms represent delayed hypersensitivity (24 hr) responses to a specific *Francisella* sensitin. Agglutinating antibody titers to *F tularensis* develop *after* sharp decline in liver and spleen viable counts. Data from Kostiala, A.A.I., McGregor, D.D., Logie, P.S. *Immunology* 1975; 28:855–869.

usually result from skin contamination with blood or infected rabbit tissue. A severe typhoidlike disease develops after ingestion of inadequately cooked meat contaminated with the organism. Local Peyer's patch involvement accompanied by severe toxemia and high fever can occur in untreated cases. The mortality rate is as high as 30%.

Host Defenses

Immunity following naturally acquired tularemia is long-lasting and effective. Immune serum is not highly protective, and killed vaccines are not generally effective. A live attenuated vaccine has been developed and is widely used in experimental studies of tularemia in rats and mice; because the risk of laboratory infections is high with virulent strains of *F tularensis*, the vaccine strain is recommended for experimental studies.

Diagnosis

Smears from pathologic material must be stained with specific fluorescent antibodies. Cultivation from pathologic material is difficult unless a cysteine-glucose-blood agar medium is used. Growth is slow, and the plates should be incubated at 37 C for 3 weeks before being discarded as negative. Hemagglutinins appear in the serum after about 10 days, and slowly increase in titer for about 8 weeks. A rising titer is always diagnostic of active disease. Infected animals develop a characteristic delayed skin hypersensitivity following the injection of sterile culture filtrates (see Figure 45-3).

Control

F tularensis is sensitive to streptomycin, tetracycline, and chloramphenicol. Relapses are not unusual, especially if treatment is stopped before all organisms have been eliminated. Successful control requires elimination of the insect vector, as well as precautions such as wearing gloves to protect against contamination of skin with infected rabbit blood during skinning and dressing of carcasses. Rabbit meat always should be well cooked before it is eaten.

PASTEURELLA

The genus *Pasteurella* contains two species of considerable veterinary importance. *P multocida* causes fowl cholera in chickens and turkeys, as well as shipping fever in calves. *P hemolytica* also causes hemorrhagic (shipping) fever in cattle.

Distinctive Properties

Morphologically, the two species are small, nonmotile coccoid rods, frequently showing bipolar staining (see Figure 45-1). They can be readily cultured on most laboratory media, although growth of *P hemolytica* may require the addition of blood or hemin. Many strains produce a capsule, and these colonies take on a mucoid appearance; most virulent strains tend to produce smooth irridescent colonies, with no demonstrable capsule, although they do contain the capsular antigens used in typing. Strains lacking capsular antigens cannot be typed. Metabolically, they are all weakly fermentative and catalase-positive.

Pathogenesis

Reports of human infections from *P multocida* have increased. Most human infections occur as localized abscesses associated with cat or dog bites (Table 45-1). *Pasteurella* organisms are extraordinarily invasive and can easily gain entry through minor cuts and abrasions to the skin. Less frequently, respiratory tract involvement occurs, apparently caused by aerogenic infections from infected cattle. Following aerogenic inoculation of *P multocida* into the lungs of normal mice, immediate logarithmic growth by the organisms occurs with no initial lag phase, no indication of early phagocytosis, and no inactivation of even a portion of the inoculum (Figure 45-4). In fact, the animal's normal host defenses seem incapable of controlling the growth of the bacilli in any of the tissues. Within hours of challenge, gram-negative bacilli can be distinguished readily in blood smears, and growth continues throughout the body until death of the animal occurs, usually within 24 hours of infection. Fortunately, most of the animal strains do not seem to be particularly pathogenic for humans, although cat and dog strains can give rise to stubborn abcesses following bites.

Host Defenses

P multocida produces capsular and somatic antigens. The former can be readily identified by slide agglutination. Four capsular types (A, B, D, and E) have been described. Type A strains are associated primarily with fowl cholera; type B are cattle

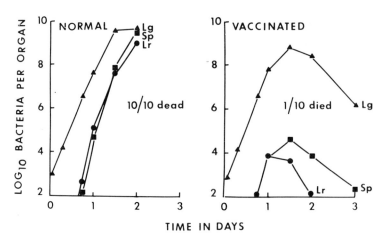

Figure 45-4 Left, Growth of *P multocida* strain 5A in the lungs (Lg), spleens (Sp), and livers (Lr) of C57Bl × DBA F1 (B6D2) hybrid mice. All the aerogenically challenged nonvaccinated mice were dead within 3 days. Right, Growth of *P multocida* in aerogenically challenged B6D2 mice that had been vaccinated intravenously with two doses of heat-killed *P multocida* (10^8 cells in 0.2 mL of saline) given 7 days apart. Only 1 mouse out of 10 died as a result of the challenge. Early growth of *P multocida* in the lungs of vaccinated and unvaccinated mice was almost identical. From Collins, F.M., Woodruff, W.H., 1979, unpublished data.

pathogens. Most human isolates are type A. The capsular groups can be further subdivided by means of agglutination tests involving a number of somatic antigens exposed only after the capsule has been removed by acid hydrolysis. Rough variants of *P multocida* without capsules make up a substantial proportion of clinical isolates.

P multocida normally multiplies extracellularly in the blood or tissue fluids; the infecting microorganisms are inactivated rapidly once they have been taken up by normal polymorphonuclear leukocytes. Acquired resistance is humorally mediated and is transferred to normal recipients by hyperimmune serum, but not by spleen cells. As a result, killed whole-cell vaccines have produced excellent levels of specific immunity in mice (see Figure 45-4). In field trials using commercial multivalent, killed vaccines, however, much less consistent results have been obtained, even when adjuvants are used. The relatively large number of antigenically distinct serotypes responsible for fowl cholera and shipping fever outbreaks may make these commercial vaccines less effective under field conditions. Live attenuated vaccines are currently under experimental evaluation.

Diagnosis

Both organisms may be readily cultured on commercial laboratory media. On blood agar, they usually form small nonhemolytic gray colonies. Most strains can be O antigenically typed, although many wild-type strains seem to be untypeable due to the absence of capsular antigens.

Control

Most strains of *P multocida* are sensitive to ampicillin and tetracycline. Human infections tend to become chronic, but usually can be controlled effectively with penicillin. Vaccination using killed whole-cell vaccines (bacterins) is a widespread farming practice in many parts of the United States and Canada, despite questions regarding its overall efficacy.

References

Bottone, E.J.: *Yersinia enterocolitica:* a panoramic view of a charismatic micro-organism. *CRC Crit Rev Microbiol* 1977; 5:211-241.

Carter, G.R.: Pasteurellosis: *Pasteurella multocida* and *Pasteurella hemolytica. Adv Vet Sci* 1967; 11:321-379.

Collins, F.M.: Mechanisms of resistance to *Pasteurella multocida* infection: A review. *Cornell Vet* 1977; 67:103-138.

Eigelsbach, H.T., et al.: Murine model for study of cell mediated immunity: Protection against death from fully virulent *Francisella tularensis* infection. *Infect Immun* 1975; 12:999-1005.

Kostiala, A.A.I., McGregor, D.D., Logie, P.S.: Tularemia in the rat. 1. The cellular basis of host resistance to infection. *Immunology* 1975; 28:855-869.

Meyer, K.F.: Effectiveness of live and killed plague vaccines in man. *Bull WHO* 1970; 42:653-666.

Meyer, K.F., et al.: Live attenuated *Yersinia pestis* vaccine: virulent in non-human primates, harmless to guinea pigs. *J Infect Dis* 1974; 129 (Suppl):S85-120.

Une, T., Brubaker, R.R.: In vivo comparison of avirulent Viva- and Pgm- or Pst^r phenotypes of Yersiniae. *Infect Immun* 1984; 43:895-900.

Walker, D.L., et al.: Studies on immunization against plague. V. Multiplication and persistence of virulent and avirulent *Pasteurella pestis* in mice and guinea pigs. *J Immunol* 1953; 70:245-252.

46 *Haemophilus*

Daniel M. Musher, MD

General Concepts
Distinctive Properties
Pathogenesis
  Meningitis
  Cellulitis and Epiglottitis
  Respiratory Disease
  Miscellaneous

Host Defenses
Epidemiology
Diagnosis
Control

General Concepts

The genus *Haemophilus* includes a number of bacterial species that cause a wide variety of infections, but share a common morphologic structure and a requirement for blood-derived x and v factors during growth that has given the genus its name. *Haemophilus influenzae*, the major pathogenic bacterium in this genus, causes a broad spectrum of clinical disease, especially meningitis and respiratory infections.

H influenzae are divided into six serologic types (a, b, c, d, e, and f), based upon the antigenic structure of the capsular polysaccharide. Nonencapsulated strains are classified as nontypable. *H influenzae* also are divided into six biotypes (I-VI), based upon several biochemical reactions. The pathogenesis of *H influenzae* infections is not completely understood, but production of the polysaccharide capsule enhances virulence. The organisms can penetrate the epithelium of the nasopharynx and invade the meninges directly. Production of exotoxins associated with virulence has not been reported. *H influenzae* colonize and produce infections in immunologically normal individuals. Nontypable *H influenzae* are found in the nasopharynx of normal individuals, but *H influenzae* type b, a frequent cause of meningitis in children, in only 1%-2% of normal children. Attempts to prevent serious outbreaks of *H influenzae* infections have included vaccination with purified capsular polysaccharide, as well as

---

prophylactic use of rifampin. Treatment of *Haemophilus* infections has been complicated by production of β-lactamase.

Other *Haemophilus* sp cause disease less frequently. *H parainfluenzae* is sometimes implicated as a cause of pneumonia and is a rare cause of bacterial endocarditis. *H ducreyi* causes a venereal disease that is characterized by a painful, relatively nonindurated genital ulcer, which must be distinguished from the primary lesion of syphilis. *H aphrophilus* is part of the normal flora of the mouth and is rarely implicated as a casue of bacterial endocarditis. *H aegypticus* and *H haemolyticus* used to be identified on the basis of their ability to agglutinate or lyse red blood cells, but they are now considered to be nontypable *H influenzae*.

Distinctive Properties

Haemophilus sp are gram-negative coccobacilli that have ultrastructural features common to all gram-negative bacilli. They contain lipopolysaccharide in their cell walls, but generally have not been shown to make toxins or other extracellular products that would account for their ability to produce infection. These organisms require hemin (x factor) or nicotinamide adenine dinucleotide (v factor) or both for growth. The former is released into the culture medium by red blood cells and is always present in blood agar; the latter is present in red blood cells but is not released into the medium unless the cells are broken up, as in chocolate agar. *H influenzae* requires both x and v factors; accordingly, it grows on chocolate but not on blood agar (Figure 46-1), although it may

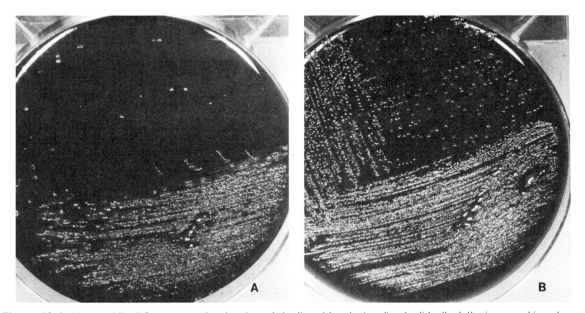

Figure 46-1 *Haemophilus influenzae* requires hemin and nicotinamide adenine dinucleotide; the latter is present in red blood cells, but is released into the medium only when cells are damaged. **A,** Sputum streaked on blood agar shows growth of "normal" flora (left). **B,** The same specimen on chocolate agar (which contains disrupted red blood cells) reveals *H influenzae* to be the overwhelmingly predominant organism.

appear on a blood agar plate in tiny satellite colonies surrounding colonies of bacteria that have lysed red blood cells. The long prevailing notion that *H ducreyi* grows only in clotted rabbit blood has been dispelled by recent studies that show slow growth of this organism in Mueller–Hinton agar containing 5% sheep blood. All *Haemophilus* sp grow more readily in an atmosphere enriched with CO_2; *H ducreyi* and some nontypable *H influenzae* will not form visible colonies on culture plates unless grown in a CO_2-enriched atmosphere.

H influenzae are classified as either serotypable, if a capsular polysaccharide has been recognized by immunologic assessments, or nontypable, if such a capsule is not detected. The word type, as applied to *H influenzae*, refers to this serotyping scheme. There are six recognized types: a, b, c, d, e, and f. A seventh type has recently been designated type e' because of the close molecular relation of its polysaccharide to type e; antiserum to type e' is not yet routinely available. These types may be identified by an agglutination reaction that uses antisera raised in rabbits. Cross-reactions with somatic antigens may lead to nontypable strains being designated erroneously as typable. This kind of error is eliminated by the use of counterimmunoelectrophoresis, because the electric current carries proteins and capsular polysaccharides in opposite directions. The presence of a capsule is an important virulence factor, in that it renders *H influenzae* resistant to phagocytosis by polymorphonuclear leukocytes in the absence of specific anticapsular antibody. Another virulence factor, susceptibility or resistance to the bactericidal effect of serum, depends upon as yet undetermined antigenic sites. Capsular material, outer membrane proteins, and lipopolysaccharide are all possible loci. *H influenzae* type b is plainly the most virulent of the *Haemophilus* sp; 95% of serious *Haemophilus* infections in children are due to this organism. In adults, nontypable strains of *H influenzae* cause more than one-half of serious infections, with type b isolates causing most of the rest.

H influenzae also are classified into six biotypes (I–VI), based on a series of biochemical reactions. Most *H influenzae* type b fall into biotypes I or II, whereas most nontypable *H influenzae* fall into biotypes II–VI. Two interesting clinical correlations have emerged: first, biotype I isolates appear to have a predilection for causing pneumonia; and second, nearly all genital isolates of *H influenzae*, as well as isolates from the bloodstream of infected neonates or women with puerperal sepsis, are biotype IV. In addition, biotype III, which agglutinates red blood cells in vitro and used to be called *H aegypticus*, has been implicated as a common cause of conjunctivitis. No explanation for these clinically observed associations is yet available.

Pathogenesis

Meningitis

The pathogenesis of meningitis due to *H influenzae* type b has been well studied. These organisms colonize the nasopharynx and spread from one human being to another by direct contact or droplets. As a result of mechanisms that are not understood, they penetrate unbroken epithelium; extend to the meninges by direct penetration, presumably via lymphatic drainage of the nasopharynx; and then cause bacteremia with seeding of a number of end organs, including the highly vascular choroid plexus. *H influenzae* type b is the most common cause of bacterial meningitis in children between the ages of

6 months and 2 years. In contrast, *H influenzae* is an uncommon cause of meningitis in adults, probably because a protective antibody develops in individuals in early childhood. This notion is supported by the finding that patients with hypogamma-globulinemia are susceptible to infection with this organism.

Most cases of *H influenzae* meningitis in adults are caused by nontypable strains. The pathogenesis of these infections is different. These causative organisms are unencapsulated, and, therefore, less virulent, and they are unable to penetrate directly to the lymphatic drainage system or to blood vessels. Instead, they gain entry to the central nervous system by direct extension, often through trauma involving the skull and sinuses. Thus, about one-half of adults with *H influenzae* meningitis have a history of head trauma, with or without a documented cerebrospinal fluid leak, and another 25% have chronic otitis media. Further support comes from the fact that *H influenzae* is second only to *Streptococcus pneumoniae* as a cause of recurring meningitis, an unusual syndrome attributed to a connection between the sinuses and the subarachnoid space, usually through a tear in the dura. Clinically, meningitis caused by typable or nontypable *H influenzae* is similar to that caused by *Streptococcus pneumoniae*. Because *Haemophilus* sp do not produce substances that damage mammalian tissues, disease is probably produced by bacterial replication, with triggering of the complement cascade by classical and alternative pathways, followed by accumulation of inflammatory cells.

Cellulitis and Epiglottitis

The pathogeneses of cellulitis and epiglottitis are probably quite similar. Both disorders are caused by *H influenzae* type b, are associated with bacteremia, and occur more often in children than adults. Epiglottitis can be regarded as a cellulitis of the loose tissues of the epiglottis. It begins with a sore throat that progresses rapidly to shortness of breath, obstruction of the airways, and respiratory arrest. Local extension from the colonized nasopharynx through soft tissues probably produces the epiglottitis. Cellulitis often involves the face or neck, sometimes seeming to start at the buccal mucosa and extending outward, supporting the idea that this condition probably also results from local extension.

Respiratory Disease

Nontypable *H influenzae* is a common colonizer, and a major pathogen of the human respiratory tract; it is often aspirated from acutely infected nasal sinuses or from behind an infected tympanic membrane. Its role in bronchopulmonary disease is much more unclear. For many years, British investigators believed that nontypable *H influenzae* caused chronic bronchitis. Even allowing for a multifactoral etiology, the data are remarkably difficult to interpret. Nontypable *H influenzae* may be cultured from the nasopharynx of about 33%-66% of normal adults. These organisms can also be isolated from the sputum of about 50%-66% of patients with chronic bronchitis. Higher rates of isolation are attained both for normal persons and for patients with bronchitis if serial cultures are done. Studies of whether *H influenzae* also colonizes the lower airways in patients with chronic bronchitis have yielded conflicting results. The older literature is based on bronchoscopy and is probably best disregarded, as it is well known that bronchoscopy carries mouth and pharyngeal discharge into the trachea and bronchi.

Using transtracheal aspiration, one group of investigators found that nontypable *H influenzae* is present distal to the larynx in 75% of patients with chronic obstructive pulmonary disease whereas another group found none of these organisms in such patients. This difference probably resulted from patient selection; the second study excluded patients with purulent sputum.

Whether the presence of nontypable *H influenzae* in purulent secretions means that these bacteria are causing, contributing to, or only reflecting the presence of inflammation is difficult to say. Bacterial infection is generally not responsible for increased shortness of breath in the absence of fever and leukocytosis in patients with chronic bronchitis, as shown by the response of such patients to medical regimens that do not include antibiotics; at the same time, some patients with chronic bronchitis do have infections, and exacerbations of chronic obstructive pulmonary disease are best treated with a regimen that includes antibiotics.

H influenzae probably runs a distant second to the pneumococcus as the cause of bacterial pneumonia in adult men, especially in populations that include a substantial proportion of long-time smokers; nontypable strains are responsible for 85% of cases. Aging, alcoholism, and debilitating diseases appear to increase susceptibility to *H influenzae* pulmonary infections, as does infection with influenza virus. Except for a tendency toward a subacute onset (mean duration of symptoms before seeking medical attention is 5-6 days), pneumonia due to nontypable *H influenzae* usually cannot be distinguished clinically from that due to any other organism. Even in patients who have acute, purulent, febrile tracheobronchitis due to *H influenzae,* the syndrome can be distinguished from pneumonia only by a radiographic evaluation that indicates the absence of a pulmonary infiltrate.

Miscellaneous

H influenzae type b is a relatively common cause of septic arthritis in children; infection results from hematogenous dissemination. Interestingly, this organism only rarely causes osteomyelitis; the reasons for this discrepancy are unknown.

Some patients have *H influenzae* bacteremia without an apparent focus of infection. Evidence indicates that if this occurs in children and is not treated, a focus of infection (for example, meningitis) will become apparent within 24-48 hours; type b organisms are responsible. In adults, a syndrome of bacteremia due to nontypable *H influenzae* can occur in which a focus never becomes apparent. Puerperal fever and neonatal sepsis also may be caused by nontypable *H influenzae.* Studies have revealed that biotype IV isolates tend to colonize the female genital tract. These organisms may cause a relatively mild puerperal sepsis or fulminating sepsis in the newborn infant. Whether nontypable *H influenzae* biotype IV has special virulence beyond the factor(s) that promote adherence to vaginal epithelial cells is unknown.

Host Defenses

For many years, it was believed that bactericidal antibody directed against the polyribosyl ribitol phosphate capsule (PRP) of *H influenzae* type b was entirely responsible for host resistance to infection. More recent studies have shown, however, that antibody to PRP is not the only determinant of resistance to infection and have stressed that antibody to somatic antigens is involved. Antibody to PRP can often be detected in the serum of children when they are admitted to the hospital with sepsis due to *H influenzae* type b. In addition, adsorption of immune serum with PRP alone does not remove its protective capabilities whereas adsorption with whole organisms does, and immunization of animals with ribosomes is protective. Separation of the outer membrane of *H influenzae* type b into its many protein constituents by polyacrylamide gel electrophoresis, as well as analysis of antibody responses during infection, has suggested that antibody to individual membrane proteins may be associated with immunity. This finding gives support, on a molecular basis, to the potential importance of antibody to noncapsular antigens in immunity to *H influenzae* type b infection. Similar studies of lipopolysaccharides extracted from *H influenzae* type b suggest that these substances might also serve as an effective immunogen.

Recent studies of nontypable *H influenzae* have shown that bactericidal antibody (presumably to outer membrane proteins, as these organisms lack capsules) develops in infants after otitis media due to these organisms. Normal adults have both bactericidal and opsonizing antibody directed against these organisms. Although levels of opsonizing antibody may be low in adults who develop acute infection from nontypable *H influenzae*, these patients have substantial levels of bactericidal antibody. Investigators do not yet understand why disease should occur despite the presence of antibody; in some instances, a blocking effect by IgA might be responsible.

Epidemiology

Haemophilus sp colonize and produce disease in immunologically normal human subjects. Organisms spread directly among humans without known contribution from environmental sources or animal reservoirs. Nontypable *H influenzae* are found in the nasopharynx of many or most normal persons, depending on the intensity of the search to find them. In contrast, *H influenzae* type b is found in only 1%–2% of normal children, and its spread to previously uncolonized children in the early years of life is associated with a substantially increased risk of infection. Day care centers have been shown to be important sources for dissemination of these organisms.

Diagnosis

The clinical presentation, findings on physical examination, and cerebrospinal fluid abnormalities in patients who have *H influenzae* meningitis do not allow the disease to be distinguished from meningitis due to other common bacterial pathogens. The cerebrospinal fluid in patients with untreated infection contains an average of 2×10^7 bacteria per mL, so that microscopic examination, especially in the absence of prior antibiotic therapy, should be distinctive. Detection of capsular material in the cerebrospinal fluid by counterimmunoelectrophoresis is helpful in cases in which the Gram stain appearance is not distinctive, a problem in children who have received enough antibiotic to suppress the growth of organisms in the cerebrospinal fluid, but not enough to cure the meningitis.

The bacteriologic diagnosis of pneumonia or acute febrile purulent tracheobronchitis due to *H influenzae* is made by finding myriad small, somewhat pleomorphic, gram-negative coccobacilli in gram-stained sputum (Figure 46-2) and by finding *H*

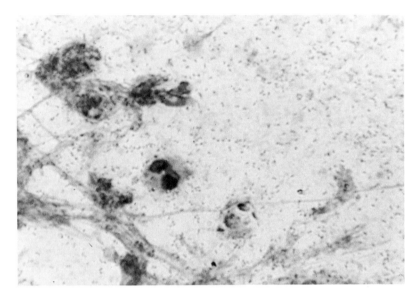

Figure 46-2 Gram-stained sputum showing profuse numbers of gram-negative coccobacilli with no other bacterial forms seen (original magnification ×440). Cultures showed nontypable *H influenzae* as the overwhelmingly predominant isolate. Quantitative culture showed 7×10^8 colony-forming units per milliliter of sputum.

influenzae to be the overwhelmingly predominant isolate in culture. The mean number of viable organisms per mL of infected sputum is about 5×10^8. Blood cultures may be positive in 15% of patients with pneumonia, but are negative in those with acute febrile tracheobronchitis.

Endocarditis due to *H parainfluenzae* tends to be associated with large vegetations that embolize; the etiologic diagnosis of endocarditis is established by blood culture. Soft chancres caused by *H ducreyi* may be confused with primary syphilitic chancres, traumatic lesions of the penis, eruptions caused by drugs, or ulcerated herpetic lesions. The diagnosis is established by culturing the causative organism on Mueller-Hinton agar supplemented with 5% sheep blood and incubated for 96 hours in a CO_2-enriched atmosphere.

Control

Two approaches to preventing outbreaks of serious infection due to *H influenzae* type b are vaccination and prophylactic therapy. Initial trials of vaccination with PRP from *H influenzae* type b have failed because, in its pure form, this polysaccharide is not immunogenic in infants, the population that is most in need of immunization. More recent studies have shown that injection of PRP along with another vaccine such as tetanus toxoid, which serves as an adjuvant, produces good antibody responses in infants. Clinical trials of this type of immunization in human subjects are in progress.

Once an outbreak of *H influenzae* type b infection has been documented, infants and young children who are in intimate contact with colonized or infected individuals have a greatly increased, albeit still small, likelihood of developing serious infection. Rifampin has been recommended as prophylactic treatment to prevent naspharyngeal colonization, or to eradicate it if colonization has occured. This recommendation is controversial, however, because widespread application of this approach may select for the emergence of rifampin-resistant organisms. In addition, the cost per each possible case of meningitis prevented is considered to be quite high.

The mainstay of therapy for infection due to *H influenzae* used to be ampicillin, because isolates were uniformly susceptible to 0.5 mcg/mL. In the last few years, an increasing proportion of *H influenzae* isolates have been found to produce β-lactamase; thus, 25%-30% of type b isolates, and a smaller percentage of nontypable isolates, are now resistant to penicillin or ampicillin.

Until recently, chloramphenicol was considered to be the drug of choice for *H influenzae* meningitis caused by a penicillin-resistant strain. Trimethoprim/sulfamethoxazole has also been used. Third-generation cephalosporins such as moxalactam, ceftriaxone, or cefoperazone, which have a good bactericidal effect against *H influenzae* and penetrate the meninges well, also have been shown to be effective in treating *H influenzae* meningitis.

Spread of soft chancre due to *H ducreyi* is best prevented by use of a condom during sexual intercourse. Two-thirds of isolates of *H ducreyi* produce β-lactamase. All isolates are susceptible in vitro to erythromycin and excellent clinical results have been achieved with this drug.

References

Hammond, G.W., et al.: Epidemiologic, clinical, laboratory, and therapeutic features of an urban outbreak of chancroid in North America. *Rev Infect Dis* 1980; 2:867-876.

Mason, E.O., et al.: Serotype and ampicillin susceptibility of *Haemophilus influenzae* causing systemic infections in children: 3 years of experience. *J Clin Microbiol* 1982; 15:543-6.

Musher, D.M., et al.: Opsonizing and bactericidal effects of normal human serum on nontypable *Haemophilus influenzae*. *Infect Immun* 1983; 39:297-304.

Musher, D.M., et al.: Pneumonia and acute febrile tracheobronchitis due to *Haemophilus influenzae*. *Ann Intern Med* 1983; 99:444-450.

Oberhofer, T.R., Back, A.E.: Biotypes of *Haemophilus* encountered in clinical laboratories. *J Clin Microbiol* 1979; 10:168-74.

Schreiber, J.R., et al.: Decreased protective efficacy of reduced and alkylated human immune serum globulin in experimental infection with *Haemophilus influenzae* type b. *Infect Immunol* 1985; 47:142-148.

Sell, S.H., Wright, P.F., (editors): *Haemophilus influenzae:* Epidemiology, immunology, and prevention of disease. New York: Elsevier Biomedical, 1982.

Shenep, J.L., et al.: Further studies of the role of noncapsular antibody in protection against experimental *Haemophilus influenzae* type b bacteremia. *Infect Immun* 1983; 42:257-63.

Wallace, R.J., et al.: Nontypable *Haemophilus influenzae* (biotype 4) as a neonatal, maternal, and genital pathogen. *Rev Infect Dis* 1983; 5:123-36.

47 *Bordetella*

Horst Finger, MD

General Concepts
Distinctive Properties
Pathogenesis
Host Defenses
Epidemiology
Diagnosis
Control

General Concepts

Within the genus *Bordetella* are three species (*B pertussis, B parapertussis,* and *B bronchiseptica*) of serologically related bacteria with similar morphology, size, and staining reactions. These bacteria cause whooping cough (pertussis) or similar respiratory syndromes in humans and animals. The pathogenesis of whooping cough may involve toxins and endotoxin that impair the ciliary function of respiratory epithelial cells. According to Bergey's *Manual of Determinative Bacteriology*, the genus *Bordetella* belongs to the gram-negative aerobic rods and cocci and has been placed in the group of genera of uncertain affiliation. This indicates that the genus *Bordetella* does not fit in with any of the five families of the gram-negative rods and cocci.

B pertussis was first isolated in pure culture in 1906 and was for a long time believed to be the sole causative agent of whooping cough. Later, studies revealed that this disease also can be caused in mild form by *B parapertussis* and occasionally by *B bronchiseptica*. Control of whooping cough has involved vaccination with a killed-cell preparation. Unvaccinated individuals may be protected by prophylactic administration of ampicillin or erythromycin.

Distinctive Properties

B pertussis is a small (approximately 0.8 μm by 0.4 μm), rod-shaped, coccoid or ovoid gram-negative bacterium that is encapsulated and does not produce spores. It is a strict aerobe. The organism, being arranged singly or in small groups, cannot be easily distinguished with certainty from species of the genus *Haemophilus*. Whereas *B pertussis* and *B parapertussis* are nonmotile, *B bronchiseptica* possesses peritrichous flagella.

Numerous antigens and biologically active structural components have been demonstrated in *B pertussis*, although their exact chemical structure and location in the bacterial cell are known only in part. The agglutinogens are surface antigens that are responsible for agglutination of the cells in the presence of their corresponding antibodies. To date, eight different agglutinogens have been distinguished. Six are restricted to the species *B pertussis;* the remaining two are demonstrable in *B parapertussis* and *B bronchiseptica* as well.

Heat-stable toxin is an endotoxic lipopolysaccharide that cannot be distinguished from the structure, chemical composition, and biologic activity of other endotoxins produced by gram-negative bacteria. Endotoxin from *B pertussis* is serologically different from corresponding preparations of *B parapertussis* and *B bronchiseptica*. The heat-labile dermonecrotic toxin is a proteinaceous material, localized in the protoplasm, which possibly contributes to the pathogenesis of whooping cough by causing tissue damage in the respiratory tract. Like many other bacteria, *B pertussis* possesses hemagglutinating activity, as expressed by its capacity to agglutinate directly red cells from chickens and other animals. Two distinct filaments can be distinguished: the filamentous hemagglutinin, which appears as fine filaments (about 2 nm in diameter and 40 to 100 nm in length), and the fimbrial filaments, which represent the carrier of the serotype agglutinogens.

Various immunologic, physiologic, and pharmacologic effects are induced by killed *B pertussis* cells in mice and other experimental animals—for example, increased sensitivity to histamine and serotonin, as well as active and passive anaphylaxis. Adjuvant activity, leukocytosis, splenomegaly, cell proliferation, hypoglycemia, and hypoproteinemia also occur. Many additional features, such as increased sensitivity to endotoxins, X-irradiation, infection, cold stress, pollen extracts, peptone shock, metacholine, increased resistance to infection, increased capillary permeability, and accelerated production of experimental "allergic" encephalomyelitis, have been described.

The various biologic activities of *B pertussis* were assumed to be due to different products and structural components of the bacteria designated, for example, the histamine-sensitizing factor, the lymphocytosis-promoting factor, pertussis toxin, or islet-activating protein. But there is increasing evidence that all these biologic activities are caused by a single biologically active protein produced by *B pertussis*, pertussigen, which has been prepared in crystalline form. Unfortunately, the crystalline substance still contained trace amounts of contaminants from the *B pertussis* cell. To avoid confusion caused by the many different names for this protein, the uniform term, pertussis toxin, was proposed by Pittman. Pertussis toxin is a protein exotoxin secreted during in vivo and in vitro growth. It has a molecular weight about 120,000 Dalton; it consists of two distinct components, neither of which is active when separated. Their mode of action is in accordance with the A-B model of toxins. Pertussis toxin was found to react with different cell types and to display its influence on different cellular regulatory processes. It interferes with the regulation of cyclic AMP-mediated events. Treatment of rat adipocytes with pertussis toxin increased the levels of cyclic AMP twentyfold. A further protein that interferes with cyclic AMP regulation is, however, also produced by *B pertussis*, the extracytoplasmic adenylate cyclase (ECAC). The ECAC-mediated increase in intracellular cyclic AMP was found to be associated with the inhibition of phagocytic cell oxidative reactions and natural killer cell activity. ECAC also appears to play a role in *B pertussis* virulence.

Pathogenesis

Whooping cough is an acute respiratory disease in which the agent is primarily transmitted through droplets. Infection results in colonization and rapid multiplication of the bacteria on the mucous membranes of the respiratory tract. In the past, conflicting results were obtained in studies investigating whether the ciliated regions of the respiratory tract serve as the exclusive target for *B pertussis* organisms. Both exclusive attachment of *B pertussis* to the ciliated portions of the respiratory epithelium and adherence to a variety of nonciliated cell types were observed. However, electronmicroscopic studies have demonstrated that phase I strains of *B pertussis* adhered to only the tuft of ciliated cells in the mucosa of the human respiratory tract. Attachment to nonciliated epithelial cells was not observed in these investigations. The bacteria adhered to the cilia either by direct apposition or by connection with filamentous material.

Bacteremia does not occur in whooping cough infections. The pertussis toxin irritates the superficial cell layers, probably impairing the normal action of the cilia of epithelial cells in the trachea and bronchi. In one study, phase I isolates of *B bronchiseptica* produced almost complete ciliostasis within 3 hours in ciliated epithelial cell outgrowths from canine tracheal explants. In humans, an initial local peribronchial lymphoid hyperplasia occurs, accompanied or followed by necrotizing inflammation and leukocytic infiltration in parts of the larynx, trachea, and bronchi. Usually, peribronchiolitis and variable patterns of atelectasis and emphysema also develop.

The frequent occurrence of leukocytosis in whooping cough, characterized by absolute lymphocytosis, is a remarkable phenomenon, because absolute lymphocytosis is unusual in bacterial infections. The development of blood leukocytosis evidently is due to the exotoxin produced by *B pertussis;* therefore, it is not surprising that lymphocytosis is regularly produced in humans and animals by injection of killed *B pertussis* vaccines. On the basis of the findings in mice showing that the lymphoid organs, bone marrow, thymus, lymph nodes, and spleen were deprived of small lymphocytes after the injection of *B pertussis* cells, it was suggested that *B pertussis*-induced blood lymphocytosis may be due to the release of small lymphocytes into the circulation rather than to the new formation of cells. This conception has not been generally accepted, however, because strong deprivation of small lymphocytes also is found regularly after injection of bacterial endotoxins without being associated with blood lymphocytosis. Nevertheless, *B pertussis*-mediated blood lymphocytosis must be considered a thymus-dependent process, because this phenomenon is not observed after injection of *B pertussis* organisms into thymectomized mice or into nude mice with congenital aplasia of the thymus.

Clinically, whooping cough is characterized by a spasmodic cough that usually lasts 6 weeks. Even though coughing may persist for a longer time, after the sixth week of the disease the patient can be considered noninfectious. Apart from frequent pulmonary sequelae such as bronchitis and pneumonia, the neurologic involvement, **encephalopathy**, is of special importance. This toxic manifestation is sometimes observed after immunization with *B pertussis* vaccines. Although not yet precisely defined, the spasmodic cough typical of the disease also is thought to be caused neurologically. In mice, localized respiratory and brain infections, but not peritoneal and blood infections, can be produced experimentally.

Host Defenses

The person who recovers from whooping cough develops substantial immunity to the disease that usually lasts many years; second infections rarely occur. Immunity acquired after infection with *B pertussis* does not protect against disease caused by another member of the genus *Bordetella*. Which structural components of *B pertussis* represent the protective antigen that induces immunity following infection or immunization is still not known. Conflicting results have been obtained by different laboratories. At first, the filamentous hemagglutinin and the pertussis toxin were identified as essential protective antigens. Most recently, it was suggested that the filamentous hemagglutinin, the fimbriae, and a variety of outer membrane proteins of *B pertussis* may be protective antigens. The activity of these antigens is increased significantly in the presence of pertussis toxin. This synergism indicates that the pertussis toxin could function as an adjuvant to a variety of protective antigens of *B pertussis*.

Apart from experimental diseases produced in monkeys, diseases in animals caused by *B pertussis* do not resemble whooping cough. Evidence suggests that the numerous biologically active structural components of *B pertussis* cells are involved in the pathogenesis of whooping cough as well as in the defense mechanisms of the host. These defense mechanisms are both nonspecific (local inflammation, macrophages, and induction of interferon) and specific (B and T lymphocytes). The basis of immunity in whooping cough is, however, incompletely understood. That the circulating antibody might take part in immunity is indicated by the correlation between protection of human vaccinees and their serum agglutinin titers. However, effective immunity does not necessarily depend on the presence of serum agglutinins. Thus, immunity to whooping cough may be mediated essentially by cellular mechanisms. This cell-mediated immunity may be considered as the crucial carrier of long-term immunity, *and specific humoral antibodies may diminish over the years*. This may be the reason why infants usually do not benefit significantly from maternal antibody.

Epidemiology

The mucous membranes of the human respiratory tract are the natural habitat for *B pertussis* and *B parapertussis*. Although *B pertussis* organisms can survive outside the body for a few days and thus may be transmitted by contaminated objects, most infections occur after direct contact with diseased persons specifically by inhalation of bacteria-bearing droplets expelled in cough spray. The patient is most infectious during the early catarrhal phase when clinical symptoms are relatively poor and noncharacteristic and have not yet been recognized as whooping cough. Subclinical cases may have similar epidemiologic significance.

Healthy carriers of *B pertussis* or *B parapertussis* are assumed to play no significant epidemiologic role. The natural habitat of *B bronchiseptica* is the respiratory tract of smaller animals, such as rabbits, cats, and dogs. Therefore, human infections with *B bronchiseptica* are extremely rare and occur only after close contact with carrier animals.

Whooping cough, as a highly communicable infection of worldwide significance, was once a common and dangerous disease killing many thousands of children per year. Widespread vaccination has effected a continuous decrease in incidence and mortality over the years, but large numbers of fatal whooping cough cases still occur in countries where vaccination is insufficiently administered. Whooping cough is mainly an infection of infants, although susceptibility is general. The disease is especially dangerous within the first 6 months of life. Both morbidity and mortality rates are higher in girls than in boys. Neither season nor climate seems to affect the morbidity rate.

Diagnosis

After an incubation period of 7-14 days, whooping cough begins with the catarrhal phase. Lasting 1-2 weeks, this phase is usually characterized by low-grade fever, rhinorrhea, and progressive cough. The patient is highly infectious in this stage. The subsequent paroxysmal phase, lasting 2-4 weeks, is characterized by severe and spasmodic cough episodes. At the end of the catarrhal phase, a leukocytosis with an absolute and relative lymphocytosis usually begins, reaching its peak at the height of the paroxysmal stage. At this paroxysmal stage, the total blood leukocyte levels may resemble those of leukemia ($>100,000/mm^3$), with 60%-80% of these being lymphocytes. The convalescent phase, lasting 1-3 weeks, is characterized by continuous decline of the cough before the patient returns to normal.

A rapid diagnosis is possible by the fluorescent antibody procedure using nasopharyngeal smears. For cultural isolation, the Bordet-Gengou agar, containing blood, potato extract, and glycerin, is still used today, although minor modifications regarding blood concentration, addition of penicillin, and nicotinamide have been recommended. Effective cultivation can also be achieved using charcoal agar. Growth of the *B pertussis* organisms occurs aerobically in phases I-IV, showing that the bacteria of the antigenically competent smooth and virulent form (phase I) are capable of mutating to the antigenically incomplete and nonvirulent rough form (phase IV). Phases II and III are intermediate forms. The three members of the genus *Bordetella* do not need X and V factors.

For collection of specimens, two different procedures are mainly employed. The cough-plate method is still widely used by physicians. During a paroxysm of coughing, the patient is asked to cough directly on the opened plate held in front of the mouth at a distance of about 15 cm. More effective is the nasopharyngeal swab method, in which the swab is introduced through one of the nostrils into the nasopharynx. Once taken, the material must be streaked immediately on Bordet-Gengou agar or placed in a suitable transport medium.

Growth of *B pertussis* at 37 C usually occurs after 3-4 days' incubation. The colonies appear as small transparent droplets indistinguishable from those of *B bronchiseptica* and usually are smaller than those of *B parapertussis*. All three members of the genus *Bordetella* undergo hemolysis. Biochemically, they are relatively inert and do not ferment carbohydrates or produce H_2S and indole. An important characteristic of *B parapertussis* is its capacity to produce brown pigmentation on blood-free peptone agar. As shown in Table 47-1, differentiation of the three *Bordetella* species is already possible on the basis

Table 47-1   Differential Characteristics of the Genus *Bordetella**

	B pertussis	*B parapertussis*	*B bronchiseptica*
Motility	−	−	+
Growth on blood-			
free peptone agar	−	+	+
Pigment production	−	+	−
Nitrate reduction	−	−	+
Urea hydrolysis	−	+	+
Oxidase reaction	+	−	+

* +, present; −, absent.

of certain biochemical and cultural differentiating characteristics. In addition, slide agglutination tests are recommended.

Circulating antibodies, occurring as late as during the third week of illness and reaching their maximum the eighth to tenth week, have been demonstrated by agglutination and complement-fixation tests. The agglutination test is applied mainly in epidemiologic studies. Although no direct relationship has been shown between the agglutinin concentration and the degree of protection, high agglutinin titers ($\geq$1:320) are assumed to be correlated with protection from disease.

Modern techniques have been introduced for the serological diagnosis of whooping cough. Also, modern serological techniques based on the principle of "sandwich" radioimmunoassay and enzyme-linked immunoassay (ELISA) were used to detect IgM, IgG, and IgA antibodies to *B pertussis*. In accordance with other serological methods, seroconversion could be observed only 2-4 weeks after the onset of the disease. The detection of specific IgA and IgM, however, was found to be indicative of recent infection and is useful for the differential diagnosis of pertussiform syndromes of longer duration. To demonstrate acute infection, another method may be of great importance: the enzyme-linked immunosorbent assay for detection of pertussis immunoglobulin A (PsIgA) in nasopharyngeal secretions. PsIgA is produced during natural human infection; it usually appears in nasopharyngeal secretions during the second or third week of illness, and persists for at least 3 months. It is remarkable that PsIgA evidently does not arise as a result of parenteral vaccination. This finding is in accordance with recent results obtained by using the ELISA assay in studies in which the serological response (IgM, IgG, and IgA) to the filamentous hemagglutinin and the pertussis toxin was measured both in subjects who had been immunized during the first weeks of life, and in patients with laboratory-acquired pertussis infection. No IgA antibodies were found in vaccinees, but IgA antibodies were found in patients recovering from infection.

Control

Susceptible children (unimmunized children who have not had whooping cough) should not have any contact with pertussis patients during the first 5 weeks of illness, although preventing contact of the patient with other family members is often impractical. In the United States, 4 weeks usually is considered to be the infectious period of untreated persons, whereas a patient treated with erythromycin or ampicillin may be contagious for only 5-10 days. Exposed, immunized children younger than 4 years of age are given booster doses of pertussis vaccine. Exposed, unimmunized children are given ampicillin or erythromycin for 10 days after contact is discontinued (or after the case ceases to be contagious).

For vaccine production, only smooth forms (phase I) are suitable. Because the disease runs a relatively mild course, and because there are occasional neurologic complications after vaccination, many specialists believe general vaccination is no longer justified; however, in the United States, general pertussis vaccination of children still is recommended. During the past years much progress has been made regarding the development of effective acellular vaccines. Such preparations composed of endotoxin-free supernatant culture fluid treated with formaldehyde for the inactivation of pertussis toxin are currently employed in Japan. No definite evaluation of vaccine efficacy can be made at this time. Human hyperimmune pertussis globulin is still used occasionally in severely ill infants, but no reliable data support its efficacy.

Although *B pertussis* is sensitive in vitro to several antibiotics (ampicillin, tetracycline, erythromycin, and chloramphenicol), their efficacy in vivo is not convincing. Indeed, patients are usually free from *B pertussis* after antibiotic therapy within a few days, but this has no influence on the course of the disease.

References

Arai, H., Munoz, J.J.: Crystallization of pertussigen from Bordetella pertussis. *Infect Immun* 1981; 31:495-499.

Bemis, D.A., Kennedy, J.R.: An improved system for studying the effect of *Bordetella bronchiseptica* on the ciliary activity of canine tracheal epithelial cells. *J Infect Dis* 1981; 144:349-357.

Burstyn, D.G., et al.: Serological response to filamentous hemagglutinin and lymphocytosis-promoting toxin of *Bordetella pertussis*. *Infect Immun* 1983; 41:1150-1156.

Finger, H., et al.: Uber Struktur und biologische Aktivitat von Bordetella pertussis-Endotoxin. *Zbl Bakt Hyg I Abt Orig A* 1976; 235:55-64

Finger, H., et al.: Reversion of dextran sulfate-induced loss of antibacterial resistance by Bordetella pertussis. *Infect Immun* 1978; 19:950-960.

Finger, H., et al.: Zur Entstehung der Lymphozytose beim Keuchhusten. *Zbl Bakt Hyg I Abt Orig A* 1976; 235:65-70.

Goodman, Y.E., Wort, A.J., Jackson, F.L.: Enzyme-linked immunosorbent assay for detection of pertussis immunoglobulin A in nasopharyngeal secretions as an indicator of recent infection. *J Clin Microbiol* 1981; 13:286-292.

Lautrop, H., Lacey, B.W.: Laboratory diagnosis of whooping-cough or Bordetella infections. *Bull WHO* 1960; 23:15-35.

Manclark, CH.R.: 1976. Serological response to Bordetella pertussis. In: *Manual of clinical immunology*. Rose, N.R., Friedman, H., (editors). Washington, D.C.: American Society for Microbiology, 1976.

Munoz, J.J., Bergman, R.K.: Bordetella pertussis. *Immunology Series*, vol. 4. New York and Basel: Marcel Dekker, 1977.

Pittman, M.: Pertussis toxin: the cause of the harmful effects and prolonged immunity of whooping cough. A hypothesis. *Rev Infect Dis* 1979; 1:401-412.

Pittman, M.: The concept of pertussis as a toxin-mediated disease. *Pediat Infect Dis* 1984; 3:467-486.

Robinson, A., Irons, L.I.: Synergistic effect of Bordetella pertussis lymphocytosis-promoting factor on protective activities of isolated Bordetella antigens in mice. *Infect Immun* 1983; 40:523-528.

Sato, Y. et al: Separation and purification of the hemagglutinins from *Bordetella pertussis*. *Infect Immun* 1983; 41:313-320.

Tuomanen, E.I., Hendley, O.: Adherence of *Bordetella pertussis* to human respiratory epithelial cells. *J Infect Dis* 1983; 148:125-130.

Wirsing v. Koenig, C.H., Finger, H.: Detection of IgG antibodies against Bordetella pertussis with ^{125}I-protein A. *Med Microb Immunol* 1981; 169:83-89.

48 *Corynebacterium, Mycobacterium,* and *Nocardia*

Lane Barksdale, PhD

General Concepts

In the microbial world, the genera *Corynebacterium, Mycobacterium,* and *Nocardia* (the CMN group) are placed in the family *Mycobacteriaceae* in the order *Actinomycetales.* Several members of this group are infectious for humans and animals and cause some acute and numerous chronic infections such as diphtheria, tuberculosis, leprosy, and nocardiosis.

Morphologically, the CMN microbes are gram-positive, nonmotile, non–endo-spore-forming, catalase-producing bacteria whose shapes range from rodlike to filamentous. Cells taken from old cultures are irregular in shape and contain granules rich in polyphosphate and globules of fat. Corynebacteria have been described as pleomorphic rods and sometimes show rudimentary branching. Mycobacteria are generally regarded as irregularly shaped rodlike bacteria; however, their shapes range from the pleomorphic rods of *M tuberculosis* to the filamentous forms of *M farcinogenes.* Nocardias are filamentous organisms that fragment into individual rods and coccoid forms when touched with a bacteriologic loop.

Members of the CMN group produce characteristic α-branched, β-hydroxylated long chain fatty acids, generally termed mycolic acids, which have the following general formula:

$$\overset{\beta}{}\quad\overset{\alpha}{}$$

$$R\!-\!\underset{|}{CH}\!-\!\underset{|}{CH}\!-\!COOH$$

$$OH\quad R_1$$

where R and R_1 are carbon chains of varying lengths, corynomycolic and corynomycolenic acids, C_{28}–C_{40} (*Corynebacterium*); nocardic or nocardomycolic acids, C_{40}–C_{56} (*Nocardia*); and mycolic acids, C_{60}–C_{90} (*Mycobacterium*). (For a comparison of these CMN-group fatty acids, see Figure 48-1.) Mycolic acids, in cord factors, are medically

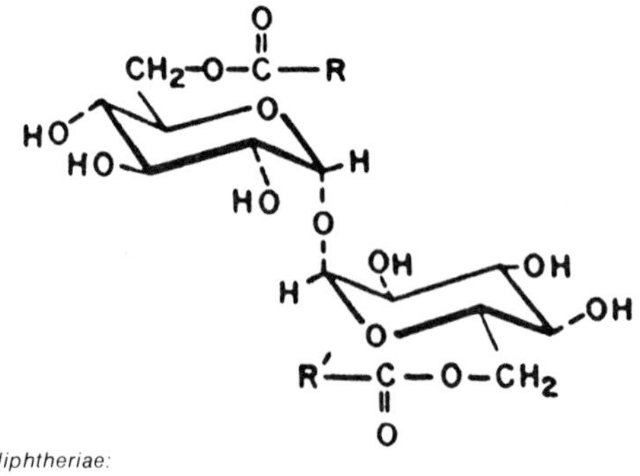

C. diphtheriae:
 R = $C_{15}H_{31}$-CHOH-CH-[COOH], corynomycolic acid
 $\phantom{R = C_{15}H_{31}\text{-CHOH-CH-[COOH]},}\underset{}{C_{14}H_{29}}$

 R' = C_6H_{13}-CH = CH-(CH_2) $_7$-CH-[COOH], corynomycolenic acid
 $\phantom{R' = C_6H_{13}\text{-CH = CH-(CH}_2)\ _7\text{-CH-[COOH]},}\underset{}{C_{14}H_{29}}$

M. tuberculosis:
 R and R' = $C_{60}H_{121}$-CHOH-CH-[COOH], mycolic acid
 $\phantom{R and R' = C_{60}H_{121}\text{-CHOH-CH-[COOH]},}\underset{}{C_{24}H_{49}}$

Figure 48-1 Trehalose dimycolates (cord factors) of *Corynebacterium diphtheriae* and *Mycobacterium tuberculosis.* Note that mycolic acids generally occur as a family of chain lengths, so above formulas represent averages.

significant because they are immunoadjuvants and they or their adducts are involved in the organism's invasive capacity. Fatty acid synthesis in these microorganisms is associated with a particulate system of interacting enzymes designated as fatty acid synthetase I. The cell walls of the CMN microbes contain mesodiaminopimelic acid and a characteristic polysaccharide, arabinogalactan. Properties unique to each of the three genera are discussed in the following pages.

CORYNEBACTERIUM: C DIPHTHERIAE

Distinctive Properties

C diphtheriae (coryne, or club, refers to the club-shaped bacterium of the pseudomembranous condition) includes *C diphtheriae* var *mitis,* var *intermedius,* var *gravis, C ulcerans,* and a gradient of entities that link *C diphtheriae* to *C pseudotuberculosis (ovis),* the cause of chronic, purulent infections in sheep, goats, horses and, rarely, humans. The cells of all diphtheria bacilli have certain features in common: when growing in tissue, their cell walls contain thin spots that leak the Gram stain (gram-variable); old cells store inorganic phosphate as polymetaphosphate, localized as intracellular metachromatic granules; and bacilli with thin spots tend to balloon out at one end of the cell (assume a shape like a club) (Figure 48-2). These properties in bacteria taken from lesions of the throat suggest *C diphtheriae,* but no one property is unique to diphtheria bacilli.

Pathogenesis

Diphtheria is a contagious disease of humans in which *C diphtheriae* colonizes the mucous membranes of the fauces and the pharynx and sometimes extends to the larynx and the trachea. These forms of the infection are called, respectively, faucial, pharyngeal, laryngeal, and tracheal diphtheria. When colonization occurs on the mucous membranes of the skin, cutaneous diphtheria results. The exudate that develops in conjunction with invasion by *C diphtheriae* often adheres so tenaciously to the mucosal surface that it has been called a pseudomembrane.

Diphtheria bacilli may be found in a fraction of any human population; however, their presence does not necessarily indicate disease. When diphtheria bacilli carry a gene called tox^+, they synthesize a toxin lethal for humans and various animals. In the absence of the gene tox^+, no toxin is made. Three major interactions are possible between diphtheria bacilli and the human host: a) infection leading to toxemic diphtheria; b) infection leading to nontoxemic diphtheria (sometimes a serious disease of infants); and c) infection leading to establishment of *C diphtheriae* as a member of the throat flora with or without any apparent disease. Healthy individuals who harbor *C diphtheriae* are termed carriers.

Colonization of Mucous Membranes

Limited information exists regarding the properties of *C diphtheriae* that adapt it to living on the mucous membranes of throat and skin. *C diphtheriae* produces a sialidase or neuraminidase (NAN-ase) that not only cleaves N-acetylneuraminic acid (NAN)

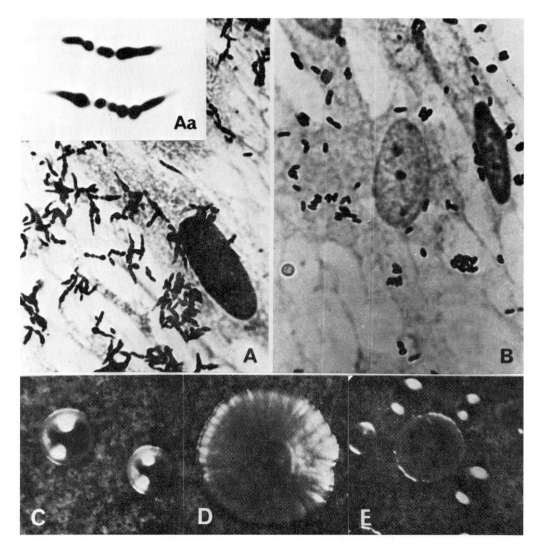

Figure 48-2 A, Cells of *C diphtheriae* var *mitis* growing with mammalian cells in tissue culture (×3000). **Aa,** As in **A** (×5200). **B,** Cells of *C diphtheriae* var *gravis* (×3000). C, Smooth colony of *C diphtheriae* var *mitis*. **D,** Colony of *C diphtheriae* var *gravis*. **E,** Four dwarf smooth colonies of *C diphtheriae* var *intermedius* surrounding a colony of irregular shape. Special clinical significance has been ascribed to these varieties of *C diphtheriae* when each produces diphtherial toxin. For example, among 25,000 cases of diphtheria studied in England, the fatalities among clinically mild cases infected with toxinogenic *C diphtheriae* var *mitis* was 7.2% of 6807; among more severe cases from whom were isolated toxinogenic *C diphtheriae* var *gravis*, 8.1% of 11,492; and in the case of toxinogenic *C diphtheriae* var *intermedius* strains, 2.6% of 6852. (Courtesy K-S. Kim.)

residues from cell surfaces and intracellular mucins, but also splits NAN into its component pyruvate and *N*-acetylmannosamine. Pyruvate is an active stimulator of growth for members of the CMN group. Cord factor (6,6′-dimycoloyl-α,α′-D-trehalose) (see Figure 48-1), a dimycolate of trehalose with the specific capacity for inactivating the mitochondrial membranes of mammalian cells, is a surface component of diphtheria bacilli. Its effect on the mammalian immune system will be discussed in relation to the cord factor of *M tuberculosis* (page 564). Among the proteases produced by *C diphtheriae* is diphthin, which inactivates immunoglobulin A. Plasma cells derived from tonsillar tissue have been shown to produce dimeric IgA (lacking a secretory piece) against antigens from *C diphtheriae*. More remains to be discovered about the role of diphthin and IgA in diphtheritic infections.

Diphtherial Toxin

Figure 48-3 shows clearly that diphtherial toxin is not required for infection by *C diphtheriae*. Infection with a toxinogenic strain can lead to a much more virulent manifestation of diphtheria than infection with a nontoxinogenic strain. In fact, the cause of nonobstructive, toxic death in toxemic diphtheria is diphtherial toxin made by diphtheria bacilli that carry the gene *tox*⁺. Toxic myocarditis is commonly fatal. The gene *tox*⁺ resides in certain temperate corynebacteriophages. When such phages lyse or lysogenize a sensitive, nontoxinogenic strain of *C diphtheriae*, diphtherial toxin is produced. The integration of *tox*⁺-carrying prophages into the genome of *C diphtheriae* is stable and so, by such lysogenization, new lines of toxinogenic *C diphtheriae* may come into being. Diphtherial toxin is lethal for humans and certain animals in amounts of 130 ng/kg body weight. It consists of a single polypeptide chain, mol. wt. 62,000, cross-linked by two disulfide bridges (Figure 48-4). At the bend, indicated by the arrow, is a trypsin-sensitive region containing three arginines. Although the amino-terminal amino acid is known to be glycine, the carboxy-terminal amino acid has not been determined. Nicking the peptide chain with trypsin at the arrow point and then reducing disulfide bonds in the presence of dithiothreitol liberates the A fragment (indicated by squiggley line, Figure 48-4). The solid line represents the B fragment.

The killing action of diphtherial toxin is ascribed to the capacity of fragment A to inactivate elongation factor 2 (EF 2). Most preparations of toxin contain some free

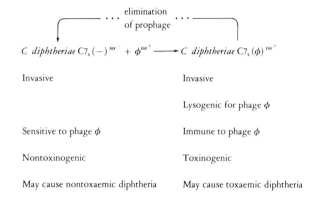

C diphtheriae C7$_s$ (−) $^{tox^-}$ + ϕ^{tox^+} $\longrightarrow$ *C diphtheriae* C7$_s$ (ϕ) $^{tox^+}$

Invasive   Invasive

                                                  Lysogenic for phage ϕ

Sensitive to phage ϕ Immune to phage ϕ

Nontoxinogenic   Toxinogenic

May cause nontoxaemic diphtheria   May cause toxaemic diphtheria

Figure 48-3 The conversion of nontoxinogenic *C diphtheriae* to lysogenic toxinogenic *C diphtheriae* with concomitant changes in bacterial genome.

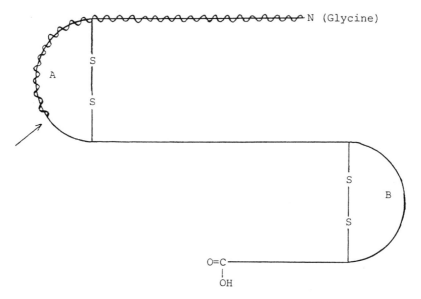

Figure 48-4 Diagrammatic representation of molecule of diphtherial toxin. A, fragment A;B, fragment B. For details, see text.

fragment A. Fragment A is a nicotinamide adenine dinucleotidase (NADase, DPNase) with the capacity to transfer and covalently link the adenine diphosphoribosyl moiety of NAD to EF 2. At physiologic pH, the reaction is irreversible, with the result that EF 2 becomes inactive. Inactivation of molecules of EF 2 blocks protein synthesis. The overall reaction involves the stoichiometric release of nicotinamide and a proton: $NAD^+ + EF\ 2 \rightarrow ADP - ribosyl - EF\ 2 + nicotinamide + H^+$. In the intoxication of mammalian cells by diphtherial toxin, the toxin molecule is thought to fix to the cell by its B portion. Proteolytic and reductive steps by the sensitive cell free the incoming fragment A with subsequent inactivation of EF 2. Fragment A consists of 193 amino acids; position 1 is occupied by glycine and position 193 by an arginine. Its active site involves a tryptophan residue at position 153. In theory, antitoxin protects against toxin because it prevents the B portion of the toxin molecule from attaching to toxin-sensitive mammalian cells.

Host Defenses

Repeated outbreaks of diphtheritic infections in the same population indicate that many serologic types of C *diphtheriae* exist. The differences in these types were first observed in toxinogenic strains at a time when nontoxinogenic strains were regarded as diphtherialike bacilli. These differences were obvious because they represented differences in colonial morphology, which reflected variations in cell shape and structure. Such differences directly affect the way bacteria pile up to form a colony (see Figure 48-2) and the structures responsible for the differences are, of course, antigenic. Each of the colonial categories (*gravis, mitis,* and *intermedius*) contains numerous serologic types and phage types. Thus, C *diphtheriae* sp have the potential to accommodate to the defenses of the human host against invasiveness, much as do group A streptococci and pneumococci.

The first evidence indicating a role for antibacterial immunity in diphtheria came from the finding that antiserum prepared against toxin produced by *gravis* strains seemed more effective in treating individuals infected with *C diphtheriae* var *gravis* than antitoxin made in response to immunization with toxin produced by *mitis* strains. The San Antonio outbreak in 1970 revealed a clear separation of antibacterial and antitoxic immunity, because a number of persons carrying a toxinogenic *gravis* strain became superinfected with a toxinogenic *intermedius* strain. Extrapolating from animal experiments and from delayed hypersensitivity reactions to the Schick test, it is clear that carriers of *C diphtheriae* manifest delayed hypersensitivity (cell-mediated immunity) to a variety of corynebacterial products. This is to be expected, as whole corynebacteria and such corynebacterial products as cord factor induce cell-mediated immunity in experimental animals. Antitoxin is not involved in this manifestation of antibacterial immunity, just as antiscarlatinal immunity is not involved in a succession of infections by nonscarlatinal streptococci of group A.

Diagnosis

Laboratory confirmation of the presence of *C diphtheriae* in a throat specimen requires adequate material for culture and for preparation of smears. Most diphtherial membranes adhere tightly, and material for culture cannot be readily obtained from them by merely swabbing the affected area. A sterile bacteriologic loop (Nichrome wire) transformed into a hook is more likely to loosen enough of the fibrinous exudate to provide adequate material for culture and smears. Material so obtained can be used to inoculate a blood agar plate (a slant of Loeffler's medium enriched with 2.5 g K_2HPO_4/L and a Mueller–Miller tellurite or Tinsdale tellurite agar plate); to prepare smears for a Gram stain; and to stain with alkaline methylene blue. Unstained smears can be set aside in case further tests are needed. Figure 48-2 shows clearly that the tapered ends of *C diphtheriae mitis* found in tissues are more exaggerated than *C diphtheriae gravis* (or *intermedius* strains, not shown).

When associated with the corresponding biochemical patterns shown in Table 48-1, the types of colonies shown in Figure 48-2C, D, E may be called var *mitis* (C), var *gravis* (D), or var *intermedius* (E). Figure 48-2 shows var *intermedius* to be a characteristically smooth colony type (four colonies and a rare rough mutant are shown). Following the isolation in pure culture of the suspected *C diphtheriae*, final identification rests on obtaining the characteristic reactions presented in Table 48-1.

Tellurite Agar

Most corynebacteria and some other bacteria, including certain mycobacteria, certain staphylococci, and some members of the genus *Bacillus* and some of the yeasts grow in the presence of 100 μg of potassium tellurite per mL to form grayish to jet black colonies. The growth of most streptococci, some staphylococci, and other members of the flora of the human throat is inhibited on tellurite agar plates. Because of this inhibition, tellurite agar is widely regarded as a selective medium to screen for the

Table 48-1 Biochemical Properties Useful in Distinguishing Members of Genus *Corynebacterium* Isolated from Human Oropharynx and Nasopharynx*

Strain	Production of					Fermentation of				
	Metachromatic Granules	Catalase	Pyrazin-amidase	Gela-tinase	Urease	Lactose	Maltose	Tre-halose	Starch†	Glucose
C diphtheriae										
var *mitis*	+	+	−	−	−	−	+	−	−	+
var *gravis*	+	+	−	−	−	−	+	−	+	+
var *intermedius*	+	+	−	−	−	−	+	−	−	+
C ulcerans	+	+	−	⊕	⊕	−	+	⊕	⊕	+
C pseudotuberculosis (ovis)‡	+	+	−	−	+	−	+	−	−	+
C pseudodiphtheriticum	+	+	+	−	+	−	−	−	−	−
C xerosis	+	+	+	−	−	−	⊖	−	−	+

*+, 100% strains tested positive; ⊕, rare negative strains may be found; −, 100% strains tested negative; ⊖, rare positive strains may be found.

†Because soluble starch contains some glucose, laundry starch is used for "starch fermentation tests."

‡*C pseudotuberculosis (ovis)* is only rarely found in the human throat. From Barksdale, L., et al: *J Clin Microbiol* 1981; 13:335.

presence of *C diphtheriae.* When black colonies are found on tellurite agar (surrounded by brown-black halos on Tinsdale tellurite agar), they must be examined microscopically for the presence of gram-positive rods exhibiting a degree of taper from one end of the cell. From those colonies that are suspected of being corynebacteria, the bacteria must be isolated in pure culture and identified by the procedures described in the preceding section.

Test for Toxin Production

Small amounts of diphtherial toxin cause necrosis of the skin (see discussion of the Schick test on page 556) of human subjects, birds, guinea pigs, rabbits, and numerous other animals. Of all the specific tests for toxin, the skin test measures the neutralizing capacity of antitoxin and is therefore not complicated by reactions between other antibodies in the antitoxic serum and corynebacterial products other than toxin. Because skin tests in animals can be performed with cultures of bacteria (cell-free preparations are not required), and because such tests alone measure toxicity and neutralization of toxicity by antitoxin, skin tests are considered the method of choice to assess toxinogenic capacity of *C diphtheriae.*

Tests for Specific Neutralization of Diphtherial Toxin by Antitoxin in Rabbit and Guinea Pig Skins

When one or two organisms are to be tested, a guinea pig is the best choice; when more are to be tested, the rabbit is preferred. The backs of the test animals are sheared and depilated, leaving the skin unblemished. At time zero, 0.1 mL amounts of suspensions of each organism are injected intracutaneously at numbered test sites. Subcutaneous injections are useless. After 3 hours, the animal is given antitoxin intravenously (in the case of the guinea pig, intraperitoneally, if finding a femoral vein is difficult). One-half hour later (3½ hours after time zero), 0.1 mL of each culture is injected at another site. Observations are made over a period up to 4 days. A positive lesion consists of a central necrotic zone surrounded by an area of erythema. When diphtherial toxin is responsible for the necrosis at the test site, that necrosis will have been neutralized by antitoxin at the corresponding control site. When severe reactions occur at both sites, the responsible organism has produced toxic substances antigenically distinct from diphtherial toxin (for example, toxin of *C pseudotuberculosis [ovis]*).

Detection of Diphtherial Toxin by Formation of Toxin-Antitoxin Precipitates in Agar Gels

To detect diphtherial toxin diffusing from *C diphtheriae* growing on agar plates, a horse serum agar plate (Petri dish) is poured; before the agar has hardened, a strip of filter paper (1.6 × 8 cm), previously dipped into horse antitoxin (500 au/mL) and drained of excess liquid, is placed across the center of the agar surface. Cotton swabs, soaked in heavy bacterial cultures and then freed of excess liquid by expression against the sides of the culture tubes, introduce each of the bacterial cultures onto the dried surface of the agar perpendicular to the strip of paper. Each unknown organism is streaked parallel to and well separated from a known toxinogenic control. For this purpose, the most satisfactory strain of *C diphtheriae* is the Park–Williams No. 8 strain (PW8) used internationally for production of diphtherial toxin (which is then used to produce the toxoid). As the growth and production of diphtherial toxin by the PW8 strain occur on the antitoxin-containing agar plate, a line of toxin-antitoxin (TAT) precipitate in the vicinity of that growth becomes apparent. If an unknown strain growing adjacent to the PW8 strain also produces toxin, its line of TAT precipitate also becomes visible. Where the two TAT precipitates meet, an arc of fusion shows the identity of the two TAT precipitates. Usually, when proteins *other* than toxin form antigen-antibody precipitates (OAgn · Ab) close to the TAT precipitate of the PW8 strain, no fusion of lines occurs. Instead, the OAgn · Ab line crosses the TAT line. If a cross-reaction occurs between toxin and an OAgn, partial fusion, or spur formation, is observed (see Chapter 5).

Epidemiology

Diphtheria is ever with us (for example, outbreaks occurred in Miami, 1969; San Antonio, 1970; Manchester, 1971; Delhi, 1973-1974; Montreal, 1974; Wurzburg, 1975; Seattle, 1972-1975; Bonn, 1976; and Lusaka, Zambia, 1977). In each outbreak, the involved physicians and public health personnel attempted to assess the degree of immunity to diphtherial toxin existing in the community through the use of the Schick test. Approximately 0.0006 μg of toxin protein nitrogen (one-fiftieth the minimal amount required to kill a guinea pig weighing 250 g) is injected into the forearm, the test site; 0.0124 μg formalized toxoid is injected at a control site. Readings are made at 48 and 96 hours. Necrosis at the test site indicates insufficient circulating antitoxin to neutralize the test dose of toxin. Originally designed to assess immunity to diphtherial toxin, the test is also valuable in demonstrating the number of persons with circulating antitoxin who also exhibit cell-mediated immunity to various corynebacterial products. Although the toxin and toxoid used in the test are purified preparations, they are not free from other corynebacterial products. Much confusion has resulted from assuming toxoid to be a single antigen rather than multiple antigens, or elicitins, or both.

Over the years, examination of human populations with the Schick test has provided various insights into immunobiology. First, any population tested contains individuals showing antitoxic immunity and cell-mediated immunity to corynebacterial products. Second, carriers of *C diphtheriae* do not necessarily have detectable levels of circulating antitoxin and that circulating antitoxin per se does not prevent diphtheritic infection. Third, the Schick test examination has led most recently to the discovery that about 1.5%-2% of the human population cannot respond to immunizing doses of toxoid with the production of detectable levels of circulating antitoxin. As long as this 1.5%-2% exists, and as long as diphtheria bacilli continue to be carried in populations immunized with toxoid, occasional deaths from diphtheria probably will occur.

Control

The greatest advance in the efforts to eliminate deaths from diphtherial toxin came with the discovery that toxin, after incubation with formaldehyde at 37 C under alkaline conditions, could be rendered into a nontoxic substance. This nontoxic substance, diphtherial toxoid, could induce production of antitoxic antibodies in human subjects. Toxoid has a remarkable immunizing capacity, although it lacks the capacity to fix to toxin-sensitive mammalian cells and cannot be separated into A and B fragments. Formalinized toxoid is one component of the widely used DPT (diphtheria, pertussis, tetanus) vaccine.

The basic immunizing course for infants consists of three primary doses, 0.5 mL each, beginning at 2 months of age and spaced at 4-8 week intervals, followed by a fourth reinforcing dose, 0.5 mL, approximately 1 year after the last primary dose. Efficacy of antitoxic immunity is approximately 97%. In the immunization of adults, an occasional severe reaction should be expected as a result of preexisting circulating corynebacterial antibodies.

Passive immunization with diphtherial antitoxin (horse) has always carried with it the risk of serum sickness. Among those patients treated with antitoxin in the San Antonio outbreak, 8.6% suffered from serum sickness. The ever present danger of serum sickness could be obviated were human antitoxic immunoglobulins available for passive immunotherapy.

Table 48-2 presents data concerning use of antitoxin in the treatment of toxemic diphtheria. Four days after disease onset, antitoxin administration no longer appears to affect the outcome of the disease. During the first days of the disease, the amount of toxin produced is related directly to the increase in numbers of diphtheria bacilli. Toxin must penetrate the patient's cells to exert its lethal effect. Antitoxin can prevent penetration, but does not affect toxin that has reached an intracellular location.

Penicillin, its congeners, and erythromycin have been used as part of the treatment of cases of diphtheria and of carriers of *C diphtheriae*. Although antibiotic therapy does not affect toxin action if offered soon enough, it can markedly limit the final amounts of toxin produced by killing diphtheria bacilli. In a recently reported outbreak of 598 cases of diphtheria in Delhi, the case fatality rate was 17%. About 16% of strains of *C diphtheriae* from 223 bacteriologically positive cases were resistant to penicillin; fewer, to ampicillin. The only antibiotic to which all strains (337 strains accumulated from 1972-1975) were sensitive was gentamicin.

Table 48-2   Early Administration of Antitoxin and Case Fatality Rates Among Patients Receiving Antitoxin*

Probable Day of Disease Antitoxin Administered	Total Cases Treated	Case Fatality Rate (%)
1	225	0
2	1441	4.2
3	1600	11.1
4	1276	17.3
5 or > 5	1645	18.7

*After Russell WT: *Medical research council special report series* 1943; 247:6.

OTHER CORYNEBACTERIA

Those species and varieties of *Corynebacterium* listed in Table 48-1 include corynebacteria that may cause lesions in the human oropharynx and sometimes in the skin along with the two apparently inoffensive organisms, *C pseudodiphtheriticum* and *C xerosis*. Note that these and most other species of corynebacteria can be distinguished readily from *C diphtheriae*, *C ulcerans*, and *C pseudotuberculosis* (*ovis*) by the pyrazinamidase reaction. *C diphtheriae*, *C ulcerans*, and *C pseudotuberculosis* (*ovis*) lack the ability to hydrolyze pyrazinamide.

Rare infections with *C pseudotuberculosis* have been reported in human subjects who work closely with animals. Other corynebacteria significant in veterinary medicine include *C renale* (the cause of pyelonephritis in cattle) and *C kutscheri* (found in overt and latent infections of mice). A group of corynebacteria associated with human genitourinary tract infections has been named *C genitalium*.

Gram-positive pleomorphic rodlike bacteria, sometimes confused with corynebacteria, include the lactose-positive actinomycete *A pyogenes* and the anaerobic-to-microaerophilic *Propionibacterium*, sometimes called *C acnes*. *A pyogenes* often causes pharyngitis and ulcers of the skin in humans and suppurative lesions in cattle, sheep, pigs, and goats. *P acnes* (*C parvum*), commonly found on human skin, has aroused interest among immunologists in recent years because of its ability (as a killed vaccine) to stimulate the reticuloendothelial system of certain experimental animals and sometimes to inhibit tumor growth in them. Anaerobic *P acnes* sometimes may be associated with deep-seated infections.

MYCOBACTERIUM: M TUBERCULOSIS AND *M BOVIS*

Distinctive Properties

The genus *Mycobacterium* includes numerous species, some of which cause chronic infections of the lung and others of which give rise to a variety of disseminated infections in human beings. For the bacteriologist, the hallmark of members of this genus is their capacity to retain dyes such as carbolfuchsin following decolorization with acidic ethanol; this capacity is called **mycobacterial acid-fastness.** Another property shared by many members of *Mycobacterium* is a tendency to grow very slowly. Thus, whereas a mean generation time for *mitis* strains of *C diphtheriae* is 60 minutes, the H37Rv strain of *M tuberculosis* requires at least 300 minutes to divide; as a result, three or more weeks may be required to obtain visible growth from small inocula of *M tuberculosis* in, for example, its cultivation from sputa. Because a few mycobacteria such as *M smegmatis* grow more rapidly, growth rates have been found useful for characterizing mycobacteria (see list).

Properties used for identifying mycobacteria differ somewhat from those employed in identifying other gram-positive microbes (see list). Most mycobacteria have relatively simple growth requirements: *M tuberculosis*, for example, grows satisfactorily in a medium containing trace metals, asparagine, and glycerol. The way mycobacterial cells growing on solid media pile up to form a colony or produce carotenoid pigments varies

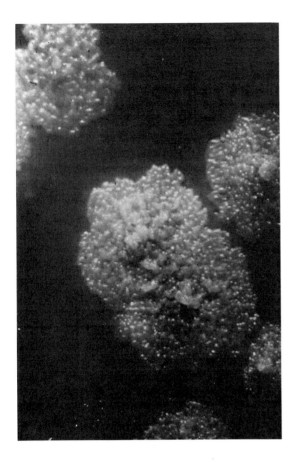

Figure 48-5 Colonies of *Mycobacterium tuberculosis* strain H37Rv exhibiting serpentine cords. Courtesy of George Kubica.

among species. For example, *M kansasii* typically forms entire round, smooth, waxy, orange-yellow colonies, whereas *M tuberculosis* forms irregular, waxy, glittering, whitish colonies (Figure 48-5).

Properties Commonly Used to Distinguish Species of Mycobacteria

1. Rate of growth (S = slow; F = fast)

2. Secretion of niacin

3. Reduction of nitrate ($NaNO_3$)

4. Semiquantitative test for hyperproduction of catalase (column of gas bubbles >45 mm)

5. Stability of catalase to 68 C, 20 min

6. Carotenogenesis constitutive (scotochromogenic)

7. Carotenogenesis photoinducible (photochromogenic)

8. Hydrolysis of Tween 80 after 10 days

9. Reduction of tellurite (KTeO$_2$), 3 days

10. Growth on media containing 5% (w/v) NaCl

11. Hydrolysis of tripotassium phenolphthalein disulfate by arylsulfatase, 3 days

12. Growth on MacConkey agar

Application: Slow-growing *M bovis* and *M tuberculosis* share many properties but differ as to secretion of niacin (positive in 70–99% of strains of *M tuberculosis*) and hydrolysis of Tween 80 (positive in 15%–69% of strains of *M tuberculosis*). Slow-growing smooth-colony-forming *M scrofulaceum* produces pigmented (yellow) colonies when grown in the dark; slow-growing smooth-colony-forming *M kansaii* develops its maximum pigment only following exposure to light. More information useful for identifying mycobacteria may be found in Chapman (1977), Vestal (1975), Barksdale and Kim (1977), and Youmans (1979).

Acid-fastness is the capacity of a cell or compound to bind a dye so as to resist decolorization (loss of dye) by dilute mineral acid or acidic ethanol. In a strict sense, mycobacterial acid-fastness must be defined as a resistance to decolorization with acid ethanol, as a number of corynebacteria and nocardias grown on specific media containing glycerol are resistant to decolorization by dilute (1%–10%) mineral acid. Mycobacterial cells that have taken up fuchsin, crystal violet, or auramine 0 in phenol water (as carbolfuchsin, carbol crystal violet, or carbol auramine 0) usually resist decolorization by acidic ethanol as applied in the Ziehl–Neelsen stain.

Mycobacterial Cell Wall and Resistance to Physical Agents

The cells walls of mycobacteria are unusual in that 80% of the cross-linking of the peptidoglycan occurs through D-alanyl-D-meso-DAP and meso-diaminopimelyl-meso-diaminopimelic acid linkages. The mycolic acids of the CMN group reach their most elaborate development in mycobacteria (C$_{60}$–C$_{90}$) and are linked to the insoluble macromolecular rigid cell wall peptidoglycan by phosphodiester bridges to *N*-glycolyl muramic acid and as glycolipids esterified to arabinogalactan. The outer envelope of the walls of mycobacteria varies from species to species, containing a variety of glycolipids or peptidoglycolipids whose serologic specificities are determined by such sugars as 0-methylrhamnose, fucose, and others (see Figures 48-6 and 48-7). Also important are the dimycolates of trehalose, called cord factors because their presence appears related to the pattern of growth of some mycobacterial species on solid media as serpentine cords (for example, *M tuberculosis;* see Figure 48-5). Mycobacterial sulfolipids also are strung on a core of trehalose. They have the capacity to bind the dye neutral red (the neutral red binding capacity of mycobacteria) and are related in some way to virulence.

The lipoidal nature of the mycobacterial cell wall appears to contribute to survival of mycobacteria by rendering them resistant to drying and acid or alkaline conditions. Old cultures often remain viable for several months. Cells of dried, sputum-coated *M tuberculosis* may remain viable for as long as 10 days. Being coated with sputum also enables tubercle bacilli to resist dry heat up to 100 C for 1 hour. Most mycobacteria resist 4% sulfuric acid, 4% sodium hydroxide, or 5% oxalic acid for 15–30 minutes or 15 minutes in *N*-acetyl-L-cysteine in 2% NaOH-1.45% sodium citrate. This kind of

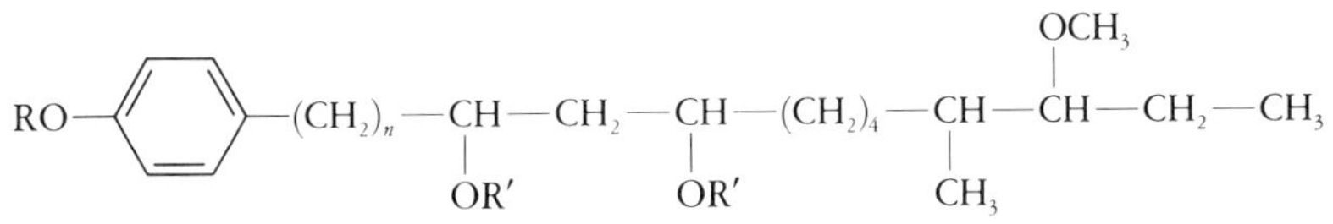

Phenolic Aglycone

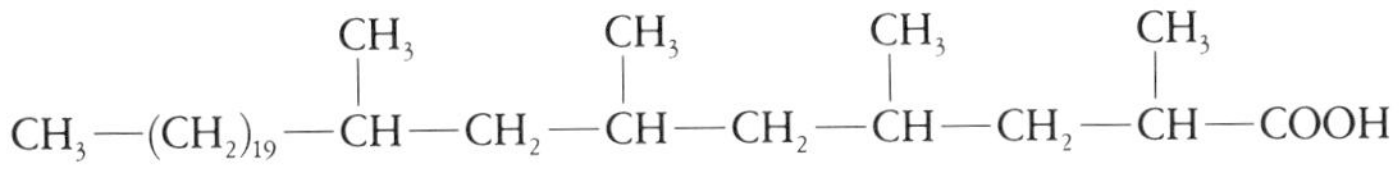

$$CH_3-(CH_2)_{19}-\underset{\underset{CH_3}{|}}{CH}-CH_2-\underset{\underset{CH_3}{|}}{CH}-CH_2-\underset{\underset{CH_3}{|}}{CH}-CH_2-\underset{\underset{CH_3}{|}}{CH}-COOH$$

A C_{32} Mycocerosic Acid

$$Ch_3\,(CH_2)_{14}\,COOH$$

Palmitic Acid

Figure 48-6 The phenolic glycol chain is the backbone of the phenolic glycolipids of the outer envelopes of *M tuberculosis, M bovis, M kansasii, M marinum,* in-armadillo-grown *M leprae* (TBKML-mycobacteria), and certain other mycobacterial species. The phenolic glycolipids are glycosides in which the sugar moiety (R) is linked in the para position of the phenol of the glycol chain whose hydroxyls (R′) are esterified with straight and branched chain fatty acids such as palmitic and mycocerosic acids shown above. For example, in *M bovis,* R′ = palmitic and mycocerosic acids; R = 2-0-methylrhamnose and n = 14, 15, 16, 17, and 18. *Note:* in the well-known mycobacterial product, phthiocerol, the phenol (above) is replaced by CH_3^-.

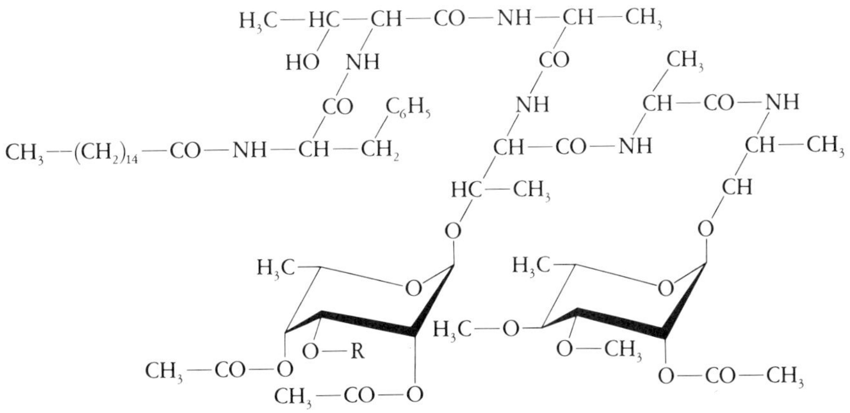

R = H or CH₃

Figure 48-7 A model peptidoglycolipid (Mycoside C_2) from the outer envelope of *Mycobacterium avium* as reported by Voiland and associates (see Barksdale and Kim, 1977, p. 278). In the pentapeptide portion of a molecule of this class is the aminoalcohol L-alaninol to which is linked 3,4-di-0-methyl-L-rhamnose. The sugar terminal to allothreonine is 6-deoxytalose or its 3-0-methyl derivative. The lipid moiety, R, of this peptidoglycolipid (PGL) consists of a complex mixture of fatty acids containing palmitic acid. Peptidoglycolipids of differing lengths of peptides and differing oligosaccharides are known for a number of serotypes of *M avium, M intracellulare, M scrofulaceum* (MAIS-mycobacteria), and related species. Compare these PGLs with the phenolic glycolipids of the TBKML-mycobacteria considered in the text and in Figure 48-6.

resistance is exploited in the routine isolation of mycobacteria from sputum, urine, or feces where the large amounts of other microorganisms present would offer a serious problem as fast-growing contaminants were those organisms not killed by alkali or acid.

Adjuvant Action of Mycobacterial Cell Wall

Folklore of long ago said that persons suffering from tuberculosis seemed to have an enhanced resistance to other infections. When this idea was put to a test in guinea pigs over a half century ago, animals infected with *M tuberculosis* responded to other injected antigens with enhanced synthesis of antibody and with development of delayed hypersensitivity. In essence, the adjuvant action of myobacteria means that living mycobacteria catalytically enhance humoral and cell-mediated responses to various antigens. Dead mycobacteria injected into animals do not produce an adjuvant effect unless they are suspended in an emulsifier plus mineral oil (Freund's complete adjuvant). When the mycobacterial component is omitted, the mixture is called incomplete Freund's adjuvant.

An international community of scientists has attempted to identify the smallest component of the mycobacterial cell wall that can produce an adjuvant effect. The cell wall fragment N-acetyl-muramyl-L-alanyl-D-isoglutamine (MurNAc-L-Ala-D-isoGln) suspended in incomplete Freund's adjuvant and administered to animals with an antigen such as egg albumin has been shown to induce antibody synthesis and delayed type hypersensitivity to egg albumin. The stereo configuration of the MurNAc-L-ala-D-isoGln (MDP) is essential for this activity. Normal peritoneal macrophages from guinea pigs or rats are inhibited in their migration by MDP. This inhibition is unrelated to macrophage migration inhibition factor (MIF) and requires the same stereospecificity of MDP as is required for adjuvant action. The presence of MDP in the peptidoglycan of many bacteria raises a question why most bacteria are not good adjuvants. The answer may be that many bacteria have not been examined for their adjuvant action, that some bacteria such as those that produce endotoxins may contain components that negate MDP action, and that members of the CMN group, because of their mycolic acids, may present MDP to the host in just the right way to assure its adjuvant action. The adjuvant action of *living* mycobacteria (LM) or such products as MDP may be conveniently summarized: LM plus Antigen X leads to the enhancement of both humoral immunity (HI) and cell-mediated immunity (CMI) to Antigen X. In such an equation (and in practice), BCG (see *M bovis*) is often the *living* mycobacterium and any of a number of antigens serve as Antigen X, including certain lines of tumor cells.

Pathogenesis

In 1868, Jean-Antoine Villemin demonstrated that material from humans with tuberculosis could produce a comparable disease in rabbits. (Some individuals with whom he dealt undoubtedly were infected with *M bovis;* see Table 48-3.) Sixteen years after publication of his findings, the remarkable German physician-microbiologist, Robert Koch, isolated *M tuberculosis* from the sputum of tuberculous human subjects and showed that pure cultures of those tubercle bacilli of human origin would cause a fatal

Table 48-3   Susceptibility of Man and Animals to Various Mycobacterial Species*

Species	Guinea Pig[†]	Rabbit[†]	Mouse[†]	Chick[†‡]	Humans[‡]
M tuberculosis	+	−	+	−	Tuberculosis
M bovis	+	+	+	−	Tuberculosis
M avium	−	+	±	+	Tuberculosis (rare)
M kansasii	−	−	±	−	Tuberculosislike
M marinum	−	−	Cool areas	−	Swimming pool granuloma and subcutaneous abscesses
M scrofulaceum	−	−	−	−	Lymphadenitis in children
M gordonae	−	−	−	−	No disease
M intracellulare[§]	+	−	+	±	Tuberculosislike in adults; lymphadenitis in children
M ulcerans	−	+	+	−	Extensive necrosis and ulceration of skin
M triviale, M terrae, M gastri	−	−	−	−	No disease
M xenopi	−	−	−	−	Tuberculosislike
M fortuitum	−	−	+	−	Local abscess, rarely tuberculosislike
M smegmatis, M phlei	−	−	−	−	No disease

*Data from Pan American Health Organization. *Leprosy: Cultivation of the etiologic agent, immunology, animal models.* PAHO Scientific Publication No. 342. Washington, D.C., 1977.
[†]Infection resulting from inoculation with syringe and needle.
[‡]Infection acquired by natural route.
[§]Although the type strain of *M intracellulare* (from a human case of generalized granulomatous disease) was pathogenic for the guinea pig and mouse (and not the chick), most strains subsequently isolated from human sources have induced no reactions in guinea pigs and mice, although a number of strains could produce disease in the chick.

tuberculosis infection in guinea pigs. Pure cultures isolated from those guinea pigs could initiate infections in other guinea pigs. He astutely observed that guinea pigs infected with *M tuberculosis* at a site such as the left inguinal region responded 2 weeks later to superinfection at a fresh site in the opposite inguinal region by showing a capacity to contain or limit the spread of the second infection. This accelerated response to superinfection was associated with marked hypersensitivity of the delayed type to products of *M tuberculosis*. Such an acquired partial immunity to *M tuberculosis* in the guinea pig came to be known as the Koch phenomenon and is a classic example of cell-mediated immunity.

Virulence Factors

The search has been long and arduous for factor(s) present in the standard virulent strain of *M tuberculosis*, H37Rv, and absent in the relatively avirulent strain, H37Ra. In 1984, Myrvik and associates at the Bowman Gray School of Medicine found that the H37Rv strain possesses the capacity to disrupt the phagosomal membranes of alveolar macrophages derived from the lungs of certain lines of rabbits. Avirulent bacilli (H37Ra) lacked this capacity. The virulent bacilli first adhere to the membrane; thereafter the membrane fragments and disintegrates leaving cells of H37Rv free in the cytoplasm of the macrophage. The membrane-destroying factor is readily inactivated when cells of H37Rv are heated to 56 C for 30 minutes.

The cord factors, also called mycosides or trehalose dimycolates, of the CMN group can inactivate the mitochondrial membranes of phagocytes and other cells exposed to them. Figure 48-1 shows formulas for cord factors of *C diphtheriae* and *M tuberculosis*. Although these two cord factors differ markedly in their molecular weights, they exhibit similar lethal effects on cells and animals. When used in small doses as immunostimulants in mice subsequently challenged with injections of living bacteria (for example, *Klebsiella pneumoniae* or *Listeria monocytogenes*), the cord factors of *C diphtheriae* and *M tuberculosis* are equally effective in inducing nonspecific antibacterial immunity (see Chapter 7). Cord factors administered to animals with a protein antigen in a water-in-oil emulsion induce delayed hypersensitivity and an enhanced antibody response. Under such conditions, cord factors are immunologic adjuvants.

Host Defenses

Organisms that have reached bronchioles and alveoli may undergo a few divisions before being engulfed by phagocytes. Once inside the phagocyte, a number of bacilli remain viable and multiply. The phenotype of intracellular bacilli differs from that of bacilli grown in a test tube. For example, within the macrophage, the bacilli have access to cholesterol, with which they esterify their mycolic acids. Whether this makes the mycobacteria more tolerable to the macrophage is not known. The bacilli may find their way through the lymphatics to regional lymph nodes and through the bloodstream to distant organs. Within 14 to about 60 days following infection, delayed hypersensitivity to tuberculin develops and, with it, an immunity adequate to limit further multiplication of the bacilli (Figure 48-8). There is no evidence that antibacterial antibodies, though present, play any role in this acquired immunity. In most cases, the granulomatous lesions heal.

The granulomatous lesion develops as an outpost of the reticuloendothelial system in the following way: bacilli continue to multiply within macrophages. Some macrophages die and liberate bacilli. More macrophages enter the lesion, scavenging bacteria and debris. An initial granulomatous infection is then underway. This particular granuloma is usually called a tubercle (tuberculous granuloma). Its center soon is occupied by a core or aggregate of plump, rounded macrophages that appear somewhat like epithelial cells (epithelioid cells). Marginal to these epithelioid cells are multinucleate giant cells derived from the fusion of macrophages. Peripheral to this growing aggregation is a zone of cells, some resembling fibroblasts and the remainder being lymphocytes. As this hard tubercle persists, its central zone becomes necrotic, yielding a residuum of cheesy consistency, the caseation necrosis regarded by pathologists as the most characteristic feature of the tubercle. Eventual calcification of the tubercle may terminate the infection. On the other hand, within weeks or even years after initial infection, breakdown of tuberculous lesions may permit spread of *M tuberculosis*, producing widespread disease (see Figure 48-8 and Table 48-4).

Many individuals for whom acquired immunity is not enough to arrest infection may represent various exceptional conditions (for example, resistance may have been lowered by concurrent disease such as diabetes mellitus, silicosis, and certain infections or by corticosteroid therapy and immunosuppression).

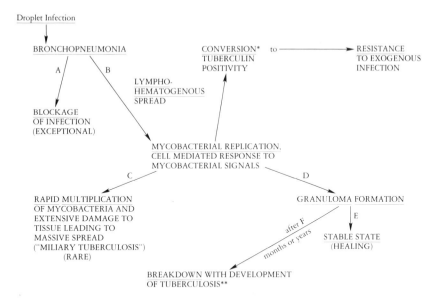

Figure 48-8 The cough, the sneeze, and the air conditioner. *, Detected using the tuberculin skin test. **, Confirmed by acid-fast staining of smears (from sputum) and subsequent cultivation of *M tuberculosis* (from sputum). About 5–15% of subjects exposed to *M tuberculosis* develop disease. Even when fed virulent tubercle bacilli in large numbers, only 66% of subjects succumbed to disease; see Table 48-4. Thus, the subject's genetic makeup is very important relative to outcome of disease.

Table 48-4   Essential Data From the Lübeck Disaster (1929–1930)

Inoculum: Oral BCG vaccine inadvertently contaminated with virulent M tuberculosis, Keil Strain	
Number of children in study:	412
Number of children receiving vaccine:	251
Number of children dying from tuberculosis:	72
Number of children developing clinical tuberculosis:	135
Number becoming tuberculin-positive but failing to manifest disease:	44
Number of control group developing tuberculosis (412 − 251 = 161):	0.00
Of the 72 coming to postmortem:	
Post-primary lesions in stomach:	27
Cervical glands involved:	69
Primary lesions in intestine:	71
Primary lung complex:	15

Epidemiology

The white plague, tuberculosis, has been a sometime deadly disease of the human race since ancient times, and still poses a serious health problem for numerous societies in the modern world. *M tuberculosis*, the infectious unit of human tuberculosis, is carried from one human subject to another by airborne droplet infection. Successful transmission requires that bacilli-laden droplets penetrate deep into the respiratory tree. Transmission can be minimized by frequently changing fresh air in the room of the infected subject, by maintaining the subject on a regimen of chemotherapy likely to reduce the bacilli load in the expectorate, thus reducing the number of infectious droplets, by limiting the amount of emitted aerosol, by covering the mouth and nose with paper handkerchiefs when coughing or sneezing, and by ultraviolet irradiation of the air near the ceiling of the room.

Diagnosis

For individuals suffering from a prolonged and productive cough and suspected of having tuberculosis, examination of their sputa for acid-fast bacilli, and of their chest roentgenograms for areas of involvement, may be supplemented with a skin test (the tuberculin test, a test for delayed hypersensitivity to certain mycobacterial products called tuberculins [or elicitins]). These are low-molecular-weight materials such as glycopeptides and perhaps peptidolipids and peptidoglycolipids purified from broth cultures of mycobacteria; they can elicit delayed hypersensitivity reactions in previously sensitized individuals infected with homologous and related mycobacteria, but they cannot by themselves induce sensitization. Koch prepared the first tuberculins as boiled filtrates from broth cultures of *M tuberculosis* (Old Tuberculin). To meet the need for purified material for skin testing, the American microbiologist, Florence Seibert, produced a purified protein derivative (PPD-S) from Old Tuberculin. PPDs have been prepared from a variety of mycobacteria (Table 48-5).

The tuberculin test (skin testing with PPD-S) can be a valuable diagnostic aid, especially in countries where vaccination with the Bacille Calmette–Guerin (BCG) strain is not widely practiced (see page 567). The American Lung Association considers the tuberculin test useful in examining adults and children. The test is based on the fact that infection with *M tuberculosis* produces sensitivity to certain of its products. Intracuta-

Table 48-5   Elicitins (PPDs) Prepared from Various Strains of Mycobacteria and Used for Skin Testing Recruits in United States Navy*

Mycobacterium (Elicitin Source)	*Elicitin Designation*	*Number Tested*	*Reaction of 2 mm or More*	
			%	*Mean Size (mm)*
M. avium	PPD-A	10,769	30.5	6.7
M. fortuitum	PPD-F	3,415	7.7	4.8
M. intracellulare	PPD-B	212,462	35.1	7.7
M. kansasii	PPD-Y	13,913	13.1	6.2
M. phlei	PPD-ph	15,229	23.1	6.4
M. scrofulaceum	PPD-G	29,540	48.7	10.3
M. smegmatis	PPD-sm	14,239	18.3	5.7
M. tuberculosis	PPD-S	212,462	8.6	10.3

*From Barksdale, L., and Kim, K.-S. 1977. *Bacteriol Rev* 41:291. The standard dose was 0.1 μg of the indicated PPD. Data adapted from Edwards LB: *Ann New York Acad Sci* 1963; 106:32.

neous injection of tuberculin into sensitized persons produces an area of induration (with or without surrounding erythema). Size of the induration varies according to sensitivity of the subject and size of the dose of injected material. Although those sensitive to tuberculin are designated reactors, not all reactors are infected with *M tuberculosis*. As Table 48-5 shows, cross-reactions with other mycobacteria are likely to occur. For example, in some countries, sensitivity to *M avium* is common. Those persons manifesting an *M avium* infection show a larger reaction to PPD-A than to PPD-S.

To administer the intracutaneous (Mantoux) test, a glass or plastic tuberculin syringe equipped with a 26- or 27-gauge intradermal bevel needle is used to inject 0.1 mL PPD-S containing 5 tuberculin units. Other methods, such as the multiple puncture test (Tine test), are not recommended because they often lead to ambiguities that must be resolved by the Mantoux test.

The following interpretations of the tests are those of the American Lung Association:

10 mm or more of induration = positive reaction

This is interpreted as positive for past or present infection with *M tuberculosis*.

5-9 mm of induration = doubtful reaction

Reactions in this range indicate sensitivity that may result from infection with other mycobacteria (see Table 48-5) or with *M tuberculosis*. If the subject is known to have been in close contact with a person having tuberculosis, that subject should be regarded as probably infected with *M tuberculosis*.

0-4 mm of induration = negative reaction

In the absence of clinical evidence of tuberculous infection or recent contact with a tubercular individual, this reaction should be taken as reflecting a lack of tuberculin sensitivity.

M bovis, the tubercle bacillus of cows, ceased to threaten public health in the so-called developed countries once pasteurization of milk and drastic tuberculosis control programs for cattle had been instituted. Although airborne infection with *M bovis* can occur, probably the major route of infections for humans always has been ingested milk containing large numbers of bacilli, which subsequently invade lymphatic tissue. The list on pages 559-560 and Table 48-3 show how *M bovis* species can be distinguished from *M tuberculosis*. Because a number of investigators have reported 100% homology between the DNA of *M bovis* and the DNA *M tuberculosis*, the differences between them would seem to involve only a few genetic markers (see list on pages 559-560).

Control

Identifying cases of tuberculosis and rendering them noninfectious is a first measure of control.

Seven decades ago, the French mycobacteriologists Calmette and Guérin succeeded in isolating an attenuated strain of *M bovis* for use as a live vaccine against tuberculosis.

They employed resistance to certain concentrations of bile as a means of selection. The strain finally obtained, from which BCG vaccine is prepared, was of low virulence, although it could grow in human tissue. Vaccination with BCG has been practiced in many countries throughout the world, converting tuberculin-negative individuals to a tuberculin-positive state. Facts assembled from a broad series of analyses of BCG vaccination trials indicate that when the amount of *M tuberculosis* in the population is high (15.6 cases/1000/year), percentage protection from BCG can be as high as 80%; when the amount of *M tuberculosis* in the population is low (0.11 cases/1000/year), the percentage protection from vaccination appears to be nil (Barksdale and Kim, 1977). This effect of BCG would seem to be another example of the adjuvant action of living mycobacteria. Because BCG vaccination often leads to PPD-S positivity (see Table 48-5), its use in countries where the incidence of tuberculosis is low may jeopardize the diagnostic value of the tuberculin test.

The drug commonly used in prophylaxis against *M tuberculosis* has been isonicotinic acid hydrazide (isoniazid). Before the availability of rifampin, the next most used drugs were streptomycin and *p*-aminosalicylic acid (PAS), followed by ethambutol. To treat new cases of the disease, drug sensitivity tests with *M tuberculosis* usually were not needed; however, the emergence of primary drug resistance in *M tuberculosis* indicates the need to establish drug sensitivity patterns for all strains of mycobacteria responsible for mycobacterioses. The drugs generally used for various mycobacterial infections include PAS, capreomycin, cycloserine, ethambutol, ethionamide, erythromycin, isoniazid, kanamycin, pyrazinamide, rifampin, streptomycin, and sulfonamides. A number of these compounds, administered in large doses, can produce serious side effects in patients.

A recent survey of drug resistance among strains of *M tuberculosis* from patients not previously treated revealed that primary drug resistance occurred in 8.6% of 3146 cultures. Of 271 cultures containing resistant organisms, 68.6% showed resistance to a single drug, 17% to two drugs, and 14.4% to three or more drugs. The specific drugs to which organisms were most frequently resistant were ethambutol, 0.7%; isoniazid, 4.4%; PAS, 1.3%; rifampin, 0.3%; and streptomycin, 5.1%

OTHER MYCOBACTERIA IMPORTANT IN HUMAN INFECTIONS

Table 48-3 indicates that, of a broad range of species, humans are most susceptible to various mycobacterial infections. Many mycobacteria to which they are susceptible are insensitive to such commonly employed antituberculous drugs as isonicotinic acid hydrazide, streptomycin, and PAS. Exact identification of these mycobacterial species seems essential. In the past, they have been called atypical mycobacteria to distinguish them from *M tuberculosis*. As there are so many of them, and as commonly, *when isolated from the wild*, they grow as smooth colonies, it is convenient to refer to them as smooth-colony-forming mycobacteria (in contrast to *M tuberculosis*, see Fig. 48-5).

M kansasii is a slow-growing photoinducibly chromogenic, smooth-colony-forming bacterium, having structures in its outer envelope that distinguish it from *M avium*, *M intracellulare*, and *M scrofulaceum* (see pages 559–560). *M kansasii* may cause a pulmonary infection resembling tuberculosis in human subjects. It occurs in dust, and human infections probably are acquired by inhalation of dust-laden air. No evidence suggests that infections by *M kansasii* are acquired from other infected human subjects. Studies of *M kansasii* infections have emphasized the role of individual genetics in susceptibility to mycobacterial infections. Thus racial groups that show an enhanced susceptibility to *M tuberculosis* (for example, blacks) may be relatively insusceptible to *M kansasii;* the converse also appears to be true. Strains of *M kansasii* isolated from patients can be serotyped. The serological specificity resides in trehalose-containing lipooligosaccharides. All strains appear to have a tetraglucose core to which are attached sugar residues such as xylose, 3-0-Methyl rhamnose, fucose, and others. The lipid moieties of the lipooligosaccharide are phenolic aglycones (see Figure 48-6).

M avium and *M intracellulare* along with *M scrofulaceum* comprise the avium-intracellulare group, which contains over 35 distinct serologic types. The macromolecules responsible for these types are peptidoglycolipids (PGLs) in whose sugar molecules reside the antigenic uniqueness of each. For example, serotype 20 from this group is characterized by 6-d-talose linked to the trisaccharide: rhamnose-2-0-methyl-fucose-2-0-methyl rhamnose (see Fig. 48-7). To appreciate the value of this sort of information in the investigation of human diseases, see the section about *Mycobacterium leprae.*

M avium causes tuberculosis in chickens and other birds. Human infections do occur, especially among poultry workers associated with infected flocks. In areas where infected birds and soil rich in bird droppings are common, conversion to PPD-A (see Table 48-5) may be widespread. A small proportion of those conversions may progress to active disease. Some animals living in common areas with infected birds also become infected. Although pulmonary disease may be the more common manifestation of avian infections, disseminated infections also occur. These same general observations apply to *M intracellulare,* the type species isolated from a child suffering from a systemic granulomatous infection. Pulmonary infections with *M intracellulare* in a group of patients ranging in age from 30-76 years and observed over a 5-year period showed a cumulative rate of relapse of 19%.

M scrofulaceum is a constitutively chromogenic microbe often associated with cervical adenitis in children. Commonly, the submandibular lymph nodes are involved; sometimes epitrochlear, femoral, or inguinal nodes may be singular sites of infection. Such patients, when tested with PPD-G and PPD-S (see Table 48-5), show a more marked response to PPD-G than to PPD-S or other PPDs.

M ulcerans, the cause of Buruli ulcer, has been isolated from necrotic lesions of the skin and subcutaneous tissue of affected individuals in Australia, Africa, Mexico, New Guinea, Bolivia, and the United States (from individuals coming by air from Africa). The extensive ulcerating necrosis of the skin and subcutaneous tissue characteristic of *M ulcerans* infections are thought to result from a toxic phospholipoprotein polysaccharide complex that can be recovered from broth cultures of *M ulcerans.* The toxic material produces necrosis in the skin of guinea pigs and cytopathic effects in mouse fibroblasts in culture (L929 cells). Almost all strains of *M ulcerans* studied show a narrow range of temperatures at which growth is optimal (around 33 C); they do not grow at 25 C or 37 C.

M leprae: over 100 years ago in Bergen, Norway, the disfiguring chronic granulomatous disease, leprosy, was a major public health problem. Approximately 11 million cases exist in the world today, mostly in tropical climates. Leprosy (Hansen's disease) manifests itself differently in different human subjects. At one extreme is the less disfiguring form of the disease, tuberculoid leprosy; at the other, lepromatous leprosy, characterized by nodular swellings and ultimate disfigurement related to slow fibrosis of peripheral nerves. The anesthesia that results leads to shortening of toes and fingers in response to repeated unfelt traumata. Armauer Hansen, physician and pathologist of Bergen, first observed that the lesions in lepromatus leprosy often were teeming with rodlike bacteria. In his day, these bacteria took on a brownish color in tissues fixed with osmium tetroxide; later, these rods were shown to be acid-fast, weakly retaining fuchsin in the Ziehl–Neelsen acid-fast stain. More recently it has been found that the acid-fastness of leprosy bacilli can be extracted with pyridine, whereas the acid-fastness of *M tuberculosis* and other mycobacteria are stable to pyridine. Today pyridine extractability of acid-fastness is used as a routine diagnostic aid for distinguishing *M leprae* from all other mycobacteria, including the obligate intracellular parasite, *M lepraemurium.*

No acid-fast organism recognized by leprologists as *M leprae* has been cultivated from patients with leprosy. For this reason, *M leprae* has been called a noncultivable mycobacterium. When inoculated into the nine-banded armadillo, macerated tissue from cases of human lepromatous leprosy causes a transmissible infection suggestive of human leprosy. A more restricted "infection" occurs in the footpad of the mouse. The challenge regarding leprosy for the microbiologist today is analogous to the challenge met by Koch in 1882 when he isolated *M tuberculosis:* the time has come for *M leprae* to be isolated in pure culture.

Within the last decade, a disease indistinguishable from human leprosy has been found in armadillos in several counties in Louisiana and in separate populations of armadillos in West Texas. DNA homology studies between DNA of leprosy bacilli harvested from leprous armadillos and DNA from leprosy bacilli obtained from naturally (sylvatic) infected armadillos suggests that the two groups of leprosy bacilli are identical.

Analyses of cell walls from leprosy bacilli grown experimentally in armadillos has yielded a trisaccharide that specifically interacts with sera from a number of leprosy patients in enzyme-linked immunosorbent assays. This 3,6-di-0-methyl glucopyranosyl $(1 \xrightarrow{\beta} 4)$ 2, 3-di-0-methyl rhamnopyranosyl $(1 \xrightarrow{\alpha} 2)$ 3-0-methyl rhamnopyranose is α-linked through a phenol to a branched glycolic chain whose hydroxyls are esterified with straight and branched chain fatty acids (see Fig. 48-6). At least three distinct such glycolipids have been found in leprosy bacilli. Synthesis of the more seroactive triglycosyl terminus of the three should greatly enhance immunological studies in leprosy. For further information, see Hunter and Brennan (1983) and Cho and associates (1983) and related references.

Lepromin, a skin test material derived from autoclaved macerates of lepromata, is employed by leprologists as a diagnostic aid. When lepromin is injected into the skins of healthy subjects living in areas where leprosy does not occur or in individuals with tuberculoid leprosy, a palpable bump (hypersensitivity type granuloma) develops in 85% of healthy subjects and in most with tuberculoid leprosy. This reaction is recorded as Mitsuda-positive, but must be confirmed with histologic methods. Patients with lepromatous leprosy do not respond to the Mitsuda test with formation of a hypersensitivity granuloma. Instead, at best, they mount a nonimmulogic response, developing a foreign body granuloma called a Mitsuda-negative reaction. From these and other data it seems that persons manifesting the lepromatous form of leprosy do not have the same degree of immunocompetence as does 85% of the general population and those persons having tuberculoid leprosy. When persons with lepromatous leprosy and with tuberculoid leprosy are skin tested with various autoclaved mycobacteria such as BCG, they form a hypersensitivity granuloma. This suggests that if an immunologic idiosyncrasy is responsible for the lepromin-negative reaction in cases of lepromatous leprosy, that idiosyncrasy does not relate to most mycobacterial antigens.

Today, persons suffering from leprosy are no longer segregated from society, and treatment often occurs on an outpatient basis. Both forms of leprosy respond to rifampin; however, its cost is so great that, in most cases, treatment is accomplished through the prolonged administration of the disulfone 4,4'-sulfonylbisbenzamine (dapsone), a much less expensive drug.

NOCARDIA ASTEROIDES AND NOCARDIOSES

Distinctive Properties

The most widely known species of nocardia, *Nocardia asteroides,* commonly inhabits soil and sometimes infects human subjects. When found in purulent lesions or on old agar slants, *N asteroides* appears as branching, filamentous growth containing numerous acid-fast beads (Figure 48-9). Like other members of the CMN group, *N asteroides* is gram-positive. When filaments are examined from old slants of *N asteroides,* they fragment into coccobacillary forms. These threads of nocardial growth (*bacterionemata*) should not be mistaken for the ramified, tubular fungal structures known as mycelia. The nocardial filaments found in tissue range from 0.5–1.0 μm in diameter and may be many micrometers long (Figure 48-9). Cross walls may be evident when growth is active. When first isolated, most strains of *N asteroides* assume a dull white appearance. From these isolates, orange-red outgrowths are common. Data for distinguishing three of the many nocardial species comprise Table 48-6.

Pathogenesis

Beaman investigated factors that affect the virulence of *N asteroides,* employing cultured rabbit alveolar macrophages as well as certain strains of mice. He found that a more virulent genotype of *N asteroides* exhibits a singular capacity to grow rapidly within unstimulated, nonimmune alveolar macrophages. Further, whereas the environment of the macrophage tends to cause an avirulent strain to produce many L-forms, the more virulent strain does not lose its essentially nocardial morphology when growing intracellularly. Also, nocardial inoculum for virulence studies of a given strain appears much more virulent if prepared from cells in the logarithmic phase of growth than when prepared from stationary phase cells. Log phase cells are found to be heavier than stationary phase cells.

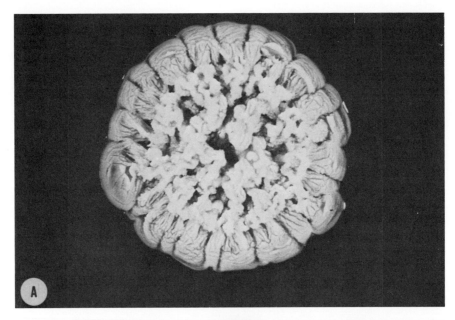

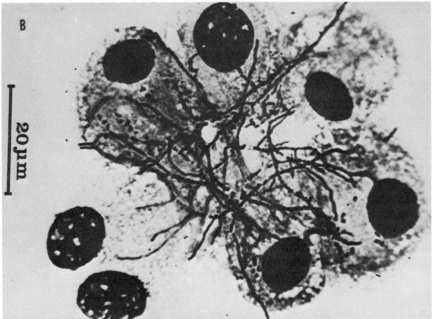

Figure 48-9 A, Colony of *Nocardia asteroides* after 3 weeks' growth at 37 C on brain heart infusion agar (×11). **B,** Interaction of *N asteroides,* virulent strain 14795, with seven (rabbit) alveolar macrophages (some in process of fusing) 24 hours postinfection. At 3 hours postinfection, only rod-shaped, intracellular forms were apparent. At 6 hours postinfection, elongation into filaments was evident. Some bacterionemata shown here are intact, and others are fragmenting. Gram-stained cover slip preparation. (**A,** Courtesy Cynthia Vistica and Blaine L. Beaman, **B,** from Beaman, B.L.: *Infect Immun* 1977; 15:934.)

Table 48-6   Distinguishing Properties of Nocardial Species Important in Animal and Human Infections*

Nocardia	Hydrolysis of				Acid from			*Growth in 7% NaCl*
	Xanthine	*Tyrosine*	*Casein*	*Urea*	*Inositol*	*Mannitol*	*Galactose*	
N asteroides	−	− (99)	−	+ (96)	−	− (95)	−	−
N brasiliensis	−	+	+	+ (95)	+	+ (81)	+	+
N caviae	+ (99)	− (86)	−	+	+	+	−	−

*+, 100% of strains give positive response; −, 100% of strains give negative response. Number under − or +, percent of strains giving indicated response when not 100%. For additional information on exceptional reactions see Mishra, S.K., Gordon, R.E., Barnett, D.: *J Clin Microbiol* 1980; 11:728.

Diagnosis

Nocardiosis due to *N asteroides* is principally a disease of humans, cows, and dogs. Characteristically, the primary pulmonary lesion in humans may be transient and subclinical or chronic, spreading through the bloodstream to various organs. In disseminated infections, the central nervous system often is involved with pyogenic lesions developing in the brain and meninges. Pulmonary nocardiosis commonly presents with loss of weight, malaise, low-grade fever, night sweats, and pleurisy. Once a productive cough occurs, *N asteroides* can be demonstrated in smears of sputum. Its isolation in pure culture carries the same implications as isolation of *M tuberculosis* from tuberculous patients. Delayed hypersensitivity develops in many such cases and, although skin testing is seldom employed as a diagnostic aid, the value of elicitins prepared from *N asteroides, N brasiliensis,* and *N caviae* has been demonstrated at the Danish State Serum Institute. Cross-reactions occur between the delayed hypersensitivity to noncardial antigens and to mycobacterial antigens. For example, experimental animals infected with *N asteroides* give a positive response to Old Tuberculin. Also, *N asteroides* may be involved in chronic, localized conditions known as mycetoma.

Nocardiosis in the dog often manifests itself as a systemic disease with lesions developing in the liver, spleen, kidney, lung, myocardium, and bones and joints. Mastitis in cattle due to *N asteroides* is not uncommon. No ill effects have been reported in human subjects following ingestion of milk containing *N asteroides.*

OTHER NOCARDIAL SPECIES

Actinomycetomata (see also discussion of mycetoma in Chapter 49) caused by *N brasiliensis* are localized, swollen lesions at a site of trauma where skin, subcutaneous tissue, fascia, and bone become involved. The infected area develops a multiplicity of granulomata and abscesses, which drain through tracts of sinuses as they break down. The pus contains granular concentrations of the invading nocardia. These clusters of nocardial growth are apparent in smears and wet mounts of expressed pus. *N brasiliensis* sometimes may be responsible for infections of the kinds described for *N asteroides.*

N caviae (*N otitidis-caviarum*), an agent associated with otisis in the guinea pig, may sometimes be involved in actinomycetomatous infections of humans and in mastitis in cattle. As with *N brasiliensis*, *N caviae* sometimes is responsible for pulmonary infections and may cause generalized nocardiosis.

Nocardial infections have long been treated with sulfonamides. In prolonged treatment, sulfonamides in combination with erythromycin have been reported effective. All three species of nocardia discussed here have been found resistant to penicillin and to rifampin. In vitro studies provide evidence that nocardial species are susceptible to some antibiotics: *N asteroides, N brasiliensis,* and *N caviae,* to gentamicin (10-50 μg/mL) and miconazole (50-100 μg/mL); *N asteroides* and *N brasiliensis,* to tobramycin (10-50 μg/mL; and *N caviae,* to kanamycin (10-50 μg/mL).

References

Corynebacterium

Andrewes, F.W., et al.: *Diptheria, its bacteriology, pathology and immunology.* London: His Majesty's Stationery Office, 1923.

Asselineau, C., Asselineau, J. Trehalose containing glycolipids. *Prog Chem Fats Lipids* 1978; 16: 59-99.

Barksdale, L.: *Corynebacterium diphtheriae* and its relatives. *Bacteriol Rev,* 1970; 34: 378-422.

Barksdale, L.: The immunobiology of diphtheria. In: *Immunology of human infection.* Nahmias, A.J., O'Reilly, R.J., (editors). Vol 8 of *Comprehensive Immunology.* Good, R.A., (editor). New York: Plenum Press, 1981.

Barksdale, L.: The genus *Corynebacterium.* In: *The prokaryotes.* Starr, M.R., et al., (editors). Berlin: Springer-Verlag, 1981.

Collier, R.J.: Diptheria toxin: mode of action and structure. *Bacteriol Rev* 1975; 39: 54-85.

Marcuse, E.K., Grand, M.G.: Epidemiology of diptheria in San Antonio, Tex., 1970. *JAMA* 1973; 224: 305-310.

Pappenheimer, A.M., Jr.: Diphtheria toxin. *Ann Rev Biochem* 1977; 46: 69-94.

Mycobacterium

Asselineau, C., Asselineau, J.: Lipides specifique des mycobacteries. *Ann Microbiol* (Inst Pasteur) 1978; 129A:49-69.

Barksdale, L.: Leprosy vaccines. *Int J Leprosy* 1983; 51:107-110.

Barksdale, L., Kim, K-S.: Mycobacterium. *Bacteriol Rev* 1977; 40:212-372.

Chapman, J.S.: *The atypical mycobacteria and human mycobacterioses.* New York and London: Plenum Medical Book Co., 1977.

Cho, S.N., et al.: Serological specificity of phenolic glycolipid I from *Mycobacterium leprae* and use in serodiagnosis of leprosy. *Infec Immun* 1983; 41:1077-1083.

Dannenberg, A.M., Ando, M., Shima, K.: Macrophage accumulation, division, maturation, and digestive and microbiocidal capacities in tuberculous lesions. *J Immunol* 1972; 109:1109-1121.

Diagnostic standards and classification of tuberculosis and other mycobacterial diseases. New York: The American Lung Association, 1981.

Glassroth, J., Robbins, A.G., Snider, D.E., Jr.: Tuberculosis in the 1980's. *N Engl J Med* 1980; 302:1441-1450.

Goren, M.B., Brennan, P.J.: Myobacterial lipids: Chemistry and biologic activities. In: *Tuberculosis.* Youmans G.P., (editor). Philadelphia: W.B. Saunders Publishing Co, 1979.

Hunter, S.W., Brennan, P.J.: Further specific extracellular phenolic glycolipid antigens and a related diacylphthiocerol from *Mycobacterium leprae. J Biol Chem* 1979; 258: 7556-7562.

Myrvik, Q.N., Leake, E.S., Wright, M.J.: Disruption of phagosomal membranes of normal alveolar macrophages by the H37Rv strain of *Mycobacterium tuberculosis. Am Rev Respir Dis* 129:322-328.

Pan American Health Organization: *Leprosy: cultivation of the etiologic agent, immunology, animal models.* PAHO Scientific publication No. 342. Washington, D.C., 1977.

Pan American Health Organization: *The armadillo as an experimental model in biomedical research.* PAHO Scientific publication No. 366. Washington, D.C., 1978.

The tuberculin skin test. New York: The American Lung Association, 1981.

Vestal, A.: *Procedures for the isolation and identification of mycobacteria.* U.S. Department of Health, Education and Welfare Publication No. (CDC) 75-8230. Atlanta, 1975.

Nocardia

Beaman, B.L.: Possible mechanisms of nocardial pathogenesis. In: *The biology of the Nocardiae.* Goodfellow, M., Brownell, G.H., Serrano, J.A., (editors). New York: Academic Press, 1976.

Beaman, B.L., et al.: Nocardial infections in the United States, 1972-1974. *J Infect Dis* 1976; 134:286-289.

Emmons, C.W., et al.: *Medical mycology.* Philadelphia: Lea and Febiger, 1977.

Mishra, S.K., Gordon, R.E., Barnett, D.: Identification of nocardiae and streptomycetes of medical importance. *J Clin Microbiol* 1980; 11:728-736.

49 *Actinomyces, Arachnia,* and *Streptomyces*

Mary Ann Gerencser, PhD

General Concepts

Actinomyces, Arachnia, and *Streptomyces* belong to the order Actinomycetales, a large group of gram-positive bacteria possessing some tendency toward mycelial growth. These organisms were once thought to be fungi, but are now firmly placed among the bacteria because they are prokaryotes with a typical bacterial cell wall and are susceptible to antibacterial antibiotics. The order may be divided into two major groups: proactinomycetes and euactinomycetes. The proactinomycetes have a limited ability to produce a mycelium and do not produce specialized spores. *Actinomyces* and *Arachnia* are proactinomycetes, both of which are common residents of the oral flora. Euactinomycetes more closely resemble fungi morphologically than do proactinomycetes, as they have a well-developed substrate mycelium, may produce an aerial mycelium, and produce a variety of specialized spores. *Streptomyces* is the largest genus of the euactinomycetes and has more than 400 species.

Actinomyces and *Arachnia* cause the disease actinomycosis in humans and animals and may play a role in human periodontal disease (see Chapter 114). Actinomycosis is characterized by the production of chronic destructive abscesses or granulomas that eventually discharge a viscid exudate containing minute yellow sulfur granules. The pathogenic mechanism by which these organisms cause disease is not clear. Diagnosis is facilitated by Gram stain of abscess material as well as culture. Infections respond readily to treatment with penicillin. *Streptomyces* occasionally cause mycetomas (subcutaneous invasive abscesses) in humans, but are probably of greater medical significance as producers of antibiotics.

ACTINOMYCES AND ARACHNIA

In the eighth edition of *Bergey's Manual of Determinative Bacteriology,* the genus *Actinomyces* has five species: *A israelii, A naeslundii, A viscosus, A odonlyticus,* and *A bovis.* Recently the specific epithet *A meyeri* has been revived, the species *Corynebacterium pyogenes* has been transferred to *Actinomyces,* and three new animal species, *A denticolens, A howellii,* and *A hordeovulneris,* have been described. *A israelii* is the major human pathogen, but infections caused by *A naeslundii, A viscosus,* and *A odontolyticus* are being recognized with increasing frequency. Although *A israelii* is usually associated with human actinomycosis, the second most common cause of this disease is probably *Arachnia propionica.* This organism (formerly *Actinomyces propionicus*) is morphologically identical to *A israelii* but differs in metabolism and cell wall composition. *A bovis* is the common agent of lumpy jaw in cattle, but it does not cause disease in humans. *A pyogenes* is best known as an animal pathogen that causes pyogenic infections in domestic animals. It also causes disease in humans.

Distinctive Properties

Actinomyces and *Arachnia* are gram-positive, non–acid-fast, nonmotile bacteria that occur as diphtheroidal rods and filaments with or without branching (Figure 49-1). Like other gram-positive bacteria, the cell wall peptidoglycan contains muramic acid, N-acetyl-glucosamine, glutamic acid, and one or two additional amino acids. *A israelii, A naeslundii, A viscosus,* and *A odontolyticus* have identical peptidoglycans that contain lysine and ornithine, whereas *A bovis* peptidoglycan contains lysine and aspartic acid and has a different type of interpeptide bridge. The peptidoglycan of *A pyogenes* contains

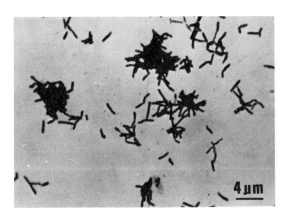

4 μm

Figure 49-1 *Actinomyces israelii.* Gram stain showing diphtheroidal rods and short branching filaments.

alanine, glutamic acid, and lysine. Its detailed structure is not known. *Arachnia propionica* peptidoglycan contains L-diamino-pimelic acid and glycine.

Actinomyces and *Arachnia* grow well on most rich culture media. They are best described as aerotolerant anaerobes. The species vary in oxygen requirements from *A viscosus,* which grows best aerobically with added carbon dioxide, to *A israelii,* which requires anaerobic conditions for growth. Both genera obtain energy from the fermentation of carbohydrates. The major end products of glucose fermentation by *Actinomyces* are acetic, lactic, formic, and succinic acids, whereas *Arachnia propionica* produces propionic, acetic, and formic acids from glucose.

The chemical composition and cellular location of *Actinomyces* antigens are being studied intensively. Antigens studied include cell wall carbohydrate antigens that are nonmobile electrophoretically and pronase-resistant and an amphipathic antigen that differs chemically from the teichoic and lipoteichoic acids found in most gram-positive bacteria.

Pathogenesis

Actinomycosis is an infection of endogenous origin that occurs when organisms normally found in the mouth are introduced into the tissues. It is divided into three clinical types: cervicofacial, thoracic, and abdominal, although primary infections can occur in other areas. Secondary spread of the disease, which may involve almost any organ, usually occurs by direct extension of an existing lesion. Hematogenous spread of the disease can occur.

Cervicofacial infections usually follow an injury to the mouth or jaw such as tooth extraction or other dental manipulation. Pulmonary infection may result from aspiration of bits of infectious material from the teeth. Abdominal actinomycosis has been associated with abdominal surgery, accidental trauma, or an acute perforative gastrointestinal disease. The organisms involved are probably oral organisms that have been swallowed. The role of the oral flora in actinomycosis is confirmed by documented cases of infection with both *A israelii* and *Arachnia propionica* following a human bite. Pelvic infections associated with the presence of an IUD (intrauterine device) are reported frequently.

Actinomyces sp and *Arachnia propionica* are generally accepted as the etiologic agents of actinomycosis. In the past, the frequent isolation of other bacteria along with the actinomycete led to the conclusion that these associated bacteria were essential for disease production. Recent studies of human disease and the production of typical lesions in animals by pure cultures of *Actinomyces* do not support this idea. However, considering the source of the infection, most natural infections probably are mixed. Considerable evidence suggests that *Actinomyces* are involved in periodontal disease and in root surface caries.

Actinomycosis is a chronic, granulomatous, and suppurative disease characterized by abscesses or indurated masses with fibrous walls surrounding a soft central area containing pus. These lesions spread directly to adjacent tissue, and eventually draining sinuses develop through the skin. These sinuses discharge pus containing the organisms. In long-standing cases, the organisms are found in firm, yellowish "sulfur" granules (Figure 49-2) that consist of a mass of filaments with a fringe of hyaline clubs. Draining

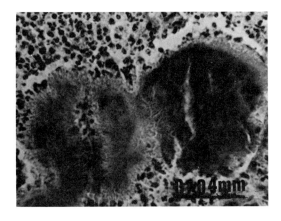

Figure 49-2 Sulfur granule from human actinomycosis tissue section (H & E stain). From Slack, J.M., Gerencser, M.A.: *Actinomyces, filamentous bacteria: biology and pathogenicity.* Minneapolis: Burgess Publishing Co., 1975, p. 95. Used by permission.

sinuses and sulfur granules are usually considered characteristic of actinomycosis, but the disease may occur without either or both.

The mechanism by which *Actinomyces* produce disease is not clear. These organisms do not produce exotoxins or other known toxic substances. Studies of oral disease suggest that pathogenicity results from the ability of *Actinomyces* to activate various cell-mediated host immune responses. *Actinomyces* are known to be chemotactic, to activate lymphocyte blastogenesis, and to stimulate the release of lysosomal enzymes from polymorphonuclear leukocytes and macrophages.

Host Defenses

Circulating antibodies to *Actinomyces* can be demonstrated in some healthy individuals and in individuals with gingivitis and periodontitis as well as in those with clinical actinomycosis. This humoral response probably does not play a major role in defense against actinomycosis. An intact mucosa is the first line of defense because *Actinomyces* and *Arachnia*, like other anaerobes of the normal flora, must gain access to tissue with an impaired blood supply to establish an infection. Once the organism has gained access to tissue, the cell-mediated immune response of the host may limit the extent of the infection but may also contribute to tissue destruction.

Diagnosis

A search for *Actinomyces* and *Arachnia* usually is based on a tentative clinical diagnosis of actinomycosis, but these bacteria should be considered whenever a direct Gram stain of pus or suppurative exudate shows gram-positive, non–acid-fast rods in diphtheroidal arrangement with or without branching. Specimens are first examined for the presence of granules, which are then crushed, Gram stained, and examined for gram-positive rods or branching filaments. Washed, crushed granules or well-mixed pus are cultured on a rich medium such as brain heart infusion blood agar and incubated anaerobically and aerobically with added carbon dioxide. Plates are examined after 24 hours and after 5-7 days for the characteristic colonies of *Actinomyces* (Figure 49-3). Isolates morphologically

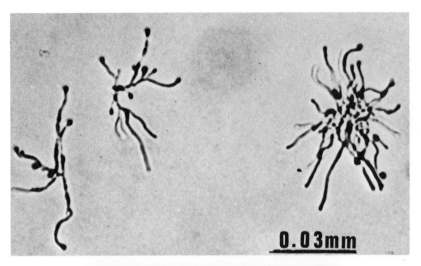

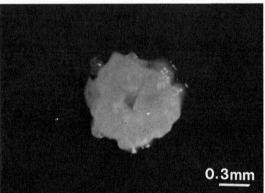

Figure 49-3 Characteristic colonies of *Actinomyces israelii*. **A,** Microcolony at 24 hours. BHI agar shows branching filaments with no distinct center—a "spider" colony. **B,** Mature colony at 14 days. BHI agar shows rough, heaped colony with central depression. From Slack, J.M., Landfried, S., Gerencser, M.A.: *J Bacteriol* 1969; 97:873

resembling *Actinomyces* are identified by determining the metabolic end products using gas-liquid chromatography and by a series of biochemical tests.

Actinomyces can be separated from *Arachnia* serologically using immunofluorescence tests. In addition, the species of *Actinomyces* can be identified by immunofluorescence, and each species can be separated into at least two serologic types. Serologic identification is rapid and reliable and can be used to identify organisms in direct smears or in sections of infected tissue. Unfortunately, satisfactory reagents for this procedure are not generally available.

EPIDEMIOLOGY

A israelii, A naeslundii, A viscosus, A odontolyticus, A pyogenes, and *Arachnia propionica* are normal inhabitants of the human mouth and are found in saliva, on the tongue, in dental plaque, in gingival crevice debris, and frequently in tonsils in the absence of clinical disease. *A bovis* is not found in humans. The extent to which these actinomycetes occur in animals has not been systematically investigated. *A bovis* is found in cattle, *A viscosus* in rodents, and *A naeslundii* and *A viscosus* have been isolated from zoo animals including primates and herbivores. *A pyogenes* is found in cattle, sheep, goats, and other domesticated animals. *Actinomyces* and *Arachnia* are not found in the soil or on vegetation.

Actinomycosis is worldwide in distribution. No relationship to race, age, or occupation has been noted, but the disease appears more often in men than in women. Except for human bite wounds, no evidence exists to support person-to-person or animal-to-human transmission.

Control

Actinomyces are susceptible to various antibiotics, including penicillin, chloramphenicol, tetracycline, and streptomycin. Penicillin is the antibiotic of choice. Successful treatment requires surgical drainage or excision of damaged tissue and antibiotics given for a long period.

STREPTOMYCES

Streptomyces sp have an extensive substrate mycelium that does not fragment and aerial hyphae with chains of spores produced by hyphal segmentation. Colonies are smooth at first, but become powdery or cottony as the aerial mycelium and spores develop. *Streptomyces* sp produce various pigments and have been divided into seven groups, based on the color of the mature aerial mycelium. All species are strictly aerobic and grow best at a temperature of 25 C.

Cell wall peptidoglycan structure and the types of sugars in whole cell hydrolysates are used extensively to characterize aerobic actinomycetes. *Streptomyces* have a type 1 cell wall containing L-diaminopimelic acid and glycine and do not have a characteristic sugar pattern.

S somaliensis and perhaps other species can cause an actinomycotic mycetoma indistinguishable from that caused by *Nocardia* sp (see Chapter 48). *S scabies* causes a plant disease called potato scab.

Streptomyces are abundant in damp soil and cause its characteristic earthy odor. Human infection from *Streptomyces* results from contamination of wounds by soil. This genus produces many of the commonly used antibiotics and its members are also of economic importance as scavengers and contributors to soil fertility.

References

Brown, D.A., Fischlschweiger, W., Birdsell, D.C.: Morphological, chemical and antigenic characterization of cell walls of the oral pathogenic strains *Actinomyces viscosus* T14V and T14AV. *Arch Oral Biol* 1980; 25:451–457.

Brown, J.R.: Human actinomycosis; a study of 181 subjects. *Human Pathol* 1973; 4:319–330.

Causey, W.A.: Actinomycosis. In: *Handbook of clinical neurology,* Vol 35. Vinken, P.V., Bruyn, G.W., (editors). Amsterdam: North Holland Publishing Co, 1978.

Coykendall, A.L., Munzenmaier, A.J.: Deoxyribonucleic acid hybridization among strains of *Actinomyces viscosus* and *Actinomyces naeslundii. Int J Syst Bacteriol* 1979; 29:234-240.

Hinshaw, H.C., Murray, J.F.: *Diseases of the chest,* 4th ed. Philadelphia: W.B. Saunders Co, 1980.

Lerner, P.I.: *Actinomyces* and *Arachnia* species. In: *Principles and practices of infectious diseases.* Mandell, G.I., Douglas, R.G., Jr, Bennett, J.E. (editors). New York: John Wiley and Sons, 1980.

Lopatin, D.E., et al.: In-vitro evaluation in man of immuno-stimulation by subfractions of *Actinomyces viscosus. Arch Oral Biol* 1980; 25:23-29.

Reddy, C.A., Cornell, C.P., Fraga, A.M.: Transfer of *Corynebacterium pyogenes* (Glage) Eberson to the genus *Actinomyces* as *Actinomyces pyogenes* (Glage) comb. nov. *Int J Syst Bacteriol* 1982; 32:419-429.

Slack, J.M., Gerencser, M.A.: *Actinomyces, filamentous bacteria: biology and pathogenicity.* Minneapolis: Burgess Publishing Co, 1975.

Sykes, G., Skinner, F.A., (editors). *Actinomycetales: characteristics and practical importance.* New York: Academic Press, 1973.

50 *Leptospira, Borrelia* (Including Lyme Disease), and *Spirillum*

Russell C. Johnson, PhD

General Concepts

Leptospira, Borrelia, and *Spirillum* are spiral-shaped organisms that cause disease characterized by clinical stages with remissions and exacerabations. *Leptospira* are very thin, tightly coiled, obligate aerobic spirochetes characterized by a unique flexuous type of motility. The genus is divided into two species: the pathogenic leptospires *L interrogans* and the free-living leptospires *L biflexa*. Serotypes of *L interrogans* are the causative agents of leptospirosis, a zoonotic disease. The primary hosts for this disease are wild and domestic mammals, and the disease is a major cause of economic loss in the meat and dairy industry. Pathogenic leptospires are shed in the urine of infected animals, and susceptible hosts become infected through contact with this urine or urine-contaminated environs such as moist soil and surface water. Humans are accidental hosts in whom this disseminated disease varies in severity from subclinical to fatal. The first human case of leptospirosis was described in 1886 as a severe icteric illness and was referred to as Weil's disease; however, most human cases of leptospirosis are nonicteric and are not life-threatening. Recovery usually follows the appearance of a specific antibody.

In contrast to the pathogenic leptospires, serotypes of *L biflexa* exist in water and soil as free-living organisms. Although *L biflexa* have been isolated from mammalian hosts on occasion, no pathology has been associated with these isolates, and they do not infect experimental animals. Because of the widespread distribution of *L biflexa* in fresh water and the capability of leptospires to pass through 0.45–0.22 μm pore size sterilizing filters, they have been found as contaminants of filter-sterilized media.

Members of the genus *Borrelia* are responsible for a febrile disease characterized by remittant fever. The *Borrelia* are primarily transmitted to humans by lice or ticks. *B recurrentis* is responsible for the louse-borne or epidemic type of relapsing fever. In the United States, *B hermsii* and *B turicatae* are the most frequent causes of tickborne or endemic relapsing fever, with *B hermsii* responsible for most human cases, which occur primarily in the western states. Antibody development in the host is important in their elimination. A newly recognized species of *Borrelia, B burgdorferi,* is the causative agent of Lyme disease. The primary hosts for this spirochete appear to be the white-footed mouse and the white-tailed deer. The spirochete is transmitted within the animal population and to humans by the ixodid ticks. In humans, the disease is characterized by distinctive skin lesions, erythema chronicum migrans, and involvement of the joints, nervous system, and heart. Lyme disease is named after Lyme, Connecticut where most of the patients in the original studies resided. The disease has now been reported in at least 17 states in the United States and in Europe and Australia.

A single member of the genus *Spirillum, S minor,* is pathogenic for humans. *S minor* causes one type of rat-bite fever, which is characterized by recurrent fever. The pathogenesis of the organism is obscure, but the host can produce a spirillicidal antibody.

LEPTOSPIRA

Distinctive Properties

The *Leptospira* possess the general structural characteristics that distinguish spirochetes from other bacteria. The outermost structure of the cell is a multilayered outer membrane or envelope. Located beneath the outer membrane are the flexible, helical-shaped peptidoglycan layer and the cytoplasmic membrane; these encompass the cytoplasmic contents of the cell. The structures surrounded by the three- to five-layer outer membrane are collectively referred to as the protoplasmic cylinder. An unusual feature of the spirochetes is the location of the flagella, which lie between the outer membrane and the peptidoglycan layer. They are referred to as periplasmic flagella. The periplasmic flagella are attached to the protoplasmic cylinder at a subterminal position of each cell end, and the free ends of the periplasmic flagella extend toward the center of the cell. The number of periplasmic flagella per cell varies among the spirochetes. The slender (0.1 × 8-20 μm) leptospires are tightly coiled, flexible cells (Figure 50-1) and, in liquid media, one or both ends are usually hooked. Because of their narrow diameter, leptospires cannot be visualized with the bright-field microscope, but are clearly seen by

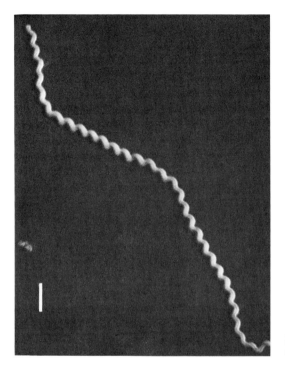

Figure 50-1 Electron micrograph of *Leptospira interrogans* serovar *icterohaemorrhagiae.* Bar equals 0.5 μm.

dark-field or phase microscopy. They are not readily visualized after staining with aniline dyes.

The leptospires contain two periplasmic flagella, each originating at opposite ends of the cell. The free ends of the periplasmic flagella extend toward the center of the cell, but do not overlap as they do in other spirochetes. The basal bodies of *Leptospira* periplasmic flagella resemble those of gram-negative bacteria, whereas those of other spirochetes are similar to the basal bodies of gram-positive bacteria. The motility of bacteria with external flagella is impeded in viscous environments; however, that of the leptospires is enhanced. The *Leptospira* also differ from other spirochetes in that they lack glycolipids and have diaminopimelic acid rather than ornithine in their peptidoglycan.

The leptospires have relatively simple nutritional requirements; long-chain fatty acids and vitamins B_1 and B_{12} are the only organic compounds known to be necessary for growth. When cultivated in media with a pH of 7.4 at 30 C, their average generation time is about 12 hours. Aeration is required for maximal growth. They can be cultivated in plates containing soft agar (1%) medium in which they primarily form subsurface colonies. The leptospires are the most readily cultivable of the pathogenic spirochetes.

The two species of leptospires, *L interrogans* and *L biflexa,* are further divided into serotypes based on their antigenic composition. Within the species *L interrogans,* over 180 serotypes have been identified. The most prevalent serotypes in the United States are *canicola, grippotyphosa, hardjo, icterohaemorrhagiae,* and *pomona.* Genetic studies have demonstrated that serologically diverse serotypes may be present in the same genetic group. At least seven genetic groups are known to exist in this genus.

Pathogenesis

The mucosa and broken skin are the most likely sites of entry for the pathogenic leptospires. A generalized infection ensues, and bacteremia occurs during the acute phase, often referred to as the leptospiremic phase of the disease. A lesion does not develop at the site of entry of the leptospires. The host responds by producing antibodies that, in combination with complement, are leptospiricidal. The leptospires are rapidly eliminated from all host tissues except for the brain, eyes, and kidneys. Little, if any, multiplication of leptospires surviving in the brain and eyes occurs; however; in the kidneys, multiplication takes place in the convoluted tubules, and leptospires are shed into the urine with a density as high as 10^7 leptospires per mL. This is referred to as the leptospiruric phase of the disease. The leptospires may persist in the host for weeks to months and, in the case of rodents, may be shed into the urine for the lifetime of the animal. The leptospiruric urine is the vehicle of transmission for this disease.

The mechanism by which leptospires cause disease remains unresolved, as neither endotoxin nor exotoxins have been associated with it.

The marked contrast between the extent of functional impairment and the scarcity of histologic lesions suggests that most damage occurs at the subcellular level. Damage to the endothelial lining of the capillaries, and subsequent interference with blood flow, appears to be responsible for the lesions associated with leptospirosis. The most notable feature of severe leptospirosis is the progressive impairment of hepatic and renal function. Renal failure is the most common cause of death from this disease. The lack of substantial cell destruction in leptospirosis is reflected in the complete recovery of hepatic and renal function in survivors of severe leptospirosis. Although abortion is a common feature of leptospirosis in animals such as cattle and swine, only recently has a human case of fatal congenital leptospirosis has been documented.

The host's immunologic response to leptospirosis is thought to be responsible for lesions associated with the late phase of this disease, which helps explain the ineffectiveness of antibiotics once symptoms of the disease have been present for 4 or more days.

Host Defenses

Nonspecific host defenses appear to be ineffective against the virulent leptospires. Leptospires are rapidly killed in vitro by the antibody-complement system; virulent strains are more resistant to this leptospiricidal activity than are avirulent strains. Immunity to leptospirosis is primarily humoral; cell-mediated immunity does not appear to play an important role in immunity to leptospirosis but may be responsible for some of the late manifestations of this disease. Immunity to leptospirosis is serotype-specific and may persist for years. Immune serum has been used to treat human leptospirosis and passively protects experimental animals from the disease. Survival of leptospires within the convoluted tubules of the kidney may be related to the ineffectiveness of the antibody-complement system at this site. Previously infected animals can become serologically negative and continue to shed leptospires in their urine, possibly because of the lack of antigenic stimulation by leptospires at this anatomic site.

Epidemiology

Leptospirosis is a zoonosis that is worldwide in distribution and encompasses a broad spectrum of animal hosts. The primary reservoir hosts are wild mammals such as rodents, which can shed leptospires throughout their lifetimes. Domestic animals may also be an important source of human infections. Presently, the dog is the major source of human leptospirosis in the United States. Leptospires have been isolated from approximately 160 mammalian species in the temperate zone. The disease is more widespread in tropical countries, where the infectious agent may be one of many serotypes carried by a large variety of hosts.

Direct or indirect contact with urine containing virulent leptospires is the major means by which leptospirosis is transmitted. As previously mentioned, leptospires from urine-contaminated environments such as water and soil enter the host through the mucous membranes and small breaks in the skin. Moist environments with a neutral pH provide suitable conditions for survival of leptospires outside the host. Urine-contaminated soil can remain infective for as long as 14 days. The cellular structure of leptospires causes them to be susceptible to killing by adverse conditions such as drying, exposure to detergents, and temperatures above 50 C. Most cases of leptospirosis occur during summer and fall.

Diagnosis

Clinical manifestations of leptospirosis are those associated with a general febrile type disease and are not sufficiently characteristic for a diagnosis of leptospirosis. As a result, leptospirosis often is initially misdiagnosed as meningitis or hepatitis. Typically, leptospirosis is a biphasic disease with an acute leptospiremic phase followed by the immune leptospiruric phase. The three organ systems most frequently involved are the central nervous system, kidney, and liver. After an average incubation period of 7-14 days, the leptospiremic acute phase is evidenced by an abrupt onset of fever, severe headache, muscle pain, and nausea that persist for approximately 7 days. Jaundice occurs during this phase in more severe infections. With the appearance of antileptospiral antibodies, this phase of the disease subsides and leptospires no longer can be isolated from the blood. Following an asymptomatic period of several days, the immune leptospiruric phase appears, manifested by a fever of shorter duration and central nervous system involvement (meningitis). Leptospires appear in the urine during this phase and are shed for periods of time that vary with the host. The more severe form of leptospirosis is frequently associated with infections with serotype *icterohaemorrhagiae* and is often referred to as Weil's disease.

Because clinical manifestations of leptospirosis are too variable and nonspecific to be diagnostic, microscopic demonstration of the organisms, serologic tests, or both are necessary for diagnosis. The microscopic agglutination test is most frequently used for serodiagnosis of this disease.

Control

Human leptospirosis can be controlled by reducing its prevalence in wild and domestic animals. Although little can be done about controlling the disease in wild animals, leptospirosis in domestic animals can be controlled through vaccination with inactivated whole cells or an outer membrane preparation. If vaccines do not contain a sufficient immunogenic mass, the resulting immune response protects the host against clinical disease but not against development of the renal shedder state. Because a multiplicity of serotypes may exist in a given geographic region and the protection afforded by the inactivated vaccines is serotype-specific, use of polyvalent vaccines is recommended. Vaccines for human use are not available in the United States.

Although the leptospires are sensitive to the action of penicillin and tetracycline in vitro, use of these drugs in the treatment of leptospirosis is controversial. If treatment is initiated within the first week of disease onset, the general belief is that it can be effective. Later in the disease, immunologic damage may already have begun, rendering antimicrobial therapy ineffective. Doxycyline has been used successfully as a chemoprophylaxic agent for military personnel training in tropical areas.

BORRELIA

Distinctive Properties

The *Borrelia* have morphologic characteristics similar to those of the *Leptospira*, except that the average cell dimensions are 0.2-0.5 × 4-18 μm and they have fewer coils (Figure 50-2). In addition, they have 7-20 periplasmic flagella originating at each end and overlapping at the center of the cell. In contrast to the *Leptospira*, their peptidoglycan contains ornithine rather than diaminopimelic acid, and basal bodies of their periplasmic flagella resemble those found in gram-positive bacteria. Because of their wider diameter,

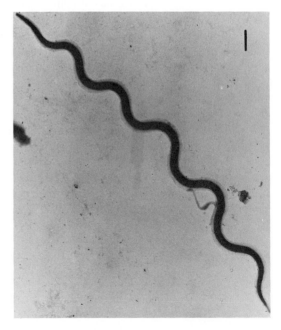

Figure 50-2 Electron micrograph of *Borrelia hispanica*. Bar equals 1 μm.

they are more readily stained with aniline dyes than are other spirochetes. The lipid components of *Borrelia* are unusual in that they include cholesterol; this substance has been reported in only one other bacterial genus, *Mycoplasma.*

The nutritional requirements of the *Borrelia* are more complex than those of the *Leptospira.* Glucose, amino acids, long-chain fatty acids, N-acetylglucosamine, and several vitamins are some of their required organic nutrients. The *Borrelia* are microaerophilic organisms. *B hermsii* has a generation time of 12 hours when cultivated in artificial media at 35 C compared to only 6-10 hours in the mouse.

Pathogenesis

Once borreliae have entered the host, they cause a generalized infection, apparent after an incubation period of approximately 1 week. The onset of the disease is abrupt, with fever, headache, and muscle pain that persist for 4-10 days, followed by an afebrile period of 5-6 days. Usually, a single relapse occurs in louse-borne relapsing fever. The clinical features of relapsing fever are not diagnostic and resemble those of leptospirosis. The case fatality rate of untreated epidemic relapsing fever can be higher than 40%, and myocarditis probably is the most common cause of death.

The tick-borne relapsing fever is similar to that of the louse-borne disease, but is less severe (case fatality rate 0%-8%), and several relapses of decreasing intensity are commonly experienced. The relapses are due to the ability of these *Borrelia* to undergo multiple cyclic antigenic variations. As antibodies for the predominant antigenic type multiplying within the host appear, the organisms "disappear" from the peripheral blood and are replaced by a different antigen variant within a few days. This process may repeat several times in an untreated host, depending on the infecting strain of *Borrelia.*

Lyme disease is characterized by a migrating annular lesion, erythema chronicum migrans (ECM), which is frequently accompanied by fever, headache, stiff neck, muscle aches, joint pain, and fatigue. These symptoms may last for several weeks and some patients develop neurologic or cardiac abnormalities weeks to months later. Subsequently, many of these patients develop intermittent attacks of arthritis that can develop into chronic arthritis with erosion of cartilage and bone. Lyme disease also is present in Europe and Australia, but in Europe chronic neurologic involvement, rather than arthritis, is the most common sequela of the disease.

No toxins are known to be produced by *Borrelia,* and the mechanism by which they cause disease remains unresolved.

Host Defenses

Borrelia appear to be resistant to nonspecific host defense mechanisms; antibody is important in their elimination from the host.

Epidemiology

Borrelia are transmitted to humans by the body louse or ticks. *B recurrentis,* the cause of louse-born (epidemic) relapsing fever is carried by the human louse, *Pediculus humanus.* The louse ingests *Borrelia* while feeding on a borrelemic host. The organisms multiple in the hemolymph and central ganglion of the louse. Because other organs are not invaded, transovarial transmission does not occur in the louse. In addition, *Borrelia* are released only when the louse is injured by host activities such as scratching. Accordingly, one louse can infect only a single host. The louse is infective for its entire life, which averages 1 month. Thus, humans rather than the louse are the reservoir of this disease. The louse-borne disease is called epidemic relapsing fever because it can be rapidly disseminated under conditions of overcrowding and poor personal hygiene such as those that occur during wars and natural disasters. Relapsing fever, which depends on the aforementioned conditions favoring the multiplication and transfer of the human louse, has disappeared from the United States with the exception of imported cases.

The tick-borne relapsing fever is called endemic relapsing fever because it occurs whenever humans are exposed to infected ticks. The soft ticks *Ornithodoros hermsi* and *O turicata* most frequently transmit the disease in the United States. These ticks often obtain their blood meal at night and because the tick bite is usually painless and feedings are short (5–20 min), people may not be aware of having been bitten. The speciation of *Borrelia* is based on the vector they are associated with (for example, *B hermsii* is associated with *O hermsi*). Genetic studies have shown that this basis for speciation is incorrect. The three North American species, *B hermsii*, *B parkeri*, and *B turicatae*, were found to represent a single species. The ticks usually become infected by feeding on borrelemic rodents. In contrast to the louse, all tissues of the tick are invaded, resulting in transovarial transmission and the presence of *Borrelia* in salivary and coxal (basal segment of appendage) secretions. These spirochetes in the salivary and coxal secretions enter the host through the bite wound while the tick is feeding (less than 1 min may be required for transmission). The largest outbreak of tick-borne relapsing fever in the western hemisphere occurred on the north rim of the Grand Canyon in 1973. Sixty-two persons who stayed in log cabins developed the disease.

Lyme disease is transmitted by members of the *Ixodes ricinus* complex (hard ticks). In the northwest and the midwest of the United States, the illness is transmitted by the deer tick, *I dammini*, whereas *I pacificus* is the primary vector in the western part of the country. The ixodid ticks transmit the newly recognized spirochete, *B burgdorferi*. This spirochete does not undergo antigenic change and only one species, *B burgdorferi*, appears to be responsible for the disease in the United States and Europe. Transovarial transmission of the spirochete does not occur in ixodid ticks. Within endemic areas of Lyme disease, 19%–61% of the *I dammini* ticks collected have been found to be carriers of *B burgdorferi*. The spirochete has been isolated from a variety of animals including the white-footed mouse and white-tailed deer, and the disease occurs in areas in which deer are present. Lyme disease is now an important public health problem. In the United States, the number of cases is increasing rapidly, whether this increase reflects an increased awareness and reporting of the disease or an actual increase in the number of cases is not yet known.

Diagnosis

Clinical features of *Borrelia* relapsing fever infections are not diagnostic. Diagnosis of the relapsing fevers is based primarily on demonstration of the spirochetes in the patient's blood by dark-field examination, the use of stained blood smears, or mouse inoculation. No satisfactory serologic test is available.

Lyme disease usually begins with a characteristic red skin lesion, erythema chronicum migrans (ECM); 50% of patients have multiple, annular secondary lesions. Lesions are not found in all cases of Lyme disease. The patient usually experiences malaise and fatigue, headache, fever and chills, generalized achiness, and enlargement of regional lymph nodes. Lyme disease can be diagnosed serologically with the indirect immunofluorescence assay. Cross-reactions have been found in sera of patients with syphilis, but the disease can be distinguished with the nontreponemal tests for syphilis.

Control

The best way to prevent the relapsing fevers and Lyme disease is to avoid their vectors. It is important to be aware of endemic areas and to take proper precautions when in these areas. Vaccines are not available for these diseases. Tetracycline is the drug of choice for the relapsing fevers and Lyme disease. Early treatment of Lyme disease shortens the early course of the disease and can prevent major late complications, such as neurologic and cardiac abnormalities and arthritis. The late complications of Lyme disease can be treated successfully with tetracycline, an observation that suggests the spirochete persists in infected persons.

SPIRILLUM

The spirilla differ from the spirochetes in possessing the rigid cell wall and external flagella typical of gram-negative bacterial morphology. A single member of this genus, *S minor*, is pathogenic for humans. It is the etiologic agent of one type of rat-bite fever, referred to as spirillar fever to distinguish it from that caused by *Streptobacillus moniliformis* (streptobacillary fever). *S minor* is an aerobic, short, spiral-shaped, gram-negative rod (0.2-0.5 × 3-5 μm) with 2-3 coils and bipolar tufts of flagella. It has not been cultivated successfully on an artificial medium.

Rat-bite fever is primarily a disease of wild rodents. Human infection follows the bite of a rodent or rodent-ingesting animals. After an incubation period of about 2 weeks, the site of the bite becomes inflamed and painful, and a chancrelike ulceration may occur. Associated with this eruption is an inflammation and enlargement of the adjacent lymphatics and lymph nodes, fever, headache, and a rash radiating from the wound site and lasting about 48 hours. In the untreated person, the symptoms subside, only to reappear in 3-9 days. This relapsing fever may last for weeks to months. Because of the low incidence of this disease, little is known of its pathogenesis. Diagnosis of the disease is established by demonstrating *S minor* in dark-field preparation of lesion and adjacent lymph node exudates or blood. If this fails, laboratory animals free of spirilla are inoculated and examined for the development of a spirillemia. The disease has been successfully treated with streptomycin and penicillin. Improvement of sanitary conditions to minimize rodent contact with humans is the best preventive measure for rat-bite fever.

References

Alexander, A.D.: *Leptospira*. In: *Manual of clinical microbiology*. Balows, A., Hausler, W.J., Jr., Truant, J.P., (editors): Washington, D.C.: American Society for Microbiology, 1980.

Burgdorfer, W., et al.: Lyme disease: A tick-borne spirochetosis? *Science* 1982; 216:1317-1319.

Canale-Parola, E.: Physiology and evolution of spirochetes. *Bacteriol Rev* 1977; 41:181-204.

Felsenfeld, O.: *Borrelia: strains, vectors, human and animal borreliosis*. St. Louis: Warren Green, 1971.

Holt, S.C.: Anatomy and chemistry of spirochetes. *Microbiol Rev* 1978; 42:114-60.

Hyde, F.W., Johnson, R.C.: Genetic relationship of Lyme disease spirochetes to *Borrelia, Treponema* and *Leptospira. J Clin Microbiol* 1984; 20:151-154.

Johnson, R.C., (editor): *The biology of parasitic spirochetes*. New York: Academic Press, 1976.

Johnson, R.C.: The spirochetes. *Ann Rev Microbiol* 1977; 31:89-106.

Smibert, R.M.: Spirochaetales: a review. *CRC Crit Rev Microbiol* 1973; 2:491-552.

Steere, A.C., et al.: The spirochetal etiology of Lyme disease. *N Engl J Med* 1983; 308:733-740.

51 *Treponema*

Thomas J. Fitzgerald, PhD

General Concepts
Distinctive Properties
Pathogenesis
Host Defenses
Epidemiology
Diagnosis

Control
Other Treponematoses
Yaws
Pinta
Endemic Syphilis

General Concepts

The genus *Treponema* contains both pathogenic and nonpathogenic species. Human pathogens cause four treponematoses: syphilis (*T pallidum*), yaws (*T pertenue*), pinta (*T carateum*), and endemic syphilis (*T pallidum* variant). The only known animal pathogen causes venereal syphilis in rabbits (*T paraluis-cuniculi*). Nonpathogenic treponemes may be part of the normal flora of the intestinal tract, the oral cavity, or the genital tract; at least seven such species have been identified.

Syphilis has widely diverse clinical manifestations that mimic many other bacterial or viral infections. Yaws, pinta, and endemic syphilis also involve highly variable manifestations. All infections by these four treponemes are characterized by distinct clinical stages. Multiplication of the organisms at the initial site of entry produces the primary stage (localized infection). The dissemination of treponemes to other tissues, and their multiplication, results in the secondary stage. After relatively prolonged periods, in some cases 20-30 years, the tertiary or late stage evolves. *T pallidum* is the most invasive organism; it produces highly destructive lesions in almost any tissue of the body. *T carateum* is the least invasive, and remains within the dermal and epidermal regions. *T pertenue* and *T pallidum* variant are intermediate in invasiveness and cause destructive lesions in bones and soft tissues.

Table 51-1 Characteristics of the Four Treponematoses

	Syphilis	*Yaws*	*Pinta*	*Endemic Syphilis*
Epidemiology				
Agent	*T pallidum*	*T pertenue*	*T carateum*	*T pallidum?*
Other names	Venereal syphilis	Framboesia, pian	Carate, cute	Bjel, dichuchwa
Prevalence	Worldwide	Hot, humid areas	Hot, humid areas	Hot, dry areas
Locations	Worldwide	Tropics	Central and South America	Deserts
Age group	Adults	Children	Children, adolescents	Children, adults
Spread	Venereal	Skin	Skin	Mucous membranes
Congenital infection	Yes	No	No	Rarely
Disease Characteristics				
Incubation period	10-90 days	14-28 days	2-6 months	?
Invasiveness	High	Intermediate	Low	Intermediate
Perivascular (cuffing)	Yes	No	Yes	Yes
Tissues	All	Skin, bones, soft tissues	Skin	Mucous membranes, skin, muscles, bones
Predominant cellular infiltrate	Lymphocytes, plasma cells	Mostly plasma cells	Mostly lymphocytes	Lymphocytes, plasma cells
Destructive lesions	Yes	Yes	No	Yes
Granulomas	Yes	Yes	No	Yes
Gummas	Yes	Yes	No	Yes
Condylomata lata	Yes	Yes	No	Yes

The pathogenic treponemes have identical morphologies, biochemical capabilities, and physiologic criteria. Specific antigenic differences have not yet been identified, and serologic reactions positive for one disease are also positive for the other three. Differentiation of the treponematoses relies primarily on geographic location and clinical manifestations (Table 51-1). Similarities in treponemal infections include their generalized nature, regional and general lymphadenopathy, chronicity, spontaneous healing, asymptomatic periods, relatively painless symptoms, and nonfatal outcome, except for tertiary and congenital syphilis.

Cross-reacting antigens are quite common, and untreated infection confers partial protection against the other treponemal diseases. In areas in which yaws is endemic, the incidence of syphilis is low. After effective campaigns to eradicate yaws, the incidence of syphilis increases greatly. Similar epidemiologic observations have been made after local eradication of pinta and endemic syphilis. The contagious nature of the treponematoses is indicated by their tendency to occur in epidemic proportions. Syphilis is distributed throughout the world, yaws is widespread in the tropics, pinta is highly endemic in Central and South America, and endemic syphilis is present in desert regions. Diagnosis of syphilis relies on clinical manifestations, darkfield microscopy, and serologic tests. Penicillin remains the antibiotic of choice for treatment of the treponemal diseases. *T pallidum* is the type species for the genus *Treponema*.

Distinctive Properties

T pallidum is a helically coiled, corkscrew-shaped organism, 6–15 μm long and 0.1–0.2 μm wide (Figure 51-1). Treponemes are readily stained, but their thinness approaches the limits of resolution of light microscopy. These gram-negative microorganisms can be visualized with the silver impregnation method of Krajian. In this procedure, the diameter of the treponemes is increased by depositing precipitates of silver on the surface of the organisms. Live treponemes can be visualized by using darkfield microscopy. *T pallidum* exhibits characteristic motility that consists of rapid rotation about its longitudinal axis and bending, flexing, and snapping about its full length. Organisms from syphilitic lesions containing viscous mucoid material also exhibit smooth translational movement, gliding rapidly forward and backward.

The structure of treponemes differs slightly from other bacteria. Figure 51-2 is a transmission electron micrograph of a cross-section of *T pallidum*. The organism has a coating of glycosamino-glycans that contains N-acetyl-D glucosamine and N-acetyl-D galactosamine. This coating may be either host-derived material adhering to the treponemal surface or capsular material synthesized by the treponemes. Just below this coating is an outer membrane (outer envelope) that is responsible for structural integrity;

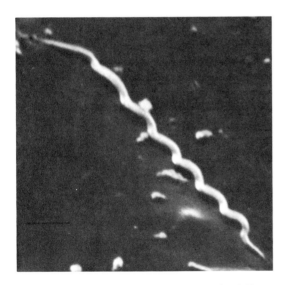

Figure 51-1 Scanning electron micrograph of *Treponema pallidum*. From Fitzgerald, T.J.J., et al.: *J Bacteriol* 1977; 130:1333.

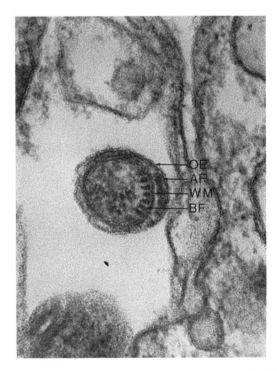

Figure 51-2 Transmission electron micrograph of cross-section of *Treponema pallidum*. (OE, outer envelope [membrane]; AF, axial filament; WM, cell wall membrane; BF, body fibrils.) From Johnson, R.C., et al.: *Infect Immun* 1973; 8:294.

susceptibility to penicillin indicates a peptidoglycan cell wall structure. This membrane covers three flagella (axial filaments) that wind around the surface of the organism. These flagella, which contain amino acids, arise at each end of the treponeme and extend halfway down the organism, overlapping at the midpoint. A cytoplasmic membrane (wall membrane) that acts as an osmotic barrier covers the protoplasmic cylinder; six to eight cytoplasmic tubules (body fibrils) are located on the inner surface of this membrane. These tubules also arise at each end and wind around the organism to the midpoint. The cytoplasm contains ribosomes, mesosomes, and a nuclear region.

T pallidum is a delicate organism that exhibits narrow optimal ranges of pH (7.2-7.4), eH (-230 to -240 mV), and temperature (30-37 C). It is rapidly inactivated by mild heat, cold, desiccation, most disinfectants, and osmotic changes. Since this organism was discovered in 1905, it has been considered a strict anaerobe. Recent evidence, however, indicates that it is microaerophilic and requires low concentrations of oxygen (1%-4%).

Multiplication occurs through binary transverse fission. No life cycle involving different forms of *T pallidum* has been observed. The in vivo generation time is relatively prolonged; in rabbits, it is 30-33 hours. Despite intense efforts over the past 75 years, *T pallidum* has not been successfully cultured and passaged in vitro. The organisms can be maintained for 18-21 days in complex media containing serum-reducing agents, vitamins, cofactors, amino acids, and salts.

The nonaqueous composition of *T pallidum* is approximately 70% proteins, 20% lipids, and 5% carbohydrates. The lipid content is relatively high for bacteria. Sixty-eight percent of the lipids are phospholipids, primarily phosphatidylcholine, sphingomyelin, and cardiolipin; 32% of the lipids are neutral lipids, primarily cholesterol. Nonpathogenic treponemes such as *T phagedenis,* biotypes Kazan and Reiter, have a defect in fatty acid synthesis; they are unable to synthesize, β-oxidize, or desaturate fatty acids.

Antigenic analysis of *T pallidum* is hampered by the inability to grow this organism in vitro, and by the presence of host material associated with the treponemal surface. Antigenic makeup is complex, as evidenced by the development of many different antibodies during infection. A genus-specific antigen is shared with nonpathogenic treponemes. A species-specific antigen exclusive for *T pallidum* has not been found. Many antigens are shared with the other pathogenic treponemes; in fact, *T pallidum, T pertenue,* and *T carateum* are at present antigenically indistinguishable. The natural course of syphilitic infection (if uninterrupted by antibiotic therapy) confers solid immunity. The protective immunogens responsible for the immunity have not been isolated.

Other antigens have been detected. Cardiolipin has recently been shown to be part of the treponemal structure. This antigen elicits Wassermann antibodies, which form the basis for a group of serologic tests. Cardiolipin is also found in human and animal tissues as part of the mitochondrial membrane. In addition, newer methodologies involving gel electrophoresis and immunoblotting have revealed over 100 distinct protein antigens.

Pathogenesis

T pallidum infects almost every tissue of the body, resulting in a wide variety of clinical manifestations. For this reason, it is called the great imitator. Syphilis is a painless, slowly evolving chronic granulomatous disease that fluctuates between short symptomatic stages and rather prolonged asymptomatic stages. The host–parasite relationship is constantly changing; multiplication of organisms results in disease (primary, secondary, and tertiary stages); host responses, in turn, produce healing. Humans are the only natural host for *T pallidum*. The rabbit provides a good animal model that mimics primary and secondary syphilis. Minimal clinical manifestations occur after inoculation of guinea pigs or hamsters; other animals are not susceptible. There are no avirulent strains (more appropriately called isolates) of *T pallidum*. Some isolates, however, are more virulent than others; these isolates produce more intense lesions that last longer and spread rapidly to other tissues.

T pallidum infects humans through person-to-person contact. The organisms gain entry by directly invading mucous membranes or through miniscule breaks or abrasions in the skin. After entering the host, organisms localize at the site of entry and begin to multiply. The incubation period before initial clinical manifestations is 10–90 days. As demonstrated by rabbit studies, this variability is associated with the number of treponemes that are transmitted. *T pallidum* enters the blood and lymphatics minutes after initial penetration and disseminates to other tissues. Thus, from the outset syphilis is a disseminated disease. As the organisms pass through the blood, they attach to the inner surface of endothelial cells of the vessel walls. Splitting these cells provides *T pallidum* with access to the perivascular areas. Target tissues include lymph nodes, skin, mucous membranes, liver, spleen, kidneys, heart, bones, joints, larynx, eyes, meninges, brain, and central nervous system. In women, the initial lesion is usually situated on the labia, the walls of the vagina, or the cervix, and in men on the shaft or glans of the penis. A primary lesion may also occur on lips, tongue, tonsils, anus, or other skin areas.

The most prominent feature of syphilitic infection is vascular involvement, especially arterioles and capillaries. Periarteritis (proliferation of adventitial cells and cuffing), endarteritis (swelling and proliferation of endothelial cells that reduce the vessel lumen), and infiltration of lymphocytes and plasma cells are characteristic of syphilitic histopathology. Infected areas contain numerous treponemes and accumulations of mucoid material. Large numbers of organisms are required to produce tissue histopathology. In rabbits, dermal lesions first become apparent when the infected area contains approximately 10^7 treponemes; in testicular infections, only minimal pathology is detectable even when 10^9 organisms are present. These observations indicate that *T pallidum* lacks potent toxins. It has been suggested that a large portion of syphilitic histopathology results from activation of host defenses. Treponemes readily attach to components within the extracellular matrix and the basement membrane. Antibodies, in association with complement or macrophages that interact with attached organisms, may indirectly damage the host tissues. Some of the tissue histopathology also may be attributed to the treponemal hyaluronidase. This enzyme breaks down the tissue glycosaminoglycans that provide partial structural support for vessels, contributing to vessel collapse.

The glycosaminoglycan coating of *T pallidum* may play a role in the infective process. It does not appear to restrict antibody access to treponemal components, but rather is anticomplementary. With certain serologic tests for syphilis (immobilization [TPI], agglutinin, fluorescent antibody [FTA-ABS]), prior incubation is required before positive responses are detectable. It has been postulated that surface antigens must dissipate before seroreactivity is possible. In addition, immunosuppression of host defenses occurs in syphilis, and may be the basis for the exacerbation of the infection and induction of the next stage of the disease. Evidence indicates that treponemal antigen-antibody complexes are responsible for this immunosuppression.

Clinical manifestations of syphilis are complex and widely diffuse, and time periods associated with each stage vary greatly; Figure 51-3 depicts averages. As the number of treponemes increases, clinical manifestations are seen; as the number decreases due to effective host responses, asymptomatic periods occur.

After an incubation period of 3 weeks, extensive multiplication of treponemes at the site of entry produces erythema and induration. A papule forms that eventually progresses to a superficial ulcer with a firm base, which is the **hard chancre** of the primary stage. (*Haemophilus ducreyi* causes soft chancre, which differs in being flat, centrally umbilicate, tender, and painful.) Numerous treponemes are present in this highly contagious, open lesion. Regional lymph nodes enlarge, and after 2-6 weeks, host defenses evolve that cause healing, leaving remnants of scar tissue.

After an asymptomatic period of 2-24 weeks, the secondary stage begins. Organisms multiply in many different tissues. Clinical manifestations include slight fever, generalized lymphadenopathy, malaise, and a mucocutaneous rash that is initially apparent on the palms and soles and eventually spreads to other areas. This rash may be macular, papular, follicular, papulosquamous, or pustular. On mucous membranes of the mouth, vagina, or anus, white mucoid patches of moist papules, or condylomata, occur. These patches and draining skin lesions teem with treponemes and are highly contagious. Although less severe clinical manifestations occur within other tissues, they are not easily detected because they are painless. If the kidney is involved, immune complexes of treponemal antigens and host antibodies may be deposited on the glomerular basement membrane, resulting in a nephrotic syndrome. After 2-6 weeks of secondary syphilis, host defenses bring about healing. About 25% of patients experience one to three relapses of this secondary stage.

The period between secondary and tertiary syphilis, termed latency, may last 3-30 years. **Early latency** refers to the first 4 years; **late latency** is beyond 4 years. No clinical manifestations are apparent. The patient, however, harbors infectious organisms,

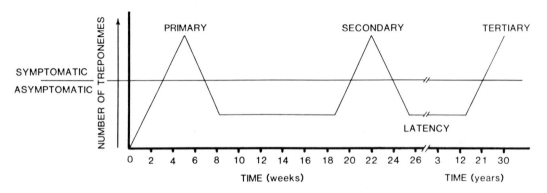

Figure 51-3 Average time periods of clinical manifestations of syphilis.

especially in the spleen and lymph nodes. Blood serology remains positive throughout this period.

Tertiary syphilis can affect almost any tissue and can be fatal. Approximately 80% of the fatalities are caused by cardiovascular involvement; most of the remaining 20% are from neurologic involvement. Cardiovascular problems are attributed to multiplication of treponemes within the aorta. The subsequent aortitis produces complications such as stenosis, angina, myocardial insufficiency, and aneurysms. Neurologic syphilis is meningovascular or parenchymatous. If the parenchymatous form involves the brain, it is called general paresis; if it involves the spinal column, it is called tabes dorsalis. Complications of neurosyphilis are paralytic dementia, amyotropic lateral sclerosis, seizures, or blindness from optic atrophy.

Gummas are highly destructive lesions of tertiary syphilis that usually occur in skin and bones but may also occur in other tissues. Gummas are large granulomas with extensive caseation necrosis. These lesions contain numerous lymphocytes, giant cells, epithelioid cells, and few treponemes. Delayed hypersensitivity similar to that found in tuberculosis may be responsible.

Besides the three stages of disease in adults, *T pallidum* also damages fetuses. In primary, secondary, or latent syphilis, the organism passes through the placenta after the fifteenth to eighteenth week of gestation and infects most organs and tissues of the fetus. Approximately 50% of fetuses abort or are stillborn; the remaining 50% exhibit diverse syphilitic stigmata. **Early congenital syphilis** refers to syphilis that is apparent at birth or up to age 2 years. Its manifestations include cutaneous lesions, mucous membrane lesions, osteochondritis (especially within the long bones), anemia, and hepatosplenomegaly. In **late congenital syphilis,** an infected child may appear normal past age 2 years and then exhibit syphilitic manifestations such as interstitial keratitis and blindness, tooth deformation (notched incisors and moon molars), eighth-nerve deafness, neurosyphilis, rhagades (fissures at mucocutaneous junctions), cardiovascular lesions, Clutton's joints (fluid accumulation on knee), and bone deformation of the legs, nose septum, and hard palate. Combinations of these stigmata usually occur. In late congenital syphilis, three commonly observed manifestations, called **Hutchinson's triad,** are interstitial keratitis, notched incisors, and eighth-nerve deafness.

Host Defenses

Immunity develops in untreated syphilis. In the nineteenth century, experiments involving reinoculation of syphilitic patients demonstrated that an infected individual was somewhat resistant to a second full-blown attack. The Oslo study, begun in the early 1900s, involved 1000 untreated patients that were observed for 30-50 years. Approximately 25% of these patients developed secondary syphilis; 13% developed tertiary syphilis; and 75% of the patients did not progress beyond primary syphilis, indicating a degree of immunity. The Sing-Sing and Tuskegee studies involving humans, in addition to experimental syphilitic infection in rabbits, confirm these observations. (The ethics of performing such studies, in which syphilis victims are not treated, is now a highly controversial issue.) Immunity is slow to evolve; as the duration of infection increases, the degree of immunity correspondingly increases. In rabbits, solid immunity to challenge infection requires at least 3 months of infection and, once established, remains for the duration of the animal's life.

The precise contribution of humoral antibodies to host defenses in syphilitic infection is not well defined. Within lesions, *T pallidum* exhibits a predilection for perivascular areas. A lymphocyte (including B cells) and plasma cell infiltration occurs early in infection and is especially prominent in perivascular areas. The presence of organisms and antibody-synthesizing host cells in identical tissue areas suggests some role for antibodies.

Syphilis generates a wide variety of antibodies that are the basis for numerous diagnostic tests. None of these antibodies, however, is directly responsible for the solid immunity that evolves in untreated syphilis. In support of this interpretation, passive transfer of immune serum in experimental syphilis of the rabbit does not confer protection against challenge inoculation, although some modification of treponemal lesions occurs. Injection of immune serum followed by *T pallidum* challenge causes extended incubation periods, less severe lesions, and more rapid healing responses. Thus, antibodies appear to be partially but not solely responsible for healing and immunity.

The precise contribution of cell-mediated immunity to host defenses in syphilitic infection is also not well defined. Treponemal antigens invoke delayed hypersensitivity skin reactions in late secondary, latent, and tertiary syphilis. Experimental observations using blast transformation and macrophage migration inhibition and histologic observations of lymphocyte depletion in lymph nodes and spleens have provided additional evidence that cell-mediated immunity is operative in syphilis. The cellular response is initially suppressed when clinical manifestations of the primary stage first appear. As the infection progresses, suppression is overcome, and the cellular response is activated. At this time, healing of the chancre becomes apparent. Immunosuppression of host defenses may be responsible for the exacerbation of the infection that results in the secondary and tertiary stages.

Due to lack of large numbers of healthy, inbred rabbits, only a few studies involving adoptive transfer of immune lymphocytes have been attempted. As with passive transfer of immune serum, partial protection against *T pallidum* challenge followed transfer of immune cells. Quite likely, immunity in syphilis is due to humoral and cellular mechanisms acting in concert.

Epidemiology

T pallidum is distributed worldwide and occurs in epidemic proportions in virtually every country. Humans are the only source of this highly contagious infection. In almost all cases, syphilis is transmitted through sexual contact. It is not restricted to prostitutes or homosexuals. Infectivity rates correspond to those age groups that are most active sexually. Highest rates occur in the 20-24 year age group; slightly lower rates occur in the 15-19 year age group, followed by rates for the 25-29 year age group.

In the late 1940s, penicillin was found to be effective in eradicating syphilis in each of its three clinical stages, in latent infections, and in congenital infections. As shown in Figure 51-4, peak incidence was observed in 1946-1947. The number of cases continually decreased until 1958. Since then, the trend has reversed, and a steady increase has

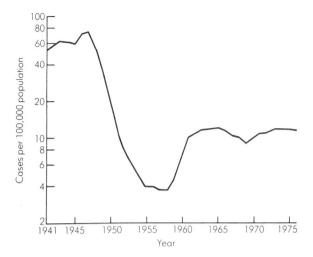

Figure 51-4 Reported cases of primary and secondary syphilis per 100,000 population in civilians in the United States from 1941–1975. From *Morbidity Mortality Weekly Report* 1973; 22:60.

occurred. Fortunately, during these years, the incidence of late manifestations has greatly declined, probably because of the widespread use of penicillin to treat many other nonsyphilitic diseases and better surveillance methods involving routine serologic tests. In addition, approximately 10% of patients with gonorrhea may also have concurrent syphilitic infection. Because gonorrhea has a shorter incubation period (2-8 days) and has painful symptoms, the patient seeks treatment before syphilitic lesions develop. Penicillin therapy of gonorrhea eradicates incubating syphilis before it becomes clinically apparent.

Diagnosis

Definitive diagnosis of syphilis is complicated by the inability to cultivate *T pallidum* in vitro. Clinical manifestations, demonstration of treponemes in lesion material, and serologic reactions are used for diagnosis. In most cases, clinical manifestations are sufficiently characteristic. If manifestations include exudative lesions, treponemes should be detectable within lesion material. Dark-field microscopy is used to demonstrate organisms.

Serologic tests are important to diagnosis, especially in cases in which clinical manifestations are confusing or exudative material is not present. The more than 200 serologic tests that have been developed fall into two general categories. Nontreponemal tests measure Wassermann antibody, which is elicited in response to cardiolipin antigens, presumably from host tissue; many variations of these tests are used. Treponemal tests measure antibodies that are elicited in response to antigenic components of *T pallidum;* these include the fluorescence of treponemes (FTA-ABS), *T pallidum* immobilization (TPI), agglutinin, and hemagglutinin tests.

Serologic reactions vary with the stage of the disease. Nontreponemal tests usually parallel the infection. The titers are high during clinical infection and decrease during subclinical infection (latency) or following antibiotic therapy. The treponemal tests may not become positive until well after the initial clinical manifestations; titers may remain high in latency and following treatment.

Two terms relevant to serologic testing are **sensitivity** and **specificity.** The perfect test, not yet developed, would detect 100% of the treponemal infections and would be nonreactive in all other diseases. Sensitivity refers to the ability to detect the tested variable, in this case syphilis. A biologic false-negative occurs when serum from a syphilitic patient fails to react; for example, the FTA-ABS test is serologically nonreactive early in the primary stage. Specificity refers to the ability to recognize when the variable is not present, that is, exclude syphilis in nonsyphilitic patients. A biologic false-positive occurs when serum from a nonsyphilitic patient reacts positively; for example, serum from patients with leprosy, tuberculosis, malaria, infectious mononucleosis, collagen disorders, systemic lupus erythematosus, rheumatoid arthritis, and thyroiditis frequently shows positive reactions. Pregnancy, old age, and drug abuse are also associated with false-positive results.

The World Health Organization recommends screening sera with the venereal disease research laboratory (VDRL) test, rapid plasma reagenic (RPR) test, or automated reaginic test (ART), and confirming positive sera with the FTA-ABS test. A group of hemagglutination tests also have been developed that are easier to perform and appear to be equivalent to the FTA-ABS test.

One other comment is pertinent to serologic testing. Congenital syphilis of the newborn is somewhat difficult to diagnose. Maternal antibodies (IgG) pass through the placenta and enter fetal circulation. At birth, the baby is serologically positive. Maternal antibodies disappear after 3 months. Quantitative VDRL or RPR tests should be performed monthly over the first 6 months. If the titer increases or stabilizes and does not decrease, congenital syphilis is indicated, and the baby should be treated accordingly.

Control

The current worldwide epidemic of syphilis emphasizes the need for developing preventive measures. Unfortunately, few effective measures are available. The condom remains the method of choice. Topical application of antibiotics, chemicals, creams, or lotions, or thorough washing with soap and water after sexual contact, are highly ineffective. A vaccine appears to be the only hope for future control of syphilis. Despite intense research in this area, only limited progress has been made. Two other control measures are important. The first is educating people about the early clinical manifestations of primary syphilis, so that they can seek treatment before infecting others. The second, for which epidemiology programs have been established, is to trace contacts of syphilitic patients; these contacts are then treated prophylactically before onset of clinical manifestations.

Penicillin remains the drug of choice for treating syphilis because penicillin-resistant strains have not yet emerged. Long-acting penicillin is used to maintain high serum levels for 7-10 days. Infection may be treated with any one of the following: procaine penicillin G, clemizole penicillin, procaine penicillin G with 2% aluminum monostearate (PAM), or benzathine penicillin G. If allergy to penicillin exists, tetracycline, erthromycin, or cephaloridine are alternative choices. Dosage depends on the stage of infection. Each clinical stage, latency, and congenital syphilis in utero and after birth are readily amenable to antibiotic therapy.

A Jarisch-Herxheimer reaction occasionally follows treatment of secondary or tertiary syphilis. This focal and systemic reaction is associated with rapid death of *T pallidum*. Two to 12 hours after antibioitc therapy, headache, malaise, slight fever, chills, muscle aches, and intensification of syphilitic lesions occur. These manifestations resolve in fewer than 12 hours. This benign reaction requires no prophylactic measures and indicates effective therapy.

Both Wassermann and treponemal antibodies remain detectable for long periods, even after effective treatment. The recommended procedure for testing cure involves detection of Wassermann antibodies, which disappear more rapidly than treponemal antibodies. Cases of primary syphilis should be Wassermann seronegative 6-12 months after treatment; cases of secondary syphilis should be Wassermann seronegative 12-18 months after treatment. Test of cure is difficult to assess if infection has endured beyond 2 years; in these infections, Wassermann and treponemal antibodies may be detected 12-25 years after treatment.

Other Treponematoses

Yaws

Yaws, caused by *T pertenue*, predominates in the tropical areas of Africa, South America, India, Indonesia, and the Pacific Islands. Its highly contagious nature is indicated by an estimated 50 million cases worldwide. Transmission occurs through human-to-human nonsexual contact. Most cases are in children and adolescents. In endemic areas, 75% of the population contract yaws before age 20 years.

The primary lesion, or mother yaw, develops within 2 to 4 weeks at the site of skin entry as a painless erythematous papule or group of papules. Lesions enlarge and ulcerate, exuding a serous fluid with a bloody tinge that is swarming with organisms. Healing occurs within one to several months, leaving an atrophic, depressed scar. The treponemes disseminate and, within 1 to 12 months, secondary lesions evolve that are quite similar to the mother yaw. Crops of these lesions develop initially on the face and moist areas of the body, and then spread to the trunk and arms. Infection of the soles and palms is characteristic as it is in syphilis. Elevated granulomatous papules may enlarge to a diameter of 5 cm, and then heal, leaving areas of depigmentation. Successive crops of these lesions occur for many months. Histopathology is similar to that observed in syphilis, with minimal vascular changes and no endothelial cell proliferation. The late destructive stage, sometimes called tertiary, involves treponemal infection of the bones and periosteum, especially the long bones of legs and forearms, and the bones of the feet and hands. Pathologic findings are similar to those seen in the tertiary stage of syphilis. Highly destructive gummas also may occur within the bones and soft tissues.

Diagnosis relies on geographic location, clinical manifestations, demonstration of treponemes within exudates, and positive serology. In areas in which syphilis and yaws coexist, tertiary infections are extremely similar and differentiation can be made only by inoculating laboratory animals. *T pallidum* infects rabbits, hamsters, and guinea pigs, whereas *T pertenue* infects rabbits and hamsters, but not guinea pigs. Penicillin readily eradicates each stage of yaws.

Pinta

Pinta, caused by *T carateum,* is endemic in the tropical areas of Central and South America. Recently, the number of cases has been estimated to be 500,000. Transmission occurs through human-to-human nonsexual contact. Most cases occur in children and adolescents.

The primary lesion develops within 2 to 6 months at the site of skin entry as a flat, erythematous papule or group of papules. These lesions and occasional satellite lesions enlarge over several months and produce plaques with scaly surfaces. Secondary lesions occur after 2-18 months, or longer, and involve ulceration and hyperchromic patches. Typically the hands, feet, and scalp are infected. Late stages of pinta involve patches of hyperchromia and achromia, irregular acanthosis, and epidermal atrophy. Lesions heal initially with hyperpigmentation. Then, with scarring, lesions become depigmented and hyperkeratotic. The treponemes disturb normal melanin pigmentation and produce the characteristic skin manifestations within 2 to 5 years.

The different stages of this disease are not clearly separated, and overlap of manifestations is common. Diagnosis relies on geographic location, clinical manifestations, demonstration of organisms in exudates, and positive serology. Differentation from yaws and syphilis is somewhat difficult and is based on laboratory injection of animals. *T carateum* does not infect rabbits, hamsters, or guinea pigs, but does infect chimps. Penicillin is the antibiotic of choice. Contrary to syphilis and yaws, in which the lesions heal rapidly following treatment with penicillin, pinta lesions may require 1 year to resolve fully. After primary or early secondary manifestations, skin pigmentation returns to normal. In later manifestations, however, pigmentation remains altered permanently.

Endemic Syphilis

Endemic syphilis, caused by *T pallidum* variant, is found in the desert areas of the Middle East, Central Africa, and South Africa. Transmission is through human-to-human nonsexual contact. The majority of cases are contracted by young children past the age of 2 years. Transmission of endemic syphilis, like that of yaws and pinta, is associated with poor hygiene.

Clinical manifestations can be quite similar to those of syphilis and yaws. The site of entry usually is the mucous membranes of the eyes and mouth. The primary lesion, a small papule, is detectable in only 1% of cases. After 2-3 months, secondary lesions or plaques develop in mucous membranes, skin, muscles, and bone. These oozing papules erode, harden, become condylomatous, and eventually heal. Clinical manifestations are then not apparent for 5-15 years (latency). Late endemic syphilis develops in the skin and skeletal system. Skin lesions may be superficial, nodular, or tuberous, or of a highly destructive deep gummatous type. Destructive bone lesions frequently localize in the tibia.

Diagnosis depends on geographic location, clinical manifestations, treponemes in the exudate, and positive serology. Penicillin eradicates endemic syphilis effectively.

References

Crissey, J.T., Denenholz, D.A.: Syphilis. *Clin Dermatol* 1984; 2:1-166.

Fitzgerald, T.J.: Pathogeneses and immunology of *Treponema pallidum. Ann Rev Microbiol* 1981; 35: 29-54.

Hovind-Haugen, K.: Determination by means of electron microscopy of morphological criteria of value for classification of some spirochetes, in particular treponemes. *Acta Pathol Microbiol Scand* [Suppl] 1976; 255: 1-41.

Johnson, R.C., (editor): *The biology of parasitic spirochetes.* New York: Academic Press, 1976.

Lomholt, G.: *Textbook of dermatology,* vol. 1. Oxford: Blackwell Scientific Publications, 1972.

Miller, J.N.: Value and limitations of non-treponemal and treponemal tests in the laboratory diagnosis of syphilis. *Clin Obstet Gynecol* 1975; 18: 191-203.

Moskophidis, M., Muller, F.: Molecular analysis of immunoglobulin M and G. Immune response to protein antigens of *Treponema pallidum* in human syphilis. *Infect Immun* 1984; 43:127-132.

Turner, T.B., Hollander, D.H.: Biology of the treponematoses. *Bull WHO* 1957; 35: 1-277.

United States Department of Health, Education, and Welfare: *Syphilis; a synopsis.* Public Health Service Publication No. 1660: 1-133, 1968.

Vegas, F.K.: *Clinical, tropical dermatology.* Oxford: Blackwell Scientific Publications, 1975.

Willcox, R.R., Guthe, T.: *Treponema pallidum. A bibliographical review of the morphology, culture and survival of T. pallidum and associated organisms. Bull WHO* [Suppl] 1966; 35:1-169.

52 Mycoplasmas

Shmuel Razin, PhD

General Concepts

Mycoplasmas are the smallest and simplest self-replicating bacteria. The mycoplasma cell contains only the minimum set of organelles essential for growth and replication: a plasma membrane, ribosomes, and a double-stranded DNA molecule (Figure 52-1). The relative simplicity of mycoplasmas has made them most useful tools for studying basic problems in cell biology. Unlike all other prokaryotes, the mycoplasmas have no cell walls and are placed accordingly in a separate class: Mollicutes (*mollis,* soft; *cutis,* skin). The common term mycoplasmas is used rather loosely to denote any species included in the class Mollicutes, whereas the common names acholeplasmas, ureaplasmas, spiroplasmas, and anaeroplasmas are used to refer to members of the corresponding genera, rather than to defined species within the genera (Table 52-1).

All mycoplasmas cultivated and identified so far are parasites of humans, animals, plants, and arthropods. Primary habitats of animal mycoplasmas are the mucous surfaces of respiratory and urogenital tracts and the joints in some animals. Although some

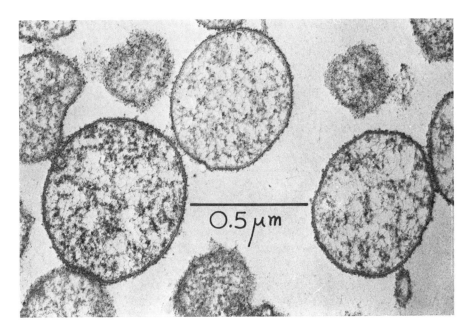

Figure 52-1 Electron micrograph of thin sectioned mycoplasma cells. Cells are bounded by a single membrane showing in section the characteristic trilaminar shape. Cytoplasm contains thin threads representing sectioned chromosome and dark granules representing ribosomes. Courtesy R.M. Cole.

Table 52-1 Taxonomy and Properties of Organisms Included in the Class Mollicutes

Classification	Number of Recognized Species	Genome Size (× 10⁸ daltons)	G+C Content (%)	Cholesterol Requirement	Characteristic Properties	Habitat
Mycoplasmataceae						
Mycoplasma	about 70	5	23–41	+	—	Animals and humans
Ureaplasma	2	5	28	+	Urease activity	Animals and humans
Acholeplasmataceae						
Acholeplasma	9	10	27–35	—	—	Animals and humans
Spiroplasmataceae						
Spiroplasma	4	10	26–30	+	Helical filaments	Arthropods and plants
Genus of uncertain taxonomic position						
Anaeroplasma	2	ND	29–34	Some + some −	Anaerobic; some digest bacteria	Rumens of cattle and sheep

mycoplasmas belong to the normal flora, most species are pathogens, causing various diseases that tend to run a chronic course. In humans, one species, *Mycoplasma pneumoniae,* has been established as the agent of primary atypical pneumonia; another species, *Ureaplasma urealyticum,* probably is associated with nongonococcal urethritis. Many mycoplasma species are established pathogens of farm animals, causing contagious pleuropneumonia and mastitis in cattle and goats and chronic respiratory diseases and arthritis in swine, chicken, and laboratory animals. In plants, mycoplasmas inhabit the phloem tissue and cause a large variety of economically important diseases in crops.

The pathogenic mechanisms of mycoplasmal infections are not clearly understood, but adherence to host cells by protein adhesins appears to be involved. The role of toxic factors (H_2O_2, NH_3) in the disease process is under investigation. Infection with *M pneumoniae* occurs worldwide and is transmitted by respiratory droplets, whereas *U urealyticum* is transmitted by sexual contact. Mycoplasmal infections can be treated effectively with broad-spectrum antibiotics such as tetracycline.

Mycoplasmas have been nicknamed the crabgrass of cell cultures because their infections are persistent, difficult to cure, and frequently difficult to detect and diagnose. Contamination by mycoplasmas presents serious problems in the production of viral vaccines in cell cultures. The origin of contaminating mycoplasmas is in components of the cell culture medium, particularly serum, or from the mycoplasma flora of the technician's mouth, spread by droplet infection.

Distinctive Properties

Morphology and Reproduction

The coccus is the basic form of all mycoplasma cultures. The diameter of the smallest cocci capable of reproduction is about 300 nm. Hence, many of the minute and plastic cells can be squeezed through membrane filters of 450 nm pore diameter. In most mycoplasma cultures, elongated or filamentous forms (up to 100 μm long and about 0.4 μm thick) also can be observed (Figure 52-2). The filaments tend to produce truly

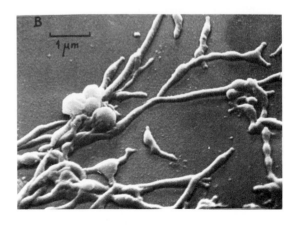

Figure 52-2 Scanning electron micrograph of a *M pneumoniae* culture, showing characteristic morphologic elements, including chains of cocci, branched filaments, and elongated cells with tapered tips (specialized tip structures). From Biberfeld, G, Biberfeld, P.: *J Bacteriol* 1970; 102: 855.

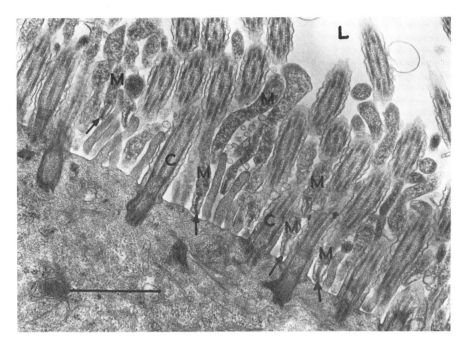

Figure 52-3 Electron micrograph of *M pneumoniae*-infected human fetal trachea after 48 hours in organ culture. **M,** mycoplasma; **C,** cilia; **L,** lumen; **arrows,** tip attachment structure. Bar = 1 μm. From Collier, A.M.: In: *The Mycoplasmas.* Vol 2. Barile, M.F., et al., (editors). New York: Academic Press. 1979.

branched mycelioid structures, hence the name mycoplasma (*myces,* a fungus; *plasma,* a form). In the case of spiroplasmas, the filaments are helical, usually 2-5 μm long and 0.1-0.2 μm thick. Mycoplasmas reproduce by binary fission, but cytoplasmic division frequently may lag behind genome replication, resulting in formation of multinuclear filaments.

A few *Mycoplasma* sp possess unique attachment organelles shaped as a tapered tip in *M pneumoniae* and a pear-shaped bleb in the avian *M gallisepticum.* These two mycoplasmas are pathogens of the respiratory tract, adhering to the respiratory epithelium primarily through the terminal attachment structures (Figure 52-3). Interestingly, these mycoplasmas exhibit gliding motility on liquid-covered surfaces. The direction of movement always is led by the terminal structure, again indicating its importance in attachment.

One of the most useful distinguishing features of mycoplasmas is their peculiar fried-egg colony shape, consisting of a central zone of growth embedded in the agar and a peripheral zone on its surface (Figure 52-4). Among the prokaryotes, only the wall-less bacterial L-forms produce a similar fried-egg colony.

Nutrition and Energy-Yielding Mechanisms

The mycoplasmas have limited biosynthetic abilities, probably reflecting their small genome and parasitic mode of life. Consequently, they require complex media

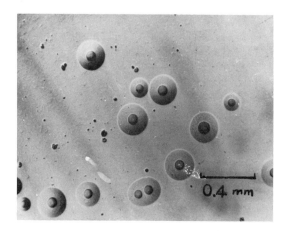

Figure 52-4 "Fried-egg" colonies of mycoplasmas. A 4-day culture on solid medium. From Razin, S., Oliver, O.: *J Gen Microbiol* 1961; 24: 225.

containing serum for growth. The serum provides fatty acids and cholesterol for membrane synthesis in an assimilable, nontoxic form. The requirement of most mycoplasmas for cholesterol (Table 52-1) is unique among prokaryotes, although cholesterol can also be found in *Borrelia* cells and is apparently required for growth of *Treponema hyodysenteriae* (see Chapter 50). Cholesterol is incorporated into the cell membrane in large quantities and appears to function as a regulator of membrane fluidity. It must be stressed that the culture media now available are inadequate for cultivation of all mycoplasmas. Nevertheless, the continuing developments in culture media have allowed identification of a number of new species, including *Mycoplasma genitalium*, which was isolated from the human genital tract.

Glucose and other metabolizable carbohydrates are possible energy sources for the fermentative mycoplasmas possessing the Embden–Meyerhof–Parnas glycolytic pathway. All mycoplasmas examined so far possess a truncated flavin-terminated respiratory system, which rules out oxidative phosphorylation as an ATP-generating mechanism in mycoplasmas. Breakdown of arginine by the arginine dihydrolase pathway has been proposed as the major source of ATP in nonfermentative mycoplasmas. Ureaplasmas show the unique requirement among living organisms for urea. Because they are nonglycolytic and lack the arginine dihydrolase pathway, it has been suggested that ATP is generated in these organisms through an electrochemical gradient produced by the ammonia liberated during the intracellular hydrolysis of urea by the organism's urease.

Molecular Biology and Phylogenetic Status

The mycoplasma genome typically is prokaryotic, consisting of a circular, double-stranded DNA molecule. The *Mycoplasma* and *Ureaplasma* genomes are the smallest recorded for any self-reproducing prokaryote; the value of 23%–25% guanine plus cytosine (G + C) content found for the DNA of some mycoplasmas is also the lowest recorded (Table 52-1). Only one or two copies of ribosomal RNA genes exist in the mycoplasma genome, compared to seven in that of *E coli,* a finding that may explain the relatively slow growth rate of mycoplasmas. The protein synthesis machinery in mycoplasmas is prokaryotic, so antibiotics such as chloramphenicol and tetracyclines inhibit protein synthesis and growth. Although it is too early to conclude whether mycoplasmas evolved from cell-wall-covered bacteria or vice versa, the repeated failure to show any genetic relationship between mycoplasmas and cell-wall-covered bacteria by DNA hybridization techniques contradicts the notion that mycoplasmas represent stable L-forms of existing cell-wall-covered prokaryotes.

The Cell Membrane

The lack of cell walls and intracytoplasmic membranes facilitates isolation of the mycoplasma membrane in a relatively pure form. The isolated mycoplasma membrane resembles that of other prokaryotes in being composed of approximately two-thirds protein and one-third lipid. The mycoplasma lipids resemble those of other bacteria, apart from the large quantities of cholesterol in the sterol-requiring mycoplasmas.

Membrane proteins, glycolipids, and lipoglycans exposed on the cell surface are the major antigenic determinants in mycoplasmas. Antisera containing antibodies to these components inhibit growth and metabolism of the mycoplasmas and, in the presence of complement, also cause lysis of the organisms. These properties are utilized in various serologic tests that differentiate between mycoplasma species and serotypes and detect antibodies to mycoplasmas in sera of patients (see Diagnosis section, page 615).

Some mycoplasmas are covered by capsules. In *M mycoides,* the contagious bovine pleuropneumonia agent, the capsule is made of galactan, a polymer possessing toxic properties. Electron microscopy has demonstrated capsules stained by ruthenium red in various mycoplasma species pathogenic to humans and animals. The possibility that capsules play a role in pathogenesis, by inhibiting phagocytosis of the organisms or by facilitating their adherence to host cell surfaces, remains to be studied.

Pathogenesis

Mycoplasmal Pneumonia

The term primary atypical pneumonia was coined in the early 1940s to describe pneumonias different from the typical lobar pneumonia caused by pneumococci. Several common respiratory viruses, including influenza and adenoviruses, were shown to be responsible for a significant number of these pneumonias. From other cases, many of which developed antibodies agglutinating red blood cells in the cold (cold agglutinins), an unidentified filterable agent was isolated by Eaton and associates and, accordingly, named Eaton agent. Identification of this agent as a new mycoplasma species was achieved in 1962, after its successful cultivation on cell-free media by Chanock, Hayflick, and Barile. This mycoplasma, named *M pneumoniae,* was the first clearly documented mycoplasma pathogenic for humans.

The effects of *M pneumoniae* on humans range from subclinical infection to upper respiratory disease to bronchopneumonia. The majority of human infections do not progress to a clinically evident pneumonia. When pneumonia occurs, the onset generally is gradual, and the clinical picture is one of a mild to moderately severe illness, with early complaints referrable to the lower respiratory passages. Radiographic examination frequently reveals evidence of pneumonia before physical signs are apparent. Involvement is usually, but not always, limited to one of the lower lobes of the lungs, and the pneumonia is interstitial or bronchopneumonic. The course of the disease varies; remittent fever, cough, and headache persist several weeks. One of the most consistent clinical features is a long convalescence, which may extend 4-6 weeks. Few fatal cases have been reported. Several unusual complications have been noted, including hemolytic anemia, central nervous system illness such as the Guillain-Barré syndrome, polyradiculitis, encephalitis, and aseptic meningitis. In addition, pericarditis and pancreatitis have been observed in some cases. These sequelae may be related to the suspected immunopathology of *M pneumoniae* disease (see pages 612-614).

Nongonococcal Urethritis and Salpingitis

Growing evidence suggests that *U urealyticum* may cause nongonococcal urethritis in persons free of *Chlamydia trachomatis,* an established agent of nongonococcal urethritis. The wide occurrence of *U urealyticum* in sexually active, symptom-free adults hampers research in this field. Evidence is primarily based on the production of nongonococcal urethritis symptoms in ureaplasma-free and chlamydia-free volunteers by intraurethral inoculation of *U urealyticum* and on a report that this disease could be cured in a chlamydia-free man only when he and his partner were treated simultaneously with tetracycline, which eliminated *U urealyticum* from both. It has been suggested, but still not proven, that the newly discovered *M genitalium* accounts for the tetracycline-responsive nongonococcal urethritis cases in which chlamydia and ureaplasmas cannot be isolated (about 20% of all cases). Ureaplasmas have also been associated with chorioamnionitis, habitual spontaneous abortion, and low birth weight infants. *M hominis,* a common inhabitant of the vagina of healthy women, becomes pathogenic once it invades the internal genital organs, where it may cause pelvic inflammatory disease, such as tuboovarian abscess or salpingitis.

Disease Mechanisms

Most mycoplasmas infecting humans and animals are surface parasites, adhering to the epithelial linings of the respiratory and urogenital tracts. Adherence is firm enough to prevent the elimination of the parasites by mucous secretions or urine. The intimate association between the adhering mycoplasmas and their host cells provides an environment in which local concentrations of toxic metabolites excreted by the parasite build up and cause tissue damage (see next page). Moreover, because mycoplasmas lack cell walls, the possibility of fusion between the membranes of the parasite and host has been suggested, but experimental evidence for it is insufficient. Several studies suggest that the parasite and host membranes exchange antigenic components, an event that may help the parasite to evade the host immunologic response and perhaps also trigger autoimmune reactions. As attachment of *M pneumoniae* and of the avian respiratory pathogens *M gallisepticum* and *M synoviae* is affected by pretreatment of the host cells by neuraminidase, it appears that sialoglycoproteins or sialoglycolipids of the host cell membrane are receptor sites for these mycoplasmas. Evidence indicates that several *M pneumoniae* membrane proteins act as adhesins, and that they have high affinity for the specific receptors for *M pneumoniae* on host cells. Monoclonal antibodies to one of these proteins, protein P1 (mol. wt. 165,000), inhibit attachment of the parasite. Ferritin labeling of the antibodies has shown that P1 concentrates on the tip structure of the mycoplasma, a finding that provides further support for the theory that the tip structure serves as an attachment organelle.

Tracheal organ cultures from the human fetus or from the Syrian hamster have been extensively used as experimental models to study the interaction of *M pneumoniae* with respiratory epithelium. Reduction of ciliary activity followed by complete ciliostasis is the most pronounced manifestation of injury to the tracheal or oviduct explants by mycoplasmas. As the infection progresses, the cilia are distorted and lost, and the superficial epithelial cells undergo desquamation. The histologic manifestations of tissue damage reflect pronounced alterations in the metabolism of the infected organ cultures, as reflected by decreased oxygen consumption and by decreased RNA and protein synthesis.

The nature of the toxic factors damaging the organ explants infected by mycoplasmas is still unclear. Toxins are rarely found in mycoplasmas. Consequently, researchers considered the possibility that the end products of mycoplasma metabolism may be responsible for tissue damage. Hydrogen peroxide, the end product of respiration in mycoplasmas, has been incriminated as a major pathogenic factor ever since it was shown to be responsible for the lysis of erythrocytes by mycoplasmas in vitro; however, the production of H_2O_2 alone does not determine pathogenicity, as the loss of virulence in *M pneumoniae* is not accompanied by a decrease in H_2O_2 production. For the H_2O_2 to exert its toxic effect, the mycoplasmas must adhere close enough to the host cell surface to maintain a toxic, steady-state concentration of H_2O_2 sufficient to cause direct damage, such as lipid peroxidation, to the cell membrane. The accumulation of malonyldialdehyde, an oxidation product of membrane lipids, in cells exposed to *M pneumoniae* supports this notion. Moreover, *M pneumoniae* has been found to inhibit host cell catalase. This would be expected to cause the accumulation of H_2O_2 at the site of parasite–host cell contact.

Ammonia is another end product of mycoplasma metabolism that may become toxic when produced in large quantities, as during urea hydrolysis by ureaplasmas. Hydrolysis of arginine by mycoplasmas possessing the arginine dihydrolase pathway also yields ammonia as an end product. In this case, however, the depletion of the essential amino acid, rather than the toxicity of the end product, is to blame for many of the symptoms in cell cultures contaminated by arginine-splitting mycoplasmas. Obviously, arginine depletion is unlikely to occur in the infected animal.

Evidence suggests that in *M pneumoniae* pneumonia, both organism-related and host-related factors are involved in pathogenesis. The host may be largely responsible for the appearance of pneumonia by mounting a local immunocyte and phagocytic response to the parasite. Syrian hamsters inoculated intranasally by *M pneumoniae* show patchy bronchopneumonic lesions consisting of infiltration of mononuclear cells. The ablation of thymic function before the experimental infection prevents development of the characteristic pulmonary infiltration, but lengthens the period during which the organisms can be isolated from the lung. Allowing the animals to recover and then reinfecting them produces an exaggerated and accelerated pneumonic process. Epidemiologic data also can be interpreted to show that repeated infections in humans are required before symptomatic disease occurs. Thus, serum antibodies to *M pneumoniae* can be found in most children 2-5 years of age, although the illness occurs with greatest frequency in individuals 5-15 years of age.

An immunopathologic mechanism also may explain the complications affecting organs distant from the respiratory tract in some *M pneumoniae* patients. Various autoantibodies have been detected in the serum of many of these patients, including cold agglutinins reacting on the erythrocyte I antigen, antibodies reacting with lymphocytes, smooth muscle antibodies, and antibodies reacting with brain and lung antigens. Serologic cross-reactions between *M pneumoniae* and brain and lung antigens have been demonstrated, and these antigens probably are related to the glycolipids of *M pneumoniae* membranes, which are also found in most plants and in many bacteria. Clearly, host reaction varies markedly, as only about one-half the patients develop cold agglutinins, and complications are rare, even among individuals with antitissue globulins.

Host Defenses

Infection with *M pneumoniae* induces development of antibodies in the serum that fix complement, inhibit growth of the organism, and lyse the organism in the presence of complement. Generally, the first antibodies produced are of the IgM class, whereas later in convalescence the predominant antibody is IgG. Secretory IgA antibodies also develop and appear to play an important role in host resistance. The first infection in infancy usually is asymptomatic and generates a brief serum antibody response. Recurrent infections, which occur at approximately 2-4 year intervals, generate a more prolonged systemic antibody response and increasing numbers of circulating antigen-responsive lymphocytes. By late childhood, clinically apparent lower respiratory disease, including pneumonia, becomes more common. Thus, mycoplasma respiratory disease manifestations appear to vary, depending on the state of local and systemic immunity at the time of reinfection. One hypothesis holds that local immunity mediates resistance to infection and that systemic immunity contributes substantially to the pulmonary and systemic reactions characteristic of *M pneumoniae* pneumonia.

The relative importance of humoral and cell-mediated immunity in resistance to mycoplasma infections of the respiratory tract is still unclear. For many mycoplasma infections, such as bovine pleuropneumonia, resistance can be transferred with convalescent serum. Although these results indicate that antibody can mediate resistance to mycoplasma infections of the respiratory tract, this may not be true for all mycoplasma respiratory diseases. Thus, resistance of rats to pulmonary disease induced by *M pulmonis* can be transferred only with spleen cells obtained from previously infected animals. Although IgA antibody may be important in upper respiratory tract resistance to mycoplasmas, other factors seem to be involved in resistance to pulmonary disease and these factors may not be the same for all mycoplasma infections.

Epidemiology

One of the most puzzling features of *M pneumoniae* pneumonia is the age distribution of patients. In a survey conducted between 1964 and 1975 of more than 100,000 individuals in the Seattle area, the age-specific attack rate was highest among the 5-9 year old children. Rates of *M pneumoniae* pneumonia in the youngest age group, 0-4 years old, were about one-half those of school-age children, but considerably higher than among adults. *M pneumoniae* pneumonia was rarely observed in infants under the age of 6 months, suggesting maternally conferred immunity. *M pneumoniae* accounts for as much as 8%-15% of all pneumonias in young school-aged children. In older children and young adults, the organism is responsible for approximately 15%-50% of all pneumonias. Infection with *M pneumoniae* is worldwide and endemic and occurs all year round but shows a predilection for the colder months, apparently because of greater opportunity for transmission by droplet infection. *M pneumoniae* appears to require close personal contact to spread; successful spreading usually occurs in families, schools, and institutions. The incubation period is relatively long, ranging from 2-3 weeks.

U urealyticum is acquired primarily through sexual contact. Colonization has been linked to the frequency of sexual intercourse and the number of sexual partners. Women may serve as asymptomatic reservoirs of infection, so simultaneous treatment of both sexual partners is necessary to cure men suffering from nongonococcal urethritis caused by *U urealyticum*.

Diagnosis

Diagnosis on the basis of microscopy alone is equivocal; therefore, cultivation is essential for definitive diagnosis.

Cultivation

A routine mycoplasma medium consists of heart infusion, peptone, yeast extract, salts, glucose or arginine, and horse serum (5%-20%). Fetal or newborn calf sera are preferable to horse serum. To prevent the overgrowth of the fast-growing bacteria that usually accompany mycoplasmas in clinical materials, penicillin or thallium acetate or both are added as selective agents. To cultivate ureaplasmas, the medium is supplemented with urea, and its pH is brought to 6.0. Ureaplasmas and *M genitalium* are relatively sensitive to thallium, so this inhibitor is omitted from their culture media. To isolate *M pneumoniae*, nasopharyngeal secretions are inoculated into a selective diphasic medium (pH 7.8) made of mycoplasma broth and agar and supplemented with glucose and phenol red. When *M pneumoniae* grows in this medium, it produces acid, causing the color of the medium to change from purple to yellow. Broth from the diphasic medium is subcultured to mycoplasma agar when a color change occurs, or at weekly intervals for a minimum of 8 weeks.

Identification

Colonies appearing on the plates can be identified as *M pneumoniae* by staining directly on agar with homologous fluorescein-conjugated antibody, or by demonstrating that a specific antiserum to *M pneumoniae* inhibits their growth on agar. Colonies of ureaplasmas are usually minute (less than 100 μm in diameter); because of urea hydrolysis and ammonia liberation, the pH of the medium becomes alkaline. When manganous sulfate is added to the growth medium, the colonies of ureaplasmas stain dark brown. More detailed characterization of isolates can be achieved by a variety of routine biochemical and serologic tests, supplemented when required by more sophisticated tests, including electrophoretic analysis of cell proteins, crossed immunoelectrophoresis of cell proteins, DNA hybridization tests, and DNA cleavage pattern evaluations by use of restriction endonucleases.

Serodiagnosis

Serodiagnosis basically consists of demonstrating antibodies in the patients' sera that inhibit growth and metabolism of the organism or fix complement with mycoplasmal antigens. Antibody response in mycoplasmal pneumonia is most easily demonstrated by complement fixation, reacting acute- and convalescent-phase sera with intact organisms or their lipid extract as antigen. A fourfold or greater antibody rise is considered indicative of recent infection, whereas a sustained high antibody titer may not be significant, because a relatively high level of antibody may persist for 1 or more years after infection. The cold agglutinin test is less useful because only about one-half of patients develop cold agglutinins, and because these antibodies also are induced by a great many other conditions.

Present techniques for laboratory diagnosis of *M pneumoniae* infections are of little use to the clinician because recovery and identification of the mycoplasmas cannot be accomplished in less than 1-2 weeks. Development of methods for rapid laboratory diagnosis, such as direct demonstration of organisms in the sputum by immunofluorescence, electron microscopy, or the ELISA technique, will be of great value.

Control

Prevention

Chemoprophylaxis of mycoplasma infections is not recommended, because it does not cure the infection, although it may modify the secondary cases to subclinical disease. Attempts at control by immunoprophylaxis fail in most cases. Prior natural infection appears to provide the most effective resistance; however, evidence shows that *M pneumoniae* infections in humans recur at intervals of several years. These observations suggest that immunity to a single natural infection is relatively short-term, particularly in children, and it may be unrealistic to expect more, or even as much, from artificially induced immunity.

Attenuation of mycoplasma strains tends to reduce virulence and immunogenicity. In most cases, attenuated viable vaccines do not reach the level of protective efficiency required from a commercial vaccine. *M mycoides* is an exception, because subcutaneous inoculation of live organisms in the tail protects cattle effectively against contagious bovine pleuropneumonia. Killed *M pneumoniae* vaccines administered intranasally to hamsters are relatively ineffective unless boosted by parenteral inoculation of vaccine. Intranasal immunizations may be ineffective because the antigenic mass is not retained for a sufficient time in the lung. On the other hand, parenteral killed vaccines, particularly if combined with adjuvant, do produce adequate protection by reducing pneumonia, although a minimal effect on the number of organisms growing in the lungs can be demonstrated. A similar protective effect can be achieved briefly by inoculation of hyperimmune serum.

In summary, a single dose of vaccine in a form suitable for clinical use is unlikely to produce lasting immunity to mycoplasma infection. Stimulation of systemic antibodies may prevent the clinical manifestations of pneumonia, but additional local stimulation with live or killed organisms may be necessary to evoke resistance to colonization. An approach worth pursuing is the preparation of vaccines made of antigenic components specifically related to the mycoplasma–host cell interaction, such as components of the mycoplasma membrane responsible for attachment of the parasites to the epithelial cell surface.

Treatment

The mycoplasmas are sensitive to most broad-spectrum antibiotics such as tetracyclines and chloramphenicol but are resistant to antibiotics that specifically inhibit bacterial cell wall synthesis. Tetracycline combined with erythromycin therapy has been definitely shown to reduce duration of fever and pulmonary infiltrations in *M pneumoniae* patients. Effective treatment of the disease symptoms, however, usually is not accompanied by eradication of the organism from the infected host. To prevent recurrence of nongonococcal urethritis caused by *U urealyticum*, sex partners should be treated simultaneously with tetracyclines.

References

Almagor, M., Yatziv, S., Kahane, I.: Inhibition of host cell catalase by *Mycoplasma pneumoniae*: A possible mechanism for cell injury. *Infect Immun* 1983; 41: 251-256.

Barile, M.F, et al. (editors): *The mycoplasmas.* New York: Academic Press, 1979.

Cassell, G.H., Cole, B.C.: Mycoplasmas as agents of human disease. *N Engl J Med* 1981; 304: 80-89.

Hu, P.C., et al.: *Mycoplasma pneumoniae* infection: Role of surface protein in the attachment organelle. *Science* 1982; 216: 313-315.

Razin, S.: The mycoplasmas. *Microbiol Rev* 1978; 42: 414-470.

Razin, S., Freundt, E.A., (editors): Special issue on biology and pathogenicity of mycoplasmas. *Isr J Med Sci* 1984; 20:749-1027.

Tully, J.G, et al.: A newly discovered mycoplasma in the human urogenital tract. *Lancet* 1981; 1: 1288-1291.

Wise, K.S., Cassell, G.H., Acton, R.T.: Selective association of murine T-lymphoblastoid cell surface alloantigens wth *Mycoplasma hyorhinis*. *Proc Nat Acad Sci (USA)* 1978; 75: 4479-4483.

53 *Rickettsia*

Mary Lou Clements, MD, MPH
Theodore E. Woodward, MD

General Concepts

Rickettsiae are small, obligate, intracellular gram-negative bacteria that characteristically infect arthropods and mammals; the latter may serve as vectors and reservoirs for incidental human infection. The rickettsiae belong to the family Rickettsiaceae, which consists of three genera. The genus *Rickettsia* is divided into three groups of antigenically and morphologically similar rickettsiae that are pathogenic for human diseases: spotted fever, typhus, and scrub typhus. *Rochalimaea quintana* (formerly designated *Rickettsia quintana*) is the agent of trench fever, and *Coxiella burnetii* is the cause of Q fever. *Rochalimaea quintana* is genetically and antigenically related to typhus rickettsiae but differs from rickettsiae in its ability to grow on cell-free media. In contrast, *Coxiella burnetii* is similar to rickettsiae in its obligate, intracellular, and parasitic nature, but differs genetically, antigenically, morphologically, and metabolically. In addition, its resistance to physical and chemical agents is greater than that of rickettsiae.

The rickettsial diseases, particularly epidemic typhus and, to a lesser extent, Rocky Mountain spotted fever, have caused human mortality and morbidity in many parts of the world for centuries. During World War I, *Rickettsia prowazekii* infected 30 million inhabitants in eastern Europe with epidemic typhus and caused about three million deaths. A similar epidemic occurred during World War II, particularly among persons in concentration camps and other louse-infested populations. Although improved socio-economic conditions and better hygiene have decreased its incidence worldwide, epidemic typhus continues to be a problem in some less developed countries, such as Ethiopia where up to 17,000 cases are reported annually. In the United States today, a mild form of epidemic typhus occurs occasionally as a recrudescence manifested as Brill–Zinsser disease or as a result of contact with squirrels. Other rickettsial diseases that occur in the United States include Rocky Mountain spotted fever and Q fever, which are the most common, rickettsialpox, and murine typhus (Table 53-1). Control of these infections depends on limitation of exposure to infected arthropods and use of personal protective measures such as insect repellents.

The rickettsial agents usually gain access to the body through the skin by an arthropod vector, except for *Coxiella burnetii*, which is acquired by inhalation. All rickettsiae probably enter vascular endothelial cells by inducing phagocytosis. Multiplication takes place within host cells. After the rickettsiae are released from the host cells, phospholipase A may help them to penetrate other cells. Endotoxin is presumed to be involved in tissue damage produced by rickettsiae.

Distinctive Properties

Rickettsiae are small, pleomorphic, coccobacilli that are less than 0.7 μm in diameter and 2 μm in length. Rickettsiae stain gram-negative and bright red by the Giménez method. Immunofluorescent techniques with specific antisera can be used to distinguish rickettsiae from other gram-negative bacteria in tissue.

The morphologic structure and chemical composition of rickettsiae are typical of gram-negative bacteria. They possess a cytoplasmic membrane, a cell wall, and a coat (halozone or slime layer) of variable thickness that is external to the outer leaflet of the cell wall and the microcapsular layer. With the exception of *R tsutsugamushi*, the outer envelopes of different species of rickettsiae are similar in overall size and structural components (Figure 53-1). The presence of the slime layer does not appear to be associated with virulence or the ability to survive intracellularly or extracellularly. The

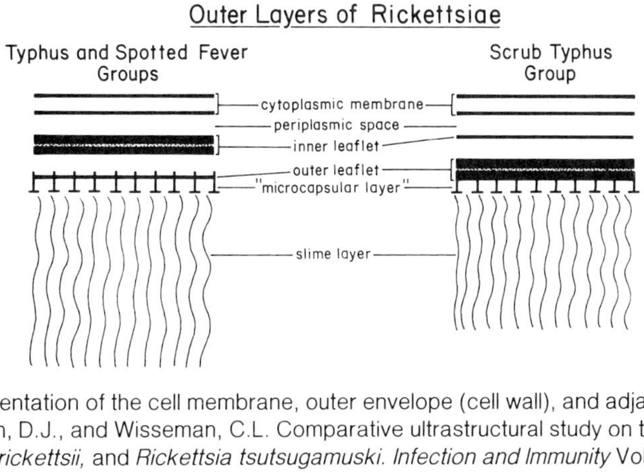

Figure 53-1 Diagrammatic representation of the cell membrane, outer envelope (cell wall), and adjacent extracellular layers of rickettsiae. From Silverman, D.J., and Wisseman, C.L. Comparative ultrastructural study on the cell envelopes of *Rickettsia prowazekii, Rickettsia rickettsii,* and *Rickettsia tsutsugamuski. Infection and Immunity* Vol. 21. 1978.

Table 53-1 Distinguishing Characteristics of Rickettsial Diseases

Disease	Organism	Natural Cycle		Geographic Area	Rash Distribution	Eschar	Serological Diagnosis	
		Insect Vector	Animal Reservoir				Confirmatory Test*	Weil-Felix Reaction
Genus Rickettsia								
Spotted Fever Group								
Rocky Mountain spotted fever	R rickettsii	Tick	Dogs, ? rodents	Western hemisphere	Extremities to trunk	Seldom	IFA, ELISA, LA, IHA, MA, CF	
Boutonneuse fever	R conorii	Tick	Rodents, dogs	Africa, Mediterranean, India	Trunk, extremities, face	Yes	IFA	Positive OX 19 OX 2
Queensland tick typhus	R australis	Tick	Rodents, marsupials	Australia	Trunk, extremities, face	Yes	IFA	
North Asian tick typhus	R sibirica	Tick	Rodents	Siberia, Mongolia	Trunk, extremities, face	Yes	IFA	
Rickettsialpox	R akari	Mite	Mouse	N. America, Soviet Union, Korea, Africa	Vesicular; trunk, extremities, face	Yes	CF	Negative
Typhus Group								
Epidemic typhus	R prowazekii	Louse	Human, flying squirrel	Highland areas of S. America, Africa, Asia, Eastern United States	Trunk to extremities	No	IFA, ELISA, CF, MA	Positive OX 19
Murine typhus	R typhi	Flea	Rodents	Worldwide	Trunk to extremities	No	IFA, ELISA, CF, MA	Positive OX 19
Scrub Typhus Group								
Scrub typhus	R tsutsugamushi	Mite	Rodents	S. Pacific, Asia, Australia, Soviet Union	Trunk to extremities	Yes	IFA, ELISA	Positive OX K
Genus Rochalimaea								
Trench fever	R quintana	Louse	Human	N. America, Mexico, Europe, Africa	Trunk	No	IHA, ELISA, CF	Negative
Genus Coxiella								
Q Fever	C burnetii	? Ticks	Cattle, sheep, goats	Worldwide	None	No	CF, MA, IFA, ELISA (Phase I and II antigens)	Negative

*Confirmatory tests include indirect fluorescent antibody (IFA), microagglutination (MA), complement fixation (CF), latex agglutination (LA), indirect hemagglutination (IHA), and enzyme-linked immunosorbent assays (ELISA).

layer may function, however, as the locus of major group-specific antigens, and it may be involved in the attachment of rickettsiae to potential host cells.

Rickettsiae possess both RNA and DNA and divide by transverse binary fission. Comparison of the properties of rickettsial DNA reveals that only small genetic differences exist between the typhus group (*R prowazekii* and *R typhi*) and the spotted fever group (*R rickettsii*) (Table 53-2). Both groups are related to *Rochalimaea quintana*. In contrast, the genetic properties of *C burnetii* are distinctly different from those of the other rickettsiae.

Rickettsia, Coxiella, and *Rochalimaea* differ in several other aspects. *Rickettsia* replicates primarily within the cytoplasm (Figure 53-2) and sometimes in the nucleus of

Table 53-2   Properties of the DNA of Selected Rickettsiae

Organism Genus, and Species	*Genome Size ($\times 10^7$ daltons)*	*Guanine Plus Cytosine Content (mol%)*	*Percent DNA–DNA Hybridizations Between Species**			
			R	*P*	*T*	*Q*
Rickettsia						
R rickettsii	130	33	—	38	27	—
R prowazekii	110	29	53	<u>97</u>	73	32
R typhi	108	29	36	73	<u>101</u>	32
Rochalimaea						
R quintana	103	39	—	—	—	<u>95</u>
Coxiella						
C burnetii	104	43	—	—	—	—

Adapted, with permission, from the *Annual Review of Microbiology*, vol. 36. c 1982 by Annual Reviews Inc.
*Initials represent the first letter of the species. Homologous reactions are underlined. Tests not performed are indicated by —.

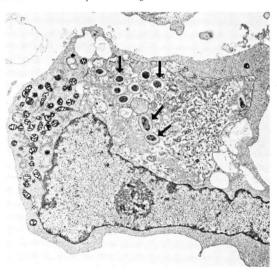

Figure 53-2   Electron micrograph shows *R rickettsii* (R) localized in the cytoplasm and nucleus of a human vascular endothelial cell. Courtesy David J. Silverman.

the host cells, unbounded by phagosomal or phagolysosomal membranes; *Coxiella* multiplies only in the phagolysosome. *Rochalimaea* grow well in cell culture (as well as on blood agar), but adhere to the outer surface of eukaryotic cells. Glycolytic enzymes are present in *Rickettsia* and in *Rochalimaea* but not in *Coxiella*. Unlike rickettsiae, *C burnetii* appears to undergo a complex developmental cycle involving two types of cells that may represent vegetative and sporelike stages of differentiation (Figure 53-3). The

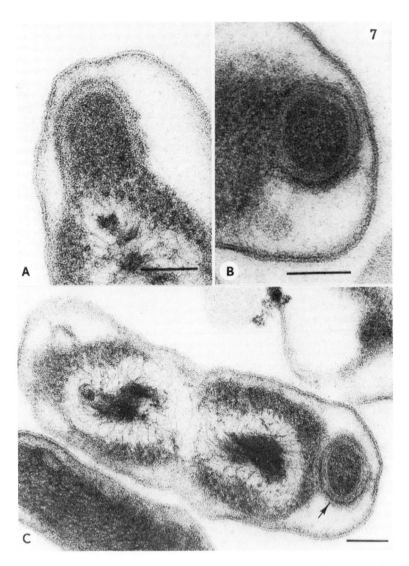

Figure 53-3 Electron micrograph of thin sections showing a putative progression of endospore formation in large cell variants (LCV) of *C burnetii*. Bar = 0.1 μm. **A**, Initial stages of spore formation within the LCV. **B**, The spore has completed its development but remains within the cytoplasm. **C**, Illustration of the complete formation of the endospore (arrow) in a LCV concurrently undergoing cell division. Courtesy Jim C. Williams.

sporelike bodies (small cell variants or endospores) may allow the organism to survive in environments that destroy nonsporulating bacteria.

Pathogenesis

Infection develops after the entry of rickettsial organisms through the skin, conjunctiva, mucous membranes, respiratory tract, gastrointestinal tract, or systemic circulation. Agents of typhus, spotted fever, and trench fever are introduced into the skin by an arthropod vector or, occasionally, in the laboratory by autoinoculation. Humans usually acquire Q fever, and occasionally other rickettsial diseases, by inhalation of contaminated aerosols or by ingestion of infected milk or food.

Within minutes, the rickettsiae enter human endothelial cells, probably by inducing their own phagocytosis by the host cells. After phagocytosis, *Rickettsia* organisms escape from the phagosome or phagolysosome and replicate within the cytoplasm or nucleus of the host cell; *Coxiella* organisms remain within the phagolysosome throughout their life cycle and multiply. The generation time of rickettsiae is approximately 9 hours. The rickettsiae proliferate within the infected cell until it bursts and releases the organisms, which then infect other cells. The enzyme phospholipase A may aid in rickettsial penetration and thereby play a role in the pathogenesis of host cell injury by the organisms.

Initially, the rickettsiae multiply locally at the original site of entry; some species produce a characteristic primary cutaneous lesion or eschar at that site (seen in scrub typhus; rickettsialpox; spotted fevers in Europe, Asia, Africa, and Australia; and occasionally in Rocky Mountain spotted fever). When disseminated hematogenously, the rickettsiae invade and damage endothelial cells, smooth muscle cells, or both, of small blood vessels at several locations. The basic lesion caused by rickettsiae is a vasculitis characterized by the presence of rickettsiae within the cytoplasm of endothelial and smooth muscle cells; endothelial swelling; perivascular infiltrate of mononuclear cells, plasma cells, and macrophages; thrombosis; microinfarcts; and occasionally vascular and perivascular necrosis. The character and evolution of the rash, the skin necrosis and gangrene, and the pathologic changes that may occur in the lung, myocardium, liver, kidney, and brain are attributed to the vasculitis. Direct cell injury by rickettsiae may cause an increase in capillary permeability with varying degrees of tissue edema, hemorrhage, and peripheral circulatory failure. Pathophysiologic abnormalities also may result from endotoxins released by rickettsiae, immune complex reactions, or cellular immune (hypersensitivity) reactions. Activation of the kallikrein-kinin system may account for the disseminated intravascular coagulopathy seen in severe rickettsial infections.

Clinically, the widespread vasculitis produces the classic triad of rickettsial diseases: fever, headache, and rash, with the exception of Q fever in which no rash occurs. The rash is initially macular or maculopapular; in severe cases, it progresses to petechiae, ecchymoses, and necrosis with infarction. Biopsy of early skin lesions reveals a typical vasculitis; special immunofluorescent staining techniques permit rickettsiae to be visualized in endothelial and other tissue cells.

Different species of rickettsiae cause varying pathophysiologic manifestations of disease. Severe vasculitis may occur with Rocky Mountain spotted fever and epidemic typhus. Myocarditis occurs more commonly with scrub typhus. Patients with Q fever present with respiratory symptoms similar to those of atypical pneumonia or influenza.

Epidemiology

Although rickettsioses differ in their hosts, vectors, and geographic sources (Table 53-1), some general statements can be made. With the exception of trench fever and louse-borne epidemic typhus, all rickettsial diseases are zoonoses, often occurring in limited geographic areas. Mammals and arthropods are natural hosts of most rickettsiae and they maintain a cycle that perpetuates the diseases. In addition, rickettsiae that cause spotted fevers and scrub typhus are maintained in succeeding generations of ticks and mites, respectively, by transovarian passage from infected arthropod to progeny. In contrast, the insect vector (body louse) of epidemic typhus dies of the infection. In each rickettsial life cycle, vertebrates serve as reservoirs. Rodents and, sometimes, dogs fulfill this role in rickettsialpox, murine typhus, scrub typhus, and spotted fever; appropriate arthropod or insect vectors become infected by ingesting blood or tissue from these animals. Humans are the reservoir for trench fever and louse-borne epidemic typhus. The flying squirrel has been identified as a natural reservoir for epidemic typhus in the eastern United States. The typical reservoirs of *C burnetii*, the agent of Q fever, are cows, sheep, and goats; ticks also harbor the infection.

In all rickettsial infections other than trench fever and louse-borne epidemic typhus, humans are only incidental, terminal hosts of infection. Except for Q fever, rickettsial infections may be transmitted to humans by infected insects (lice and fleas) or arachnids (ticks and mites). In contrast, *C burnetii* usually is transmitted to humans by the aerosolization of infected dusts or droplets. The airborne route, by which organisms gain entry through the conjunctiva or respiratory tract, is the most common mode of transmission of laboratory-acquired rickettsial infections.

Diagnosis

A febrile illness in a person exposed to ticks, lice, mites, fleas, flying squirrels, or livestock, or to aerosols from animal dusts in endemic areas, should raise the possibility of Rocky Mountain spotted fever, typhus, murine typhus, rickettsialpox, or Q fever. Failure of a physician to recognize rickettsial diseases such as Rocky Mountain spotted fever or typhus, and thus delay specific therapy, could lead to serious complications and even death. Delay in diagnosis and treatment is largely responsible for the unacceptably high mortality rate in Rocky Mountain spotted fever.

Diagnosis of rickettsioses can be confirmed by: microscopic identification by immunofluorescence of rickettsiae in biopsy specimens of skin or other tissue; isolation of rickettsial organisms from blood or tissue specimens; or demonstration of serum antibody titers to the causative rickettsia. With the exception of immunofluorescent techniques, which can demonstrate rickettsiae (especially *R rickettsii*) in cutaneous lesions as early as the fourth day of illness, these laboratory methods are not useful for diagnosis in the acute phase of illness. Isolation of rickettsiae involves inoculation of blood or tissue specimens into laboratory animals or tissue culture and at least 4-7 days of observation. The procedure is extremely hazardous for laboratory personnel, however, and, thus, should be attempted by only experienced technicians in a well-equipped reference laboratory. Serologic confirmation by standard tests usually is not possible until 10-14 days after the onset of illness. A fourfold rise in titer of antibody between paired acute and convalescent serum specimens generally is accepted as evidence of recent infection; occasionally, a single high titer is diagnostic if compatible with the clinical findings.

Traditionally, the Weil-Felix test has been used to identify rickettsial infections, as persons convalescing from certain rickettsial diseases produce serum agglutinins against the O antigen of the *Proteus* strains OX 19, OX 2, and OX K (Table 53-1). The test has major drawbacks. It is unreliable because agglutinations are often absent in cases of proven disease. Moreover, the test results are always negative in cases of Q fever, trench fever, and rickettsialpox, and are frequently negative or nondiagnostic in cases of Brill-Zinsser disease (recrudescent typhus). Furthermore, Weil-Felix reactions are nonspecific: positive reactions occur in pregnant patients, as well as in individuals with *Proteus* urinary tract infections, leptospirosis, borreliosis, or liver disease. Because strain-specific antigens and more sensitive tests—indirect fluorescent antibody, latex agglutination, indirect hemagglutination, microagglutination, complement fixation tests, and enzyme-linked immunosorbent assays (ELISA)—are available, the Weil-Felix test should not be used as the sole diagnostic test. Nevertheless, the Weil-Felix text remains a useful screening tool in the serodiagnosis of major rickettsial diseases, because it is commercially available and easy to perform.

The indirect fluorescent antibody test is used widely for most of the human rickettsioses. Like the ELISA, which is available mainly in research laboratories, it is highly sensitive and specific for diagnosis of specific rickettsial infections; both tests can be used to quantitate IgM and IgG responses, which is helpful in differentiating primary typhus infections from typhus vaccination or recrudescent typhus. Latex agglutination tests, which are also highly sensitive and specific, are employed by some reference laboratories for confirmation of Rocky Mountain spotted fever. The complement fixation test can be used for serodiagnosis of all rickettsial diseases except scrub typhus, for which the requirement that multiple strains of *R tsutsugamushi* be used makes the test impractical. The main limitation of the complement fixation test is its lack of sensitivity. Complement fixation is positive in less than one-half of cases clearly identified as Rocky Mountain spotted fever by other serologic tests. Reasons for false negative results include a slow rise in complement-fixation antibody titer and suppression of the antibody response by antibiotics.

The rickettsiae, with the exception of *C burnetii* and *R tsutsugamushi*, share antigens with other rickettsiae. Whenever possible, washed, purified, species-specific rickettsial antigens should be employed in serologic tests to minimize the possibility of cross-reacting antibodies.

Control

Effective treatment of the rickettsioses can be achieved with tetracycline or chloramphenicol; both of these antibiotics are rickettsiastatic, not rickettsiacidal. Chronic Q fever infections, such as endocarditis, require prolonged therapy. Chemoprophylaxis with tetracycline or chloramphenicol is not recommended, because administration of the drug before an immunologic response has developed will only delay the onset of disease, not prevent it. Prevention of rickettsial diseases requires control of the arthropod vectors and rodent reservoirs in endemic areas. In the case of murine typhus, it is important that flea control precede rat control. Prevention of spotted fever depends mainly upon personal protection by the use of repellents or special clothing to avoid tick infestation. At present, no vaccine for any rickettsial disease is commercially available in the United States.

Rocky Mountain Spotted Fever

Rocky Mountain spotted fever is the most severe and most common rickettsiosis in the United States, accounting for more than 90% of all cases of rickettsial diseases reported. *R rickettsii,* the etiologic agent, was first isolated and identified by Dr. Howard Taylor Ricketts, who was from the mountainous area of western Montana and Idaho; hence the name Rocky Mountain spotted fever. The term has become a misnomer as the disease is now widely distributed throughout most of the continental United States and, in fact, most cases occur in the southeastern United States. In 1982, less than 2% of cases were reported from the Rocky Mountain region, whereas 65% were reported from North Carolina, South Carolina, Virginia, Oklahoma, Tennessee, Georgia, and Maryland. Since 1959, the incidence of Rocky Mountain spotted fever increased steadily, from 0.11 cases per 100,000 to 0.52 cases per 100,000 (1,192 total cases) in 1981; it then dropped slightly to 0.42 cases per 100,000 (981 total cases) in 1982. The disease occurs most often in children and young adults, in males, and between mid-April and mid-September.

R rickettsii is transmitted to humans by various species of ixodid ticks: *Dermacentor variabilis* (dog tick) in the eastern states; *D andersoni* (wood tick) in the western states; and probably *Amblyomma americanum,* the Lone Star tick, in the southwestern states. Ticks become infected by feeding on infected animal hosts such as dogs and rodents, or by transovarial infection (passage of the organism from infected female ticks to their offspring). Thus, ticks may serve as both vectors and reservoirs for *R rickettsii.*

Humans usually acquire the infection through the bite of an infected tick or occasionally, by accidental self-inoculation by scratching or rubbing infectious tick feces into the skin. Laboratory personnel generally acquire the infection by inhalation of aerosolized, infected specimens. After an incubation period of 3-12 days, the illness begins abruptly with fever, severe headache, and myalgia. A rash, which is usually noticed 3-5 days after the onset of fever, but may appear earlier or even be absent, characteristically appears on the palms, soles, and other areas of the extremities as erythematous macules or maculopapules, and spreads centripetally to the trunk. The rash may become petechial and, in severe cases, it develops into large purpura and ecchymoses. The widespread vasculitis that characterizes this disease accounts for its multisystem manisfestations: gastrointestinal symptoms such as abdominal pain, nausea, vomiting, and diarrhea; ophthalmologic findings such as conjunctival suffusion and photophobia; neurologic problems such as headache, lethargy, meningismus, convulsions, and coma; cardiovascular abnormalities such as hypotension, arrhythmias, occasional heart failure, and shock; digital gangrene; hepatomegaly; pneumonitis; and renal failure. Activation of platelets and the kallikrein-kinin system may occur and result in thrombocytopenia and disseminated intravascular coagulation with subsequent hemorrhage. Facial and pedal edema secondary to capillary leakage usually develop. Clinical manifestations of untreated spotted fever generally last for 2 or more weeks; death due to renal failure and shock may occur at the end of the second week.

Treatment with tetracycline or chloramphenicol, which should be given early in the disease or not later than the sixth day of illness, generally is followed by prompt recovery. At present, however, the case fatality rate remains 3%-8%, largely due to a delay in diagnosis and administration of inappropriate therapy. It is essential, therefore, to consider the differential diagnosis of Rocky Mountain spotted fever in any patient with an acute febrile illness in which headache and myalgia are prominent, particularly if the illness occurs in a young person from an endemic or wooded area during the spring or summer. Generally, a presumptive diagnosis of spotted fever is based on clinical findings. A history of tick exposure is obtained in 60%-80% of patients. Headache is usually severe and frontal. A characteristic rash provides an important clue, but it may not be present, or it may be mistaken for measles, meningococcemia, viral exanthem, or drug eruption. After a clinical diagnosis of Rocky Mountain spotted fever has been established, prompt treatment with tetracycline or chloramphenicol should be initiated before confirmation by laboratory tests. Other antibiotics, such as the penicillins, cephalosporins, aminoglycosides, and erythromycin are ineffective against this disease. The clinician should be aware that patients who are treated very early in the course of the illness may experience a febrile relapse of spotted fever after discontinuation of the rickettsiastatic drug.

A clinical diagnosis can be confirmed by isolation and identification of the causative organism or by serologic tests. A highly specific (100%) and moderately sensitive (70%) procedure for early diagnosis involves the identification of *R rickettsii* in a biopsy specimen of a skin lesion by specific immunofluorescent techniques. By use of this method, the diagnosis of Rocky Mountain spotted fever can be confirmed about 4 hours after the biopsy specimen is taken, and as early as day 3-4 of illness, whereas diagnostic confirmation by isolation techniques or serologic tests cannot be made during the acute illness. The difficulty and hazards involved in the isolation of *R rickettsii* from patients preclude its general use as a diagnostic test.

For serologic confirmation of Rocky Mountain spotted fever, the CDC now requires the use of one of five specific tests that detect antibodies to *R rickettsii* antigens: indirect fluorescent antibody, indirect hemagglutination, latex agglutination, microagglutination, or complement fixation tests. Detectable antibodies usually appear by the end of the second or third week of illness. Early treatment with effective antibiotics may delay the increase in complement-fixation antibody titers although they may appear eventually. Overall, the indirect fluorescent antibody and latex agglutination tests, as well as the immunoglobulin class-specific ELISA, are the most sensitive, whereas the complement fixation is the least sensitive; all of the tests are highly specific. Each test can be used to differentiate diseases of the spotted fever group from those of the other rickettsial groups; thus, if type-specific, washed *R rickettsii* antigens are employed, Rocky Mountain spotted fever can be distinguished from other spotted fevers. Since 1981, the CDC has classified cases in which clinical manifestations are accompanied by a fourfold rise in Proteus OX 19 or OX 2 titer, or a single titer ≥1:320 obtained by the Weil-Felix test as "probable" cases. Although the *Proteus* test is widely available, it lacks specificity and reliability and its results should be confirmed by specific serologic tests.

At present, no vaccines are commercially available for prevention of Rocky Mountain spotted fever. The disease can be be prevented by eliminating tick infestations from dogs and by avoiding wooded, grassy areas in which infected ticks are prevalent. The use of insect repellents and special protective clothing, and frequent inspection of the skin and clothing for ticks, particularly in children, are other important measures. Careful removal of the tick, including the mouth parts that are embedded in the skin, may be accomplished by gentle traction with a pair of forceps. Care should be taken to avoid contaminating the fingers with potentially infected tick products. Touching a tick with a swab impregnated with gasoline, lighter fluid, or alcohol may loosen its attachment.

Rickettsialpox

Rickettsialpox is a mild illness characterized by the appearance of a cutaneous lesion or eschar at the site of a mite bite, which is followed by fever, headache, and a disseminated papulovesicular rash. The disease, caused by *R akari*, was first recognized in a housing development in New York City in 1946. Although the disease is reported to health authorities infrequently, epidemiologic investigations suggest that it may be common in cities.

The infection is transmitted to humans by the bite of a mite (*Allodermanyssus sanguineus*) that has fed on an infected house mouse. The primary lesion, which appears within 24–48 hours after the patient is bitten, is an erythematous papule which is usually asymptomatic. A central vesicle soon develops, which eventually dries, and leaves a brown or black eschar in the center of the indurated lesion. Lymph nodes that drain this area become enlarged. Nine to 14 days after the bite, systemic symptoms and fever appear; 2–3 days later, a sparse rash of erythematous, nonpuritic papules appears on the face, trunk, and extremities. These lesions usually develop a small central vesicle or pustule; hence the term rickettsialpox. The disease can be confused with a variety of illnesses, including other rickettsial diseases and chickenpox.

Serum antibody against *R akari* can be detected by complement fixation or indirect fluorescent antibody tests, but these antibodies cross-react with antibodies to *R rickettsii*. A specific serologic diagnosis of rickettsialpox can be made by first using a cross-absorption technique and then testing the absorbed sera by an immunofluorescent antibody test. Rickettsialpox is a nonfatal and usually mild illness, even if no therapy is given. Treatment with tetracycline or chloramphenicol, however, will shorten the duration of symptoms.

Epidemic Typhus and Brill–Zinsser Disease

Typhus (typhus fever, louse-borne typhus, epidemic typhus) caused by *R prowazekii* is a severe rickettsial disease that classically involves a human-body louse-human cycle of infection. It is now known, however, that extrahuman reservoirs of *R prowazekii* also exist; in the eastern United States, for example, natural infection of *R prowazekii* is widespread in the southern flying squirrel (*Glaucomys volans volans*) and its ectoparasites. Strains of rickettsiae isolated from flying squirrels are indistinguishable from the strains of *R prowazekii* that infect humans, when compared by serologic, biochemical, and DNA homology techniques.

Of all the rickettsioses, typhus is the only disease that occurs in explosive epidemics in humans. In the past, extensive epidemics have been associated with wars, famines, or other calamities that promote louse infection. Typhus remains a major communicable disease in some countries, particularly in the highlands of Africa, Central and South America, and Asia. In Europe and elsewhere, typhus persists as Brill-Zinsser disease. In the eastern United States, more than 30 indigenous human cases of squirrel-related acute typhus (sylvan typhus) were identified between 1977 and 1982.

Humans acquire epidemic typhus by rubbing infected feces deposited by the human body louse (*Pediculus humanus*) or the flying squirrel louse into abraded skin. Squirrel-acquired sylvan typhus also may be transmitted to humans by the bite of an infected flea or by aerosol transmission of infected squirrel louse feces. After an incubation period of 5-23 days (average 11 days), epidemic typhus begins with fever, headache, and myalgia. Conjunctivitis with photophobia often occurs. Five to 9 days after these symptom first occur, a generalized maculopapular rash appears in the axilla and spreads peripherally to the entire body, except for the face, palms, and soles. Complications involving the central nervous system, lungs, kidneys, and myocardium may develop; when no treatment is given, the illness generally lasts 2-3 weeks. The case fatality rate ranges from less than 10% to more than 40%. In contrast to classic epidemic typhus, squirrel-acquired sylvan typhus is milder, although life-threatening cases may occur. This disease is also characterized by fever and headache, but the rash may not be present. Cases of both louse-borne typhus and sylvan typhus occur most frequently during the cold months.

Diagnosis of epidemic or sylvan typhus can be confirmed by isolation of *R prowazekii* or by serodetection of antibodies to *R prowazekii* by several techniques (indirect fluorescent antibody, ELISA, complement fixation, and microagglutination). When a battery of tests is performed using ether-extracted, washed *R prowazekii* antigen, antibodies to epidemic typhus can be distinguished from those of other rickettsiae of either the typhus group or the spotted fever group. Tetracycline and chloramphenicol are effective treatments for typhus. Prevention is accomplished mainly by louse control and by avoiding flying squirrels and their ectoparasites. An inactivated rickettsial vaccine that provided effective protection against typhus is no longer available in the United States.

In 1910, Brill reported a mild typhuslike disease that Zinsser and others determined to be recurrent epidemic typhus fever. After the primary illness, the rickettsiae remain viable, probably within the reticuloendothelial system. Years later, when an individual's resistance to infection is diminished by stress or other factors, the rickettsiae may multiply and cause a relapse that is manifested by clinical illness and rickettsemia. Brill-Zinsser differs from primary epidemic typhus in several ways: the illness is milder, shorter in duration, and occurs occasionally without a rash; the specific antibody that appears in high titer after several days of recurrent illness is of the IgG class, not the IgM, which is the usual antibody response observed after the initial attack; and patients who are recovering from recurrent illness generally have low or negative titers to *Proteus* OX 19 antigens, whereas high titers develop after the primary attack. Diagnosis of Brill-Zinsser disease is confirmed by complement fixation or by immunoglobulin class-specific IgG (and absent IgM) IFA response. Tetracycline and chloramphenicol are effective treatments.

Murine Typhus

Murine (endemic) typhus, caused by *R typhi,* has a worldwide distribution, but its importance as a human disease probably is underestimated. Murine typhus is often unrecognized (and not reported) because it occurs sporadically and typically as a mild febrile illness with or without a characteristic rash. Although the incidence of this disease has declined gradually in the United States since 1950 as a result of effective rat control measures, a persistent endemic focus remains in the South Texas Rio Grande Valley area. In 1982, 45 cases of murine typhus were reported to the CDC. These cases occurred mainly in residential areas, in children and elderly persons from all socioeconomic classes.

A natural infection of rats, and occasionally of cats, opposums, or rabbits, *R typhi* is transmitted by feeding to the rat flea (*Xenopsylla cheopis*) and possibly to the cat flea (*Ctenocephalides felis*) in Texas. Rickettsiae multiply in the epithelium in the gut of the flea and are shed in the feces. Humans are infected, not via the flea bite, but by scratching and rubbing infected feces into the skin or by inhalation or conjunctival contamination with airborne rickettsiae. After an incubation period of 7-14 days, illness begins with fever, headache, nausea, and myalgia; 60%–80% of infected patients develop a maculopapular rash that usually originates on the trunk and may involve the abdomen, back, shoulders, arms, and thighs. In contrast to Rocky Mountain spotted fever, with which murine typhus is commonly confused, the palms or soles rarely are involved. Signs and symptoms caused by neurologic, pulmonary, and renal involvement may occur and, without treatment, the illness may last for 10-14 days. Fatalities are unusual, even in untreated cases.

Murine typhus can be distinguished from epidemic typhus by use of ether-treated, washed *R typhi* antigens and a combination of techniques, such as the complement fixation, microagglutination, and indirect fluorescent antibody tests. Differentiation between these two antigenically related rickettsiae also can be accomplished by the mouse-toxin neutralization test or by isolation of the organism in animals. Antimicrobial therapy with tetracycline or chloramphenicol should be initiated when the disease is suspected. Prevention of murine typhus depends on controlling the flea and rat populations.

Q Fever

Coxiella burnetii, the infectious agent of Q fever, differs sufficiently from other rickettsiae to be classified as a separate genus (*Coxiella*) in the family *Rickettsiaceae.* This organism is small enough to be filterable; stains variably by the Gram technique; has a DNA base composition different from that of the other rickettsiae; grows intracellularly within vacuoles or phagolysosomes rather than in the cytoplasm of host cells; possesses a broad range of glycolytic enzymes; has a developmental cycle consisting of a vegetative and spore-like differentiation (Figure 53-3); and is highly resistant to heat, cold, sunlight, drying, and chemicals. Unlike the other rickettsia, *C burnetii* displays host-controlled antigenic changes, referred to as phase variation, that resemble the rough-to-smooth variations of bacteria. The organisms exist under natural conditions (and in laboratory animals) only in phase I; when cultivated in chick embryos, they shift to phase II.

Since Q fever was first reported in 1937 in Australia, it has been recognized throughout the world. Results from serological surveys in the United States and elsewhere indicate that many more cases of Q fever occur each year than are recognized or reported. This is not surprising, as the disease resembles other respiratory illnesses, its diagnosis requires special tests, and, in most states, it is not a notifiable disease. *Coxiella* infections may be harbored naturally in domestic livestock (cattle, sheep, and goats), in wild animals, and in ticks; however, disease transmission from ticks to humans is uncommon. Instead, the disease usually is transmitted to humans in three ways: by airborne dissemination in aerosols or dust contaminated with organisms from birth tissues or excreta of infected animals; by processing of animal products (wool and hides); or by ingestion of infected raw milk or food. Outbreaks at medical research centers in California and Colorado have provided evidence that *C burnetii* infections can be acquired by persons who have only casual exposure to infectious aerosols. Because of occupational exposure, abbatoir workers, dairy and farm workers, veterinary personnel, woolsorters, tanners, and some laboratory research workers are at risk for acquiring Q fever infection.

Q fever usually becomes apparent 2–4 weeks after exposure to the causative agent. The severity of illness ranges from a subclinical infection to a febrile flulike illness accompanied by respiratory symptoms, severe headache, arthralgia, and myalgia. Pneumonia, resembling a viral or primary atypical pneumonia, occurs in about 50% of patients. Liver involvement, with hepatomegaly and abnormal results on liver function testing, is detected in at least two-thirds of patients. The characteristic rash of other rickettsial diseases does not occur. Usually, Q fever is a self-limited disease that has a mortality rate of less than 1%. Untreated illness generally lasts for 2–3 weeks, but fulminating pneumonia and chronic infections in the form of lipogranulomatous liver disease and endocarditis may complicate its course. To prevent these complications, all patients with acute Q fever should be treated with tetracycline or chloramphenicol.

Endocarditis may occur up to 20 years after acute Q fever and affect previously damaged aortic or mitral values or prosthetic valves. A diagnosis of Q fever endocarditis should be considered in all cases of culture-negative endocarditis. Prolonged therapy with tetracycline, usually in combination with a rickettsiacidal drug (lincomycin or trimethoprim/sulfamethoxazole), is required. Surgery for valve replacement is indicated in patients experiencing hemodynamic difficulties or persistent or relapsing infection. Even with proper treatment, the case fatality is high, ranging from 31% to 56%.

Attempts to isolate *C burnetii* in the laboratory are hazardous and should be avoided. The diagnosis of Q fever can be confirmed serologically by significant increases in complement fixation, microagglutination, or indirect fluorescent antibody levels to phase I or II antigens. Temporal differences in the production of these antibodies, with phase II antibodies appearing early and phase I antibodies appearing later in the course of infection, make it possible to differentiate acute infections from persistent or recrudescent infections. In general, elevated or rising titers of phase II antibody alone are characteristic of acute Q fever, and persistently elevated titers of phase I and II antibody are evidence of chronic Q fever, usually endocarditis. In contrast to other rickettsial diseases, patient reactions on the Weil-Felix test are negtive in Q fever.

An effective vaccine for Q fever is no longer available. New vaccines prepared from phase I *C burnetii* antigens have been developed and are being evaluated in humans. Until an effective vaccine is available, persons at risk should be monitored serologically at regular intervals and during respiratory or influenzalike illnesses. If Q fever is diagnosed, treatment should be instituted promptly to prevent the serious complications that can develop after Q fever.

References

Baca, O.G., Paretsky, D.: Q fever and *Coxiella burnetii:* A model for host-parasite interactions. *Microbiol Rev* 1983; 47:127-149.

Brettman, L.R., et al: Rickettsialpox: Report of an outbreak and a contemporary review. *Medicine* 1981; 60:363-372.

Clements, M.L., et al: Serodiagnosis of Rocky Mountain spotted fever: Comparison of IgM and IgG enzyme-linked immunosorbent assays and indirect fluorescent antibody test. *J Infect Dis* 1983; 148:876-880.

Centers for Disease Control: Rocky Mountain spotted fever—United States, 1982. *Morb Mortal Weekly Report* 1983; 32:229-232.

Duma, R.J., et al: Epidemic typhus in the United States associated with flying squirrels. *JAMA* 1981; 245:2318-2323.

McDade, J.E., et al: Evidence of *Rickettsia prowazekii* infections in the United States. *Am J Trop Med Hyg* 1980; 29:277-284.

Meikeljohn, G., et al: Cryptic epidemic of Q fever in a medical school. *J Infect Dis* 1981; 144:107-113.

Tobin, M.J., Cahill, N., Gearty, G.: Q fever endocarditis. *Am J Med* 1982; 72:396-400.

Weiss, E.: The biology of rickettsiae. *Ann Rev Microbiol* 1982; 36:345-370.

WHO Working Group on Rickettsial Diseases: Rickettsioses: A continuing disease problem. *Bull WHO* 1982; 60:157-164.

Woodward, T.E., et al: Prompt confirmation of Rocky Mountain spotted fever: Identification of *Rickettsia rickettsii* in cutaneous lesions. *J Infect Dis* 1976; 134:297-301.

54 *Chlamydia*

Yechiel Becker, PhD

General Concepts

The chlamydiae are prokaryotic, obligate intracellular parasites of eukaryotic cells. The agents are classified in the order Chlamydiales and family Chlamydiaceae. The genus consists of two species (*Chlamydia trachomatis* and *C psittaci*), which cause disease in humans and animals. Less than 10% homology exists between the DNA of members of the two species. The principal diseases affecting humans caused by *C trachomatis* are oculourogenital diseases such as trachoma, inclusion conjunctivitis, nongonococcal urethritis, epididymitis, proctitis, cervicitis, salpingitis, and lymphogranuloma venereum. *C psittaci* produces systemic infections, including psittacosis, ornithosis, and pneumonitis. The unusual developmental cycle of this organism, involving formation of elementary and reticulate bodies in cytoplasmic vesicles in host cells, contributes to its pathogenicity and protects against host defenses. In addition, some strains are widespread in nature and carried by many domestic animals, aiding transmission of the chlamydiae to humans.

Distinctive Properties

Developmental Cycle

The chlamydiae exist in nature in two forms: infectious particles called elementary bodies, which are released from infected cells and can be transmitted from one individual to another, and intracytoplasmic forms called reticulate bodies, which represent essential steps in the growth cycle of the agent (Figures 54-1 and 54-2). The elementary bodies, which are enveloped by a cell wall, contain a DNA genome with a molecular weight of 660×10^6 daltons (about one-quarter of the genetic information present in the DNA of *Escherichia coli*). In addition, the elementary bodies contain an RNA polymerase responsible for transcription when the elementary bodies enter the host cell and initiate their growth cycle. Ribosomes and ribosomal subunits also are present in the elementary bodies. Throughout the developmental cycle, the agent's DNA genome, proteins, and ribosomes are retained in membrane-bound prokaryotic cells (reticulate bodies) inside inclusion bodies or vacuoles in the cytoplasm of the infected eukaryotic cell. The reticulate bodies may increase in size and number relative to the stage in the growth cycle, but the prokaryotic type of cell division is preserved.

A complex series of events occurs during the developmental cycle of the chlamydiae. These and the effects on the host cell are summarized in Table 54-1. Studies on the growth cycle of *C trachomatis* and *C psittaci* in cell cultures in vitro (Figure 54-3) reveal that the infectious elementary bodies develop into noninfectious reticulate bodies (0.5-0.6 μm) after infection. There is an eclipse phase of about 20 hours during which no infectious particles can be found in the cells. The reticulate bodies divide by binary fission to form the new infectious elementary body progeny (0.25-0.3 μm) with maximal yields 36–50 hours after infection.

Antigens of Chlamydiae

Several distinct antigenic components have been recognized in *C trachomatis* and in *C psittaci*, some of which are group-specific and others of which are species-specific. Antigens have been extracted with deoxycholate, trypsin, and ether, but elementary bodies as well as reticulate bodies can serve as antigens.

A polysaccharide of large molecular weight that appears to be associated with the cell wall has been extracted from both chlamydial species and is the group-specific antigen. This antigen is heat-stable, fixes complement, and has been identified as a 2-keto-3-deoxyoctanoic acid. The species-specific antigen, common to all *C trachomatis* immunotypes but not to *C psittaci* strains, is a heat-labile protein. Certain *C trachomatis* strains share type-specific antigens that are subspecies determinants and are located on the surface of the elementary bodies. Fifteen separate immunotypes of *C trachomatis* have been identified by the microimmunofluorescence test. *C psittaci* includes many unidentified immunotypes. By using monoclonal antibodies to *C trachomatis* antigens, researchers have found that the genus-specific antigen is a heat-stable, pronase-resistant, periodate-sensitive liposaccharide, mol. wt. 10,000. The species-, subspecies-, and type-specific antigens are heat-labile, pronase-sensitive, and periodate-resistant proteins. The monoclonal antibodies that detected species and subspecies antigens reacted

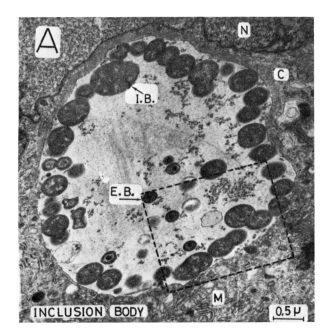

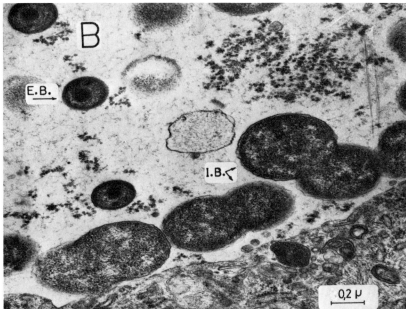

Figure 54-1 A, Electron micrograph of *C trachomatis* inclusion body in cytoplasm (C) of infected cell. Part of nucleus (N) and mitochondria (M) can also be seen. **B,** A section of inclusion body showing elementary bodies (EB) and reticulate (initial) bodies (IB) has been enlarged. Courtesy Becker, Y., unpublished data.

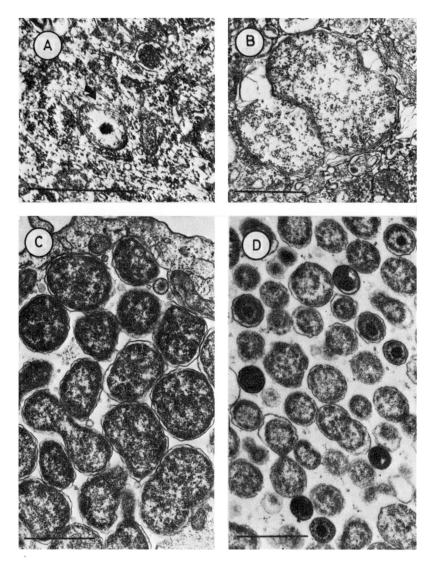

Figure 54-2 Uninhibited developmental cycle of *C psittaci* in L cells. Bar equals 1 μm. **A,** Two and one-half hours after infection. Arrow points to small chlamydial cell that has just begun to differentiate into a large cell (×36,000). **B,** Twelve hours after infection (×23,000). **C,** Twenty hours after infection (×23,000). **D,** Thirty hours after infection (×23,000). From Tribby, I.I.E., Friis, R.R., Moulder, J.W.: *J Infect Dis* 1973; 127:158.

predominantly with the 40K outer membrane protein. The citrachomatis gene that codes for the 19K antigen was cloned and expressed in *E coli*.

Toxin and Hemagglutinin

Toxic material was obtained from cells infected with *C trachomatis* strains which differ antigenically. A hemagglutinin was found in homogenates of *C trachomatis* elementary bodies, possibly the group-specific antigen similar to that of *C psittaci*.

Table 54-1   Summary of Various Stages in Developmental Cycle of Chlamydiae

Agent	*Host Cell*
Stage 1. Dormant phase. Elementary bodies have no or little metabolic activity, contain a DNA genome (600 genes), ribosomal subunits, cytoplasm, cell membrane, and cell wall.	Host cell can be in any phase of its growth cycle at infection.
Stage 2. Initiation of elementary body metabolism. Adsorption to host cell membrane. Organization of elementary body cell wall changes.	Duration: 0-12 hrs after infection. Cell phagocytizes elementary bodies. Cell forms vacuole around elementary body.
Elementary bodies utilize mitochondrial functions.	Mitochondria support elementary body development.
Elementary bodies adsorb to host cells, utilize glucose-6-phosphate as substrate.	Cellular enzyme in glucose metabolic pathway is utilized by elementary body.
DNA in elementary body changes its conformation from compact organization to loose arrangement, possibly for transcription process.	Host cell nucleic acid metabolism continues.
DNA-dependent RNA polymerase molecules, attached to DNA genome, are activated and transcribe the genome. At this stage, development of elementary body becomes sensitive to rifampin.	Nucleotides in host cell pool are available for parasite.
Protein synthesis with existing ribosomes begins.	
Low level of DNA synthesis in elementary body is detected since development is sensitive to 5×10^{-4} M hydroxyurea.	
Elementary bodies increase in mass due to above-mentioned process.	Cell responds to enlargement of elementary body by increasing size of vacuole in which agent develops.
Stage 3. Development of elementary body into reticulate body.	Duration: 12-35 hrs after infection.
Rate of DNA biosynthesis increases. DNA is replicated by a DNA-dependent DNA polymerase coded by chlamydial genome. Replication of DNA is semiconservative, with synthesis of short Okazakilike fragments on the DNA template.	
DNA synthesis accompanied by endogenous synthesis of thymidine, probably from deoxycytidine precursor. DNA synthesis is inhibited by folic acid analogs and hydroxyurea.	Host cell can supply some of the nucleotide precursors.
DNA-dependent RNA polymerase transcribes ribosomal genes of chlamydial DNA. Precursors of rRNA are synthesized and processed to yield two ribosomal RNA species, 1.1×10^6 and 0.55×10^6 daltons, respectively.	
rRNA species assemble into 50S and 30S ribosomal subunits by combining with ribosomal proteins synthesized according to genetic information in DNA.	Inhibition of protein synthesis on cytoplasmic polyribosomes by chloramphenicol.

Table 54-1 Summary of Various Stages in Developmental Cycle of Chlamydiae* (cont.)

Agent	*Host Cell*
Glucose 6-phosphate is catabolized by agent's enzymes. In *C. trachomatis* only, glycogen is synthesized and deposited in vacuole, where reticulate bodies develop.	
Syntheses of DNA, ribosomes, and proteins are coupled with the formation of new reticulate bodies by a binary fission-like process. At this stage the cytoplasmic vacuoles are filled with reticulate bodies.	The cytoplasmic vacuole containing the reticulate bodies is markedly enlarged. In *C. psittaci* the vacuole fills most of the cytoplasm. In *C. trachomatis* the vacuole is more rigid and defined.
Chlamydial enzymes are involved in the biosynthesis of the reticulate body–limiting membranes.	
Chlamydial enzymes synthesize cell walls of the reticulate bodies.	
Stage 4. Maturation of reticulate bodies, formation of elementary bodies.	Duration from 20–48 hrs after infection.
DNA synthesis in reticulate body is coupled with division of particles into two smaller daughter cells (pre-elementary bodies).	DNA synthesis in the nucleus affected.
Internal organization in pre-elementary body particles: The DNA genome is condensed in center of particle, with cell wall loosely arranged around particles.	Vacuole is disrupted and cell death is inevitable.
Cell wall synthesis leads to compact particle tightly attached to limiting membrane. At this stage, elementary bodies are formed and life cycle is completed. The elementary bodies are released from the cells.	

*From Becker, Y.: *Microbiol Rev* 1978; 42:299.

Pathogenesis

Spread of Agents

The spread of *C trachomatis* from person to person may cause trachoma, inclusion conjunctivitis, or lymphogranuloma venereum. *C psittaci* causes human pneumonitis, psittacosis, and feline and ovine pneumonitis. Transmission of *C trachomatis* from the urogenital tract to the eyes and vice versa occurs through contaminated fingers or towels, or by infection of newborns during passage through the birth canal. These diseases appear in epidemic form in populations with low standards of hygiene. On the other hand, the *C psittaci* agents are transmitted from infected birds or animals to humans through the respiratory tract, which may lead to epidemics of pneumonia in humans. Other strains of *C psittaci* can cause abortions in animals.

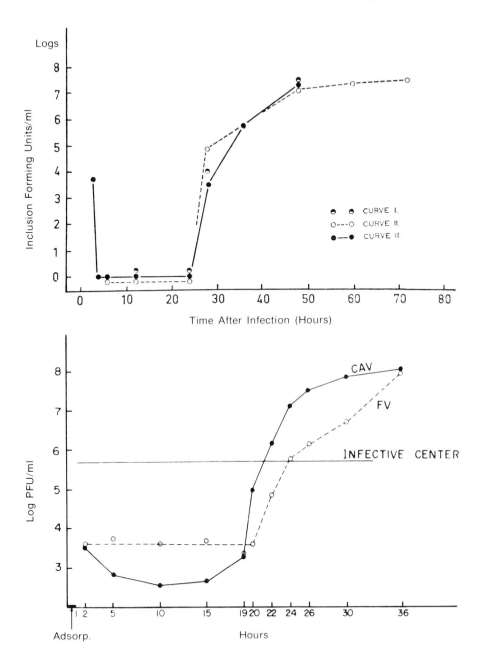

Figure 54-3. A, Three growth curve experiments carried out with the T'ang strain of trachoma in human amnion cell cultures. **B,** Growth of Cal 10 strain of meningopneumonitis virus in suspended culture of strain L mouse cells. FV, fluid virus; CAV, cell-associated virus. **A,** from Bernkopf H., Mashiah P: *J Immunol* 1962; 88:571. **B,** from Higashi, N., Tamura, A., Iwanaga, M.: *Ann NY Acad Sci* 1962; 98:104.

Clinical Manifestations

Diseases caused by chlamydial agents are summarized in Table 54-2.

Trachoma, an infection of the conjunctival epithelial cells by *C trachomatis,* causes subepithelial infiltration of lymphocytes leading to the development of follicles. The infected epithelial cells contain cytoplasmic inclusion bodies. As a result of damage to the epithelial cells, fibroblasts and blood vessels invade the infected area and a pannus forms; that is, the cornea becomes vascularized and clouded. The eyelids become scarred and malformed, causing trichiasis, an abnormal inward growth of the eyelashes. Continual scraping of the cornea by the eyelashes leads to corneal opacification.

Inclusion conjunctivitis, an eye disease occurring in children or adults that is milder than trachoma, also is caused by *C trachomatis.* It consists of a purulent conjunctivitis that heals spontaneously without scarring.

Sexually transmitted genital and rectal nongonococcal infections are caused by *C trachomatis.* The frequency of *C trachomatis* infections in men may equal or exceed the frequency of gonorrhea. Nongonoccocal urethritis, epididymitis, and proctitis in men can result from infection with *C trachomatis.* Superinfection of gonorrhea patients with *C trachomatis* also occurs. Acute salpingitis and cervicitis in young adult women can be caused by an infection with *C trachomatis* ascending from the cervix. A high rate of double genital tract infection by *C trachomatis* in women with gonorrhea has been reported.

Lymphogranuloma venereum is a venereal disease in humans caused by *C trachomatis* strains that differ from the agents of trachoma (see Table 54-2). The disease usually occurs in men and involves inguinal lymphadenopathy. Signs of infection with lymphogranuloma venereum appear within a few days after venereal exposure. The initial lesions, or vesicles, appear in the urogenital tract in men and women. If the disease does not heal spontaneously, regional lymph nodes become involved.

Polyarthritis in lambs, calves, and possibly humans also may be caused by *C trachomatis.*

C psittaci infects birds through the respiratory tract. Humans exposed to infected birds (dead or alive) may develop fever, a mild influenzalike disease, or toxic fulminating pneumonitis after an incubation period of 2-4 weeks.

Table 54-2 Human Diseases Caused by *Chlamydia**

Species	Serotypes	Disease
C trachomatis	A, B, Ba, C	Trachoma (hyperendemic) (a leading cause of blindness in humans)
	D, E, F, G, H, I, J, K	Inclusion conjunctivitis (adult and newborn); nongonococcal urethritis; cervicitis; salpingitis; proctitis, epididymitis, and pneumonia of newborns
	L-1, L-2, L-3	Lymphogranuloma venereum
C psittaci	Many unidentified	Psittacosis

*Modified from Schachter, J.: *N Engl J Med* 1978; 298:429.

Latent and inapparent infections of humans, animals, and birds are sometimes caused by chlamydial organisms. The agent of lymphogranuloma venereum, for example, may persist in infected humans for years before the disease becomes apparent. Individuals may develop acute trachoma many years after leaving areas endemic for trachoma.

Host Defenses

Nonspecific Responses

Infections with chlamydial agents evoke responses from the blood vessels (ocular trachoma), connective tissue (scars in *C trachomatis* infections), and lymphocytes. The mechanisms that trigger migration of lymphocytes or connective tissue to the site of infection are not known. Elevated temperature has been seen in pneumonitis infections caused by *C psittaci*.

In cultured cells, chlamydial agents induce the production of interferon. Because these agents are sensitive to interferon, their development is inhibited if the infected cells are treated with interferon.

Immune Response

All chlamydial infections induce synthesis of antibodies of the IgM, IgG, IgA, and IgE classes; however, patients who have recovered from these infections are not immune to reinfection. Secretions from trachomatous eyes contain specific antitrachoma IgG and IgA antibodies: nevertheless, the *C trachomatis* infection in the eye is not affected by their presence. Similar classes of antibodies can bind to *C trachomatis* elementary bodies under experimental conditions, but the infectivity of such elementary bodies in cultured cells is not affected. Addition of anti-γ-globulin to antibody-treated elementary bodies neutralizes their infectivity. The precise role of cell-mediated immunity is unknown. Most patients with *C trachomatis* infections have antibodies that react with *C trachomatis* proteins that have mol. wt. 67K, 60K, 40K, 19K, and 16K. The 40K protein is the major outer membrane protein and is the species-specific antigen.

Epidemiology

Trachoma is still prevalent in Africa and Asia, and sporadic cases occur all over the world. The disease flourishes in hot and dry areas, where there is a shortage of water and where conditions are poor. The agent is spread by flies, dirty towels, fingers, or cosmetic eye pencils. The initial infection usually occurs in childhood, and the active disease eventually appears (usually by 10–15 years of age). Trachoma may leave a residuum of permanent lesions that can lead to blindness.

The inclusion conjunctivitis agent resides in the genital tract, the cervix, and the urethra of adults. The eyes of newborns are infected during passage through the birth canal; the eyes of adults may become infected while swimming in unchlorinated pools. Lymphogranuloma venereum is a venereal disease that persists in the genital tract of infected persons. As *C trachomatis* is able to infect both the eyes and the urogenital tract, antitrachoma campaigns involving only ocular treatment are futile.

Psittacosis is carried by wild and domestic birds and by poultry. People handling birds can be infected by inhalation, possibly through the gastrointestinal tract, and through bite wounds. Psittacosis in humans has been considerably reduced by the agent's sensitivity to antibiotics.

Diagnosis

Most diseases caused by the chlamydiae can be diagnosed on the basis of their clinical manifestations. The damage to the eye caused by *C trachomatis* is typical, as are the vesicles in the infected urogenital tract. Diagnosis of pneumonitis requires laboratory testing.

Infections caused by *C trachomatis* can be identified microscopically in scrapings from the eyes or the urogenital tract. Inclusion bodies in scraped tissue cells are identified by iodine staining. To isolate the agent, cell homogenates that contain the chlamydial elementary bodies are centrifuged into the cultured cells (for example, irradiated McCoy cells). After incubation (Figure 54-4), typical cytoplasmic inclusions can be seen in the cells stained with Giemsa stain or iodine. Staining with iodine can distinguish between inclusion bodies of *C trachomatis* and *C psittaci,* as only *C trachomatis* inclusion bodies contain glycogen, which stains with iodine. Identification of each chlamydial agent also can be accomplished using specific immunofluorescent antibodies prepared against either *C trachomatis* or *C psittaci.* Homogenates, or exudates, of infected tissues also have been used to isolate the agent in the yolk sac of embryonated eggs.

Sera and tears from infected humans are used to detect anti-*Chlamydia* antibodies by the complement-fixation test or microimmunofluorescent test. The latter is useful for identifying specific serotypes of *C trachomatis;* however, even detection of anti-*C trachomatis* antibodies of the IgM class cannot be used diagnostically for genital infections because similar antibodies are found in *Chlamydia*-negative patients. Fluorescent monoclonal antibodies are used to stain *C trachomatis* EB in urethral and cervical exudates.

Control

Attempts to use *C trachomatis* vaccines for prophylaxis and treatment of trachoma have failed. The course of trachoma is more severe in immunized than in nonimmunized individuals. Specific antitrachoma antibodies fail to neutralize chlamydial elementary bodies in vivo.

Tetracycline and erythromycin are the antibiotics commonly used to treat chlamydial infections in humans. Penicillin is not effective against these infections.

Patients with trachoma have been treated effectively with erythromycin, rifampin, sulfonamides, chloramphenicol, and tetracyclines. Repeated cycles of long-acting sulfonamides have also been used in local or systemic treatment of trachoma infections. In trachoma patients with trichiasis, corrective surgery is necessary. Patients with inclusion conjunctivitis usually are not treated, because the infection is self-limiting and relatively mild.

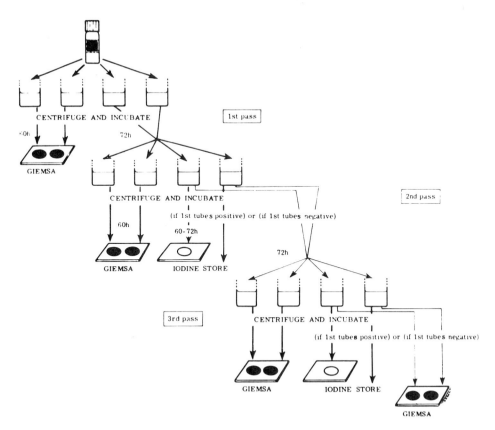

Figure 54-4. Standard three-passage technique of irradiated McCoy cell cultures for isolation of *Chlamydia*. From Darouger, S., Kinnison, J.R., Jones, B.R.: In: *Trachoma and related disorders caused by Chlamydial agents.* Nichols, R.L., (editor). Excerpta Medica International Congress Series No. 223. Amsterdam: Excerpta Medica, 1971, p. 66.

Tetracyclines or sulfonamides sometimes are effective in patients with lymphogranuloma venereum, but treatment does not always improve the patient's condition. Tetracycline treatment of gonorrhea in patients infected with gonococcus or *Chlamydia* is more effective against postgonococcal urethritis than is treatment with penicillin.

References

Becker, Y. *The agent of trachoma.* Monographs in Virology, Vol. 7. Basel: S. Karger, 1974.

Becker, Y.: The *Chlamydia:* molecular biology of procaryotic obligate parasites of eucaryocytes. *Microbiol Rev* 1978; 42:274-306.

Darouger, S., Kinnison, J.R., Jones, B.T.: Simplified irradiated McCoy cell culture for isolation of *Chlamydia.* In: *Trachoma and related disorders caused by chlamydial agents.* Nichols, R.L., (editor). Excerpta Medical Int. Congr. Series, No. 223. Amsterdam: Excerpta Medica, 1971.

Dhir, S.P., et al: Immunochemical studies on chlamydial group antigen (presence of a 2-keto-3-deoxy-carbohydrate as immunodominant group). *J Immunol* 1972; 109:116-122.

Hourihan, J.T., Rota, T.R., MacDonald, A.B.: Isolation and purification of a type-specific antigen from *Chlamydia trachomatis* propagated in cell culture utilizing molecular shift chromatography. *J Immunol* 1980; 124:2399-2404.

Paavonen, J.: Chlamydia infections. Microbiological, clinical and diagnostic aspects (review article). *Med Biol* 1979; 57:152-164.

Schachter, J.: Chlamydial infections (a review in three parts). *N Engl J Med* 1978; 298:428-435, 490-495, 540-549.

Schachter, J.: Chlamydiae: exotic and ubiquitous. *West J Med* 1980; 132:238-240.

Stephens, R.S., et al: Monoclonal antibodies to *C trachomatis:* Antibody specificity and antigen characterizations. *J Immunol* 1982; 128:1083-1089.

Wenman, W.M., Lovett, M.A.: Expression in *E coli* of *C trachomatis* antigen recognized during human infection. *Nature* 1982; 296:68-70.

Yong, E.C., et al.: Reticulate bodies as single antigen in *Chlamydia trachomatis* serology with microimmunofluorescence. *J Clin Microbiol* 1979; 10:351-356.

55 *Legionella pneumophila*

Albert Balows, PhD

General Concepts
Distinctive Properties
Pathogenesis
Host Defenses
Epidemiology
Diagnosis
Control

General Concepts

Legionella pneumophila is the genus and species designation proposed for the etiologic agent of a multisystem disease commonly referred to as "Legionnaires' disease," an appellation developed by the news media to identify the outbreak of an acute illness (primarily a pneumonia) associated with a convention held in Philadelphia in July and August 1976 for members of the Pennsylvania Department of the American Legion.

Almost 200 individuals were involved, each of them met the clinical and epidemiologic criteria of the disease, and 29 died. These criteria were onset between July 1 and August 18, 1976 of an illness consisting minimally of a cough and temperature of at least 38.9 C or of fever and radiologic evidence of pneumonia. An intensive epidemiologic and laboratory investigation was conducted; although a massive amount of clinical, epidemiologic, pathologic, and laboratory data was generated, the etiology of this strange disease eluded detection until McDade reexamined some of his earlier work and was ultimately successful in isolating the responsible microorganism. Subsequent studies indicated that the same or a strikingly similar organism was also responsible for several previously unsolved outbreaks as far back as 1965, and for sporadic cases as far back as 1947. The same organism has also been incriminated in an acute febrile nonpneumonic illness referred to as Pontiac fever. (One report suggests that Pontiac fever may be a hypersensitivity pneumonitis to free-living amebae, coupled with a mild infection with *L pneumophila*).

L pneumophila is a unique and previously unrecognized bacterium. The guanine plus cytosine (G + C) content of the chromosomal DNA of this organism is 39%, and the genome size is estimated at 2.5×10^9 daltons. These figures are well within the ranges established for bacteria and tend to exclude *Rickettsia, Mycoplasma,* and *Chlamydia.* In an effort to classify this organism, DNA hybridization studies have been conducted on many different gram-negative mesophilic bacteria. The DNA-relatedness data (essentially negative for all known genera and species tested and 80% or more related for 13 of the original isolates of *L pneumophila*) and data on the cellular fatty acid composition, antigenic composition, growth requirements, peculiar morphologic and growth patterns, and biochemical reactions indicate that this bacterium is a previously unclassified genus and species.

Although the organism is novel, the disease, which is peculiar in many respects, is not clinically distinctive; understandably, the physician is often not able to make a diagnosis without supporting or discriminatory serologic, microbiologic, and possibly pathologic data. In the early and late stages of the disease, the symptoms and clinical impressions are indeterminant and may be readily mistaken for viral, chlamydial or mycoplasmal pneumonia. Pneumonia caused by *Mycoplasma pneumoniae* and influenza are much more prevalent; therefore, the physician is urged to rely on a decision analysis approach and use the predictive value of the positive in making a diagnosis.

From the outbreak in Philadelphia in July 1976 through the end of 1978, over 1000 cases of Legionnaires' disease (legionellosis) have been reported in outbreaks and as sporadic illnesses. This and other surveillance activities suggest that between 1%–4% of all previously undiagnosed cases of pneumonia may be caused by *L pneumophila*, or about 45,000 cases and about 6000 deaths per year in the United States. Failure to isolate and identify the organism readily, the nondiscriminatory clinical picture, and incomplete knowledge of the pathogenesis, mode of acquisition (droplets from contaminated water sources), host-parasite interaction, therapy (usually erythromycin), prevention, and control are major problems that have been given wide attention. The possibility that this new organism may reveal new vistas in terms of "new" bacterial agents for "old" diseases is a challenging and to some extent frightening prospect that appears to be realized with increasing frequency.

Distinctive Properties

L pneumophila is a fastidious organism. It was isolated from guinea pigs injected with homogenized lung tissue taken at autopsy from a victim of the Philadelphia outbreak. Guinea pig spleen and liver were injected into the yolk sacs of embryonated hens' eggs; Gimenez stains of guinea pig tissue and harvested yolk sacs showed pleomorphic rod-shaped microorganisms—presumably a bacterium. Attempts to cultivate the yolk sac material on routine bacteriologic media were finally successful when Mueller-Hinton agar base supplemented with 1% hemoglobin and 1% IsoVitaleX was used. Subsequently, other media formulations were developed, including a charcoal yeast extract (CYE) agar, Mueller-Hinton agar base supplemented with L-cysteine HCl and soluble ferric pyrophosphate, and, more recently, a buffered CYE agar with and without α-ketoglutarate. This organism has not been cultivated on any medium that does not contain iron and L-cysteine or L-glutathione, which reportedly can substitute for cysteine.

The following outline presents the salient growth requirements, growth and staining characteristics, and biochemical reactions useful in bacteriologic identification of *L pneumophila*.

Growth, Morphologic, and Biochemical Characteristics of *Legionella pneumophila*

A. *Growth Media for Primary Isolation*
   1. Mueller-Hinton agar base supplemented with 1% hemoglobin and 1% IsoVitaleX.
   2. Mueller-Hinton agar base plus L-cysteine HCl · H_2O (0.4 g/L) and ferric pyrophosphate, soluble, or Fe NO_3 · 9 H_2O (0.25 g/L).
   3. Charcoal yeast-extract agar (CYE)
Yeast-extract (Difco)	10.0 g
Activated charcoal (Norit A)	1.5 g
L-cysteine HCl · H_2O	0.4 g
Ferric pyrophosphate, soluble, or Fe No_3 · 9 H_2O	0.25 g
Agar	17.0 g
Distilled H_2O	1.0 L
   4. The pH of all media is critical; adjust to pH 6.9 by adding 1.0 N KOH.
   5. Incubate at 35 C. Better growth in candle extinction jar or 2.5% CO_2. Will grow at 30 C but not as well. Grows slowly at 25 C and rather well at 42 C on CYE; no growth in anaerobic environment.
B. *Colony and Microscopic Morphology*
   1. Small, pinpoint colonies at 3 days; after 5-7 days, isolated colonies are 3-4 mm in diameter, convex, circular, with an entire edge, and have a gray, glistening appearance.
   2. Areas of confluent growth appear moist, and a brown soluble pigment is observed within 3-4 days on a clear medium such as described in A-2.
   3. With ultraviolet light (366 nm), dull-yellow fluorescence of growth and surrounding medium is seen.
   4. Gram-negative bacilli (leave safranin on slide 2 min. for better staining) 0.5-0.7 μm wide and 2-20 μm long (filamentous forms are seen in culture but seldom in tissue).
   5. Fresh isolates often appear vacuolated and stain with Sudan black B as used in the fat staining technique.
   6. Organisms are motile, and flagella can be demonstrated by modified Liefson flagella stain.
C. *Biochemical Reactions*
   1. No growth or acid production observed in commonly used carbohydrate utilization media
   2. Urease-negative on Christensen's urea agar slants
   3. Gelatin digestion: positive after 48-72 hrs with strips of Kodak Plus-X film or heavy inoculum in API gelatin cuplet
   4. Nitrate reduction: negative after 7 days' incubation

5. Oxidase production: weakly positive in 10 sec with Kovac's method; some cultures negative
6. Catalase production: strongly positive with 72 hour cultures on CYE agar
7. β-lactamase production: positive
8. Hippurate hydrolysis: positive

This bacterium is a gram-negative organism the cell wall of which typically is composed of diaminopamelic acid, but with a high cross-linkage, small amounts of 2-keto-3-deoxyoctonate, and chemically detectable peptidoglycan, although initial electron microscopy failed to show an observable peptidoglycan layer (Figure 55-1). Analysis of cellular extracts by gas-liquid chromatography does not yield the fatty acids characteristic of lipid A of classical gram-negative endotoxin. Characterization of extractable antigens of *L pneumophila* has yielded lipid-protein-carbohydrate complexes and a possible protein antigen obtained by extraction with dilute hydrochloric acid. Some of these antigens have been shown to be nontoxic and to elicit production of protective antibodies in laboratory animals.

Immunofluorescent studies (with strain-specific antibody conjugated with fluorescein isothiocyanate [FITC]) have produced conjugates that are specific in identifying cultures and in detecting the presence of *L pneumophila* or other species of *Legionella* in tissue sections, tissue scrapings, pleural fluid, and respiratory tract secretions (sputum and transtracheal aspirations). These studies therefore provide a useful rapid diagnostic aid in selected instances (Figure 55-2). In additional direct fluorescent antibody work, eight distinct serogroups were identified among the cultures of *L pneumophila* in the collection at the CDC. All eight recognized serogroups have been involved in human disease. It is likely that other serogroups will be found; 23 other *Legionella* species have been recognized,; as of this writing, 9 named species have been implicated in human disease. It is also probable that other genera in time will be identified and placed in the now accepted family designation, *Legionellaceae*.

Results of gas-liquid chromatography studies of over 100 isolates of *L pneumophila* reinforce previous findings that the cellular fatty acid compositions of strains within the species are essentially identical and that the *L pneumophila* isolates analyzed differ from other gram-negative bacteria in that they contain more than 80% branched-chain fatty acids. Furthermore, although the branched-chain fatty acid profiles of all isolates studied may show some quantitative differences, they are qualitatively so similar that an unknown gram-negative bacillus can be identified presumptively as *L pneumophila* with gas-liquid chromatography on the same day that a pure culture is obtained.

Several species of *Legionella* produce one or more hemolysins in vitro when grown on guinea pig, sheep, or dog blood agar plates, and 4-day-old cultures growing on a clear agar medium produce a brown diffusible pigment. These cultures show a dull-yellow fluorescence under a 366 nm ultraviolet light. Reports suggest that the brown pigment produced when the organism is grown on a medium containing tyrosine or phenylalanine is melanin; a lecithinaselike activity also has been suggested. These suggestions are based on preliminary observations; proof is lacking that melanin and lecithinase are indeed the metabolic end products or that they exhibit any in vivo

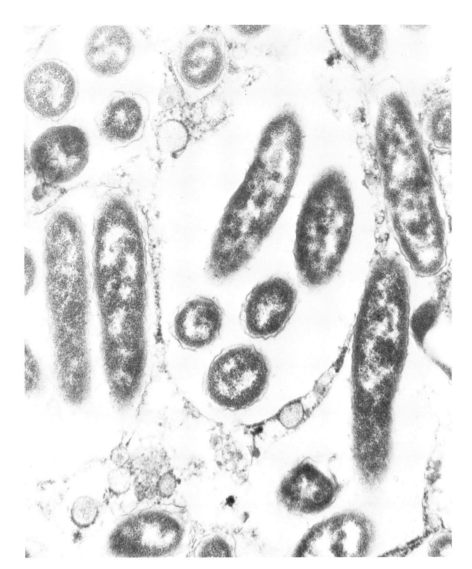

Figure 55-1 Electron micrograph of *L pneumophila* in lung tissue of infected animal. (Courtesy F.M. Chandler, Centers for Disease Control.)

toxicity. At this point, no evidence indicates production of a typical endotoxin; however the production or elaboration of other toxins (cytolytic exotoxin, phospholipase C, and small peptides that destroy monocytes) and of substances with toxinlike activity have been reported. *L pneumophila* cells are able to survive phagosomal engulfment and to multiply within the phagosome and ultimately destroy the macrophage, releasing several hundred bacterial cells, which repeat the process. Similarly, *L pneumophila* multiplies within human peripheral blood monocytes; how this sequence of intracellular events is orchestrated by legionellae remains to be determined.

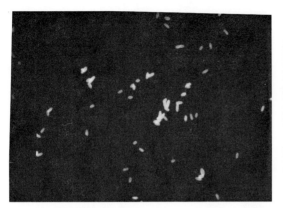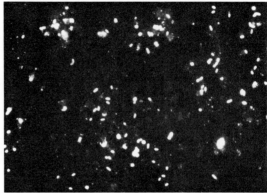

Figure 55-2 Fluorescent staining of *L pneumophila* with subgroup 1 antiserum (×1480). Left, Cells grown in culture. Right, Cells in lung scraping. (Courtesy R. McKinney.)

Pathogenesis

Early clinical manifestations of pulmonary or systemic legionellosis are headache, malaise, and myalgia, accompanied by an often dramatic temperature rise within 24 hours or less, followed by chills or rigor. A nonproductive cough is common, and about 50% of the patients produce mucoid bronchial secretions (frank purulent or mucopurulent sputum is relatively uncommon, but may provide an excellent specimen for diagnosis by direct fluorescent antibody technique). Diarrhea or abdominal pain or both are fairly common symptoms that may precede the organizing pneumonia. Chest roentgenograms usually indicate patchy infiltrates, which may progress to extensive nodular consolidation involving one or both lungs. About 25% of patients may have neurologic findings such as confusion, delirium, and occasionally ataxia.

The pneumonia is best described as a bronchopneumonia that is frequently confluent and may resemble lobar pneumonia. Complete autopsies reveal that the only consistent pathologic findings are in the lungs; extrapulmonary involvement has been demonstrated histologically. The pathology is that of an acute, purulent, fibrinous, lobar pneumonia; the alveolar spaces contain large amounts of fibrin and numerous macrophages and neutrophils. Occasionally, this exudate displays excessive necrosis; one or two observers have reported cavity formation. Nodular infiltrates have been noted often with pleural involvement in disease caused by *L micdadei*. The extent of inflammatory cell necrosis varies, so that an intact lung parenchyma may accompany an extensively necrotic inflammatory exudate. Many patients also show clinical or laboratory signs of moderate-to-severe impaired renal function, mental confusion, obtundation, and delerium. Death is usually preceded by shock or respiratory failure. In spite of the acute and occasionally fulminant course of this disease, it is difficult to diagnose on a clinical basis; however, the diagnosis should be suspected in a middle-aged or older man with a history of cigarette smoking and moderate or greater alcohol consumption, whose early stages of illness include diarrhea, rapid elevation of fever, myalgia, nonproductive cough, and chest roentgenograms showing early infiltrates that rapidly progress to areas of consolidation. Patients with renal disease or a moderate-to-severe immunocompromised state are prime targets for nosocomial legionellosis. Hospital-incurred outbreaks of legionellosis have been reported throughout the world, and medical centers remain one of the major focal points for *Legionella* infections. *L pneumophila* has also been associated with a much less severe illness (Pontiac fever) characterized by a short incubation period (6–48 hours), fever, headache, myalgia, and dry cough but no clinical or radiographic evidence of pneumonia. This form has occurred in outbreaks and, presumably, as sporadic cases. In both instances, it appears to be a self-limiting disease, not associated with documented mortality. The outbreaks of Pontiac fever that have been studied in some detail suggest that this nonpneumonic usually occurs at the work site. Species other than *L pneumophila* may cause Pontiac fever.

All available evidence points to waterborne or airborne transmission of *Legionella* infections; serologic tests of the headquarters hotel employees in the Philadelphia outbreak indicated that 42% had titers ≥64 and 17% had titers ≥128 that might be considered a protective level of antibody resulting from previous (or continuous?) exposure to the organism at unknown times. There is no clear documentation of person-to-person spread. In these respects, legionellosis is similar to histoplasmosis—an airborne infection caused by an organism that exists in nature. The lungs are the target organ, but the disease ranges from inapparent infection to an acute, severe, and possibly fatal illness. No clear evidence of secondary transmission exists in either recognized form of the disease.

Host Defenses

Information on the type or extent of specific and nonspecific host defense mechanisms is still sparse. Both humans and experimental animals produce antibody, and preliminary evidence in animals and suggestive evidence in humans indicate that some of the antibody is protective. Additionally, the organism is subject to the bactericidal effect of complement; this bactericidal activity is enhanced when bacterial suspensions are exposed to specific antibody-containing sera, but it appears to be serogroup-specific. Several reports also indicate that opsonization by specific antibody enhances phagocytosis of legionellae by monocytes in the circulating blood.

The intraalveolar exudate of neutrophils and macrophages described in the histopathology of involved lung tissue indicates that an intense cellular interaction with the invading bacterium occurs, but the nature of this interaction remains to be elucidated. Further, the cellular infiltration of other organ systems in the absence of detectable microorganisms suggests a cellular defense mechanism, which may or may not be overwhelmed during the disease. Delayed hypersensitivity to legionellae can be induced in the sensitized guinea pig model, and blastogenic and migration-inhibition factor responses can be induced in vitro. It is not known if these demonstrations of cellular immunity are protective or are related to resistance to the microorganisms.

Epidemiology

More than 50 legionellosis outbreaks were investigated in the United States and abroad from August 1976 through 1983. In some, the disease was strongly associated with the central air conditioning systems; in others, aerosolized water in various forms (shower heads, nebulizers, cooling towers, whirlpool baths, drinking water, and waste water) were incriminated; and in one, an association with recent excavation was suggested. Outbreaks occurred in which no single focal source was identified, the common thread being that all victims were in a defined geographic area before or during a given outbreak. Sporadic cases have been reported in all of the United States and at least 50 additional countries representing six of the seven continents. Although sporadic cases seem to occur primarily in warmer months, cases have been reported throughout the year. Legionnaires' disease undoubtedly will continue to be diagnosed with increasing frequency as clinicians, microbiologists, and pathologists become aware of the disease and the means of identifying it. To date, the disease has not been reported in domestic or wild animals, but no appropriate serologic or other surveys have been conducted.

The epidemiologic evidence strongly supports the concept that legionellae exist in nature; extensive attempts to isolate the organism have been successful with selected environmental samples such as cooling tower water, water from central air conditioning condensing pans, shower heads, aerosol nebulizers, fresh water streams, lakes (including newly formed lakes from the eruptions of Mount St. Helens in 1980), and mud samples. Direct fluorescent antibody examination of homogenates of some soil insects and earthworms has revealed large numbers of positively fluorescing bacteria, suggesting that *L pneumophila* or antigenically related bacteria are widely dispersed. The existence of at least eight serogroups of *L pneumophila* and at least nine additional species, along with the variety of sources that have yielded positive cultures, lend support to the theory that *L pneumophila* and other legionellae are widely distributed in nature and represent just one of several groups of naturally occurring bacteria that "accidentally" produce disease in humans.

Diagnosis

Although cultural methods exist for diagnosing viral pneumonias, psittacosis, and atypical pneumonia caused by *Mycoplasma pneumoniae*, each disease is most commonly diagnosed by serologic test results obtained with paired sera; the laboratory diagnosis of Legionnaires' disease currently fits into this category. The indirect immunofluorescent antibody test on paired sera is currently the serologic test of choice. Serum specimens collected soon after onset of the disease and again about 3 weeks later that show a fourfold rise in titer to at least 128 provides a laboratory basis for diagnosis. The immunofluorescent antibody test is not without its problems: skill and experience are required to perform it and to read the results, and cross-reactions have been reported with other disease agents. A titer of ≥ 256 on a single serum is compatible with a diagnosis of legionellosis in a patient whose clinical history and physical findings are also consistent with the laboratory result.

A rapid and inexpensive microagglutination test (MAT) also has been developed and evaluated. A semiautomatable procedure has also been described. The MAT appears to have good specificity but, as is true with other agglutination tests, the MAT detects essentially IgM antibody; the test is a potentially useful diagnostic procedure, but requires standardization of reagents and procedure.

When applied to respiratory secretions (pleural fluid, sputum, or pulmonary biopsy material), the direct fluorescent antibody test has demonstrated remarkable specificity; the sensitivity of this direct visualization of the organism is good but not exceptional. This is because adequate specimens for testing are not readily available and because the organisms may be absent or present in too few numbers to be seen by the direct fluorescent antibody method.

Cultural methods have been successful on a limited basis for the reasons just mentioned. The feasibility of demonstrating the organism in blood cultures is consistent with techniques for diagnosing bacterial pneumonias, and reports of positive blood cultures are increasing. The development of charcoal yeast extract agar and subsequent improvements of this agar medium have greatly improved the isolation of legionellae from various clinical specimens. Data obtained with the ELISA indicate the test's capability of demonstrating the presence of group-specific antigens of *L pneumophila* and other species in urine collected during the initial stages of the disease, a valuable diagnostic technique. This approach may also be of value in testing sputum or transtrachial aspirates for antigens of *L pneumophila;* however, much additional work must be done and standardized reagents must be commercially available before ELISA becomes a routine diagnostic procedure for legionellosis.

Surgical or autopsy histopathologic sections of diseased lung and other tissues can be stained with a modified Dieterle's silver impregnation method to demonstrate the organism vividly but nonspecifically. This observation, when coupled with the microscopic pathology of the lung or other tissues, provides an aid to the diagnosis of legionellosis.

Control

The established widespread occurrence in nature of *L pneumophila*, the definition of 23 species, and the available incidence data on outbreaks and sporadic cases of legionellosis indicate that certain containment measures may be effective. Although supporting data are not available at present, apparently the most effective of these measures is the regular maintenance of central air conditioning or air-handling systems to assure effective air filtration, and the incorporation of suitable biocidal compounds into water cooling towers at frequent intervals, especially during warm months. Hyperchlorination of water supplies, especially in hospitals in which nosocomial *Legionella* infections have occurred, may be helpful. (The engineering service should be consulted first, as corrosion of the pipes may occur.) Preliminary data on the induction of serogroup-specific immunity in animal models injected with highly purified and nontoxic antigens point to possible development of a vaccine for human use; however, feasibility studies, including clear definition of the groups at risk, must be conducted before large-scale immunization programs are undertaken. Data also exist on the protection conferred to white mice passively injected with IgG from hyperimmunized goats and challenged by injection with viable organisms of the same serogroup.

Therapy for patients suspected of having legionellosis is supportive and specific. Careful surveillance and appraisal of the patients' pulmonary, renal, and circulatory systems allow the nature and degree of appropriate supportive measures to be determined. In some cases, oxygen supplementation is indicated; in others, vasoactive drugs and renal dialysis have prevented death. Specific antibiotic therapy generally cannot await laboratory results. Laboratory studies, including in vitro minimal inhibitory concentration tests and in vivo experiments in which infected guinea pigs and embryonated hens' eggs were treated with various antibiotics, have provided useful guidelines in selecting antibiotics for therapy. The organism appears to have varying degrees of in vitro susceptibility to all classes of antibiotics, with the notable exception of vancomycin. On the basis of available laboratory evidence and clinical experience, erythromycin is the antibiotic of choice; however, a combination of erythromycin and other antibiotics may be indicated by clinical and laboratory data.

Although *L pneumophila* is exquisitely susceptible to rifampin, this antibiotic has not been used extensively in treating patients with legionellosis because, historically, resistance to rifampin develops quickly in other bacteria; its use has not been recommended except in unusual situations, such as for patients with a confirmed diagnosis who fail to respond to erythromycin. The possible hepatotoxicity of rifampin—and to a much lesser degree of erythromycin—also must be taken into consideration. Prompt use of the proper dosage of erythromycin has been associated with the lowest fatality rates among patients who received one or more of various antibiotics. It has been noted that the survival rate among patients given a cephalosporin is significantly lower than among those treated with erythromycin or tetracycline. The contraindication to therapy with cephalosporin may be associated with the fact that *L pneumophila* produces a β-lactamase that is more active on certain cephalosporins than on penicillins. Sulfatrimethoprim may be a suitable therapy in patients in whom erythromycin is contraindicated, or in immunocompromised patients with an undiagnosed pneumonia.

Legionellosis is a prime example of a newly recognized form of pneumonia caused by a recently discovered bacterium; however, it is not a new disease in the strict sense, because evidence suggests that the bacterium was isolated from blood of patients with a febrile illness as far back as 1947. This situation dramatically illustrates the continuing need for communication between clinicians and clinical microbiologists, and for a positive attitude toward interdisciplinary collaboration in the diagnosis, treatment, and control of infectious diseases.

As mentioned previously, species other than *L pneumophila* have been associated with human disease, and nine additional species have now been named: *L bozemanii, L micdadei, L dumoffii, L gormanii, L longbeachae, L jordanis, L oakridgensis, L wadsworthii,* and *L feelei.* At least 12 additional distinct species also have been recognized, but are as yet unnamed. Like *L pneumophila,* the other species are fastidious and have essentially the same growth requirements, demonstrate similar reaction patterns, and appear to have similar natural habitats, mode of distribution, and disease potential in humans. These species differ in their abilities to produce soluble pigment, in the color of fluorescence of growth on agar, and in β-lactamase production and hippurate hydrolysis. All species are antigenically distinct, giving species-specific reactions with direct and indirect immunofluorescence test reagents. The fatty acid profiles as determined by gas-liquid chromatography are also species-distinctive, and the DNA-relatedness studies show clear differences among all species. The bulk of current information on legionellosis is derived from *L pneumophila,* and the full spectrum of illness associated with all legionellae, the host-parasite interactions, and mode of acquisition of illness are not known with certainty. Physicians and scientists both should investigate unexplained clinical manifestations that may be associated with infection by *Legionella* sp.

References

Balows, A., Fraser, D.W., (editors): Proceedings of the Symposium on Legionnaires' Disease. *Ann Intern Med* 1979; 90:491-713.

Balows, A., et al.: Legionellosis (Legionnaires' disease). In: *Diagnostic procedures for bacterial, mycotic, and parasitic diseases,* 6th ed. Balows, A., Hansler, W.J., Jr., (editors). Washington, D.C.: American Public Health Assn., 1981.

Balows, A., Brenner, D.J.: The genus *Legionella.* In: *The prokaryotes: a handbook on habitats, isolation and identification of bacteria.* Starr, M.P., et al., (editors). New York: Springer-Verlag, 1981.

Chandler, F.W., Hicklin, M.D., Blackmon, J.A.: Demonstration of the agent of Legionnaires' disease in tissue. *N Engl J Med* 1977; 297:1218-1220.

Cherry, W.B., et al.: Detection of Legionnaires' disease bacteria by direct immunofluorescent staining. *J Clin Microbiol* 1978; 8:329-338.

Edelstein, P.H., Meyer, R.D., Finegold, S.M.: Laboratory diagnosis of Legionnaires' disease. *Am Rev Resp Dis* 1980; 121:317-327.

Fraser, D.W., et al.: Legionnaires' disease: Description of an epidemic of pneumonia. *N Engl J Med* 1977; 297:1189-1197.

Kirby, B.D., et al.: Legionnaires' disease: report of sixty-five nosocomially acquired causes and review of the literature. *Medicine* 1980; 59:188-205.

McDade, J.E., et al.: Legionnaires' disease: Isolation of a bacterium and demonstration of its role in other respiratory diseases. *N Engl J Med* 1977; 297:1197-1203.

Thornsberry, C., Baker, C.N., Kirven, L.A.: In vitro activity of antimicrobial agents on Legionnaires' disease bacterium. *Antimicrob Agents Chemother* 1978; 13:78-80.

Thornsberry, C., et al., (editors): Legionella: *proceedings of the 2nd international symposium, 1984.* Washington, D.C.: American Society for Microbiology, 1984.

Winn, W.C., Jr., Myerowitz, R.L.: The pathology of the *Legionella* pneumonias. A review of 74 cases and the literature. *Hum Path* 1981; 12:401-422.

SECTION

 MYCOLOGY

Introduction

C. P. Davis, PhD

Johnny W. Peterson, PhD

Most fungi are harmless saprophytes; some, however, have economic importance as plant pathogens, and a few others infect animals as well as humans. Only about 50 of the approximately 100,000 recognized species of fungi can cause disease in humans. The common fungal diseases of healthy humans tend to be relatively benign. Life-threatening fungal diseases are not frequently encountered, although fungal disease is an increasing problem because of widespread use or misuse of antibacterial antibiotics, radiation, and immunosuppressive agents. Individuals with reduced defense mechanisms are more likely to contract opportunistic fungal infections such as candidiasis. Consequently, this group of microorganisms constitutes an important topic in medical microbiology.

Fungi are eukaryotes and as such have a nucleus enclosed by a nuclear membrane. Some aspects of their structure, including their cell walls, endoplasmic reticula, and mitochondria, closely resemble those of plant and animal cells and are substantially different from those of bacteria. There is evidence, however, that fungi evolved from bacteria. Host defenses are similar to those utilized against bacterial diseases, except that the role of circulating antibodies is not clear. Nonspecific immunity and cell-mediated immunity seem to be the most important means for humans to resist or eliminate fungal pathogens.

Superficial and systemic mycoses comprise the two major categories of fungal diseases. Fungi in the superficial mycoses category often cause the patient cosmetic problems, but these infections are seldom life threatening. Diseases caused by the majority of these fungi are usually controllable by topical agents. In contrast, systemic mycoses frequently cause more serious infections and are usually more difficult to treat.

This section begins with a general presentation of the biology of fungi, followed by two chapters that discuss the pathogenesis and host defenses in fungal infections. These chapters describe the interplay of host-parasite mechanisms. Subsequent chapters describe the two large groups of fungal infections: superficial mycoses and systemic mycoses. Fungal infections can be treated and prevented; the final chapter in this section discusses effective forms of treatment.

56 Structure, Growth, Physiology, Metabolism, and Taxonomy of Fungi

George S. Kobayashi, PhD

Gerald Medoff, MD

General Concepts

The science of mycology encompasses the study of a diverse group of eukaryotes called fungi, which have been recognized as a special class of living organisms since antiquity. Fungi exhibit diverse morphologies ranging from microscopic unicellular organisms to macroscopic mushrooms. The growth cycle of most fungi involves two phases—vegetative and reproductive. The orderly study of these organisms is scarcely 250 years old, and originated with the work of P. Antonio Michelli. He observed many groups of fungi and showed that under appropriate conditions of culture, the spores gave rise to the same species of fungi from which they originated.

Fungi have a major influence on the health and livelihood of people throughout the world. They cause widespread destruction of food and fabrics, are implicated in diseases of plants and animals, serve as the source of potent toxins, and produce some secondary metabolites that seem to be carcinogenic. Fungi are also beneficial to humans in many ways. They provide the industrial basis for production of organic acids, vitamins, antibiotics, and enzymes; they are also used as condiments and in the production of foods such as leavened bread, alcohol, cocoa, and various cheeses.

Structure

Historically, the fungi have been classified as plants and studied mainly by botanists and hobbyists. In fact, they are not plants but are a heterogeneous group of microorganisms characterized by the absence of chlorophyll. They have a well-defined nucleus enclosed by a nuclear membrane, organelles such as mitochondria, a membranous endoplasmic reticulum that ramifies throughout the cytoplasm, and ribosomes that are bound to the endoplasmic reticulum (Figure 56-1). The cell membrane enclosing this complex cytoplasm contains ergosterol, in addition to lipids and glycoproteins, unlike animal cell membranes, which contain cholesterol. Immediately adjacent to the fungal cell membrane is a rigid cell wall, the backbone of which is chitin or, in some primitive forms, cellulose. In some of the more primitive fungi, such as the gametes of aquatic forms, the cell wall may be absent; these cells exist, at least transiently, as protoplasts.

Fungi exhibit a wide diversity of morphologies, ranging from simple, microscopic, and unicellular yeasts to highly organized, multicellular, and macroscopic mushrooms. In comparison to cells of most bacteria, cells of fungi are extremely large, ranging from 2-7 μm at their smallest diameter.

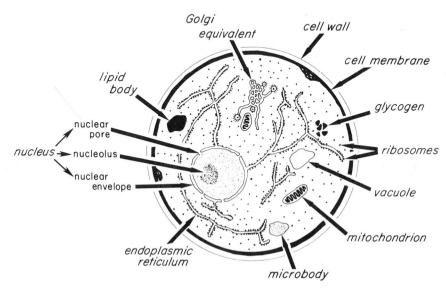

FIGURE 56-1 Diagram of the ultrastructure of a fungal cell. Features not included are flagella and associated kinetoplasts, found in aquatic Phycomycetes, and polysaccharide capsular material associated with some yeastlike fungi, *Cryptococcus neoformans*.

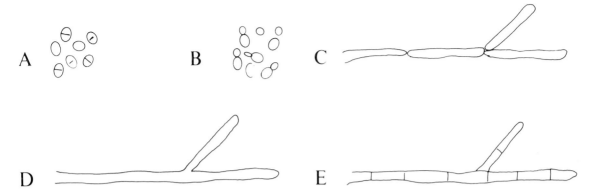

FIGURE 56-2 Diagram of vegetative morphology of fungi: **A,** Yeast (fission). **B,** Yeast (blastospore). **C,** Pseudohyphae. **D,** Coenocytic hyphae. **E,** Septate hyphae.

Growth Cycle

Vegetative Phase

Two phases—vegetative (assimilative) and reproductive (asexual or sexual)—characterize the growth cycle of most fungi. The vegetative phase of fungi is haploid, generally involving little or no structural or functional differentiation; the growth process involves simple nuclear division by mitosis. The gross appearance of fungi undergoing this process varies, depending on the unit structures involved in the division (Figure 56-2). In yeasts, which are unicellular ovoid-to-spherical cells, division is characterized by budding (blastospore formation) or by formation of a transverse septum (fission). Most fungi, however, exist as masses of intertwining filaments, **hyphae,** which typically branch and grow by apical extension and are called **molds.** The hyphae, which comprise the main body (**mycelia**), may be hollow and multinuclear (coenocytic) or compartmentalized (septate).

In some fungi, the morphology is not so clearly defined. Species of fungi belonging to the genus *Candida* may exist as oval cells, filamentous, elongated cells (pseudohyphae) linked in much the same fashion as sausages, or they may be filamentous and septate (true hyphae). Some fungi, in particular the agents of systemic disease (see Chapter 60), possess a phenotypic duality of cell shape that depends on environmental influences. Within tissue or at 37 C, these organisms exist as unicellular spherule or yeast fungi; in nature or at 25 C, they are multicellular molds. The term used to describe this changeable life form in fungi is **dimorphism.**

Reproductive Phase

In the reproductive phase, reproduction occurs by an asexual (mitotic) or sexual (conjugative) process. Spores, the result of these processes, are often highly differentiated and are characteristic for the various classes and subclasses of fungi. The reproductive phase may coincide with the vegetative phase, or it may occur late in the vegetative phase. It terminates with production of spores by an asexual process or a sexual process that involves **plasmogamy** (cytoplasmic fusion), **karyogamy** (formation of diploid nucleus), and meiosis (reduction division). The characteristic sexual structures formed by meiosis distinguish the taxonomic classes of some fungi.

Physiology and Metabolism

Because fungi lack chlorophyll, they are heterotropic and satisfy their energy requirements by living on dead or living plant and animal materials as saprobes or parasites. Most can be cultivated in **axenic** (free from other living organisms) **cultures** on defined media. Their nutritional requirements vary: a rich nitrogen source, growth factors, and sugar may be necessary for optimum growth; however, some fungi can grow on minimal media containing only ammonium (NH_4^+) or nitrate (NO_3^-), acetate ($H_3C_2OO^-$), and a few essential minerals.

In nature, fungi obtain nutrients by secreting enzymes that digest the tissues being parasitized. Fungi produce unique structures to accomplish this process. Some plant parasites produce specialized hyphae (**haustoria**), which penetrate the plant cell, obtain nutrients directly from its protoplasm, and are detrimental to the host. Other fungi form a symbiotic, or mutually beneficial, relationship between fungi and the roots of plants. This relationship, called **mycorrhiza,** is specific for fungi and plants. Some fungi obtain nutrients in a predatory manner, using specialized hyphal structures to attract and trap

Table 56-1   Classes and Distinctive Features of Fungi

Class	Distinctive Features	Examples
Mastigomycetes	Produces motile spores (zoospores)	*Allomyces macrogynus* *Blastocladiella emersonii*
Zygomycetes	Asexual reproduction by nonmotile spores (aplanospores), which develop sacs (sporangium); sexual reproduction by gametangial copulation; hyphae coenocytic (multinucleate)	*Mucor racemosus* *Rhizopus stolonifer* *Entomophthora muscae*
Ascomycetes	Products of sexual conjugation (ascospores) develop within a sac (ascus)	*Emmonsiella capsulata* *Neurospora crassa* *Saccharomyces cerevisiae* *Morels*
Basidiomycetes	Characteristic sporebearing structure (basidium) resulting from sexual conjugation; externally developed spores (basidiospores)	*Ustilago maydis* *Cryptococcus neoformans* *Mushrooms*
Deuteromycetes*	No sexual stage; spores of many types asexually produced and characteristic for genus	*Coccidioides immitis* *Alternaria* *Candida*

*This is a form (artificial) class, employed taxonomically only as a convenience to classify fungi in which no sexual phase has been observed. If such a stage is observed, the fungal isolate is transferred to its proper class and the nomenclature adjusted accordingly, although the original classification may remain in common use.

their prey, which they then invade. These fungi are collectively called **predacious fungi,** and they feed on nematodes, rotifers, and protozoa. Finally, an interesting nutritional relationship exists between fungi and algae. This symbiotic relationship results in the formation of lichens. These alga-fungus combinations are specific and environmentally important, not only to the organisms but ecologically. In nature, lichens grow on bare rocks and by chemical and physical action convert the rocks into soil. Despite the fact that lichens are composed of fungi and algae, they are classified separately from these two forms of life.

Taxonomy

Between 20,000 and 100,000 species of fungi have been described. They belong to the third major category of living organisms—the Protista. Taxonomic classification of fungi is based on mode of sexual reproduction, morphology, life cycle and, to some extent, physiology. Whereas mycological literature previously recognized four major classes of fungi (Phycomycetes, Ascomycetes, Basidiomycetes, and Deuteromycetes), current convention subdivides the heterogeneous class Phycomycetes into two major groups, creating five recognized classes of fungi. These are listed in Table 56-1 with a summary of the distinctive features that define each class.

References

Ainsworth, C.G.: *Introduction to the history of mycology.* London: Cambridge University Press, 1976.

Alexopoulos, C.J., Mims, C.W.: *Introductory mycology,* 3rd ed. New York: John Wiley and Sons, 1979.

Baum, G.L.: *The nematode-destroying fungi.* Guelph, Ontario: Canadian Biological Publication, 1977.

De Vroey, C.: Ecological and epidemiological aspects in dermatophytoses. *Zentralbl Bakteriol Mikrobiol Hyg [A]* 1984; 257:234-239.

Margulis, I.: *Origin of eukaryotic cells.* New Haven, Conn.: Yale University Press, 1970.

Moore-Landecker, E.: *Fundamentals of the fungi.* Englewood Cliffs, N.J.: Prentice-Hall, 1972.

Raper, J.R., Esser K.: The fungi. In: *The cell,* Vol. 4. Brachet, J., Mirsky, A.E. (editors). New York: Academic Press, 1964.

Smith, J.E., Berry, D.R. *The filamentous fungi,* Vol. 1. *Industrial mycology.* New York: John Wiley and Sons, 1975.

van den Ende, H.: *Sexual interactions in plants: the role of specific substances in sexual reproduction.* New York: Academic Press, 1976.

Wasson, R.G.: *Soma: divine mushroom of immortality.* New York: Harcourt Brace Jovanovich, 1968.

Webster, J.: *Introduction to fungi,* 2nd ed. London: Cambridge University Press, 1980.

57 Pathogenesis, Epidemiology, and Evolution of Fungi

Michael R. McGinnis, PhD

General Concepts
Pathogenesis
Epidemiology
Evolution of Fungi

General Concepts

Pathogenesis is the sequence of events in the development of a disease. In the disease process, a dynamic interaction occurs between host and pathogen. The pathogenicity of a fungus is a reflection of its ability to produce a disease state within a particular host. This ability to incite pathologic changes is expressed in terms of virulence. A **virulent** isolate is pathogenic, whereas an **avirulent** fungus lacks the ability to cause disease.

Epidemiology of the mycoses is concerned with the incidence, distribution, and control of fungal infections; it also includes those factors that regulate the presence or absence of infections and their etiologic agents. Except for dermatophyte and some yeast infections, fungal infections are not contagious. Most mycoses are sporadic and occur randomly throughout the world.

Evolution is a continuous, dynamic process that usually produces a complex organism from a simpler one. Because anatomic detail is limited in immature fungal reproductive structures, the concept that ontogeny recapitulates phylogeny is essentially useless in mycology. The ultimate goal of mycology is to achieve a clear understanding of the phylogenetic relationships among fungi.

Pathogenesis

Development of a fungal infection is affected by numerous factors, including the physiologic state of the host (age, pregnancy, stress), pathologic conditions (reticuloendothelial disease, cancer, defective cellular immunity, diabetes), prolonged chemotherapy (antimicrobic, immunosuppressive), medical and surgical procedures (catheters, surgery, transplantation of organs), and physical factors (radiation exposure, burns). These factors often predispose the host to aspergillosis, candidiasis, cryptococcosis, zygomycosis, and similar diseases. The host protects itself against virulent fungal pathogens by a series of barriers, including the skin and mucosal membranes, acid pH reaction, fatty acids, desiccation and desquamation properties of the skin, ciliary action of the upper respiratory tract, secretion of IgA in the upper respiratory tract and lower gastrointestinal tract, macrophages in the lungs, bile and acid pH reaction in the upper gastrointestinal tract, and the presence of a normal flora.

During the disease process (described in Chapters 59 and 60), fungi may cause any of three basic tissue responses. First, as seen in zygomycosis, the tissue response is **chronic inflammation,** which is characterized by fibrous tissue proliferation (scarring) and an accumulation of lymphocytes, histiocytes, and plasma cells. Second, **granulomatous inflammation** is typified by collections of modified histiocytes (epithelioid cells) surrounded by, or mixed with, primarily lymphocytes and plasma cells. The areas of inflammation contain giant cells resembling Langhan cells. This form of tissue reaction is often seen in blastomycosis, candidiasis (often with microabscess formation), and coccidioidomycosis (especially around spherules), cryptococcosis, histoplasmosis (often with caseation), mycetomas, and paracoccidioidomycosis. The third type of tissue response is **acute suppurative inflammation,** commonly seen in aspergillosis (with necrosis, blood vessel invasion, thrombosis, and infarction), blastomycosis, candidiasis, coccidioidomycosis (around arthroconidia), mycotic keratitis, histoplasmosis, mycetoma, sporotrichosis, and zygomycosis. Acute suppurative inflammation is marked by vascular congestion, exudation of plasma proteins, and the accumulation of polymorphonuclear leukocytes.

The actual pathogenic mechanisms of the fungal disease process have not been studied adequately. The mode of action of some fungi appears to be through production of mycotoxins, which are fungal metabolites that are toxic to the host. The presence of tissue necrosis in front of the advancing hyphae in some cases of aspergillosis indicates that some type of metabolite is probably involved. Study of *Aspergillus fumigatus* has confirmed that mycotoxins are produced by some isolates. Some of these mycotoxins are toxins resembling endotoxin, Asp-hemolysin (polypeptic endotoxins), and tremorgens. The toxin resembling endotoxin is a lipopolysaccharide-protein complex similar to bacterial endotoxins physicochemically, immunologically, and biologically. Asp-hemolysin, a hemolytic toxin consisting of a sugar-containing protein, causes lethal toxicity, hemolysis, and hemorrhagic lesions in animals. Tremorgenic mycotoxins, such as fumitremorgin A and B, may cause sustained tremors, convulsions, and death in experimental animals. Of special interest are fumitoxins A, B, C, and D, but especially A, which is apparently a steroid (molecular formula, $C_{31}H_{42}O_8$).

Medically important *Aspergillus* sp other than *A fumigatus* also may produce mycotoxins. Human deaths have been attributed to fatal hepatitis induced by aflatoxin. Some researchers believe that one mode of action of *Rhodotorula rubra* in fungemia is through a mycotoxin, but this hypothesis has not been confirmed by adequate investigations. Considerable information is beginning to accumulate regarding canditoxin, a simple protein produced by *Candida albicans*. Canditoxin has an amino acid composition similar to bacterial toxins such as those produced by *Clostridium botulinum*, *C tetani*, *C perfringens*, and *Staphylococcus aureus*. Animal studies show canditoxin is injurious to murine spleen lymphoid cells. Other mycotoxins have also been isolated from *C albicans*. Study of these and similar substances will greatly enhance understanding of some aspects of the pathogenesis of fungal infections.

Recent data suggest that hormonal factors may play an important role in diseases such as paracoccidioidomycosis where the male:female ratios in countries such as Colombia are approximately 48:1. Some hypothesize that sex hormones may affect the in vivo fungus. It has been shown that fungi such as *C albicans* and *Coccidioides immitis* may be influenced by mammalian hormones.

Epidemiology

Dermatophytes occasionally are transmitted from one individual to another by personal contacts, on combs, hairbrushes, furniture, and towels, resulting in small, restricted outbreaks of ringworm. Many instances are recorded in which *Microsporum audouinii* and *Trichophyton tonsurans* have caused epidemics of tinea capitis (ringworm of the scalp) in groups of children attending the same school. Tinea capitis also occurs in isolated families. Epidemics of tinea pedis (athlete's foot) and tinea cruris (jock itch) caused by *T mentagrophytes* occasionally are seen among individuals who serve on ships at sea and those who frequent gymnasiums. The yeast *C albicans* may also occasionally be contagious. It is part of the normal flora of the genitourinary tract and is passed at birth from mother to child. The organism is usually abundant in the mother, because vulvovaginitis is frequently associated with pregnancy. *C albicans* also may be sexually transmitted.

Age is a factor in some fungal infections. Once a child has reached puberty, a natural resistance to tinea capitis caused by fungi such as *M audouinii* apparently develops. Coccidioidomycosis, which is caused by *C immitis*, is much milder in early childhood. In contrast to coccidioidomycosis, disseminated or fatal histoplasmosis and blastomycosis tend to have higher incidence in children and older individuals. In major endemic areas for mycetomas, such as the Sudan, young adults are infected more frequently. This frequency is probably related to exposure and not age. Patients with paracoccidioidomycosis tend to be older adults. This disease frequently occurs in the subtropical forest areas of Mexico and Central and South America.

Sex and race often play a role in a few of the mycoses. Allergic reactions to *C immitis* occur much more frequently in white adult women than in any other group. Filipinos, black people, and pregnant women have a great frequency of severe coccidioidomycosis. Men typically have a higher incidence of chromoblastomycosis, sporotrichosis, mycetomas, blastomycosis, and histoplasmosis than do women. This difference is probably due to frequency of exposure rather than to a difference in susceptibility between men and women.

Occupation may play an important role in some mycoses. Individuals working with or near woody plant material, such as gardeners, farmers, and nursery workers, have a higher incidence of sporotrichosis. The etiologic agent, *Sporothrix schenckii*, normally is associated with woody plants and is introduced by trauma (splinters and thorns). Transient agricultural workers, and residents of some semiarid regions in North, Central, and South America, have a high incidence of coccidioidomycosis. The arthroconidia (arthrospores) are inhaled along with the dust that is typically abundant in these regions. Dark-skinned individuals tend to have more severe cases of this disease. Heavy-equipment operators and laborers working around soil enriched with avian fecal material, especially from chickens and starlings, may develop severe pulmonary histoplasmosis. Small epidemics have been associated with community cleanup events during which parks and similar areas are cleaned during the spring. These areas typically have a bird roost nearby. People who explore caves may develop histoplasmosis if *Histoplasma capsulatum* is present in the bat or bird dung that has accumulated there.

Skin testing has become a valuable tool for defining endemic areas of coccidioidomycosis and histoplasmosis. Based on skin test data and case reports, histoplasmosis in the United States occurs primarily along the Mississippi River Valley, Ohio River Valley, and various areas in the Appalachian Mountain region. In some regions, 80% or more of the population have a positive skin test. At least 500,000 new infections are estimated to occur yearly in the United States. Coccidioidomycosis is associated with the Lower Sonoran life zone, characterized by high summer temperatures, mild winters, and limited rainfall. In the endemic areas, 60%-90% of the skin-tested population are positive. At least 100,000 new infections are estimated to occur yearly in the United States. Unfortunately, a skin test antigen is not available for blastomycosis. Based on cases reported, the endemic area in the United States for *Blastomyces dermatitidis* is located in the Mississippi and Ohio River basins and the Central Atlantic states, especially Kentucky, North Carolina, Mississippi, Arkansas, and Tennessee. Both histoplasmosis and blastomycosis are worldwide diseases.

Geographic variation in some pathogenic fungi have been observed. The minus mating type or strain of *Ajellomyces capsulatus*, the sexual form of *H capsulatum*, is eight times more frequent than the plus mating type or strain found in clinical specimens. The A, B, C, and D serotypes of *Cryptococcus neoformans* vary from one region to another. Serotypes A and D are typically associated with pigeon droppings, whereas B and C are not. A significant antigenic variation appears in isolates of *H capsulatum* and *B dermatitidis*.

Except for yeasts such as *C albicans*, etiologic agents of the mycoses are normally associated with soil, plants, and similar substrates. Fungi that cause aspergillosis, chromoblastomycosis, phaeohyphomycosis, mycetomas, mycotic keratitis, and zygomycosis are usually associated with plant material, soil, or both. *C immitis* and *H capsulatum* var *capsulatum* normally occur in soil; *C immitis*, in alkaline soil; and *H capsulatum* var *capsulatum*, in soil enriched with avian or bat fecal material. *Cryptococcus neoformans* often is recovered from pigeon droppings, as well as from fruit juices and flowers. Many dermatophytes and lipophilic yeasts, such as *Malassezia furfur*, live and grow only on humans and lower animals. Some dermatophytes, such as *Microsporum gypseum*, grow naturally in soil. The natural habitats for the agents of blastomycosis, lobomycosis, and rhinosporidiosis are unknown.

Evolution of Fungi

The earth originated approximately 4.6×10^9 years ago, and the oldest known sediments were deposited about 1.2×10^9 years later. Life, in the form of bacteria and blue-green algae, first appeared nearly 3.1 to 3.3×10^9 years ago. From these early prokaryotic life forms, eukaryotic organisms probably evolved 1.3 to 1.5×10^9 years ago, with fungi first appearing about 8.0×10^8 to 1.0×10^9 years ago. Unfortunately, the fossil record does not contain numerous organisms whose size and morphology resemble the fungi known today (Figure 57-1). The true nature of the oldest fossil microorganisms is somewhat equivocal, because it has been shown recently that many artifacts intrude during the fossilization process. These artifacts primarily cause extreme variations in size and morphology of preserved cells.

New fungi evolve from genetically plastic groups but not normally from climax groups. Plastic groups are less specialized, genetically variable, heterogeneous assemblages of fungi that represent the parental lineage to the stable, specialized climax groups. As a result, the connecting links between groups of fungi do not usually survive, because nonsuccessful fungi disappear before they have the opportunity to become stable. Because the environment is concurrently changing, new niches are being created constantly. Thus, new genetically plastic groups of fungi are continuously arising to occupy these new niches.

Two theories based on comparative morphology have dominated mycologic thought concerning the origin and evolution of fungi. The first theory hypothesizes that the fungi arose from an ancestral flagellate and developed monophyletically into the present groups of fungi. A second theory postulates that the Chytridiomycetes and Zygomycetes evolved from unicellular algae and that the Ascomycetes arose from the red algae, eventually giving rise to the Basidiomycetes.

In light of available morphologic, biochemical, and fossil data, it appears that the fungi developed polyphyletically from flagellated or similar ancestors. The Chytridiomy-

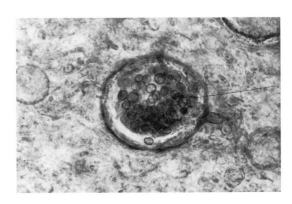

FIGURE 57-1 Fossil sporangium containing sporangiospores. Rhynie chert, Middle Devonian Period, Scotland.

cetes, which produce posterior uniflagellate cells, are apparently the most primitive fungi. These fungi and the Zygomycetes are morphologically and biochemically similar; some scientists suggest they did not originate from the Oomycetes, but developed parallel to them. Some mycologists find the proposal that the Zygomycetes gave rise to the Ascomycetes difficult to endorse. For these investigators, structural similarities support the theory that the Ascomycetes probably gave rise to the Basidiomycetes.

The Fungi Imperfecti, or Deuteromycetes, are excluded from phylogenetic schemes because most of them probably are asexual forms of Ascomycetes and, less commonly, of Basidiomycetes. Lichens also are not considered in discussions of the origin of fungi, because they represent a specialized growth relationship with algae. Because of the inadequate fossil record, it is often assumed that contemporary groups of fungi must have evolved from each other. It is important, however, to remember the limitations of the present day perspective when viewing events that occurred over evolutionary time.

References

Ainsworth, G.C., Sussman, A.S. (editors): *The fungi: an advanced treatise,* vol. 3. New York: Academic Press, 1968.

Ajello, L.: Comparative ecology of respiratory mycotic disease agents. *Bacteriol Rev* 1967; 31:6-24.

Hay, R.J.: Managing fungal infections. *Br J Hosp Med* 1984; 31:278-282.

Howard, D.H.: *Fungi pathogenic for humans and animals. Part B. Pathogenicity and detection: 1.* New York: Marcel Dekker, 1983.

Iwata, K. (editor): *Recent advances in medical and veterinary mycology.* Baltimore: University Park Press, 1977.

McGinnis, M.R.: *Laboratory handbook of medical mycology.* New York: Academic Press, 1980.

Ragan, M.A., Chapman, D.J.: *A biochemical phylogeny of the protists.* New York: Academic Press, 1978.

58 Host Defenses Against Fungi

Jim E. Cutler, PhD

General Concepts
Nonspecific Immunity
  Physical Factors
  Chemical Factors
  Acute Inflammatory Response—Phagocytic
    Cells

Normal Flora
Specific Acquired Immunity
  Antibody
  Cell-Mediated Immunity

General Concepts

Clinical observations and animal experimental studies have added to the understanding of host-fungal interactions. It is becoming recognized that host defense against fungal disease is multifactorial and may vary, depending on the etiologic agent. The mechanisms of resistance are not well defined in most instances, but various innate barriers and cell-mediated immune responses seem to be of primary importance. At this time, the role of antibody in resistance is uncertain. Clearly, debilitation of innate defenses and of cell-mediated immune responses can increase an individual's susceptibility to severe fungal disease from opportunistic agents such as *Cryptococcus neoformans* and species of *Candida* and *Aspergillus*, as well as from fungal pathogens such as *Histoplasma capsulatum* and *Coccidioides immitis*. The difficulty in gaining a complete understanding of the critical host defenses has been further complicated by many studies that show fungi may affect various host immune functions adversely. Although it is too early to evaluate the clinical importance of many of these experimental findings, investigators have demonstrated that fungi impair neutrophil function, induce IgE responses, and cause suppression of cell-mediated immune responses.

Host changes likely to be associated with increased susceptibility may be accidentally induced, as in traumatic injuries (such as burns or puncture wounds);

self-induced, as in chronic alcoholism; naturally occurring, as in diabetes mellitus, various congenital immune deficiencies, collagen diseases, lymphoreticular neoplastic disease, and other types of tumors; or iatrogenically induced by instrumentation (such as catheterization), surgical procedures (such as open heart surgery), or by use of cytotoxic drugs (as in an attempt to prevent graft rejection and to treat neoplastic disease), corticosteroid therapy, and long-term use of broad-spectrum antibiotics.

Nonspecific Immunity

A high degree of nonspecific immunity (or innate resistance) to most fungal diseases exists in healthy individuals before contact with fungal agents. These resistance factors are partly a reflection of the genetic constitution of humans and include physical, chemical, and cellular components; they are partly due to competing microorganisms that make up the normal flora found on body surfaces (Figure 58-1).

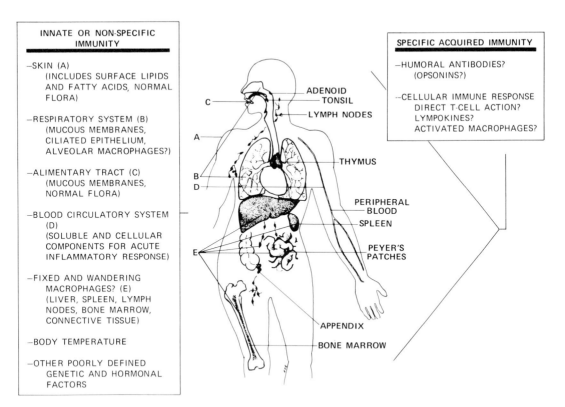

Figure 58-1 Summary of proposed host defenses against fungi. Some factors listed are important in resistance to most fungi; others are known to affect only a few fungal agents. Host defenses followed by a question mark are factors believed to be important for which definitive data are lacking.

Physical Factors

Physical factors important in resistance to fungal diseases are body temperature, skin, mucous membranes, and ciliated epithelia. Normal body temperature is high enough to prevent most fungi in the environment from becoming pathogens. This form of natural defense also may partially explain restriction of certain mycotic agents, such as dermatophytes (agents of ringworm) and *Sporothrix schenckii* (the cause of sporotrichosis), to cooler areas of the body. Resistance to fungal diseases like simple cutaneous candidiasis, dermatophytoses, sporotrichosis, and mycetoma depends to a large extent on the integrity of intact skin. The ciliated mucous membranes of the respiratory system continuously prevent fungi from gaining access to other body tissues. Damage to these membranes may allow infection and invasion by several species of fungi.

Chemical Factors

Chemical factors that aid resistance to fungal diseases are poorly defined. Knowledge of these substances is based primarily on circumstantial evidence at the clinical level and in vitro observations at the experimental level. Hormonally associated increases in lipid and fatty acid content on the skin occurring at puberty have been correlated with increased resistance to tinea capitis caused by the dermatophyte *Microsporum audouini,* although pubescent changes are not the sole factors in resistance. Substances in serum, cerebrospinal fluid, and saliva may limit growth of *Cryptococcus neoformans,* and basic peptides in body fluids have been shown to inhibit *C albicans.*

Results of clinical and experimental studies indicate that *C albicans, C neoformans, Aspergillus fumigatus,* and *C immitis* activate the alternative pathway of the complement cascade. Because of the polysaccharide nature of fungal cell walls, it is expected that all medically important fungi activate complement. Such activation may be important in defense against some mycoses; a positive correlation has been demonstrated between animals deficient in late-acting complement components (C3–C9) and increased susceptibility to fungi such as *C neoformans* and *C albicans.* Assuming that phagocytic cells are important in resistance to fungi, complement activation may play a role by provoking an acute inflammatory response on generation of complement fragments C3a and C5a, and by coating the fungal elements with opsonic fragments C3b and C3d for ingestion by phagocytic cells (Figure 58-2).

Acute Inflammatory Response—Phagocytic Cells

Over the past several years, data have accumulated indicating that the acute inflammatory response to fungal invasion has beneficial aspects for the host. When strains of dermatophytes that usually are associated with soil (geophilic) or animals (zoophilic) infect humans, the lesions tend to be intensely suppurative and the individual may quickly recover. On the other hand, dermatophytes passed primarily from person to person (anthropophilic) often produce lesions that are less inflamed, and the disease tends to be chronic; however, many cases may be acute, suggesting host factors play a role. Similarly, acute inflammation typifies the tissue responses in an animal that recovers from infection with an unencapsulated strain of *C neoformans,* whereas little if any tissue

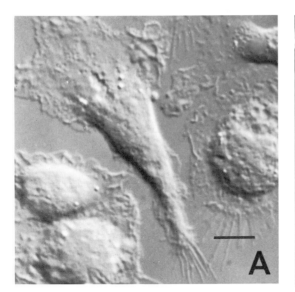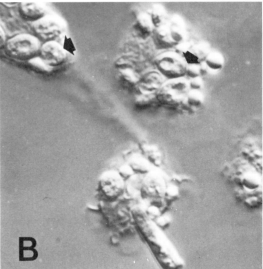

Figure 58-2   The ability of phagocytes to ingest fungal cells is illustrated by these photomicrographs using interference contrast optics. **A,** Mouse macrophages and neutrophils that adhered to and spread onto cover glass. **B,** When yeasts and hyphal fragments of *Candida albicans* are added and incubated at 37 C, phagocytic cells readily ingest fungal particles (arrows). Ingestion of these particles occurs best in presence of serum containing antibodies specific for *C albicans* or serum containing a functional alternative complement pathway. (Bar = 5 μm.)

response may occur in animals that succumb to infection with encapsulated strains (Figure 58-3). Although the capsular material is antiphagocytic, some investigators speculate that the infecting unit from nature is an unencapsulated organism, and that phagocytic cells usually prevent clinically apparent cryptococcosis. Individuals who develop disease may have defective phagocytic cells, or may have been infected with an encapsulated strain of *C neoformans* or with an unencapsulated strain that converted to capsule production in vivo.

Persons who cannot mount a normal inflammatory response are at risk of developing a fungal disease. Patients treated systemically with antiinflammatory agents such as corticosteroids have increased susceptibility to opportunistic fungal diseases. These individuals also run a greater risk of developing systemic disease by fungi considered as true pathogens, such as *C immitis*, although the risk also may relate to the suppressive effect of corticosteroids on cell-mediated immune responses. Granulocytopenia and impaired neutrophil function have been positively correlated with cases of disseminated mucormycosis and invasive aspergillosis. Defective neutrophil function has also been noted in patients with diabetes mellitus, a disease that predisposes an individual to candidiasis and other fungal diseases. In experimental animals, *Candida albicans* has been shown to suppress neutrophil release of H_2O_2, which is one of the important fungicidal components of these phagocytic cells. It is not known if other fungi produce this effect, or if suppression of H_2O_2 release occurs in human fungal infections.

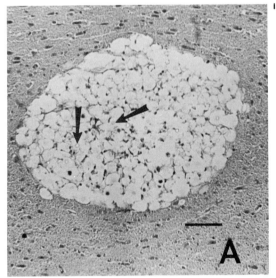

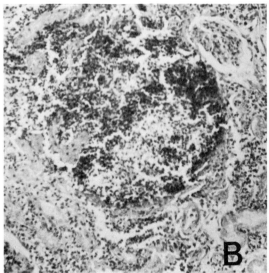

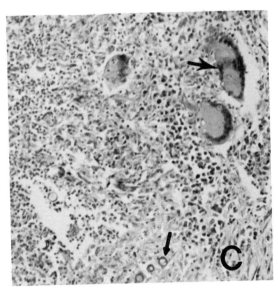

Figure 58-3 Types of tissue reactions that may occur in response to fungal invasion depicted by photomicrographs of hematoxylin and eosin stained sections of infected tissues. **A** shows typical lack of cellular response occurring in brain tissue to infection with an encapsulated *Cryptococcus neoformans* (arrows point to yeast cells). The capsular material is antiphagocytic and induces immunologic tolerance in experimental animals. **B** shows acute inflammatory reaction occurring in kidney infected with *Candida albicans*. This response may be due to activation of complement, tissue damage, and fungal products that attract neutrophils. **C** shows chronic inflammatory reaction that may occur to any fungal disease and to bacteria such as *Mycobacterium tuberculosis*. Classically, this reaction occurs because of infection by *Coccidioides immitis* (as in this case; small arrows denote spherules), *Blastomyces dermatitidis*, *Histoplasma capsulatum,* and *Paracoccidioides braziliensis*. Large arrow points to a giant cell. (Bar = 100 μm.)

Normal Flora

The importance of normal flora in resistance to certain opportunistic invaders such as *C albicans* has been shown repeatedly in experimental and clinical situations. An antagonism exists between some organisms that are part of the normal flora and *C albicans*, which prevents the fungus from overgrowing and invading mucous membranes. Although the antagonistic mechanisms are not well understood, certain gram-negative rods that are commonly part of the normal flora in humans have been shown in vitro to inhibit *C albicans*. Alterations of normal flora may occur in patients receiving long-term doses of broad-spectrum antibacterial agents such as tetracyclines.

These individuals are susceptible to oral, intestinal, and vaginal overgrowth of *C albicans* along with possible tissue invasion by the fungus.

Specific Acquired Immunity

Antibody

Fungal infections, clinically apparent or not, may induce formation of antibodies specific for fungal cell wall and cytoplasmic antigens. In cases of coccidioidomycosis, histoplasmosis, and paracoccidioidomycosis, precipitin antibodies specific for fungal antigens usually are present in the patient's serum only during acute phases of active disease and are therefore diagnostically useful; however, antibodies to some fungal cell wall antigens, such as *C albicans*, often are found in healthy persons and thus are not diagnostically useful.

The role of antibody in resistance to fungal disease is speculative and controversial. Certain specific antibodies are known not to be protective. For example, in some diseases such as coccidioidomycosis and histoplasmosis, a rising complement-fixation titer indicates that the disease is disseminating. Several investigations suggest that production of high antibody titers to mycotic agents suppresses antifungal cell-mediated immune responses that are believed to play an important role in resistance. Specific IgE responses occur in experimental animals infected with *C albicans*, and increased IgE levels have been demonstrated in patients with candidiasis, histoplasmosis, and coccidioidomycosis. However, a correlation between disease severity and IgE production has not been demonstrated conclusively.

Other clinical examples indicate that antibodies are protective. Some patients with cryptococcosis who developed severe disease or experienced relapse following antimycotic therapy were found negative for antibody to cryptococcal antigen, whereas antibody titers were present in those who recovered readily. A positive correlation has also been noted between production of anti-*Candida* secretory IgA and resistance to vaginal candidiasis. It is possible that toxic substances produced by fungi (for example, substances resembling endotoxin from *C albicans* and *C neoformans* as well as toxins that may be produced and contribute to tissue damage in aspergillosis and blastomycosis) are neutralized by specific antibodies. Also, specific antibodies may opsonically promote phagocytosis, which may be especially important in patients unable to generate complement factor C3b.

Cell-Mediated Immunity

On recovery from many fungal diseases, an otherwise healthy individual is in at least a transitory state of enhanced resistance to reinfection. With some diseases, such as coccidioidomycosis, recovery confers a high degree of long-lasting immunity. Most experimental and clinical evidence shows that this acquired immune state is T cell dependent and fits current concepts of cell-mediated immunity. The protective mechanisms have not been well defined but probably involve a combination of factors such as activated macrophages, direct attack of fungi by sensitized T cells, and production by T cells of fungitoxic lymphokines (see Figure 58-1). Cell-mediated immunity not only confers a degree of protection against reinfection, but also seems important in containing a fungus once it has traversed the innate barriers.

Many clinical examples substantiate the importance of cell-mediated immunity as a host defense mechanism against fungi. Although dermatophytoses usually are limited to keratinized areas such as skin and hair, a few cases of disseminated disease have been associated with individuals who have compromised cell-mediated function. In immunologically normal individuals, resistance to reinfection is associated with a type IV (delayed type) hypersensitivity to dermatophyte (trichophytin) skin test antigens. Chronic mucocutaneous candidiasis occurs almost exclusively in individuals who have general dysfunction of cell-mediated immunity or are compromised only in their ability to respond to *Candida* antigens. Progressive disease in cases of histoplasmosis and coccidioidomycosis is more likely to occur in individuals such as pregnant women and others with an immune imbalance who do not respond normally to appropriate fungal skin test antigens. Remission of chronic mucocutaneous candidiasis and disseminated coccidioidomycosis has been induced in some patients by combining amphotericin B with therapy such as thymosin or transfer factor to restore T cell function.

Researchers also have considered whether defective cell-mediated immunity can be a consequence, rather than a cause, of a disseminated fungal disease. Some patients who are nonreactive to fungal skin test antigens during dissemination convert to positive reactivity during antifungal therapy. A few investigators have speculated that fungus-specific antibodies may enhance fungal growth by masking surface antigens, thus preventing recognition of the fungus by the cell-mediated immune system. Interesting clinical evidence also indicates that suppressor T cells, which prevent mitogenic responses of normal T cells, may be found in patients with disseminated fungal disease. Although *C albicans* may cause enhanced antibody responses to unrelated particulate antigens, the fungus appears to induce suppression of cell-mediated immunity.

References

Ajello, L. (editor): *Coccidioidomycosis: Current clinical and diagnostic status.* Miami: Symposia Specialists, 1977.

Brahmi, Z., Liantaud, B., Marill, F.: Depressed cell-mediated immunity in chronic dermatophytic infections. *Ann Immunol (Inst Pasteur)* 1980; 131 C:143–153.

Calderon, R.A., Hay, R.J.: Cell-mediated immunity in experimental murine dermatophytosis. I. Temporal aspects of T-suppressor activity caused by *Trichophyton quinckeanum. Immunology* 1984; 53:457–464.

Cox, R.A., Arnold, D.R.: Immunoglobulin E in coccidioidomycosis. *J Immunol* 1979; 123:194–200.

Cutler, J.E., Lloyd, R.K.: Enhanced antibody responses induced by *Candida albicans* in mice. *Infect Immun* 1982; 38:1102–1108.

Grappel, S.F., Bishop, C.T., Blank, F.: Immunology of dermatophytes and dermatophytosis. *Bacteriol Rev* 1974; 38:222–250.

Hilger, A.E., Danley, D.L.: Alteration of polymorphonuclear leukocyte activity by viable *Candida albicans. Infect Immun* 1980; 27:714–720.

Kauffman, C.A., et al: Histoplasmosis in immunosuppressed patients. *Am J Med* 1978; 64:923–932.

Kozel, T.R., Gulley, W.F., Cazin, J.: Immune response to *Cryptococcus neoformans* soluble polysaccharide: immunological unresponsiveness. *Infect Immun* 1977; 18:701–707.

Rives, V., Rogers, T.J.: Studies on the cellular nature of *Candida albicans*-induced suppression. *J Immunol* 1983; 130:376–379.

Rogers, T.G., Balish, E.: Immunity to *Candida albicans. Microbiol Rev* 1980; 44:660–682.

Stobo, J.D., et al: Suppressor thymus-derived lymphocytes in fungal infection. *J Clin Invest* 1976; 57:319–328.

Winterrowd, G.E., Cutler, J.E.: *Candida albicans*-induced agglutinin and immunoglobulin E responses in mice. *Infect Immun* 1983; 41:33–38.

59 Superficial Mycoses: Cutaneous and Subcutaneous

Edward Balish, PhD

General Concepts

Fungal infections of the keratinized body areas (skin, hair, and nails) are known collectively as **dermatomycoses.** When the stratum corneum, hair, or nails are infected by fungi of the genera *Trichophyton, Microsporum,* or *Epidermophyton,* the infections are more properly called **dermatophytoses.** Dermatomycoses are among the most common human infectious diseases. Although chronic fungal infections of the skin and its appendages are not life threatening, they cause considerable discomfort, stress, and frustration to the patient. Dermatomycoses often cause serious cosmetic problems that can interfere with the patient's psychologic and social development. Fungal infections of the skin are troublesome because of the lack of low-toxicity antimicrobial therapy and knowledge of the basic aspects of these host-parasite interactions. Chronic dermatophytoses usually are treated with oral griseofulvin; however, numerous other agents (for example, miconazole) also are available for treatment of dermatophytoses.

Because other skin diseases can mimic dermatomycoses, it is important to establish the fungal etiology of a suspected dermatomycosis. Laboratory identification of these

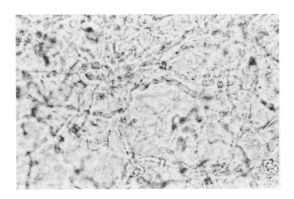

Figure 59-1 Branching septate hyphae and arthro-spores in a 10% KOH digest of infected human skin (×400).

agents should routinely entail microscopic examination of a potassium hydroxide (KOH), 10%–30%, slide preparation of infected tissue (skin, hair, or nails), and culturing the infected tissue on a medium that will support the growth of fungi (Sabouraud's dextrose agar). Use of a growth medium that inhibits the overgrowth of skin bacteria by incorporating antibacterial antibiotics into the growth medium (mycosel agar) also is desirable.

Fungal etiology usually can be established quickly by verifying the presence of hyphae with or without arthrospores in the KOH preparation (Figure 59-1). Specific identification takes longer (one to several weeks), because it can be accomplished only by observing the colonies that grow on the inoculated media for gross morphology and pigmentation, asexual spores (microaleuriospores and macroaleuriospores), and special hyphal structures (such as racquet hyphae, spiral or coiled hyphae, and antlerlike hyphae called favic chandelier). Speciation of pathogenic fungi is accomplished by identifying their morphologic characteristics; few biochemical tests are available to identify and classify them.

Dermatomycoses occur worldwide; however, some manifest geographic and host limitations (Table 59-1).

Dermatomycoses also can be categorized by the keratinized tissue they infect. Superficial dermatomycoses occur in the most superficial areas of the skin and hair shaft. The cutaneous dermatomycoses are caused by fungi that infect stratum corneum, hair, and nails. Subcutaneous mycoses constitute infections of viable tissues beneath the stratum corneum and frequently involve the lymphatics, bone, and fascia.

SUPERFICIAL DERMATOMYCOSES

An interesting ecologic niche is occupied by fungi that cause superficial mycoses known as **piedra.** These fungi invade only the external hair shaft; the resulting disease is primarily a cosmetic problem, because it does not evoke any apparent immune or cellular response by the host. Black piedra, caused by *Piedraia hortai*, is a fungal infection of the hair that results in hard, black nodules of fungi on the hair shaft. White piedra, caused by *Trichosporin beiglii*, is characterized by soft, white nodules of fungi on the hair shaft. Black piedra and white piedra rarely occur in the United States, but they

Table 59-1   Characteristics of Dermatophytoses

Dermatophyte	Source in Nature	Geographic Distribution	Tinea Capitis	Tinea Corporis	Tinea Barbae	Tinea Cruris	Tinea Pedis	Tinea Unguium	Shaft Invaded	Ecto-thrix	Endo-thrix	Fluore-scence†
			*Clinical Manifestations**						*Hair Infections*	*Spores*		
Trichophyton sp												
T mentagrophytes	Humans, animals‡	Worldwide	+	+	+	+	+	+	+	+	−	+
T tonsurans	Humans	Worldwide	+	+	+			+	+	−	+	Rare
T schoenleini	Humans	Africa, Asia, Europe‖	+ (favus)§	+	+		+	+	+	−	+	−
T violaceum	Humans	Africa, Asia, Europe‖	+	+	+				+	−	+	−
T rubrum	Humans	Worldwide	−	+	+	+	+	+	−	−	−	−
T concentricum	Humans	Asia, South America, Polynesia	−	+ (Tinea imbricata)				+	−	−	−	−
T verrucosum	Humans, animals	Worldwide		+	+				+	+	−	−
T megninii	Humans	Europe		+	+			+	+	+	−	−
T gallinae	Fowl	Worldwide	+									
Microsporum sp												
M audouinii	Humans	Worldwide	+	+				−	+	+	−	+
M canis	Dogs, cats	Worldwide	+	+	+			Rare	+	+	−	+
M gypseum	Soil	Worldwide	+	+				Rare	+	+ (few)	−	−
M nanum	Soil (swine)	Worldwide	+	+				−	+	+ (few)	−	−
M fulvum	Soil	Worldwide	+	+				−	+	+ (few)	−	−
M ferrugineum	Humans	Africa, Asia, Europe‖	+	+				−	+	+	−	−
Epidermophyton												
E floccosum	Humans	Worldwide		+		+	+	+	−	−	−	−

*See Table 59-2.

†Wood's light.

‡T. mentagrophytes var. interdigitalis is anthropophilic, whereas T. mentagrophytes var. mentagrophytes is zoophilic; however, both can cause disease in humans.

§Favus: concentrated masses of mycelia and epithelial debris, cause chronic scalp infections that are characterized by the presence of yellowish cup-shaped scutula.

‖Endemic areas in United States are also known.

are common in South America and the Orient. These hair shaft infections are sometimes self-inflicted by South American natives for cosmetic purposes. They sleep with their uncoiled hair in an earth depression to encourage the hair shaft infections.

Pityrosporon orbiculare (formerly called *Malassezia furfur*) is a yeastlike microorganism, isolated from the skin and scalp of healthy humans. *P orbiculare* can multiply dramatically in the superficial regions of the stratum corneum and cause a disease known as pityriasis (tinea) versicolor. The reason for the organism's switch from commensal to pathogen is as yet unknown. The disease is primarily a cosmetic problem. Usually, brownish red, scaly patches of skin are observed on the neck, trunk, and arms. A KOH preparation of skin scrapings or a yellow fluorescence of the affected area with a Wood's light can help establish a diagnosis. Both yeast and hyphal forms of *P orbiculare* can be seen in a KOH preparation of infected skin. Although the disease is most common in the tropics, cases also occur commonly in the United States.

Selenium sulfide has been effective in treating pityriasis versicolor; however, some toxicity is associated with its use (skin irritation in body folds), and the infection often recurs.

Tinea nigra is another superficial dermatomycosis whose causative agent, *Cladosporium werneckii*, fills an interesting ecologic niche. *C werneckii* infects the stratum corneum and is characterized by brown-to-black nonscaly macules that usually occur on the palmar surfaces. When treated daily with Whitfield's ointment, tincture of iodine, 2% salicyclic acid, or 3% sulfur, the lesions usually clear and do not recur.

CUTANEOUS DERMATOMYCOSES: DERMATOPHYTOSES

Distinctive Properties

The **dermatophytes** are a group of 37 closely related fungi that can utilize keratin and invade the stratum corneum, hair, and nails of humans and animals. Dermatophytes have many properties in common. The primary property that differentiates dermatophytes from a large number of keratinolytic soil fungi is their capacity to utilize keratin that is still present on a host in the form of skin, hair, and nails. With rare exceptions, dermatophytes are unable to invade the host's viable tissue. In keratinized tissue, all dermatophytes grow as branching septate hyphae with or without arthrospores formed by a hyphal fragmentation. On culture medium (Sabouraud's dextrose agar) at room temperature, dermatophyte growth is moldlike. Morphology and pigmentation of the colony along with the formation of asexual spores (microaleuriospores and macroaleuriospores) and specialized hyphal structures (for example, antlerlike hyphae called favic chandeliers, spiral or coiled hyphae, and racquet hyphae) are used to identify the fungi. Some dermatophytes are now known to have sexual cycles and are classified with the *Ascomycetes* (for example, *Nannizzea* and *Arthroderma*). In contrast, because asexual spores and hyphal structures are key factors in identifying most dermatophytes that have no readily discernable sexual stages, these fungi are still classified in the clinical literature

Table 59-2   Dermatophytoses

Tinea	*Body Area Affected*	*Most Frequent Cause* *(United States)*
Capitis	Scalp, head hair, eyebrows, eyelashes	*M audouini, T tonsurans, M canis, M ferrugineum*
Favus	Scalp, head hair (yellow, cup-shaped scutula)	*T schoenleini, T violaceum*
Corporis	Glabrous skin	All dermatophytes can cause tinea corporis; *T rubrum* and *T mentagrophytes* are common etiologic agents
Barbae	Bearded area of face	*T mentagrophytes, T verrucosum*
Cruris	Groin (jock itch)	*E floccosum, T rubrum, T mentagrophytes*
Pedis	Feet (toe webs and soles)	*T mentagrophytes, T rubrum, E floccosum*
Manus	Hands and fingers	*T mentagrophytes, T rubrum, E floccosum*
Unguium	Nails (hands and toes)	*T mentagrophytes, T rubrum, E floccosum*

as genera (*Trichophyton, Microsporum,* and *Epidermophyton*) of the fungi imperfecti (Deuteromycetes).

Pathogenesis

Clinical Disease

Dermatophytes can be categorized by the clinical diseases they cause. Dermatophyte infections are known as **tineas,** because these infections were originally thought to be caused by larvae (Table 59-2). They are also called **ringworm** because of the circular, spreading skin lesions they cause.

The dermatophytes differ in their capacities to invade different parts of the body. All dermatophytes can cause tinea corporis, and nearly all species have been isolated from cases of tinea unguium. Generally, dermatophyte infections of the body are caused by those fungi that are endemic in the area and may have already caused dermatophytoses of the head or feet. Some dermatophytes (for example, *T mentagrophytes* and *T tonsurans*) can invade skin, hair, and nails and can cause tinea infections on almost all keratinized body areas (see Table 59-2). *T tonsurans* and *T violaceum* cause endothrix tinea capitis. *T schoenleini* is the major cause of favus, a chronic ringworm infection of the scalp that destroys hair follicles, causes scarring, and results in permanent hair loss. *T rubrum* is a common cause of tinea unguium, tinea pedis, tinea cruris, and tinea corporis, but it usually does not cause tinea capitis. *Microsporum* sp are most frequently associated with tinea capitis; they can also cause tinea corporis, but they usually do not cause tinea unguium. *M audouini,* a common cause of tinea capitis in children, is frequently associated with gray-patch ringworm epidemics in children; the dermatophytosis usually disappears spontaneously. Individuals beyond the age of puberty usually do not contract these infections. *M canis,* primarily a parasite of domestic animals (dogs and cats), also is a frequent cause of tinea capitis. *Epidermophyton* is a monotypic genus. *E floccosum* causes infections of the body, groin, and feet.

Pathogenic Mechanisms

Hyphae, arthrospores, or conidia can initiate dermatophytoses in humans and laboratory animals. The infectious form of these fungi in naturally occurring infections is not yet known; in fact, little is known about the initial interactions that take place between the dermatophyte and the host. Experimental infections can be initiated on occluded human skin with one spore. The spore germinates in the humid atmosphere on the occluded skin, and the hypha penetrates the stratum corneum. The branched, septate hyphae spread radially from the inoculation site through the stratum corneum and, if hair is present and the fungus is capable of invading it, the fungus penetrates the hair shaft and grows down to the area where viable cells are present in the hair shaft (Adamson's fringe). The hyphae in the hair shaft then fragment and form spores, either within (endothrix) or outside (ectothrix) the hair shaft. In the stratum corneum, the branching, septate hyphae also usually fragment and form arthrospores, but the hyphae never penetrate into living tissues that lie below the stratum corneum.

The first sign of disease usually is scaling, crusting, or eczematous reactions on the surface of the skin. On glabrous (hairless) skin, a circular inflamed area becomes prominent about 3 weeks after infection. Skin scrapings, digested with KOH, reveal that hyphae, arthrospores, or both are prevalent at the inflamed radiating border of the ringworm lesion. The central, noninflamed area of the lesion is usually free of hyphae and arthrospores. The degree of inflammation varies with the dermatophyte causing the lesion. Generally, anthropophilic fungi (*M audouini, T mentagrophytes* var *interdigitale, T rubrum, T tonsurans,* and *E floccosum*) cause chronic diseases that evoke little tissue reaction. Zoophilic species (*M canis, M gallinae, T verrucosum, T equinum, T mentagrophytes* var *mentagrophytes*) cause acute inflammation, vesiculation, and even some suppuration when they invade the keratinized body area of humans. Dermatophytoses caused by zoophilic dermatophytes are also usually acute and highly inflammatory; the infection usually resolves over a period of several months.

Many dermatophytes that invade hair form compounds (thought to be pteridines) that fluoresce green when exposed to ultraviolet light (Wood's light). Ultraviolet light is used frequently to identify infected children during *M audouini* epidemics, and although it is useful, not all dermatophytes fluoresce in infected hair (for example, *M gypseum* and *M fulvum* do not).

Host Defenses

Although dermatophytes cannot invade the hosts' nonkeratinized living tissues, they can induce antibody formation and a hypersensitive state in humans. Intradermal injections of trichophytin, a complex nonspecific dermatophyte antigen, can elicit immediate and delayed (24-48 hr) hypersensitivity skin reactions. These skin reactions to trichophytin can occur in individuals who show no clinical signs of dermatophytoses. This suggests that although infection with dermatophytes may be a relatively common event, clinically evident dermatophytoses occur in a small percentage of the infected population.

Many attempts have been made to immunize humans and animals against dermatophytoses, but the immunizations have not had great success. At best, a shortened infection course is observed in so-called immune individuals. Research is currently underway to elucidate basic mechanisms of host resistance and susceptibility to dermatophytoses, and to evaluate the relative contributions of antibody- and cell-mediated immunity in human resistance to these infectious agents.

Dermatophytids (**ids**) are papular, bullous, or pustular (rare) lesions that develop on skin that is distant to the infected area. The ids are sterile (no hyphae) hypersensitivity reactions thought to be caused by circulating dermatophyte antigens.

Epidemiology

Dermatophytoses occur worldwide, but some dermatophytes have endemic areas (for example, *T schoenleinii* in Mediterranean countries; *T concentricum* in South America and the South Seas; *M ferrugeneum* in Japan). Because of jet travel and migrating human populations, it is not surprising to see fungal infections once thought to be rare or geographically limited occur outside that endemic area. (For example, *T tonsurans*, once the primary cause of tinea capitis in Mexico and Puerto Rico, now is prevalent in the United States; *T schoenleinii*, although most prevalant in Mediterranean countries and Central Europe, now occurs in the United States in areas settled by immigrants from endemic European areas.)

Dermatophytes also manifest an interesting ecology. Some species are present in the soil (geophilic), others have animals as their primary reservoir in nature (zoophilic), and still others are closely associated with humans (anthropophilic). Identification of a dermatophyte frequently can lead to epidemiologic information about the source of the etiologic agent. *M canis* infections are usually traced to direct contact with an infected cat or dog, whereas *M audouini* infections of the scalp are usually caused by direct contact with infected children.

Diagnosis

Clinical diagnosis of ringworm usually can be made by an experienced clinician. Because many skin diseases can mimic dermatophytoses, especially in the early stages of infection, a KOH slide preparation of infected hair, nails, or skin should be prepared and examined for hyphae or arthrospores and for endothrix or ectothrix spores in infected hairs. Care should be taken to take skin specimens from the inflamed edge of the lesion in glabrous skin. The infected hair or tissues also should be inoculated onto Sabouraud's dextrose agar (with and without antibacterial antibiotics). The laboratory personnel who examine the growth that occurs on the inoculated plate to rule out nonpathogenic fungi must be experienced enough to observe the fungal growth for gross morphology, pigmentation, asexual spores (size, shape, and surface of microaleuriospores and macroaleuriospores), and special hyphal configurations such as favic chandeliers, racquet hyphae, and coiled hyphae. An experienced mycologist often has trouble speciating these pathogenic fungi.

Control

Antibacterial antibiotics are of no use in treating dermatophytoses. As is true of mycoses in general, therapy available for dermatophytoses is inadequate. Griseofulvin is still the primary agent that is given orally to treat chronic dermatophytoses. It is absorbed into the circulation and then appears to concentrate in keratinized body areas. The dermatophyte is unable to survive in keratinized areas where griseofulvin is deposited. Oral therapy with ketoconazole also has been successful in treating chronic dermatophytoses; however, as occurs with most oral antifungal agents, liver toxicity has been reported in patients treated with ketoconazole.

Numerous compounds and formulations are available for topical treatment of dermatophytoses. Tolnaftate, haloprogin, and miconazole appear to be the most effective topical agents in use today.

The role of *C albicans* as a systemic pathogen is described in Chapter 60; this versatile pathogen also can infect skin and mucous membranes, and it is a prevalent cause of dermatomycoses. Treatment with nystatin or amphotericin B often is an effective therapy for mucocutaneous candidosis (candidiasis).

SUBCUTANEOUS MYCOSES

Several fungi can cause chronic diseases of subcutaneous tissues following traumatic implantation of their spores or hyphae caused by thorns, splinters, soil, and possibly animal or insect bites. These fungi are usually soil-inhabiting species common to decaying vegetation; subclinical infection may be prevalent in those areas where the fungi are found. Malnutrition, immunologic defects, or exposure to large numbers of spores can interfere with or overcome host defense mechanisms and allow these fungi to cause chronic, disfiguring, infectious diseases in humans.

Sporotrichosis

Sporotrichosis is a disease of people who have close contact with the soil (farmers, horticulturists, and gardeners). The fungi are implanted in the skin, usually as a result of trauma. An abscess develops at the site of the trauma, and subcutaneous nodules may subsequently develop along the draining lymphatics. This is referred to as the cutaneous-lymphatic form of the disease, and about 75% of the cases are of this type. The subcutaneous nodules can persist for years; they also can ulcerate. Although not as common as the cutaneous-lymphatic form, disseminated sporotrichosis also has been reported after inhalation of spores.

The causative agent of sporotrichosis is *Sporothrix schenckii*, a dimorphic fungus. In tissue, it exists in the form of oval-to-cigar-shaped yeast cells (3-5 μm in diameter) that are not numerous. When infected tissue, wound exudates, or pus are inoculated onto Sabouraud's dextrose agar and incubated at 25-27 C, a mold colony grows. The color of the colony can vary from white (young colony) to black, brown, or yellow. Microscopically, the mold is composed of septate, branching hyphae (2 μm in diameter). Multiple oval conidia (2-3 μm to 2-6 μm) in the shape of a palm tree or a flowerblossom arise from conidiophores that branch at right angles from the hyphae. In older colonies, the spores also arise at the sides of the conidiophores and the hyphal branches. The yeast phase of *S schenckii* can be induced by culturing the microorganism at 37 C in blood agar tubes.

The cutaneous-lymphatic form of the disease is probably the most common disease manifestation. The lesion usually begins on the hand or fingers as a small ulcer or subcutaneous nodule.

Therapy for sporotrichosis is oral potassium iodide, systemic treatment with amphotericin B, or both.

Chromomycosis

Although worldwide in occurrence, chromomycosis primarily occurs in residents of the tropics. This disease also is caused by the implantation of soil fungi into the skin, usually on hands or feet. An erythematous papule develops at the site of the inoculation. With time (months to years), a new crop of raised (1-3 mm) lesions appears, and some peripheral spreading of the lesion occurs. Pedunculated, warty lesions (resembling cauliflower) eventually develop. This clinical syndrome is the most typical form of the disease, called verrucous dermatitis (chromoblastomycosis). Many clinical variations occur. The involved areas on the hands and feet often are damaged; they ulcerate and frequently become infected with bacteria. The lesions may have a purulent exudate associated with them. For the most part, chromomycosis involves only the subcutaneous tissues. The verrucose, pedunculated lesions often spread along the lymphatics. Dissemination of these fungi to the brain has been reported.

Etiologic agents of this disease are slow-growing soil fungi that are difficult to identify and classify. Some of the etiologic agents have been identified as *Fonsecaea pedrosoi, F. compactum, F dermatitidis, Cladosporium carrionii,* and *Phialophora verrucosa.* Potassium hydroxide digests of infected tissue or aspirated lesion debris may reveal the presence of brown-pigmented, branching hyphal strands (2-6 μm wide). The hyphae in pus are often distorted (3-8 μm wide). Often, pleomorphic brown bodies (up to 20 μm in diameter) and thick-walled, round cells (6-10 μm in diameter) that are dark brown and exhibit planate (single plane) division can be seen in pus from cysts and in biopsies of infected tissues.

At 25 C, the organism grows as a mold. The formation of asexual spores is used to identify the genus and species of the fungus.

In early stages of the disease, surgical excision usually is recommended. Oral treatment with 5-fluorocytosine or thiabendazole has had limited success in therapy.

Maduromycosis

Mycetoma is the generic term used to describe swollen, deforming, suppurative, granulomatous lesions that have draining sinuses and usually occur on the hands or feet. If the etiologic agent is a fungus, the term **maduromycosis (eumycotic mycetoma)** is used. If the causative agent is a bacterium such as *Nocardia, Actinomyces,* or *Streptomyces,* the term **actinomycotic mycetoma** is applied (see Chapters 48 and 49). Maduromycosis usually originates after trauma or injury to people residing in the tropics. The fungus is implanted into the subcutaneous tissues. Multiple burrowing sinuses are formed in the soft tissue; these sinuses penetrate to the skin surface and drain pus containing grains, or granules, that are hyphal strands of fungi. The size (0.5-2 mm), texture, color, and shape of these grains can be used to identify the etiologic agent. With time (months to years), the bones, fascia, subcutaneous tissues, and skin of the hands or feet can all be involved. The result is a gross, swollen, and deforming lesion that usually does not disseminate beyond the hand or foot. Some fungi commonly isolated from maduromycosis are *Allescheria (Petriellidium) boydii, Madurella grisea, M mycetomii, Acremonium kiliense, Lepotosphaeria senegalensis,* and *Phialophora jeanselmii.* These fungi grow as molds at room temperature and are still the subject of considerable taxonomic debate.

It is important to differentiate between an actinomycotic mycetoma and maduromycosis. The former disease can be treated with antibacterial antibiotics such as penicillin and sulfadiazine, because the etiologic agents are bacteria (see Chapter 26). Mycetomas of fungal etiology, however, are consistently resistant to treatment, even with those antifungal agents that show some success in other fungal diseases.

References

Al-Doory, Y.: *Laboratory medical mycology.* Philadelphia: Lea & Febiger, 1980.

Emmons, C.W., et al: *Medical mycology.* Philadelphia: Lea & Febiger, 1977.

Gentle, T.A., Warnock, D.W., Eden, O.B.: Prevalence of oral colonization with *Candida albicans* and anti-*C. albicans* IgA in the saliva of normal children and children with acute lymphoblastic leukaemia. *Mycopathologia* 1984; 87(1-2):111-114.

Grappel, S.F.: Immunology of surface fungi. In: *Comprehensive immunology. Part I: Mycoplasmae, Chlamydiae, and fungi.* Nahmias A.J., O'reilly, R.J. (editors). New York: Plenum, 1981.

Howard, N.H.: Ascomycetes: the dermatophytes. In: *Fungi pathogenic for humans and animals.* Howary, D.H., Howard, L.F. (editors). New York: Marcel Dekker, 1983.

Koneman. E.W., Roberts, G.D., Wright, S.E.: *Practical laboratory mycology,* 2nd ed. Baltimore: Williams and Wilkins Co., 1979.

Rebell, G., Taplin, D.: *Dermatophytes: their recognition and identification,* 2nd ed. Coral Gables, Fl.: University of Miami Press, 1970.

Rippon, J.W.: *Medical mycology: the pathogenic fungi and the pathogenic actinomyces,* 2nd ed. Philadelphia: W.B. Saunders Co., 1982.

Ross, I.K.: *Biology of the fungi.* New York: McGraw Hill Book Co., 1979.

60 Systemic Mycoses

Richard A. Calderone, PhD

John P. Utz, MD

General Concepts
Distinctive Properties
Pathogenesis
Host Defenses
Epidemiology
Diagnosis
Control

General Concepts

The systemic mycoses of humans and other animals are caused by some fungi that are pathogenic and cause disease in the healthy host, and by other fungi (opportunistic pathogens) that are usually innocuous but cause disease in patients whose immune defenses are impaired. Some of these fungi may be saprophytes in nature (soil, bird droppings), whereas others are a part of the normal human flora (commensals). In no case are humans the solitary or necessary host.

An example of a soil saprophyte is *Histoplasma capsulatum,* which commonly causes infection in endemic areas; 80%-90% of adults react positively to histoplasmin in delayed cutaneous hypersensitivity tests. An example of an opportunistic pathogen is *Candida albicans,* normally present in the oral cavity, gastrointestinal tract, and probably the skin. In the patient with acute leukemia, however, *C albicans* is commonly present in blood, causing a fulminant, usually fatal, septicemia. Other opportunistic infections are seen in patients with diabetic acidosis (mucormycosis) and Hodgkin's disease (for example, cryptococcosis and histoplasmosis). The pathogenesis of these organisms is obscure, but cell-mediated immunity of the host seems to be essential for a good prognosis.

Distinctive Properties

A striking feature of some fungi is dimorphic growth. In tissue and in the laboratory at 37 C, they grow as yeasts; in the laboratory at 22-33 C, as filamentous forms. This property is possessed by *Blastomyces dermatitidis, H capsulatum,* and *Paracoccidioides brasiliensis. Coccidioides immitis,* another temperature-dependent dimorphic fungus, differs from yeastlike fungi because it does not reproduce by budding. Instead, it reproduces in tissue by endogenous spore formation. *C albicans* also is dimorphic, but transition between growth forms is influenced by nutrition as well as temperature.

The regulation of dimorphism has been studied in *H capsulatum* in great detail. Cystine is taken up by yeast and hyphae, but a reduced nicotinamide adenine dinucleotide-dependent cystine reductase is detectable only in the yeast. Parachloromercuriphenylsulfonic acid, an inhibitor of cystine reductase, also prevents the transition of hyphae to yeast. Thus, reduced sulfhydryl groups provided by cystine reductase may be critical in regulating cell differentiation. The concentration of cyclic adenosine monophosphate (cAMP) is five times greater in the hyphal form. Because phosphodiesterase, the enzyme that catabolizes cAMP, requires a reducing substance, high concentrations intracellularly of sulfhydryl groups may affect levels of cAMP and thus control genesis of one form. *Mucor* sp grow as yeasts in an anaerobic environment and as hyphae in an aerobic one. When cAMP is included in the medium, yeasts remain yeasts, even when shifted to an aerobic environment, suggesting cAMP plays a role in differentiation.

Pathogenesis

Except for *C albicans,* which can invade the body through the gastrointestinal tract, these fungi usually enter through the respiratory tract. Fungi that reach the terminal bronchi and alveoli are phagocytosed by alveolar macrophages. Growth intracellularly continues, however, and the processing of antigen attracts T lymphocytes. As macrophages degenerate from the fungal multiplication, they are transformed into epithelioid cells or, by loss of their cell membrane (to produce a syncytium), into giant cells (Langhans or foreign body type). The process is eventually walled off by fibrous tissue, occasionally with calcification, which forms the classical granuloma. With some fungi (such as *B dermatitidis*), suppuration also occurs.

Fungi engulfed by macrophages are transported by the lymphatics to the regional (hilar and paratracheal) lymph nodes; the infected lung and lymph node together form the Ghon complex, similar to that of tuberculosis. From the peripheral or lymph node sites, fungi disseminate hematogenously to distant organs in patterns characteristic for each fungus. For example, *H capsulatum* disseminates to liver, spleen, and adrenal glands, whereas *Cryptococcus neoformans* disseminates to the meninges and the kidney.

Adherence of *Candida albicans* to host epithelial cells has been studied extensively. The nature of the *Candida* receptor has not been identified fully, but it appears to be a mannan-protein. Nonpathogenic *Candida* do not adhere as readily as *C albicans*. Protease activity in *C albicans* seems to be at least partly responsible for virulence. Little information exists about the nature of the virulence factors of the other pathogenic fungi, although the polysaccharide capsule of *C neoformans* may impede phagocytosis.

The patient with a systemic mycosis usually has one or more generalized symptoms or findings of inflammatory or infectious disease. Low grade fever (37.5-38.5 C) is probably the most common. Usually, no recognizable diurnal pattern occurs. Chilliness or shaking chills occur in patients with blastomycosis and *Candida* sp septicemia. Sweating, usually at night, is frequently severe enough to require the patient to change night clothes or bed linen, sometimes more than once. Loss of fluid and salt contributes to the generalized malaise and exhaustion. The patient's appetite almost always disappears early in the illness, which often leads to weight loss. Flat affect and depression are common.

Even though the portal of entry of the fungus is respiratory and the original focus of infection is the lung, symptoms may be absent or minimal. Only in blastomycosis, and then rarely, do early acute and later consolidated pneumonia appear. In one form, aspergillosis is accompanied by wheezing, transient infiltrates, and local and peripheral eosinophilia.

When disease disseminates, the findings vary according to the organ or system affected. Skin lesions are characteristic of blastomycosis and paracoccidioidomycosis, but rarely of cryptococcosis. Meningitis in cryptococcosis and coccidioidomycosis is manifested by headache, impaired vision, and mental and behavioral changes. *Candida* sp are the commonest causes of fungal endocarditis, which is manifested by heart murmur and emboli, often in large vessels. Phycomycosis (zygomycosis, mucormycosis) may take the form of an acute, fulminant infection developing from ocular or nasal cellulitis and usually leading to death. The manifestations of histoplasmosis are less dramatic: weakness, hepatosplenomegaly, and lymphadenopathy.

With the few exceptions already cited, the classic course of illness is chronic with symptoms stable or increasing slowly over a period of many weeks to many months.

Host Defenses

Most evidence supports the critical role of cellular, rather than antibody-mediated, immunity in protection. For example, in coccidioidomycosis, the development of delayed cutaneous hypersensitivity (cell-mediated) to coccidioidin or spherulin is correlated with an effective body defense and good prognosis, whereas the presence of antibody, measured by complement-fixation or precipitin techniques, is correlated with an ineffective body defense and a poor prognosis. Experimental studies in laboratory animals support these observations in human disease, showing protection by transfer of cells (splenic, lymph node), not of serum, from other immunized animals. However, in candidiasis, experimental animal studies indicate that the degree of resistance to *C albicans* in nude, or thymectomized, mice is similar to normal mice. Thus, innate immunity may be more important in certain forms of candidiasis (systemic), whereas it is of lesser importance in other forms (chronic mucocutaneous candidiasis). Fungi are facultative, intracellular microorganisms, and may survive in macrophages or polymorphonuclear leukocytes to a considerable extent (see Chapter 57).

Epidemiology

The saprophytic existence in environment and the geographic distribution of conditions favorable to growth of these fungi are major factors in epidemiology. For example, *H capsulatum* grows in soil enriched by chicken, bird, or bat excreta, and thus is worldwide in distribution; however, in the United States infection occurs more frequently in the Mississippi and Ohio river valleys and in the middle eastern states. *C immitis*, in contrast, grows in an environment described as the Sonoran life zone, with infection common in the San Joaquin Valley of California and in Arizona, New Mexico, Nevada, Utah, and Texas. Age and sex also are important; disease is more common and more severe in men than in women infected with almost any of these fungi. Workers whose occupations expose them to infected soil (highway construction, archeology) develop more severe coccidioidomycosis by virtue of a greater inoculum. For unknown reasons, persons with darker skin are also more prone to severe coccidioidomycosis. Disease from the opportunistic fungi is not geographically dependent, but occurs instead in the patient whose host defenses are impaired.

Diagnosis

In the epidemiologic and clinical settings described above, fungal disease may be strongly suspected; however, diagnosis is confirmed unequivocally by culturing the causative fungus from appropriate patient specimens and by identifying it with proper laboratory methods. Exceptions are candidiasis and aspergillosis, in which the causative fungi are commensals; their cultures (for example, from sputum) must be interpreted with caution.

In all these diseases, diagnosis is strongly supported by finding the fungi on microscopic examination of specially stained tissue sections. The tissue reaction, as such, is not diagnostic, but the great microscopic differences in morphology do permit identification and distinction of the fungi and diseases.

Direct microscopic examination, with and without staining, of fresh patient specimens (sputum, pus, urine, cerebrospinal fluid) may not produce as certain a diagnosis, but when fungi are seen, the time saved is often critically important. Microscopic appearance of these fungi in tissue and in culture is presented in Table 60-1 and Figures 60-1 to 60-8.

Serologic methods have formerly received considerable emphasis in diagnosing systemic mycoses. These techniques include detecting antigen (cryptococcosis) and antibodies (coccidioidomycosis) in serum, and detecting fungal forms in tissue, by using fluorescent antibody (histoplasmosis, blastomycosis). Widespread use of these methods in laboratories has been hampered by the absence of standardized reagents, varying cross-reactions of specific sera to other fungal antigens, and the frequency of false-positive and false-negative results.

Skin testing is a useful means of measuring rates of infectivity in geographic and epidemiologic studies; however, it is not satisfactory in diagnosis because many healthy inhabitants in an endemic area are positive, and because a positive skin test may convert a serologic test to positive or raise the titer falsely to an otherwise diagnostically helpful degree (fourfold).

Table 60-1   Cultural and Histopathologic Description of Major Systemic Mycoses Fungi

Fungus	Cultural	Histopathologic
Aspergillus fumigatus (aspergillosis)	Most common disease-producing specis of *Aspergillus;* grows at 50 C; Colony color white, becoming gray-green; columnar mass of conidia attached to conidiophore expanded at tip, forming vesicle to which spores attach by phialides	Septate hyphae with abundant dichotomous branching; sporophores within pulmonary cavity
Blastomyces dermatitidis (blastomycosis)	Large (8-14 μm), thick-walled multinucleate yeast cells with wide pores (4-5 μm) between bud and parent cell at 37 C; at 30 C, hyphae with conidiophores arising at 90-degree angle	Similar to 37 C culture phase
Candida albicans (candidiasis)	Spherical macroconidia (chlamydospore) 8-12 μm in diameter and germ tube formation; fermentation and carbon-nitrogen assimilation tests differentiate other *Candida* species	Blastospores and pseudohyphae
Coccidioides immitis (coccidioidomycosis)	Arthrospores formed at 25-37 C in vitro	Multinucleate sporangia (30-60 μm in diameter), filled with sporangiospores at maturity
Cryptococcus neoformans (cryptococcosis)	Spherical cells (4-20 μm in diameter) at budding (37 C); polysaccharide capsule; nitrate and fermentation negative; assimilates sucrose, maltose, dulcitol	Same as cultural; capsule often larger in tissue; cells may appear eccentric due to invagination of cell wall
Histoplasma capsulatum (histoplasmosis)	Large (8-14 μm), tuberculate macroconidia (30 C)	Intracellular yeasts (2-4 μm) within macrophages, giant cells, or polymorphonuclear leukocytes
Mucor, Absidia, Rhizopus sp (mucormycosis, zygomycosis, phycomycosis)	Abundant growth with sporangia containing sporangiospores; broad hyphae with few septa; sporophore morphology varies with species and genus	Broad hyphae with few cross walls or septa
Paracoccidioides brasiliensis (paracoccidioidomycosis)	Spherical or elliptical cells (a few 30 μm in diameter); single or multiple buds (37 C)	Similar to cultural

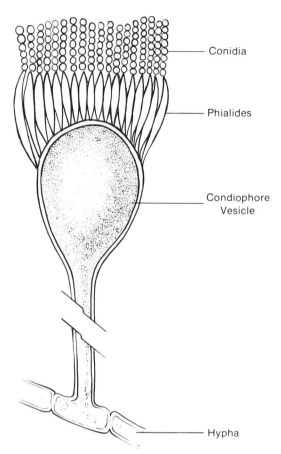

Conidia

Phialides

Condiophore
Vesicle

Hypha

Figure 60-1 *Aspergillus fumigatus* in culture. Organism
occurs occasionally in pulmonary cavities.

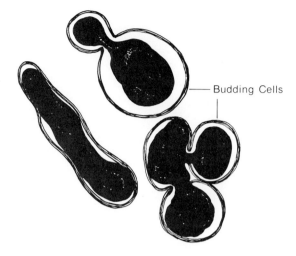

Budding Cells

Figure 60-2 *Blastomyces dermatitidis* (tissue phase).

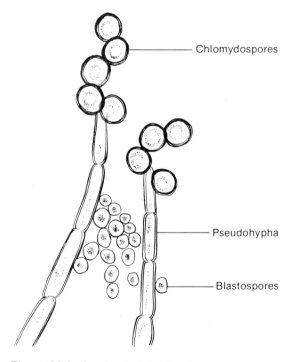

Chlomydospores

Pseudohypha

Blastospores

Figure 60-3 *Candida albicans* in culture.

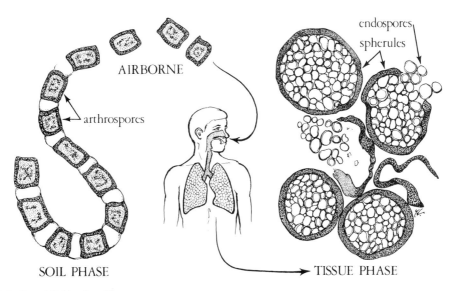

Figure 60-4 *Coccidioides immitis.*

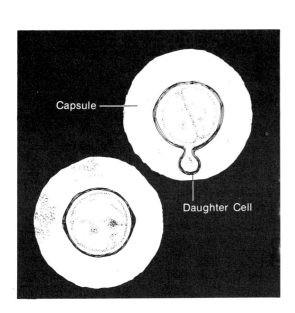

Figure 60-5 *Cryptococcus neoformans* (India ink preparation) in cerebrospinal fluid.

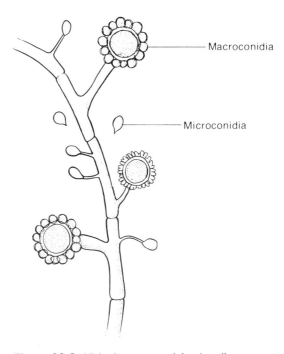

Figure 60-6 *Histoplasma capsulatum* in culture.

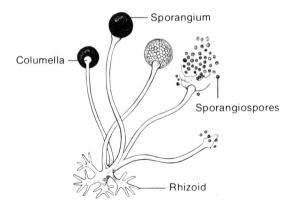

Figure 60-7 *Rhizopus* sp in culture.

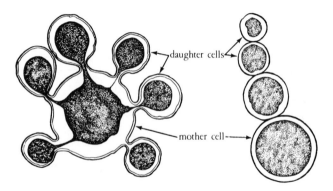

Figure 60-8 *Paracoccidioides brasiliensis* (tissue phase).

Control

Eliminating these fungi from soil has been attempted rarely and has had little success. Masks to prevent infection also have been notoriously unsuccessful. Neither active vaccines nor passive immune serum immunization has been sufficiently successful to result in commercially available preparations.

Treatment of active disease may be symptomatic (for example, pain relief), sometimes surgical (resection of irremedially damaged tissue and correction of hydrocephalus), and, most successfully, chemotherapeutic (Table 60-2). Agents presently used are hydroxystilbamidine isethionate, amphotericin B, 5-fluorocytosine (flucytosine), miconazole, and ketoconazole. Response to these drugs varies according to the fungus, type of disease, and course of illness. For example, response is good in most *B dermatitidis* infections, but is poor in most diseases caused by *A fumigatus*. Response is better for skin lesions caused by *B dermatitidis* than for meningitis due to *C immitis;* response is better in chronic cryptococcosis than in fulminant candidiasis. (For more detail, see Chapter 61.)

Table 60-2   Chemotherapeutic Agents for Systemic Mycoses

Disease	First Choice	Second Choice
Aspergillosis	Amphotericin B	Ketoconazole
Blastomycosis	Amphotericin B	Hydroxystilbamidine isethionate
Candidiasis	Amphotericin B	Flucytosine or ketoconazole
Coccidioidomycosis	Amphotericin B	Ketoconazole
Cryptococcosis	Amphotericin B, flucytosine	Either drug alone*
Histoplasmosis	Amphotericin B	Ketoconazole*
Mucormycosis	Amphotericin B	Miconazole*
Paracoccidioidomycosis	Amphotericin B	Sulfonamides, Ketoconazole*

*Depending on minimal inhibitory concentration necessary for the fungus.

References

Conant, N.F. et al: *Manual of clinical mycology,* 3rd ed. Philadelphia: W.B. Saunders, 1971.

Emmons, C.W. et al: *Medical mycology,* 3rd ed. Philadelphia: Lea and Febiger, 1977.

Hazen, E.L., Gordon, M.A., Reed, F.C.: *Laboratory identification of pathogenic fungi simplified,* 3rd ed. Springfield, Ill.: Charles C Thomas, Publisher, 1973.

Lee, J.C., King, R.D.: Characterization of *Candida albicans* adherence to human vaginal epithelial cells *in vitro. Infect Immun* 1983; 41:1024-1030.

Odds, F.C.: *Candida and candidosis.* Baltimore: University Park Press, 1979.

Rippon, J.W.: *Medical mycology.* Philadelphia: W.B. Saunders, 1974.

Rogers, T.J., Balish, E.: Immunity to *Candida albicans. Microbiol Rev* 1980; 44:660-682.

Stevens, D.A.: *Coccidioidomycosis.* New York: Plenum Press, 1980.

Vanbreuseghem, R., de Vroey, CH., Takashio, M.: *Practical guide to medical and veterinary mycology.* New York: Masson, 1978.

61 Chemotherapy of Fungi

George S. Kobayashi, PhD
Gerald Medoff, MD

General Concepts
Antifungal Agents that Affect Membranes
   Polyenes
   Imidazoles
Agents that Act Intracellularly

General Concepts

In addition to attempts to domesticate fungi for their beneficial properties, efforts have also been directed toward eradicating those with harmful effects. For example, there is intense interest in the use of systemic fungicides such as oxathins, pyrimidines, and benzimidazoles to control plant pathogens. Similarly, much concerted effort has been expended in search of agents useful in treating fungal infections of humans. As a result, many compounds have been isolated and shown to have antifungal activity, but problems associated with solubility, stability, absorption, and toxicity have limited the therapeutic value of most of them in human infections. The most useful antifungal antibiotics fall into one of two categories: those that affect fungal cell membranes and those that are taken up by the cell and interrupt vital cellular processes such as RNA, DNA, or protein synthesis. Table 61-1 lists some useful antifungal agents and their mechanisms of action.

Table 61-1   Some Useful Antifungal Agents, Their Chemical Classification, and Their Mechanisms of Action

Class	Compounds	Mechanism
Polyene	Amphotericin B Nystatin	Interacts with sterols (ergosterol) in fungal cell membrane, rendering cells selectively permeable to the outflow of vital constituents, e.g. potassium
Imidazole	Miconazole Clotrimazole Ketoconazole	Inhibits demethylation of lanosterol thus preventing formation of ergosterol, a vital component of fungal cell membrane; also has a direct cidal effect on fungal cells
Pyrimidine	5-Fluorocytosine	Is taken up and deaminated by susceptible cell to form 5-fluorouracil, which in turn inhibits RNA synthesis; also thought to inhibit thymidylate synthetase and DNA synthesis
Grisan	Griseofulvin	Binds to tubulin and inhibits microtubule assembly
3-Arylpyrrole	Pyrrolnitrin	Appears to inhibit terminal electron transport between succinate or NADH and coenzyme Q
Glutaramide	Cycloheximide	Inhibits protein synthesis at 80S ribosomal level, preventing transfer of aminoacyl tRNA to the ribosome

Antifungal Agents that Affect Membranes

Polyenes

The polyene macrolide antibiotics are secondary metabolites produced by various species of *Streptomyces*. Several common features of these compounds are useful in classifying the more than 80 different polyenes that have been isolated. All are characterized by a macrolide ring, composed of 26–38 carbon atoms and containing a series of unsaturated carbon atoms and hydroxyl groups. These features of the molecule contribute to the polyenes' amphipathic properties (those relating to molecules containing groups with different properties, for example, hydrophilic and hydrophobic). The ring structure is closed by the formation of an internal ester or lactone bond (Figure 61-1). The number of conjugated double bonds varies with each polyene, and the compounds are generally classified according to the degree of unsaturation.

Toxic effects of polyenes are dependent on their binding to cell membrane sterols. Thus, they bind to membranes of fungus cells as well as to those of other eukaryotic cells (human, plant, and protozoa), but not to bacterial cell membranes, which do not contain membrane sterols. The exact nature of the lesions produced by the polyene-sterol interaction is not known, but the resulting membrane perturbations induce leakage of cellular constituents and ultimately cell death.

The usefulness of an antibiotic is measured by the differential sensitivity of the pathogen and host. Two agents, nystatin and amphotericin B, are relatively specific for fungi and have therapeutic usefulness in humans. The relative specificity of these two polyenes is based on their greater avidity for ergosterol, the principal sterol of fungal membranes, compared to cholesterol, the principal sterol of human cell membranes.

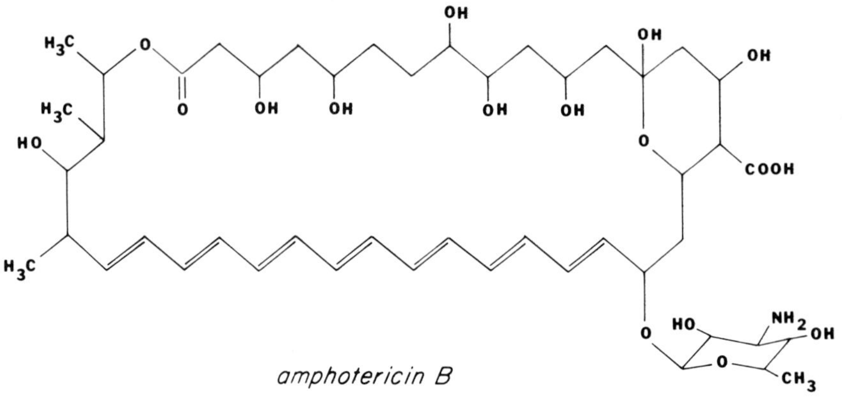

Figure 61-1 Chemical structures of amphotericin B and nystatin showing common structural features of macrolide ring with several hydroxyl groups and a conjugated double-bond system. Nystatin differs structurally from amphotericin B only in that the conjugated portion of the ring is interrupted to yield a diene and tetraene.

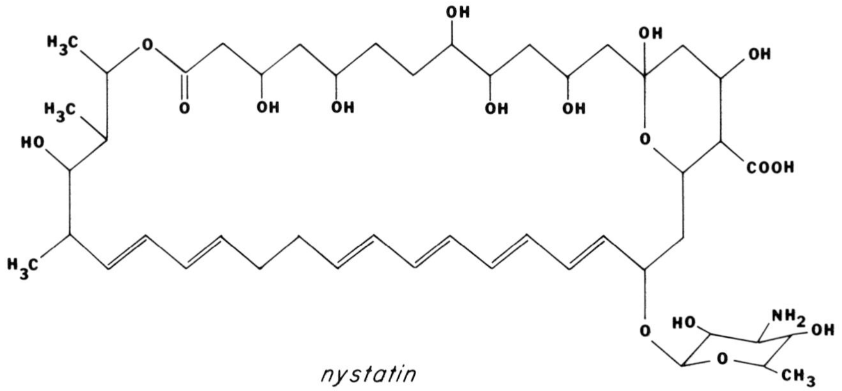

Amphotericin B is a heptaene macrolide with seven resonating carbon bonds (see Figure 61-1). The compound was first isolated from broth filtrates of *S nodosus* in 1956. Like other polyene macrolide antibiotics, amphotericin B is insoluble in water. The problem of its solubility has been circumvented by combining the antibiotic with sodium deoxycholate and sodium phosphate and hydrating the mixture with 5% dextrose solution. Amphotericin B is the only polyene antibiotic sufficiently nontoxic to humans that it can be used parenterally at effective doses against various fungi.

Nystatin, first isolated from *S noursei*, is structurally related to amphotericin B, but is not classified as a pentaene because the conjugated portion of the ring is interrupted and thus forms a tetraene and a diene (see Figure 61-1). Tolerated well both orally and topically, the drug is not available for intravenous use because of its presumed high toxicity. Nystatin is available as oral tablets (500,000 units) or as an ointment for topical use (100,000 units/g). It is used in the management of cutaneous and mucocutaneous candidiasis.

Imidazoles

The antimicrobial activity of imidazoles is effective against fungi, several species of gram-positive bacteria, and certain parasitic protozoa. The imidazole derivatives are believed to act by interfering with sterol biosynthesis at the level of C-14 of lanosterol, resulting in accumulation of 24-methylene dihydrolanosterol and obtusifoliol. This rate-limiting step prevents formation of ergosterol, a vital component of the cell membrane of fungi. The first imidazole described as an effective agent for treating cutaneous candidiasis and various dermatophyte infections was 1-chlorobenzyl-2-methylbenzimidazole.

Several other imidazole derivatives have since been synthesized; some show promise as extremely effective antifungal agents. Chemical substitutions at the R_1, R_2, or R_3 position of the methyl group on the imidazole nucleus can be varied (Figure 61-2); these substitutions alter the pharmacokinetic and antimycotic properties of the molecule.

The chemical structures of three imidazole derivatives (clotrimazole, miconazole, and ketoconazole) found to be effective in topical treatment of dermatophyte infections and cutaneous candidiasis are shown in Figure 61-2. Clotrimazole is highly toxic to animals and humans and therefore is unavailable for parenteral use in treating the systemic mycoses. Miconazole is available as a parenteral and topical agent and is effective in treating a variety of fungal infections. Ketoconazole, a new imidazole that has been tested extensively, is absorbed well from the gastrointestinal tract and therefore is effective when taken orally. Clinical trials show that it has low toxicity in humans and that it is effective in treatment of many systemic mycoses.

Agents that Act Intracellularly

Several agents effectively inhibit vital cellular processes in fungi, but problems associated with toxicity or permeability preclude their use in controlling human mycotic infections. For example, cycloheximide, produced by *S griseus* and a potent inhibitor of protein synthesis, is an effective antifungal agent against *Cryptococcus neoformans* and various saprophytic fungi, but is ineffective against most pathogens when cultured at 25 C. In addition, cycloheximide is toxic for humans; for this reason, it is not used therapeutically and is employed mainly in agriculture to control fungal diseases of plants. Also, cycloheximide is used in culture media as a selective agent to isolate various pathogenic fungi.

Another antifungal agent with limited therapeutic usefulness and interesting biologic properties is griseofulvin, a phenolic, benzofuran cyclohexane produced by various species of *Penicillium*. Taken orally, it acts against various species of dermatophytes and has been the drug of choice for chronic ringworm infections. Although its exact mechanisms of activity are unknown, data indicate that griseofulvin binds to the subunit proteins of microtubules and interferes with microtubular assembly.

The drug 5-fluorocytosine is a pyrimidine analog, first synthesized in 1957 for use as an anticancer agent; however, it proved to be ineffective against human cancer cells but active against fungi (Figure 61-3). Its spectrum of activity includes various yeastlike

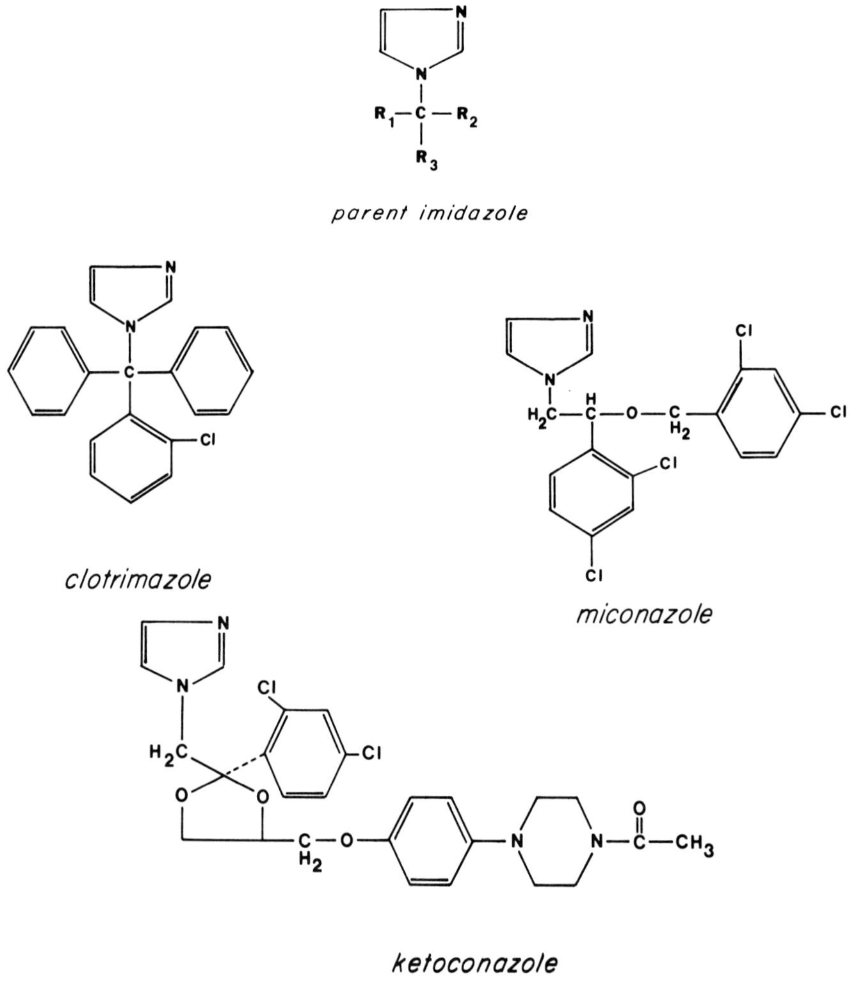

parent imidazole

clotrimazole

miconazole

ketoconazole

Figure 61-2 Chemical structure of the parent imidazole nucleus and three imidazole derivatives: clotrimazole, miconazole, and ketoconazole.

organisms belonging to the genera *Cryptococcus, Candida,* and *Torulopsis.* It also has limited antifungal activity against isolates of *Aspergillus* and has been effective in treating chromomycosis caused by *Fonsecaea pedrosoi;* it is not effective, however, in treating histoplasmosis, blastomycosis, or coccidioidomycosis. Physicians are reluctant to use this agent to treat candidiasis and cryptococcosis because resistant strains emerge; however, data indicate that when 5-fluorocytosine is used in combination with amphotericin B, an additive or synergistic effect occurs and the treatment is effective against candidiasis, cryptococcosis, and aspergillosis. A recent study has shown that this combination of amphotericin B and 5-fluorocytosine is the best treatment for cryptococcal meningitis.

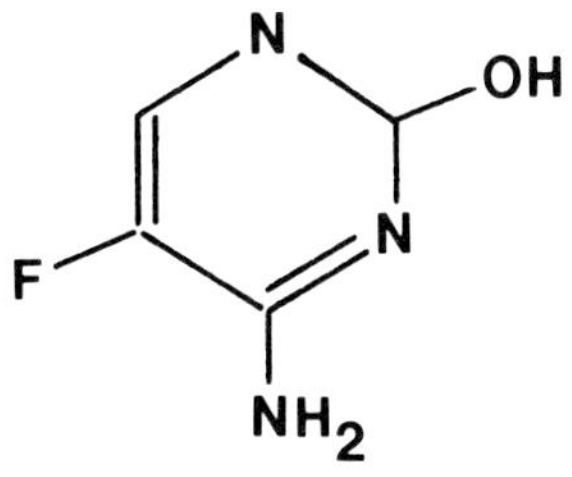

Figure 61-3 Chemical structure of pyrimidine analog, 5-fluorocytosine.

Many other compounds are available for topical use in the management of superficial and cutaneous mycotic diseases. These include tolnaftate, haloprogin, sodium thiosulfate, and selenium sulfide. One final agent worth mentioning is potassium iodide. From a historic point of view, iodides are one of the oldest compounds used in treating fungus infections. Empirically, as a saturated solution of potassium iodide taken orally, it is the drug of choice for treating subcutaneous lymphangitic sporotrichosis. It has been used in other fungus infections but without apparent effectiveness. The mechanism of its action is unknown.

Many undesirable side effects are associated with currently available antifungal agents. More specific compounds with minimal or no toxicity for humans are urgently needed.

References

Bennett, J.E.: Chemotherapy of systemic mycoses. *N Engl J Med* 1974; 290:30-32, 320-323.

D'Arcy, P.F.: Inhibition and destruction of moulds and yeasts. In: *Inhibition and destruction of the microbial cell.* Hugo, W.B. (editor). New York: Academic Press, 1971.

Dickinson, A., Tschen, J.A., Wolf, J.E., Jr.: Coccidioidomycosis with cutaneous involvement. *South Med J* 1984; 77:1464-1465.

Kobayashi, G.S., Medoff, G.: Antifungal agents: recent developments. *Ann Rev Microbiol* 1977; 31:291-308.

Medoff, G., Kobayashi, G.S.: Strategies in the treatment of systemic fungal infections. *N Engl J Med* 1980; 302:145-155.

Medoff, G., et al: Antifungal agents useful in therapy of systemic fungal infections. *Ann Rev Pharmacol Toxicol* 1983; 23:303-330.

Norman, A.W., Spielvogel, A.M., Wong, R.G.: Polyene antibioticsterol interaction. *Adv Lipid Res* 1976; 14:127-170.

Oster, K.A., Woodside, R.: Fungistatic and fungicidal compounds. In: *Disinfection, sterilization and preservation.* Block, S.S. (editor). Philadelphia: Lea and Febiger, 1977.

Petranyi, G., Ryder, N.S., Stutz, A.: Allylamine derivatives: new class of synthetic antifungal agents inhibiting fungal squalene epoxidase. *Science* 1984; 224:1239-1241.

Shadomy, S., Espinel-Ingroff, A.: Susceptibility testing with antifungal drugs. In: *Manual of Clinical Microbiology,* 3rd ed. Lennette, E.H., et al (editors). Washington, D.C.: American Society for Microbiology, 1980.

Shadomy, S., Mayhall, C.G.: Chemotherapeutics, antimycotic and antirickettsieae. In: *Encyclopedia of chemical technology,* Vol. 5, 3rd ed. Kirk, R.E., Othmer, D.F. (editors). New York: John Wiley and Sons, 1979.

IV VIROLOGY

Introduction

Thomas Albrecht, PhD

Ferdinando Dianzani, MD

Samuel Baron, MD

Recent epidemiologic reports show that viral infections in developed countries are the most common cause of acute disease that does not require hospitalization. In developing countries, viral diseases also exact a heavy toll in mortality and permanent disability, especially among infants and children. Now that antibiotics effectively control most bacterial infections, viral infections pose a relatively greater, uncontrolled threat to human health. Some data suggest that the already broad gamut of established viral diseases soon may be expanded to include other serious human ailments such as juvenile diabetes, rheumatoid arthritis, various neurologic and immunologic (for example, AIDS) disorders, and some tumors.

Viruses can infect all forms of life (bacteria, plants, protozoa, fungi, insects, fish, reptiles, birds, and mammals); however, Section IV covers only viruses capable of causing human infections, even though some of these viruses also have animal reservoirs and vectors. The fundamental concepts and genetics of bacteriophages (viruses of bacteria) are presented in Chapter 20. The omission of a separate bacteriophage chapter does not belittle the fundamental contribution made by the study of these viruses to the advancement of animal virology; rather, it reflects the fact that research on animal viruses has become an autonomous discipline with its own problems, techniques, and solutions.

Like other microorganisms, viruses may have played a role in the natural selection of animal species. A documented example is the natural selection of rabbits resistant to virulent myxoma virus during several epidemics deliberately induced to control the rabbit population in Australia. Indirect evidence suggests that the same selective role was played by smallpox virus in humans. Another possible, though unproved, mechanism by which viruses may affect evolution is by introducing viral genetic material into animal cells by mechanisms similar to those that govern gene transfer by bacteriophages. For example, genes from avirulent retrovirus integrated into genomes of chickens or mice produce resistance to reinfection by related, virulent retroviruses. The same relationship may exist for human retroviruses, since a human leukemia-causing retrovirus has been reported.

Viruses are small, subcellular agents that are unable to multiply outside a host cell (**intracellular obligate parasitism**). The assembled virus (virion) is formed by only one type of nucleic acid (RNA or DNA) and, in the simplest viruses, a protective protein coat. The nucleic acid contains the genetic information necessary to program the synthetic machinery of the host cell for viral replication. The protein coat serves two main functions: first, it protects the nucleic acid from extracellular environmental insults such as nucleases; second, it permits attachment of the virion to the membrane of the host cell, the negative charge of which repels the naked nucleic acid. Once the viral genome has penetrated and thereby infected the host cell, virus replication mainly depends on host cell machinery for energy and synthetic requirements.

The various virion components are synthesized separately within the cell and are later assembled, somewhat as in a jigsaw puzzle, to form progeny particles. This assembly type of replication is unique to viruses and distinguishes them from all other small, obligate, intracellular parasites. The basic structure of viruses can cause them to be simultaneously adaptable and selective. Many viral genomes are so adaptable that once they have penetrated the cell membrane under experimental conditions, viral replication can occur in almost any cell. On the other hand, intact viruses are so selective that most virions can infect only a limited range of cell types. This selectivity exists largely because penetration of the nucleic acid usually requires a specific reaction for the coat to attach to the host cell membrane.

Another important feature of viral infections is that most viruses, unlike most other microorganisms, cannot establish a mutual relationship with the host. In fact, although some viruses may establish some forms of silent infection, their multiplication usually causes cell damage or death; however, since viruses must depend on host survival for their own survival, they tend to establish mild infections in which death of the host is more an aberration than a regular outcome.

Viruses are distinct among microorganisms in their extreme dependence on the host cell. Since a virus must grow within a host cell, the virus must be viewed together with its host in any consideration of pathogenesis, epidemiology, host defenses, or therapy. The bilateral association between the virus and its host imposes specific conditions for pathogenesis. For example, rhinoviruses require a temperature not exceeding 34 C; this requirement restricts their growth to only those cells in the cool outer layer of the nasal mucosa, thereby preventing spread to deeper cells where temperatures are higher.

The intracellular location of the virus often protects the virus against some of the host's immune mechanisms; at the same time, this location makes the virus vulnerable because of its dependence on the host cell's synthetic machinery, which may be altered by even subtle physical and chemical changes produced by the viral infection (inflammation, fever, circulatory alterations, and interferon).

Epidemiologic properties depend greatly on the characteristics of the virus–host association. For example, some arthropod-borne viruses require a narrow range of temperature to multiply in insects; as a result, these viruses are found only under certain seasonal and geographic conditions.

Viruses are difficult targets for chemotherapy because they replicate only within host cells, mainly utilizing many of the host cell's biosynthetic processes. The similarity of host-directed and virus-directed processes makes it difficult to find antiviral agents specific enough to exert a greater effect on viral replication in infected cells than on functions in uninfected host cells. It is becoming increasingly apparent, however, that each virus may have a few specific steps of replication that may be used as targets for highly selective, carefully aimed chemotherapeutic agents. Therefore, proper use of such drugs requires a thorough knowledge of the suitable targets, based on a correct diagnosis and a precise understanding of the replicative mechanisms for the offending virus.

Knowledge of the pathogenetic mechanisms by which virus enters, spreads within, and exits from the body also is critical for correct diagnosis and treatment of disease and for prevention of spread in the environment. Effective treatment with antibody-containing immunoglobulin requires knowing when virus is susceptible to antibody (for example, during viremia spread) and when virus reaches target organs where antibody is not effective. Many successful vaccines have been based on knowledge of pathogenesis and immune defenses. Comparable considerations govern treatment with interferon.

Clearly, viral infections are among the most difficult and demanding problems a physician must face. Unfortunately, some of these problems still lack satisfactory solutions, although tremendous progress has been made during the last several decades. Many aspects of medical virology are now understood, others are being clarified gradually, and many more are still completely obscure. Knowledge of the properties of viruses and the relationships they establish with their hosts is crucial to successful investigation and clinical management of their pathologic processes.

Our plan for conveying this knowledge is to present, first, concepts of viral *structure*, and then relate them to principles of viral *multiplication*. Together these concepts form the basis for understanding how viruses are *classified*, how they *effect cells*, and how their *genetic* system functions. These molecular and cellular mechanisms are combined with the previously presented concepts of immunology to convey viral pathogenesis, nonspecific defenses, persistent infections, epidemiology, evolution, and control. Each of the important families of viruses is then discussed. Having studied the virology section, the reader should be able to use most principles of virology to explain individual manifestations of virus infection and the processes that bring them about.

62 Structure

Carl F. T. Mattern, MD

General Concepts

Because they are obligate intracellular parasites, viruses do not need the complicated structure required to carry out the multiple functions of eukaryotic and prokaryotic cells. The only function the virus must perform is delivery of its **genome** (nucleic acid) into the host cell so that the genome can be expressed (translated and transcribed) by the host's synthetic machinery.

A fully assembled infectious virus is called a **virion.** The simplest virion consists of two basic components: **nucleic acid** (single- or double-stranded RNA or DNA) and a protein coat or **capsid,** which protects the viral genome from nucleases and attaches the virion to the host cell membrane. Coat proteins are specified by the virus genome, but the limited amount of genomic nucleic acid can code for only the few structural proteins that form the capsid. Units that consist of only one or a few structural proteins must therefore **self-assemble** to form the continuous coat structure. Such self-assembly arrangements follow two basic patterns: **helical symmetry,** in which the protein subunits and nucleic acid are arranged in a helix, and **icosahedral symmetry,** in which protein subunits assemble into symmetric shells covering viral cores of nucleic acid or nucleoprotein. Some of the larger viruses have more complex structures.

Virions with these symmetries may also have an additional covering or **envelope,** usually derived in part from the host cell membranes. Lipid is usually present in viral envelopes as a bilayer in contact with virus-coded proteins internally and with glycosylated proteins externally. Under electron microscopic examination, viral envelopes often appear to be studded with glycoprotein spikes (projections). In those viruses that complete their assembly by budding from the plasma or other cell membrane, the lipid composition of the viral envelope frequently reflects that of the host cell membrane. Envelope glycoproteins are important in adsorption of viruses to cells, and thus in the determination of viral host range.

The diameters of virions range from 20 to 300 nm. Extremes of diameter differ by a factor of about 15; however, masses or volumes differ about 500-fold. Viruses form well-defined anatomic groups that are quite distinct from each other. These morphologic variations may reflect different phylogenetic origins and evolutionary adaptations that permit viruses to infect different host cells or to survive hostile extracellular environments. Viruses that cause human disease reflect only a small part of the morphological spectrum.

Helical Symmetry

In the replication of viruses with helical symmetry, identical protein units (**protomers**) self-assemble into a helical array surrounding the nucleic acid, which follows a similar spiral path deep within the protein capsid. The entire structure (nucleic acid within capsid) is referred to as a **nucleocapsid.** Such structures appear as rigid, highly elongated rods or as flexible filaments; in either, details of the capsid structure are difficult to discern by electron microscopy. In addition to classification as flexible or rigid and naked or enveloped (by membrane), helical nucleocapsids are characterized by length, width, pitch of the helix, and number of protomers per helical turn. The most extensively studied helical virus is tobacco mosaic virus (Figure 62-1). Many important structural features of this plant virus have been detected by x-ray diffraction studies.

Viruses With Helical Symmetry

All viruses with both helical symmetry and pathogenicity for humans are enveloped and contain RNA (Figures 62-2 and 62-3). This group of viruses includes orthomyxoviruses and paramyxoviruses, which are the etiologic agents of influenza, some upper respiratory infections, mumps, and measles.

A variant helical structure is seen in the rhabdoviruses (rodlike viruses), which are rounded on one end and flattened on the other (see Figure 62-3). Rhabdoviruses are shorter and wider than simple helical nucleocapsids and contain a short, broad, helical nucleocapsid within a lipid-containing envelope. Rabies is caused by a rhabdovirus.

Enveloped RNA Viruses of Uncertain Symmetry

Other major groups of viruses that infect humans are enveloped and may have helical nucleocapsids. These include the coronaviruses, which cause respiratory disease, and the arenaviruses, etiologic agents of lymphocytic choriomeningitis, hemorrhagic fever, and

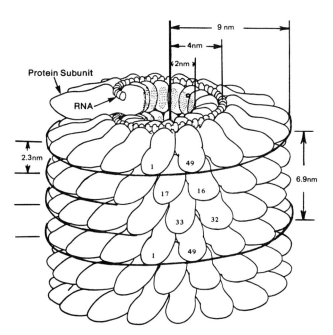

Figure 62-1 Model of a rigid, helical tobacco mosaic virus (about 5% of the length depicted). Individual protein subunits (17,400 mol. wt.) assemble in a helix with an axial repeat of 6.9 nm (49 subunits in 3 turns). Each turn contains a nonintegral number of subunits (16⅓) producing a pitch of 2.3 nm. The RNA (2×10^6 mol. wt.) is sandwiched internally between adjacent turns of capsid protein forming an RNA helix of the same pitch, 8 nm in diameter, and extending the length of the virus, with three nucleotide bases in contact with each subunit. Some 2130 subunits per virion cover and protect the RNA. The complete virus is 300 nm long and 18 nm in diameter, with a hollow cylindrical core 4 nm in diameter. From Mattern (1977), courtesy of Marcel Dekker, Inc., as modified from Caspar, D.L.D. *Adv Protein Chemistry* 1963; 18:37.

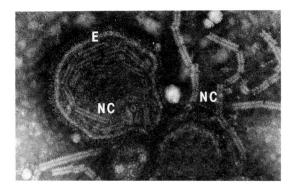

Figure 62-2 Fragments of flexible helical nucleocapsids (NC) of Sendai virus, a paramyxovirus, are seen either within the protective envelope (E) or free, after rupture of the envelope. The intact nucleocapsid is about 1000 nm long and 17 nm in diameter; its pitch (helical period) is about 5 nm. (Courtesy A. Kalica, National Institutes of Health. × 200,000.)

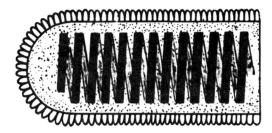

Figure 62-3 Scheme of typical rhabdovirus, 180 nm long, 60 nm in diameter, and consisting of an internal helix of RNA and protein (nucleocapsid) covered with a lipid membrane (envelope) that is studded with externally projecting spikes.

Lassa fever. Coronaviruses are notable for their prominant envelope spikes, which impart a coronal effect to negatively stained viruses on electron microscopic examination.

The retroviruses constitute a large viral group that infects vertebrates and causes a variety of neoplastic and chronic diseases. They now are known to be significant in human disease. Human T cell lymphotropic viruses (HTLV-I, HTLV-II) are leukemia-lymphoma viruses. Another retrovirus, HTLV-III, is probably the etiologic agent of AIDS through its lytic effect on helper T cells. Retroviruses often appear to have a polyhedral core component.

Icosahedral Symmetry

An **icosahedron** is a polyhedron having 20 equilateral triangular faces and 12 vertices (Figure 62-4). Lines through opposite vertices form axes of fivefold *rotational symmetry;* all structural features of the polyhedron repeat five times within each 360 degrees of rotation about the fivefold axis. Lines through the centers of opposite triangular faces form axes of threefold rotational symmetry; twofold rotational symmetry axes are formed by lines through midpoints of opposite edges. Icosahedra (polyhedral or spherical) with fivefold, threefold, and twofold axes of rotational symmetry (see Figure 62-4) are defined as having 532 symmetry (read as 5,3,2). Because 32 symmetry also is exhibited by the cubic or isometric crystal system, the terms **cubic** and **isometric** also are employed to describe 532 symmetry of viruses.

Viruses were found to have 532 symmetry first through x-ray diffraction studies and subsequently by electron microscopy employing negative staining techniques. Several icosahedral viruses have protomers (protein subunits) conveniently arranged in relatively large clusters called capsomers, which are readily delineated by electron-dense stain (Figure 62-5). The arrangement of capsomers into icosahedral symmetry (compare Figure 62-5 with the upper right model in Figure 62-4) permits the classification of such viruses by capsomer number. Such classification requires the identification of a closest pair of vertex capsomers (those through which the fivefold symmetry axes pass) and the distribution of capsomers between them.

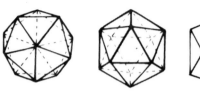

Figure 62-4 Icosahedral models seen, left to right, on fivefold, threefold, and twofold axes of rotational symmetry. These axes are perpendicular to the plane of the page and pass through the centers of each figure. Both polyhedral (upper) and spherical (lower) forms are represented by different virus families.

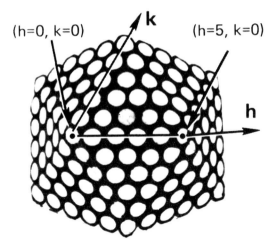

Figure 62-5 Adenovirus model. Capsomers are depicted as circles delineated by an electron-dense stain. The inclined axes, h and k, are indicated, the second vertex has the indices $h = 5$, $k = 0$. The total number of capsomers: $C = 10 (h^2 + hk + k^2) + 2 = 252$. Capsomer organization also is expressed by the triangulation number, T, the number of unit triangles on each of the 20 faces of the icosahedron. A unit triangle is formed by lines joining the centers of any three adjacent capsomers. $T = (h^2 + hk + k^2) = 25$ for adenoviruses and $C = 10T + 2$. Adenoviruses also have 12 antennalike protein structures (pentons); one projects from each of the 12 vertex capsids (not shown; see Chapter 87). Protomers are the smallest protein units of which capsomers are assembled and are usually not delineated by negative staining.

DNA Viruses With Icosahedral Symmetry

Adenoviruses.   In the adenovirus model in Figure 62-5, one of the capsomers on a fivefold axis is arbitrarily assigned the indices $h = 0$, $k = 0$ (origin), where h and k are the indicated axes of the inclined (60 degree) net of capsomers. The net axes are formed by lines of the closest-packed neighboring capsomers. In adenoviruses, the h and k axes also coincide with the edges of the triangular faces. Any second neighboring vertex capsomer has indices $h = 5$, $k = 0$ (or $h = 0$, $k = 5$). The capsomer number (C) can be determined to be 252 from the h and k indices and the equation: $C = 10 (h^2 + hk + k^2) + 2$. This number of capsomers is found in all members of the adenovirus group. Some members of this virus group are responsible for respiratory infections and conjunctivitis in humans; others are indigenous to a variety of nonhuman vertebrate species.

Herpesviruses.   In herpesviruses, the indices of a second vertex capsomer are $h = 4$, $k = 0$; thus, according to the preceding equation, herpesviruses are constructed of 162 capsomers. These viruses are enveloped. In humans, members of this group are associated with herpes simplex disease complex, varicella, herpes zoster, infectious mononucleosis, and possibly Burkitt's lymphoma and carcinoma of the cervix and nasopharynx. Herpes viruses also are associated with adenocarcinomas of the kidney in frogs, lymphomas in monkeys, and Marek's disease (neural lymphomatosis) in chickens.

Papovaviruses. The papovaviruses (*pa*pilloma, *po*lyoma, *va*cuolating viruses) important in human disease are JC virus, which has been isolated from patients with multifocal leukoencephalopathy; BK virus, isolated from patients with immunosuppression states; and human papilloma virus, isolated from the lesions of patients with common, plantar, and genital warts, laryngeal papillomas, and epidermodysplasia verruciformis. Other viruses in this group produce papillomas and malignant tumors in various animals. Members of this group have indices for the second vertex capsomer of $h = 1, k = 2$, or $h = 2, k = 1$. In all icosahedral viruses in which neither the h nor the k index is 0 and h and k are not equal, dextro ($h < k$) or levo ($h > k$) forms may exist. Both forms are known to exist within the papovavirus group; their capsomer number is 72.

Other DNA Viruses. *Parvoviruses* are small (about 22 nm diameter), single-stranded DNA viruses of which only the adeno-associated virus (AAV) can replicate in humans, provided that adenovirus infection is also present. AAV has not been associated with human disease. It probably has icosahedral symmetry, but its surface structure has not been determined. In contrast, surface structure of the bacterial parvovirus ϕX 174 has been found to be icosahedral.

Members of the poxviruses (variola, vaccinia, and molluscum contagiosum viruses) are among the largest viruses known; they are brick-shaped (240 × 300 nm), enveloped, and have a complex structure not yet clearly defined. They contain about 50 times more nucleic acid than do the smallest viruses.

RNA Viruses With Icosahedral Symmetry

Picornaviruses. Picornaviruses (*pico-RNA-viruses*) constitute a major group of small (25–30 nm) RNA viruses that are not enveloped. Of the human pathogens (polio, Coxsackie, Enteric Cytopathic Human Orphan [ECHO], Hepatitis A, and rhinoviruses), only poliovirus has been demonstrated by x-ray diffraction to have 532 symmetry. The surface structure of these viruses is difficult to visualize; their surfaces may be complex and may not consist simply of 32 capsomers ($h = 1, k = 1$), as do those of some plant picornaviruses.

Caliciviruses. Caliciviruses have been reported to cause gastroenteritis in a number of mammals. These agents are 32–39 nm diameter RNA viruses variously seen by negative staining electron microscopy as presenting surface spikes or 32 surface depressions ($h = 1, k = 1$). Morphologically similar isolates associated with gastroenteritis in humans have been documented, but their structure has not been fully elucidated.

Togaviruses. Togaviruses comprise a large number of encephalitis-producing viruses and rubella virus. The structure of these agents has not been determined. They are enveloped and probably have icosahedral symmetry.

Bunyaviruses. The bunyavirus family contains a large number of viruses that are transmitted to humans by arthropods and cause disease ranging from mild febrile infections to serious illness with significant mortality. These viruses are enveloped and have an icosahedral nucleocapsid that in some members appears to contain 122 capsomers ($h = 2, k = 2$).

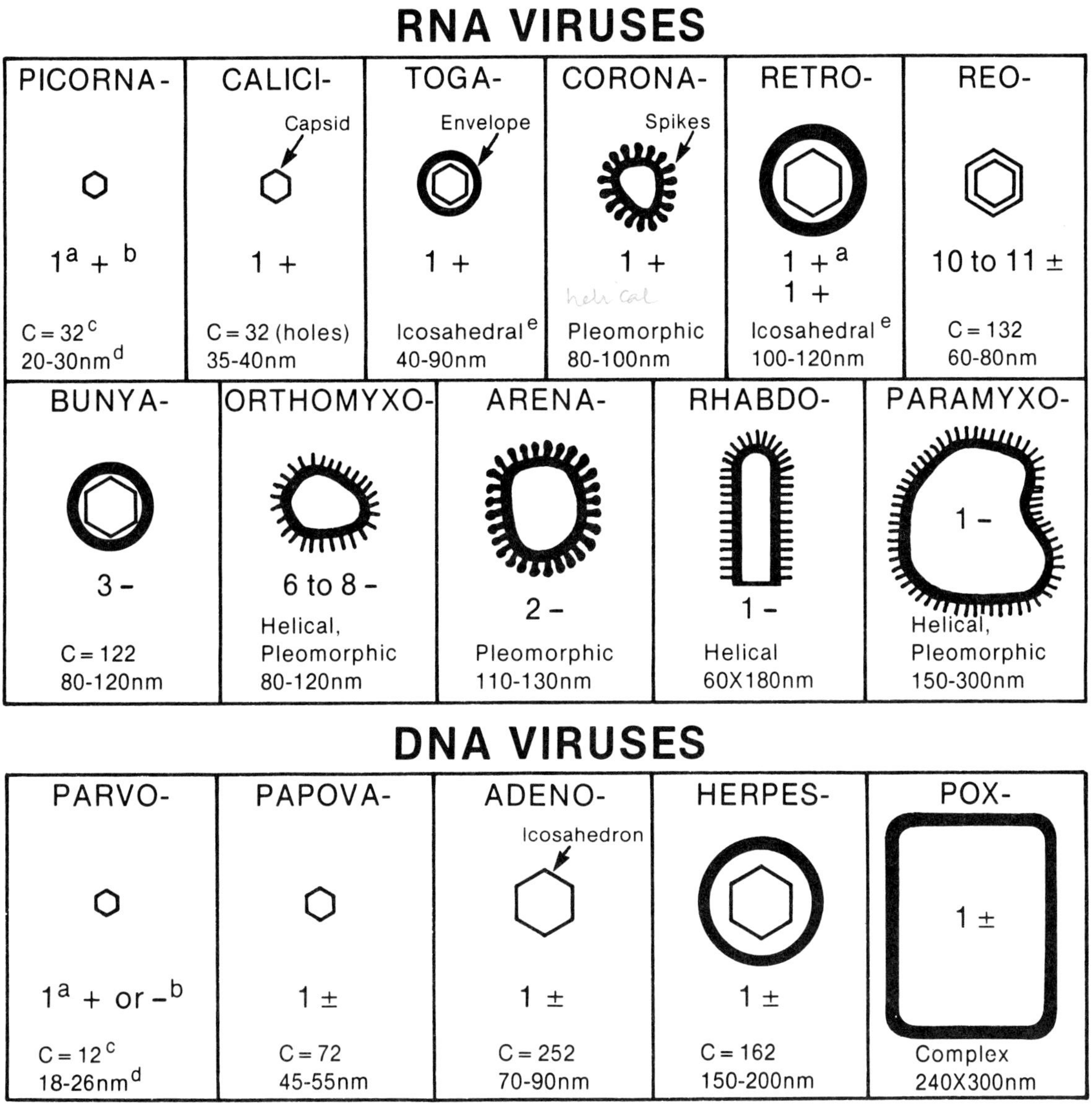

RNA VIRUSES

DNA VIRUSES

Figure 62-6 Structural features of viral pathogens of humans. Hexagons denote capsids with icosahedral symmetry. Envelopes are indicated by heavy boundaries some of which present projecting glycoprotein spikes. a, Number of different genome segments (retroviruses have two identical RNA genomes). b, Polarity of nucleic acid (RNA or DNA): +, positive; −, negative; ±, double stranded; + or −, either one.) c, Symmetry: icosahedral (denoted by capsomer number C, when known), helical, pleomorphic, or complex. d, Size in nanometers (figures about $10^5\times$ virus size). e, Capsomer number unknown.

Reoviruses.   Three groups of reoviruses (*r*espiratory, *e*nteric, *o*rphan) produce disease in humans: reoviruses (which usually cause mild illness), rotaviruses (which cause gastroenteritis that is often severe in children), and orbiviruses (which cause Colorado tick fever). These viruses are unusual in that their RNA is double-stranded, their genomes exist as 10–12 separate segments, and they apparently possess a double capsid. The inner capsid of some members is icosahedral with 132 capsomers ($h = 3, k = 1$). The structure of the outer capsid is not known; earlier reports of its having 92 depressions filled with stain may have been due to artifactual images.

Virus Core Structure

With the exception of helical nucleocapsids, little is known about the packaging or organization of viral nucleic acid (RNA or DNA) within the virion core. It has been found, however, that some virions are simple nucleocapsids and that others have a core containing nucleic acid and basic protein(s) surrounded by capsid protein. Recent developments in preparation of specimens for electron microscopy coupled with optical diffraction of their images hold promise for elucidating viral core structure.

RNA Virus Genomes

The genomes of many RNA viruses show remarkable variations. In addition to existing as single-stranded or double-stranded molecules, they may exist as single molecule genomes or as two or more separate molecules (**segmented genomes**). In addition, single-stranded RNA may be either a **plus strand,** which is **messenger RNA** (mRNA), or a **minus strand,** which is **complementary** to the plus strand and has no messenger (protein translation) function. Purified plus strand viral RNA alone induces infection in appropriate cells because it is mRNA and initiates translation of a viral-coded enzyme (**polymerase**) necessary for the initiation of RNA replication. Viruses with minus strand RNA must contain this polymerase (*RNA-dependent RNA polymerase*) to initiate transcription of plus strand RNA, which is necessary for the continued synthesis of viral components. Purified minus strand RNA (free of RNA polymerase), therefore, is not infectious.

Double-stranded RNA viruses such as the reoviruses contain 10 or 11 separate genome segments, each consisting of complementary plus and minus strands that are hydrogen bonded into linear double-stranded molecules. The replication of these viruses is complex: only the plus RNA strands are released from the infecting virion to initiate replication.

Retroviruses represent a unique RNA virus group. Their genome consists of two identical, single-stranded, plus strand RNA molecules that are noncovalently linked over a short terminal region. These viruses contain a **reverse transcriptase** (RNA-dependent DNA polymerase) by which a double-stranded, circular proviral DNA is transcribed. This DNA becomes covalently bonded into the DNA of the host cell to make possible the transcription of the plus RNA strands that form the progeny retrovirus virions.

DNA Virus Genomes

Most DNA viruses contain single genomes of double-stranded, linear DNA. The papovaviruses, however, have circular DNA genomes. Double-stranded DNA serves as a template both for mRNA translation and for self-transcription. Because the plus strand RNA is complementary to only one of the DNA strands, that strand is called the minus DNA strand.

Single-stranded, linear DNA is found in the small viruses of the parvovirus group. The AAV subgroup produces progeny virions of which equal numbers contain either plus DNA or minus DNA. These viruses are replication-defective, requiring coinfection with adenovirus or herpesvirus for the production of AAV progeny virions.

Structural Features of 16 Virus Families

Figure 62-6 summarizes many of the known structural features of the 16 virus families that are known to be pathogenic for humans. Included are their size, symmetry or shape, capsomer number (where reasonably well established), presence or absence of an envelope and spikes, and properties of the viral genome.

References

Adrian, M. et al: Cryo-electron microscopy of viruses. *Nature* 1984; 308:33-36.

Bridger, J.C., Hall, G.A., Brown, J.F.: Characterization of a calici-like virus (Newbury agent) found in association with astrovirus in bovine diarrhea. *Infect Immun* 1984; 43:133-138.

Caspar, D.L.D.: Design principles in virus particle construction. In: *Viral and rickettsial infections in man,* 4th ed. Horsfall, F.L., Tamm, I., (editors). Philadelphia: J.B. Lippincott, 1975.

Compans, R.W., Klenk, H-D.: Virus membranes. In: *Comprehensive virology,* vol 13. Fraenkel-Conrat, H., Wagner, R.R., (editors). New York: Plenum Press, 1979.

Fisher, H.W.: Use of electron microscopy in virology. In: *Comprehensive virology,* vol 17. Fraenkel-Conrat, H., Wagner, R.R., (editors). New York: Plenum Press, 1981.

Holmes, I.A.: Rotaviruses. In: *Reoviridae.* Joklik, W.K., (editor). New York: Plenum Press, 1983.

Jacrot, B: Structural studies of viruses with x-rays and neutrons. In: *Comprehensive virology,* vol 17. Fraenkel-Conrat, H., Wagner, R.R., (editors). New York: Plenum Press, 1981.

Joklik, W.K.: Reoviruses. In: *Reoviridae.* Joklik, W.K., (editor). New York: Plenum Press, 1983.

Mattern, C.F.T.: Symmetry in virus architecture. In: *Molecular biology of animal viruses.* Nayak, D.P., (editor). New York: Marcel Dekker, 1977.

Popovic, M., et al.: Detection, isolation and continuous production of cytopathic retroviruses (HTLV-III) from patients with AIDS and pre-AIDS. *Science* 1984; 224:497-500.

Schaffer, F.L.: Caliciviruses. In: *Comprehensive virology,* vol 14. Fraenkel-Conrat, H., Wagner, R.R., (editors). New York: Plenum Press, 1979.

63 Multiplication

Bernard Roizman, ScD

General Concepts

Viral diseases result from the expression of viral genes in infected cells or from the reaction of the host to infected cells expressing viral genes. In most instances, acute viral diseases can be directly related to the destruction of the infected cell during multiplication of the virus. The key to understanding how viruses multiply is a set of concepts and definitions.

For a virus to multiply, it must first infect a cell. Infection is the presence in cells of viral genetic material. **Susceptibility** refers to the capacity of a cell to become infected. The **host range** of a virus describes both the kinds of cells and the animal species it can infect and in which it can multiply; the host range of viruses varies greatly.

In the course of infection, the virus brings into the cell its genetic material—RNA or DNA—accompanied in some instances by essential proteins. The size, composition, and gene organization of viral genomes vary enormously. Viruses have evolved by many different independent routes, and no single evolutionary line seems to have prevailed. In consequence, two concepts must be stressed. First, the ability of the virus to multiply and the fate of the infected cell hinge on the synthesis and function of viral gene products—the proteins. The diversity of the viral genomic structures is reflected in the diversity of the mechanisms by which viruses ensure that their proteins are made. Second, although viruses differ considerably in the number of genes they contain, all viruses can be said to encode three sets of functions that are expressed by the proteins they specify: viral proteins ensure the replication of viral genomes, package the genome into virus particles—the virions—and alter the structure and function of the infected cell. In most instances (for example, herpesviruses) it is the viral proteins that replicate the viral genome. In a few instances (for example, papovaviruses), the viral proteins merely insure that host enzymes replicate the viral genome. In all instances, it is the viral proteins that package the genome into virions. Lastly, the effects of viral multiplication on the host cell range from cell death to subtle but potentially significant changes in function and in antigenic specificity.

Knowledge of the reproductive cycles of viruses stems from analyses of the events occurring in synchronously infected cells in culture; little is known about viruses that have not yet been grown in cultured cells. The reproductive cycles of all viruses exhibit several common features (Figure 63-1). First, immediately after penetration of the virus into the cell and for several hours thereafter, little or no infectious virus can be detected. Known as the **eclipse phase,** this interval signals that the viral genomes are exposed to host or viral machinery necessary for their expression, but that no progeny virus has yet been assembled. An interval follows in which viral progeny accumulate in the cell or in the extracellular environment at exponential rates. This interval is known as the **maturation phase.** After several hours, cells infected with viruses cease all metabolic activity and disintegrate. Cells infected with other viruses may continue to synthesize viruses indefinitely. The reproductive cycle of viruses ranges from 6 to 8 hours (picornaviruses) to more than 40 hours (some herpesviruses). The virus yields per cell range from more than 100,000 poliovirus particles to several thousand poxvirus particles.

Infection of a susceptible cell does not automatically ensure that viral multiplication will ensue and that viral progeny will emerge. Awareness of this fact is by far the most important conceptual development in virology to emerge in the last decade and should

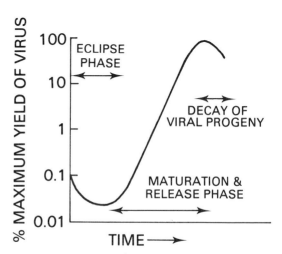

Figure 63-1 Schematic representation of reproductive cycle of viruses infecting human and animal cells.

be considered in some detail. Infection of susceptible cells may be productive, abortive, or restrictive. **Productive infection** occurs in **permissive cells** and is characterized by production of infectious progeny. **Abortive infection** can occur for two reasons. Although a cell can be susceptible to infection, it may be **nonpermissive** in that, for reasons mostly unknown, it allows only a few of the viral genes to be expressed. Abortive infection also may result from infection of permissive or nonpermissive cells with **defective viruses** that lack a full complement of viral genes. Lastly, cells can be only transiently permissive, with the consequences that either the virus persists in the cell until the cells become permissive or that only a few of the cells in a population produce viral progeny at any time. This type has been defined as **restrictive infection.** The significance now placed on nonpermissive cells and the abortive infection that occurs in them stems from the observation that cytolytic viruses, which normally destroy the permissive cell during productive infection, may merely injure but not destroy abortively infected permissive or nonpermissive cells. The consequences of this injury may be the expression of host functions that transform the cell from normal to malignant. An additional consequence of restrictive and abortive infections is the persistence of the viral genomes.

Initiation of Infection

To infect a cell, the virus must adsorb to the cell surface, penetrate the cell, and become sufficiently uncoated to make its genome accessible to viral or host enzymes for transcription or to the translation machinery of the cell.

Adsorption

Adsorption constitutes specific binding of a virion protein (the **antireceptor**) to a constituent of the cell surface (the **receptor**). The hemagglutinin of influenza virus (orthomyxovirus) is an example of an antireceptor molecule. Antireceptors are scattered throughout the surface of viruses infecting human and animal cells. Complex viruses such as vaccinia (a poxvirus) and herpes simplex virus (herpesviruses) may have more than one type of antireceptor molecule. Furthermore, antireceptor molecules may have several domains, each of which may react with different receptors. Mutations in the genes specifying antireceptors may cause virions to lose the capacity to interact with certain receptors. For example, the wild type poliovirus can infect cells in both the gastrointestinal tract and in the central nervous system, whereas the attenuated vaccine strains have retained the capacity to infect the former but not the latter.

The cellular receptors identified so far are largely glycoproteins. Adsorption requires cations but is largely temperature- and energy-independent. The susceptibility of a cell is defined on the basis of availability of receptors, and not all cells in an otherwise susceptible organism express receptors. Human cells in the kidney lack receptors for poliovirus, but receptors are readily made when renal cells are propagated in cell culture. Susceptibility should not be confused with permissiveness; thus, chick cells are insusceptible to poliovirus because they lack receptors, but they are fully permissive in that they will replicate the virus following infection with the intact RNA extracted from poliovirus particles.

Adsorption of viruses to cells in many instances leads to irreversible changes in the structure of the virion. In other instances, when penetration does not ensue, the virus can detach itself and readsorb to a different cell. Viruses that can detach and readsorb are orthomyxoviruses and paramyxoviruses, which carry a neuraminidase on their surface. These viruses can elute from the receptor by cleaving the sialic acid in the polysaccharide chains of the receptor.

Penetration

Penetration is an energy-dependent step. It occurs almost instantaneously after adsorption and involves one of three mechanisms: translocation of the virus across the plasma membrane, pinocytosis of the viral particle resulting in accumulation of viral particles inside cytoplasmic vacuoles, and fusion of the plasma membrane with the virion envelope. Nonenveloped viruses penetrate by the first two mechanisms. For example, in the course of adsorption of the poliovirus particle to the cell, VP4 becomes modified, the particle loses its structural integrity, and the RNA protein complex is translocated into the cytoplasm. Myxoviruses and herpesviruses are examples of viruses that penetrate as a consequence of fusion of their envelopes with the plasma membrane. In these examples, the envelope of the virus remains in the plasma membrane, whereas the internal constituents spill into the cytoplasm. Fusion of the viral envelope with the plasma membrane requires the function of specific viral proteins in the envelope of the virus.

Uncoating

Uncoating is a general term applied to the events that occur after penetration and set the stage for the viral genome to express its functions. In the case of papovaviruses, adenoviruses, and herpesviruses, the capsid is disaggregated—most likely by cellular enzymes with the participation of viral structural proteins—and only viral DNA or a DNA protein complex remains of the virus particle before expression of viral functions. In cells infected with reoviruses, only portions of the capsid are removed and the viral genome expresses all its functions, even though it is never fully released from the capsid. The poxviruses genome is uncoated in two stages; whereas in the first stage, the outer covering is removed by host enzymes, the release of viral DNA from the core appears to require the participation of viral gene products made after infection.

Mechanisms of Replication

In the course of their evolution, viruses have developed several strategies to deal with encoding and organization of viral genes, expression of viral genes, the replication of viral genomes, and assembly, and maturation of viral progeny. Before considering each of these in detail, it is worth reiterating that the synthesis of viral proteins by the cellular protein-synthesizing machinery is the key event in viral replication. Irrespective of the size, composition, and organization of its genome, the virus must present to the protein-synthesizing machinery of the eukaryotic cell a messenger RNA (mRNA) that the cell can recognize and translate. In this regard, the cell imposes two sets of constraints on viruses. First, the cell synthesizes its own mRNA in the nucleus by transcription of its DNA, followed by posttranscription processing of the transcript. The cell therefore lacks the enzymes necessary to synthesize mRNA from a viral RNA genome either in the nucleus or in the cytoplasm and the enzymes capable of transcribing viral DNA in the cytoplasm. The consequence of this constraint is that only viruses with genomes that consist of DNA and reach the nucleus can take advantage of cell transcriptases to synthesize their RNA. All other viruses had to develop their own enzymes to generate mRNA. The second constraint is that the eukaryotic cell's synthesizing machinery is equipped to translate only monocistronic messages, since this machinery does not recognize internal initiation sites within mRNA. The consequence of this constraint is that viruses must synthesize a separate mRNA for each gene (monocistronic messages) or an mRNA encompassing several genes and specifying a large precursor polyprotein, which is then cleaved into individual proteins.

Encoding and Organization of Genomes

Viral genes are encoded into RNA or DNA genomes. Further, these genomes can be single- or double-stranded. In addition, they can be **monopartite** (all genes linked in a single chromosome) or **multipartite** (viral genes distributed in several chromosomes that together constitute the viral genome). Multipartite genomes often are called **segmented** genomes.

Among the RNA viruses, reovirus is the only family containing a double-stranded genome; this genome is multipartite and consists of 10 segments or chromosomes. The single-stranded RNA viruses can be monopartite (piconaviruses, togaviruses, paramyxoviruses, rhabdoviruses, and retroviruses) or multipartite (orthomyxoviruses, arenaviruses, and bunyaviruses). All RNA genomes are linear molecules. Some, like picornaviruses, contain a covalently linked polypeptide or an amino acid at the 5' end of the RNA.

All DNA viruses contain a monopartite genome. Except for parvoviruses, all are double stranded. Although the individual parvovirus virions contain single-stranded DNA, both complementary strands of the DNA may be packaged in separate virions. The papovavirus DNA is circular and supercoiled; the hepatitis B virus DNA also is circular, but contains a gap in each of its strands; and the DNAs of herpesviruses and adenoviruses are linear.

Expression and Replication of RNA Viral Genomes

The single-stranded RNA viruses form three groups. The first comprises picornaviruses and togaviruses. These genomes have two functions (Figure 63-2); the first is to serve as a messenger RNA. By convention, viruses with genomes that can and do serve as messengers are known as plus (+) strand viruses. Following entry into the cell, picornavirus RNA binds to ribosomes and is translated in its entirety. The product of this translation—the polyprotein—is then cleaved into smaller polypeptides. The second function of the genomic RNA is to serve as a template for synthesis of a complementary minus (−) strand RNA by a polymerase derived from the products of cleavage of the polyproteins. The (−) strand RNA then serves in turn as a template to make more (+) strands. The progeny (+) strands can then serve as mRNA, templates to make more (−) strands, and constituents of progeny virus.

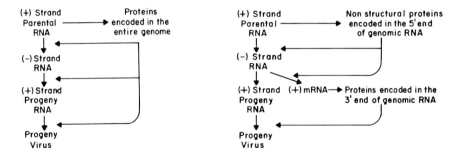

Figure 63-2 Schematic diagram of flow of events during replication of picornaviruses (left) and togaviruses (right). The RNAs of these two (+) strand virus families function as mRNA after infection.

Togaviruses differ in only one respect from picornaviruses. Specifically, only approximately one-half of the genomic RNA is translated in the first round of protein synthesis (see Figure 63-2). The function of the resulting products is to transcribe the genomic RNA. A (−) strand is then synthesized, and this RNA in turn serves as a template for two classes of (+) strand molecules. The first class is mRNA encompassing the region of the genomic RNA not translated in the first round. The resulting polyprotein is cleaved into proteins whose main function is to serve as structural components of the virion. The second class consists of full-size (+) strands, which are packaged in the virion.

Central to replication of (+) strand viruses is the capability of the genomic RNA to serve as mRNA after infection. This capability has three consequences. First, the enzymes responsible for the transcription of the genome are made after infection and are not brought into the infected cell by the virion. Second, because all (+) strand genomes are monopartite and therefore have all their genes linked in a single chromosome, the products of translation are necessarily polyproteins, which must be cleaved to yield the individual gene products. Thirdly, naked RNA extracted from virions is infectious.

The second group of single-stranded RNA viruses, defined as the minus (−) strand viruses, is composed of myxovirus, paramyxoviruses, bunyavirus, arenaviruses, and rhabdoviruses. Characteristically, their genomic RNAs serve only one function, that of a template for transcription. Because they must be transcribed to make mRNA and the cell lacks the appropriate enzyme, all (−) strand viruses package into the virion a transcriptase along with the viral genome. Transcription of the viral genome is the first event after entry of the virus into the cells. Both the multipartite and the monopartite RNA genomes are transcribed in two phases. The first phase yields monocistronic mRNAs, each specifying a single protein. The second yields full-length, (+) strand RNAs, which in turn serve as templates for the synthesis of (−) strand genomic RNA (Figure 63-3).

Central to the replication of the (−) strand viruses is that the genomic RNAs function only as templates for transcription. There are three consequences: first, the virus must bring into the infected cell the transcriptase to make (+) strand RNA to function as mRNA; second, naked RNA extracted from virions is not infectious because the cell lacks the suitable transcriptases; third, each mRNA specifies a single polypeptide. However, splicing of transcription product may yield several mRNAs encoding different proteins off the same template. Consequently, the individual

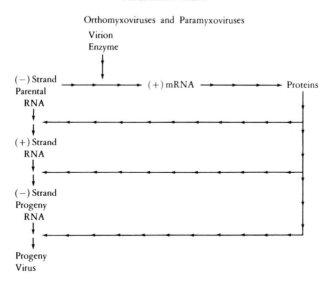

Minus Strand Viruses

Orthomyxoviruses and Paramyxoviruses

Figure 63-3 Schematic diagram of flow of events during replication of orthomyxoviruses and paramyxoviruses.

chromosomes of multipartite genomes may each encode more than one protein and the (+) strand RNA transcripts that function as mRNA may differ in length and spliced-out portions from the (+) strand transcript that functions as the template for the synthesis of the progeny genomic (−) strand RNA. The advantage of specifying monocistronic mRNA is that the virus can control the abundance of the individual proteins; they need not be made in equimolar amounts.

Retroviruses comprise the third group of RNA viruses. Characteristically, retrovirus genomes are monopartite but diploid, and the two strands are either partially hydrogen-bonded to another macromolecule or base-paired in a fashion as yet unknown. The sole function of genomic RNA is to serve as a template for the synthesis of viral DNA. Since the eukaryotic cells lack enzymes competent to perform this function, the virion contains, in addition to the genome, an RNA-dependent DNA polymerase (reverse transcriptase) as well as a mixture of host transfer RNAs, one of which serves as a primer. The key steps in the reproductive cycle (Figure 63-4, right) are binding of the transfer RNA (tRNA)–reverse transcriptase complex to genomic RNA; synthesis of a DNA complementary to the genomic RNA across the two ends of the RNA molecule to produce a circular, single-stranded DNA molecule hydrogen-bonded to the linear genomic RNA; digestion of genomic RNA by a nuclease that attacks only RNA in DNA-RNA hybrids (ribonuclease H, also packaged in the virion); and the synthesis of the complementary copy of the viral DNA. The circular, double-stranded DNA is then translocated into the nucleus, where it integrates linearly into the host genome. Viral gene expression does not always follow; when it occurs, the integrated viral DNA is transcribed by a host transcriptase. The RNA transcripts can be genome-length or shorter. Each RNA directs the synthesis of one of several polyproteins. The polyproteins are then cleaved to yield the individual viral proteins. Only the

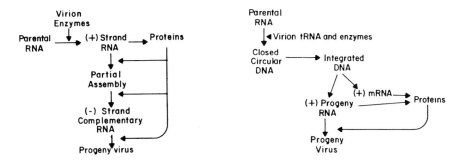

Figure 63-4 Schematic diagram of flow of events during replication of reoviruses (left) and retroviruses (right).

genome-length transcript is packaged into virions with the reverse transcriptase and tRNA molecules.

The double-stranded, multipartite reovirus genome is transcribed within the partially opened capsid by a polymerase packaged into the viron, and ten different mRNA (+ strands) species are extruded through the exposed vertices of the capsid. The mRNA has two functions (see Figure 63-4, left). First the mRNAs are translated as monocistronic messages to yield the viral proteins. Second, one molecule of RNA of each of the ten species assembles within a precursor particle; the ten assembled molecules then serve as templates for synthesis of the complementary strands.

Expression and Replication of DNA Genomes

The DNA viruses can be split into four groups. Papovavirus, adenovirus, and herpesvirus genomes are transcribed and replicated in the nucleus and therefore can utilize the transcriptional enzymes of the host to generate mRNA (Figure 63-5). Consistent with this, the DNAs of those viruses are infectious. The transcriptional program consists of at least two cycles of transcription for papovaviruses, and at least three for herpesviruses and adenoviruses. In each instance, the structural or virion polypeptides are made from mRNA that is generated from the last cycle of transcription.

The poxviruses constitute the second group. Although poxvirus DNAs have been detected in the nucleus, at least the initial transcription and most of the events in the

Figure 63-5 Schematic diagram of flow of events during replication of adenoviruses and herpesviruses. In both instances, parental genome is transcribed by host polymerase in at least three coordinately regulated, sequentially ordered cycles. The polypeptides in each cycle have been designated by various names (for example, α, β, and γ; immediately early, early, and late; or pre-early, early, and late). The function of early polypeptides is not known. The middle polypeptides are usually directly involved in the replication of viral DNA. Late proteins are usually the structural polypeptides of the virion. In papovaviruses, the early and middle cycles are compressed in one.

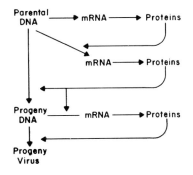

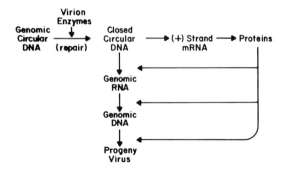

Figure 63-6 Schematic diagram of the flow of events
in the replication of hepatitis B virus.

reproductive cycle appear to take place in the cytoplasm. The initial transcription occurs
in the core of the virion. Many questions concerning the reproductive cycle of this virus
remain unresolved.

Parvoviruses constitute the third group. The only parvovirus that infects humans
and for which information is available—the adenovirus-associated virus—is a "defective" virus and requires adenoviruses as helper viruses for its multiplication. The
synthesis of the DNA strand complementary to the single-stranded genomic DNA in
the nucleus appears to precede transcription of the genome.

Hepatitis B virus is a member of the fourth group (see Figure 63-6). The DNA of
this virus is first repaired and converted into a supercoiled molecule by a DNA
polymerase package in the virion, and then transcribed into two mRNAs that specify
proteins and a genomic RNA that serves as a template for the synthesis of genomic
DNA by reverse transcriptase.

Assembly, Maturation, and Egress from Infected Cells

Viruses have evolved two fundamental mechanisms for their assembly, maturation
(acquisition of the capacity to infect), and egress from the infected cell. The first,
exemplified by picornaviruses, reoviruses, papovaviruses, parvoviruses, adenoviruses,
and poxviruses, involves intracellular assembly and maturation. In picornaviruses, 60
copies each of virion proteins designated as VP0, VP1, and VP3 assemble in the
cytoplasm into a procapsid. Viral RNA then wraps around the procapsid; in the process,
VP0 is cleaved to yield two polypeptides, VP2 and VP4. The cleavage probably causes a
rearrangement of the capsid into a thermodynamically stable structure in which the
RNA is shielded from access by nucleases. Poxvirus and reoviruses also assemble in the
cytoplasm. In contrast, adenoviruses, papovaviruses, and parvoviruses assemble in the
nucleus. As a general rule, all viruses that assemble and acquire infectivity inside the cell
depend on the disintegration of the infected cell for their egress. Accumulated evidence
implicates the structural proteins of these viruses in the inhibition of host macromolecular metabolism and in the ultimate disintegration of the infected cell.

The second mechanism employed by enveloped viruses is exemplified by all $(-)$
strand RNA viruses, togaviruses, and retroviruses. This mechanism combines assembly
with egress from the infected cell. Specifically, some of the virus proteins insert
themselves into the inner and outer surfaces of the plasma membrane or other

cytoplasmic membranes; the proteins projecting from the outer surface become glycosylated. The membrane proteins aggregate into patches, displacing the host proteins. RNA-protein complexes (minus strand viruses) or capsids (togaviruses and retroviruses) bind to inner surface proteins in these patches and become wrapped by the patch. In the process, the nascent virion is extruded, or buds, into the extracellular environment. In some instances (for example, orthomyxoviruses and paramyxoviruses), cleavage and rearrangement of the surface proteins occur during extrusion and enable the newly formed virion to infect cells. Virus assembly and maturation by extrusion from the cell surface provides a more efficient mechanism of egress because it does not depend on disintegration of the infected cell. Indeed, viruses that mature and egress in this fashion vary considerably in their effects on host-cell metabolism and integrity. They range from highly cytolytic (togaviruses, ortho- and paramyxoviruses, rhabdoviruses) to virtually noncytolytic (retroviruses); however, by inserting viral glycoproteins into the cell surface, these viruses impart upon the cell a new antigenic specificity, and the infected cell can and does become a target for the immune mechanisms of the host.

The herpesvirus nucleocapsid is assembled in the nucleus. Unlike other enveloped viruses, its envelopment and maturation occur at the inner lamella of the nuclear membrane. The enveloped virus accumulates in the space between the inner and outer lamellae of the nuclear membrane and in the cisternae of the cytoplasmic reticulum and vesicles carrying the virus to the cell surface. The enveloped virus is shielded from contact with the cytoplasm. Herpesviruses are cytolytic and invariably destroy the cells in which they multiply. Like other enveloped viruses, herpesviruses impart to the infected cell a new antigenic specificity.

Variability in Genomes

A major focus of current research in virology is the role of genetic variation within various species of viruses, defective viruses, and restrictive and abortive infections in human disease. Interest in these phenomena stems from observations that the spectrum of clinical disease caused by many viruses infecting humans varies considerably in severity and symptomatology. Moreover, many years after primary infections, individuals may exhibit symptoms of recurrent infections, chronic debilitating diseases of the central nervous system, and malignancy that is apparently related to that infection. The relationship of these phenomena to the various manifestations and sequelae of virus infection is summarized in the following discussion.

Viruses belonging to the same species and family may differ enormously. For example, no two epidemiologically unrelated strains of herpes simplex virus are identical with respect to the fine structure of their genomes. The notion that some naturally occurring strains are more likely to cause severe illness than others is more anecdotal than proven, but is not far-fetched.

This chapter defines two groups of defective viruses. Viruses in the first group lack one or more essential genes and therefore cannot replicate without a helper virus. Interest in this group stems from the experimental demonstration that specific types of defective viruses (papovaviruses, adenoviruses, and herpesviruses) can transform permissive cells from normal to neoplastic. Viruses in the second group contain mutations and deletions that prevent them from replicating in an efficient fashion. Interest in this second group stems largely from the suspicion that chronic debilitating infections of the central nervous system might in some fashion be related to viruses that are sluggish in their replication, in their ability to destroy the infected cells, or in their ability to alter the infected cell sufficiently to make it a target for the immune system of the host.

Restrictive and abortive infections are of interest chiefly because the cell may survive and carry the viral genome indefinitely for the life of the host. The cell restrictively infected with competent virus may become a latent reservoir of virus that can replicate and disseminate the virus when the cell is triggered to become permissive. A cell abortively infected with a defective virus may also survive and, given the appropriate stimulus, become malignant.

To reiterate, the roles of these phenomena in human disease are not proven. Undoubtedly, they will be the focus of investigation for many years to come.

References

Baltimore, D.: Expression of animal virus genomes. *Bacterial Rev* 1971; 35:235-241.

Huang, A.S.: Defective interfering viruses. *Ann Rev Microbiol* 1973; 27:101-117.

Nayak, P., (editor): *The molecular biology of animal viruses,* Vol. 1. New York: Marcel Dekker, 1977.

Nayak, P., (editor): *The molecular biology of animal viruses,* Vol. 2. New York: Marcel Dekker, 1978.

Palesi, P, Roizman, B., (editors): Genetic variation of viruses. *Ann NY Acad Sci* 1980; 354:1-507.

64 Classification

Nathalie J. Schmidt, PhD

General Concepts
Classification
Nomenclature

General Concepts

Viruses currently are classified on the basis of chemical composition, morphology, and mode of replication.

Viruses of vertebrates are grouped into **families** with names ending in **-viridae** and **genera** with names ending in **-virus.** Rather than binomial nomenclature, vernacular names, such as "measles virus," are still used for individual members of viral genera. These individual members are the equivalent of species.

The current classification and nomenclature of viruses were developed by the International Committee on the Taxonomy of Viruses (a committee of the Section on Virology of the International Association of Microbiological Societies) and by various international study groups dealing with individual virus families.

Classification

Viruses are grouped into families and genera solely on the basis of their chemical composition, morphology, and mode of replication; their host range or pathogenic properties are not considered. The first major division of viruses is based on possession of a **DNA or RNA genome.** The viral capsid proteins and the antigenic composition of these proteins are direct expressions of the nucleotide sequences of the viral genome. Antigenic characteristics serve to separate further viruses within genera.

Viral morphology is the integrated expression of the viral genes; it provides a basis for grouping viruses into major **taxons,** or families. A virus family may consist of members that replicate only in vertebrates, only in invertebrates, only in plants, or only in bacteria; certain families contain viruses that replicate in more than one of these hosts. This section concerns only those virus families and genera that infect vertebrate hosts because these include viruses of medical importance.

Several factors pertaining to the **mode of viral replication** play a role in classification: the configuration of the nucleic acid (single- or double-stranded, linear or circular), whether the genome consists of one or several molecules of nucleic acid, and whether single-stranded viral RNA can serve as mRNA (positive or + sense) or whether it is complementary RNA that requires a transcriptase in the virion to transcribe mRNA (negative or − sense). Also considered in classification are the **site of viral capsid assembly** and, in enveloped viruses, the **site of nucleocapsid envelopment.**

Table 64-1 lists the major chemical and morphologic properties of families containing animal viruses.

Nomenclature

The use of latinized names ending in -viridae for virus families and ending in -virus for viral genera has gained wide acceptance. Wherever subfamilies exist, their names end in **-virinae.** Less support exists for latinized binomial nomenclature, and vernacular names continue to be used to describe the viruses within a genus. In this text, the latinized endings for families and subfamilies usually are not used. Table 64-2 shows the current classification of the major groups of animal viruses.

From the early 1950s until the mid-1960s, when new animal viruses were being discovered at a rapid rate, it was popular to compose virus names from **sigla** (abbreviations derived from a few or initial letters). Thus, the name for Picornaviridae is derived from pico (small) and RNA; the name for Reoviridae is derived from *r*espiratory, *e*nteric, and *o*rphan viruses, because the agents were found in both respiratory and enteric specimens and were not related to other classified viruses. Although the current rules for nomenclature do not prohibit the introduction of new sigla, they require that the sigla be meaningful to workers in the field and be recognized by international study groups. The names of other families containing animal viruses are derived as follows: Parvoviridae (parvo means small); Papovaviridae (derived from *pa*pilloma, *po*lyoma, and *va*cuolating agent SV-40); Adenoviridae (adeno [gland]; that is, the adenoid tissue from which the viruses were first isolated); Herpesviridae (herpes [creeping] describes the nature of the lesions); Poxviridae (pock means pustule); Togaviridae (toga [cloak] refers to the viral envelope); Orthomyxoviridae (ortho [true] and myxo [mucus], for which the viruses have an affinity); Paramyxoviridae (para [closely resembling] and myxo [mucus]); Rhabdoviridae (rhabdo [rod] describes the shape of the viruses); Retroviridae (from *r*everse *t*ranscriptase); Arenaviridae (arena [sand] describes the sandy appearance of the virion); Coronaviridae (corona [crown] describes the appearance of the peplomers protruding from the viral surface); Bunyaviridae (from Bunyamwera, the place in Africa where the type-species was isolated); Iridoviridae (irido [iridescent], from the appearance of infected larval insects and pelleted virions); and Calicivirus (calici [cup or goblet] from

Table 64-1   Chemical and Morphologic Properties of Animal Virus Families

Family	Nucleic Acid Genome		Shape**	Diameter (nm)	Enveloped***	Virion			Transcriptase Present in Virion
	Type and Configuration*	MW × 10⁶				Capsid Symmetry	No. Capsomeres#	Site of Capsid Assembly	
Parvoviridae	ssDNA; + or − sense	1.5–2.0	S	18–26	0	Cubic	32	Nucleus	None
Papovaviridae	dsDNA; circular	3–5	S	45–55	0	Cubic	72	Nucleus	None
Adenoviridae	dsDNA	20–25	S	70–90	0	Cubic	252	Nucleus	None
Herpesviridae	dsDNA	80–150	S	120–200	+	Cubic	162	Nucleus	None
Iridoviridae	dsDNA	100–250	S	125–300	+	Cubic	ca. 1500	Cytoplasm	DNA-dependent; RNA polymerase†
Poxviridae	dsDNA	85–240	X	240 × 300	+	Complex	—	Cytoplasm	DNA-dependent; RNA polymerase
Hepadnaviridae (proposed)	dsDNA; circular; one ss region	1.6–2.3	S	40–50	0	?	—	?	DNA-dependent; DNA polymerase
Picornaviridae	ssRNA; + sense	2.5	S	22–30	0	Cubic	32	Cytoplasm	None
Caliciviridae	ssRNA; + sense	2.6–2.8	S	35–39	0	Cubic	32	Cytoplasm	None
Togaviridae	ssRNA; + sense	4	S	40–70	+	Cubic	?	Cytoplasm	None
Reoviridae	dsRNA; 10–12 pieces	12–20	S	60–80	0	Cubic	32 or 92	Cytoplasm	RNA-dependent; RNA polymerase
Orthomyxoviridae	ssRNA; 8 molecules, − sense	5	S††	80–120	+	Helical	—	Cytoplasm	RNA-dependent; RNA polymerase
Paramyxoviridae	ssRNA; mostly − sense	5–7	S††	150–300	+	Helical	—	Cytoplasm	RNA-dependent; RNA polymerase
Rhabdoviridae	ssRNA; − sense	3.5–4.6	U	60 × 180	+	Helical	—	Cytoplasm	RNA-dependent; RNA polymerase
Bunyaviridae	ssRNA; 3 molecules, − sense	6–7	S	90–100	+	Helical	—	Cytoplasm	RNA-dependent; RNA polymerase
Coronaviridae	ssRNA; + sense	5.5–6.1	S	75–160	+	Helical	—	Cytoplasm	None
Arenaviridae	ssRNA; 5 molecules, 2 virus-specific	3–5	S	50–300	+	?	—	Cytoplasm	RNA-dependent; RNA polymerase
Retroviridae	ssRNA; inverted dimer of + sense strand	6–7	S	80–100	+	?	—	Cytoplasm	RNA-dependent; DNA polymerase
Filoviridae (proposed)	ssRNA; − sense	4.2	Pleomorphic	80 × 800–900	+	Complex	—	Cytoplasm	?

*ss, single stranded; ds, double-stranded.

**S, spherical; X, brickshaped or ovoid; U, elongated with parallel sides and a round end.

***Most enveloped viruses are sensitive to lipid solvents; however, some members of the Poxviridae are resistant to ether, and conversely, some members of Reoviridae (Orbiviruses) are only partially resistant to lipid solvents.

#Applicable to viruses with cubic (icosahedral) symmetry.

†Some members, including African swine fever virus.

††Filamentous forms also occur.

Table 64-2 Current Classification of Major Groups of Animal Viruses

Family	Genera (or Subfamilies)	Vernacular Name of Type Species or Typical Member	Species Shown to Produce Infection in Humans
Parvoviridae	Parvovirus	Latent rat virus	Possibly virus associated with erythema infectiosum and aplastic crisis of sickle cell anemia
	Dependovirus	Adeno-associated virus type 1	Defective viruses, infect humans in the presence of a "helper" adenovirus
Papovaviridae	Papillomavirus	Rabbit papilloma virus	Human papilloma (wart) virus
	Polyomavirus	Polyoma virus (mouse)	JC and BK viruses, simian virus 40
Adenoviridae	Mastadenovirus	Human adenovirus type 2	≥40 human adenovirus serotypes (species)
	Aviadenovirus (Subfamilies)	CELO virus (fowl)	None
Herpesviridae	Alphaherpesvirinae	Herpes simplex virus	Herpes simplex virus types 1 and 2, varicella-zoster virus
	Betaherpesvirinae	Cytomegalovirus	Human cytomegalovirus
	Gammaherpesvirinae	Epstein-Barr virus	Epstein-Barr virus
Iridoviridae	Iridovirus	African swine fever virus	None
Poxviridae	Orthopoxvirus	Vaccinia virus	Vaccinia, variola, cowpox, monkeypox viruses
	Parapoxvirus	Orf virus	Orf, bovine pustular stomatitis, milker's node viruses
	Avipoxvirus	Fowl pox virus	None
	Capripoxvirus	Sheep pox virus	None
	Leporipoxvirus	Myxoma virus	None
	Suipoxvirus	Swinepox virus	None
	Not yet allocated	—	Molluscum contagiosum and tanapox viruses
Hepadnaviridae (proposed)	Not yet defined	—	Hepatitis B virus
Picornaviridae	Enterovirus	Poliovirus type 1	67 enterovirus serotypes, hepatitis A virus
	Rhinovirus	Human rhinovirus type 1	Over 100 rhinovirus serotypes
	Aphthovirus	Foot-and-mouth disease virus	Foot-and-mouth disease virus (rarely)
Caliciviridae	Calicivirus	Vesicular exanthem (swine)	Human gastroenteritis viruses
Togaviridae	Alphavirus	Sindbis virus	Various group A arboviruses
	Flavivirus	Yellow fever virus	Various group B arboviruses
	Rubivirus	Rubella virus	Rubella virus
	Pestivirus	Mucosal disease virus (cattle)	None
Reoviridae	Reovirus	Reovirus type 1	Reovirus types 1, 2 and 3
	Orbivirus	Bluetongue virus	Colorado tick fever virus
	Rotavirus	Human rotavirus	Human rotavirus

Table 64-2   Continued

Family	Genera (or Subfamilies)	Vernacular Name of Type Species or Typical Member	Species Shown to Produce Infection in Humans
Orthomyxoviridae	Influenzavirus	Influenza virus type A, strain A/WS/33 (HON1)	Influenza type A and type B viruses
	Probable separate genus	Influenza virus type C	Influenza virus type C
Paramyxoviridae	Paramyxovirus	Newcastle disease virus (NDV)	Parainfluenza virus types 1–4, mumps virus, NDV
	Morbillivirus	Measles virus	Measles virus
	Pneumovirus	Respiratory syncytial virus	Respiratory syncytial virus
Rhabdoviridae	Vesiculovirus	Vesicular stomatitis virus (VSV)	VSV and Chandipura virus
	Lyssavirus	Rabies virus	Rabies, Mokola, Duvenhage viruses
Bunyaviridae	Bunyavirus	Bunyamwera virus	Various arthropod-transmitted viruses
	Phlebovirus	Sandfly fever (SF) Sicilian virus	Sandfly fever virus, Rift Valley fever virus
	Nairovirus	Crimean-Congo hemorrhagic fever virus	Crimean-Congo hemorrhagic fever virus, Nairobi sheep disease virus
	Uukuvirus	Uukuniemi virus	None
Coronaviridae	Coronavirus	Avian infectious bronchitis virus	Human coronaviruses, several types
Arenaviridae	Arenavirus	Lymphocytic choriomeningitis virus	Lymphocytic choriomeningitis virus, Lassa viruses, viruses of the Tacaribe complex
Retroviridae	(Subfamilies)		
	Oncovirinae	Type B and type C oncoviruses	Human T cell leukemia viruses
	Spumavirinae	Foamy virus group	Human foamy virus
	Lentivirinae	Maedi/visna virus group	Probably virus(es) associated with acquired immunodeficiency syndrome
Filoviridae (proposed)	Filovirus	Marburg virus	Marburg virus, Ebola virus

cup-shaped depressions on viral surfaces). Nomenclature for the proposed Hepadnavirus family is based on replication of the viruses in hepatocytes and their DNA genomes, and the name for the proposed Filoviridae family is based on the Latin *filo*, meaning thread or filament, which describes the morphology of this group. In the early days of virology, it was also popular to name viruses after their discoverers; however, current rules indicate that persons' names shall no longer be used in viral nomenclature.

Several viruses of medical importance remain unclassified. Some are difficult or impossible to propagate in standard laboratory host systems and thus cannot be obtained in sufficient quantity to permit more precise characterization. The hepatitis A virus is now classified as a picornavirus, and a new family, Hepadnaviridae, has been proposed to include human hepatitis B virus and related viruses from other species. The family Filoviridae has been proposed for classification of the pleomorphic Marburg and Ebola viruses, which are etiologic agents of African hemorrhagic fever, and do not appear to fit into any of the currently classified groups of animal viruses. The Norwalk virus and similar agents that cause nonbacterial gastroenteritis in humans are now recognized to be more similar to caliciviruses than to parvoviruses. The viruses that cause degenerative diseases of the central nervous system in animals and humans (scrapie in sheep and kuru and Creutzfeldt-Jakob disease in humans) have been likened to viroids because of their resistance to certain chemical and physical agents, particularly to ultraviolet irradiation; they are also similar to "prions," a name coined for replicating agents that have no demonstrable nucleic acid. Their properties do not fit completely into either of these categories, however, and they are still considered to be unconventional viruses within the group of organisms that cause the subacute spongiform viral encephalopathies.

References

Gajdusek, D.C.: Unconventional viruses and the origin and disappearance of kuru. *Science* 1977; 197:943-960.

Kiley, M.P., et al.: Filoviridae: A taxonomic home for Marburg and Ebola viruses? *Intervirology* 1982; 18:24-32.

Matthews, R.E.F.: Classification and nomenclature of viruses. Fourth report of the International Committee on Taxonomy of Viruses. *Intervirology* 1982; 17:1-199.

Melnick, J.L.: Taxonomy and nomenclature of viruses, 1982. *Prog Med Virol* 1982; 28:208-221.

Melnick, J.L.: Classification of hepatitis A virus as enterovirus type 72 and of hepatitis B virus as hepadnavirus type 1. *Intervirology* 1982; 18:105-106.

Siegl, G.: The human parvovirus. In: *The parvoviruses.* Berns, K.I. (editor). New York: Plenum Press, 1984.

65 Effects on Cells

Jose Costa, MD
Alan S. Rabson, MD
Thomas Albrecht, PhD

General Concepts
Cytocidal Infection
Steady-State Persistent Infection
Carrier-Culture Persistent Infection
Latent Persistent Infection
Transformation

General Concepts

In most cases, the disturbances of bodily function that are manifested as the signs and symptoms of viral disease result from the effects of viruses on cells. Knowledge of the biologic and biochemical effects of viruses on cells is essential for understanding the pathophysiology of viral disease and for developing accurate diagnostic procedures and effective treatment.

Virus–host cell interactions (Table 65-1) may produce either **cytocidal infections,** in which the virus kills the cell, or **persistent infections,** in which the virus resides in some or all of the cells without killing most of them. Four types of persistent infection have been identified in cell cultures: in **steady-state infection,** essentially all cells are infected, and they continuously produce noncytocidal (nonlytic) virus; in **carrier-culture infection,** only a fraction of cells are infected at any one time, and multiplication is restricted to a few cells that may undergo cell lysis; in **latent infection,** only a fraction of cells are infected, and infectious virus is produced only sporadically; in **transformation,** the virus does not kill the cell, but produces morphologic, biochemical, and biologic changes that may result in the acquisition of malignant properties by the cell (malignant transformation) (see Chapter 70). The mechanisms of **persistent infection** in animals or humans appear to be similar to those of carrier-culture, latent, and steady-state infections in vitro.

Cytocidal Infection

Many viruses kill the cells in which they reproduce. The first effects of the replication of cytocidal viruses on cells to be described are the morphologic changes known as **cytopathic effects (CPE).** Cell monolayers that are infected by viruses develop morphologic changes, which can be observed easily in unfixed, unstained cultures under a light microscope. Characteristic CPE may be caused by certain virus types; thus, observation of these effects (Figure 65-1) is an important tool for virologists concerned with isolating and identifying viruses from infected animals or humans.

Many types of CPE can occur. In some diseased tissues, intracellular structures called **inclusion bodies** appear in the nucleus and/or cytoplasm of the infected cells. Inclusion bodies were first identified by light microscopy in smears and stained sections of infected tissues, but their composition has been clarified by electron microscopy. In an adenovirus infection, for example, crystalline arrays of adenovirus capsids accumulate in the nucleus to form an inclusion body. In other infections, the inclusions are not aggregates of viral particles; rather, they are host-cell structures altered by the virus (for example, in reovirus-infected cells, virions associate with the microtubules, giving rise to the crescent-shaped perinuclear inclusion). Some characteristics of inclusion bodies produced by various viruses are listed in Table 65-2.

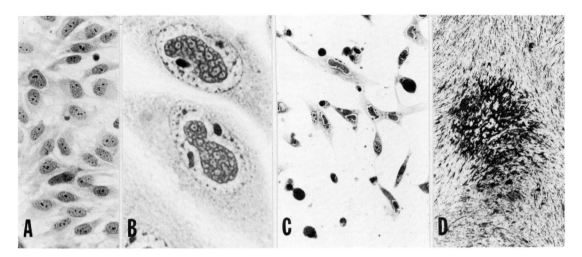

Figure 65-1 Development and progression of viral cytopathology. Human embryo skin muscle cells were infected with human cytomegalovirus and stained at selected times to demonstrate **A,** uninfected cells; **B,** late virus cytopathic effects (nuclear inclusion, cytomegaly); **C,** cell degeneration; **D,** foci of infected cells in a cell monolayer—i.e., a plaque. Bouins fixative. Hematolylin and eosin stain. A, ×255; B, ×900; C, ×225; D, ×20.

Table 65-1   Virus–Cell Interactions

Type of Infection	Fraction Cells Infected	Fate of Infected Cell	Release of Infectious Virus	Schematized Mechanism*	Disease Examples	Controlling Mechanism
Cytocidal	Variable	Death	Yes		Smallpox Poliomyelitis Togavirus encephalitis	None
Persistent steady-state	All	Survival	Yes		Rubella LCM	Noncytocidal viruses
Carrier culture	Few	Death	Yes		Adenovirus infections	Antiviral substances (e.g., antibody, interferon)
Latent	Few	Survival (during latency)	Sporadic		Herpesvirus infections	Not known
Transformation	Few	Survival	Variable		Cancer	New genes in cells

*   ⬤ , cell;   o   or   ⊛ , virus

Table 65-2 Viral Inclusion Bodies in Some Human Diseases

	Location in Cell*		
Virus	Nucleus	Cyto- plasm	Eponym
Herpes simplex	+	0	Cowdry type A
Cytomegalovirus	+	+	
Rabies	0	+	Negri bodies
Vaccinia	0	+	Guarnieri bodies
Adenovirus	+	0	
Measles	+	+	
Papovaviruses	+	0	

* +, present; 0, absent.

A particularly striking effect of some viral infections is the formation of *syncytia*, or *polykaryocytes*, which are large cytoplasmic masses that contain many nuclei (*poly*—many, *karyon*—nucleus) and are produced by fusion of cells infected by the virus. The mechanism of cell fusion during viral infection is not well understood, but it probably results from the interaction between viral gene products and host cell membranes. Cell fusion may be a mechanism by which virus spreads from cell to cell.

Replication of viruses may alter the morphologic characteristics of the cellular chromosomes. Chromatids often break and fragment, or pulverization of chromosomes can take place. The chromosomal breaks may occur in a nonrandom fashion, since they most often affect chromosomes that have been damaged by radiation or radiomimetic drugs.

Many morphologic alterations have biochemical correlates. Biochemical research has shown that protein synthesis often is inhibited during the replicative cycle of cytocidal viruses. The inhibition occurs in characteristic ways. In poliovirus or herpesvirus infections, for example, selective inhibition of host protein synthesis occurs at the same time that the virus protein synthesis is proceeding at a vigorous rate. The mechanism of selective inhibiton (host shutdown) is not understood completely, but it appears to depend on an early viral-coded protein and it probably varies according to the type of virus.

Viral products also can nonselectively inhibit protein and nucleic acid synthesis (total shutdown). For example, certain adenovirus proteins (such as the fiber antigen) inhibit DNA, RNA, and protein synthesis in cell cultures. Total shutdown may occur when excess viral products accumulate in the cell late in the replicative cycle. Some picornaviruses may specify a protein that causes cell damage independent of the viral proteins that inhibit cell macromolecular synthesis.

In herpes simplex infections, cell mRNA is not bound with ribosomes to form polyribosomes; only viral-specific mRNA is bound. How this selectivity is achieved is not known. Most cytolytic viruses inhibit cell DNA synthesis. Since protein synthesis is required for cell DNA synthesis, the inhibition of DNA synthesis is, in most cases, secondary to inhibition of protein synthesis. Reoviruses may be exceptional in that they cause a decrease in cell DNA synthesis before a substantial decline in protein synthesis occurs.

Most events that damage or modify the host cell during lytic infection are difficult to separate from viral replication but, in some cases, the effect is not linked directly to the manufacture of progeny virions. Interferon, for example, is a cellular product that is not normally synthesized by the cell, but is induced during viral infection (see Chapter 68).

Steady-State Persistent Infection

In steady-state infections, infected cells produce virus continuously; however, viral replication and release do not drastically affect cellular protein, RNA, and DNA synthesis, and the infected cells can divide and grow. DNA viruses do not produce steady-state infections, whereas some RNA viruses (such as paramyxoviruses) often do. For example, SV-5, a simian paramyxovirus, is a common contaminant of cultures of kidney cells from rhesus monkeys. The virus multiplies in the cells, producing abundant progeny but almost no discernible CPE. In many cases of steady-state infection, the progeny virus is released by budding through the cell membrane (Figure 65-2). The effect of budding on cell membrane turnover and movement is poorly understood. Budding of virions through the membrane often is preceded by insertion of viral peptides (after glycosylation by host enzymes) in or at the cell membrane. The viral peptides associated with the membrane are thought to provide a recognition site at which budding of the viral capsid takes place (see Chapter 63).

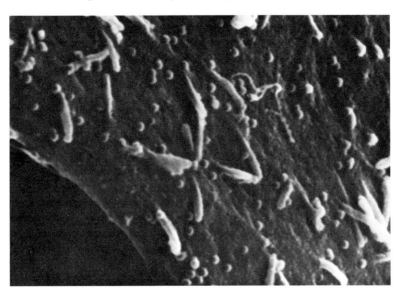

Figure 65-2 Scanning electron micrograph of retrovirus virions budding (round objects) from surface of cell.

Budding virions and viral peptides associated with the cell membrane change the antigenic characteristics of the cell, so that the immune system of the infected person will recognize the cell as foreign (see Chapter 69). The cell then may be attacked by the humoral and cellular immune system of the host, and will die even though it was infected by a noncytocidal virus.

In addition to this type of immune response to infected cells, the constant release of virus in a steady-state infection leads to antibody production by the host. This production may explain the lifelong persistence of antibody to some viruses. The immune response also may cause formation of circulating antigen-antibody complexes composed of viral antigens bound to their antibodies. These complexes may deposit in the kidney and lead to renal disease, as has been described in infections by lymphocytic choriomeningitis virus in mice.

Steady-state infections are detected in cultures by several techniques: staining of cells with labeled antibody to viral antigens; adsorption of red blood cells to viral antigens at the cell surface (hemadsorption); inhibition of replication of a second, superinfecting virus (interference); and transfer of virus to susceptible cells that will manifest cytopathic effects.

Carrier-Culture Persistent Infection

In carrier-culture infection, a small number of cells are infected and the infecting virus may produce CPE; however, host factors such as interferon, natural inhibitors, and antibody can limit the spread of infection to only a few cells. The small number of cells that die are replaced by cell division.

Latent Persistent Infection

In latent infection, infectious virus is seldom detected. Relatively few cells are infected, and virus replication usually is restricted in these cells so that the biosynthetic events required for formation of progeny virus are not completed. Current data suggest that the virus may be associated with the latently infected cells for years (for example, varicella-zoster virus may survive for decades in cells of the dorsal root ganglia) and that virus is released sporadically from these cells (see Chapter 70). Although it has been suggested that integration of the virus genome into the cell DNA is a mechanism of latency, this hypothesis has not been proved. Researchers also have postulated that latently infected cells may express some virus proteins that modify the infected cells and thus produce chronic disease. Although some limited evidence has been obtained in support of this concept, much more is needed. We do know that, in the case of certain herpesviruses, the latent infection provides a mechanism in nature to maintain the virus in one generation of humans, until another susceptible (nonimmune) generation is available.

Transformation

A fourth type of persistent virus-cell interaction is **oncogenic transformation,** a term that implies a malignant change in the cell. In fact, the term *transformation* is used by several fields of science and each field has its own definition. Here, oncogenic transformation refers to the process by which the control of cell proliferation is modified in at least two important aspects; first, the cell gains the capacity for unlimited cell division in culture (**immortalization**), and second, the transformed cells acquire the ability to produce a tumor in an appropriate host. The second process is associated with cell multiplication. Immortalization is necessary for oncogenic transformation, but it cannot produce such transformation by itself, since some immortalized cells are not oncogenic.

Other types of transformation of cells can include biochemical, antigenic, morphologic, and physiologic alterations and their various combinations (Table 65-3). These four types of transformation are not sufficient individually to produce oncogenic transformation, which appears to require a combination of transformation events. These pleiotypic responses suggest that carcinogenesis may be effected by agents that act on several different loci within cells, possibly by different mechanisms. For example, polyomavirus middle T protein alone can transform immortalized cells to malignant cells, whereas both the large T and middle T polyomavirus proteins are required to transform nonimmortalized cells.

Current data indicate that transformation occurs in cumulative steps and that it results in modification of the control of cell proliferation, and eventually, the development of a fully malignant cell. For example, in the first step, the cell may undergo changes that result in immortalization; in the second step, one of these cells

Table 65-3   Cellular Effects of Transformation

Cell Growth
Reduced serum requirement for cell growth
Growth in semisolid media (anchorage independency)
Growth in a less oriented manner
Loss of contact inhibition of growth
Growth on monolayers of normal cells
High saturation density
Tumor formation upon injection into susceptible animals

Metabolic or Structural Changes
Increased rate of sugar transport
Increased agglutinability by lectins
Decrease or absence of fibronectin (a high-molecular-weight cell-surface glycoprotein)
Increased depolymerization of cytoskeletal proteins
Changes in membrane glycolipid and glycoprotein composition
Induction of fetal antigens
Release of proteases and protease activators

Detection of Virus or Its Products
Viral-specific transplantation antigens present on surface
Intracellular viral antigens detectable
Virus DNA sequences present
Virus mRNA present
Transforming virus rescued by helper virus or fusion with susceptible cell

may gain the capacity to produce benign tumors; and the third step, one or more of these cells may gain the capacity to produce metastatic tumors. During each of these steps, different agents (chemical, physical, viral) may act in the initiation and promotion of transformation.

Results from experiments in animals may be helpful in understanding the transformation process. In the first transformation step (**initiation**), a laboratory animal is exposed to a dose of chemical carcinogen (**initiator**) that does not induce a tumor. This exposure, however, does produce heritable changes in affected cells, but the cells often are not recognized because of the absence of tumor formation. In the second step, exposure to a second (**promoter**) agent results in tumor formation, even though the promoting agent would not induce tumors if used alone. Here, tumor viruses, chemicals, and radiation serve as carcinogens. Promotion is thought to include two steps: the fixation of the genetic changes through a process of genetic rearrangements, and the clonal multiplication of the transformed cells to produce the tumor mass. In general, single-point mutations at multiple specific sites alone have not appeared to be sufficient for the production of malignant transformations, since subsequent promotional genetic rearrangements appear to be crucial events in the fixation of genetic damage and carcinogenesis. Recent reports, however, suggest that multiple point mutations leading to serial activation of oncogenes may induce such transformations. Some agents are referred to as *complete carcinogens* because they are capable of both initiation and promotion. The term *progression* is often used for the multiple steps of *promotion* that cause the transformed cells and the tumors derived from these cells to manifest increased malignancy.

As noted above, various types of agents may cause the genetic alterations that lead to transformation, but here we will focus on viruses. Many tumors of animals have been shown to be induced by virus infection. Both DNA viruses (herpesviruses, adenovirus, poxviruses, papovaviruses, and perhaps hepadnavirus) and RNA viruses (retroviruses) may transform cells. Since, in natural hosts, multiplication of DNA viruses usually results in lysis of the infected cells, transformation with DNA viruses is detectable only under conditions that restrict virus replication and permit survival of infected cells (for example, in nonlytic infections of selected cell types or unnatural animal hosts, or in infection with damaged virions). As a consequence of the requirement for restricted virus replication, infectious DNA viruses seldom can be isolated from the cells they transform. In contrast, RNA viruses, because their replication is noncytocidal, can cause oncogenic transformation in their natural hosts, and viral products are produced whether or not virus is released.

Transforming viruses often integrate all or part of their genome into the cell DNA (in the case of RNA tumor viruses, a DNA copy of the RNA genome is integrated). Herpesvirus and bovine papilloma virus DNA are maintained in transformed cells as *episomes*, which are separate from the host genome. Current information suggests that the integration is random, but it is not clear if all integration sites permit expression of the virus *oncogenes* and result in the generation of tumor cells (see Chapter 82). Indeed, some experimental results suggest that integration of a defective retrovirus adjacent to a cellular oncogene may activate it to transform the cell. Basically, however, oncogenic transformation requires an altered expression of the oncogenes of virus or cell origin that modify control of cell proliferation. As noted, genetic rearrangements after integration may be an important aspect of the expression of the oncogene. One of the major unanswered questions of modern oncology and molecular biology is: How does the expressed oncogene modify the affected cell and cause it to exhibit a transformed phenotype?

Some viruses (for example, papovaviruses such as SV40) have been particularly valuable in studying the mechanisms of transformation because of the relatively small size of their DNA. In cells transformed by SV40, a single virus protein (the large T-antigen; Figure 65-3) is associated with the maintenance of a transformed phenotype. The large T-antigen may be considered to be a product of the SV40 oncogene. Although the large T-antigen has a number of recognized activities (including binding to DNA, which indicates that T-antigen might affect initiation of cell DNA synthesis and thus initiate and maintain cell transformation), only two (an ATPase activity and the ability to form a complex with, and to stabilize, a cell protein of about 53,000 daltons) have been consistently found to be required for maintenance of transformation. The 53,000 dalton host cell protein, often referred to as p53, is a normally short-lived phosphoprotein that is consistently associated with protein kinase activity and is believed to have a regulatory effect on normal cell proliferation. Thus, the stabilization of p53 by complex formation with SV40–large T protein may result in the cellular modifications associated with a transformed phenotype. Such an interpretation is attractive, although not all data support it.

Some of the products of the cellular and retrovirus oncogenes (for example, pp60^{src}; see Chapter 82) also appear to be protein kinases that have the relatively uncommon ability to phosphorylate tyrosine residues (in contrast to serine or threonine). In addition, current hypotheses suggest that other oncogene products may be related to cellular growth factors or their receptors. For example, the avian erthroblastosis virus oncogene (erb B) recently has been found to be related closely to the receptor for epidermal

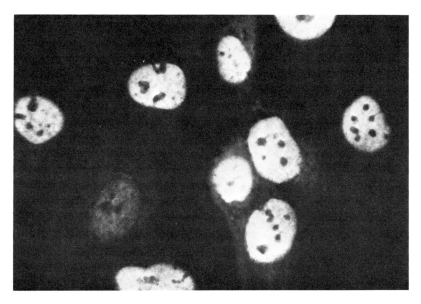

Figure 65-3 Transformed cells have been stained by immunofluorescence to demonstrate intranuclear T antigen of human papovavirus (×600).

growth factor (one of a class of cellular proteins that induce cell division). Moreover, both the organization of the simian sarcoma virus oncogene, and the amino acid sequence of its product, have been observed to be similar to those of human platelet-derived growth factor. These findings support the hypothesis that carcinogenesis results from the enhanced expression of cellular (or viral) genes that code for proteins with regulatory or growth-factorlike activities. Additional evidence is needed to verify this hypothesis.

References

Fenner, F.J., White, D.O.: *Medical virology,* 2nd ed. New York: Academic Press, 1976.

Hiatt, H.H., Watson, J.D., Winsten, J.A. (editors): *Origins of human cancer: Book B—Mechanisms of carcinogenesis.* Cold Spring Harbor, NY.: Cold Spring Harbor Laboratory, 1977.

Luria, S.E., et al., (editors): *General virology,* 3rd ed. New York: John Wiley and Sons, 1978.

Klein, G. (editor): *Viral oncology.* New York: Raven Press, 1980.

Slamon, D.J., et al.: Expression of cellular oncogenes in human malignancies. *Science* 1984; 224:256–262.

Stewart, T.A., et al.: Spontaneous mammary adenocarcinomas in transgenic mice that carry and express MTV/myc fusion genes. *Cell* 1984; 38:627–637.

Tooze, J., (editor): *Molecular biology of tumor viruses,* 2nd ed. Part 2, *DNA tumor viruses.* Cold Spring Harbor, N.Y.: Cold Spring Harbor Laboratory, 1980.

66 Genetics

David W. Kingsbury, MD

General Concepts
Sources of Variation in Viruses
   Mutation
   Gene Rearrangements
   Rearrangements of Virus Genes and Cell Genes
Interactions Between Virus Gene Products
New Research Tools

General Concepts

Genetics, the study of variation and its inheritance in living organisms, is as important for understanding and controlling viruses as it is for the rest of microbiology (see Chapter 20). In turn, virus research has made important contributions to the development of modern genetic concepts. For example, the demonstration that the DNA of bacteriophage (bacterial virus) T4 contains all of the genetic information in the organism, and the discovery that the isolated RNA of tobacco mosaic virus is infectious, helped to prove that genes are nucleic acids. Viruses continue to be favored subjects for fundamental genetic research because they are far less complex than cells, although they obey the same chemical and biologic ground rules. The most complex viruses, such as herpesviruses and poxviruses, contain as many as a few hundred genes; the simplest, like picornaviruses, papovaviruses, and togaviruses, possess only a handful. Moreover, viruses are almost universally *haploid* organisms; that is, they possess only one copy of each gene, which simplifies genetic analysis further.

This chapter reviews the impact on virus behavior of mutation, gene rearrangements, and interactions between gene products (proteins) (Table 66-1). Mutations and gene rearrangements (*recombination* and *reassortment*) are changes in the genetic material

Table 66-1 Genetic Phenomena

Changes in Genetic Material	Interactions Between Gene Products During Dual Infection
Mutation (change of genome of one virus)	Complementation (one virus provides a missing gene product for replication of a second defective virus)
Recombination (exchange of genes between two genomes during dual infection of a cell)	Phenotypic mixing (genotype from one parent but phenotype from two parents)
Reassortment (exchange of gene segments between two segmented genomes during dual infection)	

that are heritable and therefore of primary importance in nature, since they determine whether a virus is transmissible from host to host, capable of replicating in a given host, and virulent. This chapter compares the biologic effects of heritable changes in genetic materials with nonheritable interactions between gene products (*complementation* and *phenotypic mixing*) that may occur in mixed infections (see Table 66-1). It also describes how live virus vaccines have been developed by selection of favorable mutants and how scientists employ other types of mutants to study the organization of viral genomes and functions of viral gene products. New research tools are rapidly advancing virus genetics, promising better control of virus diseases in the future.

Sources of Variation in Viruses

Mutation

Frequency of Mutation. Mutation of genetic material is the basis of variation in all organisms, including viruses. Rate of mutation is determined mainly by chemical properties of the nucleic acids (see Chapter 10), so it is not surprising that mutations occur in viruses at frequencies comparable to other organisms: about once every 10^7–10^8 nucleotide duplications. Since genomes of the most complex viruses contain no more than 2×10^5 nucleotide pairs, several hundred rounds of accurate virus genome duplication generally occur between mutational events. In most virus infections, however, thousands of genome duplications occur in a single cell, making the generation of one or more mutants practically inevitable. Most mutations appear to be neutral (without effect on behavior) or disadvantageous to the point of being lethal, so that most types of viruses ordinarily display limited biologically significant variation (a notable exception is influenza virus; see Chapter 78).

Practical Application of Selective Pressure. A change in environment, as when a virus infects a new host, brings a new set of selective pressures to bear. Under the new conditions, a selective advantage may be conferred by a mutation that was neutral or even deleterious in the former environment. Experience has shown that full adaptation to a new host is progressive, involving the cumulative effects of many mutations, each conferring a slight additional replication advantage. The trade-off that generally occurs is a diminished ability to proliferate and cause disease in the original host. If the surface antigens of the virus are not altered in this process, the passaged virus has been attenuated into a potentially useful live vaccine. This was first achieved by Pasteur, who painstakingly passed rabies virus repeatedly in rabbits. In recent times, cell cultures have supplanted animals in this work, as in the development of the polio virus and measles virus vaccines. Such vaccine strains are stable enough to be used in human populations because they have sustained too many mutations for a reversion to virulence to be probable (see Chapter 72).

Another example of the consequences of a change in a virus host is the evolution of myxoma virus (a poxvirus) that has been observed in Australia. This virus, which is endemic but nonvirulent in wild rabbits in South America, was introduced into Australia in 1950 to control an infestation by European rabbits. Although the rabbits in Australia suffered high mortality from infection with the virus, in a few years, variants of the myxoma virus appeared that were less virulent and allowed infected rabbits to survive as virus carriers for weeks (instead of days). This lengthened survival of the host animals increased the probability that the variant viruses would be transmitted to uninfected rabbits, thereby giving those viruses a selective advantage over the original virulent strain. (At the same time, resistant variants in the rabbit population were selected by the pressure of myxoma virus infection.) This experiment in nature illustrates how mutual adaptation of a host and a pathogen can increase the survival of both parties.

Mutants as Research Tools.   In fundamental research, mutants are employed as probes of virus genome organization and gene functions. **Deletion mutants** contain less genetic information than parental types. They arise spontaneously and in some cases with high frequency (herpesvirus, papovavirus, influenza virus, rhabdoviruses, and paramyxoviruses).

Since organisms with genomes as small as those of viruses rarely possess nonessential genes and since a deletion of part of a gene almost always inactivates it, deletion mutants usually are defective (unable to replicate). However, if the genome of the defective virus retains the restricted set of nucleotide sequences that are recognized normally by the genome-replicating machinery of the nondefective parental virus, the defective virus can be helped to replicate by the nondefective virus (in a mixed infection). Yet, if the defective virus genome appropriates too large a share of the replicating machinery provided by the helper virus, reproduction of the helper may be hindered. Thus, some deletion mutants have been termed **defective-interfering (DI)**. In animals and in cultured cells, the addition of DI mutants can change an acute, lethal infection into a chronic infection. Thus, it has been proposed that DI mutants may alter the outcome of viral diseases in the same way (see Chapter 70).

Investigators employ chemical and physical *mutagens* as well as site-specific substitution of nucleotides (Chapter 20) to generate various mutants for genetic studies. Readily identified mutant phenotypes that have been exploited include changes in virulence or plaque (lesion) morphology in cell cultures, alterations in virion surface properties, antigenic structure, host range, or sensitivity to inactivating substances.

Most of these phenotypes, however, involve a narrow spectrum of virus genes. More versatile and widely used in animal virology are **conditional-lethal** mutants of the temperature-sensitive type. These mutants are selected for ability to grow in a permissive (low temperature) condition, but their replication is blocked at nonpermissive (high temperature) conditions by conformational changes in the mutant gene product.

Because any protein species can, in theory, undergo a **temperature-sensitive mutation** any kind of virus function can be affected. The conditional nature of this type of mutation facilitates the identification of altered functions. The investigator can shift infected cells to nonpermissive conditions at any stage of the virus replication cycle and observe the consequences. For example, if a mutation resides in an enzyme required for viral nucleic acid synthesis, incorporation of a radioactive precursor into viral nucleic acid will decrease as the temperature increases.

Temperature-sensitive mutants offer prospects for rational and rapid construction of live vaccines, because a temperature-sensitive mutation in a gene responsible for virulence is not likely to affect surface antigens that elicit a protective antibody response. To reduce the chance of reversion to virulence in the population, however, it is prudent to introduce additional mutations into the vaccine strain, recreating the result that occurs spontaneously during attenuation. (The effects of added mutations are, at least in theory, dramatic, because of the multiplication of probabilities: if the probability of reversion at a single gene locus is 10^6, the probability that two loci will revert is 10^{12}.)

This principle was recently applied by Chanock and coworkers, who developed several reassortant influenza viruses with temperature-sensitive mutations in two of the three genes that specify the proteins required for viral RNA synthesis (see Chapter 78). Although all of these reassortants were attenuated and genetically stable in hamsters, one of them reverted unexpectedly to temperature-insensitivity when given to a human subject. Analyses showed that the temperature-sensitive phenotypes of both genes had been suppressed by compensating mutations, a finding that may reflect a special facility of influenza virus to mutate, an inappropriate choice of attenuated genes, or an instability of the temperature-sensitive phenotypes. Other types of attenuating mutations now are being tested in attempts to prevent this suppression by mutations.

Gene Rearrangements

Recombination, an exchange of genes between two genomes, occurs during replication of most types of DNA viruses and is detected in the laboratory by characterizing the phenotypes of a large number of offspring from a mixed infection with a pair of mutants of a single virus. Recombination frequencies depend largely on distances between genes, as in higher organisms, and these frequencies can be used to deduce a genetic map (Figure 66-1).

RNA viruses exhibit a wider range of nucleic acid interactions, reflecting their disparate life cycles. Some types give no evidence of an ability to recombine, despite careful searches (togaviruses, rhabdoviruses, and paramyxoviruses). Some types recombine but at low efficiencies (picornaviruses); other recombine efficiently (retroviruses).

Influenza virus and reovirus are special in that their genomes are **segmented,** with each gene contained in a separate piece of nucleic acid. In mixed infection, reassortment of these segments readily occurs. In nature, many variants of influenza virus are distributed widely in domestic and wild animals. The hypothesis that genetic reassortments among these variants and existing human influenza viruses generate new epidemic strains explains in part why influenza viruses are exceptionally variable. The term *genetic reassortment* is preferable to *genetic recombination* in describing gene interchanges of this kind, since it signifies the special mechanism involved. Since no physical linkage of the genes in these viruses occurs, their genes cannot be mapped in the conventional sense.

A.   FREQUENCY OF RECOMBINATION BETWEEN NEAR AND DISTANT MARKERS

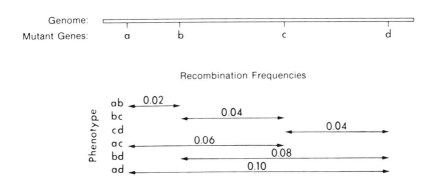

B.   MARKER RESCUE WITH DNA

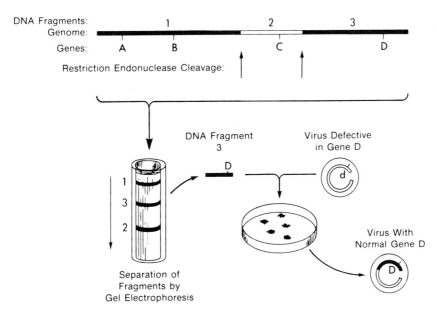

Figure 66-1 Two methods of genetic mapping. **A,** Genetic mapping by recombination frequencies. The frequency of recombination of two mutations is proportional to their separation in genome. **B,** Genetic mapping with restriction enzyme fragments. This example employs marker rescue (recombination between a DNA fragment and a mutant viral genome). Fragment 3 from wild-type virus recombines with DNA of a mutant defective in gene D during mixed infection, rescuing the mutant.

Rearrangements of Virus Genes and Cell Genes

Instead of destroying its host cell, a virus may form a stable relationship with it. Of paramount importance in the induction of cancer by viruses is the **genetic integration** of all or, more commonly, part of a virus genome into a cellular chromosome (retroviruses, papovaviruses, and adenoviruses). Sometimes, as with herpesviruses, a virus may take up residence as an unintegrated *episome* (a genetic element that can replicate autonomously). In either case, persistent expression of virus genes that stimulate cell proliferation produces a transformed state (see Chapter 65).

Interactions Between Virus Gene Products

Other interactions between viruses are nonheritable. When two different mutants infect the same cell, **functional complementation** may occur between them; that is, if each mutant possesses a normal counterpart of the gene that is defective in its partner, the normal gene products (proteins) can cooperate to support the replication of both parents (Figure 66-2). The genes of the parents are not usually redistributed in this process. By systematically crossing all the mutants in a collection, an investigator can sort them into complementation groups. Members of a complementation group are defective in the same gene, so they do not complement each other, but they will complement members of other complementation groups. Thus, the number of complementation groups that can be obtained reflects the number of genes that a virus possesses.

When complementation involves viral structural proteins, phenotypic mixing can occur in virus assembly, producing virions with structural characteristics of both parents, but containing the genome of only one parent. Phenotypic mixing also occurs between nondefective mutants and even between unrelated but structurally analogous viruses, as in mixed infections with an influenza virus and a paramyxovirus. The progeny are called **mosaics** if structural proteins of both parental types are distributed randomly among them; if the genome (or nucleocapsid) of one virus is enclosed within a capsid (or envelope) specified completely by the other parent, the progeny form a **pseudotype.** Within a pseudotype, a virus genome acquires new surface properties that can alter its host range.

New Research Tools

Recombinant DNA technology and rapid nucleic acid sequencing methods are accelerating the pace of discovery in viral genetics, as in all of molecular biology. The complete nucleotide sequences of many virus genomes have been determined already, and more such assessments are being made all the time. We are obtaining detailed information about the structure of genes and about the nucleotide sequences that signal gene transcription, genome replication, and the regulation of these functions. Mutagenesis can now be directed by the experimenter to a specific site within a gene; a sequence can be deleted, rearranged, or duplicated; the altered gene can be produced in abundant quantities; and the functional consequences of the genetic alteration can then be examined.

An example of the power of this technology for gaining fundamental information is given in Figure 66-1b. A bacterial **restriction endonuclease** cleaves a double-stranded

A. NORMAL INFECTION

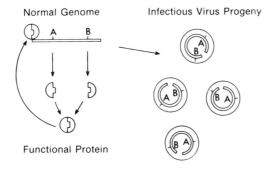

Normal Genome   Infectious Virus Progeny

Functional Protein

B. SEPARATE INFECTIONS WITH MUTANT VIRUSES

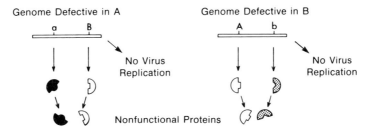

Genome Defective in A   Genome Defective in B

No Virus Replication   No Virus Replication

Nonfunctional Proteins

C. MIXED INFECTION WITH MUTANT VIRUSES

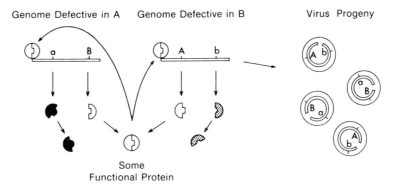

Genome Defective in A   Genome Defective in B   Virus Progeny

Some
Functional Protein

Figure 66-2 Example of complementation. **A,** Normal products of genes A and B form a protein needed for virus replication. **B,** In separate infections, products of mutant genes a and b cannot complement their normal partners. Lacking essential protein, neither mutant virus can replicate. **C,** In mixed infections, each mutant virus contributes a complementing gene product. The essential protein is made, and viruses replicate. Note parental genotypes in progeny. Although a protein with two subunits is illustrated, the principle also applies to proteins that do not interact directly. For example, a mutant defective in an enzyme may be complemented by a mutant defective in a structural protein. Uppercase letters represent nondefective genes; lowercase letters denote defective genes.

viral DNA molecule in a limited number of specific locations. The resulting fragments usually differ significantly in size, making possible their separation by electrophoresis in agarose or polyacrylamide gels. Such fragments can be used directly or after amplification as inserts in a bacterial plasmid clone (see Chapter 20) to map the virus genome. Fragments are located on the genetic map, and genes are located within fragments in various ways: hybridization with virus RNA species (which may be translated in vitro to identify their gene products); rescue of a mutant by an endonuclease fragment from wild-type (see Figure 66-1b); detection of functional changes produced by directed mutagenesis in a specific fragment; and infection of cells with individual fragments that may express a limited spectrum of viral functions, such as the ability to induce cell transformation. The technology is versatile and new approaches are continually being developed.

Moreover, practical applications of recombinant DNA technology to virus vaccine development are being made rapidly. DNA segments that represent the major type-specific (neutralizing) antigens of a herpesvirus, a rabies virus, several influenza virus strains, and a hepatitis B virus have been inserted into plasmids and expressed in bacteria. Once in the form of recombinant DNA, such virus genes can be modified in the test tube to specify a protein suitable for use as a subunit vaccine. For example, in studies in which nucleotide sequences encoding the membrane-anchoring domains of influenza virus and rabies-virus glycoproteins were deleted, water-soluble antigens were obtained when the genes were expressed. Another approach to vaccine development that has great potential is the identification of antigenic regions in the viral protein and the chemical synthesis of the relevant peptides for use as immunogens. For example, two peptides of the VP1 protein of foot-and-mouth disease virus (a picornavirus), which represented amino acid residues 151 to 160 and 200 to 213, were found to be protective as vaccines when coupled to a carrier protein. Similar experiments have been done with influenza virus and hepatitis virus antigens.

Experimental tools like these are providing an understanding of virus genetics of such scope that we can anticipate rapid development of rational controls of all important virus infections.

References

Bittle, J.L., et al.: Protection against foot-and-mouth disease by immunization with a chemically synthesized peptide predicted from the viral nucleotide sequence. *Nature (London)* 1982; 298:30–33.

Burge, B.W., Pfefferkorn, E.R.: Complementation between temperature-sensitive mutants of Sindbis virus. *Virology* 1966; 30:214–223.

Fenner, F., Ratcliffe, F.N.: *Myxomatosis*. London: Cambridge University Press, 1965.

Hirst, G.K.: Genetic recombination with Newcastle disease virus, poliovirus and influenza. *Cold Spring Harbor Symp Quant Biol* 1962; 27:303–308.

Huang, A.S., Baltimore, D.: Defective viral particles and viral disease processes. *Nature (London)* 1970; 226:325–327.

Jones, N., Shenk, T.: Isolaton of deletion and substitution mutants of adenovirus type 5. *Cell* 1978; 13:181–188.

Tolpin, M.D., et al.: Genetic factors associated with loss of the temperature-sensitive phenotype of the influenza A/Alaska/77-*ts*-1A2 recombinant during growth *in vivo*. *Virology* 1981; 112:505–517.

Yelverton, E., et al.: Rabies virus glycoprotein analogs: Biosynthesis in *Escherichia coli*. *Science* 1983; 219:614–620.

67 Pathogenesis

Samuel Baron, MD

General Concepts

General Concepts
Sequence of Virus Spread in the Host
    Implantation at Portal of Entry
    Local Replication and Local Spread
    Dissemination from Portal of Entry

Replication in Target Organs
Shedding of Virus
Congenital Infections

General Concepts

Pathogenesis is a process by which a virus infection in a host leads to disease. Pathogenic mechanisms include implantation of virus at a body site (the **portal of entry**), replication at that site, and then spread to, and replication within, sites where disease (**target organs**) or shedding of virus into the environment occurs. Most viral infections are subclinical, suggesting that body defenses against viruses arrest most infections before disease symptoms become manifest. Knowledge of subclinical infections comes from serologic studies that show sizeable portions of the population have specific antibodies to viruses even though the individuals have no history of disease. These inapparent infections have great epidemiologic importance: they constitute major sources for dissemination of virus through the population, and they confer immunity (see Chapter 71).

Many factors affect pathogenic mechanisms. An early determinant is the extent to which body tissues and organs are accessible to virus. Accessibility is influenced by physical barriers such as mucous and tissue barriers, by the distance to be traversed within the body, and by natural defense mechanisms. If virus reaches an organ, infection occurs only if cells capable of supporting virus replication are present. Cellular susceptibility requires a cell surface attachment site (receptor) for the virions and also an intracellular environment that permits virus replication and release. Even if virus initiates infection in a susceptible organ, replication of sufficient virus to cause disease may be prevented by host defenses (see Chapters 68 and 69).

Other factors that determine whether infection and disease occur are the many virulence characteristics of the infecting virus. To cause disease, the infecting virus must have the appropriate set of characteristics to overcome the inhibitory effects of physical barriers: distance, host defenses, and differing cellular susceptibilities to infection. These inhibitory effects are genetically controlled and therefore may vary among individuals and races. Virulence characteristics enable the virus to initiate infection, spread in the body, and replicate enough to impair the target organ. Virulence factors include ability to replicate under certain circumstances: during inflammation, during the febrile response, in migratory cells, and in the presence of natural body inhibitors and interferon. Extremely virulent strains often occur within virus populations; occasionally, these strains become dominant as a result of selective pressures (see Chapter 71). The viral proteins and genes responsible for specific virulence functions are being identified.

Fortunately for the survival of humans and animals (and for the infecting virus), most natural selective pressures favor the dominance of less virulent strains; because these strains do not cause severe disease or death, their replication and transmission are not impaired. Mild or inapparent infections can result from absence of one or more virulence factors. For example, a virus that has all the virulence characteristics except the inability to multiply at elevated temperatures is arrested at the febrile stage of infection, therefore causing a milder disease than its totally virulent counterpart. Live virus vaccines are composed of viruses deficient in one or more virulence factors; they thus cause only inapparent infections and yet are able to replicate sufficiently to induce immunity.

Disease does not always follow successful virus replication in the target organ. Disease occurs only if enough virus is replicated to damage essential cells directly, cause the release of toxic substances from infected tissues, or damage organ function indirectly as a result of the body's immune response to the presence of virus antigens. Damage of cells by replicating virus and damage by the immune response are considered in Chapter 65, Effects on Cells, and Chapter 69, Immune Defenses, respectively.

Affinity for specific body tissues by most viruses is implied by the tissue specificity, or tropism. This specificity is determined by selective susceptibility of cells, physical barriers, local temperature and pH, and host defenses. Many examples of tissue tropism by viruses occur. Polioviruses selectively infect and destroy certain nerve cells, which have a higher concentration of surface receptors for the viruses than do virus-resistant cells. Rhinoviruses multiply exclusively in the upper respiratory tract, because they are adapted to best multiply under local low temperature and pH and high oxygen tension. Enteroviruses can multiply in the intestine, partly because they resist inactivation by digestive enzymes, bile, and acid. Similarly, rabies virus selects the brain and salivary glands; hepatitis virus, the liver; herpes simplex virus, mucosal surfaces and nerve ganglia; and wart virus, the skin. In all these cases, however, the precise mechanisms for affinity are not known.

As a group, viruses use all conceivable portals of entry, mechanisms of spread, target organs, and sites of excretion. This abundance of possibilities is not surprising considering the occurrence of astronomic numbers of viruses and their variants (see Chapter 71).

Sequence of Virus Spread in the Host

Implantation at Portal of Entry

Viruses may be carried to the body by all possible routes (air, food, bites, and any contaminated object). Similarly, all possible sites of implantation (all body surfaces and internal sites reached by mechanical penetration) may be used. The frequency of implantation is greatest where virus contacts living cells directly (in the respiratory tract, in the alimentary tract, and subcutaneously). With some viruses, implantation in the fetus may occur at the time of fertilization through infected germ cells.

Even at the earliest stage of pathogenesis (implantation), certain variables may influence the final outcome of the infection. For example, the dose, infectivity, and virulence of virus implanted and the location of implantation may determine whether the infection will be inapparent (subclinical) or whether the disease will be mild, severe, or lethal.

Local Replication and Local Spread

Successful implantation may be followed by local replication and local spread of virus (Figure 67-1). Virus that replicates within the initially infected cell may spread to adjacent cells extracellularly or intracellularly. Extracellular spread occurs by release of virus into the extracellular fluid and subsequent infection of the adjacent cell. Intracellular spread occurs by fusion of infected cells with adjacent, uninfected cells or through cytoplasmic bridges between cells. Most viruses spread extracellularly, but herpesviruses, paramyxoviruses, and poxviruses may spread through both intracellular

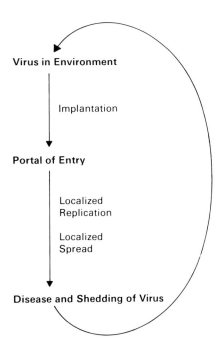

Figure 67-1 Sequence of virus spread during localized infection.

and extracellular routes. Intracellular spread provides virus with a partially protected environment because the antibody defense does not penetrate cell membranes.

Spread to cells beyond adjacent cells may occur through the liquid spaces within the local site (for example, lymphatics) or by diffusion through surface fluids such as the mucous layer of the respiratory tract. Also, infected migratory cells such as lymphocytes and macrophages may spread the virus within local tissue.

Establishment of infection at the portal of entry may be followed by continued local virus multiplication, leading to localized virus shedding and localized disease. In this way, local sites of implantation also may become the target organ and site of shedding during many infections (Table 67-1). Respiratory tract infections that fall into this category include influenza, the common cold, and those caused by parainfluenza viruses. Alimentary tract infections caused by several gastroenteritis viruses (for example, rotaviruses and picornaviruses) also may fall into this category. Localized skin infections of this type include warts, cowpox, and molluscum contagiosum. Localized infections may spread over body surfaces to infect distant surfaces. An example of this is the picornavirus epidemic conjunctivitis shown in Figure 67-2; in the absence of viremia, virus spreads from the eye (site of implantation) to the pharynx and intestine. Other viruses may spread internally to distant target organs and sites of excretion (disseminated infection). A third category of viruses may cause local and disseminated disease, as in herpes simplex and measles.

Dissemination from Portal of Entry

At the portal of entry, multiplying virus contacts pathways to the blood and peripheral nerves, the principal routes of widespread dissemination through the body. The most common route of systemic spread of virus utilizes the circulation (Figure 67-3). Viruses such as those causing poliomyelitis, smallpox, and measles disseminate through the blood but replicate initially at the portal of entry (the alimentary and respiratory tracts), where infection often causes no significant symptoms or signs of illness because the virus kills cells that are normally expendable and easily replaced. Virus progeny diffuse through the afferent lymphatics to the lymphoid tissue and then through the efferent lymphatics to infect cells in close contact with the bloodstream (for example,

Table 67-1   Pathogenesis of Selected Virus Infections: Localized Infections

Disease	*Site of Implantation*	*Route of Spread*	*Target Organ*	*Site of Shedding*
Influenza	Respiratory tract	Local	Respiratory tract	Respiratory tract
Coryza	Respiratory tract	Local	Respiratory tract	Respiratory tract
Gastroenteritis	Alimentary tract	Local	Alimentary tract	Alimentary tract
Warts	Skin and mucosa	Local	Skin and mucosa	Skin and mucosa

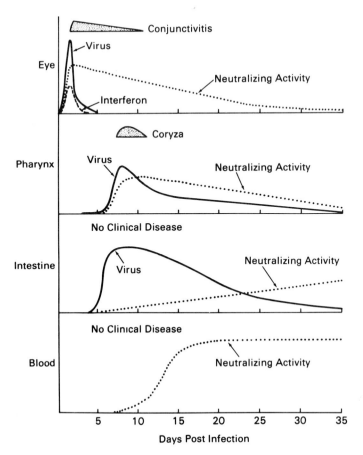

Figure 67-2 Picornavirus spread over body surfaces from eye to pharynx and intestine during natural infection. Local neutralizing activity (antibody) is shown. Adapted from Langford, M.P., et al.: *J Infect Dis* 1979; 139:653–658, and Langford, M.P., et al.: *Infect Immun* 1980; 29:995–998.

endothelial cells, especially those of the lymphoreticular organs). This initial spread may result in a brief primary viremia. Subsequent release of virus directly into the bloodstream induces a secondary viremia, which usually lasts several days and puts virus in contact with the capillary system of all body tissues. Virus may enter the target organ from the capillaries by replicating within a capillary endothelial cell or fixed macrophage and then being released on the target organ side of the capillary. Virus may also diffuse through small gaps in the capillary endothelium or penetrate the capillary wall through an infected, migrating leukocyte. The virus may then replicate and spread within the target organ or site of excretion by the same mechanisms described for local dissemination at the portal of entry. Disease may occur if the virus replicates within a sufficient number of essential cells and destroys them. For example, in poliomyelitis, the central nervous system is the target organ; the alimentary tract is both the portal of entry and the site of shedding. In some situations, the target organ and site of shedding may be the same. Table 67-2 presents other examples.

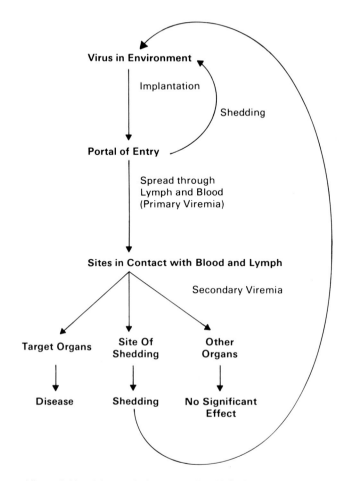

Figure 67-3 Virus spread through bloodstream during generalized infection.

The second mechanism of systemic spread, through the nerves, is second in frequency but highly important in several diseases (Figure 67-4). This mechanism occurs in rabies virus, herpesvirus, and, occasionally, poliomyelitis virus infections. For example, rabies virus implanted by a bite from a rabid animal replicates subcutaneously and within muscular tissue to reach nerve endings. Evidence indicates the virus spreads centrally in the axons and perineural cells, where virus is shielded from antibody. This nerve route leads rabies virus to the central nervous system, where disease originates. Rabies virus then spreads centrifugally through nerves to reach the salivary glands, the site of shedding. Table 67-2 shows other examples of nerve spread.

During most virus infections, no signs or symptoms of disease occur through the stage of virus dissemination. Thus, the incubation period (the time between exposure to virus and onset of disease) extends from the time of implantation through the phase of dissemination, ending when virus replication in the target organs causes disease. Occasionally, mild fever and malaise occur during viremia, but they often are transient and have little diagnostic value.

Table 67-2   Pathogenesis of Selected Virus Infections: Disseminated Infections

Disease	Common Site of Implantation	Route of Spread	Target Organ(s)	Site of Shedding
Poliomyelitis	Alimentary tract	Blood (nerve)	Central nervous system	Alimentary tract
Hepatitis A	Alimentary tract	Blood	Liver	Alimentary tract
Kuru	Alimentary tract	Blood	Brain	Brain (transmitted by ingestion)
Rubella	Respiratory tract	Blood	Skin, lymph nodes, fetus	Respiratory tract, excreta in newborn
Measles	Respiratory tract	Blood	Skin, lung, brain	Respiratory tract
Herpes simplex (type 1)				
Acute	Respiratory tract	Nerve, leukocytes	Many (e.g., brain, liver, skin)	Respiratory tract, epithelial surfaces
Recurrent	Ganglion	Nerve (to site of latency)	Skin, eye	Skin, eye
Rabies	Subcutaneously (bite)	Nerve	Brain	Salivary glands
Arbovirus	Subcutaneously (bite)	Blood	Brain and others	Lymph and blood (via insect bite)
Hepatitis B	Penetration of skin	Blood	Liver	Blood
Herpes simplex (type 2)	Genital tract	Nerve (to site of latency)	Genital tract	Genital tract

The incubation period tends to be brief (1-3 days) in infections in which virus travels only a short distance to reach the target organ (that is, in those infections in which disease is due to virus replication at the portal of entry). Conversely, incubation periods in generalized infections are longer because of the stepwise fashion by which the virus moves through the body before reaching the target organs. Other factors also may influence the length of the incubation period. Generalized infections produced by togaviruses may have an unexpectedly short incubation period because of direct intravascular injection (insect bite) of a rapidly multiplying virus. The mechanisms governing the long incubation period (months to years) of persistent infections are poorly understood. The persistently infected cell is often not lysed or lysis is delayed. Disease may result from an immune reaction to viral antigen (for example, arenaviruses in rodents) or from unknown mechanisms in those slow-virus infections during which no immune response has been detected (as in the scrapie-kuru group).

Replication in Target Organs

Virus replication in the target organ resembles replication at other body sites except that the target organ is reached late during the stepwise progression of virus through the body, and disease originates there. At each step of virus progression through the body, the local recovery mechanisms (local body defenses, including interferon, local

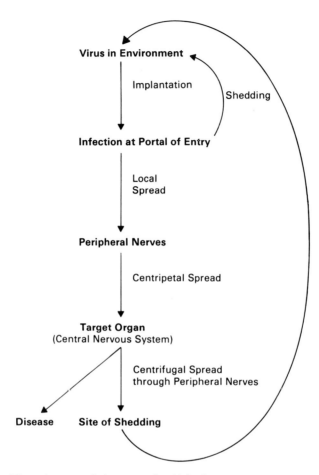

Figure 67-4 Virus spread through nerves during generalized infection.

inflammation, and local immunity) are activated; thus, when the target organ is infected, the previously infected sites have reached various stages of recovery. Figure 67-2 illustrates this staging of infection and recovery in different tissues during a spreading surface infection. Circulating interferon and immune responses probably account for the termination of viremia, but these responses may be too late to prevent seeding of virus into the target organ and into sites of shedding. Nevertheless, these systemic defenses can diffuse in varying degrees into target organs and thereby help retard virus replication and disease.

Depending on the balance between virus and host defenses, virus replication in the target organ may be sufficient to produce dysfunction manifested by disease and death. Additional constitutional disease such as fever and malaise may result from diffusion of toxic products from virus replication and cell necrosis. Viral antigens also may participate in immune reactions, leading to disease manifestations.

Different viruses may have tropisms for different target organs. The determinants of tropism are discussed in General Concepts.

Shedding of Virus

Because of the diversity of viruses, virtually every possible site of shedding may be utilized; however, the most frequent sites are the respiratory and alimentary tracts. Blood and lymph may be sites of shedding for the arboviruses, since biting insects become infected by this route. Milk may be a site of shedding for viruses such as some RNA tumor viruses (retroviruses) and cytomegalovirus (a herpesvirus). Several viruses (for example, cytomegaloviruses) may be shed simultaneously from the urinary tract as well as from other sites more commonly associated with shedding. The genital tract may serve as a site of shedding for herpesvirus type 2 and may be the route through which the virus is transmitted to sexual partners or the fetus. Saliva is the primary source of shedding for rabies virus. Cytomegalovirus is also shed from these last two sites. Finally, viruses such as tumor viruses that are integrated into the DNA of host cells may be shed through germ cells.

Congenital Infections

Infection of the fetus is a special case of infection in a target organ. The factors that determine whether a target organ is infected also apply to the fetus, but the fetus presents additional variables. The immune and interferon systems of the very young fetus may be immature. This immaturity, coupled with the placental barrier to transfer of maternal immunity and interferon, may deprive the very young fetus of important defense mechanisms. Another variable is the high vulnerability to disruption of the rapidly developing fetal organs, especially during the first trimester of pregnancy. Further, susceptibility to virus replication is influenced by the undifferentiated state of the fetal cells and by hormonal changes during pregnancy. Interestingly, although virus multiplication in the fetus may lead to congenital anomalies or fetal death, the mother may have only a mild or inapparent infection.

To cause congenital anomalies, virus must reach the fetus and multiply in it, thereby causing maldeveloped organs. Generally, virus reaches the fetus during maternal viremia by infecting or passing through the placenta to the fetal circulation and then to fetal target organs. Sufficient virus multiplication may disrupt development of fetal organs, especially during their rapid development (the first trimester of pregnancy). Although many viruses occasionally cause congenital anomalies, cytomegalovirus and rubella virus are the most common offenders. Virus shedding by the congenitally infected newborn infant may occur due to persistence of the virus infection at sites of shedding.

References

Fenner, F., White, D.O.: *Medical virology*, 2nd ed. New York: Academic Press, 1976.

Fields, B.N.: How do viruses cause different diseases? *JAMA* 1983; 250:1754-1756.

Galasso, G.J., Merigan, T.C., Buchanan, R.A., (editors): *Antiviral agents and viral diseases of man*. New York: Raven Press, 1984.

Kauffman, R.S. et al.: The sigma 1 protein determines the extent of spread of reovirus from the gastrointestinal tract of mice. *Virology* 1983; 124:403-410.

68 Nonspecific Defenses

Ferdinando Dianzani, MD

Samuel Baron, MD

General Concepts

Most viral infections are self-limited by host defenses, which enable the host to accommodate successfully to large accumulations of viruses that would have been lethal if presented initially. Although immune and nonimmune (nonspecific) defenses operate together to control viral infections, this chapter considers only nonspecific defenses. Some nonspecific defenses such as anatomic factors, nonspecific inhibitors in body fluids, and phagocytosis exist independently of infection; others (fever, inflammation, and interferon) are produced by the host in response to infection.

The intracellular site of virus replication and the ability of some viruses to spread by cell fusion protect them against such extracellular defenses as antibody, phagocytosis, and nonspecific inhibitors; however, because they replicate within the cell, viruses are vulnerable to intracellular alterations caused by host responses to infection. Nonspecific responses that alter the intracellular environment include fever, inflammation, and interferon.

These multiple defenses are made complex by their interactions with one another. This complexity is compounded by the varying effectiveness of the defenses that result from the diversity of viruses, hosts, and sites and stages of infection.

Defense Mechanisms Preexisting Infection

Anatomic Barriers

Anatomic barriers to viruses exist at the surfaces and within the body. At the body surfaces, the dead cells of the epidermis and the live cells that may lack viral receptors resist virus penetration and do not permit virus replication; however, this barrier is easily breached (for rabies virus by animal bites, for togaviruses by insect bites, and for wart virus by minor traumas). At mucous surfaces, only the mucous layer stands between invading virus and live cells. The effectiveness of the mucous layer depends on its formation of a physical barrier and its entrapment of foreign particles that are cleared by the mucous flow, as well as on the nonspecific inhibitors it contains (see following section). This mucous barrier is not absolute, however, since sufficient quantities of many viruses can infect by this route. In fact, most viruses use mucous surfaces as the portal of entry and initial replication site.

Within the body, an anatomic barrier to virus spread is formed by the layer of endothelial cells that separates blood from tissues (for example, the blood-brain barrier). Under normal conditions, these barriers have low permeability for viruses unless virus penetrates by replicating in the endothelial cells or in circulating macrophages. These internal barriers may explain in part the high level of viremia required to infect organs such as the brain, placenta, and lungs.

Nonspecific Inhibitors

A number of viral inhibitors occur naturally in most body fluids and tissues. They vary both chemically (lipids, polysaccharides, proteins, lipoproteins, and glycoproteins) and in degree and range of viral inhibition. Some inhibitors are related to the viral receptors of the cell surface, but most are of unknown origin. Almost all inhibitors protect by preventing virus attachment to cells. Whereas most of these inhibitors block only one or a few viruses, a recently described contact-blocking virus inhibitor (CVI) has a broad antiviral spectrum that also acts by blocking virus attachment. Other important properties of CVI are its molecular weight of approximately 1000 daltons, its distribution in all internal and surface fluids, and its ability to protect mice against several different viruses. There is also direct inactivation of many viruses by acid, bile salts, and enzymes in the gastrointestinal tract. Although the effectiveness of the inhibitors has not been fully established in vivo, their importance as host defenses is suggested by their antiviral activity in tissue culture and in vivo and by the direct correlation between the degree of virulence of some viruses and the degree of resistance to certain inhibitors. The presence of these inhibitors may explain the relatively high doses of virus required to initiate infection in vivo, as compared with those necessary in cell cultures.

Phagocytosis

The limited information available suggests that phagocytosis is less effective against viral infections than against bacterial infections; however, few of the factors that control uptake of virions or infected cells by phagocytes (chemical and electrical affinities) and their digestion by lysosomal enzymes have been studied systematically. The observed result of this process is that different viruses are affected differently by the various phagocytic cells. Specifically, some viruses are not engulfed, whereas others are engulfed but may or may not be inactivated. In fact, some viruses may even multiply in the phagocytes. Macrophages seem to be more effective against viruses than are granulocytes, and large viruses seem to be more affected than small viruses. An important mechanism of protection by phagocytes is the marked reduction of viremia by macrophages when the conditions are optimal. For example, the degree of virulence in several strains of herpes simplex virus correlates with their ability to survive or even multiply within macrophages. Thus, depending on the situation, macrophages in their phagocytic function may reduce virus, help spread the infection or, more commonly, have little or no effect. Macrophages in their nonphagocytic functions may be permissive or nonpermissive for multiplication of certain viruses and thereby affect the outcome of these infections (see Chapter 69).

Defense Mechanisms Evoked by Infection

Fever

Viral replication is influenced strongly by temperature. Even a modest increase can cause strong inhibition; a temperature rise from 37 C to 38 C may decrease drastically the yield of many viruses. This phenomenon has been observed in tissue culture as well as in many experimental and natural infections. The artificial induction of fever in mice infected with viruses reduces mortality rates, as compared with mortality rates in control animals maintained at normal temperature. On the other hand, the artificial lowering of temperature during the infection may increase mortality, as shown in suckling mice infected with coxsackieviruses and taken away from the warmth of their mother's nest.

Several observations suggest strongly that the same phenomenon may occur during human viral infections. Retrospective studies have shown that the incidence and severity of paralysis among children infected by polioviruses were significantly higher in patients treated with antipyretic drugs than in untreated children. Also consistent with these findings is the observation that virus strains that replicate best at fever temperature are usually virulent, whereas virus strains that replicate poorly at fever temperature are usually low in virulence and therefore often are used as live virus vaccines.

Temperatures as low as 33 C are normal at body surfaces; viruses that infect these sites and replicate optimally at these temperatures establish only local infections that do not spread to deeper tissues where body temperature is higher. For example, rhinoviruses that cause common colds replicate optimally at 33–34 C (temperatures found in normally ventilated nasal cavities); however, they are inhibited at 37 C (a temperature found when swelling of the edematous mucosa interrupts air flow). An interesting question is whether this temperature increase is important for recovery from coryza.

Probably, the same general considerations of temperature apply to other human viral infections such as measles, rubella, and mumps, although, unfortunately, suitable and controlled studies have not yet been conducted. Nevertheless, available information suggests conservative use of antipyretic drugs.

Inflammation

Several antiviral mechanisms are generated by the local inflammatory response to virus-induced cell damage. The major components of the inflammatory process are circulatory alterations, edema, and leukocyte accumulation. The resulting phenomena are elevated local temperature, reduced oxygen tension in the involved tissues, altered cell metabolism, and increased CO_2 and organic acids. All these alterations, which occur in a cascading and interrelated fashion, may drastically reduce replication of many viruses. For instance, altered energy metabolism of the infected and surrounding cells, as well as the accumulating lymphocytes, can generate local hyperthermia. When inflammation occurs at superficial sites, where temperature is normally lower, hyperthermia can be generated also by hyperemia during early stages of the inflammation. As inflammation progresses, hyperemia becomes passive, thereby greatly reducing blood flow and decreasing oxygen tension. Two factors account for this decrease in oxygen tension: limited influx of erythrocytes, and lower diffusion of oxygen through edema fluid. In turn, the decreased oxygen tension causes less ATP production (and thus reduces energy available for viral synthesis) and increases anaerobic glycolysis, which increases the accumulation of CO_2 and organic acids in the tissues. These acid catabolites may decrease the local pH further to levels that have been shown to inhibit replication of many viruses. Local acidity also may increase by accumulation and subsequent degradation of the leukocytes in the affected area; possibly other less-defined factors play significant roles.

Thus, the local inflammation resulting from viral infection clearly activates several metabolic, physicochemical, and physiologic changes; acting individually or synergistically, these changes probably are an effective barrier to virus multiplication. Although it requires further study in whole animals and humans, this interpretation is supported by the finding that treatment with antiinflammatory drugs (corticosteroids) often increases the severity of infection in animals. Therefore, this type of drug should be used with caution in treating viral diseases.

Viral Interference and Interferon

Generally, infection by one virus renders host cells highly resistant to other, superinfecting viruses. Called **viral interference,** this intriguing phenomenon occurs frequently in cell cultures and in whole animals. Although interference occurs between most viruses, it may occur between only homologous viruses under certain conditions. Some types of interference are caused by competition among different viruses for critical replicative pathways (extracellular competition for cell surface receptors or intracellular competition for biosynthetic machinery). Similar interference may result from competition between defective viruses and infective viruses that may be produced concurrently. Another type of interference, which occurs most commonly in nature, is directed by the host cells themselves; these infected cells may respond to viral infection by producing a new protein, called **interferon,** which can react with uninfected cells to render them resistant to infection by a wide variety of viruses.

The important role played by interferon as a defense mechanism is clearly documented by a number of experimental and clinical observations: in many viral infections, a strong correlation has been established between interferon production and natural recovery; inhibition of interferon production or action enhances severity of infection; and treatment with interferon protects animals against infection by various viruses. In addition, the interferon system is the earliest appearing of the known host defenses and becomes operative within hours of infection. Figure 68-1 compares the early production of interferon with antibody during experimental infection of humans with influenza virus. Clinical trials of interferon and its inducers already have shown protection against certain viruses.

Although interferon was first recognized as an extraordinarily potent antiviral agent, it was found subsequently to affect other vital cellular and body functions. For example, interferon may influence the subsequent production of interferon; enhance killing by macrophages, NK cells, and cytotoxic T lymphocytes; and affect the immune response and the expression of cell membrane antigens. Interferon also may inhibit the division of, or lyse, certain cells, influence the body's response to ionizing radiation, and cross-activate hormone functions such as those of epinephrine and ACTH.

Production of interferon occurs de novo by cellular protein synthesis. Various

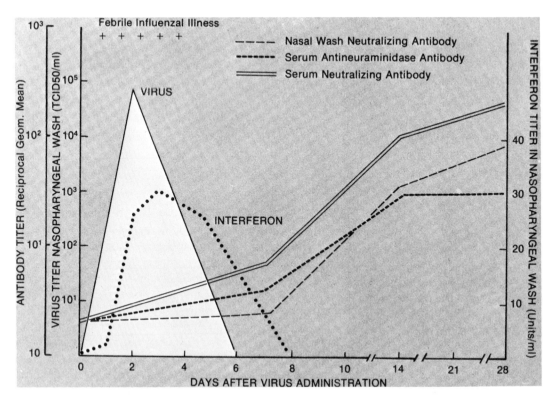

Figure 68-1 Production of virus, interferon, and antibody during experimental infection of humans with influenza wild-type virus. From a study by Drs. B. Murphy, et al, National Institutes of Health.

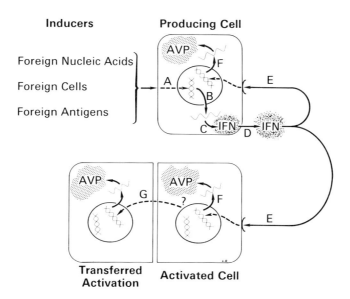

Inducers

Foreign Nucleic Acids

Foreign Cells

Foreign Antigens

Producing Cell

Transferred Activation **Activated Cell**

Figure 68-2 Cellular events of the induction, production, and action of interferon (IFN). Inducers of IFN react with cells to derepress the IFN gene(s) (**A**). This leads to the production of mRNA for IFN (**B**). The mRNA is translated into the IFN protein (**C**) which is secreted into the extracellular fluid (**D**) where it reacts with the membrane receptors of cells (**E**). The IFN-stimulated cells derepress genes (**F**) for effector proteins (AVP) that establish antiviral resistance and other cell changes. The activated cells also stimulate contacted cells (**G**) to produce AVP by a still unknown mechanism.

molecular subtypes of three interferons have been found with molecular weights ranging from 16,000–75,000 daltons. β interferon contains small amounts of associated carbohydrates. Interferons are secreted by the cell into the extracellular fluids (Figure 68-2). Usually, viral-induced interferon is produced at about the same time that the viral progeny are released by the infected cell; interferon can thus protect neighboring cells from the spreading virus.

There are three known antigenic types of interferon and a number of subtypes. Historically, the first type (fibroblast interferon or IFN β) was discovered by Isaacs and Lindenmann in viral infections of cells. Isaacs and coworkers postulated that viral and other foreign nucleic acids induced most body cells (fibroblasts, epithelial cells, and macrophages) to produce interferon. This induction mechanism has been largely confirmed and is illustrated in the top portion of Figure 68-3.

The second type of interferon (leukocyte interferon or IFN α) differs antigenically and structurally from fibroblast interferon. As shown in the middle portion of Figure 68-3, this interferon can be induced by foreign cells, virus-infected cells, tumor cells, bacterial cells and viral envelopes that stimulate B lymphocytes, null lymphocytes, and macrophages to produce leukocyte interferon. Mitogens for B cells may mimic this induction.

The third type of interferon (variously named immune interferon, T interferon, type 2 interferon, or IFN γ) differs molecularly and antigenically from fibroblast and leukocyte interferons. As shown in the lower portion of Figure 68-3, immune interferon

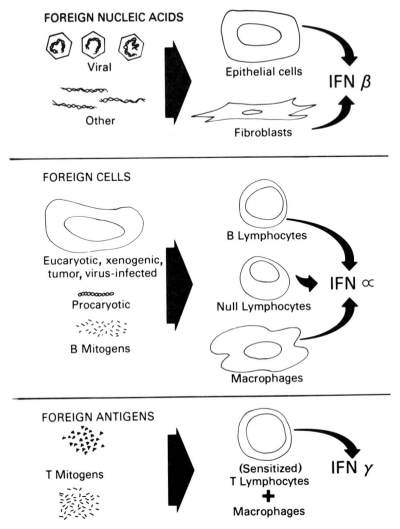

FOREIGN NUCLEIC ACIDS

Viral

Other

Epithelial cells

Fibroblasts

IFN β

FOREIGN CELLS

Eucaryotic, xenogenic,
tumor, virus-infected

Procaryotic

B Mitogens

B Lymphocytes

Null Lymphocytes

Macrophages

IFN α

FOREIGN ANTIGENS

T Mitogens

(Sensitized)
T Lymphocytes
+
Macrophages

IFN γ

Figure 68-3 Induction of fibroblast interferon (β), leukocyte interferon (α), or immune interferon (γ), respectively, by foreign nucleic acids, foreign cells, or foreign antigens.

is produced (along with other lymphokines) by T lymphocytes induced by foreign antigens to which the T lymphocytes have been presensitized. Mitogens for T cells may mimic this induction. Immune interferon has the unusual properties of: (1) exerting greater antitumor activity relative to its antiviral activity than do the other interferons, (2) exerting relatively greater immunosuppressive activity, (3) exerting relatively greater cell lytic effects, (4) potentiating the actions of other interferons, and (5) activating cells by a mechanism different from that of the other interferons.

Interferon does not inactivate virus directly. Instead, it prevents viral replication in surrounding cells by reacting with specific receptors on the cell membranes to derepress other cellular genes that encode intracellular effector antiviral proteins, which must be

Table 68-1 Biochemical Actions of Interferon

Effects Induced by Interferon	Secondary Effects	Effects on Viral Multiplication
Oligo (A) synthetase	Methylation of mRNA Cap Activation of RNase	mRNA
Protein kinase	Phosphorylation of initiation factors and ribosomal proteins	Initiation of protein synthesis
Phosphodiesterase	Degradation of tRNA	Elongation of proteins
Glycosyltransferase	Decreased protein glycosylation	Protein processing
		Virion release (or attachment)
Alteration of cell membranes	Altered cell membrane	Virion release (or attachment)
		Maturation to infectivity

synthesized before virus replication can be inhibited (Table 68-1). The mechanism of viral inhibition by the antiviral proteins probably occurs by inhibiting synthesis of essential viral proteins, but alternative or additional inhibitory mechanisms (transcription and viral release) are still being investigated. The inhibition of viral protein synthesis may occur via several biochemical alterations of cells. These alterations may, in theory, inhibit viral replication at the different steps shown in Table 68-1.

That the antiviral state may be transferred from interferon-treated cells to adjacent untreated cells without the continued presence of interferon has been shown (see Figure 68-3); this transfer mechanism may further amplify the interferon system's activity.

The interferon system is nonspecific in two ways: different viral stimuli induce the same type of interferon and different viruses are inhibited by the same interferon. On the other hand, the interferon molecule is mostly specific in its action for the animal species in which it was induced. Thus, interferon produced by animals or humans generally stimulates antiviral activity only in cells of the same or closely related animal families; that is, human interferon protects human and monkey cells but not chicken or mouse cells.

As with the other defenses, interferon is not the sole mechanism that influences recovery and, in certain virus infections, it may not be the most important. Much depends on the effectiveness of the virus in stimulating interferon production and on the susceptibility of the virus to the antiviral action of interferon. Interferon protects solid tissues during virus infection; interferon is also disseminated through the bloodstream during viremia, thereby protecting distant organs against the spreading infection.

A number of viral diseases (and cancer) in humans have the potential to be treated by application of the interferon system, including rabies, serum hepatitis, respiratory virus infections, encephalitis, and eye infections. Methods of application of the interferon system include administration of exogenous interferon or of various substances that induce body cells to produce endogenous interferon: natural and synthetic nucleic acids, avirulent viruses, several small-molecular-weight compounds, and certain highly complex biologic substances such as endotoxin and microbial products—many of which induce interferon through mitogenic activity.

Scientists have attempted to apply interferon to the control of viral diseases. The same principles that govern the effectiveness of the interferon defense control the effectiveness of applied interferon. For prophylaxis, a sufficient concentration of interferon (depending on the sensitivity of the virus) must reach the critical site. For therapy of an ongoing viral infection, the amount of exogenously administered interferon must exceed that produced endogenously.

Interferon availability has increased from large-scale production in bacteria by recombinant DNA technology as well as large-scale production in human cells, and more clinical trials are being conducted. The effectiveness of interferon prophylaxis for coryza has been demonstrated clearly. Additionally, interferon has been shown to have a therapeutic effect against human laryngeal papilloma (caused by a papovavirus). Therapeutic effects also have been reported against viral infections of the eye due to herpes simplex virus, vaccinia virus, adenovirus, hepatitis B, and disseminated varicella-zoster.

In conclusion, individual defense mechanisms assume roles of varying importance during different viral infections; in most cases, the recovery process is probably carried out not just by an isolated factor but by the simultaneous or sequential action of several mechanisms. The presence of multiple defenses helps to explain why suppression of one or several mechanisms does not entirely abrogate host resistance to viral infections; however, impairment of host defenses by medications used for symptomatic relief of viral infections conceivably may lead to more severe illness. For example, aspirin may prevent the febrile defensive response as well as reduce the interferon defense. Thus, the well-established principle of the ancient physician—"primum non nocere" (primarily do not harm)—is still valid.

References

Baron, S.: Mechanisms of recovery from viral infections. *Adv Virus Res* 1963; 10:39–64.

Baron, S., Dianzani, F., Stanton, G.J.: The interferon system. *Texas Rep Biol Med* 1982; Parts I and II: 1–715.

Baron, S., McKerlie, L.: Broadly active inhibitor of viruses spontaneously produced by many cell types in culture. *Infect Immun* 1981; 32:449–453.

Isaacs, A.: Interferon. *Adv Virus Res* 1963; 10:1–38.

Kumar, S., Baron, S.: Non-interferon cellular products capable of virus inhibition. *Texas Rep Biol Med* 1981; 41:395–401.

Kumar, S., et al.: A broadly active viral inhibitor in human and animal organ extracts and body fluids. Proc Soc Exp Biol Med 1984; 177:104–111.

Smorodintsev, A.A.: Basic mechanisms of nonspecific resistance to viruses in animal models and man. *Adv Virus Res* 1960; 7:327–376.

Wasserman, F.E.: Methods for the study of viral inhibitors. In: *Methods in virology*. Marmarosh, K., Koprowski, H., (editors), New York: Academic Press, 1968.

69 Immune Defenses

Gary R. Klimpel, PhD

General Concepts

Viral infections, which range from acute to chronic, cause numerous diseases and sometimes death. Many of these infections are controlled through natural defenses and vaccines that stimulate the host immune responses necessary for the prevention of viral diseases. In some viral infections, however, immune processes can play a major role in the pathogenesis of disease. Thus, knowledge of immune mechanisms is essential to understanding the pathogenesis and control of viral diseases.

As used in this chapter, the term *immunity* encompasses all the mechanisms by which a host may specifically recognize and react to viruses with or without injuring itself. A host's immune response may be beneficial, detrimental, or both. Immune responses first occur during the primary infection of a susceptible, nonimmune host, and they are increased during reinfection of an immune host. The individual immune responses that are effective against viruses are the T lymphocytes and cytotoxic effector T lymphocytes, antibody (with and without its interaction with complement), natural killer (NK) cells, macrophages, antibody-dependent cell-mediated cytotoxicity (ADCC), and lymphokines and monokines. Some of these host immune defenses may interact, often synergistically, with nonimmune defense mechanisms (Chapter 68).

The degree to which viral antigens are exposed to the host immune defenses is governed by the obligate intracellular replication of viruses. This exposure varies according to several virus–host cell interactions. These virus–host cell interactions are shown in Figure 69-1 and also are discussed in Chapter 65.

The most common virus–host cell interaction is the first shown in Figure 69-1, in which the virus destroys the infected cell (**cytolytic infection**). As illustrated, cytolytic infections vary in the way in which the immune system encounters virus or virus-specific antigens. Many viruses infect and replicate in cells primarily by the interactions shown in (a) and (b). In such cases, as cytolysis occurs, the virus and its antigens are released extracellularly and become exposed to the immune system. Many viruses (reoviruses, coxsackieviruses), however, can induce virus-specific antigens on the cell surface before cell death occurs and sometimes before viral multiplication is complete. In the third type of cytolytic infection (c), which is common with enveloped viruses (herpesviruses, poxviruses, paramyxoviruses), virus-specific antigens are present on the cell surface and the cells release the infectious virus for a short period before cell death. The virus is released into the extracellular fluids through a budding process at the surface of the cell membrane. Dissemination of these viruses (for example, herpesviruses, poxviruses, and paramyxoviruses) can occur by contiguous spread from cell to cell without exposure to

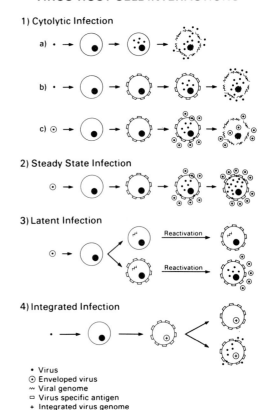

VIRUS-HOST CELL INTERACTIONS

1) Cytolytic Infection

2) Steady State Infection

3) Latent Infection

Reactivation

Reactivation

4) Integrated Infection

- • Virus
- ⊙ Enveloped virus
- ⌇ Viral genome
- ▢ Virus specific antigen
- + Integrated virus genome

Figure 69-1 The degree to which viral antigens are exposed to the host immune defenses is governed by the obligate intracellular replication of viruses. This exposure varies according to the virus–host cell interactions shown here: (1) cytolytic infection, (2) steady state infection, (3) latent infection, (4) integrated infection.

extracellular antibody. Cell-mediated immune responses are believed to be important in controlling the local spread of this type of infection.

The second type of virus-cell interaction is the **steady-state infection,** in which infected cells produce virus continuously, with little adverse effect on cellular metabolism. These cells express virus-specific antigens on their cell surface and produce abundant virus progeny, but they are not killed by the infectious process. In some steady-state infections, the progeny virus is released by budding through the cell membrane, and virus can spread from cell to cell without being exposed to the extracellular environment. DNA viruses do not produce steady-state infections, whereas some RNA viruses (paramyxoviruses, retroviruses) often do.

Latent infection is the third type of virus–host cell interaction. Herpesviruses are usually associated with such infections, which result when a virus infects a cell and is maintained within that cell for a long time (sometimes years) without giving rise to progeny virus or damaging the cell. Cells infected in this way may or may not express virus-specific antigens on their cell surface. Months to years after infection, the virus in these cells can be reactivated, the virus can replicate, and disease can occur. The mechanisms by which the virus is maintained intracellularly for such long periods of time and by which it is reactivated are not known. Interestingly, many latent infections occur in sequestered areas of the body (such as the nervous system) where recognition of infected cells by the immune system is believed to be difficult. In addition, cells that harbor virus but do not express viral antigens are not recognized by the immune system.

In the fourth type of virus–host cell interaction, **integrated virus infection,** all or part of the viral nucleic acid becomes integrated into the genome of the host cell. This type of interaction differs from the others in that, after integration, infectious virus may or may not be assembled within, or released from, the host cell. New virus-specific antigens, however, can be detected within the cell or on the cell surface. Infection with retroviruses is a classic example of this mechanism.

In most of these interactions, modification of *self* to *nonself* occurs because the virus and its antigens (nonself) may be present in varying concentrations in extracellular fluid, on the cell membrane, and within the cell. These modifications stimulate the components of the body's immune system.

Another important consideration in how viral infections trigger an immune response is the way in which a particular virus spreads in the host. Within an animal host, four general types of viral spread are recognized: (1) *local,* in which the viral infection is confined largely to a mucosal surface or organ (as in infection of the respiratory epithelium by rhinoviruses or of the gastrointestinal epithelium by rotaviruses); (2) *primary hematogenous,* in which the virus is inoculated directly into the bloodstream and then disseminates to target organs (as occurs with arboviruses); (3) *secondary hematogenous,* in which the initial virus infection and replication occur on a mucosal surface with subsequent dissemination to target organs via the bloodstream. The initial mucosal phase is often relatively asymptomatic. Examples for this type of spread are common viral exanthems, poliomyelitis, and mumps; and (4) *nervous system spread,* in which viruses (such as herpesviruses and rabiesviruses) disseminate via the nervous system. Thus, viral antigens may be present in different parts of the body depending on route of spread and phase of infection. Therefore, different immune mechanisms may be operative at the various sites of virus infection.

Consideration of type of virus spread within the host is important not only for understanding the immune response but also for vaccine development and for proper administration of a vaccine. For example, cell-mediated and humoral (IgA) immune responses take place at areas of a local infection such as the mucosal surface of the gastrointestinal or respiratory tracts; yet that local immune response does not necessarily mean that systemic immunity also will develop. The reverse is also true; systemic immunity does not always lead to local mucosal immunity. For example, the Salk poliovaccine (killed virus administered systematically) produces serum IgG as the major antibody, and little or no secretory response occurs. Although immune to systemic infection by virtue of serum antibody, the patient may become a temporary carrier, with virus persisting at the intestinal portal of entry because of the lack of secretory antibody. With the oral live Sabin poliovaccine, secretory antibody is induced in the intestine and is effective in preventing replication and subsequent mucosal penetration by the virus; therefore, it also prevents establishment of the carrier state.

Immune Response to Viral Infection

Recent studies have revealed a great complexity of host immune defenses against viral infection. This complexity arises from the multiplicity of host immune defenses and their interactions with one another. Multiplicity of defenses is not surprising in view of the diversity of viruses, hosts, routes of infection, body compartments, body cells, and mechanisms of virus multiplication and spread. The situation is further complicated by the varying effectiveness of the different host defenses during the different phases of the primary viral infection (implantation, spread to target organs, and subsequent recovery of each of the infected tissues), as well as during resistance to reinfection. Furthermore, the host defenses can actually cause disease manifestations as they react to the infection. It has become evident that a number of immune and nonimmune host defenses may operate to control viral infections or, at times, add to the disease process. The presence of multiple defenses against each infection helps explain why impairment of one defense or a few defenses does not entirely abrogate host resistance to viral infections.

Despite their complexity, many of the host immune defenses have been delineated, but determination of the relative effectiveness of each will require additional research. In this chapter, humoral immunity and cell-mediated immunity are considered separately, but, in each case, explanations are provided of how cells and cell populations from both systems interact and are essential for regulating the duration and magnitude of each type of immune response.

Humoral Immunity

B Lymphocytes

B lymphocytes respond to viral antigen introduced by immunization or infection. The exquisite specificity for the recognition of antigen by the B cells occurs through immunoglobulin on their cell surfaces. After the binding of antigen to this surface receptor and the interaction of the B cell with macrophages and T helper lymphocytes, the B cell differentiates into clones of antibody-secreting plasma cells, each of which is capable of secreting antigen-specific immunoglobulin [that is, antibody associated with the five major classes of immunoglobulins: IgG, IgM, IgA, IgD, and IgE (Chapter 4)]. The primary actions of antibody in viral defense are neutralization of virus by direct binding with virions and antibody-directed lysis of infected cells.

Antibody and Antibody-Mediated Reactions

At least three immunoglobulin classes have been demonstrated to exert antiviral activity: IgG, IgM, and IgA. These antibodies have been shown to neutralize the infectivity of virtually all known viruses. Antibody neutralization of virus can take place at the cellular level or extracellularly. At the cellular level, antibody can block the following steps associated with a virus infection: (1) virus attachment to the cell surface, (2) the penetration of the virus into the cells, and (3) the actual uncoating of the antibody–virus complex once inside the cell (Figure 69-2). Based on a number of studies, the mechanism of viral neutralization involves the binding of antibody to virus coat proteins. In most cases, this leads to an alteration of the receptor on the virus for the target cell. In some instances, antibody coating of extracellular virus may also interfere with penetration into the target cell or even with the uncoating of the virus once it has entered the cell. The exact mechanism of neutralization is unclear, but it probably involves changes in steric conformation of the virus surface. These antibody–virus interactions can take place independent of complement.

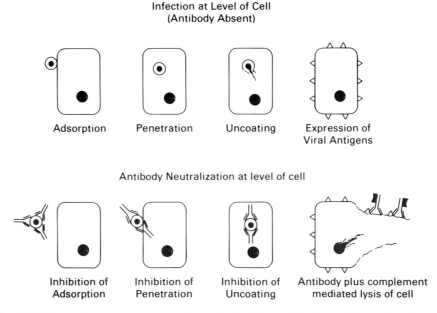

Infection at Level of Cell
(Antibody Absent)

Adsorption   Penetration   Uncoating   Expression of Viral Antigens

Antibody Neutralization at level of cell

Inhibition of Adsorption   Inhibition of Penetration   Inhibition of Uncoating   Antibody plus complement mediated lysis of cell

Figure 69-2   Mechanisms of virus neutralization by antibody at the cellular level. At the cellular level, antibody can block the following steps associated with a virus infection: (1) virus attachment-adsorption to the cell surface, (2) penetration of the virus into the cells, and (3) actual uncoating of the antibody-virus complex once inside the cell. Antibody also can act at the cellular level by recognizing virus-specific antigens on the surface of infected cells. In the presence of complement, these virally infected cells can be destroyed.

Antibody also can act at the cellular level by recognizing viral-specific antigens on the surface of infected cells. In the presence of complement, these infected cells can be destroyed. This complement-mediated lysis has been shown to occur both by the alternative complement pathway and by the classical complement pathway. Antibody-coated cells infected by virus also can be destroyed by different effector cells via antibody-dependent cellular cytotoxicity (ADCC). Alternatively, some antiviral antibodies can cap or modulate viral antigens on the surface of infected cells, thereby removing or covering antigen on the surfaces of infected cells.

Extracellularly, antibody can neutralize virus by causing aggregation (Figure 69-3), thus preventing adsorption of virus to cells and decreasing the number of infectious particles. Antibody and complement acting together also can inactivate certain viruses (in most cases, enveloped virus). Besides direct binding to virus, antibody may interact with phagocytic cells. Three types of antibody interactions with phagocytic cells are seen: direct binding of antibody to the surface of the phagocytic cells (cytophilic antibody), uptake of antigen-antibody (Ag-Ab) complexes through the Fc receptor, and uptake of antigen-antibody complement (Ag-Ab-C) complexes through the C3b receptor (see Chapters 4 and 6).

Before antibody can combine with and neutralize virus, it must reach the site of virus replication. Barriers to the distribution of antibody include the cell membrane, which excludes antibody, and anatomic tissue barriers, which limit the distribution of macromolecules into certain organs such as the central nervous system and lung.

A fixed concentration of antibody is most effective when it is present in large fluid spaces such as the serum and moist surfaces (for example, the respiratory and gastrointestinal tracts); this effectiveness is achieved because the virus is exposed to

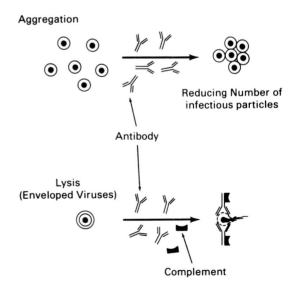

Figure 69-3   Extracellular neutralization of virus by antibody. Antibody can reduce the number of infectious particles by linking virions and thereby causing aggregation. Antibody and complement acting together can also inactivate certain viruses (in most cases, enveloped virus).

antibody for relatively long periods before the virus is able to escape into the interior of cells. Consequently, low levels of antibody in the serum are effective in terminating viremia and in preventing viremia during reinfection. For the viruses that do not use the blood plasma to spread to target organs, such as herpesviruses and rabiesviruses, relatively high levels of antibody are needed to prevent spread, since those viruses spend only a brief time traversing the small extracellular spaces between cells in solid tissue.

IgG antibodies are the most thoroughly studied and are responsible for most antiviral activity in serum. This immunoglobulin has been shown to be particularly protective in generalized viral infections with a viremic phase (for example, measles, poliomyelitis, and hepatitis), perhaps because virions in serum are not present within cells and therefore are exposed to antibody. Also, the IgG antibodies are transferred passively from mother to offspring through the placenta, and usually provide temporary protection against generalized viral infections during the first few months of life. Antibody is most protective when present before infection or during virus spread to target organs.

After immunization or infection with viruses, various classes of antibody appear sequentially; these antibodies may bind directly to virions and thereby neutralize virus. For example, with primary infection or immunization, most antigens first elicit IgM (early antibody) responses; IgA and IgG responses follow within a few days. After reinfection, most of the antibodies made are of the IgG class, although some IgM and IgA are generated. When the primary antigenic stimulation is in the respiratory or gastrointestinal tract, IgA antibody is the predominate immunoglobulin synthesized. The secretory IgA antibodies are secreted locally at mucosal sites and appear to be important in providing host protection against localized viral infections such as the common cold and influenza. Thus, when viral replication is confined to a mucosal surface, resistance to infection is determined predominantly by secretory IgA; serum IgG antibody provides less protection. In fact, viral infections that begin on a mucosal surface and then spread by hematogenous spread (for example, measles, rubella, polio) can be prevented at the mucosal stage by local secretory antibody. These diseases, which are dependent on hematogenous spread, can also be prevented by serum antibody but viral replication still may occur on the mucosal surface.

Recent information suggests that viruses acting through the induction of IgE antibodies may trigger immediate hypersensitivity responses through the release of vasoactive mediators. These observations may explain many of the apparent allergic manifestations of immediate hypersensitivity, such as wheezing and urticaria, that accompany some viral infections.

Complement is involved in the neutralization of many viruses, often through participation in increased phagocytosis of antibody-complement or complement-coated virions. Complement also is important as an adjunct to neutralization by specific antibody in that it can enhance either antibody-mediated steric changes on the virus or aggregation of the virus via antibody. In addition, complement can cause direct inactivation of antibody-coated enveloped virions.

In a small minority of patients with impaired B-lymphocyte function (hypogamma-globulinemia limited to impairment of humoral immunity), there are significantly increased frequencies of severe poliovirus and enterovirus infections of the nervous system (in addition to enhanced infection with pyogenic bacteria). This can be caused by prolongation of viremia, as has been detected in immunosuppressed animals. Interestingly, the course of most of these and other viral infections is typically benign in most of these hypogammaglobulinemic patients, indicating that other defense mechanisms may play roles that are equal to, or more important than, that played by antibody during certain viral infections. The development of normal specific resistance to reinfection in hypogammaglobulinemic patients may result, in part, from the ability of these patients eventually to produce low levels of serum antibody to virus as well as from the action of their intact cell-mediated immune system.

Cell-Mediated Immunity

The interactions between sensitized cells of the immune system and viral antigen are commonly termed *cellular* or *cell-mediated immune (CMI) reactions.* Until recently, these reactions were thought to be mediated solely by T lymphocytes, independent of antibody; however, it is now generally accepted that these reactions may be carried out by a variety of cell types, cell factors, or both. Virus-infected cells or virally transformed cells have been shown to activate strong cell-mediated immune responses. For some viral infections, cell-mediated immune reactions may be more important than antibody in early termination of viral infection and prevention of dissemination within the host. Recent evidence shows that cell-mediated immunity functions at the body surfaces, as well as internally. Cell-mediated immune responses to viral infections involve T lymphocytes, antibody-dependent cell-mediated cytotoxicity (ADCC), macrophages, natural killer (NK) cells, and lymphokines and monokines (Figures 69-4 and 69-5).

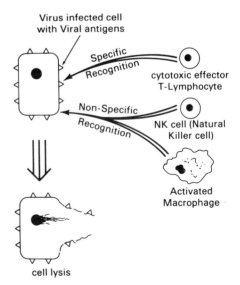

Figure 69-4   Lysis of virus-infected cells by cytotoxic effector cells. Cytotoxic effector cells that can destroy virus-infected cells include cytotoxic T cells, NK cells, and activated macrophages. Cytotoxic T lymphocytes can recognize and destroy virus-infected cells, and this recognition is virus-specific and HLA-restricted. Activated macrophages and NK cells also can recognize virus-infected cells, but this is not virus-specific or HLA-restricted.

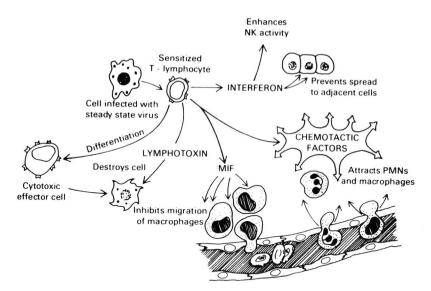

Figure 69-5 Cell-mediated events in steady-state viral infections. Soluble mediators include immune (γ) interferon, chemotactic factors, macrophage migration inhibitory factor (MIF), and lymphotoxin; other lymphokines and monokines are not depicted. Cytotoxic effector lymphocytes, macrophages, and NK cells also may play important roles in this type of infection.

T Lymphocytes

Much evidence indicates the importance of T lymphocytes in recovery from viral infections. Of the many functional subsets of T cells now recognized, those that express cytotoxic activity against virus-infected or transformed cells have aroused the most interest. The generation of virus-specific cytotoxic T lymphocytes (CTLs) is believed to be important in preventing the multiplication of virus (see Figure 69-4). Presumably, the T lymphocytes prevent virus multiplication by destroying infected cells before mature, infectious virus particles can be assembled. This hypothesis assumes that viral antigens appear on the plasma membrane before the release of virus progeny, a view that is substantiated by studies in many, but not all, systems.

The generation of CTLs is mediated by cell-associated antigens. Virus glycoproteins that can be recognized by CTLs not only are synthesized in infected cells, but also can be derived exogenously from the infecting virions whose envelopes fuse with the plasma membrane of the cell during the first stage of viral penetration. Thus, even some noninfectious or inactivated viruses can induce a CTL response.

Upon exposure to virally infected cells, T lymphocytes can differentiate into cytotoxic effector T cells, which can lyse virus-infected or virally transformed cells. These cytotoxic T cells are specific for the infecting virus, but they also exhibit specificity for self major histocompatibility antigens. Thus, these effector cells can lyse virus-infected cells only if such cells also express shared major histocompatibility complex gene products.

Activation of T lymphocytes (CTLs and other T cell populations) may be one of the earliest manifestations of an immune response. T cell activation has been shown to occur as early as 3 to 4 days after initiation of a viral infection. However, T cell responses often decrease rapidly, within 5 to 10 days of elimination of the virus (although virus-specific memory T cells remain for long periods of time). In contrast, antibodies usually become measurable later in the viral infection (after 7 days) and remain at high levels for a much longer time (often for years).

Helper T cells and T cells that mediate delayed type hypersensitivity may be as important as CTLs in the immune response against a virus infection. Helper T cells are required for the generation of CTLs and for optimal antibody production. In addition, helper T cells and T cells that mediate delayed type hypersensitivity and CTLs produce a number of important soluble factors (lymphokines) that can recruit and influence other cellular components of the immune and inflammatory responses.

A number of studies in animals have indicated that impairment of the thymus or T lymphocytes enhances infections by herpes simplex virus, poxviruses, and Sindbis virus, as well as the development of tumors induced by polyoma virus. Since the decrease of resistance to infection by specific impairment of T lymphocytes is incomplete, T lymphocytes probably are only partly responsible for the host defense against these viruses. Impairment of T lymphocytes also has been found to hinder T cell–dependent antibody production, an observation that indicates that cell-mediated immune responses and antibody production both are reduced by T lymphocyte depletion. In humans, impairment of T lymphocytes is associated mainly with increased frequency or severity of poxvirus and herpesvirus infections. Yet, despite the increases observed in the frequency of these infections, they do not develop in most individuals with T cell deficiencies, even though the prevalence of herpesviruses (and many other viruses) is great.

Antibody-Dependent Cell-Mediated Cytotoxicity (ADCC)

Effector cells for ADCC have surface receptors that recognize and bind to the Fc portion of IgG molecules. In this manner, when IgG binds to virus-specified antigens (or any other Ag) on the surface of an infected cell, it becomes a target for effector cells capable of mediating ADCC. Lysis of the virus-associated cell then occurs via attachment of these ADCC effectors to the Fc portion of IgG bound to the infected cell surface antigens. ADCC is a very efficient way of lysing virus-infected cells because it requires 10-fold to 100-fold less antibody than does antibody-complement lysis.

Lymphocytes, macrophages, and neutrophils have been shown to be capable of mediating ADCC against virus-infected cells. The lymphocytes with this ability appear to be heterogeneous. NK cells, as well as null lymphocytes with Fc receptors for IgG, appear to be able to mediate ADCC activity. Accumulating evidence indicates that ADCC of virus-infected cells occurs readily in vitro with very small amounts of antibody. Thus, this mechanism of cytotoxicity may be important in humans in vivo.

Macrophages

Macrophages are important immunospecific and nonspecific mediators against viral infections (for example, herpesvirus infections). Factors that modify their activity in one direction or another have been found to influence the outcome of an infection.

Moreover, since macrophages play key roles in T and B lymphocyte responses, any effects on macrophages also will influence the responses of those cells.

Macrophages confer protection in viral infections either through an intrinsic process, in which infectious virus is disposed of within macrophages acting either as phagocytes or as nonpermissive host cells, or through an extrinsic process, in which macrophages retard or ablate virus multiplication in neighboring cells by destroying the virus-infected cells or by producing soluble factors (interferon) that act on these cells. Phagocytosis of some viruses by macrophages decreases virus levels in body fluids (as during viremia) and thereby impedes virus spread. These effects can be produced only if the virus is destroyed or contained by macrophages. If a virus replicates in macrophages, the infected macrophages may aid in transmission of the virus to other body cells. The permissiveness of macrophages for virus replication may depend on the age and genetic constitution of the host, and the specific condition of the macrophages.

Macrophage activation mediated either by stimulating agents or by soluble factors produced by T cells can result in enhanced phagocytosis and elimination of free virus particles. Another important effector mechanism of activated macrophages is their ability to recognize and destroy virus-infected and virus-transformed cells (see Figure 69-4). In addition, activated macrophages produce interferon and can mediate ADCC against antibody-coated cells that harbor virus.

Natural Killer (NK) Cells

NK cells have been shown to exhibit cytotoxic activity against a number of tumor cell lines, particularly against virus-infected or virus-transformed cells (see Figure 69-4). NK or NKlike cells, which have been found in almost every mammalian species examined and even in some invertebrates, are identified as large granular lymphocytes that possess Fc receptors. NK cells can mediate ADCC activity; their cytotoxic activity is increased by interferon and interleukin 2 (IL2); and they can produce interferon when stimulated with virus or virus-infected cells.

Although NK cells have cytotoxic activity against virus-infected or transformed cells, they show little or no cytotoxic activity against normal cells. Unlike CTLs, NK cells are not HLA-restricted, and they do not exhibit conventional immunologic specificity. There is no conclusive evidence that NK cells play an important role in virus infections of humans, but studies in vitro and in vivo with animal model systems indicate that NK cells are involved in host defenses.

Lymphokines and Monokines

Soluble factors from T lymphocytes (lymphokines) and macrophages (monokines) have been shown to regulate the degree and duration of the immune responses generated by T lymphocytes, B lymphocytes, and macrophages. T cell growth factor (or interleukin 2; IL2) and gamma interferon (IFNγ) are two of the important factors produced by activated T cells. Interleukin 1 (IL1) is a soluble factor produced by macrophages. All three of these factors have been shown to be essential for the full differentiation and proliferation of CTLs. IL2 and IL1 are also important for antibody production by B lymphocytes.

IFNγ differs from IFNα and IFNβ not only in the type of producer cells but also in molecular structure. All interferons, however, can inhibit virus multiplication, increase NK cell activity and ADCC activity, and activate macrophages.

T lymphocytes also produce several other important lymphokines that act in both the immune and the inflammatory responses. Chemotactic factor and migration inhibitory factor (MIF), for example, can call in and retain inflammatory cells. Macrophage-activating factor and IFNγ (may be one substance) can activate macrophages to become cytotoxic toward virus-infected cells and can increase phagocytosis and degradation. Lymphotoxins produced by T cells also may participate in the destruction of virus-infected cells.

Virus-Induced Immunopathology

A host clearly has numerous mechanisms to recognize and eliminate the viruses that it encounters. In the case of viruses that persist in spite of these mechanisms, however, immune responses may become detrimental to the host and cause immunologically mediated disease. Some persistent viral infections of humans produce immunologically mediated disease in which the host sustains injury. When an antigen persists, pathologic changes and diseases result from different types of immunologic interactions, including immediate hypersensitivity; antibody-mediated immune complex syndrome; and tissue damage caused by cell-mediated effector cells and antibody plus complement. Of these mechanisms, the immune complex syndrome during viral infections has been studied most intensively. Two major complications of deposition of immune complexes are vascular damage and nephritis. Some viral infections in which immune complexes have been demonstrated are shown in Table 69-1.

CTLs have also been shown to mediate immunopathologic injury in mice infected acutely with LCMV and ectromelia virus. Both CTLs and T cells responsible for delayed type hypersensitivity have also been implicated in the pathology associated with influenza pneumonia and coxsackievirus myocarditis of mice. A delicate balance between the removal of infected cells that are the source of viral progeny versus injury to vital cells probably exists for T cells as well as for the other host immune components.

An important factor that may impair the function of sensitized T lymphocytes is illustrated by the observation that reaction with antigen or mitogen activates T cells and results in loss of their normal resistance to most viruses. Thus, these activated T lymphocytes develop the capacity to support replication of a large number of viruses, which usually leads to defects in T lymphocyte function.

Roles of Immune Components During Viral Infections

On the basis of the mechanisms described in this and the preceeding chapter, a hypothetical model can be constructed that shows how the immune components defend against viruses (Table 69-2). For a nonimmune and susceptible host, primary infection may be countered initially by the nonspecific defense mechanisms. The early, nonspecific responses consist of interferon, inflammation, fever, phagocytosis, and NK cell activity. If these succeed, infection is prevented or aborted; if not, the virus may be disseminated by local spread, viremia, or nerve spread, and may seed to a number of target organs, thereby producing a generalized infection.

Table 69-1   Viral Infections and Diseases in Which Immune Complexes Have Been Demonstrated

Species	Infection or Disease
Human	Hepatitis B
	Epstein-Barr (EB)
	Dengue hemorrhagic fever
	Subacute sclerosing panencephalitis (measles rubella)
	Multiple sclerosis
Animal	Lactic dehydrogenase
	LCM—infant mouse, adult mouse
	Oncorna viruses
	Aleutian disease
	Equine infectious anemia
	Hog cholera

Table 69-2   Host Effector Functions Important Against Viral Infections

Host Defense	Effector	Target of Effector
Early nonspecific responses	Fever	Virus replication
	Phagocytosis	Virus
	Inflammation	Virus replication
	NK cell activity	Virus-infected cells
	Interferon	Virus replication, immuno-modulation
Cell-mediated immune responses	Cytotoxic T lymphocytes	Virus-infected cells
	Activated macrophages	Virus, virus-infected cells
	Lymphokines	Virus-infected cells, immunomodulation
	Antibody-dependent cell-mediated cytotoxicity (ADCC)	Virus-infected cells
Humoral immune responses	Antibody	Virus-infected cells, virus
	Antibody + complement	Virus, virus-infected cells

The events that lead to the specific immune responses begin almost immediately after exposure and produce antibody- and cell-mediated immunity within 3 to 10 days (which is enough time to terminate viremia and limit the spread of free virus through body fluids). The disseminated antibody response in serum is predominantly IgG (preceded by IgM); the local antibody response in secretions is predominantly secretory IgA (with some IgM). The duration of IgA antibodies in secretions is much shorter (months) than the duration of IgG antibody in serum (years). The role of the IgE immunoglobulins in secretions is unknown, but they may mediate immediate hypersensitivity and amplify the immune response during infection. The antibodies may neutralize virus directly, or they may destroy virus-infected cells by ADCC or complement. Clearly, serum antibody confers protection in generalized infections (for example, measles, poliomyelitis, and hepatitis type A) in which virus must spread through the antibody-containing bloodstream; inoculation of small quantities of antibody into susceptible individuals prevents these viral diseases but may not prevent subclinical infection.

In localized surface infections, protection from infection does not correlate with serum antibody, but it does correlate with local IgA antibody, as has been shown in human studies of viruses restricted to the respiratory tract (for example, respiratory syncytial virus and influenza virus) or to the gastrointestinal tract (as in poliomyelitis). Under some conditions in which serum antibody is present but local IgA is absent, hypersensitivity may occur instead of protective immunity. Also, serum antibody may fail to protect against latent infections such as varicella-zoster and recurrent herpes simplex, because the virus may be shielded by its intracellular location and because cell-mediated immunity may be the more important defense. Antibody also may cause undesirable effects in certain chronic infections. For example, in lymphocytic chorio-meningitis in mice and in leukemia in birds, small amounts of serum antibody complex with virus and deposit in the kidney, thereby inducing immune-complex disease.

Thus, serum antibody seems to be effective in preventing infections of a generalized nature; however, in localized surface infections, the presence of local IgA antibody appears to correlate much better with protection than the presence of circulating IgG antibody. In persistent infections, serum antibody may be responsible for certain long-term sequelae.

Cell-mediated immunity plays an essential role in recovery from, and sometimes in controlling, viral infections, especially those in which oncogenic viruses are involved or in which the virus spreads from cell to contiguous cell. In these situations, antibody cannot reach the virus, but virally induced antigens on the surface of the infected cell can be recognized by different effector cells (see Figure 69-5).

If virus reaches target organs, it is more difficult to control. The host defenses that may play important roles in target organs are inflammation, fever, interferon, and probably cell-mediated immunity.

In some situations, cell-mediated immunity may develop before antibody production begins. For example, cytotoxic effector T cells have been found in bronchial washings 3 to 4 days after initiation of intranasal infection in mice; at this time, antibody cannot yet be detected.

Cell-mediated immune responses can cause tissue damage; the lung lesions produced in influenza may be examples of a result of this process. The lethal effects of LCMV in mice have been shown to be mediated by cytotoxic effector T cells. The rash of many exanthems (such as measles) is thought to represent a cell-mediated attack on virus localized within cells of the dermis and its vasculature.

In summary, a host immune response to virus involves complex interactions between nonspecific factors and cell-mediated and humoral immunity. These interactions vary according to the type of virus and viral spread, the portal of entry, and the immune state of the host. An encounter between the host immune defense system and an invading virus can have one of the following results: the host mounts an effective defense and eliminates the virus; the immune response fails to meet the challenge and the virus becomes persistent, injurious, or both; or the immune response is excessive and produces immunologic injury to the host, thus causing or enhancing the symptoms of the disease.

References

Ada, G.L., Leung, K.-N., Erty, H.: An analysis of effector T cell generation and function in mice exposed to influenza A or Sendai viruses. *Immunol Rev* 1981; 58:5-24.

Baron, S., et al.: Mechanisms of action and pharmacology: The immune and interferon systems. In: *Antiviral agents and viral diseases of man.* Galasso, G., (editor). New York: Raven Press, 1984.

Herberman, R.B., Ortaldo, J.R.: Natural killer cells: Their role in defenses against disease. *Science* 1981; 214:24-30.

Hirsch, R.L., Winkelstein, J.A., Griffin, D.E.: The role of complement in viral infections. III. Activation of the classical and alternative complement pathways by Sindbis virus. *J Immunol* 1980; 124:2507-2510.

Mogensen, L.A.: Role of macrophages in natural resistance to virus infections. *Microbiol Rev* 1979; 43:1-26.

Ogra, P.L., Morag, A., Tiku, M.L.: Humoral immune response to viral infections. In: *Viral immunology and immunopathology.* Notkins, A.L., (editor). New York: Academic Press, 1975.

Oldstone, M.B.A.: Immune responses, immune tolerance and viruses. In: *Comprehensive virology,* Vol. 15. Fraenkel-Conrat, H., Wagner, R.R., (editors). New York: Plenum Press, 1979.

Sissons, J.G.P., Oldstone, M.B.A.: Antibody-mediated destruction of virus-infected cells. *Adv Immunol* 1980; 29:209-260.

70 Persistent Infections

David D. Porter, MD

General Concepts

For many decades, medical practitioners and virologists viewed viral diseases as acute self-limited episodes. Those patients who recovered usually developed life-long immunity to the same disease; in some patients, however, disease recurred (for example, herpes cold sores) or became chronic (as in chronic hepatitis). Investigators gradually recognized that recurrent and chronic disease as well as tumors may be caused by viruses that persist in the host. As more acute viral infections have been controlled by vaccines and other measures, persistent viral infections have become a relatively greater problem.

The continued presence of virus in a host for more than 1 month after primary infection is defined as **persistent infection**. The nomenclature applied to persistent infections in vivo is useful for classification, which is undergoing continuous change as new knowledge of the mechanisms involved becomes available. Table 70-1 presents a classification scheme with characteristics of the principal types of persistent infections in vivo. **Latent infection** is characterized by little or no demonstrable infectious virus between episodes of recurrent disease. **Chronic infection** is characterized by continued presence of virus following recovery from primary infection and may include chronic or recurrent disease. **Slow infection** is characterized by a prolonged incubation period

Table 70-1   Types of Persistent Infection in Humans

Type of Persistent Infection	Characteristics			Virus
	Primary Acute Infection*	State of Persistent Virus	Subsequent Disease	
Latent	Yes†	Noninfectious	Recurrent with reactivated virus	Herpes simplex Varicella-zoster Epstein-Barr Cytomegalovirus
Chronic	Yes†	Usually infectious	Chronic or recurrent	Hepatitis B Cytomegalovirus Subacute sclerosing panencephalitis (measles)
Slow	No	Infectious	Progressive	Kuru Creutzfeldt-Jakob
Integrated (transformation)	Yes‡	Infectious or noninfectious	Tumors	Retrovirus

*Primary acute infection is defined as initial rapid multiplication of virus with or without disease.
†Clinical or subclinical disease.
‡A possible exception is transmission of integrated virus through germ cells.

followed by progressive disease. Unlike latent and chronic infections, slow infection does not begin with an acute primary infection. In **integrated infection,** a DNA copy of the viral genome becomes integrated into the host cell DNA.

Pathogenesis

Persistent infections are caused by a wide variety of viruses and produce many strikingly different diseases. Although the mechanisms by which any of these viruses produce persistent infection are not completely understood, some common factors have been identified.

Mechanisms of Persistence

Many viruses causing persistent infection avoid the nonspecific and immune defenses in several ways. Some viruses, such as herpes simplex, cytomegalovirus, and varicella-zoster, persist in sites (cells of the nervous system and those lining body lumina) that are separated from the immune defenses by physiologic and anatomic barriers. Other viruses (those causing Aleutian disease, equine infectious anemia, and lymphocytic choriomeningitis) may alter the immune response by replicating in cells of the immune system. Diseases produced by these viruses are associated with the production of nonneutralizing antibody, defective cell-mediated immunity, or tolerance. At least two retroviruses (equine infectious anemia and visna-maedi) change antigenically during infection. Kuru and Creutzfeldt-Jakob viruses appear to be nonimmunogenic and may not induce interferon. Persistent lymphocytic choriomeningitis infection of some rodents provides a model of infection in which an immunologically immature (newborn) or immunosuppressed host results in an immunologically tolerated infection or an altered immune response.

Several other mechanisms may contribute to persistence of viruses. Retroviruses can cause an integrated infection, thereby avoiding immune and nonspecific defenses. Some viral mutations (for example, temperature-sensitive mutants) are associated with persistent infections at the nonpermissive body temperature. The production of defective interfering virus particles aids the establishment of persistent infections in vitro and addition of these particles to standard virus may convert a lethal acute reovirus infection in mice into a chronic infection. Further work is required to define the relative importance of various mechanisms in the initiation and maintenance of persistant viral infections in humans and animals.

Reactivation of Persisting Viruses

For disease to recur during a latent infection, multiplication of infectious virus must be reactivated. Some factors associated with reactivation are infection with other viruses (as in herpes simplex cold sores), nerve trauma (herpes facialis following surgery of the trigeminal ganglion), physiologic and physical changes (fever, menstruation, and sunlight), and immunosuppression (as in herpes zoster, cytomegalovirus disease). Papovavirus encephalitis in immunosuppressed patients may represent reactivation of a chronic infection.

Persistent Infections in Cell Culture

Although multiplication of many viruses in cell culture destroys all the cells, in some instances, the cell culture survives in a state of persistent infection. Persistent infection usually occurs in cell culture through one of three ways, which function also in vivo. First, in carrier cultures, only a fraction of the cells are infected (typically with a cytocidal virus) at any one time; multiplication is restricted to a few cells by a limited number of susceptible cells or by the presence of soluble inhibitors such as antibody, interferon,

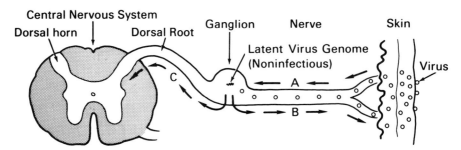

Figure 70-1 Establishment (**A**) and reactivation (**B** and **C**) of latent herpesvirus infections. **A,** Establishment of herpes simplex or varicella-zoster virus latency in ganglia after primary infection of skin or mucosa. **B,** Reactivation of virus in ganglion and spread through nerves to skin or mucosa to cause surface lesions. **C,** Reactivation of virus in ganglion and spread through nerves to central nervous system to cause encephalitis (infrequent).

and nonspecific inhibitors. A probable example is persistent adenovirus infection of the human adenoids. Second, in steady-state infections, essentially all cells in a culture are infected and continuously produce noncytocidal (nonlytic) virus. An example is the continuous production of rubella virus by the cells of congenitally infected infants. Finally, in integrated infection, the virus genome is integrated with the cell DNA, resulting in a persistent infection in which the virus genome is replicated and segregated to daughter cells within the chromosomes (vertical transmission). Examples include retrovirus infections resulting in no disease, slow disease, or tumors (see Chapter 65).

Persistent Infections of Humans

Latent Infections

The most important latent infections are those caused by the herpesviruses, all of which can cause life-long persistent infections. Characteristics of several latent herpesvirus infections appear in Table 70-2.

Herpes simplex virus type 1 commonly infects humans in childhood (see Chapter 88). The primary infection is usually silent. Months to many years after the primary infection, virus may be reactivated; this reactivation leads to formation of vesicles, commonly called cold sores or fever blisters, that appear on the skin of the face, especially at the mucocutaneous junction of the lips. Many stimuli (fever, other infections, physiologic imbalances, and sunlight) are believed to cause reactivation of the virus. Clinically apparent reactivation occurs in less than one-half of individuals harboring the virus; relatively few individuals experience frequent lesions. Recurrent shedding of virus in saliva and tears is not always accompanied by disease. Experimental evidence suggests that the virus resides in sensory ganglia in a latent form between recurrences. The mechanisms (discussed earlier under Pathogenesis) involved in the

Table 70-2   Latent Herpesvirus Infections of Humans

Virus	Usual Site of Primary Disease	Site of Reactivated Disease	Site of Latency
Herpes simplex type 1	Mouth, eye	Mucocutaneous junction and conjunctiva	Trigeminal and autonomic ganglia
Herpes simplex type 2	Genitalia	Genital skin or mucosa	Sacral ganglia
Varicella-zoster	Generalized	Skin in a dermatome* distribution	Sensory spinal ganglia
Epstein-Barr	Generalized (infectious mononucleosis)	Lymphoid tissue	B lymphocytes
Cytomegalovirus	Generally asymptomatic (occasionally mononucleosis and cytomegalic inclusion disease)	Many	Not established

*Area of skin supplied with afferent nerve fibers by a single posterior spinal root.

restriction of virus to a latent state are not definitively established; possibilities include host defenses, impaired virus replication, and integration of virus DNA with the DNA of the cell. Type 2 (genital) strains of herpes simplex virus seem to behave in a similar fashion, except that the primary infections do not often occur until the onset of sexual activity and the site of latency may be the sacral ganglia (Figure 70-1).

Varicella-zoster virus causes chickenpox in children. The virus apparently remains dormant for decades in sensory ganglia and is occasionally reactivated, causing herpes zoster (shingles) with vesicles usually limited to an area of skin innervated by a single sensory ganglion. Although herpes zoster may appear spontaneously, it often is associated with lymphoid neoplasms, irradiation, or the administration of immunosuppressive drugs.

Cytomegalovirus infection of children is usually asymptomatic, and the sites of latency are not established. Reactivation may occur during immune suppression (induced by, for example, neoplasia and drug therapy) or spontaneously. Reactivation may account for virus shedding during pregnancy and lactation.

Epstein-Barr virus infection of children also is usually asymptomatic. The site of latency is thought to be B lymphoid cells. Reactivation has been associated with Burkitt's lymphoma, nasopharyngeal carcinoma, and immunosuppression.

Chronic Infections

A wide variety of chronic viral infections occurs in humans and animals. Table 70-3 lists representative viruses that can cause these infections. (The pathogenic mechanisms are discussed in Chapter 69.)

Rubella virus infection of a mother and fetus during the first trimester of pregnancy may result in congenital defects such as cataracts, deafness, or heart disease in the baby. Some of these babies have the rubella syndrome with virus present in some of the cells of various organs for months to years. The infected cells have reduced growth potential, and clones of these cells eventually appear to die. This process may leave the child's organs with fewer cells than normal, explaining the mental and physical retardation associated with the syndrome.

Table 70-3   Chronic Virus Infections

Virus	Virus Family	Host	Disease
Rubella	Togavirus	Humans	Rubella syndrome (intrauterine infection)
Measles	Paramyxovirus	Humans	Subacute sclerosing panencephalitis
Hepatitis B	Unclassified	Humans	Chronic hepatitis (occasionally)
JC	Papovavirus	Humans	Usually none, progressive multifocal leuko-encephalopathy
Aleutian disease	Parvovirus	Mink	Glomerulonephritis, arteritis
Equine infectious anemia	Retrovirus	Horse	Anemia, glomerulonephritis
Visna-maedi	Retrovirus	Sheep	Demyelinating disease, chronic pneumonia
Lymphocytic choriomeningitis	Arenavirus	Mouse	Glomerulonephritis
Murine leukemia	Retrovirus	Mouse	Often none, glomerulonephritis, leukemia
Avian leukosis	Retrovirus	Chicken	Often none, lymphomas

Subacute sclerosing panencephalitis is a rare consequence of measles infection, occurring several years after recovery from the acute disease. The virus persistently infects many cells of the central nervous system with severe effects and eventual death. Although much virus antigen is present in brain cells, little or no infectious virus is demonstrable and high levels of antibody are present. A defect in expression of M protein (the measles virus inner membrane protein) may occur in subacute sclerosing panencephalitis.

After a clinical or subclinical infection by hepatitis B virus, viral antigen persists in about half the infected individuals; variable amounts of infectious virus appear in the serum for months to years. A few persistently infected individuals develop chronic liver disease, glomerulonephritis, or polyarteritis nodosa, perhaps due to immune complexes.

The primary infection with papovaviruses is usually asymptomatic. Occasionally, in individuals who are immunosuppressed by disease or therapy, papovaviruses related to JC virus infect oligodendroglia in the central nervous system and cause severe demyelinating lesions (progressive multifocal leukoencephalopathy). Current studies are assessing whether viruses also may be involved in other neurologic disorders such as multiple sclerosis. In many individuals, a benign tumor (wart) may be caused by wart (papilloma) papovaviruses.

Slow Infections

Spongiform encephalopathy agents that cause human kuru, human Creutzfeldt-Jakob disease, sheep scrapie, and mink encephalopathy have prolonged incubation periods before the appearance of progressive and fatal central nervous system disease.

Integrated Infections

Some viruses form long-term (life-long in many cases) infections in which the virus genetic information or a DNA copy of it is integrated into the host DNA. Retroviruses are an example of agents forming these types of infections, which may be associated with oncogenic transformation of the host cell (see Chapter 65). These infections may or may not be productive of virions.

Persistent Infections of Animals

A number of chronic viral infections are of economic importance to animal husbandry and may be analogs of important human diseases. These include Aleutian disease, equine infectious anemia, and visna-maedi.

The parvovirus that causes chronic Aleutian disease of mink is naturally temperature-sensitive in its replication. The infection results in extremely high levels of nonneutralizing antibody; deposition of virus-antibody-complement complexes in glomeruli and arteries causes severe disease and death. The host and viral genetic types determine the extent of disease. Some aspects of this disease resemble those of human collagen diseases.

Equine infectious anemia retrovirus causes intermittent attacks of concurrent fever and viremia. Lesions are caused by immune complexes. The virus appears to change antigenically in a single host under the pressure of antibody.

The visna-maedi retrovirus can cause a slowly progressive pneumonia or a demyelinating condition of the central nervous system in affected sheep. A DNA copy of the RNA viral genome appears to be integrated into infected cells. This virus also changes antigenically with time during infection of a single host.

When the lymphocytic choriomeningitis arenavirus infects adult mice, it produces an acute, fatal disease mediated by T cell immunity. If mice are immunosuppressed or infected as immunologically immature newborns, they have life-long (chronic) viremia and viruria. The virus circulates as infectious complexes with antibody; some strains of mice develop severe immune complex glomerulonephritis during the chronic infection. It appears likely that defective interfering virus particles are involved in the persistent infection in vivo. Related arenaviruses (Junin, Machupo, and Lassa fever) also are perpetuated in nature by chronic infection of their rodent hosts. Occasionally, these viruses cause acute and severe infections in humans.

Leukemia and leukosis retroviruses are perpetuated in nature largely by DNA copies of the RNA genome; the DNA copies are integrated into the host cell genome, including the genome of germ cells. Laboratory strains and, rarely, natural strains of these viruses can cause horizontal infection as well. Under most conditions, the infection is silent or, at most, causes a mild immune complex disease. Leukemia, lymphoma, or sarcoma is an uncommon final result, except with laboratory strains of high virulence virus or when certain susceptible inbred lines of hosts are infected. The avian and murine viruses are the best characterized, but similar viruses are widespread in the animal kingdom. In addition, the recently described human T cell leukemia viruses are similar to the other viruses in this group (see Chapter 82).

References

Gajdusek, D.C.: Unconventional viruses and the origin and disappearance of kuru. *Science* 1977; 197:943-960.

Holland, J.J., et al.: Defective interfering RNA viruses and the host-cell response. In: *Comprehensive virology*, Vol. 16. Fraenkel-Conrat, H., Wagner, R.R., (editors). New York: Plenum Press, 1980.

Johnson, R.T.: *Viral infections of the nervous system.* New York: Raven Press, 1982.

Jordan, M.C., et al.: Latent herpesviruses of humans. *Ann Intern Med* 1984; 100:866-880.

Lehmann-Grube, F., et al.: Persistent infection of mice with the lymphocytic choriomeningitis virus. In: *Comprehensive virology*, Vol. 18. Fraenkel-Conrat, H., Wagner, R.R., (editors). New York: Plenum Press, 1983.

Norkin, L.C.: Papovaviral persistent infections. *Microbiol Rev* 1982; 46:384-425.

Porter, D.D., Larsen, A.E., Porter, H.G.: Aleutian disease of mink. *Adv Immunol* 1980; 29:261-286.

Rapp, F.: The challenge of herpesviruses. *Cancer Res* 1984;44:1309-1315.

Stevens, J.G.: Latent characteristics of selected herpesviruses. *Adv Cancer Res* 1978; 26:227-256.

ter Meulen, V., Stephenson, J.R., Kreth, H.W.: Subacute sclerosing panencephalitis. In: *Comprehensive virology*, Vol. 18. Fraenkel-Conrat, H., Wagner, R.R., (editors). New York: Plenum Press, 1983.

Youngner, J.S., Preble, O.T.: Viral persistence: evolution of viral populations. In: *Comprehensive virology*, Vol. 16. Fraenkel-Conrat, H., Wagner, R.R., (editors). New York: Plenum Press, 1980.

71 Epidemiology and Evolution

Frank Fenner, MD

General Concepts

Within the field of virology, pathogenesis (Chapter 67) concerns the behavior of viruses in individuals; epidemiology is the study of the transfer and persistence of viruses in human populations. Epidemiology and evolution are linked because epidemiologic mechanisms of transfer determine the natural selection component of viral evolution. Because survival of a virus depends largely on its ability to circulate among its natural hosts, natural selection tends to favor those viruses with the most efficient mechanisms of transmission. Efficient transmission generally requires an active host who can spread large amounts of virus widely for a sufficiently long time. Thus, as viruses adapt to a host over time, they tend to produce less acute and less lethal diseases. This concept, which will be further examined, is crucial to understanding the epidemiologic pattern of most viral infections. Also, viruses multiply only within cells, so their epidemiology is not complicated by their multiplication in food, water, or soil. This chapter describes the ways in which human viruses survive in nature and cause illness in infected individuals.

For the most part, epidemiology is concerned with viral transfer between physically separate animals of the same or different species. This has been called **horizontal transmission,** to differentiate it from **vertical (congenital) transmission** that may occur through the ovum or across the placenta. Important human congenital infections include rubella and cytomegalovirus. Perinatal transmission, either during the birth process or through mother's milk, also can be regarded as vertical transmission.

Recently recognized in humans and common in other animals, vertical infection is produced by the retroviruses, which cause leukemia in many animals and, perhaps, in humans. In these infections, transfer occurs with the germ plasm, the viral genome being incorporated in the host genome as an integrated DNA copy.

Viruses gain entry to the body via its surfaces. Human disease-causing viruses can survive as infections of other animals (viral zoonoses). The transmissibility of viruses is determined chiefly by excretion, environment, and immunity. The epidemiologic control of viral infections requires knowledge of transmissibility, incubation period, period of communicability, seasonal incidence, and immune status of the population. Viruses undergo genetic changes as a result of evolutionary pressures; for example, new serotypes of respiratory viruses are developing continuously.

Routes of Entry and Exit

The human body presents three large epithelial surfaces to the environment (the skin, the respiratory mucosa, and the alimentary tract) and two lesser surfaces (the eye and the genitourinary tract) (Figure 71-1). To gain entry to the body, viruses must infect cells in one of these surfaces or otherwise breach the surface (by trauma, including arthropod or animal bite) or bypass the surface by congenital transmission. The same considerations apply to the escape of virus from the body.

Infection in the Skin or Oral Mucosa

Intact skin, which protects the body from infection, is frequently breached by **trauma** or by **inoculation** (Table 71-1). The significance of trauma is obvious. Injection by

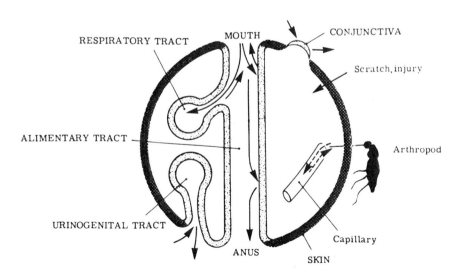

Figure 71-1 Body surfaces as sites of viral infection and shedding. From Mims, C.A.: *The pathogenesis of infectious diseases.* London: Academic Press, Inc., 1976.

Table 71-1   Viruses That Initiate Infection in Humans by Mechanical Penetration of Skin or Mucosa

Route	Family	Virus	Disease Examples
Minor trauma	Papovaviridae	Wart	Warts
	Herpesviridae	Herpes simplex types 1 and 2, Epstein-Barr virus	Oral and genital herpes Mononucleosis
	Poxviridae	Molluscum contagiosum, cowpox, orf, milkers' nodes	
Bite of vertebrate	Herpesviridae	B virus	Ascending myelitis
	Rhabdoviridae	Rabies virus	Rabies
Arthropod bite			
Mechanical	Poxviridae	Tanapoxvirus	Local skin lesion
Propagative (arboviruses)	Togaviridae	Alphaviruses	Eastern and Western equine encephalitis
		Flaviviruses	Yellow fever, dengue
	Bunyaviridae	Bunyaviruses	California encephalitis
	Reoviridae	Orbiviruses	Colorado tick fever
Artificial introduction (injection, inoculation, transplantation)	Herpesviridae	Cytomegalovirus	Cytomegalovirus infection
	Hepadnaviridae	Hepatitis B	Hepatitis B

arthropod bite is important for the large number of viruses that also multiply in arthropods (the **arboviruses,** which include most togaviruses, the *Orbivirus* genus of the reoviruses, and all bunyaviruses except Hantaan virus, the causative agent of Korean hemorrhagic fever and related diseases). All these infections are zoonoses, that is, infection is usually maintained in nature by transfer from one nonhuman animal host to another, and humans are usually infected only occasionally and in a manner irrelevant to the survival of the virus in nature. Dengue and urban yellow fever are partial exceptions in that human-to-human infection is important, but not vital, in ensuring survival of the virus.

The other mode of transmission, artificial inoculation (injection or transfusion), has become prevalent through new practices in medical technology, or social practices such as the parenteral administration of addictive drugs. In Western society, hepatitis B usually is transmitted this way; less often, cytomegalovirus, Epstein-Barr virus, and other viruses may be transferred in this manner. In the past in western society, and still in some parts of the world, hepatitis B was transferred by minor "surgical" procedures like tattooing, dentistry, ear piercing, and even arm-to-arm vaccination. In much of Africa and Asia, perinatal transfer of hepatitis B virus is important because it is relatively common and often produces a persistent infection that may lead to primary hepatocellular carcinoma (see Chapter 90).

In contrast to the many viruses that enter the body through the skin, only a few are shed through it. Smallpox (now an extinct disease) was shed in pharyngeal secretions, but also in the scabs of skin lesions, the virus remaining viable on fomites for weeks. Herpes zoster lesions usually shed little virus, but they are epidemiologically important in that adults shedding virus may initiate chickenpox in susceptible children, thus spanning the human generation gap. Some viruses that infect humans by the respiratory route may be shed from superficial lesions of the oral mucosa.

Infection Through the Respiratory Tract

The respiratory tract is by far the most common route of viral infection in our society. The average adult human samples about 600 L of air hourly; small suspended particles ($< 2 \mu$m diameter) pass down the pharynx and a few reach the alveoli. If they attach to cells of the respiratory tract, viruses in such droplets may initiate infection. Many respiratory viruses are also transferred by contact with contaminated fingers or fomites. Some viruses, commonly grouped as the respiratory viruses, multiply only in the respiratory tract and cause colds, pharyngitis, bronchiolitis, and pneumonia; others produce generalized infections (Table 71-2).

A large variety of viruses is shed from the respiratory tract; indeed, this constitutes the main route of excretion for all the viruses that initiate infection by this route. Herpes simplex and chickenpox are exceptions, because the vesicles on the skin contain virus (although the oropharynx is a more important source of virus), as are rubella and cytomegalovirus, which may be transmitted transplacentally.

Infection Through the Alimentary Tract

Although the large surface of the alimentary tract is potentially exposed to a great number and variety of viruses, it is protected against many of these by the harsh conditions that prevail in the stomach and duodenum. For instance, viruses that have a lipid-containing envelope are readily inactivated by lipid solvents present in the intestine.

Table 71-2   Human Viruses That Initiate Infection of the Respiratory Tract

Producing Local Respiratory Symptoms
Orthomyxoviridae (influenza A and B)
Paramyxoviridae (parainfluenza, respiratory syncytial virus)
Coronaviridae (many serotypes)
Adenoviridae (many serotypes)
Picornaviridae
    Rhinovirus (many serotypes)
    Enterovirus (a few serotypes)

Producing Generalized Disease, Usually Without Initial Respiratory Symptoms

Herpesviridae	Varicella, herpes simplex, cytomegalovirus, Epstein-Barr virus
Poxviridae	Smallpox
Togaviridae	Rubella
Paramyxoviridae	Mumps, measles
Arenaviridae	Lymphocytic choriomeningitis, lassa virus
Bunyaviridae	Korean hemorrhagic fever and related diseases

Therefore, infection of the intestinal tract is initiated by viruses from feces, which are resistant to the acids, bile salts, and enzymes that occur in the gut (Table 71-3). After excretion in feces, these viruses usually are relatively resistant and may thus cause water- and food-borne epidemics.

Infection of the Conjunctiva or Genitourinary Tract

Compared with other routes of entry, the conjunctiva and genitourinary tract are less important. Several kinds of virus occasionally cause conjunctivitis by direct infection (Table 71-4), although when conjunctivitis occurs in generalized diseases such as measles, the virus reaches the eye through the bloodstream. Sexually transmitted viral diseases (herpes simplex type 2, genital warts) have become more prevalent because of changing social mores.

Several viruses are shed in the urine of humans (or, in arenavirus infections, of animals) and may then cause infection by inhalation of infected dust from dried urine.

Table 71-3   Human Viruses That Initiate Infection of the Alimentary Tract

Family	Viruses	Disease Examples
Picornaviridae	Enteroviruses	Most: nil
	Polioviruses	Poliomyelitis
	Hepatitis A	Hepatitis
Reoviridae	Rotaviruses	Diarrhea
Adenoviridae	Several types	Gastroenteritis (rare)
Unclassified (Calcivirus?)	Norwalk agent	Diarrhea

Table 71-4   Viruses That Initiate Infection of the Eye or Genitourinary Tract of Man or Are Excreted in Urine

Infection	Family	Virus	Disease
Ocular	*Adenoviridae*	Human type 8 and several others	Conjunctivitis
	Herpesviridae	Herpes simplex type 1	
	Poxviridae	Accidental vaccinia	
	Picornaviridae	Enterovirus type 70 and coxsackie A24	
	Paramyxoviridae	Newcastle disease	
Venereal	*Herpesviridae*	Herpes simplex type 2, cytomegalovirus	Genital herpes
	Papovaviridae	Wart	Genital warts
	Hepadnaviridae	Hepatitis B	Hepatitis
Excretion in urine (viuria)	*Herpesviridae*	Cytomegalovirus	Various
	Togaviridae	Rubella	Rubella
	Paramyxoviridae	Measles, mumps	Measles, mumps
	Hepadnaviridae	Hepatitis B	Hepatitis

Vertical Transmission

Vertical transmission refers to the transfer of virus from an individual of one generation to its offspring and then to the offspring's progeny, and so on. The most important routes of vertical transmission are via the ovum, across the placenta to the fetus, or to the newborn infant via the mother's milk. Several viruses cross the human placenta and multiply in the fetus; the consequences range from fetal death and abortion (smallpox) through teratogenic effects (rubella), to severe neonatal disease (rubella and cytomegalovirus). Congenital infections may also be asymptomatic.

Cytomegalovirus can be transmitted "vertically," by a different mechanism; virus can spread from a nursing mother to her susceptible infant through her milk. Herpes simplex virus, as well as cytomegalovirus, can be transferred by parents to infants through salivary contamination. Then, because of its long latency and periodic recurrence, the same virus may again be transferred to the next human generation. In small, isolated human populations, zoster-chickenpox may constitute a similar cycle of vertical transmission.

The classical examples of vertical transmission in animals involve lymphocytic choriomeningitis virus of mice and retroviruses: avian leukosis, murine leukemia, and the mammary tumor virus of mice. The retroviruses may be transmitted with the germ plasm, as an integrated DNA copy of the viral RNA genome, and in birds, as infectious virions via the egg.

Viral Zoonoses

A wide range of viruses that can cause human diseases survive in nature as infections of other animals; humans are only occasionally infected, and such infection is usually unimportant for viral survival. These infections are called **zoonoses** (Table 71-5).

Epidemiologic Features of Common Viral Diseases in Humans

Some major epidemiologic features of viral diseases are listed in Table 71-6. Mode of transmission has already been discussed. The control of infections requires knowledge of the incubation period, period of communicability, and seasonal incidence. Not all infections cause disease; inapparent infection (which may nevertheless be responsible for new cases) is the rule with many viruses, especially enteroviruses and some of the herpesviruses. In only a few diseases (smallpox and measles) does virtually every infection of a susceptible individual cause disease.

Humoral immunity greatly affects the behavior of viral infections in human populations, as it does in individuals; the level of immunity in a population is sometimes called **herd immunity.** Generalized viral diseases usually are associated with life-long immunity; therefore, in the absence of an animal reservoir or of recurrent infectivity, these diseases survive only in large populations and die out in small isolated communities. For example, measles and poliomyelitis do not occur as endemic infections in Eskimos and the Pacific island populations.

In superficial infections of the respiratory and alimentary tracts, humoral antibodies are less important than secretory antibodies (IgA), which, however, are effective for a shorter period. Further, the effect of antibody in respiratory and enteric infections often

Table 71-5   Viruses Responsible for Viral Zoonoses

Family	Species	"Reservoir" Host	Mode of Transmission
Poxviridae	Cowpox, milkers' nodes, orf	Cattle, sheep, goats	Contact, through skin abrasions
	Monkeypox	?Monkeys	Contact (?eating)
	Tanapox	?Monkeys	?Mosquitoes
Togaviridae			
Alphavrius	Several species	Birds and mammals	Mosquitoes
Flavivirus	Several species	Birds and mammals	Mosquitoes, ticks, rarely milk
Bunyaviridae	Several species	Birds and mammals	Mosquitoes, Phlebotomus, Culicoides
	Hantaan virus	Rodents	Contact
Reoviridae			
Orbivirus	Several species	Mammals	Mosquitoes, Culicoides, ticks
Rhabdoviridae	Rabies	Canines, felines, bats	Animal bite; respiratory
Orthomyxoviridae	Influenze A	Horse, swine, birds	Respiratory
Paramyxoviridae	Newcastle disease	Birds	Contact through conjunctiva
Arenaviridae	LCM, Machupo, etc.	Rodents	Respiratory

Table 71-6   Epidemiologic Features of Some Common Human Viral Diseases

Disease	Mode of Transmission	Incubation Period* (days)	Period of Communicability†	Incidence of Subclinical Infections‡	Season of Maximum Incidence
Influenza	Respiratory	1-2	Short	Moderate	Winter
Common cold	Respiratory§	1-3	Short	Moderate	Spring, autumn
Bronchiolitis, croup	Respiratory§	3-5	Short	Moderate	Winter
A.R.D. (adenovirus)	Respiratory	5-7	Short	Moderate	Winter
Dengue	Mosquito bite	5-8	Short	Moderate	Summer
Herpes simplex	Salivary	5-8	Long	Moderate	Nil
Enteroviruses diarrhea	Alimentary	6-12	Long	High	Summer
Rotavirus diarrhea	Alimentary	2-4	Moderate	Moderate	Winter
Norwalk diarrhea	Alimentary	2-4	Moderate	Moderate	Nil
Poliomyelitis	Alimentary	5-20	Long	High	Summer
Measles	Respiratory	9-12	Moderate	Low	Spring
Chickenpox	Respiratory	13-17	Moderate	Moderate	Spring
Mumps	Respiratory§	16-20	Moderate	Moderate	Spring
Rubella	Respiratory	17-20	Moderate	Moderate	Spring
Mononucleosis	Salivary	30-50	?Long	High	Nil
Hepatitis A	Alimentary	15-40	Long	High	Summer
Hepatitis B	Inoculation	50-150	Very long	High	Nil
Rabies	Animal bite	30-100	Nil	Nil	Nil
Warts	Contact	50-150	Long	Low	Nil

*Until first appearance of prodromal symptoms. Diagnostic signs, e.g., rash or paralysis, may not appear until 2-4 days later.
†Most viral diseases are highly transmissible for a few days before symptoms appear. Long = >10 days; short = <4 days.
‡High = >90%; low = <10%.
§Also by contact.

is circumvented by the great number of serotypes of most viruses that cause superficial infections.

In conclusion, the main variables that determine the transmissibility of viruses are excretion (manner of excretion, quantity of virus excreted, duration of excretion, and infectivity of the virus excreted); environment (stability of the virus in the environment and the chance of contact with a new host); and immunity (the level of herd immunity among possible hosts). Control of many viral diseases has been achieved by altering some of these variables to prevent viral contact with susceptible hosts. This topic is covered in Chapter 72.

Evolution

For the practicing physician, the evolution of viruses may appear to be an academic matter, because evolutionary changes generally occur over a time scale that is long compared with human life; however, many genetic changes may occur rapidly as a consequence of certain evolutionary pressures. For instance, the highly virulent myxoma virus introduced into Australia to control the wild rabbit population evolved in a few years toward a much more attenuated strain, enabling infected rabbits to survive for weeks instead of days, thereby increasing chances for viral transmission. Also, antigenic variation toward decreased affinity for preexisting neutralizing antibodies may occur among influenza viruses during the course of an individual outbreak. Thus, evolutionary pressures tend to select for viruses of lower virulence, higher transmissibility, lower susceptibility to antibody, and greater ability to persist. Also, the virus's capacity to produce reactions that promote excretion, such as coughing and sneezing in respiratory infections and diarrhea in many enteric infections, is likely to be retained.

Virus diseases may also influence the evolution of their vertebrate hosts through selection or transduction; for example, the highly lethal nature of myxomatosis within a few years selected for rabbits that were genetically more resistant to the disease. It is possible (but not proven) that diseases like smallpox may have exerted a similar effect on humans. Viruses that have a stage in which they are integrated into the host chromosomes may be involved in transduction of genetic material.

Contemporary society seems to be experiencing an explosive development of new serotypes of several kinds of respiratory viruses, because of the evolutionary potential afforded by the unprecedented numbers of individuals in and mobility of the human species. Ongoing evolution allows influenza to remain the most important human viral disease (see Chapter 78). With this disease, genetic reassortment and exchange of viruses between humans and domestic animals (producing **antigenic shift**) provide an important alternative to the process of mutation and selection (**antigenic drift**), which accounts for year-to-year variation in influenza A subtypes. Although the origin of viruses is unknown, proposed hypotheses include retrograde evolution from cellular organisms and disassociation of subcellular genetic components.

References

Evans, A.S., (editor): *Viral infections of humans: Epidemiology and control,* 2nd ed. New York: Plenum Press, 1982.

Mims, C.A.: *The pathogenesis of infectious diseases,* 2nd ed. London, Academic Press, 1982.

White, D.O., Fenner, F.: *Medical Virology,* 3rd ed. New York, Academic Press, 1985.

72 Control

Harry M. Meyer, Jr., MD
Hope E. Hopps
Paul D. Parkman, MD

General Concepts
Immunoprophylaxis
Sanitation and Vector Control
Antiviral Substances
    Chemotherapy
    Interferon and Interferon Inducers

General Concepts

Viral diseases range from the trivial infections to plagues that have altered the course of history. Because of the enormous variations in the viruses themselves, their epidemiology and their pathogenesis, there is no single, magic bullet approach to control. Each virus presents its own set of problems to those seeking solutions. This chapter concerns methods useful to varying degrees in controlling selected viral diseases. The most spectacular progress so far has involved the concept of immunoprophylaxis. Vector control and sanitation have both contributed greatly. Antiviral drugs hold exciting future promise, but, to date, efficacy has been shown in only a few instances.

Immunoprophylaxis

Immunoprophylaxis is a virus-specific approach to control. Protection is achieved by immunization with a vaccine prepared from a virus (**active immunity**) or by inoculation of a serum or globulin preparation containing antibodies against the virus (**passive**

immunity). The viral vaccines available for use in the United States are listed in Table 72-1; available immunoglobulins are listed in Table 72-2. Use of a vaccine generally provides immunity that lasts many months or years; the passive immunity conferred by antibody injection is transient, lasting only weeks. Vaccination evokes an antibody response that is, in turn, a measure of the vaccine's effectiveness in stimulating B lymphocytes. Antiviral antibodies can be classified as IgA, IgM, or IgG and can be measured by various techniques (virus neutralization, hemagglutination-inhibition, complement fixation, hemadsorption-inhibition, precipitation, fluorescence, radioimmunoassay, and ELISA). Some categories of antiviral antibodies (IgA and IgM) are abundant in respiratory and intestinal secretions; others (mainly IgG) are confined primarily to the circulatory system. Vaccines also stimulate T lymphocytes, and the cellular immunity thus induced may also be of consequence in protection. Antiviral antibody assays are now fairly routine laboratory procedures, but measuring cellular immunity in vitro usually requires research laboratory facilities. Fortunately, in spite of the complexities of the immune system, resistance to the vaccine-preventable viral diseases correlates well with the presence of circulating antiviral antibodies, which are easily measured.

Vaccines may be **live** or **killed.** Live vaccines contain viruses that have been attenuated by laboratory manipulation. These modified viruses can infect and immunize

Table 72-1 Viral Vaccines Available for General Use in the United States*

Disease	Live Virus Vaccine	Inactivated Virus Vaccine
Smallpox	Yes	No
Rabies	No	Yes
Yellow Fever	Yes	No
Influenza	No	Yes
Poliomyelitis	Yes	Yes
Measles	Yes	No
Mumps	Yes	No
Rubella	Yes	No

*Certain products are available to special high-risk groups; e.g., laboratory workers can receive smallpox vaccine.

Table 72-2 Commercially Available Products Currently Used for Passive Immunization and Immunotherapy Against Viral Disease

Product	Source	Use
Immune globulin	Pooled human plasma	Modification or prevention of measles; prevention of hepatitis A; immunoglobulin deficiency
Rabies immunoglobulin	Pooled plasma from hyperimmunized donors	Immunotherapy of rabies
Hepatitis B immunoglobulin	Pooled plasma from donors with high antibody titers	Use in accidental needle or oral ingestion exposure to hepatitis B virus
Varicella-zoster (V-Z) immunoglobulin	Pooled plasma from donors with high antibody titers	Use in treatment of V-Z infected immunosuppressed patients

the recipient but are less able to produce disease than their unattenuated counterparts. Killed virus vaccines contain whole virus particles, inactivated by chemical or physical means, or selected antigens of the virion. Although inactivation of infectivity must be complete, the process cannot be excessive if the inactivated vaccine is to retain its immunogenicity.

To develop a live virus vaccine, it is necessary to determine if the virus is genetically stable during replication in the recipient or, if not, to what extent progeny revert to virulence. It is also necessary to study and quantify the virologic events attending recipient immunization. What is the optimum dose? To what degree does the attenuated virus replicate and in what tissues? Is the virus transmissible to contacts? It is important to demonstrate with the killed virus vaccine that the inactivation process extends sufficiently beyond the point of calculated zero infectivity to provide a comfortable margin of safety. Biologic processes have an unfortunate tendency toward inconsistency; to assure safety, the inactivation process must be carefully monitored. Potency is more likely to be a problem with inactivated than with live virus vaccines. Because killed virus does not replicate, the inoculum itself must provide a sufficiently large concentration of viral antigens to induce the desired immune response. Achieving this generally requires 10^8 or more killed virus particles per human dose of inactivated vaccine.

Vaccines share a number of general characteristics and have certain generic problems. Viruses are obligate intracellular parasites; therefore, any virus vaccine contains substances derived from the cells or living tissues used in virus production. Technical advances have improved production methods. One can think of **generations** of vaccines: those prepared in the tissues of an inoculated animal are the first generation (for example, smallpox vaccine from the skin of a calf), products from the inoculation of embryonated eggs are the second generation (inactivated influenza virus vaccine), and tissue culture-propagated vaccines such as poliomyelitis, measles, mumps, and rubella vaccines are third generation. The concept of vaccine generations is important to production methodology, sophistication, and relative purity. The third generation vaccines usually contain the least host protein and other extraneous constituents, but they are the most difficult to produce. The development of recombinant DNA (rDNA) technology may make a fourth generation possible. Such a vaccine for foot-and-mouth disease in cattle is being tested. This new technique may make it possible to produce inactivated vaccines of very high potency.

One vexing problem common to all viral vaccines is their theoretical potential for contamination by extraneous infectious agents indigenous to the cells or tissue-derived nutrients used in vaccine production. Known infectious agents can be excluded by appropriate tests; however, testing for an unknown virus is not possible. Consequently, in several instances, the development of new test technology has allowed recognition of extraneous agents that were previously undetectable. The presence of simian (tumor) virus-40 in the early poliomyelitis vaccines is a notable example.

A few general comments can be made about adverse reactions to vaccines. With live, attenuated virus vaccines, reactions typically mirror some portion of the clinical spectrum of illness caused by the natural disease, as when paralytic complications occur with attenuated polio vaccine administration. Reactions to inactivated virus vaccines also can be caused by the viral components, but the adverse symptoms usually do not mimic the natural disease, and the reaction is more a general response to foreign protein and viral antigens. Typically, local tenderness and inflammation occur at the injection site; systemic reactions commonly are fever, malaise, and myalgia. These reactions occur within the first 48 hours after administration of the inactivated vaccine; disease-mimicking symptoms attributable to a live vaccine inoculation occur after a longer period following many cycles of virus replication. Experience has shown that reactions to live or inactivated viral vaccines rarely can be attributed to mistakes in production; instead, these reactions generally reflect the inherent risk of the product, which is a function of the state of the art at any given time. It is important to keep in mind the difference between illnesses having a temporal association with vaccination and illnesses actually caused by vaccines. Although the reporting of temporal associations is an important first step in looking for causes, the documentation of cause-effect relationships generally requires careful study and statistical analysis.

Effectiveness, like safety, is a key concern with any vaccine. Here the standard for comparison is the immunity conferred by the natural disease. Both epidemiologic and laboratory methods are used to generate comparative data. Vaccine-induced immunity can be defined in terms of three parameters: the percent of recipients protected, the projected duration of protection, and the degree of protection. Most viral vaccines considered effective protect more than 90% of recipients, and with most, the immunity produced appears to be fairly durable; however, vaccines usually do not induce an immunologic response entirely comparable to that seen in the natural disease. Immunity to viral diseases should not be thought of as absolute; vaccinees and persons immune from the natural disease sometimes experience subclinical reinfection if exposed. Thus, evaluating the degree of protection often involves measuring the frequency and extent to which subclinical reinfection can override vaccine-induced resistance.

To develop a new vaccine, researchers must first establish which virus is causing the disease in question; they must then produce the virus in quantity under circumstances acceptable for vaccine preparation. Normally this means growth of virus in cell cultures, embryonated eggs, or the tissue of an experimental animal; however, in experimental hepatitis type B vaccines, viral antigens are harvested and purified directly from the plasma of human carriers. Finding an acceptable production system can be a real problem, especially in developing inactivated viral vaccines, because a high concentration of antigen is needed. For example, the principal barrier to developing a hepatitis type A vaccine has been lack of a good production system. Production of specific viral proteins using rDNA procedures may provide a solution to many of these problems. A final consideration is the clinical importance of the virus. Normally a virus must cause a disease of some severity and be capable of affecting a substantial proportion of the population before consideration is given to developing a vaccine. For example, coxsackie group B viruses can produce severe, sometimes fatal, disease, but they do so rarely. Thus, although developing a vaccine for any of the several group B serotypes is technically feasible, no one has proposed doing so.

In the United States, experimental vaccine or globulin preparations must be tested in clinical trials of gradually increasing size until the product can be shown to be safe and effective for its recommended use in disease prevention. The law requires these trials to be performed under the Investigational New Drug (IND) provisions of the Food, Drug and Cosmetic Act. When the trials have been satisfactorily completed, the products are licensed by the Food and Drug Administration for commercial distribution and general use.

Sanitation and Vector Control

Several early approaches to viral control deserve recognition, even though they are less dramatic than vaccination. One can be described as the **avoidance of viral exposure.** This approach is more complex than it might seem because avoidance can have many ramifications. Hospital practices directed at preventing the exposure of immunosuppressed patients to varicella and other life-threatening infections is avoidance. Blood bank testing for hepatitis B surface antigen is avoidance. A careful review of the medical history of potential donors of tissues and organs for transplantation is avoidance. Countless other examples of this approach exist.

The control of extrahuman reservoirs of viruses is another old but worthwhile approach. Unfortunately, few opportunities exist for practical application. The most notable successful use was the elimination of rabies in some countries through removal of stray dogs and quarantine of incoming pets. The control of animal reservoirs of rabies continues to be valuable in countries where the virus cannot be eradicated because of its entrenchment in sylvan reservoirs such as foxes, raccoons, skunks, and bats.

Another approach of enormous contemporary as well as historical importance is vector control; transmission of viral disease by the bite of an arthropod vector was first demonstrated by Walter Reed and his associates with their discovery that yellow fever was transmitted by mosquitoes. At the turn of the century, yellow fever was a disease of major consequence in the Americas and Africa. Immediately applying Reed's discovery, Gorgas mounted the anti-*Aedes aegypti* campaign in Havana that marked the beginning of the conquest of epidemic yellow fever. In dealing with the arthropod-borne diseases such as St. Louis encephalitis, any procedure that reduces vector populations or limits arthropod access to humans has potential value. These procedures include draining swamps, applying insecticide, screening homes, and using insect repellant or protective clothing.

The last of the older approaches is to improve sanitation. This method is applicable in a limited way to those diseases whose epidemiology involves fecal–oral transmission. The well-known link between the discharge of raw sewage into tidal waters, shellfish contamination, and type A hepatitis is an example of a situation readily reversible by improved sanitary practices.

Antiviral Substances

Chemotherapy

A newer and completely different approach to the control of viral diseases is chemotherapy. Since the early 1950s, many investigators have sought synthetic and natural substances, similar to antibiotics, that would inhibit viral multiplication. Indeed, many initially promising compounds have been found, but few offer general usefulness; most substances that significantly inhibit viruses are unacceptably toxic to host cells.

The use of antiviral compounds is beset by a variety of complex problems. The intimate involvement of virus replication with cellular functions makes it difficult to arrest virus replication chemically without harming normal host cell functions. Timing related to diagnosis and treatment is also a problem. To identify a virus as the causative agent of an illness is not always a simple matter. By the time an exact diagnosis is made, it may be too late for effective chemotherapy if the viral infection is well established and tissue damage extensive.

Despite these difficulties, some chemotherapy has been successful. Table 72-3 shows the antiviral drugs that have been proved effective in clinical trials and have been approved for clinical use.

It is unlikely that antiviral drugs will have general prophylactic use. They may someday be shown to be helpful when a high attack rate can be predicted with some confidence, as in developing pandemics of influenza, epidemics of arbovirus disease, and adenovirus infections of military recruits. Another application is after a clear high-risk exposure, as from the bite of a rabid dog or inadvertent virus inoculation by needle in the hospital or laboratory.

Finally, some viral diseases fall into the category of **persistent** (slow, latent, and chronic) infections. These allow time to establish the specific viral diagnosis before instituting chemotherapy. In fact, recurrent ocular infections with herpes simplex virus as well as herpes encephalitis have been treated successfully. Varicella-zoster and cytomegalovirus syndromes are under study. Subacute sclerosing panencephalitis, Creutzfeldt-Jakob disease, progressive multiple leukoencephalopathy, and other persistent virus diseases appear to be ideal candidates for future therapeutic trials as new antiviral compounds are developed.

Interferon and Interferon Inducers

Since the mid-1930s, scientists have recognized that under certain circumstances one virus can interfere with another. In 1957, Isaacs and Lindenman made a dramatic discovery that explained the mechanism of resistance. They found that virus-infected cells can elaborate a protein substance called interferon that, when added to normal cells in culture, protects them from viral infection. Other microbial agents (such as rickettsia and bacteria) and natural and synthetic polynucleotides were later shown to induce interferon. Subsequent research established that interferons are a group of substances

Table 72-3   Antiviral Drugs Approved for General Use in the United States

Drug	Active Against	Main Mechanism of Action	Clinical Use	Administration
Acycloguanisone (Acyclovir)	DNA viruses	Inhibits DNA polymerase	Herpes simplex, types I and II in immunocompromised adults and children; herpes genitalis in nonimmuno-compromised patients	Intravenous
Iododeoxyuridine	DNA viruses	Incorporates into replicating DNA	Herpes keratitis	Topical
Adenine arabinoside	DNA viruses	Inhibits viral DNA polymerase	Herpes encephalitis	Systemic
Amantadine	Influenza A	Inhibits viral uncoating	Prophylaxis or treatment of influenza A	Systemic
Trifluorothymidine	DNA viruses	Unknown	Herpes keratitis	Topical

that tend to have species specificity (mouse cell interferon protects mouse cells and not human cells) and are inhibitory to numerous viruses. In fact, interferon may be useful in inhibiting tumor cell growth as well as in restricting viral replication (see Chapter 68).

Quantities of human interferon sufficient for experimental studies have been produced in leukocytes (buffy coat cultures), fibroblast cell cultures, Epstein-Barr virus-transformed lymphoblasts, and more recently in bacteria through genetic engineering. Interferon has been used in preliminary clinical trials with some degree of success in preventing respiratory virus infections and in treating chronic progressive hepatitis type B. In the past several years, new techniques for improving interferon yields are making it possible to explore the full range of its prophylactic and therapeutic uses. Future studies also are likely to demonstrate diseases for which interferon is effective, thus bringing this newest approach to viral control into routine use.

References

Baron, S., Dianzani, F., Stanton, G.J., (editors): The interferon system: A current review to 1978. *Texas Rep Biol Med* 1982; 41:1-715.

Baron, S.: The interferon system. *ASM News* 1979; 75:358-366.

Downs, W.G.: Arboviruses. In: *Viral infections of humans: epidemiology and control.* Evans, A.S., (editor). New York and London: Plenum Medical Book Co, 1976.

Galasso, G.J.: An assessment of antiviral drugs for the management of infectious diseases in humans. *Antiviral Res* 1981; 1:73-96.

Galasso, G.J., Merigan, T.C., Buchanan, R.A., (editors): *Antiviral agents and viral diseases of man.* New York: Raven Press, 1984.

Krugman, S., Katz, S.L., (editors): Viral hepatitis. In: *Infectious diseases of children,* 7th ed. St. Louis: the C.V. Mosby Co, 1981.

Lennette, E.H., Schmidt, J.J., (editors): *Diagnostic procedures for viral and rickettsial infections,* 5th ed. Washington, D.C.: American Public Health Association, 1979.

Meyer, H.M., Jr, Hopps, H.E., Parkman, P.D.: Appraisal and reappraisal of viral vaccines. In: *Advances in internal medicine.* Stollerman, G.H., (editor). Chicago and London: Year Book Medical Publishers, Inc., 1980.

Shope, R.E.: Rabies. In *Viral infections of humans. Epidemiology and control.* Evans, A.S., (editor). New York and London: Plenum Medical Book Co., 1976.

Yelverton, E., et al: Rabies virus glycoprotein analogs: Biosynthesis in *Escherichia coli. Science* 1983; 219:614-620.

73 Picornaviruses

Sidney Kibrick, MD, PhD

C = 32
20-30nm

1 +

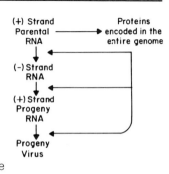

(+) Strand
Parental
RNA

Proteins
encoded in the
entire genome

(-) Strand
RNA

(+) Strand
Progeny
RNA

Progeny
Virus

The diagrams of the virion morphology and the multiplication scheme are derived from Chapters 62 and 63, respectively. The multiplication scheme applies only generally as indicated in Chapter 63.

General Concepts

The picornaviruses are small (20-30 nm), naked (nonenveloped), ether-resistant (no essential lipids), single-stranded RNA viruses with cubic symmetry. They replicate in the cytoplasm, have four structural polypeptides, and are stabilized against thermal inactivation by molar $MgCl_2$. They are divided into two subgroups that affect humans: the **enteroviruses,** found primarily in the gut; and the **rhinoviruses,** found in the upper respiratory tract.

The enteroviruses, which share common nucleotide sequences, are further subdivided into **polioviruses, coxsackieviruses** groups A and B, and **echoviruses,** formerly known as orphan viruses. Initially 67 distinct enterovirus immunotypes were recognized, but reclassifications have reduced this number to 63. Over 100 distinct rhinovirus serotypes have now been identified (Figure 73-1).

Differences between the coxsackie and echoviruses have proved to be less distinct than initially believed. As a result, new enteroviruses, discovered since 1969, have been designated only as enterovirus types, beginning with type 68. Four such serotypes, enterovirus types 68-71, have now been recognized. The coxsackie and echovirus designations and type numbers have been retained, however, for those agents classified before 1969.

No picornavirus group-specific antigen exists. Some serotypes in each subgroup, however, share complement-fixing antigens with other members of that subgroup. Certain coxsackie and echoviruses also have complement-fixing antigens in common. Identification of picornavirus serotypes is based on neutralization tests, which are specific.

The picornaviruses are relatively stable agents. They are resistant to lipid solvents and alcohol, can be preserved for years by freezing, and may survive for long periods in the presence of organic matter such as sewage. They are, however, inactivated by

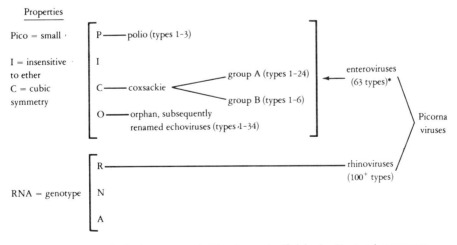

* Coxsackie virus A23 and echoviruses 8, 10, and 24 have been reclassified, leaving 63 enterovirus serotypes.

Figure 73-1 Etymology of "Picornaviruses."

pasteurization, boiling, formalin, and chlorine. The enteroviruses are resistant to gastric acidity and bile, and they are relatively stable at acid pH (3.0-5.0). By contrast, the rhinoviruses, which are found primarily in the nose and throat, are acid-labile at this pH range.

Subclinical infections with the picornaviruses are common. These agents also can cause various disorders, ranging from minor illness, respiratory infections, and skin rashes to myocarditis, pericarditis, aseptic meningitis, and paralytic disease.

POLIOVIRUSES

Distinctive Properties

The three poliovirus types are 1, 2, and 3. They share some complement-fixing antigens but are antigenically distinct in neutralization tests. Strains of each type may vary considerably in virulence. Humans are the only host in nature (Figure 73-2), although various primates and cultures of primate cells also are susceptible.

The events in poliovirus replication are similar to those in the replication of all enteroviruses. The virus attaches to specific receptor sites on the susceptible cell. In humans, these receptor sites are controlled by a gene on chromosome 19. After attachment, the virus penetrates and is uncoated. Replication occurs in the cytoplasm.

In the body, poliovirus adsorbs only to cells of the central nervous system (primarily motor neurons) and to the cells that line the intestinal tract. Other human and primate cells develop the ability to adsorb this virus only after being cultured in vitro, which results in unmasking of the receptors.

Poliovirus RNA consists of a single positive strand RNA molecule of about 7000 nucleotides, mol. wt. 2.5×10^6 daltons. It codes for four viral capsid proteins (VP1-VP4), one viral noncapsid protein (VPg), and the nonvirion proteins.

Pathogenesis

Poliovirus infection may be restricted to the intestine, may spread systemically without reaching the central nervous system, or spread systemically and reach the central nervous system. When restricted to the intestine, the infection usually is asymptomatic; when systemic, the infection may cause a mild febrile illness; when it reaches the central nervous system, the infection is symptomatic and may cause paralysis (paralytic poliomyelitis).

The virus enters through the mouth; primary replication takes place in the oropharynx and intestinal mucosa (**alimentary phase**). Virus is regularly present in the throat and feces before the onset of illness. It disappears from the throat in about 1 week, but persists in the feces for several weeks or more. Virus spreads from the oropharynx and enteric tract to the tonsils and Peyer's patches of the ilium, and from these sites to deep cervical and mesenteric nodes (**lymphatic phase**). Subsequently, further spread occurs into the blood (**viremic phase**), with additional viral multiplication in certain viscera and lymph nodes. In most cases, no further spread of virus occurs, and a subclinical infection or a minor illness results.

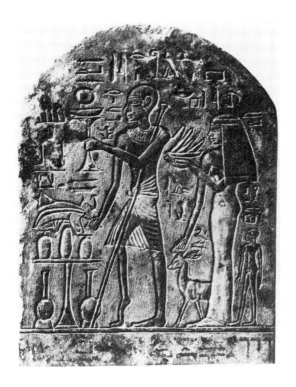

Figure 73-2 XVIIIth dynasty stele (1580–1350 B.C.) showing young man who is leaning on staff and has a withered leg characteristic of polio that was incorrectly attributed to drunkenness and trauma. From Lyons, A.S., Petracelli, R.J.: *Medicine, an illustrated history.* New York: Harry M. Abrams, Inc, 1978.

Occasionally, virus is disseminated during viremia to the spinal cord or brain stem or both (**neurologic phase**), where it attacks and destroys the anterior horn and other motor nerve cells. If only scattered nerve cells are destroyed, the patient may develop no visible sign of muscle weakness. More concentrated damage results in paralytic disease, characterized by a flaccid paralysis of muscles innervated by the affected motor nerves (Figure 73-2). Virus may also reach the central nervous system by progressing along peripheral nerves. The incubation period for minor illness is about 3-5 days, and for central nervous system involvement is about 1-2 weeks.

Clinical syndromes associated with poliovirus infection are summarized in Table 73-1. Most poliovirus infections (90%-95%) are subclinical. An additional 4%-8% are manifested by minor illness, with fever, sore throat, and headache. Nonparalytic poliomyelitis occurs in about 1% of infections. This clinical entity may be initiated by minor illness and is characterized by central nervous system involvement with fever, stiff neck, and pain and tenderness in the back and muscles. Examination of the cerebrospinal fluid reveals an increased cell count with early predominance of neutrophils, followed by a shift to mononuclear cells, elevated protein, and normal glucose levels.

Paralytic disease is uncommon, occurring in only about 0.1% of cases; about 5%-10% of these represent bulbar poliomyelitis. Paralytic disease is called **spinal** if weakness is limited to muscles innervated by motor neurons in the cord; it is called **bulbar** if the cranial nerve nuclei or medullary centers are affected. Bulbar disease is

Table 73-1   Clinical Syndromes Associated with Enteroviruses*

Clinical Syndrome	Polioviruses	Coxsackieviruses Group A	Coxsackieviruses Group B	Echoviruses
Nonspecific febrile illness	+	+	+	+
Aseptic meningitis	+	+	+	+
Paralytic and encephalitic disease	+	±	±	±
Acute respiratory disease		+	+	+
Exanthematous disease		+	+	+
Herpangina		+		
Hand, foot, and mouth disease		+		
Acute lymphonodular pharyngitis		Type 10		
Pleurodynia		±	+	±
Pericarditis, myocarditis		±	+	±
Neonatal myocarditis		±	+	
Enteritis				±
Acute hemorrhagic conjunctivitis		Enterovirus type 70 Coxsackievirus A24		

*+, commonly implicated, multiple serotypes; ±, occasionally implicated, multiple serotypes.

especially severe because it may result in swallowing dysfunction or in cardiac or respiratory failure.

Various factors that influence the severity of poliovirus infection include the virulence of the infecting virus strain, the size of the infecting dose, and the antibody status of the host. Factors predisposing to paralytic or bulbar disease include recent or previous tonsillectomy, fatigue, recent irritating inoculations (for example, diphtheria-pertussis-tetanus (DPT) immunizations), and pregnancy.

The characteristic lesions in poliomyelitis result from virus localization in motor neurons. The areas most commonly affected are the anterior horn cells of the spinal cord, the motor area of the cerebral cortex, and the motor nuclei of the medulla. The lesions reveal neuronal necrosis, neuronophagia, and loss of nerve cells. Areas of neuronal damage also show leukocytic infiltration and perivascular cuffing. In addition, a round-cell infiltrate usually is present in the leptomeninges.

Host Defenses

Poliovirus multiplication induces interferon production in infected cells shortly after infection, inhibiting synthesis of new virus. Interferon has no effect on extracellular virus. It is probably most effective as an antiviral agent early in infection when viral titers are low.

Infection with the polioviruses induces protective IgA antibodies in the enteric tract and saliva, as well as circulating neutralizing antibodies. Both IgA and circulating antibodies provide long-lasting protection against reinfection with the same virus types. The IgA antibodies decrease viral replication in the gut, as well as the oral and fecal excretion of virus; the circulating antibodies prevent viremic spread of these agents to the central nervous system. Both antibodies act by combining with extracellular virus to form virus–antibody complexes, which are then eliminated by excretion or phagocytosis.

Epidemiology

Poliomyelitis is a worldwide disease. In temperate zones, it is most prevalent in the summer and fall. Infected individuals carry the virus in their throat for about 1 week and in their feces for several weeks or more, beginning 3–5 days after exposure. Spread of the infection occurs mainly through the fecal-oral route, most commonly by feces to fingers to mouth. Some spread also occurs by the pharyngeal-oropharyngeal and, possibly, the respiratory route.

Dissemination of poliovirus to close associates is rapid. By the time a patient becomes ill, almost all other susceptible family members have been infected. Outbreaks have been traced to contamination of water supplies by sewage. Although flies and cockroaches are capable of contaminating food, their role in spreading this infection is uncertain.

In areas of poor sanitation, most infants are infected relatively early in life while still protected by maternal antibodies; they develop active immunity and, as a result, constitute a pool of immune individuals as they grow older. With improving sanitation, however, infants may escape such early contact with the polioviruses and thus may become the pool of susceptible individuals needed for an outbreak of this disease.

Diagnosis

Nonparalytic poliomyelitis cannot be distinguished clinically from aseptic meningitis caused by other agents. Poliomyelitis should be suspected in patients with aseptic meningitis accompanied by a flaccid paralysis, in ill associates and contacts of such patients, and in unimmunized patients who develop aseptic meningitis. Poliomyelitis should especially be considered when the infection is known to be present in the community.

Diagnosis may be confirmed by recovering virus from the throat or feces in cultures of human or primate cells and identifying it by neutralizing tests in tissue culture. Unlike the other enteroviruses, the polioviruses rarely can be isolated from the cerebrospinal fluid.

Serologic tests on paired sera have limited value because antibody levels may already have risen by the time the patient becomes ill and a significant increase in antibodies (fourfold or greater) is no longer demonstrable. Complement fixation tests may be helpful in demonstrating an antibody rise, however, because complement-fixing antibodies develop later than neutralizing antibodies. Neutralizing antibodies persist for years, perhaps for life. Complement-fixing antibodies decrease over a period of months; after 6 months to 1 year, they may be present only in low titer or even absent.

Control

Two types of vaccine are available: a trivalent, formalin-inactivated poliovirus vaccine given parenterally (**Salk vaccine**) and an attenuated trivalent poliovirus vaccine given orally (**Sabin vaccine**). With widespread use of these vaccines, poliomyelitis has been virtually eliminated from the United States, dropping from an average of 21,000 paralytic cases per year in 1951–1955 to about 20 such cases per year at present.

Inactivated vaccine consists of the three poliovirus serotypes, grown in monkey renal cell culture and made noninfectious by formalin treatment. The vaccine is given as a series of intramuscular injections at monthly intervals with periodic boosters to maintain adequate antibody levels. Its effectiveness depends on the stimulation of circulating antibodies that block spread of these viruses through the blood to the central nervous system. This vaccine also has some suppressive effect on viral multiplication in the pharynx but no effect on viral replication in the gut.

Trivalent oral vaccine consists of the three poliovirus serotypes, which are grown in monkey or human cell cultures using living, attenuated strains of virus. This vaccine possesses numerous advantages over the inactivated vaccine for protecting the individual and the community from paralytic disease. It stimulates natural infection, inducing neutralizing antibodies in the blood and IgA antibodies in the gut. In addition, it is administered easily and immunity is achieved quickly. Thus, trivalent oral vaccine has potential for eradicating the disease and controlling spread of epidemics by limiting intestinal dissemination of wild virus. Antibodies resulting from oral vaccine are long lasting, reducing the need for regular booster doses required with inactivated vaccine. Some spread of vaccine virus to contacts may occur, resulting in their immunization as well.

The chief disadvantage of the oral vaccine is the rare occurrence of vaccine-associated paralytic disease in persons receiving the vaccine or in their contacts. The risk of this occurrence, which is most common among adults, is less than one per several million doses.

Immunization programs are directed primarily at infants and young children because this population is the most susceptible and thus most responsible for spreading wild polioviruses.

Immunoglobulin contains poliovirus-neutralizing antibodies and, if given before the infection is acquired, it prevents spread of virus to the central nervous system; however, it does not prevent the initial infection. It is of no value after onset of clinical symptoms.

Treatment for poliomyelitis at present consists of supportive care and prompt attention to complications. After the acute stage, appropriate rehabilitative measures should be instituted.

COXSACKIEVIRUSES

Distinctive Properties

The coxsackieviruses were discovered in 1948 during attempts to use suckling mice to isolate polioviruses from feces of patients diagnosed clinically as having poliomyelitis. Because the patients whose feces first yielded these agents lived in Coxsackie, New York, the agents were named the coxsackieviruses.

Further use of suckling mice for attempted virus isolations in various disorders revealed a large number of coxsackieviruses, which are characterized by pathogenicity for suckling mice and other common properties. These viruses were subsequently divided into two groups, A and B, on the basis of the two differing types of pathology they induce in suckling mice. Group A viruses produce an extensive myositis in the skeletal muscles, resulting in a flaccid paralysis. Group B viruses produce focal muscle lesions, necrosis of the fat pads, and focal lesions in the brain and cord, often with spastic paralysis. Visceral lesions are also present occasionally.

Twenty-three coxsackie A serotypes (A1–A22 and A24) and six coxsackie B serotypes (B1–B6) are recognized (coxsackie A23 has been been dropped because it is identical with echovirus type 9). Neutralization tests reveal these agents to be antigenically distinct; that is, the neutralizing antibodies are type-specific. The group B viruses and coxsackie A9 share a common complement-fixing antigen. No common antigen exists for the coxsackie A viruses, although several are antigenically related. A number of the coxsackieviruses have been shown to hemagglutinate human or monkey erythrocytes.

Humans are the only natural host for these agents. Both group A and B viruses can be isolated and propagated in suckling mice. The group B viruses and some of the group A serotypes also can be propagated in appropriate human or monkey renal cell cultures.

The coxsackieviruses produce a variety of disorders in humans, including: respiratory disease; herpangina; hand, foot, and mouth disease; febrile rashes; pleurodynia; pericarditis; myocarditis; aseptic meningitis; and paralytic disease. Coxsackie B viruses are among the most commonly known viral causes of heart disease in humans.

Pathogenesis

The events during infection with these agents are believed to resemble those of other enteroviruses. The viruses enter the oropharynx and multiply, primarily in the pharynx and small intestine. They are found in the throat for several days early in the infection, and in the feces for 2 weeks or more. Virus is widely disseminated to various organs during viremia. Clinical manifestations may then become apparent, usually within 1 week of infection. Host response to these agents varies and covers a wide spectrum of disease, ranging from trivial to severe, based on such factors as properties of the infecting virus strain and variations in host susceptibility. As with other enteroviruses, inapparent infections are common. Not all of these agents have yet been shown to cause disease in humans. The clinical syndromes associated with coxsackievirus infection are shown in Table 73-1.

Nonspecific Febrile Illnesses

Acute febrile illnesses without distinctive features occur in the summer or fall. Both group A and B coxsackieviruses can cause this syndrome.

Acute Respiratory Disease

Numerous coxsackieviruses can induce illness manifested as the common cold. These viruses also have been etiologically implicated less frequently in various other respiratory syndromes, ranging from pharyngitis and croup to pneumonia.

Herpangina

Herpangina is caused chiefly by group A coxsackieviruses. At least nine serotypes have been implicated. Onset is acute, with fever, sore throat, vomiting, and, less frequently, abdominal pain and headache. Its distinctive feature is the presence of small (1-2 mm), scattered oropharyngeal vesicles with red areolae, most commonly in the posterior oropharynx. These progress quickly to shallow ulcers and usually are gone within 3-5 days.

Acute Lymphonodular Pharyngitis

Acute lymphonodular pharyngitis has been associated only with coxsackie A10 to date; it resembles herpangina. The lesions, however, are solid, white-to-yellow papules rather than vesicles. They develop simultaneously and resolve without ulceration in about 1 week.

Hand, Foot, and Mouth Disease

Several coxsackie A virus types, especially A16, are responsible for hand, foot, and mouth disease. Characteristic features include fever, an oral vesicular enanthema, and a sparse, symmetric, maculopapular eruption that involves the hands, feet, and occasionally other sites, and may progress to vesicles.

Exanthematous Disease

Coxsackievirus infection may be manifested by fever and rash, a condition known as exanthematous or summer rash disease. The rashes vary in type and extent, but are most commonly maculopapular. They generally begin on the face and descend to the trunk. Occasionally, they are accompanied by an oral enanthema or by aseptic meningitis. Exanthematous disease, most common in infants and children, has been often mistaken for rubella.

Aseptic Meningitis

Aseptic meningitis is a self-limited syndrome that may result from infection with a large number of agents, including the enteroviruses. Clinical features of aseptic meningitis caused by coxsackieviruses are not distinctive. Onset may be characterized by fever, headache, nausea, vomiting, and, in children, abdominal pain. A few days later, signs of meningeal irritation develop, including stiff neck and back. Cerebrospinal fluid examination reveals a pleocytosis, usually of less than 500 cells per cubic millimeter; mononuclear cells predominate, glucose level is normal; and protein levels are normal to elevated.

Paralytic and Encephalitic Disease

Illness clinically indistinguishable from paralytic or bulbar poliomyelitis or from encephalitis or other causes of cerebral dysfunction may infrequently result from infection with coxsackievirus and other nonpolio enteroviruses. These viruses should be suspected when such illness occurs in patients adequately immunized against the polioviruses.

Pleurodynia

Pleurodynia (epidemic myalgia or Bornholm disease) is an acute disease, resulting primarily from infection with group B coxsackieviruses. Onset usually is abrupt with fever, headache, and stabbing pain in the muscles of the chest or upper abdomen or both. The pain, which is intensified by respiration and movement, may persist for days to weeks. Relapses, with recurrences of fever and other symptoms, are common. Occasional complications include pleuritis, orchitis, pericarditis, and myocarditis.

Pericarditis and Myocarditis

Group B coxsackieviruses are an important cause of pericarditis and myocarditis in older children and adults. Pericarditis generally predominates. Common findings include fever, tachycardia, dyspnea, precordial pain, and occasionally pericardial friction rub. Electrocardiography and radiography are helpful in confirming these diagnoses. The prognosis for patients with pericarditis is generally good; however, this condition is more serious when myocarditis is also present.

Neonatal Myocarditis

Infection with coxsackie B viruses in the first month of life may result in severe, frequently fatal disease, characterized by myocarditis and involvement of various other organs, especially the central nervous system and liver. Onset may be abrupt, with lethargy, feeding difficulties, and often fever. Signs of cardiac or respiratory distress may follow; death may occur within days, or the infant may recover over the next few weeks. These infections generally are acquired from an infected mother or during a nursery outbreak.

Little is known about the pathology of human coxsackievirus infection, because very few patients succumb. Autopsies of neonates with fatal, generalized coxsackie B infection show focal myocarditis and inflammation. Additional findings, in order of decreasing incidence, include meningoencephalitis, hepatitis, and pancreatitis. Fatal myocarditis in older persons also is associated with focal necrosis. Patients with aseptic meningitis generally recover. Fatal cases of encephalomyelitis caused by coxsackieviruses and other enteroviruses show involvement of motor neurons in the brain stem and spinal cord. With group B coxsackieviruses, both white and gray matter may be affected.

Host Defenses

Infection with the coxsackieviruses induces bodily responses similar to those noted with poliovirus and the other enteroviruses. The first antibodies to appear are IgA. They appear in the saliva and secretions of the small intestine, and limit further viral replication and extension from these sites. In serum, the earliest antibodies, IgM, are replaced by neutralizing IgG antibodies at about 2 weeks. These prevent spread of virus through the bloodstream and provide type-specific, long-lasting immunity against the infecting agent. In addition, interferon, induced by viral multiplication, probably also plays a role by helping to limit virus replication at the target organs.

Epidemiology

The epidemiology of the coxsackieviruses is similar to that of the polioviruses and other enteroviruses. In temperate zones, peak incidence occurs in summer and fall. Young children compose the bulk of the susceptible population, and they are chiefly responsible for viral dissemination. Transmission occurs primarily by direct contact with infected individuals, usually by the fecal–oral route, but oral and respiratory spread also occur. Commonly, more than one member of a family is affected; often each person presents different clinical features. Because of their epidemiologic similarities, enteroviruses frequently occur together in nature. Occasionally, several such agents may be present in a single host at the same time.

Diagnosis

The coxsackieviruses induce a variety of clinical syndromes, many of which also may be caused by other agents. As a result, an accurate diagnosis based solely on clinical findings often cannot be made. Certain of these syndromes, however, such as herpangina; hand, foot, and mouth disease; pleurodynia; pericarditis; and myocarditis neonatorum have distinctive features that strongly implicate coxsackievirus. The presence of coxsackieviruses or their manifestations among family members or associates of the patient provides further support for diagnosis.

In patients with clinical features consistent with coxsackievirus infection, the diagnosis often can be confirmed by isolating virus from the throat or feces, identifying it in neutralizing tests with specific antisera, and demonstrating a fourfold or greater specific antibody response between acute and convalescent sera. Because subclinical infections with these agents are common, throat or fecal isolation of a virus may not always indicate that it is responsible for the patient's illness. More definitive evidence of etiology is provided by recovery of virus from parenteral sites of pathology (for example, from cerebrospinal fluid in aseptic meningitis, vesicle fluid in exanthematous disease, or pericardial fluid in pericarditis).

Coxsackie group B and some of the group A viruses can be readily isolated in rhesus renal tissue or other susceptible tissue culture systems, where they produce cytopathogenic effects characteristic of enteroviruses. All of the coxsackieviruses can be isolated in newborn or suckling mice.

Diagnosis by serologic tests alone is impractical, because so many antigenic types of virus exist; serologic tests are valuable, however, in confirming a diagnosis made by viral isolation. Neutralizing antibodies are type-specific and persist for years. Complement-fixing antibodies decrease with time and may be difficult to detect after 1 year.

Control

There is no vaccine to prevent coxsackievirus infections and no specific therapy to treat diseases induced by these agents. Treatment is entirely symptomatic and supportive.

ECHOVIRUSES

Distinctive Properties

Echoviruses are enteroviruses that have been grouped together because they produce cytopathogenic effects in cultures of various primate cells; unlike the coxsackieviruses, echoviruses generally produce no disease in suckling mice. In addition, they differ immunologically from the polioviruses.

The echoviruses were discovered through use of tissue culture in attempts to isolate polioviruses from feces. At first named **orphan viruses** because their relationship to disease was obscure, they were subsequently renamed **echoviruses** to describe their origin and behavior (*e*nteric *c*ytopathogenic *h*uman *o*rphan viruses). Although 34 distinct echovirus serotypes (types 1–34) were recognized initially, echo 8 was found to be identical to echo 1, echo 10 was reclassified as a reovirus, and echo 28 became rhinovirus type 1, leaving a total of 31 echovirus serotypes (see Figure 73-1).

No common group antigen exists for the echoviruses. Cross-reactions are demonstrable by complement fixation, however, between certain of these agents and other enteroviruses. Neutralization tests are type-specific and form the basis for classification into serotypes. A number of echoviruses can agglutinate human erythrocytes and, during infection, stimulate production of antihemagglutinins.

The echoviruses, like the coxsackieviruses, also have been associated with various disorders including respiratory illness, febrile illness (with or without rash), aseptic meningitis, and paralytic disease.

Pathogenesis

Infection with the echoviruses is believed to follow the same pattern as that with the other enteroviruses. Initial viral replication takes place in the epithelial cells and lymphoid tissue of the pharynx and of the small intestine. The agents are found in the throat for several days early in the infection and in the feces for 2 weeks or more, coinciding with the period of disease communicability. Virus is disseminated to various organs through viremia, giving rise to a variety of generally nonspecific, often overlapping syndromes indistinguishable from those caused by other enteroviruses. The incubation period is usually less than 1 week. Inapparent infections are common. As with the coxsackieviruses, the role of many of these agents in human disease remains to be determined. The clinical symptoms associated with echovirus infection are shown in Table 73-1.

Nonspecific Febrile Illnesses

Nonspecific febrile illnesses are clinically indistinguishable from those caused by various other agents, including enteroviruses.

Acute Respiratory Disease

Echoviruses, like coxsackieviruses, have been implicated in a variety of respiratory syndromes, ranging from the common cold to croup and pneumonia. Like other enteroviruses, they are not a major cause of such illness.

Exanthematous Disease

The echoviruses are an important cause of outbreaks and sporadic cases of exanthematous, or summer rash, disease. Occurring most commonly in young children, these rashes are generally maculopapular and are occasionally accompanied by an enanthema or aseptic meningitis. Rashes associated with other enteroviruses are so similar in appearance that they cannot be distinguished clinically, especially in sporadic cases. With several of the echoviruses, certain features may be helpful in establishing a diagnosis. A maculopapular eruption, occasionally with petechiae, which begins on the face, descends to the trunk, and clears last from the face suggests echo 9 virus, especially when it occurs in outbreaks. The rash seen with echo 16 virus is also known as Boston exanthem because it was first described there. The illness resembles roseola infantum in that the rash usually appears when the fever subsides.

Aseptic Meningitis

Echovirus-induced aseptic meningitis cannot be differentiated from such illness caused by other enteroviruses and additional agents. The echoviruses, however, are the commonest cause of this syndrome in temperate zones during the summer and fall.

Paralytic and Encephalitic Disease

Occasionally, muscle weakness may occur during aseptic meningitis caused by echoviruses, but permanent paralysis is rare. Infrequently, encephalitis and cerebellar ataxia may be seen.

Enteritis

Some evidence implicates certain echoviruses in enteritis, especially in young infants. Enteroviruses, however, are not an important cause of such illness.

Little is known about the pathology of echovirus infections because these agents generally produce nonlethal disease. In fatal cases with central nervous system involvement, the pathologic findings have resembled those in poliomyelitis.

Host Defenses

The body's responses to echovirus infection are similar to those described for other enteroviruses (see page 810).

Epidemiology

The epidemiology of the echoviruses is like that of the other enteroviruses. These agents are highly infectious by the fecal-oral route and spread rapidly to close contacts.

Diagnosis

Although an echovirus infection may be suspected from clinical and epidemiologic findings, laboratory confirmation usually is necessary because of the nonspecific syndromes produced by these agents. Laboratory support for such a diagnosis is provided by isolation of an echovirus from throat washings or feces or both, followed by demonstration of a fourfold or greater antibody response to this agent during the illness. Virus isolation from a parenteral source such as cerebrospinal fluid in a patient with aseptic meningitis is the most significant diagnostic finding. Human or monkey renal cell cultures are susceptible to these agents and are often used for such studies. As with the coxsackieviruses, serologic tests alone are of limited value for diagnosis in the absence of viral isolates.

Control

No vaccines are available to prevent echovirus infections. Treatment of disease is symptomatic and supportive.

NEW ENTEROVIRUS TYPES

All four of the new enterovirus types (68-71) are cytopathogenic for cultures of monkey renal cells. Enterovirus 68 has been associated with upper and lower respiratory tract disease in children; enterovirus 70 has been associated with outbreaks of acute hemorrhagic conjunctivitis; and enterovirus 71 with meningitis and encephalitis. Enterovirus 69 was recovered from an asymptomatic infection and has not yet been implicated in disease.

RHINOVIRUSES

Distinctive Properties

The rhinoviruses are picornaviruses that differ from the enteroviruses by their lability at acid pH (3.0-5.0). They are transient inhabitants of the human nose and pharynx. The usual laboratory animals, including newborn mice, are not susceptible. Cell cultures of choice to isolate these agents include various human embryonic tissues such as kidney and lung; some rhinoviruses, however, can be isolated only in organ cultures of human ciliated respiratory tissue. Optimal growth for these viruses is at 33 C, which is similar to the temperature in the nose.

No rhinovirus group antigen has been reported. Neutralizing antibodies are type-specific. More than 100 serotypes have now been identified by neutralization tests in cultures of susceptible cells.

Pathogenesis

Infection occurs through the nasopharynx or conjunctiva, chiefly by direct contact with infected secretions but also by droplets. The virus localizes and replicates in the nasopharynx, especially on the nasal mucosa, inducing inflammation and edema. Following an incubation period of several days, the patient may develop signs and symptoms of the common cold. Virus shedding begins several days after infection, peaks shortly after onset of symptoms, and may persist for a week or more. Virus is not generally present in the feces. Inapparent infections occur but are less frequent than with the enteroviruses.

Clinical syndromes associated with the rhinoviruses are shown in Table 73-1. The chief characteristic of the common cold is a prominent, profuse, nasal discharge, initially watery but subsequently mucopurulent and associated with nasal obstruction. Cough also may be present. Complications include bacterial sinusitis and otitis media. Illness may last 1-2 weeks. Fever and pharyngeal exudate usually are absent. These agents may rarely produce lower respiratory tract disease of variable severity.

Pathologic findings in the common cold consist of inflammatory changes with hyperemia, edema, and leukocyte inflammation in the ciliated columnar epithelial cells lining the nasopharynx. Desquamation of these infected cells coincides with peak virus spreading. Regeneration is completed within a few weeks.

Host Defenses

Susceptibility or resistance to rhinoviruses is influenced by the previous immunologic experience of the host. Infection stimulates production of specific IgA antibodies in nasal secretions and IgG antibodies in the blood. The IgA antibodies prevent or modify reinfection with the same virus type. The IgG antibodies are a transudate from serum IgG and also appear in nasal secretions but in relatively low titer. These IgG antibodies provide an additional defense against reinfection; however, reinfections with the same virus type may still occur. Reinfections are believed to be influenced by the levels of specific antibody in the nasal secretions.

Interferon has been found in the respiratory secretions of volunteers infected with rhinoviruses. Because recovery from colds occurs before antibodies to these agents appear, it is likely that interferon plays a role.

Gastric acidity generally prevents extension of these acid-labile agents into the gut. Normal body temperature (37 C) also helps to limit spread of the rhinoviruses; their optimal growth occurs at 33 C.

Epidemiology

Perpetuation of rhinoviruses requires continued person-to-person transmission because humans are the only reservoir in nature. The agents are most commonly spread by children. Inapparent infections occur in about one-third of cases and are associated with virus shedding. In the United States, the average person has two to four colds yearly, each generally caused by a different serotype. The peak incidence of such infections occurs in the fall and spring.

Diagnosis

Diagnosis of the common cold usually is based on clinical findings, because specific laboratory diagnosis is neither practical nor generally available. Nasal washings provide the best source for virus isolation, but throat washings and nasopharyngeal swabs are satisfactory. Virus is most readily recovered in the first few days of illness. Cell cultures of human embryonic kidney or lung are used. Diagnosis by examining paired sera for a neutralizing antibody response is impractical because of the large number of rhinovirus serotypes.

Control

No vaccine exists to prevent rhinovirus disorders, and development of an effective vaccine is unlikely because of the many rhinoviral serotypes and the transitory immunity that follows rhinoviral infection. Injections of experimental vaccines, moreover, indicate that serum antibody responses to these agents are not necessarily associated with significant titers of IgA, which appear to be most important for protection.

In one study, topical interferon repeatedly administered nasally before rhinovirus challenge reduced the incidence of colds. The frequency of these infections and the scarcity of interferon, however, make such prophylaxis impractical at present.

Treatment of rhinovirus infections consists of symptomatic relief and supportive care. Secondary bacterial infections are treated with antibiotics specific to the infecting organisms.

References

Bodian, D., and Horstmann, D.M.: Polioviruses. In: *Viral and rickettsial infections of man,* Horsfall, F.L. Jr., Tamm, I., (editors). Philadelphia: J.B. Lippincott Co., 1965.

Gwaltney, J.M., Jr.: Rhinoviruses. In: *Viral infections of humans: Epidemiology and control,* 2nd ed. Evans, A.S., (editor). New York: Plenum Press, 1982.

Jackson, G.G., Muldoon, R.L.: Viruses causing common respiratory infections in man. I. Rhinoviruses. *J Infect Dis* 1973; 127:328-355.

Krugman, S., Ward, R., Katz, S.L.: Enteroviral infections. In: *Infectious diseases of children,* 8th ed. Krugman, S., (editor). St. Louis: The C.V. Mosby Co., 1985.

Melnick, J.L.: Enteroviruses. In: *Viral infections of humans: Epidemiology and control,* 2nd ed. Evans, A.S., (editor). New York: Plenum Press, 1982.

74 Togaviruses

Philip K. Russell, MD

Philip K. Russell, MD

Envelope

1 +

Icosahedral
40-90nm

General Concepts
ALPHAVIRUSES
Distinctive Properties
Pathogenesis
Host Defenses
Diagnosis
Epidemiology
Control

FLAVIVIRUSES
Distinctive Properties
Pathogenesis
Host Defenses
Diagnosis
Epidemiology
Control

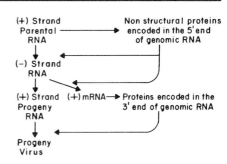

General Concepts

Togaviridae are enveloped RNA viruses containing infectious single-stranded RNA. They are small (40-70 nm) spherical viruses with nucleocapsids having cubic symmetry. The family Togaviridae has four recognized genera. The two largest genera, *Alphavirus* and *Flavivirus,* are described in this chapter; the genus *Rubivirus* is discussed in Chapter 76. The genus *Pestivirus* has no members pathogenic for humans. All alphaviruses and flaviviruses that cause disease in humans are arthropod-borne viruses (arboviruses). In an earlier classification scheme based on antigenic relationships, alphaviruses and flaviviruses were termed group A and group B arboviruses, respectively.

Most togaviruses survive in nature by alternate cycles of replication in a vertebrate host and a hematophagous arthropod (mosquitoes or, with some flaviviruses, ticks). Arthropod vectors acquire the virus infection by biting a viremic host and, after an extrinsic incubation period during which the virus replicates in the vector's tissues, they

---

The diagrams of the virion morphology and the multiplication scheme are derived from Chapters 62 and 63, respectively. The multiplication scheme applies only generally as indicated in Chapter 63.

transmit virus through salivary secretions to another verebrate host. Virus replicates in the vertebrate host, causing viremia and, rarely, illness.

The ability to infect and replicate in both vertebrate and arthropod cells is an essential quality of alphaviruses and flaviviruses. The principal vertebrate hosts for most togaviruses are various species of wild mammals or birds; the natural zoonotic cycles that maintain the virus do not usually involve humans. A few togaviruses, however, can be transmitted in a human-mosquito-human cycle; yellow fever, dengue types 1, 2, 3, and 4, and chikungunya virus have this property. As a result of being pathogenic for humans and capable of transmission in heavily populated areas, these viruses can cause widespread and serious epidemics. Because of their high transmission potential, these viruses are major public health problems in many tropical and subtropical regions of the world where appropriate mosquito vectors are present.

At least 20 alphaviruses and 59 flaviviruses have been recognized. They vary widely in their basic ecology; each virus occupies a distinct ecologic niche, often with restricted geographic and biologic distribution. Approximately 25 of the togaviruses are medically important human pathogens. As shown in Table 74-1, togaviruses can cause various syndromes, ranging from benign febrile illnesses to severe systemic diseases with hemorrhagic manifestations or major organ involvement. The neurotropic alphaviruses and flaviviruses can produce severe destructive central nervous system disease with serious sequelae. Several alphaviruses (chikungunya, Mayaro, and Ross River) cause painful arthritis that persists for weeks or months after the initial acute febrile illness. Yellow fever virus has unique hepatotropic properties that cause a clinically and pathologically distinct form of hepatitis with a hemorrhagic diathesis. The dengue viruses, which cause more human illness than all other members of their genus, may produce a serious, sometimes fatal, immunopathologic disease in which shock and hemorrhage occur.

Some of these agents are dangerous human pathogens and are highly infectious, thus requiring special containment and safety precautions in the laboratory.

ALPHAVIRUSES

Distinctive Properties

Virions of the alphaviruses consist of a nucleoprotein capsid enclosed in a lipid envelope. The RNA is a single 42S positive sense strand of approximately 4×10^6 daltons and is capped and polyadenylated. Virion RNA can function intracellularly as mRNA. The single capsid protein (C protein) has a molecular weight of approximately 30,000 daltons. The alphavirus envelope consists of a lipid bilayer derived from the host cell plasma membrane and two glycoproteins (called E_1 and E_2) of 48,000–52,000 daltons. A small third protein (E_3) of 10,000 daltons is present in some alphaviruses such as Semliki Forest virus. The only proteins in the envelope of alphavirus are the viral glycoproteins that are anchored in the lipid at the hydrophobic C-terminal end.

The known important antigenic determinants of alphaviruses are on the virion proteins. The capsid protein induces antibodies that are widely cross-reactive within the genus by complement fixation and fluorescent antibody tests. Anticapsid antibodies do not neutralize infectivity or inhibit hemagglutination. Unlike myxoviruses, the hemag-

Table 74-1   Principal Medically Important Togaviruses

Virus	Clinical Syndrome	Principal Vector(s)	Hosts	Distribution
Alphaviruses				
Chikungunya	Febrile illness, rash, arthritis	*Aedes Aegypti, Aedes* sp.	Primates, humans	Africa, India, Southeast Asia
Mayaro	Febrile illness, rash, arthritis	*Haemagogus* sp.	Primates	South America, Trinidad
O'nyong-nyong	Febrile illness, rash, arthritis	*Anopheles* sp.	Primates	Africa
Ross River	Febrile illness, rash, arthritis	*Culex* sp.	Mammals, humans	Australia, Pacific
Eastern equine encephalitis	Encephalitis	Culiseta melanura, *Aedes* sp.	Birds	Americas
Western equine encephalitis	Encephalitis	*Culex tarsalis, Culex* sp., Culiseta melanura	Birds	North America
Venezuelan equine encephalitis	Febrile illness, encephalitis	*Culex* sp., *Aedes* sp., *Mansonia* sp.	Rodents, horses	Americas
Sindbis*	Febrile illness	*Culex* sp.	Birds	Africa, Asia
Semliki Forest*	Encephalitis	*Aedes* sp.	Birds	Africa
Flaviviruses				
Dengue (four types)	Febrile illness, rash, hemorrhagic fever, shock syndrome	*A. aegypti, Aedes* sp.	Humans	Tropics, worldwide
Yellow fever	Hemorrhagic fever, hepatitis	*A. aegypti, Aedes* sp., *Haemagogus* sp., *Sabethes* sp.	Primates, humans	Africa, South America
St. Louis encephalitis	Encephalitis	*C. tarsalis, C. pipiens*	Birds	Americas
Japanese B encephalitis	Encephalitis	*Culex* sp.	Birds, pigs	India, China, Japan, Southeast Asia
Murray Valley encephalitis	Encephalitis	*Culex* sp.	Birds	Australia
West Nile	Febrile illness	*Culex* sp.	Birds	Africa, Middle East, Europe
Rocio	Encephalitis	Unknown	?Birds	South America
Tick-borne encephalitis	Encephalitis	*Ixodes* sp., *Dermacentor* sp.	Rodents	Europe, Asia
Omsk hemorrhagic fever	Hemorrhagic fever	*Dermacentor* sp.	Muskrats	Siberia
Kyasanur Forest disease	Hemorrhagic fever	*Haemaphysalis* sp.	Primates, rodents	India
Powassan	Encephalitis	*Ixodes* sp., *Dermacentor* sp.	Rodents	North America

*Sindbis and Semliki Forest viruses are not epidemiologically important human pathogens. They are included because of the extensive virologic research studies done with these agents. Both can cause human disease, and wild strains can be hazardous.

glutinin and the receptor for cells are not the same among all togaviruses. Therefore, antibodies to the hemagglutinin do not necessarily have neutralizing activity. The E_1 glycoprotein is involved in hemagglutination; antibodies to E_1 inhibit hemagglutination and cross-react to varying degrees with other viruses in the genus. The E_2 glycoprotein contains determinants that induce neutralizing antibodies. The virus neutralization reaction is specific, and virus species or serotypes are defined principally on the basis of neutralization tests.

Alphaviruses enter susceptible cells by a poorly understood but highly efficient mechanism, probably pinocytosis. Viral replication occurs in the cytoplasm. Initial translation of virion (42S) positive strand RNA produces high-molecular-weight translation products that are proteolytically cleaved into an RNA polymerase and structural proteins. Positive virion RNA is transcribed to negative strand RNA that is either transcribed to 45S positive mRNA or virion RNA. Transcription of the virion RNA through a negative strand RNA intermediate produces a 26S positive strand mRNA that contains the code for only the structural proteins, as well as additional 42S mRNA, which is incorporated into progeny virions. Translation from the 26S mRNA produces a polyprotein that is cleaved proteolytically into three proteins: C, PE_2, and E_1; PE_2 is subsequently cleaved into E_2 and E_3. Envelope proteins formed by posttranslational cleavage are glycosylated and inserted into the plasma membrane. Virion formation occurs by budding of preformed 12-14 nm nucleocapsids through regions of the plasma membrane containing E_1 and E_2 glycoproteins.

The multiplication of this virus group is depicted on the first page of the chapter and described in detail in Chapter 63.

Pathogenesis

Pathogenesis of human illness caused by alphaviruses is exemplified by three different agents that produce markedly different disease patterns. Chikungunya virus causes an acute (3-7 day) febrile illness with malaise, arthralgias, a rash, and occasionally arthritis. Mayaro, O'nyong-nyong, and Ross River viruses, which are closely related to Chikungunya virus, cause similar or identical clinical manifestations. Virus introduced by the bite of an infected mosquito replicates and causes a viremia with concomitant fever and generalized malaise; the site of virus replication is unknown. The viremia subsides in 3-5 days, and antiviral antibody appears in the blood. A macular-papular rash occurs, usually from the third to fifth days. Arthritis involving mainly the large joints occurs most commonly in adults; involved joints are red, swollen, and tender, and effusions may occur. Joint symptoms may last for weeks after the acute illness.

The pathogenesis of eastern equine encephalitis and western equine encephalitis virus infection of humans (as well as equines) similary involves percutaneous introduction of virus by a vector and development of viremia; however, in eastern and western equine infections, the viremia phase often is asymptomatic and the infection may resolve without serious manifestations of disease. In some instances, however, central nervous system invasion by the virus results in viral replication in neural tissues, which produces cytolysis, inflammation, and clinical manifestations of encephalitis or encephalomyelitis. The encephalitis may be severe, with high fever, delirium, and coma progressing to death. Convulsions, motor dysfunction, and paralysis are common. Histopathologic findings are similar to those of most other acute viral encephalitis and include inflammatory cell infiltrate, perivascular cuffing, and neuronal degeneration; all regions of the brain may be affected.

Venezuelan equine encephalitis virus infections of humans cause acute febrile illnesses, often with a superimposed central nervous system component; in the Venezuelan form the systemic manifestations are often pronounced, whereas the central nervous system disease usually is less severe than in eastern and western equine encephalitis. Venezuelan equine encephalitis infection can cause severe, sometimes fatal, systemic disease with shock and coma. The fulminant disease is thought to involve a lytic effect on lymphocytes by the virus.

Host Defenses

Alphaviruses are efficient inducers of interferon, the production of which undoubtedly plays a role in modulating or resolving the infection. Alphavirus infections usually resolve soon after antiviral antibody appears in the blood if central nervous system invasion does not occur. Antiviral antibody has been experimentally shown to play a role in suppressing an established infection, possibly in conjunction with antibody-dependent cellular cytotoxic effects on infected cells. The role of cell-mediated immunity in alphavirus infections is not well defined, but is probably significantly involved in the resolution of the infection. Protection from infection (homologous protective immunity) is related to circulation of virus-neutralizing antibody in serum.

Diagnosis

Diagnosis of alphavirus infections depends on epidemiologic knowledge, clinical suspicion, and laboratory confirmation. Infection by one of the viruses of the chikungunya-mayaro complex may be difficult to distinguish from many clinically similar illnesses such as rubella, dengue, sandfly fever, enterovirus infection, and scrub typhus; virologic or serologic diagnosis is essential. Encephalitis from one of the alphaviruses must be suspected on epidemiologic grounds and distinguished from other viral encephalitides by laboratory tests. Diagnosis of an alphavirus can be established by isolating virus from the blood during the viremic phase or by antibody determination. A variety of serologic tests, including complement-fixation, hemagglutination-inhibition, and virus neutralization, are used by public health laboratories to diagnose alphavirus infections.

Epidemiology

The two alphaviruses important in the United States are eastern and western equine encephalitis. Both are maintained in natural ecologic cycles involving birds and, principally, bird-feeding mosquitoes. Eastern equine encephalitis is enzootic in fresh water swamps in the eastern United States; it causes sporadic equine and rare human cases; small human outbreaks may occur. Western equine encephalitis virus is widespread in the United States and has been responsible for outbreaks of equine and human disease in western and southwestern states. Its principal vector, *Culex tarsalis*, is a common mosquito, especially in irrigated regions.

Eight or more subtypes of Venezuelan equine encephalitis virus exist and have differing virulence and epidemic potential. Endemic subtypes of relatively low equine virulence exist in South and Central America and Florida. Endemic strains are ecologically restricted to a small-mammal-mosquito cycle and cause only occasional human cases. Epidemic strains of Venezuelan equine encephalitis, however, may spread by an equine-mosquito cycle involving several mosquito species; in this manner, these strains have caused massive equine epizootics with associated human epidemics. A recent epizootic involved several Central American countries and spread through Mexico to Texas.

Chikungunya virus exists in Africa in a forest cycle involving baboons and other primates and forest species of mosquitoes. It can also be transmitted in a human-mosquito-human cycle by *Aedes aegypti;* by this mode of transmission, it has caused massive epidemics in Africa, India, and Southeast Asia. The virus is endemic throughout much of South and Southeast Asia. The antigenically similar Mayaro virus exists in the Amazon basin; its cycle involves new world primates and hemagogic mosquitoes and causes outbreaks of human disease through exposure to the forest cycle. Ross River virus is endemic in Australia and has spread in epidemic form to several islands of the Western Pacific.

Control

Control of alphavirus diseases in the United States is based on surveillance of disease and of virologic activity in natural hosts and, when necessary, on control measures directed at reducing populations of vector mosquitoes. The latter include larval and adult control, sometimes using ultra low volume aerial spray techniques. In some areas, insecticide resistance (for example, resistant *C tarsalis*) is a major limitation. Experimental inactivated vaccines are used to protect laboratory workers from eastern, western, and Venezuelan encephalitis. An effective live attenuated Venezuelan equine encephalitis vaccine is in use to protect laboratory workers and has been used extensively in equines as an epidemic control measure. Experimental vaccines for Chikungunya are being developed.

FLAVIVIRUSES

Distinctive Properties

Flavivirus virions are 48–55 nm in diameter and, like alphaviruses, consist of a nucleoprotein capsid enclosed in a lipid envelope. The RNA is a single 40S positive sense strand and is capped at the 5′ end but, unlike alphaviruses, has no poly A segment at the 3′ end. The virion has a single capsid or core protein (V-2) with a molecular weight of approximately 14,000 daltons. The envelope consists of a lipid bilayer, a single envelope glycoprotein (V-3) of 51,000–59,000 daltons, and a small nonglycosylated protein (V-1) of approximately 8000 daltons. Whether V-1 is exposed on the external surface of the membrane is uncertain.

The mechanism by which flaviviruses enter cells has not been determined but is probably pinocytosis. Unlike alphaviruses, which can replicate in enucleated cells, the flaviviruses probably require the presence of the cell nucleus for replication. Transcription produces a genome-size mRNA that appears identical to virion RNA. No high-molecular-weight precursor proteins have been identified in flavivirus-infected cells. Translation produces the three virion proteins and at least five (possibly eight or nine) nonstructural proteins. Molecular weights of the nonstructural proteins are approximately 5000–85,000 daltons. No specific functions have been ascribed with certainty to the nonstructural proteins, although one or more of the high-molecular-weight nonstructural proteins probably has RNA polymerase activity. The mechanism of protein translation is poorly understood, but it may involve the rapid cleavage of polyprotein, short-lived, low-molecular-weight RNAs, or multiple initiation sites on the 42S mRNA.

Virion formation occurs in the cytoplasm in association with the endoplasmic reticulum. Virions appear within cytoplasmic vacuoles and are released from the cell through exocytosis of the vacuoles. The morphogenesis of flaviviruses is completely dissimilar to that of alphaviruses; no evidence of budding has been seen in flavivirus-infected cells. The mechanism of virion assembly remains obscure. Flavivirus replication times are relatively long, and virus yields from in vitro cultures are usually low. Flavivirus infection does not effectively suppress host cell protein synthesis as in alphavirus infections. The replication of flaviviruses produces, in addition to infectious virions, a noninfectious subvirion particle approximately 14 nm in diameter called slow-sedimenting hemagglutinin; this small particle contains envelope proteins but no capsid protein or RNA.

All flaviviruses are antigenically related by sharing common or similar antigenic determinants. The V-2 (capsid) protein contains genus-specific antigenic determinants. The single envelope glycoprotein, V-3, is the viral hemagglutinin; antibodies against V-3 are involved in virus neutralization and hemagglutination inhibition. The antigenic determinants that induce neutralizing antibody are specific, and the serotypes or species of flaviviruses are distinguished principally by neutralization tests. Hemagglutination-inhibition tests reveal a broad range of cross-reactions among the flaviviruses. Monoclonal antibody studies reveal genus, group, and virus-specific epitopes on the envelope glycoprotein. The nonstructural proteins also are antigenic and are antigenically distinct from the virion proteins. At least one nonstructural protein, NV-3, contains virus-specific and cross-reactive antigenic determinants.

Pathogenesis

Flaviviruses vary widely in their pathogenic potential and mechanisms for producing human disease. Three examples are discussed here: St. Louis encephalitis, yellow fever, and dengue.

Human St. Louis encephalitis virus infections are initiated by deposition of virus in the skin through the saliva of an infected mosquito. Virus replicates locally and in regional lymph nodes and causes viremia. In most infections, no apparent disease occurs. The infection is resolved, and lasting immunity is produced. In some infections (1:800 to 1:100, depending on patient's age), central nervous system invasion occurs, and viral replication in neural and glial tissue produces a severe inflammatory process. Neuronal degeneration accompanied by lymphocytic and microglial cell infiltrates may be widespread. Clinical manifestations of encephalitis due to St. Louis encephalitis virus are fever, headache, stiff neck, convulsions, delirium, coma, tremors, and motor dysfunction. Death may follow; in nonfatal cases, neurologic sequelae are common. The pathogenetic potential of St. Louis encephalitis virus and several other flaviviruses such as Japanese B encephalitis, Murray Valley encephalitis, and tick-borne encephalitis depends entirely on their neurovirulence—that is, their ability to invade and replicate in the central nervous system. The systemic phase of infection with these mosquito- and tick-borne encephalitic agents produces negligible illness.

In contrast to the encephalitis-producing agents, yellow fever virus produces severe systemic disease. Viral replication occurs in reticuloendothelial cells in many organs and in the parenchyma of the liver, adrenal glands, heart, and kidneys. High concentrations of virus are present in the blood and involved organs. Characteristic liver damage from infection of hepatic cells is midzonal necrosis and intracellular hyaline deposits called Councilman bodies. Liver function tests become markedly abnormal, and icterus is often severe. Cellular degeneration of kidney and cardiac cells produces an acute nephritis and myocarditis. Disseminated intravascular coagulation is a major manifestation and causes the severe gastrointestinal hemorrhages characteristic of yellow fever.

The clinical course of yellow fever is that of an acute illness lasting 1 week or more. A first phase consists of fever, myalgia, headache, nausea, and vomiting, often followed by a second phase of severe toxicity, jaundice, gastrointestinal hemorrhage, anuria, and shock. Death may occur within 5–10 days; case fatality rates are 10%–50%.

Dengue viruses of all four serotypes cause two distinct syndromes: classic dengue fever and dengue hemorrhagic fever. Although caused by the same viruses, dengue and dengue hemorrhagic fever are pathogenetically, clinically, and epidemiologically distinct. Dengue viruses replicate in the skin at the site of the mosquito bite, in regional lymph nodes, and throughout the reticuloendothelial system. Viremia is concomitant with clinical illness; virus is present in the serum and in association with circulating monocytes. A severe leukopenia often is present. Fever, headache, myalgia, anorexia, and a maculopapular or petechial rash, which occurs on the third to fifth day, are the major manifestations of dengue fever. Dengue fever lasts 3–9 days, is self-limiting, and is rarely associated with hemorrhagic phenomenon or serious sequelae.

Dengue hemorrhagic fever results from additional pathogenetic processes not present in classical dengue fever; the most important of these processes are increased vascular permeability, hemoconcentration, thrombocytopenia, and disseminated intravascular coagulation. Lowered plasma volume caused by vascular permeability causes clinical shock that, if uncorrected, may be followed by acidosis, hyperkalemia, and death.

The specific pathogenetic mechanism that produces dengue hemorrhagic fever and dengue shock syndrome is not well understood, but strong evidence incriminates immunopathologic mechanisms. Ninety percent of dengue hemorrhagic fever cases occur in children who are experiencing their second infection with a dengue virus; some cases occur in infants under 6 months of age born to immune mothers. Usually, the dengue-2 serotype causes severe disease, although the other serotypes also may be involved. The immunologic processes that result from closely spaced infections with antigenically related viruses probably are responsible for the immunopathologic manifestations of dengue hemorrhagic fever. In infants, the presence of subprotective levels of maternal anti-dengue antibody has been shown to be a factor. Activation of complement and release of anaphylotoxins are usually found in patients with dengue shock syndrome. Both the classic and alternate pathways are involved. Immune complexes in circulation or on infected cell surfaces have been postulated to be the cause of this complement activation. Immune enhancement of disease also is thought to play a major role in pathogenesis. Both homologous and heterologous antibodies binding to dengue virus can markedly enhance infection of macrophages in vitro via cellular Fc receptors. Several antigenic determinants for infection-enhancing antibodies have been found on the envelope glycoprotein. Thus, it has been postulated that cross-reacting antibodies from a previous dengue infection or maternal anti-dengue antibodies in infants enhance the entry of virus into macrophages. The increased viral replication in the macrophages then contributes to the pathogenesis of complement activation, vascular permeability, and clotting abnormalities observed in patients, through the release of products from infected macrophages. These products may be released by increased destruction of infected macrophages via cellular immune mechanisms.

The clinical course of dengue hemorrhagic fever is characterized by an initial stage of 3–5 days with fever, rash, and anorexia, followed by a shock phase in which hepatomegaly, hypotension, and a hemorrhagic diathesis occur. Complement activation and thrombocytopenia typically takes place at the onset of the shock phase and reverse spontaneously after a period that ranges from hours to a few days.

Host Defenses

Other than antiviral antibody, which has an important protective role, little is known about host defenses against flaviviruses. Interferon and antibody-dependent cellular cytotoxicity probably play a role in resolving infections. Heterologous immunity is not protective, even though prominent serologic cross-reactions by hemagglutination-inhibition and complement fixation tests are present. Indeed, heterologous antibody increases the infectivity of dengue viruses for human macrophages in vitro. Natural defenses against central nervous system invasion by St. Louis encephalitis virus are most effective in children and much less effective in the elderly, resulting in much higher disease-to-infection ratios in older persons.

Diagnosis

Diagnosis of flavivirus infection is based on epidemiologic knowledge and clinical suspicion confirmed by serology and virus isolation. When a patient develops symptoms of encephalitis, virus is not present in the cerebrospinal fluid and is no longer present in the blood; viruses usually can be isolated only by brain biopsy or from the brain at autopsy. Thus, serologic tests showing antibody rise are most practical for diagnosis.

Interpretation of serologic data obtained by hemagglutination-inhibition, complement-fixation, and fluorescent antibody tests is difficult in most tropical areas where several flaviviruses are endemic. In primary infections, the virus neutralization test provides virus-specific confirmation. If a patient has had previous flavivirus infections, cross-reactions make even neutralization test results difficult or impossible to interpret. In some instances, IgM antibody can be used to make a specific serologic diagnosis because the IgM antibody, unlike IgG, is virus-specific in secondary infections. Demonstration of specific IgM antibody in the cerebrospinal fluid by antibody-capture immunoassay is an excellent way to diagnose encephalitis caused by flaviviruses. In yellow fever, dengue, and dengue hemorrhagic fever, virus is present in the blood for 4 or even 5 days after onset of fever; virus isolation in mammalian or insect cell culture is the method of choice for diagnosis. The earlier the specimen is obtained for isolation, the higher the likelihood of success.

Epidemiology

The flaviviruses compose a highly diverse genus, and their ecology is diverse and complex. Only the basic concepts are dealt with here. The mosquito-borne encephalitides—St. Louis, Japanese B, Murray Valley, and West Nile—exist in nature primarily as viruses of birds and are transmitted by species of *Culex* mosquitoes that feed readily on birds. St. Louis encephalitis virus is maintained in nature in the avian cycle; in temperate areas, the virus is maintained through the winter in infected hibernating adult mosquitoes. In the United States, human epidemics of St. Louis encephalitis are preceded by increased virus dissemination among wild birds and increases in vector populations and vector infection rates. St. Louis encephalitis virus is widespread in the United States and causes periodic outbreaks in California, Texas, the Ohio-Mississippi Valley, and the southeast. In Asia, Japanese B encephalitis virus occupies an ecologic niche similar to St. Louis encephalitis in the western hemisphere, with one major difference: it infects swine, in which it causes high viremias. Because Asian vectors of Japanese B encephalitis feed readily on swine, swine are an efficient amplifying host for this virus. As a result, Japanese B encephalitis epidemics in regions where swine are present have been frequent and severe. This virus is a major public health problem in Japan, China, India, and Southeast Asia.

The tick-borne flaviviruses are maintained by tick-mammal cycles and by vertical transovarian transmission in ticks. Humans are infected with this subgroup of flavivirus through the bite of infected ticks.

Yellow fever virus in Africa and South America has two distinct epidemiologic patterns: sylvan and urban. In South America, sylvan or jungle yellow fever is transmitted among canopy-dwelling monkeys and mosquitoes of the genera *Haemagogus* and *Sabethes*. Human disease occurs sporadically or in small outbreaks, and only in persons exposed to the forest mosquitoes. In previous years, urban yellow fever was transmitted in a highly efficient human-mosquito-human cycle by the urban mosquito *Aedes aegypti*. In the Americas, yellow fever is now confined to the Amazon Basin and adjacent savannah forest. In Africa, sylvan and rural yellow fever involves monkeys and several *Aedes* sp; the urban cycle involves *A aegypti*. Yellow fever is present in tropical sub-Sahara Africa from Senegal to Ethiopia.

Dengue viruses are distributed through the tropics and depend principally on a human-mosquito-human cycle, although primate infections occur in Asia and probably in Africa. The principal vector is *A aegypti,* but other *Aedes* sp of the subgenus *Stegomyia* may be involved in Asia and the Pacific region. Epidemiologic patterns are highly varied but may be described as epidemic, endemic, or hyperendemic. Epidemics of dengue fever are frequent in Caribbean and Pacific islands. Epidemics occur in nonimmune populations when a dengue virus is introduced and vectors are present. Endemic regions in the western hemisphere in which one or more serotypes are continuously transmitted include Jamaica, Haiti, the Dominican Republic, Cuba, Puerto Rico, Columbia,

Venezuela, El Salvador, Guatamala, and Mexico. In Africa, endemic dengue is present in Niger, Nigeria, Senegal, Kenya, and Somalia. India, Pakistan, and Bangladesh also have endemic and epidemic regions. In endemic regions, dengue fever occurs principally in children and often is unrecognized. In Southeast Asia, dengue viruses of all four serotypes are continuously transmitted, often at high rates. Under these conditions, epidemics of dengue hemorrhagic fever occur among children. Dengue hemorrhagic fever has become a major cause of death among children in hyperendemic regions, including Indonesia, Vietnam, Cambodia, Thailand, Malaysia, and Burma. In these countries, its incidence has been steadily increasing; annual rainy season epidemics involve thousands of cases; there is a 3%–10% case fatality rate.

Control

Control of disease caused by flaviviruses is based on vaccines for some viruses and on vector control. At present, formalinized killed virus vaccines are used to prevent Japanese B encephalitis in Japan and China and tick-borne encephalitis in Austria and the Soviet Union. Vaccination of school children is credited with effective control of epidemic Japanese B encephalitis in Japan. The live attenuated 17D yellow fever vaccine is an extremely effective and safe vaccine, and is widely used in South America and Africa.

Control of urban epidemics of yellow fever in the Americas was accomplished by containment and, in some regions, eradication of the *A aegypti* vectors. Vector control is not feasible to prevent jungle yellow fever; therefore, vaccines are widely used in endemic regions.

No vaccines are yet available for dengue or dengue hemorrhagic fever, although experimental attenuated vaccines have been developed. Vector control, including destroying larval habitats and spraying insecticide to kill adult mosquitoes, is the only means available to control dengue and dengue hemorrhagic fever.

St. Louis encephalitis is managed in the United States by vector control, including aerial ultra low volume spraying of insecticides in populated areas. No vaccine is available. Surveillance of St. Louis encephalitis virus activity in wild bird populations and vectors is used to monitor the risk of epidemics and to guide vector control requirements.

References

Berge, T.O.: *International catalogue of arboviruses including certain other viruses of vertebrates*. DHEW Publ. No. (CDC) 75-8301, 1975.

Monath, T., (editor): *St. Louis encephalitis*. Washington, D.C.: American Public Health Association, 1980.

Pang, T., Pathmanathan, R., (editors): *Proceedings of the International Conference on dengue/dengue hemorrhagic fever*. Kuala Lumpar: University of Malaya, 1983.

Pfefferkorn, E.R., Shapiro, D.: Reproduction of togaviruses. In: *Comprehensive virology*, vol 2. Fraenkel-Conrat H., Wagner, R.R., (editors) New York: Plenum Press, 1974.

Schlesinger, R.W.: *Dengue viruses*. Virology Monographs, vol. 16. New York: Springer-Verlag, 1977.

Schlesinger, R.W., (editor): *The togaviruses*. New York: Academic Press, 1980.

Strauss, E.G., Strauss, J.H.: Replication strategies of the single-stranded RNA viruses of eukaryotes. In: *Current topics in microbiology and immunology*. Berlin: Springer-Verlag, 1983.

Theiler, M., Downs, W.G.: *The arthropod-borne viruses of vertebrates: An account of the Rockefeller Foundation virus program, 1951-1970*. New Haven, Conn.: Yale University Press, 1973.

World Health Organization: *Guide for diagnosis, treatment and control of dengue hemorrhagic fever*. Geneva: WHO, 1980.

75 Bunyaviruses

Robert E. Shope, MD

3 -

C = 122
80-120nm

Minus Strand Viruses

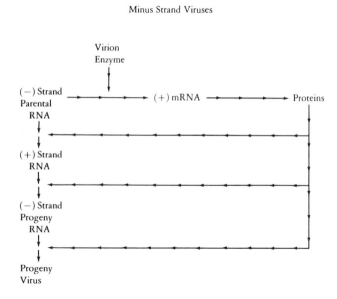

General Concepts

Bunyaviridae constitute a family of arthropod-borne viruses (arboviruses) and rodent-borne viruses that cause several diseases of human and domestic animals, including fever, hemorrhagic fever, renal failure, encephalitis, meningitis, blindness, and congenital defects. The virions of this group are 90-100 nm diameter, enveloped spheres

---

The diagrams of the virion morphology and the multiplication scheme are derived from Chapters 62 and 63, respectively. The multiplication scheme applies only generally as indicated in Chapter 63.

containing three segments of negative, single-stranded RNA. Each segment is a gene. Because the RNA is segmented, genetic reassortment can occur during infection.

The family includes 4 genera with at least 180 viruses, of which only 35, in 3 genera, are known to cause disease. Table 75-1 shows these 35 with their vectors, geographic distribution, and case fatality rates. Most bunyaviruses have a wild vertebrate host; in most cases, humans are accidental hosts. The host, which is different for each virus, usually is a small mammal, often a rodent.

Bunyaviruses are arthropod-borne except for Hantaan virus, the cause of hemorrhagic fever with renal syndrome, which has a rodent reservoir from which the virus is transmitted to humans through rodent urine or other body fluids. The viruses replicate in the arthropod, which may be a mosquito, tick, midge, or phlebotomine fly. The gut is infected initially, and after a few days or weeks, the virus appears in the saliva; the arthropod remains infective for life. When the vector takes a blood meal, the infective saliva enters the small capillaries of the human or other vertebrate host. An incubation period of a few days ensues, after which the host vertebrate develops viremia. The host may either have an inapparent infection (commonly), or become febrile and manifest the more serious signs and symptoms that are characteristic of the infecting virus. Viremia subsides with the appearance of antibody and the host recovers unless a specific target organ has been permanently damaged.

LaCrosse virus and probably several other bunyaviruses are maintained from season to season by transovarial and venereal transmission in the arthropod. This offers a unique advantage to these viruses, allowing them to survive under adverse conditions.

Most bunyavirus illnesses are self-limited fevers that last 1–4 days and are characterized by headache, muscle aches, nausea, conjunctivitis, and generalized weakness. A few are more serious illnesses: LaCrosse encephalitis is characterized by fever, convulsions, drowsiness, and focal neurological signs; Crimean hemorrhagic fever by headache, pains in arms and legs, and in severe cases, bleeding from the gums, nose, uterus, lungs, and intestines; and hemorrhagic fever with renal syndrome (Korean hemorrhagic fever) by fever, hemorrhage, and acute renal failure. Rift Valley fever may mimic the febrile, the encephalitic, or the hemorrhagic illness of other bunyaviruses and the patient may also become blind secondary to retinal vasculitis. These illnesses are significant, currently uncontrolled human diseases: LaCrosse encephalitis causes most arbovirus encephalitis in North America; thousands of cases of hemorrhagic fever with renal syndrome occur annually in Asia and Europe. Rift Valley fever has explosive potential, as shown in Egypt in 1977 when an estimated 200,000 cases, with 598 deaths, were recorded.

Distinctive Properties

Bunyaviruses have spherical enveloped particles about 100 nm diameter; Hantaan virus is somewhat smaller. Bunyaviruses contain single-stranded RNA, which has three segments and a total molecular weight of about 5×10^6 daltons. The genome is negative sense, and its segmented nature facilitates genetic reassortment. Nucleocapsid protein is associated with a large, medium, and small helical, circular nucleocapsid; two distinct surface glycoproteins are responsible collectively for neutralization of infectivity and for hemagglutination of red blood cells. The nucleocapsid is surrounded by a lipid-

Table 75-1 Diseases of Humans and Domestic Animals Caused by Viruses of the Family Bunyaviridae

Genus and Group	Virus	Disease in Humans	Disease in Animals	Vector	Where Found	Case Fatality Rate
Bunyavirus						
Bunyamwera	Bunyamwera	Fever		Mosquito	Africa	0
	Germiston	Fever		Mosquito	Africa	0
	Guaroa	Fever		Mosquito	South America, Panama	0
	Ilesha	Fever		Mosquito	Africa	0
	Wyeomyia	Fever		Mosquito	South America, Panama	0
Bwamba	Bwamba	Fever		Mosquito	Africa	0
C	Apeu	Fever		Mosquito	South America	0
	Caraparu	Fever		Mosquito	South America	0
	Itaqui	Fever		Mosquito	South America	0
	Madrid	Fever		Mosquito	Panama	0
	Marituba	Fever		Mosquito	South America	0
	Murutucu	Fever		Mosquito	South America	0
	Oriboca	Fever		Mosquito	South America	0
	Ossa	Fever		Mosquito	Panama	0
	Restan	Fever		Mosquito	Trinidad	0
California	California encephalitis	Encephalitis		Mosquito	North America	0
	LaCrosse	Encephalitis		Mosquito	North America	0.5%–1%
	Snowshoe hare	Encephalitis		Mosquito	North America	0
	Jamestown Canyon	Encephalitis		Mosquito	North America	0
	Tahyna	Fever		Mosquito	Europe	0
Guama	Catu	Fever		Mosquito	South America	0
	Guama	Fever		Mosquito	South America	0

Group / Virus	Disease	Animal disease	Vector	Distribution	Mortality
Simbu					
Akabane		Hydranencephaly and arthrogrypo-sis (sheep and cattle)	Culicoides	Japan, Australia, Israel	High in newborn
Shuni	Fever		Mosquito	Africa, Asia	0
Oropouche	Fever		Unknown	South America	0
Phlebovirus					
Phlebotomus fever					
Candiru	Fever		Unknown	South America	0
Chagres	Fever		Phlebotomine	Panama	0
Naples	Fever		Phlebotomine	Europe, Africa, Asia	0
Punta Toro	Fever		Phlebotomine	Panama	0
Rift Valley fever	Fever, encephalitis, hemorrhagic fever, blindness	Abortion, hepatitis	Mosquito	Africa	0.2%–10% in humans; high in sheep, cattle, camels
Sicilian	Fever		Phlebotomine	Europe, Africa, Asia	0
Nairovirus					
Congo					
Crimean-Congo hemorrhagic fever	Hemorrhagic fever		Tick	Africa, Asia	2%–50%
Nairobi sheep disease	Fever	Enteritis (sheep)	Tick	Africa, Asia	25%–75% in sheep
Dugbe	Fever		Tick	Africa	0
Hantaviruses					
Ungrouped					
Hantaan and related viruses	Hemorrhagic fever with renal syndrome		Rodent (reservoir)	Europe	0.5%
				Asia	5.0%

containing envelope. The antigen (nucleoprotein) responsible for eliciting the major complement-fixation response is sometimes type-specific but more often is group reactive. The antigens (glycoproteins) responsible for eliciting the neutralization and inhibition of hemagglutination responses are type-specific. Naturally occurring viruses may contain the nucleoprotein of one serotype and the glycoproteins of another serotype; these viruses presumably represent natural reassortments.

Replication occurs in the cytoplasm, and virions usually bud into the Golgi cisternae. Virus particles are liberated from the cell by plasma membrane disruption and by fusion of intracellular vacuoles with the plasma membrane.

Pathogenesis

The primary site of virus multiplication in humans is not known; it may be the vascular endothelium, the skin, or the regional lymph nodes. From there the virus is probably seeded into the bloodstream, causing viremia and the initial febrile response. Viremia terminates in a few days, coincident with appearance of humoral antibody. In some bunyavirus diseases a target organ—the liver in Rift Vally fever, the brain in LaCrosse encephalitis, the vascular endothelium in Crimean hemorrhagic fever and in hemorrhagic fever with renal syndrome, or the fetus in Akabane infection of sheep and goats—is damaged and a specific disease occurs. Although this damage is believed to result from direct invasion of the virus and not from a host-mediated antigen-antibody or antigen-lymphocyte reaction, the pathogenesis of bunyaviruses in the vertebrate host has not been well studied. The pathologic findings in the kidneys of patients who have hemorrhagic fever with renal syndrome may result from a host reaction to antigen-antibody complexes. Occasionally, permanent damage to the brain, liver, fetus or eye occurs, but usually recovery is rapid and complete.

Host Defenses

There are relatively few studies on host defenses against bunyavirus infections. Humoral antibody plays a protective role. Its appearance, either naturally or passively acquired, is associated with disappearance of virus from the blood. In addition, colostrum from immune mothers protects offspring animals from infection. Bunyaviruses also induce interferon, which may help to control the infectious process. The role of the T cell system has not been evaluated nor has the relative importance of humoral antibody and interferon been determined.

Epidemiology

Like other arboviruses, the bunyaviruses, are maintained in natural cycles involving replication in mosquitoes, ticks, *Culicoides* midges, or phlebotomine flies and a vertebrate host, usually a small mammal. Humans may become ill when infected, but their blood rarely infects biting arthropods in the natural cycle; thus humans are usually dead-end hosts. In addition to the arthropod-vertebrate-arthropod cycle, some bunyaviruses, such as those in the California and phlebotomus fever groups, are transmitted transovarially in the arthropod, and can therefore winter in the egg and be transmitted to humans in the late spring or early summer when the adult arthropod emerges. Bunyaviruses are found throughout the world, but any serotype has limited geographic distribution because it relies on one or at best a few arthropod species to maintain its natural cycle. Hemorrhagic fever with renal syndrome is maintained in a rodent reservoir and is not arthropod-borne. Transmission to humans is believed to occur by inhalation of virus excreted in rodent urine and other body fluids.

The most serious disease of bunyavirus origin in the United States is LaCrosse encephalitis. First recognized when there was a fatal case in LaCrosse, Wisconsin, in 1960, it is now recognized not only in the north central United States but also New York and Pennsylvania and in Canada. The closely related viruses California encephalitis, snowshoe hare, and Jamestown Canyon are also occasionally implicated as a cause of encephalitis. At least 800 cases of encephalitis have been reported since 1960, with a case fatality ratio of about 1:200. The disease is characterized by fever, headaches, vomiting, malaise, lethargy, and seizures. It affects children primarily. Although children usually appear to recover rapidly, sequelae such as epilepsy and more subtle learning and behavior defects are common. The vector of LaCrosse virus is a woodland, tree-hole-breeding mosquito, *A triseriatus;* consequently, the infection usually occurs after exposure in the woods when camping, or among children living in rural areas. Chipmunks and tree squirrels are amplifying hosts. Virus may also be transmitted from male to female mosquitoes venereally.

The group C and group Guama viruses cause self-limited febrile disease in humans in Central America and northern South America. The disease lasts 2–4 days and may be severe enough to put to bed even the most robust worker. Infection is usually transmitted by forest *Culex (Melanoconion)* sp mosquitoes. Forest rodents are the vertebrate hosts and infection in humans is dead-end. Bunyamwera group virus illnesses occur in Africa and South America. These are transmitted by mosquitoes and are also self-limited febrile diseases.

Naples and Sicilian phlebotomus fevers are endemic in North Africa and southern Europe, and from the Middle East to Pakistan. During World War II, severe epidemics of these diseases were recognized as febrile illnesses in troops in the Mediterranean theater. *Phlebotomus papatasii* proved to be the vector. Subsequently, related viruses such as Candiru, Chagres, and Punta Toro were discovered in the New World tropics, where a cycle of phlebotomine sandflies and forest rodents was responsible for maintaining the infection.

Oropouche virus causes a major febrile disease in Brazil and Trinidad. Tens of thousands of cases have been recorded in epidemics. The vertebrate host is not yet known; *Culicoides* midges are implicated as vectors of the virus. There is no known mortality from the disease.

Crimean hemorrhagic fever is a tick-transmitted viral disease of Bulgaria, Yugoslavia, the Soviet Union, China, Iraq, Dubai, and Pakistan. Human disease also has been recorded rarely in subSaharan Africa. The disease in the Soviet Union is characterized by fever, headache, vomiting, muscle aches, thrombocytopenia, leukopenia, and, in severe cases, by subcutaneous and gastrointestinal bleeding, which is fatal in 5%–50% of cases. The virus is transmitted by ticks, usually of the *Hyalomma* genus. Domestic and wild mammals may be amplifying and reservoir hosts. Human infection may also occur directly from contaminated blood of hospitalized patients; thus, cases should be isolated in the hospital.

Bunyaviruses also cause significant veterinary diseases. Sheep, cattle, buffalo, and camels infected with Rift Valley fever virus abort; Nairobi sheep disease causes epidemics of hemorrhagic gastroenteritis in sheep with up to 75% mortality. Akabane virus infection in pregnant sheep and cattle produces fetal abnormalities such as failure of the cerebral hemispheres to develop or contractures of joints, because the virus destroys germinal cells during the development of the brain and joints.

Bunyavirus diseases usually are restricted to focal geographic areas because of the limited distribution of their vectors or vertebrate hosts. Awareness of their geographic distribution, seasonality, and clinical syndrome may help in establishing a diagnosis. Definitive diagnosis, however, can be made only by laboratory tests. No specific treatment is available. Control depends on public health measures such as the killing of vectors and, in the case of Rift Valley fever, vaccination of sheep and cattle to prevent amplification of transmission by mosquitoes. The use of bed nets and arthropod repellents also may be effective.

Rift Valley fever appears as epizootics in sheep, cattle, camels, and goats in Africa. Massive outbreaks have been recognized in South Africa, Kenya, Uganda, Sudan, and in 1977 for the first time in Egypt. Human cases usually are restricted to veterinarians, butchers, and others in close contact with blood of domestic livestock; however, in Egypt, widespread human epidemic disease was recognized. Abortion in sheep and cattle is common; human mortality (up to 10%) is associated with jaundice and hemorrhage or with encephalitis. Some cases exhibit ocular vasculitis and retinitis leading to macular degeneration and blindness. The virus is presumably transmitted by mosquitoes.

Nairobi sheep disease virus was first isolated in 1910 from a sheep with gastroenteritis. It also produces glomerulonephritis, leukopenia, and hypoproteinemia; the mortality in sheep in some outbreaks is as high as 75%. Disease in humans is rare and mild; fever and arthralgia are the principal complaints.

Akabane virus produces a striking syndrome in sheep and cattle—arthrogryposis and hydranencephaly. Adult livestock show no signs of illness, but offspring from animals infected during the first and second months of gestation are characterized by absence of the brain and marked deformities of the spine and limbs. This virus is transmitted by mosquitoes and midges. First recognized in Japan, the disease has been recorded also in Australia and Israel. It has caused the loss of an estimated 50,000 calves in Japan since 1972, as well as killing several thousand animals in Australia.

Diagnosis

Bunyavirus illness is diagnosed by isolating the virus or by showing a fourfold or greater rise in antibody titer between acute phase and convalescent phase sera. The viruses can be isolated from blood (or from brain, liver, and other organs postmortem) during the viremic phase, but not usually after the third day of fever. Virus is propagated in baby mice or mosquitoes, or in vertebrate or invertebrate tissue cultures. Serologic tests used to diagnose bunyavirus infections include complement-fixation, fluorescent antibody, ELISA, neutralization, and hemagglutination-inhibition tests. The complement-fixation, ELISA, and fluorescent antibody tests are often group reactive; the neutralization and hemagglutination-inhibition test are type-specific. Virus also is identified using these tests with a reference immune serum. Assessments of IgM may be especially useful in establishing an early diagnosis.

Usually a bunyavirus infection cannot be diagnosed on clinical grounds. Suspicion based on travel history, exposure to arthropods or rodents, seasonal occurrence, geographical factors, and information about concurrent disease in other people or domestic animals can aid the laboratory scientist. Hemorrhagic fever with renal syndrome should be strongly suspected in a person in Europe or Asia who has fever, proteinuria, thrombocytopenia, and elevated blood urea nitrogen, especially if the patient has been exposed to wild rodents.

Control

Control of bunyavirus transmission is through control of the arthropod vector or vertebrate reservoir. Personal measures such as the use of proper protective clothing, repellants, bed nets, and house screens are effective but are often forgotten. Insecticides often are used on a community-wide basis, as well as at the breeding ground of mosquitoes or other arthropods. Rodenticides are used in outbreaks of hemorrhagic fever with renal syndrome.

Vaccines exist for Rift Valley fever and can be used in animals to stop the transmission cycle or in humans and domestic animals to prevent disease. A vaccine for sheep is available for Nairobi sheep disease. No vaccines or other specific antiviral agents for the other bunyaviruses are in use.

Patients should be protected from the bites of arthropods, usually by bed nets, if they are in the viremic phase of illness. When hemorrhage occurs, as in Crimean hemorrhagic fever, hospital personnel should wear gown and mask to prevent aerosol infection, and should take precautions with needles to prevent infection by blood. For other bunyavirus infections, no quarantine, isolation, or concurrent disinfection is needed other than the precautions noted previously.

References

Benenson, A.S., (editor): *Control of communicable diseases in man,* 13th ed. Washington, D.C.: American Public Health Association, 1981.

Bishop, D.H.L.; Shope, R.E.: Bunyaviridae. In: *Comprehensive virology,* Vol. 14. Fraenkel-Conrat H., Wagner, R.R., (editors). New York: Plenum Press, 1979.

Calisher, C.H., Thompson, W.H., (editors): *California serogroup viruses.* New York: Alan R. Liss, 1983.

Schwartz, T.A., Klingberg, M.A., Goldblum, N. (editors): *Rift Valley fever.* Basel: Karger, 1981.

Shope, R.E.: Arbovirus. In: *Manual of clinical microbiology,* 3rd ed. Lennette, E.H., et al. (editors). Washington, D.C.: American Society for Microbiology, 1980.

76 Rubella Virus

Envelope

1 +

Icosahedral
40-90nm

Paul D. Parkman, MD
Hope E. Hopps
Harry M. Meyer, Jr., MD

General Concepts
Distinctive Properties
Pathogenesis
Host Defenses
Epidemiology
Diagnosis
Control

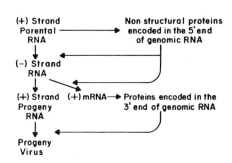

General Concepts

Rubella (German measles) is a common mild disease associated with a rash. It occurs worldwide, usually affecting children and adolescents, but not uncommonly in young adults. When rubella virus infects susceptible women early in pregnancy, it may be transmitted to the placenta and fetus, thereby producing birth defects. Humoral and cellular immunity, as well as interferon, are host defenses. Accurate diagnosis is critical in pregnancy. The virus is a member of the Togaviridae family, genus *Rubivirus*. Only one serotype has been identified, and it is genetically stable; thus, a monovalent vaccine

---

The diagrams of the virion morphology and the multiplication scheme are derived from Chapters 62 and 63, respectively. The multiplication scheme applies only generally as indicated in Chapter 63.

of constant virus composition can be used to prevent rubella. In the absence of vaccination programs, major epidemics have occurred.

Distinctive Properties

Rubella virus is a 40-80 nm diameter RNA and lipid-containing enveloped virus. The RNA is single stranded, positive, and has a molecular weight of about 3×10^6 daltons. The virus particles are spherical with spikelike surface projections and an electron-dense core. Morphologically, they resemble the togaviruses; despite this resemblance, neither serologic relationships nor transmission by arthropods have been demonstrated.

Several components (antigens) of the virus react with antibodies developing in sera from persons convalescing from rubella virus infection; the intact virus is neutralized by convalescent phase sera. Antigen preparations commonly used for diagnostic and research purposes include the hemagglutinin, complement-fixation, precipitin, and infectious antigens. Specific antisera for identification of isolates has been produced by immunizing small laboratory animals.

Humans are the only known reservoir of rubella virus. In the laboratory, subclinical infections resembling those seen in humans can be produced in rhesus and vervet monkeys; these species were used to study the pathogenesis of infection and to develop experimental vaccines.

Cell cultures are used for virus isolation, production of antigens, and preparation of vaccines. This noncytolytic virus may be detected by its interference with the cytopathic effects of other viruses added after 7-14 days of incubation of the rubella-infected cultures, the production of subtle cytopathic effects on certain cell lines, immunofluorescence, and immunoperoxidase staining. The special techniques needed for virus detection accounted for the rather late (1961) discovery of means to work with this virus in the laboratory.

Pathogenesis

The disease appears to be transmitted by the respiratory route. Although the early events are incompletely characterized, the virus almost certainly must undergo an initial period of multiplication in the upper respiratory tract before viremic spread to target organs (skin, lymph nodes, and joints) and to the sites of excretion. Approximately 1 week after infection and 1-1½ weeks before rash onset, virus appears in the blood (viremia) and respiratory tract (Figure 76-1). The highest concentration of virus in respiratory secretions is detected from 3 days before rash onset until 3 days afterward. This period corresponds with the period of maximum infectivity. If infection occurs during the first 3-4 months of pregnancy, the virus may invade the placenta and be transmitted to the fetus (Figure 76-2). After this time, the fetus is rarely infected. Fetal infection commonly results in birth defects; the virus can multiply and damage virtually any organ system. From studies in cell cultures, the virus is known to produce chromosomal abnormalities, to slow cellular growth rates, and to cause cell death in some cell types; these effects appear to produce the characteristic abnormalities of cell structure and function. A clinically recognizable pattern of defects (the rubella syndrome) involving the eye, heart, and brain may be produced in severely affected infants; multiple other derangements, both permanent and transiently present in the neonatal period, may be observed with or without the major defects. Damage to the fetus is more severe when infection occurs

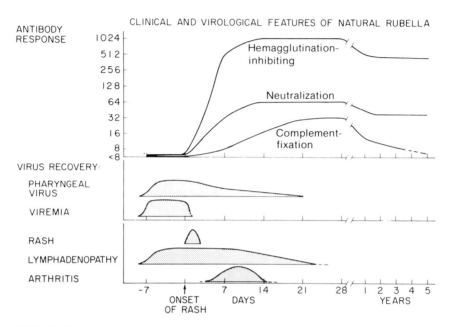

Figure 76-1 Clinical findings, virus shedding, and serologic response in postnatally acquired rubella. From *Am J Clin Pathol* 1972; 57:804.

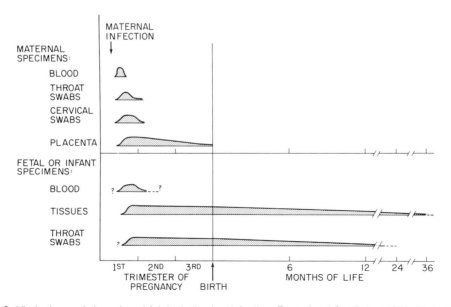

Figure 76-2 Virologic events in maternal-fetal rubella virus infection. From *Am J Clin Pathol* 1972; 57:808.

early in gestation. The virus commonly persists during the first year of life and occasionally even longer; the infant continues to shed virus in respiratory secretions and in the urine and can infect susceptible contacts.

Host Defenses

Currently, no evidence delineates the role of nonspecific factors (such as febrile response, interferon induction, or nonspecific inhibitors) in preventing rubella or in modifying its clinical course. Rubella virus induces only low levels of interferon in cell cultures; this may explain the failure to demonstrate interferon in infected experimental animals or in natural- or vaccine-induced infections. However, rubella virus is unusually sensitive to the antiviral action of interferon.

The immune system responds promptly to infection; neutralizing and hemagglutination-inhibiting antibodies appear shortly after onset of rash, reach maximum levels in 1-4 weeks, and persist for years, perhaps for life. Cell-mediated immunity also develops in convalescence. When exposed to rubella, individuals with neutralizing or hemagglutination-inhibiting antibodies are protected against the natural disease; boosts in antibody level following reexposure have been observed, suggesting limited reinfection.

Epidemiology

Because rubella appears to be less contagious than diseases such as measles and varicella, a significant proportion of the population escapes rubella infection in childhood. About 15% of child-bearing-age women in the United States lack serologic evidence of earlier rubella infection. Sporadic outbreaks of rubella occur each year and, before the availability of vaccine, major epidemics involving the entire country, or large areas of the country, were observed every 6-9 years. A seasonal pattern clearly exists, similar to that of other infections transmitted by the respiratory route, with high incidence in late winter and early spring.

Diagnosis

The incubation period is 14-20 days, averaging 17. The extent of illness varies; it can present as an illness with a rash mimicking that of measles, or it may be so evanescent as to go unnoticed. In typical cases, rash appears first on the face and neck, quickly spreading to the trunk and upper extremities, then to the legs (Figure 76-3). Generalized enlargement of the lymph nodes occurs, especially in the posterior cervical area. Unlike the clinical picture of rubeola, significant respiratory symptoms are uncommon. Joint pain and occasionally joint swelling and symptoms suggestive of peripheral neuritis occur, particularly in women. Such symptoms and signs most commonly begin several days after the appearance of rash. Rare complications include encephalitis and thrombocytopenic purpura.

The clinical features of congenital rubella vary and depend on the organ system or systems involved; for example, the eye (congenital cataract), the ear (deafness), the heart (patent ductus arteriosus, pulmonary valvular or arterial stenosis), or the brain (encephalitis, mental retardation).

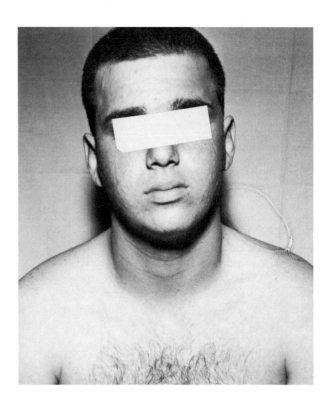

Figure 76-3 Young adult with characteristic rubella rash 24 hours after onset.

Confirmation of rubella is critical when infection is suspected during the first several months of pregnancy. Specific laboratory tests are required; common clinical laboratory tests are of little value in diagnosis. Virus can be readily recovered from respiratory tract specimens and, in infants suspected of having congenital infection, from urine specimens. Inoculation of specimens into primary African green monkey kidney cell cultures is a sensitive means for virus isolation. In this cell culture system, rubella virus can be detected by the interference it produces, after 7–14 days, with the cell-killing effect of an enterovirus selected for this purpose (for example, echovirus type 11). Interfering viruses isolated may be identified by neutralization with specific animal antisera. In 1981, an immunoperoxidase staining procedure was described that is as accurate as, but is more rapid than (10 days as compared to 17 days), the conventional interference test procedure. Because virus isolation procedures are costly and require a relatively sophisticated virologic laboratory, serologic diagnostic methods are most commonly used. Serum is collected early after exposure or as soon as possible after rash onset, and again after an interval of 6 weeks from exposure or 2–4 weeks after the onset of illness. Paired sera are assayed in the same test run because test-to-test variation in antibody titer results may be substantial. A fourfold or greater rise in antibody titer (for example, 1:16–1:64) between early and convalescent sera is considered diagnostic. The hemagglutination-inhibiting test currently is used in approximately 50% of laboratories. Other tests now available in commercial kit form include indirect hemagglutination, immunofluorescence, enzyme-linked immunofluorescence, ELISA, radioimmunoassay, and latex agglutination. Diagnosis of congenital rubella in the neonate may be accomplished by virus isolation or serologic testing. The affected neonate has circulating antibodies including transplacentally acquired maternal IgG and actively produced fetal and neonatal IgM antibodies. Thus the presence of significant amounts of rubella-specific IgM antibody early in life is evidence of congenital rubella infection. Also, the IgM procedure occasionally may be useful in the diagnosis of postnatally acquired rubella when only a single serum specimen, taken several weeks after onset of rash, is available. This type of test is now performed in many state health laboratories, as well as in research laboratories.

Control

A live virus vaccine is available to prevent rubella. In the United States, this vaccine is most often combined with live measles and mumps virus vaccines. Immunization strategy in this country calls for large-scale programs aimed at vaccination of all children over 15 months of age, and selective vaccination of adolescent girls and adult women. Rubella vaccine should not be given to pregnant women under any circumstance. If a pregnant woman is inadvertently vaccinated or if she becomes pregnant within 3 months of vaccination, she should be advised of the risk to the fetus.

With widespread use of vaccine in the United States since 1969, the number of reported cases and rubella-affected babies has declined, and no major epidemics have occurred. Since 1980, a downward trend in reported cases of rubella has been observed by the CDC. In addition, the incidence of congenital rubella syndrome has decreased markedly since 1979. Fifty-five cases of congenital rubella syndrome were reported at that time, whereas 14 cases were reported in 1980 and 9 in both 1981 and 1982. Immunization programs such as requiring proof of immunity before college entry, vaccinating susceptible women identified by premarital serologic tests, and vaccinating women after childbirth, miscarriage, or abortion could bring about a further decline in incidence of both rubella and congenital rubella syndrome.

Vaccine-induced antibody levels are lower than those produced by the natural disease, but when sensitive assay methods are used, the vaccine-induced levels show the same pattern of persistence. As with all attenuated vaccines, the duration of protection is a matter of concern, and continued monitoring will be required in future years. In 1982, the CDC reported surveillance studies on 741 of 5153 originally susceptible individuals enrolled in a vaccine study in 1969. During the first 4 years after vaccination, a drop in hemagglutination-inhibition titer of approximately 50% occurred in these persons, with generally stable titers after that time. Frequency of reversion to hemagglutination-inhibition titers of 1:10 has remained less than 0.5% per year. Measurable hemagglutination-inhibition antibody levels persisted during the 10-year period in 97% of persons vaccinated.

Immune globulin (γ-globulin) has been used in attempts to prevent rubella in pregnant women exposed to the virus. However, immunoglobulin does not appear to be highly effective; congenital infection has been observed in the infants of women given appropriately timed large doses. Thus, immunoglobulin is not routinely recommended for prophylaxis of rubella in early pregnancy. No specific chemotherapeutic measures are available for prevention or treatment.

References

Avery, G.B., et al.: Rubella syndrome after inapparent maternal illness. *Am J Dis Child* 1965; 110:444-446.

Herrmann, K.L.: Rubella virus. In: *Diagnostic procedures for viral, rickettsial and chlamydial infections,* 5th ed. Lennette, EH, Schmidt NJ (editors). Washington, D.C.: American Public Health Association, 1979.

Herrmann, K.L., Halstead, S.B., Wiebenga, N.H.: Rubella antibody persistence after immunization. *JAMA* 1982; 247:193-196.

Parkman, P.D., Hopps, H.E., Meyer, H.M., Jr.: Rubella virus: isolation, characterization and laboratory diagnosis. *Am J Dis Child* 1969; 118:68-77.

Preblud, S.R., et al.: Rubella vaccination in the United States: A ten-year review. *Epidemiol Rev* 1980; 2:171-194.

Rubella and congenital Rubella—United States, 1980-1983. Morbidity and Mortality Weekly Report 1983; 32:505-509.

Schmidt, N.J., Ho, H.H., Chin, J.: Application of immunoperoxidase staining to more rapid detection and identification of rubella virus isolates. *J Clin Microbiol* 1981; 13:627-630.

Sever, J.L., Cleghorn, C.: Rubella diagnostic tests: What is a significant result? *Postgrad Med* 1982; 71:73-77.

Shebarchi, I.C., et al.: Polycarbonate-coated microsticks as solid-phase carriers in an enzyme-linked immunosorbent assay for rubella antibody. *J Clin Microbiol* 1984; 20:305-306.

77 Arenaviruses

Charles J. Pfau, PhD

2 –

Pleomorphic
110-130nm

General Concepts
Distinctive Properties
Pathogenesis
Host Defenses
Epidemiology
Diagnosis
Control

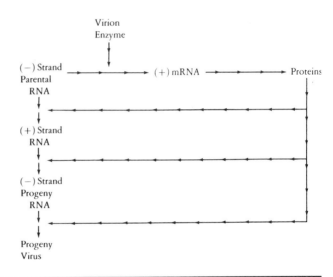

Minus Strand Viruses

General Concepts

The hallmark of the unusual family of arenaviruses is their tendency to cause persistent and silent infections in their natural hosts (rodents) and severe, often lethal, disseminated disease in humans. Arenaviruses are pleomorphic, enveloped particles, which contain

---

The diagrams of the virion morphology and the multiplication scheme are derived from Chapters 62 and 63, respectively. The multiplication scheme applies only generally as indicated in Chapter 63.

two RNA segments of virus origin and ribosomelike components. Suitable conditions for transmission of virus to humans occur in areas where humans ingest foods contaminated with rodent urine that contains virus (Figure 77-1). Persistent viremia and viruria in rodents result from a slow or insufficient immune response, resulting from infection of the immunologically immature fetus or neonate. In people, the disease is acute and may not have an immunologic cause.

In humans, who are only accidental hosts, four arenaviruses are well-known pathogens that can cause case fatality rates of up to 60%: Lassa fever virus, Junin and Machupo viruses (the causative agents of Argentine and Bolivian hemorrhagic fevers, respectively), and LCM virus. Infections are limited to areas containing the rodent host. Limited control of arenavirus infections has been achieved by various rodent control measures, but vaccines are needed for long-term control.

Distinctive Properties

Arenaviruses mature by budding from the plasma membrane of cells (Figure 77-2). In ultrathin sections, all arenaviruses appear as round, oval, or pleomorphic particles with a mean diameter of 110–130 nm (Figure 77-3). The particles have club-shaped surface projections about 10 nm long (Figure 77-3), which cover a unit membrane derived by budding from the plasma membrane of the cell. During this morphogenesis, sandy (the Latin *arena* means sand) granules resembling ribosomes are found within the unstructured interiors of nascent viruses. Indeed, highly purified arenaviruses have been found to contain 18S and 28S host ribosomal RNAs which have no required role in virus replication, and two distinct viral RNA species designated L and S. These latter RNAs appear to have no messenger function, but an RNA-dependent RNA polymerase within the virions presumably makes translatable RNA within the infected cell. All arenaviruses contain internal cross-reacting antigens that link together this family of viruses. Other

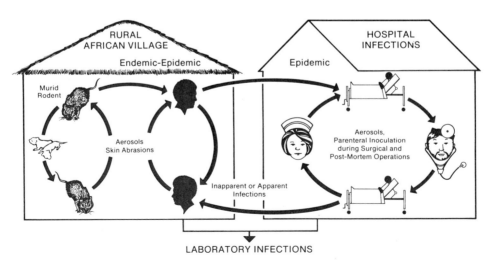

Figure 77-1 Epidemiologic transmission cycle of Lassa virus in Africa. Modified from Monath TP. *Bull WHO* 1975; 52:577.

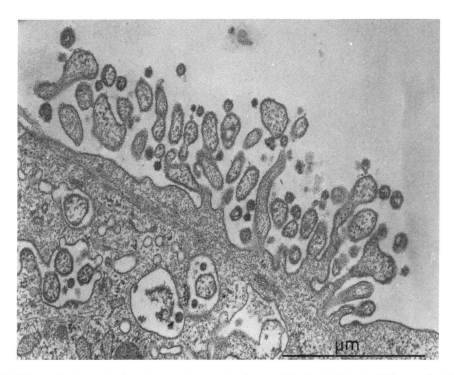

Figure 77-2 Thin-section transmission electron micrograph of mouse fibroblastic (L) cells 36 hours after infection with lymphocytic choriomeningitis virus (×55,000). Viruses are seen either released or budding from the plasma membrane. Internal granules and fuzzy surfaces caused by spikelike projections can be seen. (Courtesy Klaus Mannweiler, Heinrich-Pette-Institut, Hamburg.)

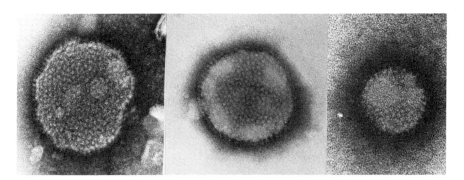

Figure 77-3 Pichinde virus negatively stained. (×180,000.) This composite shows variation in size of particles and in the degree of negative contrast penetration. Closely spaced surface projections are seen affixed to a membranous envelope without apparent symmetry. (Courtesy J. David Gangemi, University of South Carolina, Columbia, S.C.)

antigens distinct for each species are primarily structures of the envelope. In the past, intraspecies differences were recognized by pathogenicity, but now they can also be determined by oligonucleotide fingerprints. Little is known about the molecular biology of arenavirus–cell interactions.

The multiplication of this virus group is depicted on the first page of the chapter and described in detail in Chapter 63.

Pathogenesis

One of the central unresolved questions in arenavirus research is why viruses that are virtually nonpathogenic in their rodent hosts cause severe, sometimes fatal, disease in humans. The arenaviruses are not ordinarily contagious among humans; rodent-to-human infections are the usual route of infection. Although aerosol and respiratory spread are suspected, the portal of entry of these viruses as well as the time course of their systemic distribution is uncertain. Onset of the hemorrhagic fevers caused by Lassa, Junin, and Machupo viruses may be insidious, with the disease presenting itself within 7–14 days after infection simply as pyrexia, headache, sore throat, and myalgia. Virus can be recovered from the blood and serum up to 3 weeks after onset of the infection and, with Lassa, up to 5 weeks in the urine. Hemorrhagic phenomena heralded by unremitting high fever can begin after the fifth day of illness. This is followed by dehydration and hemoconcentration, shock syndrome, hemorrhagic manifestations, and cardiovascular collapse. The pantropic nature of these viruses is revealed by their presence in various dysfunctional organs.

Compared to the dramatic clinical course and mortality rate, the gross pathology is unimpressive and of little help in constructing a pathogenetic scheme. Complete autopsies have not been performed in cases of Lassa and Bolivian hemorrhagic fevers; however, autopsies performed on cases of Argentine hemorrhagic fever show a lack of deposited immunoglobulin and complement component C3 in the kidneys and small blood vessels. With no evidence for immunopathology, direct virus-induced endothelial damage leading to increased fragility and permeability of capillary beds is a distinct possibility. Although lymphocytic choriomeningitis can produce severe disease in humans characterized by prominent neurologic manifestations, pathologic lesions have not been studied extensively.

Host Defenses

Following overt human infection with arenaviruses, antibodies develop. These have been detected by complement-fixation, neutralization, and fluorescence antibody techniques. The humoral response is exceptionally slow, but ultimately a long-lasting and vigorous production of antibodies occurs. Usually, antibodies demonstrable by immunofluorescence are the first to appear, followed by complement-fixing antibodies. These complement-fixing antibodies are short-lived with titers diminishing rapidly 6-12 months after onset. In contrast, neutralizing antibodies remain detectable for many years. Although cell-mediated immunity plays a prominent role in arenavirus infections of experimental animals, its importance in human infections has not been assessed. Induction of alpha interferon has been found in patients with Argentine hemorrhagic fever. Although no apparent association between interferon levels and severity of disease has been noted, animal models have shown that interferon may actually enhance the pathogenicity of certain arenavirus infections. All evidence suggests that viral clearance in humans is complete and that chronic infection is not established. There is no evidence of reinfection in humans.

Epidemiology

The arenaviruses exist in nature as benign infections in restricted rodent hosts. The infection is usually lifelong with persistent viruria and viremia. The only exception is Tacaribe virus, which was isolated from *Artibeus* bats. In every case in which a human arenaviral disease has been studied, an interface between human activity and rodent activity has been described; the one common characteristic of these zoonotic infection patterns is human contact with rodent excreta. For example, Junin virus exposure occurs primarily when Argentine agricultural workers enter maize fields at a time when large numbers of reservoir rodents are disturbed by crop harvesting. In recent years, significant numbers of lymphocytic choriomeningitis infections have been attributed to silently infected pet hamsters and hamsters in biomedical laboratory colonies.

In humans, Lassa virus has caused explosive hospital-associated infections in Africa with case fatality rates of 30%-60%. The case fatality rates for Junin and Machupo viruses, the causal agents for Argentine and Bolivian hemorrhagic fevers, respectively, range from 5%-25%. Lymphocytic choriomeningitis virus, which is found worldwide in *Mus musculus*, is considered to be the agent in about 5% of central nervous system infections of virus origin; these infections may be debilitating but they are rarely fatal. The other arenaviruses—Amapari, Latino, Parana, Pichinde, Tacaribe, and Tamiami— can cause infections in laboratory personnel, especially when high concentrations of virus are being processed.

Diagnosis

Differential diagnosis of the arenaviral hemorrhagic fevers is complex. Consideration must be given to the arenaviruses that are prevalent in those geographic areas where infections have occurred and in those areas known to harbor reservoir rodent species. Various diseases leading to sepsis with disseminated intravascular coagulation and shock can be confused with diseases caused by arenaviruses. Other viruses also must be considered along with lymphocytic choriomeningitis in differential diagnosis of aseptic meningitis. Primary isolation of Junin and Machupo viruses is done by intracerebral inoculation of newborn hamsters. Lassa virus is regularly isolated by inoculation of Vero cells. The most sensitive method for isolating lymphocytic choriomeningitis is intracerebral inoculation of weanling mice.

All arenaviruses appear to share similar antigenic determinants in their ribonucleoproteins; however, in actual practice, positive immunofluorescent staining of acetone-fixed infected cells is definitive for more than just family identification. Thus, with limiting dilutions of antibody, old world viruses (Lassa and lymphocytic choriomeningitis) can be readily distinguished from new world viruses. Each arenavirus appears to contain unique surface glycoproteins; living cells stained by fluorescein-labeled antibodies, as well as tests based on infectivity neutralization, will differentiate species.

Control

A successful rodent control program in areas affected by Bolivian hemorrhagic fever has been described. Although this elimination of virus shedders has protected humans, few people consider it a reasonable long-term approach in other parts of the world. The need for vaccines for each of the pathogenic arenaviruses is apparent, but vaccine development is still in a formative stage. Although several classes of antiviral compounds have been found with specific in vitro activity, only one (ribavirin) has been found to be effective in animal models. Plasma from convalescent patients has become the single specific therapeutic adjunct for patients severely ill with Lassa, Bolivian, and Argentine hemorrhagic fevers. Physicians attending patients are convinced that such plasma is valuable if given during the first 5 days of disease, but more controlled trials are needed. At least 7 serologically distinct strains of Lassa fever virus have been isolated; animal studies suggest that effective therapy should involve geographic matching of immune plasma and virus strain. Early admission to the hospital with bed rest and careful attention to oral hydration, sedation, and analgesia is important. In view of the frequency of Lassa virus transmission from person to person in a hospital setting, strict measures must be taken to isolate patients who have or are suspected of having the disease. Isolation is also probably desirable in cases of the other pathogenic arenaviruses.

References

Buchmeier, M.J., et al.: The virology and immunobiology of lymphocytic choriomeningitis virus infection. *Adv Immunol* 1980; 30:275–331.

Casals, J.: Arenaviruses. In *Viral infections of humans,* 2nd ed. Evans, A.S., (editor). New York: Plenum Press, 1982.

Lehmann-Grube, F., et al.: Persistent infection of mice with the lymphocytic choriomeningitis virus. In: *Comprehensive virology,* vol 18. Fraenkel-Conrat, H., Wagner, R.R., (editors). New York: Plenum Press, 1983.

McCormick, J.B., Johnson, K.M.: Viral hemorrhagic fevers. In: *Tropical and geographic medicine.* Warren, K.S., Mahmoud, A.A.F., (editors). New York: McGraw-Hill, 1984.

Peters, C.J.: Arenaviruses. In: *Textbook of human virology.* Belshe, R., (editor). Littleton, Mass.: PSG Publishing Company, Inc., 1984.

Rawls, W.E., Leung, W.C.: Arenaviruses. In: *Comprehensive virology,* vol 14. Fraenkel-Conrat, H., Wagner, R.R., (editors). New York: Plenum Press, 1979.

78 Orthomyxoviruses

Robert B. Couch, MD

6 to 8 –

Helical,
Pleomorphic
80-120nm

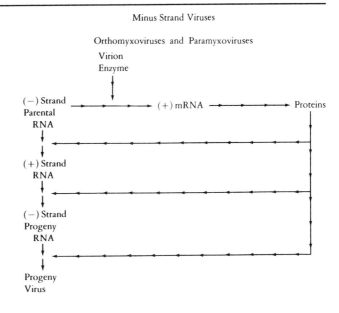

General Concepts

The orthomyxoviruses consist of one genus (the influenza viruses) and three types (species): A, B, C. These viruses are enveloped, have a nucleocapsid with helical symmetry, and contain a segmented RNA genome. The RNA is of opposite polarity to

---

The diagrams of the virion morphology and the multiplication scheme are derived from Chapters 62 and 63, respectively. The multiplication scheme applies only generally as indicated in Chapter 63.

mRNA. The influenza viruses cause influenza, an acute respiratory disease with prominent systemic symptoms. Despite a prominence of systemic symptoms, infection rarely spreads beyond the respiratory mucosa. Protection is mediated by antibody; IgG antibody is primarily responsible for preventing infection of the lower respiratory tract, whereas IgA antibody is needed for optimal prevention of infection of the upper respiratory tract. Type A viruses cause periodic worldwide epidemics (pandemics) in human populations; both types A and B cause recurring regional and local epidemics. In temperate climates, these recurring epidemics typically occur in winter and cause considerable morbidity in all age groups.

The pattern of recurring influenzal epidemics is primarily attributable to the ability of types A and B influenza viruses to exhibit antigenic variation. The surface antigens of these viruses periodically undergo change so that little or no antigenic relationship to surface antigens of earlier viruses is demonstrable. Renewed susceptibility of human populations results and, in combination with the winter factors, is the basis for epidemics. Complicating pneumonia may occur and lead to death, particularly in elderly persons with underlying chronic disease. An inactivated vaccine containing the current A and B viruses is recommended for prevention of influenza in selected population groups—notably, those at risk for a complicating pneumonia. The drug amantadine is effective for prevention and treatment of type A influenza.

Recurring epidemics and pandemics of influenza have been documented since A.D. 1173. In the past 83 years, the United States has experienced 55 epidemics accompanied by an excess of deaths over the number expected; most notable was the 1918 pandemic, which was associated with about 20 million deaths in the world and about 500,000 deaths in the United States. Prevention of this great plague constitutes one of the most significant challenges of modern medicine.

Distinctive Properties

Structure

Influenza virus particles are spherical and are 80-120 nm in diameter, although filamentous forms may also occur. A diagrammatic representation of a portion of an influenza A or B virus is shown in Figure 78-1. The nucleic acid is single-stranded (−) RNA (opposite polarity from mRNA). It occurs in eight separate segments with nucleoprotein covers and exhibits helical symmetry. The capsid is covered by a lipid bilayer. As a consequence of containing a lipid coat, the influenza viruses are rapidly inactivated by lipid solvents and surface-active agents. The two surface glycoproteins, hemagglutinin and neuraminidase, possess a hydrophobic sequence of amino acids; these glycoproteins are attached to the envelope by insertion of the hydrophobic "tail" into the lipid bilayer. The capsid contains more hemagglutinin (so named because it is the attachment unit responsible for agglutination of red blood cells by virus) than neuraminidase. Influenza C is less well studied but appears to have only 7 segments and to contain only a single glycoprotein.

Major Antigens

Three influenza viral antigens—the nucleoprotein, hemagglutinin, and neuraminidase— are useful for classification. The nucleoprotein antigen is antigenically stable and is used

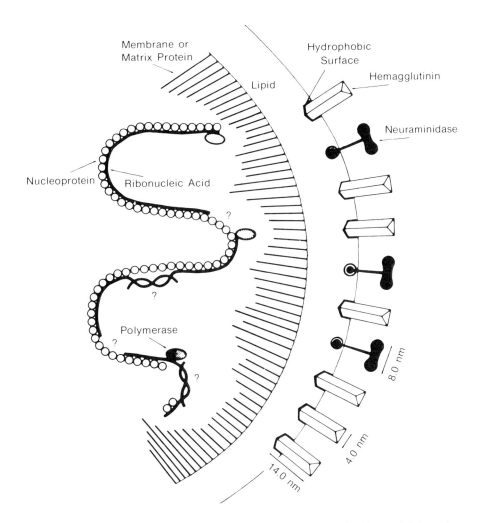

Figure 78-1 Diagrammatic representation of segment of influenza virus particle. Hemagglutinin and neuraminidase subunits, which protrude as spikes from surface of virus, are attached by their hydrophobic regions to lipid envelope. Ratio of hemagglutinin to neuraminidase spikes varies from strain to strain, but relative distribution of these on surface of virus particle is not known. Orientation of nucleoprotein RNA complex in virion has not been fully elucidated; these complexes occur in segments when extracted from virion but may be linked within virion by labile bonds. Polymerase activity has been demonstrated within core of virion. From Webster, R.G., Laver, W.G.: In: *Influenza viruses and influenza.* Kilbourne, E.D. (editor). New York: Academic Press, p. 276.

for designation of type. No serologic cross-reactions are exhibited between the nucleoprotein antigens of types A, B, and C viruses. Hemagglutinin and neuraminidase antigens exhibit antigenic variation; antibody directed against these antigens is associated with immunity to infection.

Replication

Attachment of influenza viruses to permissive cells during initiation of the infection process is mediated by the hemagglutinin subunit. Although it was formerly assumed that attachment occurred by binding to a glycoprotein receptor containing *N*-acetyl neuraminic acid similar to that found on red blood cells, more recent studies indicate that this process may be mediated through a receptor of different specificity. Penetration presumably begins by pinocytosis, and uncoating results from fusion between the lipid bilayer of the pinocytotic vesicle and the plasma membrane. Unlike other RNA viruses, orthomyxovirus replication depends on the presence of functional host cell DNA. Active transcription of host cell DNA provides a pool of newly synthesized messenger RNA that must be present because orthomyxoviruses utilize the cap structure of nascent host messenger RNA. RNA replication occurs in the nucleus, and proteins are synthesized on cytoplasmic ribosomes. The nucleocapsid is assembled in the nucleus; virion assembly takes place at the plasma membrane and mature virus is released by budding. The lipid bilayer is acquired during the budding process. Proteolytic cleavage of the hemagglutinin by host cell enzymes takes place during the assembly-budding process and is required for released particles to be infectious. Newly synthesized virions possess surface glycoproteins containing *N*-acetyl neuraminic acid as a part of their carbohydrate structure. A major function of the neuraminidase is the enzymatic removal of these *N*-acetyl neuraminic acid residues to disrupt or prevent the occurrence of aggregates and thereby increase the number of free infectious particles. The entire replicative process requires only about 6 hours. Cell death results from the infection.

Effect of Antibody on Infectivity

Antibody to the hemagglutinin binds to virions and prevents initiation of infection. If added after infection occurs, antibody reduces the number of infectious units released, presumably because divalent antibody promotes aggregation of many individual virions into one infectious unit. Antibody to nucleoprotein has no effect on virus infectivity.

Gene Reassortment

As a consequence of their segmented genome, influenza viruses exhibit a phenomenon called gene reassortment. In cells simultaneously infected with two antigenically different type A viruses, assembly of progeny virus may result in incorporation of RNA segments from both of the infecting viruses. Thus, the gene segments of progeny virus may be derived from either parental strain. This phenomenon is illustrated in Figure 78-2. This ease of gene reassortment probably accounts for the periodic appearance of new variants of type A viruses (see discussion of epidemiology). The multiplication of this virus group is depicted on the first page of the chapter and described in detail in Chapter 63.

Pathogenesis

Transmission of influenza virus infection is primarily by the airborne route. When coughing and sneezing, infected persons produce small particles of respiratory secretions that are inhaled by susceptible persons and deposited in the lower respiratory tract. The primary site of disease is the tracheobronchial mucosa, although the nasopharynx is also involved. Since virus deposits first in respiratory secretions, the

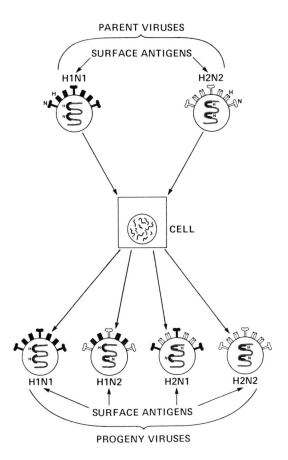

Figure 78-2 Example of reassortment of influenza virus genes for two different surface antigens leading to occurrence of progeny viruses containing surface antigen from each parent.

action of neuraminidase on the residues of *N*-acetyl neuraminic acid in mucus may produce liquefaction and, in concert with mucociliary transport, promote spread of virus throughout the respiratory tract. Infection of mucosal cells results in cellular destruction and desquamation of the superficial mucosa. Edema and mononuclear cell infiltration of involved areas occur and are accompanied by such local symptoms as nonproductive cough, sore throat, and nasal discharge. Although cough may be striking, the most prominent symptoms of influenza are fever, muscle aches, and general prostration. Viremia is rare, and other explanations of the striking systemic symptoms of influenza have not been found.

Current evidence indicates that the extent of virus-induced cellular destruction is the prime factor in determining occurrence, severity, and duration of illness. In an uncomplicated case, virus may be recovered from respiratory secretions for 3 to 8 days. Peak quantities of 10^4-10^7 infectious units per mL of secretion are detected at the time of maximal illness. After a 1 to 4 day period of peak titers, progressive reduction in titer ensues; this fall is accompanied by progressive improvement in symptomatology.

On occasion, particularly in persons with underlying heart or lung disease, viral involvement of alveolar tissues of the lung may be extensive; interstitial pneumonia, sometimes with marked accumulation of lung hemorrhage and edema, may also occur (pure viral pneumonia). Virus titers in secretions from these persons may be high and virus shedding prolonged. The illness usually is severe with a high mortality rate. Pneumonia in association with influenza is, however, more commonly caused by bacteria. In these cases, viral infection has presumably impaired the normal lung defense mechanisms, thus promoting invasion by pneumococci, staphylococci, or gram-negative bacteria.

Host Defenses

The immune mechanisms responsible for recovery from influenza have not been delineated, although several mechanisms acting in concert seem likely. Interferon appears in secretions shortly after occurrence of peak titers of virus; reduction in titers of virus in secretions follows. Antibody usually is not detected in serum or secretions until later in recovery or during convalescence; nevertheless, local antibody appears to be responsible for final clearance of virus from secretions. T cell and antibody-dependent cellular cytotoxicity probably contribute to clearance of the infection.

Antibody is the primary host defense against acquisition of infection. IgG antibody appears to be the primary mediator of resistance; it predominates in lower respiratory secretions and is derived primarily from serum. This accounts for the close correlation between serum antibody titer and resistance. IgA antibody that predominates in upper respiratory secretions, and is less persistent than IgG antibody, also contributes to the resistance. For prevention of infection, antibody must be directed against the hemagglutinin. Antibody to the neuraminidase is associated with a lessened intensity of infection and occurrence of an asymptomatic infection or mild illness. Antibody to the hemagglutinin may similarly lessen intensity of infection when insufficient for prevention.

A potent immunity to reinfection with an antigenically identical influenza virus lasts for years; the periodic reinfections that occur are attributable to antigenic change of surface antigens, which results in renewed host susceptibility.

Epidemiology

The pattern exhibited by a typical epidemic of type A influenza in an urban community is shown in Figure 78-3. In the initial phases of an epidemic, infection and illness appear predominantly in school-aged children, as indicated by a sharp rise in school absences, physician visits, and pediatric hospital admissions. These children bring the virus into the home, where preschool children and adults acquire infection. Infection and illness in adults are reflected in industrial absenteeism, adult hospital admissions, and an increase in mortality from pneumonia–influenza. An epidemic generally spans 3 to 6 weeks, although virus is present in the community for a variable number of weeks before and after the epidemic period.

The highest attack rates of illness during type A epidemics are in the 5 to 19 year age group, although high frequencies occur in preschool children and adults of all ages. Influenza B exhibits a similar epidemic pattern, although preschool children and adults usually exhibit lower attack rates, and an increase in expected numbers of deaths may not occur.

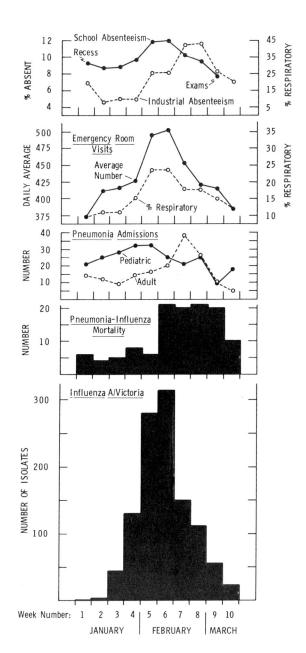

Figure 78-3 Correlation of nonvirologic indexes of epidemic influenza with number of isolates of influenza A/Victoria virus according to week, Houston, 1976. (Industrial absenteeism is indicated by percent with respiratory complaints.) Reprinted by permission from *New England Journal of Medicine,* 298:589, 1978.

Virus types A and B (and probably C) cause infections and illnesses every winter. An epidemic may not occur, however. The constellation of factors needed to cause an epidemic has not been delineated, but the most significant factor is a population susceptible to the circulating viruses.

The recurring susceptibility of populations is attributable to antigenic changes of the surface antigens of influenza viruses. When surface antigens change, a proportion (sometimes all) of the population lacks immunity to a new virus. The magnitude of the ensuing epidemic is directly proportional to the degree of antigenic change. A major change in one or both of the surface antigens so that no serologic relationship to earlier antigens is demonstrable has been called **antigenic shift.** Such changes are responsible for pandemics of influenza and have been demonstrated for type A viruses only. Repeated minor antigenic changes occur between pandemics and are responsible for epidemics of varying frequency and magnitude. These changes are called **antigenic drift,** and a serologic relationship to earlier surface antigens can be shown. This type of change has been demonstrated for types A and B viruses.

When persons are reinfected with drift viruses, serum antibody responses to surface antigens on the earlier viruses are frequently higher and of greater avidity than are responses to the new antigens. This phenomenon, which has been called "original antigenic sin," is sometimes useful in serologic diagnosis. Its role in immunity is uncertain.

Major change (shift) represents acquisition of new antigens through gene reassortment; the donor of new surface antigens is probably an animal influenza virus. Type A viruses have been identified in pigs, horses, and birds, and animal viruses with antigens closely related to those of human viruses have been described. Minor antigenic change (drift) results from selection of naturally occurring variants by the pressure of population immunity.

Since the initial isolation of influenza viruses from swine in 1931 and from humans in 1933, antigenic monitoring of human viruses has been performed. The current classification and years of prevalences of human viruses are shown in Table 78-1. As noted in the table, the recurrence of the H1N1 subtype in 1978 suggests that all possible major changes have been identified and that recycling of earlier viruses is beginning.

When a new subtype arises, it spreads around the world along transportation routes. Seeding of populations with new virus occurs during the "off season" and may cause

Table 78-1 Classification of Human Influenza Viruses*

Type	Subtype	Years of Prevalence	Selected Variants*
A	H1N1†	1918–1957‡	A/Puerto Rico/8/34
			A/FM/1/47
	H2N2 (Asian)	1957–1967	A/Singapore/1/57
	H3N2	1968–	A/Hong Kong/1/68
			A/Philippines/2/82
	H1N1	1977–	A/USSR/90/77
			A/England/333/80
B	none defined	1940–§	B/Singapore/222/79
C	none defined	1949–‖	C/JHB/2/66

*Variants (drift) are monitored by using a reference strain described by subtype/geographic origin/strain number/year of isolation.
†Earlier classifications of this subtype included separate designations for Hsw1N1, H0N1, and H1N1. All are now designated as the H1N1 subtype.
‡An influenza virus was first isolated from swine in 1931 and from humans in 1933; retrospective serologic studies indicated a swine/31-like virus became prevalent in humans in 1918.
§First isolated from humans in 1940.
‖First isolated from humans in 1949.

localized outbreaks, but epidemics generally begin in the fall after school opens or in the succeeding winter.

Diagnosis

The influenza syndrome is an illness of sudden onset with fever, malaise, headache, marked muscle aches, sore throat, nonproductive cough, and rhinorrhea. When this syndrome occurs in the winter in an adult (illnesses and etiologies are more complex in children), an influenza virus is a likely cause. If an epidemic of febrile respiratory illness is occurring in a community (excess school and industrial absenteeism), the diagnosis is more certain. Nevertheless, a diagnosis based on such information is presumptive; a definitive diagnosis requires isolation of the virus or demonstration of a significant rise in antibody titer between that occurring in the sera of patients acutely affected and that following convalescence.

Tissue cultures or chicken embryos may be used to isolate influenza virus from respiratory secretions. Virus growth in tissue cultures is detected by testing for hemadsorption, which consists of adding red blood cells to the culture and observing for red cell adherence to cells. (Red cells adhere to virus budding from the surface of infected cells.) Specific viral identification of these positive cultures must be accomplished by serologic means such as immunofluorescence with specific antisera. Fluid from the amniotic or allantoic cavity of chicken embryos is tested for the presence of newly formed viral hemagglutin; virus in positive fluids is then identified by hemagglutination-inhibition tests with specific antisera. Tests for serum antibody rise may be performed by various techniques; complement fixation, hemagglutination-inhibition, and immunodiffusion (using specific viral antigens) are most commonly used. None of these techniques will detect all infections.

Control

Prevention

Inactivated influenza viral vaccines have been used to prevent influenza for about 35 years. Virus for vaccines is grown in chicken embryos, inactivated by formalin, purified to an extent, and adjusted to a dosage known to produce an antibody response in most persons. Vaccines generally contain the types A and B viruses most likely to produce infections in the subsequent winter. They are given parenterally in the fall; one or two doses are required, depending on the immunologic experience of the population with related antigens. Protection against illness has varied from 50% to 90% in civilian populations and from 70% to 90% in military populations. Only minor local and systemic reactions occur in the first day or two after vaccination. During the national swine immunization campaign of 1976 in the United States, an increased risk of developing the Guillain-Barré syndrome accompanied vaccination; however, since then a similar risk from vaccination has not been confirmed.

Inactivated influenza virus vaccine currently is recommended in the United States for annual use in persons at risk of developing pneumonia and dying from influenza. Such high-risk persons are those over age 65 years and those with chronic underlying disease, particularly cardiovascular and respiratory disease. Live attenuated vaccines currently are being developed as alternatives to inactivated vaccine.

The synthetic drug amantadine hydrochloride effectively prevents infection and illness caused by type A, but not by type B, viruses. This drug interferes with uncoating of the virus and has been shown to prevent about 50% of infections and about 67% of illnesses under natural conditions. When administered to household contacts of a person with influenza for a 10-day period, it may protect up to 80% of persons from illness. The usual dosage is 100 mg twice daily. Side effects are limited primarily to the central nervous system.

Treatment

Specific antiviral treatment is limited to use of amantadine. If started early in the course of illness, amantadine treatment hastens the disappearance of fever and symptoms of illness caused by type A influenza viruses.

References

Beare, A.S., (editor). *Basic and applied influenza research.* Boca Raton, Fla.: CRC Press, 1982.

International Conference on Asian Influenza. *Am Rev Resp Dis* 1961; 83:1-219.

International Conference on Hong Kong Influenza. *Bull WHO* 1969; 41:335-748.

Kilbourne, E.D., (editor): *The influenza viruses and influenza.* New York: Academic Press, 1975.

Nayak, D., Fox, C.F., (editors): *Genetic variation among influenza viruses: ICN-UCLA symposia on molecular and cellular biology,* Vol. XXII. New York: Academic Press, 1981.

Pollock, R.R., et al.: Monoclonal antibodies: A powerful tool for selecting and analyzing mutations in antigens and antibodies. *Ann Rev Microbiol* 1984; 38:389-417.

79 Paramyxoviruses

Gisela Enders, MD

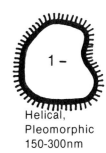

Helical,
Pleomorphic
150-300nm

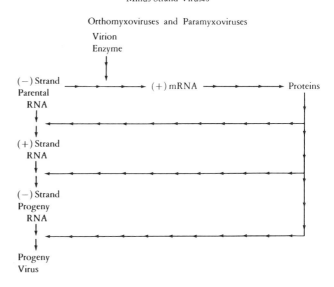

Minus Strand Viruses

Orthomyxoviruses and Paramyxoviruses

The diagrams of the virion morphology and the multiplication scheme are derived from Chapters 62 and 63, respectively. The multiplication scheme applies only generally as indicated in Chapter 63.

General Concepts

The human paramyxoviruses are important causes of respiratory and other diseases in children. For example, the parainfluenza group and respiratory syncytial viruses are responsible for most of the croup, bronchiolitis, and pneumonitis in infants and young children. The predominant features of mumps are parotitis and sometimes meningitis. Measles is characterized by conjunctivitis, coryza, and rash and is occasionally complicated by pneumonia and encephalitis; in rare instances, measles recurs as chronic encephalitis (subacute sclerosing panencephalitis). Thus, paramyxoviruses cause many of the common and severe childhood diseases (Table 79-1). Newcastle disease virus, a pathogen of the respiratory tract of chickens, may cause conjunctivitis in humans.

The family of Paramyxoviridae consists of three genera: *Paramyxovirus*, *Morbillivirus*, and *Pneumovirus* (Table 79-2). All members of the genus *Paramyxovirus* share similar properties. The separate genus of *Morbillivirus* is distinguished by the absence of neuraminidase in the virions and by the presence of common envelope and nucleocapsid antigens in the species listed in Table 79-2. Pneumoviruses lack hemagglutinin and neuraminidase activity; they also differ in morphology (diameter of nucleocapsid and surface projections) from the other members of the Paramyxoviridae family.

Structurally, the virions of the human Paramyxoviridae family are enveloped particles with an average diameter of 150–300 nm. The complete virion consists of two

Table 79-1 Diseases Caused by Paramyxoviruses*

		Disease	
Virus	*Age*	*Common*	*Less Common*
Parainfluenza 1–4	Any age	URTI, † Pharyngitis	None
1 + 2	Infants	Croup (laryngotracheobronchitis)	
3	Infants	Bronchiolitis Pneumonitis	
Mumps	Children and young adults	Parotitis Meningitis Orchitis	Pancreatitis Encephalitis Oophoritis Thyroiditis Myocarditis
Newcastle disease‡	Adults		Conjunctivitis
Measles	Young children	Measles (rash, coryza, conjunctivitis)	Otitis media Pneumonia Encephalitis SSPE§
Respiratory Syncytial	Any age Infants	URTI Bronchiolitis Pneumonitis	

*Adapted from Fenner, F., White, D. O.: *Medical virology*, 2nd ed. New York: Academic Press, Inc., p. 390, 1976.
†URTI, Upper respiratory tract infection.
‡Rare laboratory infection contracted from fowls.
§SSPE, subacute sclerosing panencephalitis.

Table 79-2   Family Paramyxoviridae

Genus	Species	Host
Paramyxovirus	Parainfluenza virus types 1, 2, 3, 4A, 4B	Humans
	Mumps virus	Humans
	Newcastle disease virus	Animals and humans
Morbillivirus	Measles virus	Humans
	Canine distemper virus	Animals
	Rinderpest virus	Animals
	Peste des petits ruminants virus (PPRV)	Animals
Pneumovirus	Respiratory syncytial virus	Humans
	Pneumonia virus of mice	Animals

components: the nucleocapsid and the envelope. The nucleocapsid is a tubelike structure with helical symmetry (Figure 79-1). It contains the genome, a nonsegmented single-stranded $(-)$ RNA (approximately 7×10^6 mol. wt.), the major structural nucleoprotein, and an RNA-dependent RNA polymerase, which is necessary for the transcription of viral RNA. The envelope is a double-layered membrane covered with spikes; it contains lipoproteins and glycoproteins and glycolipids that are mainly derived from the host cell. Also, a nonglycosylated membrane protein is attached to the underside of the envelope. The glycosylated protein, involved in hemagglutinating and neuraminidase activities, is located in the spikes. Another envelope protein is involved in hemolytic and cell-fusing activities. Virus multiplies by attaching to mucoprotein receptors of cells and penetrating the cell by fusion with the cell membrane. Replication occurs in the cytoplasm and, unlike myxoviruses, seems not to depend on functioning cellular DNA. Maturation and release of the virion takes place by budding through the cytoplasmic membrane. Virion infectivity is lost readily when the envelope is disrupted

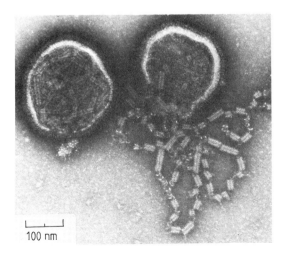

100 nm

Figure 79-1 Parainfluenza virus type 1, Sendai strain. An intact virion and a disintegrating particle with free nucleocapsid fragments. Courtesy Dr. June Almeida, The Wellcome Research Laboratories, Beckenham, England.

spontaneously or by treatment with lipid solvents and by several chemical and physical reactions.

Two main sets of antigens are present: viral and soluble. The viral antigen is associated with the envelope structures and the soluble antigen, with the nucleocapsid. Among the genera, no antigenic relationship exists. The species of *Paramyxovirus* possess distinct viral and soluble antigens but share minor common components of the viral antigens. The members of *Morbillivirus* possess common nucleocapsid and viral envelope antigens. Within the *Pneumonvirus* genus, no common viral or soluble antigens have been found. Each member of the *Paramyxovirus* and *Morbillivirus* occurs in a single serotype, whereas the respiratory syncytial virus is suspected to exist in at least two subtypes. All members of the Paramyxoviridae family are antigenically stable, and genetic recombination has not been found (Table 79-3).

Host range is mainly limited in vivo to humans and monkeys; in vitro, these viruses multiply in cell cultures and, except for respiratory syncytial viruses, in embryonated eggs (see Table 79-3). Virus multiplication in cell cultures produces lytic or presistent infections. Lytic infections begin with formation of multinucleated giant cells (**syncytia**) by the action of the cell-fusing factor, eventually leading to cell necrosis. Multiple

Table 79-3   Antigenic and Biologic Properties of Certain Human Paramyxoviridae

	Parainfluenza	*Mumps*	*Measles*	*Respiratory Syncytial*
Number of serotypes	4*	1	1	1†
Serologic cross-reactions	Mumps	Parainfluenza	—	—
Antigenic cross-reactivity	—	—	Distemper Rinderpest Peste des petits ruminants	—
Surface antigens:				
Hemagglutinin	+	+	+‡	—
Neuraminidase	+	+	—	—
Hemolysin	+	+	+‡	—
Complement fixing	+	+	+	+
Growth in eggs	(+)§	+	(+)	—
Growth in tissue culture‖	+	+	+	+
Cell fusion	+	+	+	+
Hemadsorption	+	+	+‡	—
Inclusions	Cytoplasmic	Cytoplasmic	Nuclear and cytoplasmic	Cytoplasmic
Natural disease in animals	None	Monkey¶	Monkey	Chimpanzee
With animal strains	Monkey, mice, cattle, dog, horses			Cattle, mice

*A fifth serotype is being considered.
†Two or more subtypes are reported.
‡Monkey erythrocytes only, at 37C.
§After adaption in tissue culture.
‖The hemagglutinin titer of the tissue culture harvest can be significantly increased by Tween 80 ether splittng.
¶Experimental infection.

acidophilic inclusions develop in the cytoplasm and sometimes in the nucleus of these giant syncytial cells. Some paramyxoviruses cause chromosome damage in the infected cells. In persistent infection, the virus does not mature or release virions; however, an experimental technique of fusing virus-susceptible cells with persistently infected cells allows complete virions to develop. This cell fusion technique has been used to allow measles virus (normally defective in subacute sclerosing panencephalis brain cultures [see Measles section]) to develop and be isolated.

Those species of the Paramyxoviridae family that cause important human disease (parainfluenza viruses, mumps virus, measles virus, and respiratory syncytial virus) are discussed in this chapter.

PARAINFLUENZA VIRUSES

Parainfluenza viruses account for approximately 30%-40% of all acute respiratory infections in infants and children. The spectrum of disease ranges from a mild, afebrile cold to severe, potentially life-threatening croup, bronchiolitis, and pneumonia. These viruses are the most common identifiable agents causing the croup syndrome and are exceeded only by respiratory syncytial virus as a cause of severe lower respiratory tract disease in infants. Reinfection, causing milder upper respiratory illness, is common in older children and adults.

Four human parainfluenza serotypes are presently recognized: 1, 2, 3, and 4. Type 4 occurs in two subtypes (A and B), possessing common soluble but different viral antigens. A fifth serotype infects animals.

Distinctive Properties

The parainfluenza viruses have all the properties of the family Paramyxoviridae (see General Concepts section). Antigenic relatedness exists among all paramyxoviruses in the genus (parainfluenza virus types, mumps virus, and Newcastle disease virus), as reflected in *heterotypic anamnestic antibody responses.*

Pathogenesis

The parainfluenza viruses generally initiate localized infections in the upper and lower respiratory tracts without causing systemic infection, although viremia may occur. Local and serum antibodies develop after primary infection. The resulting immunity is not adequate to prevent reinfection, but does provide some protection against disease.

Human parainfluenza viruses with appropriate tissue tropism implant in the ciliated epithelial cells of the respiratory mucosa. These viruses first infect the epithelium of the nose and throat; infection may extend to the paranasal sinuses, the middle ear, and occasionally to the lower respiratory tract. New progeny virus spreads among cells extracellularly and intracellularly. Virus is shed in the respiratory secretions over 3–16 days. Shedding starts shortly before onset of disease and ends with development of local antibody. The main pathogenic change is an inflammatory response in the superficial layers of the mucous membranes.

The most characteristic and important clinical syndromes associated with parainfluenza virus infection are croup, bronchiolitis, and pneumonia. The most severe manifestation of infection with types 1 and 2 is croup, whereas type 3 causes all three syndromes. Croup caused by parainfluenza virus is not distinguishable from that caused by other viruses such as respiratory syncytial or measles virus.

Host Defenses

Human species resist infection by animal parainfluenza viruses. Nonspecific defenses (including interferon) may contribute to resistance against human parainfluenza viruses (see Chapter 68). The immunologic events during and after natural infection with parainfluenza viruses in infants and children are not well defined. Type-specific secretory and humoral immune responses take place, but protection does not last, since reinfection with the same serotype may occur within 3 months to several years after primary infection. The degree of resistance to reinfection and, even more, to clinical disease seems to depend mainly on the concentration of secretory IgA antibodies that possess neutralizing activity. Neutralizing IgA is found in infants and young children only for a short time after primary infection. Serum antibodies usually do not play a significant role in resistance to reinfection with the nonsystemic respiratory viruses, but their presence in high titers may restrict local virus multiplication and disease manifestation. Passive maternal antibodies do not protect against infection; however, they appear to prevent disease manifestations with types 1 and 2, but not with type 3 in infants. Also maternal antibodies may suppress the immune response following primary infection. Serum antibodies induced by inactivated parainfluenza virus vaccine neither protect against nor enhance disease.

Epidemiology

The parainfluenza viruses are distributed worldwide, causing infection and illness in young children of all races, in all areas, and in all climates. In contrast to parainfluenza virus types 1, 2, and 3, infection with types 4A and 4B are somewhat less frequently encountered, perhaps due to difficulty in isolating the virus. Parainfluenza virus infections are endemic, sometimes reaching epidemic proportions (particularly with types 1 and 2) (Table 79-4).

The source of human parainfluenza virus infection is the respiratory tract of humans, and the incubation period ranges from 2 to 6 days. In primary infection, the duration of contagion ranges from 3 to 16 days, depending on the virus type and severity of disease. During reinfections, the contagious periods get progressively shorter. Transmission of the parainfluenza viruses occurs by direct person-to-person contact and by the airborne route through large droplet spread, with only a small inoculum required to infect. Being labile, however, parainfluenza viruses do not persist in the environment. These viruses are spread mainly by infants and preschool children with only mild signs of infection. Serologic surveys show that at the age of 5 years, 90%-100% of children possess antibodies for type 3; 74% for type 1; and 58% for type 2. The age-specific seropositive rates for types 4A and 4B are undetermined.

Table 79-4 Clinical and Epidemiologic Characteristics of Parainfluenza Virus Infections*

| Human Serotype | Clinical Manifestations | | Epidemic Behavior of Infection and Disease | | |
	Peak Age	Severe	Mild (Common)	Pattern	Periodicity	Peak Season
Primary Infection						
1	>6–30 mon.	Croup	Febril URTI†	Epidemic‡	Even years	Fall
2	>6–30 mon.	Croup, tracheobronchitis	Afebrile URTI	Epidemic (erratic)	Odd years	Fall/winter
3	1–24 mon	Pneumonia, bronchiolitis, croup	Febril URTI	Endemic (small outbreaks)	Throughout every year	Late spring
4 A and B	>24 mon.	NI§	URTI	Sporadic	NI§	
Reinfection	<6 yrs.					
1	Within a	Rare	Cold,			
2	few months		bronchitis			
3 high rate	to years in children and adults					

*Adapted from Glezen, W. P., Loda, F. A., Denny, F. W.: *Viral Infections of Humans, Epidemiology and Control.* Evans, A. S. (editor). New York: John Wiley and Sons, p. 344, 1976; and from Hendley, J. O.: Paramyxoviridae. In: *Principles and Practice of Infectious Disease,* Vol. 2. Mandell, G. I., Douglas, R. G., Bennett, J. F., (editors). New York: John Wiley & Sons, p. 1173, 1979.

†URTI, upper respiratory tract infection (cold).

‡Variable pattern: endemic to sharp epidemics.

§No information.

Diagnosis

Because sporadic disease caused by parainfluenza virus has no distinguishing features, etiologic diagnosis based on clinical manifestations is not possible. Laboratory diagnosis can be made by isolating the virus in tissue culture. Isolation is fairly easy with nasopharyngeal secretions taken within 4 days after onset of illness in types 2 and 3 infections. Isolation is difficult for type 1 and is particularly so for types 4A and 4B. More rapid diagnosis is accomplished by fluorescent antibody staining of nasopharyngeal cells, and by detection of viral antigens and/or antibodies in sonicated nasopharyngeal specimens by indirect radioimmunoassay and enzyme-linked immunosorbent assay (ELISA).

Serologic evidence of infection may be obtained by conventional and newer techniques (complement fixation, hemagglutination inhibition, neutralization, indirect fluorescence, RIA, and ELISA) for demonstrating significant antibody rises between two serum samples. Serodiagnosis by these means is hampered by the heterotypic anamnestic responses to previous parainfluenza and mumps virus infection. The indirect fluorescence test, the RIA, the indirect and direct ELISA, and the hemadsorption immunosorbent techniques (HIT) allow detection of class-specific antibodies in secretions and serum. A rapid and usually reliable type-specific serodiagnosis of acute infection can now be made when significant levels of the transient IgM antibodies are found in a single serum sample.

Control

Cross-infections with parainfluenza virus types 1 and 3 are common in hospital wards and children's homes. These can be prevented by strict isolation. Recent techniques that allow rapid diagnosis facilitate such control.

Active immunization against parainfluenza viruses is desirable but not yet available. Experimental killed vaccines are not effective. Experimental live virus vaccines have failed to induce protective secretory antibody levels. Passive prophylaxis with human immunoglobulin in exposed infants is not indicated because it may dampen an active serum antibody response. Chemoprophylaxis with amantadine and rimantadine has been shown to be effective in vitro against parainfluenza viruses but has not been tested clinically. No specific therapy for parainfluenza virus infection exists. Supportive care is important.

MUMPS VIRUS

Mumps is a common acute disease of children and young adults, characterized by a nonpurulent inflammation of the salivary glands, especially the parotids. Severe manifestations may include meningitis and encephalitis at any age and orchitis in postpubertal males. Most disease manifestations are benign and self-limiting. Both symptomatic and asymptomatic mumps virus infections induce life-long immunity. An effective live virus vaccine is available.

Distinctive Properties

Mumps virus belongs to the *Paramyxovirus* genus (see Table 79-2) and exhibits most characteristics of the Paramyxoviridae family (see General Concepts section). It occurs only in a single serotype and shares minor common envelope antigens with other paramyxoviruses in the genus. The commonality of these antigens results in reciprocal, heterotypic, anamnestic rises in antibody.

Pathogenesis

Mumps virus causes a systemic infection spread by viremia with target organ involvement of glandular and nervous tissues. The infecting virus probably enters the body through the pharynx or the conjunctiva. Local multiplication of the virus at the portal of entry and possibly a primary viremia precedes a secondary viremia lasting 2-3 days. The virus is carried to the main target organs (various salivary glands, testes, ovaries, pancreas, and brain), where viral replication takes place. The incubation period usually is 18-21 days. Recognizable symptoms do not appear in 35% of infected individuals.

Shedding of the virus in salivary gland secretions begins about 6 days before onset of symptoms and continues for another 5 days, even though humoral antibodies become detectable during that time. Although also found in conjunctival secretions and urine, the virus usually does not spread from these sites due to low virus titers, virus instability, and sanitation. During the first two days of illness, the virus may be recovered from blood leukocytes, where it may replicate in T lymphocytes. In cases of meningitis or encephalitis of early onset, virus can be detected in cerebrospinal fluid and cells during the first 6 days after onset of disease. The virus may persist in tissues for 2-3 weeks after the acute stage, despite the presence of circulating antibodies.

The main pathogenic changes induced by mumps virus infection in the salivary glands and the pancreas are inflammatory reactions. When the testes are involved, swelling, interstitial hemorrhage, and local areas of infarction (leading to atrophy of the germinal epithelium) may occur. Infection of the pancreas disturbs endocrine and exocrine functions, leading to diabetic manifestations and increased serum amylase levels.

The pathologic reaction to mumps virus infection of brain tissues is generally an aseptic meningitis. Altered encephalograms are uncommon, suggesting that the meninges rather than the brain are the common sites of involvement. Less often, when the infection involves the brain neurons (as in mumps encephalitis of early onset), the meningeal component is a minor aspect of the disease. Histopathologic findings are widespread neuronolysis and ependymitis, which may lead to hydrocephalus in children. The late onset (postinfectious) type of mumps encephalitis is attributed to autoimmune reactions. Histopathologic findings are characterized by perivascular accumulation of mononuclear leukocytes, demyelinization, and overgrowth of glial cells, with relative sparing of the neurons. These findings resemble those seen in postinfectious measles, rubella, and varicella encephalitis.

The most characteristic clinical feature of mumps virus infection is the edematous, painful enlargement of one or both of the parotid glands. Commonly, the submandibular salivary glands are involved and, less frequently, the sublingual glands. Pancreatitis is uncommon as a severe illness, but a mild degree of upper abdominal pain occurs frequently. A distressing clinical manifestation is epididymoorchitis, which develops in 23% of infected postpubertal males. Epididymoorchitis may lead to atrophy of the affected testicles, though rarely to total sterility. Oophoritis develops in 5% of infected postpubertal women. Other glands (thyroid, breast, prostate, and liver) are involved rarely. Mumps meningitis occurs in up to 10% of patients with or without parotitis; in 40%-50% of patients with mumps meningitis, the meningitis is the sole disease manifestation. Encephalitis has been reported to occur in 1 of 400 cases of mumps. Transient high-frequency deafness is the most common complication (4%), and permanent unilateral deafness occurs infrequently (0.005%).

Host Defenses

Mumps virus infection is followed by interferon production and by specific cellular and humoral immune responses. Interferon, which limits virus spread and multiplication, is found in detectable levels in the serum and salivary gland secretions during the first 3-4 days of acute illness. Interferon production ceases as virus levels decrease and humoral antibodies and cell-mediated immunity appear. Little is known about cell-mediated immunity to mumps virus; in contrast, the humoral antibody response is well understood. IgM class-specific antibodies to mumps antigens develop rapidly within the first 3 days after onset of symptoms and persist for approximately 2-3 months. The IgG antibodies appear a few days later and persist for life.

Circulating antibodies are responsible for the life-long protection against recurrent disease, even though inapparent reinfection with mumps virus occasionally may occur in persons with very low antibody levels. Parainfluenza virus infections cause a rise of mumps antibody titers, contributing to the life-long stability of the mumps antibody. Protective mumps antibody of the IgG class is transplacentally transferred to the newborn and persists in declining titers during the first year of life.

Epidemiology

Mumps occurs worldwide. In urban areas, the infection is endemic with a peak incidence between January and May. Local outbreaks are common wherever large numbers of children and young adults are concentrated (institutions, boarding schools, and military camps). Epidemics occur every 2-7 years. In rural areas, mumps tends to die out until enough susceptible individuals have accumulated and the virus is reintroduced. Humans are the only known hosts.

Infection is transmitted mainly by salivary gland secretions. Peak contagion occurs just before and shortly after clinical onset; in asymptomatic infections, peak contagion occurs within a similar period. Transmission of mumps virus occurs usually by direct person-to-person contact and less often by the airborne route. The main spreaders are school children 6-14 years old. Since mumps virus is less contagious than the other paramyxoviruses, transmission requires more intimate contact. Also, mumps infection is acquired later in childhood than are other paramyxovirus infections.

Serologic surveys in unvaccinated populations show that 25% of children have been infected by age 2; 45% by age 5; 80% by age 10; 90% by age 14; and 95% by age 15. As already mentioned, 35% of infections are subclinical. In remote rural areas, a much lower percentage of children may be infected. Vaccination has reduced the incidence of reported mumps and mumps complications by over 90%.

Diagnosis

Typical cases of mumps involving the salivary glands can usually be diagnosed without laboratory tests; however, an etiologic diagnosis of other clinical manifestations (for example, meningitis, encephalitis, orchitis, and oophoritis), if they occur without parotitis, require laboratory confirmation. An individual's immunity resulting from natural infection or immunization may be established by detection of specific antibody. Diagnosis of acute infections can be made by isolating the virus from saliva or urine (or CSF when appropriate), usually in tissue culture over several days or, more rapidly, by detecting specific antigen in infected specimen using immunofluorescence, ELISA, or RIA. Serologic evidence of acute infection and vaccine effectiveness may be obtained early by demonstrating IgM antibodies in the first serum specimen and later by a significant IgG antibody rise in paired sera.

Control

In view of the long period of contagion and the 35% rate of subclinical infection, isolating patients with typical symptoms does little to prevent spread. Passive prophylaxis with mumps immunoglobulin is used for individuals at high risk, for example, children with underlying disease, those in hospital wards, postpubertal males, and pregnant women. The success of this measure is questionable if the immunoglobulin is administered after viremia has occurred. New serologic techniques assess immunity in 6 hours so that immunoglobulin may be given only to exposed seronegative (susceptible) individuals.

Active immunization against mumps is recommended for all children at 15 months of age. A combined live virus vaccine is available for mumps, measles, and rubella. The mumps component contains attenuated virus grown in chick embryo tissue culture. It is well tolerated and safe and usually is effective only when maternal antibodies are absent. The vaccine-induced antibody titers are initially lower than those following natural infection; this antibody protects against clinical disease but not against reinfection. Long-term duration of vaccine-induced immunity seems to be maintained by inapparent reinfection with mumps wild-type virus and probably also by frequent parainfluenza infections.

No specific drugs or therapeutic measures are available for treatment of mumps virus infection. Management is purely symptomatic. Fortunately, disease manifestations generally are self-limited, and death is rare.

MEASLES VIRUS

Measles virus causes an acute childhood disease characterized by coryza, conjunctivitis, fever, and rash. The disease usually is benign but can be dangerous, causing pneumonia and acute encephalitis. Defective measles virus may cause subacute sclerosing panencephalitis and possibly other chronic neurologic diseases. A live vaccine has markedly reduced incidence in developed countries, but measles remains a major health problem in developing countries.

Distinctive Properties

Measles, canine distemper, rinderpest, and peste des petits ruminants viruses comprise the genus *Moribillivirus* of the family Paramyxoviridae (see Table 79-2). The virion of measles virus shares structure (see Figure 79-1) and most other properties with other paramyxoviruses but is distinguished by the lack of neuraminidase and by hemagglutination activity restricted to monkey erythrocytes. Measles and the other moribilliviruses occur only as one antigenic type, antigenically stable but cross-reactive, giving rise to heterologous antibody responses.

The natural disease is limited to humans and monkeys. The other moribilliviruses cause economically important disease resembling measles in their natural hosts (distemper in dogs, rinderpest in cattle, and peste des petits ruminants in sheep and goats) but are noninfectious for humans. In vitro, the host range of measles virus is human, monkey, and canine cell cultures and the embryonated egg (see Table 79-3).

Pathogenesis

Measles virus causes a systemic infection, disseminated by viremia, with acute disease manifestations involving the lymphatic and respiratory systems, the skin, and sometimes the brain. Inapparent infections are rare. Measles virus may persist for years in some individuals and cause subacute sclerosing panencephalitis.

Measles virus enters the host through the oropharynx and possibly through the conjunctiva. Local virus multiplication in the respiratory tract and the regional lymph nodes is followed by a primary viremia with virus spread to the rest of the reticuloendothelial system, where extensive replication takes place. A second viremia, which occurs 5-7 days later, disseminates virus to the mucosa of the respiratory, gastrointestinal, and urinary tracts, to the skin, and to the central nervous system. With development of serum antibodies, free virus is quickly cleared from the blood and body fluids but persists for varying times in lymphoid, lung, and bladder tissue. In subacute sclerosing panencephalitis patients, measles virus antigen can be identified regularly in the brain and lymph nodes, but infectious virus can be "rescued" only occasionally by cocultivation of brain and lymph node explant cultures with measles-susceptible cells.

The main pathologic change directly or indirectly attributable to viral replication in the main target organs is an inflammatory response. Virus-infected cells contain virus antigens and inclusions in cytoplasm and nuclei; the cells may fuse to form giant cells. The pathology and pathogenesis of postinfectious (allergic) measles encephalitis are the same as those characterizing other viruses.

The temporary loss of delayed skin hypersensitivity during measles may be due to virus multiplication in T and B lymphocytes. Simultaneous onset of rash with the appearance of serum antibodies suggests an allergic cause of the exanthem. Abnormal encephalograms are common during measles, suggesting frequent viral invasion of the brain.

Clinically, measles is characterized by the upper respiratory tract symptoms during the prodromal stage and the maculopapular rash during the eruptive phase. After an incubation period of 9-12 days, the prodromal stage starts with malaise, fever, coryza, cough, and conjunctivitis. At the end of this stage, the pathognomonic Koplik's spots (red spots with bluish white specks in their centers) appear in the oral mucosa opposite the second molars. One to 2 days later, the rash appears, first on the head and then spreading down the body and limbs, including the palms and soles. First erythematous and maculopapular, the rash later becomes confluent. The uncomplicated illness lasts 7-10 days. Otitis media caused by bacterial superinfection is the most frequent complication. Primary viral or secondary bacterial pneumonia is the most common complication responsible for hospitalization and fatal outcome of measles. Purely viral complications are croup, bronchiolitis, and the fatal giant-cell pneumonia; these often occur without rash in immunocompromised children.

A rare but severe form is *hemorrhagic (black) measles*. *Atypical measles syndrome* (high fever; urticarial, purpuric rash resembling varicella that begins peripherally with centripedal spread; and atypical pneumonia) tends to be severe. This syndrome is an allergic response to measles infection in adolescents and young adults who were inadequately immunized (mainly with killed measles vaccine) in childhood.

Measles encephalomyelitis has a frequency of 0.1% with a mortality rate of 20%. Permanent sequelae (neurologic disorders, epilepsy, and personality changes) follow in 20%-40% of cases. *Subacute sclerosing panencephalitis* (SSPE) is a rare, chronic, usually lethal encephalitis that develops in children and adolescents some years after the original attack of measles.

Mild (modified) measles develops in children possessing low levels of maternally derived or injected antibodies.

Host Defenses

Little natural resistance to measles virus infection exists. Nonspecific substances such as interferon appear to contribute to early limitation of virus spread. Interferon may be detected until virus-specific antibodies appear. The cell-mediated immune response is associated with recovery from primary infection and also with resistance to reinfection at the portal of virus entry. The humoral immune response helps eliminate extracellular virus during primary infection and prevents systemic or body surface reinfection. Supporting evidence is the extreme severity of measles in some patients with T cell immunodeficiency. In contrast, children with hypo-γ-globulinemia have normal disease and resist reinfection. This evidence, however, is not definitive because viral antigens require T cell help to induce antibodies and because hypo-γ-globulinemic patients produce low but effective levels of serum antibodies.

The humoral immune response (anti-V and anti-S antibodies) occurs in the three immunoglobulin classes in measles as in other paramyxovirus infections. Life-long persistence of serum antibodies may be due to persistence of virus antigen. Maternal IgG antibodies completely protect the infant for 6 months; between 6 and 12 months of age, subclinical infection or modified disease may occur.

In patients with subacute sclerosing panencephalitis, strikingly high titers of measles antibody (IgG) are present in serum and CSF. Antibodies in the CSF are oligoclonal.

Most patients with subacute sclerosing panencephalitis lack antibodies to the nonglyco-sylated membrane protein.

Epidemiology

Measles occurs throughout the world in all races and all climates with humans as the only host. The main factors accounting for the epidemiologic pattern are universal susceptibility to infection in the absence of antibody, extreme contagiousness, population density, and standard of living.

Thus, measles infection has become endemic in most areas of the world. Sporadic cases occur throughout the year with peak incidence in the late winter and early summer months. Epidemics arise every 2–4 years in developed urban areas and every 4–8 years in rural areas, when the number of susceptible persons reaches about 40% of the population. The epidemics last 3–4 months, until the percentage of susceptible persons falls below 20%. Local outbreaks occur in crowded institutional settings, even when less than 2% of the population is susceptible. Introduction of measles into a fully susceptible population results in explosive epidemics with nearly 100% becoming infected within 6 weeks.

The source of infection is the virus-containing respiratory tract secretions, either airborne or transmitted by fomites. The contagious period lasts about 6 days, beginning with the prodromal symptoms and persisting until about 2 days after rash develops, at which time antibodies first appear.

In developed societies, measles occurs between 4 and 7 years of age. In underdeveloped societies, measles occurs before age 4. By age 7 to 12 years, in all but the most isolated areas, nearly 100% of children have had measles and possess specific antibodies.

In countries using vaccine (particularly the United States), the incidence of reported disease and its complications has dropped more than 95%; as a result, decreased transmission partly accounts for a transitory shift to older teenagers. The incidence of measles encephalitis is almost twice as great in teenagers as in younger children.

Subacute sclerosing panencephalitis follows natural measles at an estimated rate of 6–20 cases for every million children developing measles. The risk of subacute sclerosing panencephalitis from live measles vaccine is one-tenth that from natural infection.

Diagnosis

Clinical diagnosis of measles is easy when the characteristic symptomatology is present. Laboratory diagnosis helps during uncharacteristic exanthems, atypical measles, pneumonia, or encephalitis after a rash, and also in suspected cases of giant-cell pneumonia and of subacute sclerosing panencephalitis.

Laboratory diagnosis may be made until about 2 days after onset of rash by demonstrating multinucleated giant cells or fluorescent antibody-staining cells in nasal secretions, urine, and skin biopsies. Isolation of measles virus in tissue culture is difficult and therefore not suitable for routine diagnosis.

More commonly, measles virus infection is diagnosed by detecting significant complement-fixing, hemagglutinin-inhibiting, or neutralizing antibody rises using two serum samples taken during the first and second weeks after the rash appears. Use of the newer solid-phase techniques (ELISA and RIA) permits serodiagnosis of acute measles infection to be made with a single serum specimen, taken as early as 3–4 days after the rash appears, by demonstrating significant levels of IgM antibodies. A specific serologic diagnosis of subacute sclerosing panencephalitis can be made by demonstrating extremely high antibody levels in the serum and CSF.

Control

Quarantine is futile because by the time the rash signals the disease, shedding has been in progress for 2 or 3 days. Passive prophylaxis with measles immunoglobulin is recommended for exposed, susceptible individuals, especially those at high risk (for example, cancer, immunosuppressed, and immunodeficient patients, infants under 1 year of age, and pregnant women). To completely prevent measles infection, an appropriate dose of immunoglobulin must be given early enough (within 3 days of exposure) to prevent viremia. Application of immunoglobulin between the fifth and ninth days after exposure no longer can prevent the secondary viremia, but will modify the disease and allow immunity to develop. Modification of disease also can be achieved within 3 days of exposure by reducing the dose of immunoglobulin. Immunoglobulin may protect recipients for about 4 weeks.

Active immunization with the combined measles-mumps-rubella live-virus vaccine is recommended for all healthy 15-month-old children. Vaccine-induced antibody develops in about 95% of the seronegative recipients and persists in declining titers for more than 16 years in the absence of further exposure to virus. Reexposure may cause an antibody booster response (without illness) only if antibody titers are low. If the prevalence of wild measles virus is reduced by vaccination, infections that boost antibody diminish in frequency, and revaccination may have to be considered; however, the present purpose of revaccination is to immunize the primary vaccine failures (about 5%). Live-virus vaccine also should be given to anyone who does not have a history of measles or who has not received live-virus vaccine since the age of 15 months.

No specific treatment for measles, measles encephalitis, or subacute sclerosing panencephalitis is available. Management is symptomatic and supportive. Bacterial superinfection should be treated with appropriate antimicrobials, but prophylactic antibiotics to prevent superinfection have no known value and are contraindicated.

RESPIRATORY SYNCYTIAL VIRUS

Respiratory syncytial virus, the major cause of bronchiolitis and pneumonia in infants under 1 year of age, is the most important etiologic agent of respiratory tract disease of early childhood. Reinfection is common in children and adults, causing mainly upper respiratory tract illness. Mounting evidence suggests that lower respiratory tract illness in infancy may predispose to chronic lung disease in later life. Respiratory syncytial virus is named for the respiratory disease it produces and for its characteristic syncytial (cell-fusing) cytopathic effect during isolation in cell culture.

Distinctive Properties

The respiratory syncytial viruses belong to a separate genus, *Pneumovirus* (see Table 79-2), because of their distinctive morphologic features (club-shaped surface projections and a nucleocapsid diameter of 13 nm rather than the 18 nm characteristic of the other genera [Figure 79-2]) and because they lack hemagglutinin and neuraminidase activity. No antigenic relationship exists between the members of the *Pneumovirus* genus. Respiratory syncytial virus behaves in the human host as a single serotype. The host range of respiratory syncytial virus is limited in vivo to humans and chimpanzees and in vitro to tissue culture (see Table 79-3).

Pathogenesis

Respiratory syncytial virus generally initiates a localized infection in the upper or lower respiratory tract or both. The degree of illness varies with the host's age and previous experience with this virus.

Initially, the virus infects the surface ciliated mucosal epithelial cells of the nose, eye, and mouth. Infection generally is confined to the epithelium of the upper

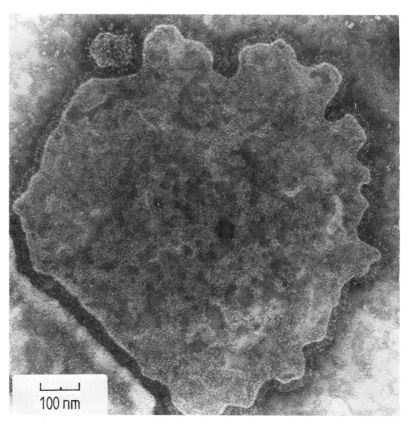

Figure 79-2 Respiratory syncytial virus, showing club-shaped spikes. Courtesy Dr. June Almeida, The Wellcome Research Laboratories, Beckenham, England.

respiratory tract, but may involve the entire lower respiratory tract. The virus spreads extracellularly after release from infected cells and also directly by fusion of cells, so that humoral antibodies that do not penetrate intracellularly cannot completely restrict infection. The virus is shed in respiratory secretions usually for about 5 days and sometimes for as long as 3 weeks. Shedding begins with the onset of symptoms and declines with the appearance of local antibody.

The most important clinical syndromes caused by respiratory syncytial virus are bronchiolitis and pneumonia in infants, croup and tracheobronchitis in young children, and tracheobronchitis and pneumonia in the elderly. Conjunctivitis, otitis media, and various exanthems involving the trunk or face or both are occasionally seen in primary and secondary infections.

During bronchiolitis, the bronchiolar epithelial cells undergo necrosis. Subsequent changes are accumulation of lymphocytes around bronchioles, plugging of small bronchioles, collapse of the corresponding portion of the lung, and obstructive emphysema. During pneumonia, the pulmonary lesions are characteristic of interstitial pneumonitis. Some morphologic alterations may persist after the acute infection.

The pathogenesis of bronchiolitis remains an open question; some support exists for the suggestion that immunopathologic (hypersensitivity) mechanisms are partially responsible. Alternatively, the severe illness in infancy and the pathogenesis of bronchiolitis can be attributed to the destructive effect of the virus on the small peripheral airways and the contributory role of immunologic immaturity (see next section).

Host Defenses

Nonspecific defenses such as virus-inhibitory substances in secretions and interferon production probably contribute to resistance to respiratory syncytial virus infection and recovery from it. Age, immunologic competence, and physical condition also appear to be important. Data on the development, persistence, and effectiveness of specific cell-mediated and secretory immunity in first and repeat infections are still fragmentary. Although secretory and serum antibody responses take place, immunity does not protect completely against reinfection and repeat illness, which may occur as early as a few weeks after recovery from the first infection. Secretory and serum antibody responses are poor in young infants.

Resistance to reinfection and repeat illness seems to depend mainly on the presence of neutralizing activity in the throat and on the concentration of the IgA secretory antibody. Preexisting serum antibody, even in high levels, is not protective. Serum antibody may be immunosuppressive or may even cause a paradoxical effect, for example, the enhanced disease associated with maternal or vaccine-induced antibodies. Breast milk that contains antibodies to respiratory syncytial virus may have some protective effect, but definite proof is lacking (see discussion of control).

Epidemiology

Respiratory syncytial virus is distributed worldwide, causing infection and illness in infants and young children of all races, in all areas, and all climates. The infection is endemic, reaching epidemic proportions every year. In temperate climates, these epidemics occur each winter and last 4-5 months with peaks mainly from January to March. Estimates for urban settings suggest that about half the susceptible infants undergo primary infection in each epidemic, the infection being almost universal by the second birthday. Reinfection may occur as early as a few weeks after recovery but usually takes place during subsequent annual outbreaks with a rate of 10%-20% per epidemic throughout childhood; in adults, frequency of reinfection is lower.

The source of human respiratory syncytial virus infection is the respiratory tract of humans; the incubation period is about 4 days. As noted earlier, in primary infections, the contagious period may range from about 5 days to 3 weeks, depending on the severity of disease. Usually, large quantities of virus are shed in the first 4-5 days after onset of symptoms. During reinfection, the contagious periods get progressively shorter. Transmission of the virus occurs by direct person-to-person contact and by the airborne route through large droplet spread, but the virus may also be transmitted from contaminated skin surfaces. Respiratory syncytial virus is probably introduced into families by school children undergoing reinfection; secondary spread is to younger siblings and parents. In hospital and institutional settings, mildly symptomatic infected adults also spread the infection. Respiratory syncytial virus readily infects infants during the first few months of life despite the presence of maternal serum antibodies. Thus, the age at which first infection takes place depends primarily on the opportunity for exposure.

Most infants exhibit upper respiratory tract symptoms and the incidence of lower respiratory tract disease varies from 15%-50%. For every 100 primary infections, one or two infants are hospitalized with bronchiolitis and pneumonia. The mortality rate in hospitalized infants is about 2%.

Sex and socioeconomic factors appear to influence the outcome of infection. Bronchiolitis and pneumonia caused by respiratory syncytial virus are more common in boys than in girls. Also, lower respiratory tract disease occurs more often and earlier in life in low socioeconomic groups and under crowded conditions.

Diagnosis

In infants with lower respiratory tract disease, respiratory syncytial virus infection can be strongly suspected based on the season of the year, the presence of a typical outbreak at the time, and the family epidemiology. Aside from this virus, only parinfluenza virus type 3 attacks infants with any frequency during the first few months of life.

Definite diagnosis of infection (of practical importance in ruling out bacterial involvement) rests on the virology laboratory. The diagnosis is made within 4-8 days by isolating the virus from nasal secretions in tissue culture or within hours by fluorescent antibody staining of infected nasal epithelial cells. Newer rapid diagnostic methods are the detection of specific antigen or secretory IgA and IgE antibodies in respiratory secretions by RIA and ELISA.

Serologic evidence of respiratory syncytial virus infection may be obtained by demonstrating seroconversion or significant antibody rises within 1-2 weeks after onset of illness. The presence of (secretory) IgA and IgE antibodies in significant concentration indicates an acute primary or secondary infection with respiratory syncytial virus.

Control

Preventing respiratory syncytial virus transmission in the home setting is nearly impossible. In hospital wards, cross-infection may be restricted by separating infected infants, washing hands, using gowns, and excluding personnel with mild respiratory tract symptoms.

Active immunization is not likely to be achieved in the near future. Inactivated vaccines induce a significant serum antibody response; however, they fail to protect and may even cause more severe disease. Research is now directed toward developing live attenuated virus vaccines to protect infants younger than 1 year of age against severe lower respiratory tract disease. Breast-feeding appears to offer the infant some protection against lower respiratory tract illness.

No specific therapy for respiratory syncytial virus infection is available. Good supportive care is essential for the severely ill child.

References

Christenson, B., Heller, L., Bottiger, M.: The immunizing effect and reactogenicity of two live attenuated mumps virus vaccines in Swedish school children. *J Biol Stand* 1983; 11:323-331.

Enders-Ruckle, G.: Frequency, serodiagnosis and epidemiological features of subacute sclerosing panencephalitis (SSPE) and epidemiology and vaccination policy for measles in the Federal Republic of Germany. *Dev Biol Stand* 1978; 41:195-207.

Evans, A.S.: *Viral infections of humans.* London: John Wiley and Sons, 1976.

Fenner F., White D.O.: *Medical virology.* 2nd ed. New York: Academic Press, 1976.

Gardner, P.S., McQuillin, J.: *Rapid virus diagnosis: application of immunfluorescence,* 2nd ed. London and Boston: Butterworths, 1980.

Hall, W.W., Lamb, R.A., Choppin, P.W.: Measles and SSPE virus proteins: lack of antibodies to the M protein in patients with subacute sclerosing panencephalitis. *Proc Nat Acad Sci USA* 1979; 76:2047-2051.

Kurstak, E., Kurstak, C.: *Comparative diagnosis of viral diseases.* Vol. 1. New York: Academic Press, 1977.

Mandell, G.L., Douglas, R.G., Bennett, J.F.: *Principles and practice of infectious diseases,* Vol. 2. New York: John Wiley and Sons, 1979.

Martin, D.B., et al.: Atypical measles in adolescents and young adults. *Ann Intern Med* 1979; 90:877-881.

Norrby, E.: In: *Virology and rickettsiology,* Vol. 1. Part 1. Hsiung, G.D., Green, R. (editors). Ft. Lauderdale: CRC Handbook Series, 1978.

Paisley, J.W., et al.: Pathogens associated with acute lower respiratory tract infection in young children. *Pediatr Infect Dis* 1984; 3:14-19.

Tyeryar, F.J.: Report of a workshop on respiratory syncytial virus and parainfluenza viruses. *J Infect Dis* 1983; 148:588-598.

Vaughan, V.C., McKay, R.J., Behrman, R.E.: *Nelson's textbook of pediatrics,* 11th ed. Philadelphia: W.B. Saunders Co., 1979.

80 Coronaviruses

Sylvia E. Reed, MB

Spikes

1 +

Pleomorphic
80-100nm

General Concepts
Distinctive Properties
Pathogenesis
Host Defenses
Epidemiology
Diagnosis
Control

General Concepts

Coronaviruses are single-stranded RNA viruses with distinctive surface projections from their envelopes. The members of this group cause a variety of infections in humans and in animals. Because human strains are difficult to isolate and cultivate, they are not well studied. Coronaviruses most commonly cause minor upper respiratory infections (colds) and are perhaps also capable of affecting the lower respiratory tract. Of the many coronaviruses affecting animals, the best known are those causing avian infectious bronchitis of chickens, mouse hepatitis, and transmissible gastroenteritis of piglets. Other coronaviruses infect rats, calves, dogs, cats, and foals. A number of the animal strains infect the intestinal tract of the host species; analogous human enteric coronaviruses have also been described.

Distinctive Properties

Coronaviruses are about 80-120 nm in diameter and tend to be pleomorphic (Figure 80-1). The particles are surrounded by a halo of club-shaped projections resembling

---

The diagram of the virion morphology is derived from Chapter 62.

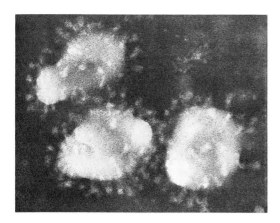

Figure 80-1 Electron micrograph showing human coronavirus 229E. The bar indicates 100 nm. Courtesy H. Davies.

spikes or petals which suggest the solar corona. These projections are longer (up to 20 nm) and usually more widely spaced than the spikes of orthomyxoviruses, to which the coronaviruses bear a slight morphologic similarity.

All coronaviruses probably share the same basic biophysical and biochemical structure, but much of the information about them derives from studies of animal strains, particularly mouse hepatitis. The internal component of coronavirus consists of RNA and protein. The nucleoprotein is coiled and forms a helical structure 9–16 nm wide that seems fragile and easily disrupted. The membrane that encloses the coronavirus particle has protein and lipid components; its club-shaped projections, called **peplomers,** are proteins. Biochemical analysis of the virions indicates that they contain polypeptides of three main classes. The first, which is phosphorylated but nonglycosylated (mol. wt. about 50,000 daltons), is associated with the internal ribonucleoprotein. The second polypeptide is glycosylated and is associated with the membrane; the third, which is also glycosylated, is associated with the peplomers. The coronaviruses of humans and of various animal species seem to differ in the number, molecular weight, and extent of glycosylation of these polypeptides. The virus particles can be destroyed by lipid solvents.

The single-stranded RNA genome (mol. wt. 6×10^6 daltons) is infectious and has a positive polarity with covalently attached polyadenylated sequences. Much of the coronavirus-specific RNA found in infected cells is of genome size, but five or six smaller classes (subgenomic RNAs) also are found. The structures of the 3' ends of all these RNAs are similar. Each RNA consists of the nucleotide sequence present in any of the smaller RNAs, plus an additional sequence, so that the genomic and subgenomic RNAs are said to form a **nested set.** These intracellular RNAs probably all act as mRNA, each directing the translation of one viral protein. It seems, therefore, that coronaviruses have an unusual and interesting replication strategy.

Coronavirus replication occurs in the cytoplasm of infected cells. The virus matures by budding into vesicles in the cell cytoplasm and is released when the cell lyses.

Although some of the animal coronaviruses can be grown relatively easily in the laboratory, human strains have very strict host cell specificities and are notoriously difficult to isolate from patients and to adapt to cell cultures. As a result, coronaviruses still pose many unanswered questions. The prototype human respiratory coronavirus, 229E, first described in 1965, and strains related to it can be grown in certain tissue cultures. Other human strains, the OC strains, are so called because most of them can be grown only in organ cultures (explants) of differentiated human respiratory epithelium originating from nasal or tracheal tissue of aborted human fetuses; the presence of virus in the culture requires confirmation by electron microscopy.

Of the human coronaviruses, strains 229E and OC43 have been studied most (Table 80-1). These two viruses are antigenically distinct. As yet, there is no definition of an antigenic type or group, and it may be difficult to make such a definition if partial sharing of antigens proves to be as common among the human coronaviruses as among coronaviruses causing infectious bronchitis of chickens. Subtypes or variants may prove to be epidemiologically important. Human coronavirus strains isolated in tissue culture all appear to be antigenically related to 229E and may thus constitute one broad type or group, and OC strains constitute at least one other such group. None of the human respiratory coronaviruses tested so far is related antigenically to the infectious bronchitis of chickens, although human strain 229E has been found to be related to certain coronaviruses of pigs, dogs, and cats, and human strain OC43 to coronaviruses of mice (mouse hepatitis), rats, and cattle. The relationship of virus structure to antigenic composition is being investigated. The surface spikes probably elicit neutralizing activity and, when it occurs, hemagglutinating activity, but definite information is sparse.

Type OC43 has been adapted to grow in brains of infant mice and also (although somewhat poorly) in tissue culture. The mouse-adapted virus, unlike other human coronavirus strains, agglutinates red blood cells so that infected tissue cultures show a weak hemadsorption known as pseudohemadsorption; these properties can be used in serologic tests. Serologic properties of the strains that grow in tissue culture can be studied by neutralization or complement fixation; neutralization tests can also be done with some difficulty in organ culture. ELISAs with 229E and OC43 antigens have been used successfully and have confirmed the antigenic difference between the two strains. All strains can be examined by the rather cumbersome techniques of fluorescent staining of viral antigen in infected cells or by immune electron microscopy.

The multiplication of this virus group is depicted on the first page of the chapter and described in detail in Chapter 63.

Table 80-1   Types of Human Coronavirus: In Vitro Cultivation and Serologic Tests

Types of Human Coronavirus	Cultivation in Vitro			Serologic Tests Available*					
	Organ Culture	Tissue Culture	Baby Mice	N	CF	IF	HI	IEM	ELISA
229E types	+	+	−	+	+	+	−	+	+
OC43	+	±†	+†	+	+	+	+	+	+
Other OC types	+	−	−	+‡	−	+‡	−	+‡	?

*N, neutralization; CF, complement-fixation; IF, immunofluorescence; HI, hemagglutination inhibition; IEM, immunoelectron microscopy; ELISA, enzyme-linked immunosorbent assay.
†After adaptation.
‡Using organ cultures.

Pathogenesis

Inoculation of human volunteers with coronaviruses has provided valuable information. Volunteers develop colds, often with profuse coryza, 2-3 days after intranasal inoculation of a coronavirus. The virus evidently multiplies in nasal epithelium and can be recovered from nasal secretions by appropriate tissue cultures or organ cultures. In adult volunteers, infections generally are brief and without pyrexia; asymptomatic infections also may occur. Natural infections with coronaviruses occur in all age groups. Lower respiratory involvement seems not to be a common feature of the infection, although coronaviruses, like rhinoviruses, have been implicated in exacerbations of asthma and chronic bronchitis.

Coronaviruses can cause chronic or persistent infections in some animals and in tissue cultures, but persistent infection in humans has not been demonstrated conclusively. Coronaviruses or coronaviruslike particles have been observed by electron microscopy in human feces, but the association of these particles with disease is not clearly established, and most attempts to cultivate the particles have not been successful.

Host Defenses

Infection may be followed by a rise in serum antibody against the infecting virus, but little is known about mechanisms of immunity to coronavirus infection. Individuals who already possess serum-neutralizing antibody may nevertheless become infected; the protective roles of nasal antibody, cell-mediated immunity, and interferon need to be investigated.

Epidemiology

Respiratory infections due to coronaviruses are most prevalent during the winter months. Accurate assessment of the overall proportion of colds and other respiratory infections caused by coronaviruses is difficult because relatively few types have so far been identified; however, the proportion approximates 15% and at times of coronavirus prevalence may be considerably higher. All age groups are affected. The infection seems to spread readily in families; spread is probably by airborne droplets, although direct evidence of this does not exist.

Diagnosis

Coronavirus infections cannot be distinguished clinically from other viral respiratory infections. Laboratory diagnosis usually is made by examining paired sera to detect rising antibody titers. Viral strain 229E is used in complement-fixation or neutralization tests and strain OC43 in complement-fixation or hemagglutination-inhibition tests. ELISA methods may supplement these. Rising antibody titers against 229E or OC43 may also be produced by infection with heterologous but related viruses.

Virus may be isolated from nasal swabs or washings by using human embryo nasal or tracheal organ cultures. Strain 229E and related strains sometimes can be isolated directly in human embryo kidney cells, diploid human embryo fibroblast lines, or other sensitive cells, but isolation may be easier after preliminary passage in organ culture. The cytopathic effect in tissue culture is not distinctive; the presence of coronavirus in the cultures is confirmed by electron microscopy and use of reference antisera. Identification of coronavirus in nasal secretions by ELISA also has been described.

Control

Neither vaccination nor chemoprophylaxis is available for human coronavirus infections.

References

Bradburne, A.F., Bynoe, M.I., Tyrrell, D.A.J.: Effects of a "new" human respiratory virus in volunteers. *Br Med J* 1967; 3:767-769.

Cukor, G., Blacklow, N.R.: Human viral gastroenteritis. *Microbiol Rev* 1984; 48:157-179.

Kapikan, A.Z., et al.: Isolation from man of "avian infectious bronchitis virus-like" viruses (coronaviruses) similar to 229E virus, with some epidemiological observations. *J Infect Dis* 1969; 119:282-290.

Monto, A.S.: Medical reviews: Coronaviruses. *Yale J Biol Med* 1974; 47:234-251.

Siddell, S., Wege, H., Ter Meulen, V.: The biology of coronaviruses. *J Gen Virol* 1983; 64:761-776.

81 Rhabdoviruses

Alice S. Huang, PhD

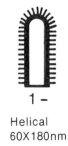

1 -

Helical
60X180nm

General Concepts
Distinctive Properties
Pathogenesis
Host Defenses
Epidemiology
Diagnosis
Control

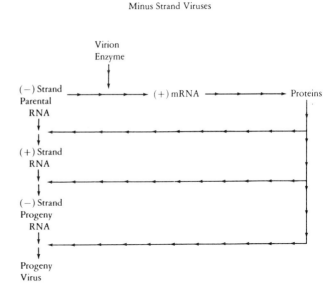

Minus Strand Viruses

General Concepts

The rhabdovirus group consists of diverse bullet- or bacilliform-shaped RNA viruses; it includes rabies virus, which is the only established human pathogen in this group, and vesicular stomatitis virus, a pathogen for cattle. Other animal rhabdoviruses cause disease in fish (Egtved virus) and in *Drosophila* (sigmavirus).

The diagrams of the virion morphology and the multiplication scheme are derived from Chapters 62 and 63, respectively. The multiplication scheme applies only generally as indicated in Chapter 63.

Rhabdoviruses have a broad host range and infect vertebrates, invertebrates, and plants. In animals, the virus is introduced into a wound through the bite of an arthropod or an animal. The encephalitis that induces aggressive biting behavior clearly plays a role in the survival of rabies virus. Rhabdoviruses are remarkably stable to freeze-drying and remain viable in the dried state for long periods of time.

Infectious rhabdovirus is bullet-shaped and measures 180 by 65 nm. Noninfectious deletion mutants occur frequently and form shorter, bullet-shaped particles, which can be physically separated from the wild-type virus. Reconstruction experiments with these mutants show that they form a special class called **defective interfering particles.** Not only are defective interfering particles noninfectious, but they interfere with replication of infectious virus. For rhabdoviruses especially, differences in the proportion of defective interfering particles during an infection may partly account for variability in host response and seriousness of the disease (see Chapter 68).

Distinctive Properties

Rhabdoviruses consist of a lipid envelope, covered on the outside with the surface glycoprotein, and associated on the inside with the matrix protein (Figure 81-1). Inside the envelope is a core composed of a single-stranded RNA genome covered with the RNA-binding nucleocapsid protein and associated with the highly phosphorylated protein and the virion-associated polymerase protein. These structural proteins range in molecular weight from 25,000 to 241,000 daltons.

The RNA of vesicular stomatitis virus has now been completely sequenced. Of the approximately 12 kilobases, 99% are utilized for coding the five structural proteins. Distributed at the ends of the genome, as well as in between the coding regions, there are a total of 117 nucleotides that control replication and gene expression (Figure 81-2).

The strategy of replication of the rhabdoviruses follows the general scheme of all negative-strand viruses. The virus attaches, penetrates, and is uncoated to the core stage. The core initiates the primary transcription of all five complementary, small RNAs utilizing the incoming RNA as template and the virion-associated RNA-dependent RNA polymerase as enzyme. Each RNA is then translated into an individual protein. Once protein synthesis is accomplished, replication of the genome RNA proceeds by the synthesis of a full-sized complementary RNA, which in turn acts as template for the synthesis of more genome RNA. These new genome RNAs can lead to amplified transcription or genome replication as well as to association with structural proteins and budding out of the cell as progeny virions.

The multiplication of this virus group is depicted on the first page of the chapter and described in detail in Chapter 63.

Pathogenesis

Rabies virus, the only rhabdovirus with medical significance in humans, usually enters the body by a bite; it may also enter by exposure of a wound to infected saliva or it may be inhaled. The virus multiplies in cells at the inoculation site and then moves toward the central nervous system. The incubation period lasts from 10 to 14 days up to several months, depending on the severity of the wound, the amount of virus inoculated, and the degree of innervation of the muscle involved. The virus spreads rapidly via nerves.

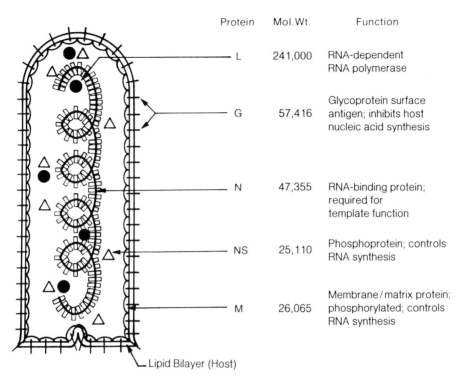

Protein	Mol. Wt.	Function
L	241,000	RNA-dependent RNA polymerase
G	57,416	Glycoprotein surface antigen; inhibits host nucleic acid synthesis
N	47,355	RNA-binding protein; required for template function
NS	25,110	Phosphoprotein; controls RNA synthesis
M	26,065	Membrane/matrix protein; phosphorylated; controls RNA synthesis

Lipid Bilayer (Host)

Figure 81-1 Vesicular stomatitis virus.

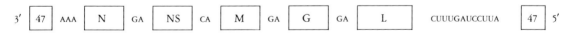

Figure 81-2 Genome of vesicular stomatitis virus. Single-stranded RNA, 12 kilobases. 47, leader noncoding nucleotides. N, NS, M, G, and L = VSV genes. See Figure 81-1, which describes the function of the gene products.

Damage to the central nervous system produces disease. Neurons of the sensory system accumulate viral ribonucleoprotein as intracytoplasmic inclusions called **Negri bodies.** Areas of the brain most vulnerable to rabies virus infection are the thalamus, the hypothalamus, and the pons. Infection of these areas causes overt disease consisting of fever, acute excitation, dilatation of the pupils, excessive lacrimation and salivation, and anxiety. Hydrophobia develops from spasms of the throat muscles, stimulated by the act or even the thought of swallowing. In contrast to **furious rabies, dumb rabies** results from ascending paralysis and depression. In humans, both forms almost always lead to death.

Host Defenses

Interferon, antibody, cell-mediated immunity, and defective interfering particles are protective when present before or during the early stages of infection; however, during the primary natural infection it is not known whether these defenses are evoked sufficiently early and in sufficient quantities to affect the outcome. Only about one-half of subjects bitten by a rabid animal contract the disease. One possible explanation for this is that the virus is not transmitted because it is not present in the animal saliva at the time of the bite, or because it is trapped in the clothing covering the bitten area. Another possibility is that, during the early phase of the infection, some defensive mechanisms may control virus infection in the nondiseased individuals. Once the disease becomes clinically evident, death occurs almost invariably, suggesting that natural defenses and current therapeutic approaches are unable to control the overt infection of the central nervous system.

Epidemiology

The only rhabdovirus now known to cause disease in humans is rabies virus; however, other viruses of this group ultimately may be found to cause human diseases. Latency and persistence of rhabdoviruses have been shown in various animal species (birds, bats, and arthropods) without causing overt disease.

Rabies virus normally resides in and causes diseases among domestic and wild animals. Dogs, cats, cattle, bats, foxes, skunks, and raccoons are common hosts; however, probably all terrestrial mammals are susceptible. In the United States, 8% of animals examined in 1981 were positive for rabies. Transmission to humans usually occurs by animal bites. However, this is not always necessary. In many instances, virus can penetrate small, preexisting wounds exposed to the saliva of an infected animal, or it can be inhaled, but this type of infection is mostly confined to spelunkers exposed to virus aerosols from asymptomatically infected bats.

Rabies in humans and dogs has virtually disappeared in certain areas of North America (for example, Massachusetts) because of required vaccination of dogs and careful monitoring of wildlife. The disease still prevails in parts of the Americas, Europe, Africa, and Asia. Eradication of rabies virus from a geographic location may not be permanent because of the uncontrolled migration of infected wild animals. More than 10,000 human cases of rabies per year are estimated to occur throughout the world.

Diganosis

Diagnosis of rabies is based on a history of exposure to a rabid animal, clinical manifestations of encephalitis, and laboratory findings. Confirmation of rabies in the offending animal (as discussed in the following section) strongly supports the diagnosis. Clinical manifestations are those of encephalitis: hyperexcitability followed by confusion, muscle spasms (hydrophobia), photophobia, paralysis, and coma. Laboratory confirmation comes from demonstrating virus or its antigens (fluorescent antibody staining) in the cornea, skin, saliva, or brain, and by demonstrating serum antibody rise in patients who have not received vaccine or immunoglobulin. In immunized patients, high levels of antibody in the spinal fluid favor the diagnosis of rabies.

Control

Postexposure treatment includes extensive cleansing of the wound, active immunization with vaccine, and passive immunization with hyperimmune globulin. Prompt cleansing of the wound reduces the number of viral particles. Cleansing consists of thorough washing with soap and water, followed by application of a mild disinfectant (for example, surfactants such as quaternary ammonium compounds that solubilize the viral membranes). Cleansing and disinfection do not protect completely because certain parts of a wound may be inaccessible.

Pasteur introduced postexposure treatment with vaccine in 1885. He developed his vaccine by intracerebral passage of rabies virus in rabbits until the virus strain lost its ability to reach the central nervous system after peripheral inoculation ("fixed" rabies virus). Pasteur's vaccine consisted of nerve tissue from an infected rabbit, desiccated for varying periods of time to inactivate the virus gradually. Thus, different levels of infectivity were achieved in different vaccine preparations by varying the length of desiccation. Starting with emulsified preparations that were desiccated the longest (little or no infectivity) and ending with preparations desiccated for only short periods (high infectivity), he gave subcutaneous injections daily for 3 weeks. This method was later modified by adding phenol or formalin, which completely inactivated the virus. This modified vaccine was undoubtedly safer, but perhaps less effective than the original. Side effects included troublesome local reactions and allergic encephalitis caused by nerve tissue antigens in the vaccine.

Another method of vaccine preparation, developed after rabies virus was adapted to replicate in duck embryo, consists of extracts of infected duck embryos fully inactivated with β-propiolactone; it is still available in the United States. Other inactivated vaccines prepared from rabies virus propagated in human diploid cell cultures have been licensed in the United States and are currently recommended for human use. These newer vaccines require fewer injections (3-5 compared to 23) and have greatly reduced the incidence of local reactions and of vaccine-induced allergic encephalitis. For immunization of dogs, a modified live virus strain grown in cells of canine origin is used. Cats are vaccinated with a killed preparation. Recent data raise the possibility that postexposure treatment with vaccine may protect by inducing not only the immune response but also interferon production.

Passive immunization is best achieved with hyperimmunoglobulin, one-half the dose administered at the site of the bite and the other one-half administered intramuscularly. Controlled field trials showed combined active and passive immunization to be more effective for postexposure treatment than either treatment administered alone.

Studies using interferon alone or in combination with the vaccine are being conducted. The results appear promising in that interferon significantly increases the protection rate in animals, including primates. One attempt in a human to reverse the fatal course with interferon, once the onset of symptoms had occurred, failed.

Because vaccine treatment is expensive and sometimes dangerous, administering it in every case of possible exposure is a questionable practice. Its use is clearly appropriate when a person is bitten or licked on an open wound or mucous membrane by a rabid animal. If the presence of rabies in the area is suspected, the first concern is whether the animal is rabid. Ideally, the animal should be captured and examined. Any wild animal must be regarded as rabid unless negative laboratory tests prove otherwise. The wild animal should be killed and tested as soon as possible for presence of rabies antigen (fluorescent antibody staining) or Negri bodies in the brain. Dogs or cats should be observed for 10 days; failure to develop disease within this time indicates the saliva

Table 81-1 Rabies Preexposure* and Postexposure** Prophylaxis Guide

	Animal Species	Condition of Animal at Time of Attack	Treatment of Exposed Person†
Domestic	Dog and cat	Healthy and available for 10 days of observation	None, unless animal develops rabies‡
		Rabid or suspected rabid	RIG§ and HDCV
		Unknown (escaped)	Consult public health officials. If treatment is indicated, give RIG§ and HDCV
Wild	Skunk, bat, fox, coyote, raccoon, bobcat, and other carnivores	Regard as rabid unless proven negative by laboratory tests‖	RIG§ and HDCV
Other	Livestock, rodents, and lagomorphs (rabbits and hares)	Consider individually. Local and state public health officials should be consulted on questions about the need for rabies prophylaxis. Bites of squirrels, hamsters, guinea pigs, gerbils, chipmunks, rats, mice, other rodents, rabbits, and hares almost never call for antirabies prophylaxis.	

Note: The above recommendations are only a guide. In applying them, take into account the animal species involved, the circumstances of the bite or other exposure, the vaccination status of the animal, and presence of rabies in the region. Local or state public health officials should be consulted if questions arise.

*Preexposure prophylaxis is now recommended at 3 doses with 0.1 mL of HCDV, intradermally, by the Centers for Disease Control. *Morbidity and Mortality Weekly Report* 31:279, June 4, 1982.

**From Centers for Disease Control. *Morbidity and Mortality Weekly Report* 29:279, June 13, 1980.

†All bites and wounds should be immediately cleansed thoroughly with soap and water. If antirabies treatment is indicated, both rabies immune globulin (RIG) and human diploid cell rabies vaccine (HDCV) should be given as soon as possible, regardless of the interval from exposure.

‡During the usual holding period of 10 days, begin treatment with RIG and vaccine (preferably with HDCV) at first sign of rabies in a dog or cat that has bitten someone. The symptomatic animal should be killed immediately and tested.

§If RIG is not available, use antirabies serum, equine (ARS). Do not use more than the recommended dosage.

‖The animal should be killed and tested as soon as possible. Holding for observation is not recommended.

probably was not infectious at the time of the bite. If these domestic animals become diseased, diagnosis should be confirmed by fluorescent antibody staining of the brain. Postexposure treatment with immunoglobulin plus vaccine is indicated if the diagnosis is established in the animal and also if the animal is unavailable. Preexposure prophylaxis with human diploid cell vaccine for persons at high risk (veterinarians, spelunkers, laboratory workers, and animal handlers) is desirable. Recommendations for pre- and postexposure prophylaxis appear in Table 81-1.

References

Bishop, D.H.: *Rhabdoviruses,* vol I–III. Boca Raton, Fl.: CRC Press, Inc., 1979.

Ferguson, C.K., Roll, L.J.: Rabies in humans. *Critical Care Update.* 1983; 10:11-16.

Howatson, A.F.: Vesicular stomatitis and related viruses. *Adv Virus Res* 1970; 16:195-256.

Huang, A.S.: Ribonucleic acid synthesis of vesicular stomatitis virus. In: *Negative strand viruses*. Barry R.D., Mahy, B.W.J. (editors). New York: Academic Press, 1975.

Huang, A.S., Baltimore D.: Defective interfering animal viruses. In: *Comprehensive virology*. vol 10. Fraenkel-Conrat, H., Wagner, R.R., (editors). New York: Plenum Press, 1977.

National Association of State Public Health Veterinarians: *Compendium of animal rabies vaccines*. 1985; 33:714–720, 725.

Shope, R.E.: Rabies. In: *Viral infections of humans: Epidemiology and control*. Evans, A.S. (editor). New York: Plenum Press, 1976.

Wagner, R.R.: Reproduction of rhabdoviruses. In: *Comprehensive virology*, vol 4. Fraenkel-Conrat, H., Wagner, R.R., (editors). New York: Plenum Press, 1975.

82 Retroviruses

George J. Todaro, MD

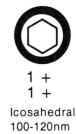

1 +
1 +
Icosahedral
100-120nm

General Concepts
Distinctive Properties
Pathogenesis
Host Defenses
Epidemiology
Diagnosis
Control

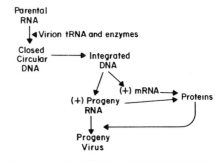

General Concepts

The various RNA-containing tumor viruses of chickens and mammals fall into a single taxonomic group known as the retroviruses (Retroviridae). The name comes from a viral enzyme, called reverse (re) transcriptase (tr), which makes DNA from viral RNA. Replication of these viruses requires making double-stranded circular viral DNA and integrating the viral DNA into host cellular DNA. These properties contribute to the retrovirus potential to recombine genetically with other related viral genomes as well as with various cellular gene sequences and to transmit the recombined information to new cells.

In general, members of this group are not cytopathic for cells they infect: viral replication and cell proliferation are not antagonistic. Since their replication proceeds

The diagrams of the virion morphology and the multiplication scheme are derived from Chapters 62 and 63, respectively. The multiplication scheme applies only generally as indicated in Chapter 63.

through a DNA intermediate from the genomic RNA, the name retrovirus has come to be applied to the whole group. Table 82-1 summarizes the characteristics of this group, which includes many viruses that are major causes of cancer in various animal species under natural and experimental conditions. In animals, these viruses cause leukemias, sarcomas, carcinomas, and a wide spectrum of other neoplastic diseases. Certain members of the group, visna virus and progressive pneumonia virus of sheep, also produce chronic neurologic disease and chronic pulmonary disease. In addition, for many members of the retrovirus group, such as the foamy virus of cats, cows, and various primates, no pathologic effects have been demonstrated.

Many mammalian species have been shown to carry genetic information for retroviruses within their chromosomal DNA. This genetic information generally is repressed but can become active spontaneously or after treatment with certain chemicals and mutagens. Viruses released from normal cells are called **endogenous viruses.** By definition, a retrovirus is endogenous to a given species if at least one copy of the virus genome is integrated in the DNA of every cell of every animal of the species. Endogenous viruses are transmitted genetically from parent to offspring and maintained as normal Mendelian genes in animal populations. These virus-related genes (**virogenes**) are found in the DNA of all somatic and germ cells of every individual of a given species. Expression of virus-related genes usually is under stringent cellular control, but virus release can occasionally occur early in life, spontaneously late in life, or after cellular transformation.

In contrast, a retrovirus is said to be **exogenous** to an animal species if viral DNA sequences can be demonstrated in the infected tissues of the diseased animal but are absent from normal tissues of the same individual. At the animal level, infection by exogenous viruses is referred to as **horizontal transmission.** Exogenous viruses are often highly oncogenic and induce a variety of tumors after infecting an animal.

The feature that most distinguishes retroviruses from other viruses is their ability to be transmitted largely as cellular genes along with the normal genetic information of the host. They can then be viewed as cellular genes rather than as viruses, although these genes have some capacity to move around within a cell, perhaps in a fashion similar to insertion sequences. They can also be transmitted between cells, between animals of a species, and even to different species. In several examples, the viral genes can be inserted into germ cells. The introduction of viral genes does not appear to perturb normal developmental processes in the recipient cells. This close relationship between the intracellular form of virus and genetic material of normal cells is the main characteristic of this group of viruses. The medical problems that arise come from this close genetic relationship and from strong transforming genes that these viruses appear to acquire by recombining with host cell genes.

In the normal cellular DNA of many vertebrates, multiple copies of viral genes exist that are closely related to infectious retroviruses that have been isolated from animals. In various rodents and in primates, as much as 0.03%–0.3% of the entire cellular genome is estimated to be composed of retroviral-related gene sequences. In many of these cases, the sequences do not appear capable of giving rise to whole virus, but in some cases, the animals do spontaneously release virus or it can be activated by certain mutagenic agents such as irradiation.

Table 82-1 Retroviridae Family

	Species	Maturation	Characteristics	Infectivity
Type A	Mouse (*Mus musculus*)	Within cisternae of endoplasmic reticulum	Contains reverse transcriptase and a large polyprotein that is not cleaved	Noninfectious
	Mouse (*Mus cervicolor*)		Nucleic acid and proteins are related to the noninfectious form of *Mus musculus*	Infectious
Type B (mammary tumor virus)	Various mouse species (related virus in guinea pigs)	Nucleoids completed in cytoplasm, bud through plasma membrane; extracellular particle has eccentric core	Several variants exist that differ in oncogenicity, host range, and serologic properties	Noninfectious
Type C (leukemia and sarcoma viruses)	Snakes, chickens, cats, rodents, primates, humans, and most other vertebrates	Assembled in cytoplasm and buds from the cell membrane; immature particles resemble type A viruses; the center of the core becomes electron dense, forming a mature particle	Life cycle includes two phases: (a) genomes exist as DNA and as integral parts of host cell chromosomes; (b) capacity to give rise to complementary RNA that can be packaged as extracellular virions and transmitted to other cells	Some infectious; some noninfectious
Type D	Rhesus monkeys, other macaques, langurs, squirrel monkeys	Nucleoid completed in cytoplasm; eccentric nucleoid in virion	"Horizontally" spread, portions also genetically transmitted in primates	Poorly infectious
Type E (visna, maedi, and progressive pneumonia virus)	Sheep	Resemble leukemia/sarcoma viruses; mature as type C particles	Slow virus infections; associated with respiratory or demyelinating diseases	Capable of chronic infection
Type F	Cats, cattle, primates	Develop as spherical particles in the cytoplasm and bud to form enveloped A particles	Foamy viruses; cause cytoplasmic vacuolization and cell destruction; remain latent in a high percentage of hosts; have no known pathogenic potential but are frequently isolated from tumors	Infectious

Distinctive Properties

Retroviruses have two main components. The outer core contains virus-specific proteins that are needed to infect new cells (Figure 82-1). The electron-dense structure known as the inner core (or nucleoid) contains the viral RNA, the reverse transcriptase enzyme, and other viral structural proteins that form the capsid or inner coat.

Retroviruses form by budding from cytoplasmic membranes. With the electron microscope, several distinct subgenera of retroviruses can be distinguished morphologically: types A, B, C, D, E, and F. Type A particles are commonly found in the cytoplasm and endoplasmic reticulum cisternae of various murine solid tumors and leukemias. Some evidence suggests that they may be immature virus particles. The viruses involved in development of mammary tumors (type B viruses) in mice differ distinctly in

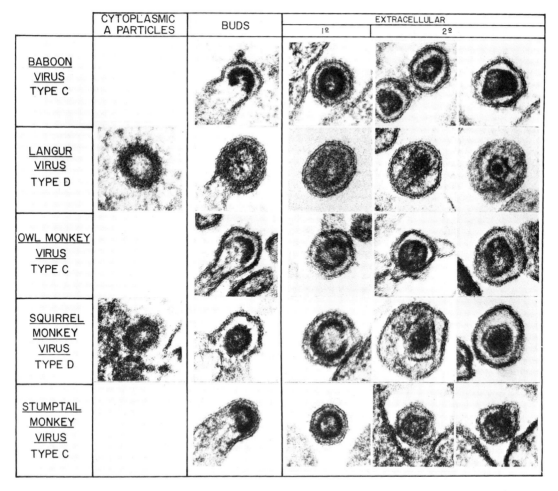

Figure 82-1 Development of types C and D primate viruses. Electron micrograph of thin sections of infected cells shows intracellular formation and extracellular maturation of virions. Courtesy G. Schidlovsky.

morphology from the viruses that produce leukemias and sarcomas (type C viruses) in the same animal. Other viruses that have reverse transcriptase include viruses that produce progressive neurologic disease in sheep and a common group of viruses called foamy viruses, which are isolated readily from cats, cattle, and various primate cell cultures. Some species commonly release endogenous type B and type C viruses, whereas in other species the complete virus is released rarely, if at all.

Figure 82-1 shows the development of five different primate retroviruses. Type D viruses are characterized by completed nucleoids free in the cytoplasm. In contrast, type C viruses form these nucleoids as they bud from the cell membrane. Outside the cell, the nucleoids condense; those of type D particles assume a cylindrical shape. All of these viruses are endogenous with DNA sequences in the normal cellular DNA of primates.

Conventional retrovirus classification schemes utilize immunologic or nucleic acid cross-reactivity in appropriate assays to determine the closeness of relationships between viruses. More distant relatedness is revealed by morphology and biochemical mode of reproduction. Estimates of relatedness and ancestral derivation are based on the chemical structure of the viral genes and their products. These chemical criteria are more sensitive indicators than are immunologic criteria.

The endogenous viruses from normal animals have little or no pathogenicity compared to laboratory strains and to some isolates obtained directly from tumor-bearing animals. Type C retroviruses may be divided by their functions into two groups: nontransforming (or weakly transforming) viruses and strong, rapidly transforming viruses. Most spontaneously appearing viruses transform weakly, if at all, but some variants that transform rapidly have been obtained from chickens, mice, rats, cows, and cats. A group of closely related type C viruses associated with leukemias and sarcomas in primates (the gibbon leukemia viruses and simian sarcoma viruses) have been shown to produce leukemias as well as sarcomas when experimentally inoculated into other primates.

All nondefective retroviruses contain three basic genes required for replication. As summarized in simplified form in Table 82-2, these genes are designated *gag, pol,* and *env* and are located in order from the 5′ end to the 3′ end of the single-stranded RNA genome. The *gag* gene codes for a precursor protein that is processed during virion maturation into the major internal structural proteins: p30 (capsid), p15, p12 and p10. The *pol* gene codes for the reverse transcriptase molecule, and the *env* gene governs the

Table 82-2 RNA Tumor Virus Genes

Gene*	Products	Action
pol	Reverse transcriptase	RNA → DNA
env	Glycoprotein (gp70)	Binding to membrane receptors
gag	p30, p15, p10, p12	Viral structural proteins
onc	Various (See Table 82-4)	Transforms cells from normal to cancer

pol, env, and *gag* are required for retrovirus replication. The different *onc* genes are picked up by recombination with cellular genes and are not required for replication.

major virion envelope glycoprotein structure, consisting of gp70 and p15E. Each gene is essential for replication of retroviruses, but these genes do not appear to be involved in the process of transformation.

At each end of the proviral DNA are long terminal repeats (LTRs), which are involved in viral replication and integration into the host. In some cases, they also contain enhancers of RNA transcription. In the case of several of the cellular oncogenes, the oncogene needs only to be attached to a transcriptionally active retrovirus LTR sequence for it to be able to transform the recipient cell.

The viral structural proteins may be produced from the *gag* gene code by two mechanisms. By the first, the *gag* gene codes for a precursor polypeptide (pr76) of 76,000 daltons; this polypeptide is processed into four small polypeptides that comprise the major viral structural proteins. Translation of pr76 utilizes the full-length 35S RNA as the message. By the second mechanism, translational "read-through" from the *gag* gene into the adjacent *pol* gene forms a 180,000-dalton second precursor polypeptide (pr180); this precursor is cleaved into pr76 (ultimately, viral structural proteins), reverse transcriptase, and some "extra" polypeptides of unknown functions. Translation of the *env* gene occurs on a smaller mRNA species, which seems to form by splicing terminal 5' leader sequences next to sequences in the 3' one-third of the viral RNA. Also, a fourth gene is essential for transformation but not for viral growth. Called *onc*, this gene has been most thoroughly studied with the avian sarcoma viruses, in which deletion mutants that lack the transforming function are available (see Chapter 65).

The genome organization of replication-defective sarcoma and acute leukemia viruses appears to differ significantly from that of avian sarcoma virus. The RNAs of these isolates lack at least portions of the *gag*, *pol*, and *env* gene sequences that characterize nondefective virus strains. All, however, contain the *onc* gene, which confers the ability to rapidly transform cells. Although the order of genes in most of the replication-defective viruses has not been determined, recent studies suggest that the *onc* gene of at least one such avian virus, MC29, maps in the 5' one-half of the viral RNA genome. Other rapidly transforming viruses that produce leukemias and sarcomas have been isolated also.

Almost all the strongly transforming (acute) viruses are defective for replication and rely on other replicating and weakly transforming (chronic) helper viruses. The helper viruses provide the essential functions needed to complete replication of the defective transforming viruses. The exception is the original avian sarcoma virus isolated from chickens by Peyton Rous. Figure 82-2 shows that analysis of the genome structure of the strongly transforming viruses (mouse sarcoma, cat sarcoma, avian erythroblastosis, and avian myeloblastosis), compared to the helper viruses, has revealed a substantial deletion of viral genetic information and replacement by genes derived from the host cell. The deletions are in the region that would code for the polymerase and the envelope genes. Both the 5' and 3' ends of the genomes of the strongly transforming viruses are homologous to those of the helper virus from which they arise. Variant viruses that produce rapid (acute) transformation of specific target tissues have been described; these variants include those that produce predominantly B cell leukemias, those that produce myeloid leukemias, others that produce sarcomas, and still others that produce only carcinomas. Comparison of acute and chronic retrovirus infections is presented in Table 82-3.

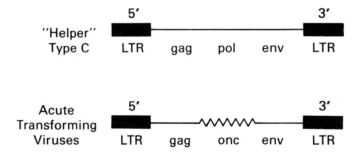

Figure 82-2 Schematic representation of the genomes of rapidly transforming DNA viruses. LTR, long terminal repeating sequences; pol, gene that codes for reverse transcriptase; gag, genes that code for structural proteins; onc, oncogene; env, genes that code for envelope proteins.

Table 82-3   Characteristics of Acute and Chronic Retrovirus Infections

	Acute Infection	*Chronic Infection*
Replication	0 *	+
Oncogene in virus genome	+	0
Direct transformation	+	0
Virus occurrence	±	+
Natural disease	0	+
Rapid onset of experimental disease	+	0
Examples	Feline sarcoma viruses	Avian, bovine and human leukemia lymphoma viruses
	Murine serum viruses	Visna/Maedi virus; feline panleukopenia virus

*Rous sarcoma virus is an exception.

Pathogenesis

Detection of a retrovirus in a tumor tissue is not proof that the virus was involved in the disease process. Proof requires establishing the origin of the virus by distinguishing between the activation of endogenous viruses whose genetic information already exists in the host and infection by exogenous viruses.

In three well-studied animal systems (avian, bovine, and feline), the major causes of cancer are infectious, horizontally transmitted viruses that are acquired congenitally or after birth. These spread in a manner similar to that of other viruses: the feline leukemia and sarcoma viruses spread primarily through the saliva and urine; the bovine lymphosarcoma virus spreads most effectively by contact with affected animals. In each of these systems, many more animals are infected than become diseased. Feline leukemia virus replication in the domestic cat results in overt leukemia in only a small fraction of the infected animals, but this virus also produces immune depression and anemias that cause more deaths than the leukemia itself. Some strains of feline leukemia virus mainly produce visceral lymphomas; others mainly produce leukemias.

In certain strains of mice such as the AKR mouse, the situation is more complex because the virus believed to be the essential etiologic agent of the leukemia may arise by recombination between two different genetically transmitted viruses, both of which are present in normal tissues. A rare recombinant virus that has a different host range and the capacity to infect thymus cells may be the etiologic agent of the thymic leukemias characteristic of inbred strains of mice like AKR and C3H that have been extensively used for experimental leukemia studies. These recombinant viruses appear to be changed primarily in their envelope region, suggesting that altered envelope proteins play a role in pathogenesis of the disease.

The strongly transforming viruses represent rare isolates from the field. Some such as the mouse and rat sarcoma viruses have arisen as variants in stocks of helper or leukemia viruses; however, some acute defective leukosis viruses (especially those of chickens) and also leukemia and sarcoma viruses of cats have been isolated on multiple occasions directly from the field.

Retroviruses have been found to pick up oncogenes from host cell DNA and transmit these genes from animal to animal. About 20 distinct oncogenes have been identified, all of which are highly conserved in evolution. These genes have been found in normal human cellular DNA and most have been mapped to specific human chromosomes. Closely related sequences have been found in all vertebrates and even have been isolated from fruit flies and found in yeast DNA. The normal cellular oncogenes may be involved in various aspects of growth regulation. Several are related structurally to one another and their gene products function as protein kinases that specifically phosphorylate tyrosine residues (Table 82-4). Several growth regulatory factors act by binding to specific membrane receptors that are also tyrosine-specific protein kinases. Examples include insulin, platelet derived growth factor (PDGF), and epidermal growth factor (EGF). Each of these facilitate cell growth and interact with a cell membrane receptor that is a protein kinase. One oncogene product, from the simian sarcoma virus, is almost identical with one of the subunits of PDGF; another, from an avian erythroblastosis virus, *erb* B, has extensive sequence homology with a portion of the EGF receptor. Many human tumors produce a growth factor, called tumor growth factor (TGF), that stimulates cell division of both normal cells and tumor cells and acts by binding to specific growth factor receptors.

Table 82-4   Functions of Viral Oncogene Products*

Class	Function
1	Tyrosine-specific protein kinases (*src, abl, fes,* etc.)
2	Growth factors and their receptors (e.g., *sis* gene product-PDGF) (*erb* B gene product-EGF receptor)
3	Guanine nucleotide binding proteins (e.g., various *ras* genes)
4	Chromatin binding proteins (*myc, myb, fos,* etc.)

*Each different oncogene is identified by a three-letter code that indicates something about its origin and function. For example, the *feline* sarcoma virus oncogene is *fes* and is a class 1 oncogene; the *simian* sarcoma virus (*sis*) oncogene is in class 2; and the *rat* sarcoma virus (*ras*) oncogene is one of several members of the class 3 oncogene family.

Another family of oncogenes, those related to the rat sarcoma virus (*ras*), produces a 21,000-dalton protein that is cell-membrane associated and binds GTP and GDP. Mutated forms of the *ras* gene have been isolated from DNA of human tumors and from DNA of chemically transformed murine tumor cells. The exact function of the *ras* gene product and how the specific mutations alter or enhance that function is not yet known. By using the cell transformation assay system, oncogenes have been isolated directly from various human tumors, including bladder cancer, lung cancer, and neuroblastomas. In some cases, these oncogenes are related closely to those found in the acute transforming animal retroviruses. This has been especially true for the *ras* oncogene family (see Table 82-4). Detailed analysis has shown that the *ras* gene in the tumor DNA differs slightly from the *ras* gene in normal cellular DNA and that the changes are not random. For example, amino acid 12 or amino acid 61 of the *ras* gene are altered in the tumor cell. This indicates that somatic mutation of normal cellular oncogenes may be important in converting a normal cell into a cancer cell. Thus, *qualitative* changes in the oncogene structure itself, as well as *quantitative* changes in the level of expression of the oncogene product, may be necessary for production of the full tumor state.

The last major group of oncogene products are the only such products that localize to the cell nucleus. Included in this group is the *myc* oncogene product that binds to chromatin and is activated in chicken leukemias and in human Burkitt's lymphoma. Cell-culture experiments have suggested that two different classes of oncogenes are necessary to transform normal cells fully: the cell membrane-associated oncogenes (classes 1 to 3, Table 82-4); and either the *myc* or another of the nuclear chromatin-associated oncogenes.

As more oncogenes are isolated and characterized, it appears that probably only a small number (perhaps less than 100 genes out of the entire genetic makeup) are responsible for changing the properties of a normal cell into a cancer cell. The awareness that the number of oncogene families is small and that their functions are coming to be understood at the molecular level makes scientists optimistic about understanding the fundamental basis of cancer. Research with the retroviruses has provided many of the critical insights that have helped us to reach the present level of understanding in this area.

Host Defenses

A possible defense against virulent, exogenous viruses is the genetic suppression mechanism that normally prevents expression of endogenous viral DNA. A similar defense is the genetic suppression mechanism by which certain lysogenic (endogenous) bacteriophages protect against virulent, exogenous, and related phages. Neutralizing antibody produced against the infectious viruses usually suffices to arrest spread and prevent development of disease. Cell-mediated immunity also plays a protective role against the development of viral-induced tumors in immunologically competent animals. Animals with a persistent viremia have a high probability of developing disease and shedding virus that can infect other animals.

Many different retroviruses have an immunosuppressive effect on their hosts. This capacity to decrease host defenses may contribute to the ability of retroviruses to persist in the host and to circumvent the immune defenses. An example of a disease in which a retrovirus exercises such an ability may be acquired immune deficiency syndrome (AIDS), a slowly progressive disease characterized by blood-related transmission and severe immunodeficiency that leads to lethal Kaposi's sarcoma or to opportunistic infections. The growing evidence that links retrovirus and AIDS includes the findings that certain retrovirus infections of animals cause severe immunosuppression and that a retrovirus or its antibody occurs in most patients with AIDS.

Although retroviruses are inhibited by sufficient quantities of interferon, they tend to be poor inducers of interferon. In mouse cells, interferon has been shown to inhibit replication of leukemia viruses and mammary tumor viruses by blocking a late step in the budding process. Viruses and viral antigens accumulate on the cell surface, but completed viral particles are not formed. Similar observations have been described of various primate viruses growing in human cells. How important this mechanism is in preventing the spread of viruses in natural populations is not yet clear.

Epidemiology

The introduction of a feline leukemia virus-shedding cat into a household of virus-negative cats is associated with a high risk of spread of the virus to the exposed animals. Since these viruses are transmitted horizontally, conventional modes of viral transmission are dominant; prevention or control is achieved by isolating the animals from contact with known carriers. The introduction of infected cows into herds greatly increases the risk of development of bovine leukemia; a similar situation exists with infected chickens introduced into flocks that are negative for leukosis virus.

The transmission of virus from an infected mother to her offspring also is associated with a high risk of disease. Milk-borne transmission of the mammary tumor virus is a major factor in the development of breast cancer in susceptible mouse strains (for example, C3H mice). In mouse strains with a high incidence of "spontaneous" breast cancer (for example, the GR mouse), the transforming genes are already integrated into the somatic cells and germ cells of all the animals. Activation of this genetically transmitted viral information leads to early breast cancer in 100% of the females. Specific transforming gene sequences in the mammary tumor virus from the GR strain are also present in normal GR mouse cellular DNA but not in C3H mice. Genetic crosses between GR and C3H mice establish that the presence of the transforming gene sequences can be used as a predictor of early breast cancer and that the sequences segregate in a Mendelian dominant pattern. Animals lacking the gene sequences are at low risk for spontaneous breast cancer but still are susceptible to milk-borne transmission.

A rare form of human leukemia, acute T cell leukemia, appears to be associated with a human retrovirus, human T cell leukemia virus (HTLV). Epidemiologic findings suggest that this virus infects a significant fraction of the population in southern Japan, the Caribbean, and the Mediterranean Basin. In fact, the distribution of this virus eventually may be found to be worldwide. At least 100 times more people are infected than develop the disease. The virus is related structurally to the bovine leukemia virus, which has a similar epidemiologic nature. The suggestion also has been made that HTLV may be involved in human acquired immune deficiency syndrome (AIDS).

Direct evidence has indicated that a type D retrovirus is the causative agent of simian AIDS. This profound immune deficiency, which leads to secondary infections and death and has been reported in at least three primate centers, is due to a family of infectious type D retroviruses (see Figure 82-1). The incubation period for monkeys inoculated experimentally with the retrovirus can be as short as a few months. At this writing there have not been any isolates of type D retroviruses from humans; nor has evidence been found that the primate type D retroviruses can be transmitted to humans.

A profound immune suppression also occurs in cats inoculated with feline leukemia virus (a type C retrovirus) and in animals inoculated with retroviruses of the "foamy" virus group. The type F foamy viruses cause a cytoplasmic vacuolization in cell cultures, but have not yet been associated with particular diseases. Such viruses can be isolated readily from various primates, cats, and cows.

Infectious viruses from outside the body can act directly by carrying in specific oncogene sequences and producing tumors rapidly in the host. Retroviruses also can insert in the DNA of a host in such a way as to facilitate the activation of a particular oncogene. For example, chicken leukemia viruses appear to act by increasing the level of the *myc* oncogene. This same oncogene is activated in human Burkitt's lymphoma, in which it is associated with a chromosomal translocation between human chromosomes 8 and 14. The infectious virus involved in that disease is a member of the herpes virus group, the Epstein-Barr virus (EBV). The human T cell leukemia virus does not appear to carry an oncogene; therefore, it may act indirectly to produce leukemia, perhaps by activating one or more of the cellular oncogenes.

Diagnosis

For those retroviruses that produce cell transformation in culture, sensitive assays are available to titer the transforming effect. Fibroblasts and epithelial cells can be used for viruses that transform cells into solid tumors; bone marrow cells can be used for leukemia viruses. Figures 82-3 and 82-4 show an early and late focus of transformed cells produced by mouse sarcoma virus infection of mouse embryo cells. Virus inoculation into the spleen of newborn mice gives a rapid and sensitive assay for spleen focus-forming virus (Friend leukemia virus). Temperature-sensitive mutants of the virus in the transforming gene establish that transformation depends on a viral-coded gene product or products. This appears to be a membrane protein and, in most cases, a phosphorylated protein that has protein kinase activity or nucleotide-binding properties associated with it (see Table 82-4). Localization of the transforming gene products in or under the cell membrane suggests that they may alter the cellular control mechanism by changing some interactions between the cell membrane and its external environment. Different transforming viruses appear to have acquired different cellular gene sequences. The DNA extracted from virus-transformed cells can, in turn, transform recipient cells, thereby directly demonstrating that the information in the virus-transformed tumor cells is contained in the form of integrated cellular DNA. The presence of reverse transcriptase activity in a biologic sample indicates the presence of retrovirus.

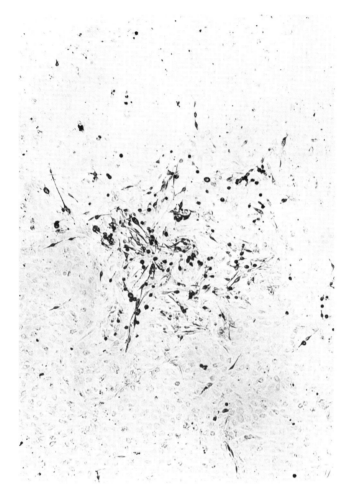

Figure 82-3 Transformed focus of BALB/3T3 cells induced by infection with Moloney murine sarcoma virus 7 days previously (×49). Multiplication of the transformed cells gives rises to the focus of proliferating cells, shown in Figure 82-4.

Control

Knowledge of the underlying mechanism of a disease can lead to effective control or prevention. An example is the eradication of bovine leukemia, an economically important disease that can severely affect whole herds. Control grew out of knowledge that transmission occurs horizontally from animal to animal, a separate natural reservoir does not appear to exist, and sensitive and reliable assays can detect infection. The knowledge led to identification and elimination of antibody-positive carrier animals. Within 1 year of initiating one such eradication program, the incidence of seropositive animals in five separate herds dropped from over 25% to well under 1%.

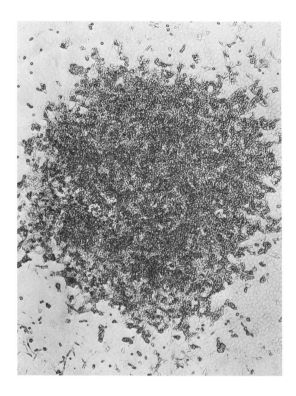

Figure 82-4 Colony of BALB/3T3 cells transformed by Moloney murine sarcoma virus 4 weeks after infection (×49).

In contrast to approaches directed toward the control of infectious viruses, measures designed to protect against activated endogenous viral genes and tumor genes require an understanding of what they are, how they produce their transforming effect, and how they are regulated by the normal host. Although cancer is a multifactorial disease and viruses act as environmental carcinogens, control of the virus, which may be the critical influence in cancer causation, may provide an approach to control of cell proliferation. Progress in this area is developing rapidly through the use of recombinant DNA technology.

References

Bishop, J.M.: Cellular oncogenes and retroviruses. *Ann Rev Biochem* 1983; 52:301–54.

Essex, M., Todaro, G.J., zur Hausen, H. (editors): 1980. *Viruses in naturally occurring cancers,* Cold Spring Harbor Conferences on Cell Proliferation, Vol. 7. Cold Spring Harbor, N.Y.: Cold Spring Harbor Press, 1980.

Klein, G. (editor): *Advances in viral oncology.* New York: Raven Press, 1982.

Popovic, M., et al.: Detection, isolation and continuous production of cytopathic retroviruses (HTLV-III) from patients with AIDS and pre-AIDS. *Science* 1984; 224:497–500.

83 Rotaviruses, Reoviruses, and Orbiviruses

10 to 11 ±

C = 132
60-80nm

Albert Z. Kapikian, MD

Robert E. Shope, MD

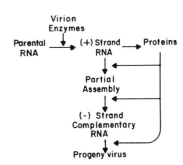

General Concepts

The family Reoviridae is composed of six distinct groups (genera): *Reovirus*, *Orbivirus*, *Rotavirus*, *Phytoreovirus*, *Fijivirus*, and an as yet unnamed group that includes the cytoplasmic polyhedrosis viruses. Certain members of the *Reovirus*, *Orbivirus*, and *Rotavirus* genera infect humans; the phytoreoviruses and Fijiviruses infect plants; and the cytoplasmic polyhedrosis viruses infect insects. This chapter concerns only those members of the Reoviridae family known to infect humans.

The diagrams of the virion morphology and the multiplication scheme are derived from Chapters 62 and 63, respectively. The multiplication scheme applies only generally as indicated in Chapter 63.

Although the reoviruses, orbiviruses, and rotaviruses share certain properties (morphology, approximate 70 nm size, and segmented, double-stranded RNA) that unite them into a common family, each differs markedly from the others in epidemiology, association with disease, and ability to propagate in the laboratory.

Rotaviruses have emerged as major etiologic agents of severe diarrhea of infants and young children in the developed and developing countries. Reovirus infections occur quite commonly in humans, although they tend to be mild or subclinical. Their importance as etiologic agents of illness in humans is unclear. Four orbiviruses cause human disease. The most serious of these is Colorado tick fever, characterized by diphasic fever, headache, muscle pain, anorexia, leukopenia, and weakness; some cases are complicated by encephalitis, hemorrhage, thrombocytopenia, or pericarditis. Death rarely occurs.

ROTAVIRUSES

Diarrheal diseases are a major cause of morbidity in infants and young children in developed countries, and a major cause of morbidity and mortality in the developing countries. For example, in a family study in the United States that included some 25,000 illnesses, infectious gastroenteritis was the second most common disease experience and accounted for 16% of all illnesses. The impact of diarrheal illnesses on infants and young children in the developing countries is staggering. An estimate of the number of diarrheal episodes in children under 5 years of age in Asia, Africa, and Latin America for a 1-year period indicated that over 450 million episodes of diarrhea would occur and that 1%–4% would be fatal, resulting in the deaths of 5–18 million children. In spite of the importance of this disease, the etiologic agents of a large proportion of diarrheal illnesses of infants and young children were not known, although it was assumed that viruses played an important role because the bacterial agents known at that time could be recovered from only about 10%–25% of cases during nonepidemic periods. In 1973, rotaviruses were discovered in duodenal biopsies obtained from pediatric patients with gastroenteritis; subsequently, the agent was detected in stools by electron microscopy, and laboratories all over the world soon began to detect the virus in stools of a large proportion of patients with gastroenteritis. Efficient and practical tests were developed to detect rotavirus from clinical specimens, thus facilitating the study of this fastidious agent, which replicates inefficiently in cell cultures from clinical specimens. Rotaviruses were soon recognized as major etiologic agents of diarrheal illness in infants and young children. Important advances in delineating the role of toxigenic *E coli* in diarrheal diseases in the developing countries are discussed in Chapter 41.

Distinctive Properties

Rotaviruses have a distinctive wheel-like shape (Figure 83-1). Complete particles have a double-layered capsid and measure about 70 nm in diameter; without the outer layer of the double capsid, they measure about 55 nm; the core has a diameter of about 37 nm. The term rotavirus is derived from the Latin word *rota,* meaning wheel, and was suggested because the sharply defined circular outline of the outer capsid resembles the

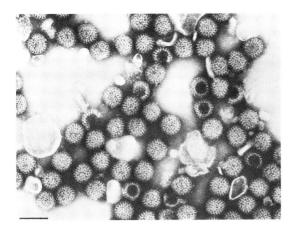

Figure 83-1 Human rotavirus particles from a stool filtrate. Particles appear to have a double-shelled capsid. Occasional "empty" particles are seen. Adapted from Kapikian, A.Z., et al. *Science* 1974; 185:1050.

rim of a wheel placed on short spokes radiating from a wide hub. Rotaviruses resemble the reoviruses and orbiviruses; however, the sharply defined circular outline of the outer capsid of rotavirus differs from the amorphous outer capsid of orbiviruses. Reoviruses also have a distinct outer capsid, although it is not as sharply defined as that of the rotaviruses; however, this distinction is not always clear-cut.

The rotavirus genome contains 11 segments of double-stranded RNA in contrast to the reoviruses and orbiviruses, both of which contain 10 segments. Colorado tick fever virus is considered an orbivirus in this chapter, although the recent finding that it has 12 segments of RNA puts its taxonomic status in doubt. The biochemical properties of human rotaviruses have not been studied extensively because, until recently, these agents have been difficult to propagate in cell culture. Reoviruses are acid- and ether-stable, whereas rotaviruses and orbiviruses are ether-stable but acid-labile. Studies of the effect of various disinfectants on simian rotavirus infectivity demonstrated that 0.95 by volume (95% v/v) ethanol was most effective for rotavirus inactivation in the laboratory.

Rotaviruses are distinct serologically from the three reoviruses and from all orbiviruses with which they have been tested. Most human rotaviruses share certain common antigens, but other antigens separate rotaviruses into serotypes and subgroups. Neutralization reveals at least four human rotavirus serotypes. Rotaviruses can also be separated into two distinct subgroups by specific complement-fixation, ELISA, and immune adherence hemagglutination assay. The neutralization and subgroup specificities are coded for by different genes. Rotaviruses also have been detected in stools of numerous animals. A few of these strains have been propagated efficiently in cell cultures. Rotaviruses of humans and animals characteristically share common complement-fixation and immunofluorescence antigens, but strains may be classified into distinct serotypes by other assays such as neutralization and solid phase immune electron microscopy. Several animal rotavirus strains (simian, canine, feline, and equine) share neutralization specificity with human rotavirus type 3, and various porcine rotaviruses are antigenically similar to human rotavirus type 4. In addition, a few human and animal rotavirus strains have been detected by electron microscopy that do not share the common antigen; these have been designated tentatively as pararotaviruses. Tested orbiviruses and reovirus (type 3) are serologically distinct from each other.

Human rotaviruses are rather fastidious agents, and for many years they could not be cultivated serially from clinical specimens with efficiency. Human rotavirus strain "Wa," a subgroup 2 virus, was propagated efficiently in African green monkey kidney cell cultures after multiple passages in an animal model. In addition, noncultivatable human rotaviruses were "rescued" following mixed infection of cell cultures with noncultivatable human rotavirus and cultivatable bovine rotavirus and the application of various selective pressures. The cultivatable reassortants had the neutralization specificity of the human rotavirus. Recently, the efficient cell culture propagation of human rotavirus strains directly from clinical material has been described.

Pathogenesis

Rotaviruses are transmitted by the fecal-oral route. Other routes of transmission, such as water-borne, food-borne or airborne (respiratory), have also been suggested. From clinical studies, the incubation period of rotavirus diarrheal illness was estimated to be less than 48 hours. Large numbers of virus are shed in the stool following multiplication in epithelial cells of the small intestine. Shedding may persist for 10 or more days after the illness, but peak shedding appears to occur within 8 days of illness. Studies in adult volunteers have demonstrated that oral administration of a rotavirus-containing suspension can induce a diarrheal illness in certain individuals. Also, human rotavirus induces a gastrointestinal illness following administration by the alimentary route in various newborn colostrum-deprived animals. Histopathologic studies of tissue from the small intestine of humans with rotavirus infection show shortening of villi and mononuclear cell infiltration of the lamina propria; electron microscopy shows sparse and irregular microvilli, distended cisternae of the endoplasmic reticulum, and mitochondrial swelling. D-xylose absorption was found to be impaired, and some patients had depressed disaccharidase levels.

Rotaviruses induce a clinical illness characterized by vomiting, diarrhea, and dehydration, which frequently results in hospitalization of infants and young children. Although milder gastroenteric illnesses that do not require hospitalization are also common, most studies of clinical manifestations of rotavirus-induced gastroenteritis rely on data from hospitalized patients. The duration of hospitalization characteristically ranges from 2–14 days with a mean of 4 days. The highest attack rate characteristically occurs in the 6–24-month-old age group, with the less-than-6-month age group usually experiencing the next highest frequency of rotavirus illness; during rotavirus infection, normal neonates usually do not develop clinical manifestations. Death from rotavirus gastroenteritis may occur as a result of dehydration and electrolyte imbalance.

Host Defenses

In volunteer studies, serum antibody was found to correlate with resistance to rotavirus-induced illness, whereas the relationship of intestinal fluid-neutralizing activity to rotavirus resistance was less clear-cut. In animal models, resistance to rotavirus-induced illness correlates with rotavirus antibody present in the intestinal lumen and not with circulating serum antibody. Little is known about other host defenses during rotavirus infection.

Epidemiology

Rotaviruses are major etiologic agents of severe gastroenteritis of infants and young children. These agents also have been associated with milder episodes of gastroenteritis that do not require hospitalization. The efficient transmission of rotavirus is evident by the presence of rotavirus antibody in most children by the age of 3 years. This high prevalence of antibody is maintained into adulthood, probably reflecting frequent reinfection. Important sources of rotavirus infection for infants are individuals of any age who shed this virus. Community outbreaks of rotavirus infection occur infrequently, probably because previous rotavirus exposure leads to protective immunity. Although rotavirus gastroenteritis occurs infrequently in adults, large outbreaks of severe gastroenteritis in adults have been associated with a pararotavirus in China.

Rotaviruses have been associated with about 35%-45% of hospitalized cases of diarrheal illness in infants and young children in various countries in the temperate climates. A striking feature of rotaviral illness in these climates is its seasonal distribution; it usually occurs in the cooler months of the year when, cumulatively, over 50% of diarrheal illnesses are associated with rotaviruses (Figure 83-2). The reason for this temporal distribution is not known; also, this striking seasonal pattern has not occurred uniformly in all settings. In tropical climates, rotavirus infections have been detected

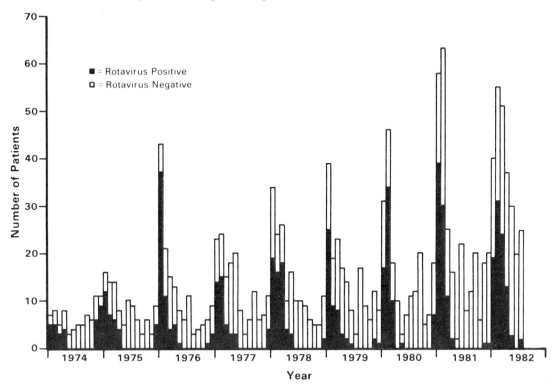

Figure 83-2 Temporal distribution of human rotavirus infections in 1537 infants and young children hospitalized with gastroenteritis at Childrens Hospital National Medical Center, Washington, D.C., January 1974 (partial) through July 1982, as demonstrated by EM, IEM, and rotavirus confirmatory ELISA. From Brandt, C.D., et al. *J Clin Microbiol* 1983; 18:71.

throughout most of the year, although less pronounced peaks can occur. In studies of newborns in nurseries, most virus-positive neonates were symptom-free. A mechanism for this relative lack of susceptibility to illness in neonates in newborn nurseries has yet to be explained satisfactorily. However, it has been shown that such neonatal infections induce significant protection against postneonatal rotavirus diarrheal illness (but not infection) for a period of about 3 years. Rotaviruses also have been associated with prolonged diarrhea in immunodeficient children and with gastroenteritis in patients undergoing bone marrow transplantation.

Rotavirus infections have been detected rarely or infrequently in patients with intussusception, gastroenteritis with rectal bleeding, Henoch-Schoenlein purpura, Reye's syndrome, central nervous system disturbances, aseptic meningitis, circulatory abnormalities, hemolytic uremic syndrome, disseminated intravascular coagulation, Kawasaki syndrome, sudden infant death syndrome, neonatal necrotizing enterocolitis, neonatal hemorrhagic gastroenteritis, exanthema subitum, pneumonia, abortions, and chronic diarrhea. Whether such varied clinical findings were associated etiologically with or were incidental to rotavirus infection needs to be clarified.

Rotaviruses also cause diarrhea in many newborn animals, including calves, mice, piglets, foals, lambs, rabbits, deer, antelopes, apes, turkeys, chickens, young goats, kittens, and puppies. No evidence exists that animal rotaviruses are transmitted to humans under natural conditions, but human rotavirus has been shown to induce a diarrheal illness in certain animals.

Diagnosis

Because the clinical manifestations of rotavirus gastroenteritis in individual cases are not distinctive enough to permit a specific etiologic diagnosis, appropriate specimens must be examined in the laboratory. This is necessary even during the cooler months of the year, when over 50% of hospitalizations due to diarrhea may be associated with rotavirus, because the illnesses associated with other agents cannot be distinguished clinically from the rotavirus illnesses.

Laboratory diagnosis of rotavirus infection requires identifying the virus in stool or rectal swab specimens or demonstrating a fourfold or greater increase in antibody to a rotavirus antigen between acute and convalescent sera. Numerous methods to detect rotavirus in stool and rectal swab specimens have been described. Some of these include electron microscopy, radioimmunoassay, counterimmunoelectroosmophoresis, centrifuging of clinical material onto tissue culture cells followed by immunofluorescence, inoculation of tissue cultures, latex agglutination, reverse passive hemagglutination assay, dot hybridization, and ELISA. ELISA has now become the mainstay in most laboratories, because it is practical, rapid, efficient, and does not require sophisticated laboratory equipment. When the number of specimens is limited, the most rapid method of rotavirus diagnosis in a hospital setting is by examination of a patient's stool by negative-stain electron microscopy. This can be accomplished in a few minutes. Human rotaviruses that do not share the common antigen with conventional rotaviruses cannot be detected by conventional serologic assays; thus, they are usually detected by electron microscopy because they are morphologically identical to conventional rotaviruses.

Serologic evidence of rotavirus infection can be detected by various techniques, including complement fixation, ELISA, immunofluorescence, and neutralization.

Treatment and Control

The primary aim of treatment of rotavirus gastroenteritis is to replace fluids and electrolytes lost by vomiting or diarrhea; intravenous or alimentary administration may be used. In patients with severe dehydration and shock, intravenous rehydration is indicated for efficient replacement of fluid loss. Virus-specific chemotherapy is not available. However, human milk that contained rotavirus antibody has been given orally to treat immunodeficient patients with chronic rotavirus infection and has been shown to be effective. Human immune serum globulin (γ-globulin) that contains rotavirus antibody was given prophylactically (orally) to low-birth-weight infants in a nursery in which recurrent rotavirus infections occurred; treatment resulted in delayed rotavirus excretion and milder symptoms. In addition, cow colostrum that contained rotavirus antibody was given prophylactically to infants and young children once a day (orally) and was shown to induce significant protection against rotavirus diarrhea; it did not have a therapeutic effect when administered to children who already had rotavirus diarrheal illness.

The importance of rotavirus as a cause of diarrheal illness in infants and young children throughout the world indicates that an effective vaccine is needed to prevent rotavirus-induced illness. An attenuated bovine rotavirus strain has been administered orally to infants and young children as an experimental vaccine; in preliminary studies, it has been found to provide protection against severe rotavirus diarrhea. Further studies are underway to evaluate the extent and duration of such protection. Because rotaviruses are highly contagious and can spread by the fecal-oral route, careful attention to hand washing, disinfection, and disposal of contaminated material may limit its spread, especially in nurseries and hospitals where nosocomial infections occur so frequently.

REOVIRUSES

The family name Reoviridae is derived from *Reovirus,* the first genus of this family to be identified. Important features of reoviruses include a diameter of 70 nm; a double capsid; ether and acid stability; a genome constituted of 10 segments of double-stranded RNA; three serotypes designated types 1, 2, and 3; and the ability to infect humans as well as various animals. The three serotypes share a common complement-fixation antigen but can be distinguished by hemagglutination-inhibition and neutralization techniques. Reoviruses grow efficiently from clinical specimens in various cell cultures, including monkey kidney.

Reovirus strains identical serologically to the human reovirus serotypes have been recovered from a wide variety of animals, including mice, dogs, cats, cattle, sheep, swine, horses, and monkeys. Avian reoviruses also have been isolated; however, with one possible exception, these are antigenically distinct from the three reovirus serotypes described previously. In addition, a reovirus possessing certain characteristics of the mammalian and avian reoviruses has been recovered from a bat.

Reovirus infections occur often in humans; most infections are mild or subclinical. The virus is detected efficiently in stools; it may also be recovered from nasal or pharyngeal secretions, urine, blood, cerebrospinal fluid, and various organs obtained at autopsy.

Despite the ease with which reoviruses may be detected from clinical specimens, their role in human disease remains uncertain. Reoviruses have been recovered from patients with fever, exanthema, upper and lower respiratory tract illnesses, gastrointestinal illness (including steatorrhea), hepatitis, meningitis, and encephalitis, and from the tumor tissue of patients with Burkitt's lymphoma. Their importance as etiologic agents of such illnesses remains unclear.

ORBIVIRUSES

Orbiviruses are a genus consisting of at least 86 serotypes of arthropod-borne viruses. These viruses cause serious diseases in humans and animals. Table 83-1 shows the four human pathogens, their diseases, vectors, and geographic distribution. The most serious of these, Colorado tick fever, is emphasized in the following discussion. Kemerovo is a tick-borne virus isolated from cerebrospinal fluid of two patients in western Siberia in 1962 during a small outbreak of febrile disease. Orungo virus was found in blood of febrile patients in tropical Africa and is believed to cause small epidemics. Changuinola virus was isolated from a patient with fever in Panama. Little more is known about the disease potential of Kemerovo, Orungo, and Changuinola viruses.

Distinctive Properties

Orbiviruses have spherical virions that contain ten (or for Colorado tick fever, 12) segments of double-stranded RNA, exhibit icosahedral symmetry, and have a diameter of 60-80 nm. The total molecular weight is about 12 million daltons. Orbivirus infectivity is destroyed at pH 3.0, unlike that of reoviruses. Orbiviruses also replicate in arthropods and are transmitted by them; reoviruses are not arthropod-associated. Except for these differences, orbiviruses are similar to reoviruses in morphology, biochemical properties, and replication. Orbiviruses have at least seven structural and two nonstructural polypeptides. Members of the 13 orbivirus serogroups cross-react within the serogroups by complement-fixation test. They are distinct by the neutralization test, which derives its reactivity from one or two outer capsid proteins.

Table 83-1   Orbiviruses Associated with Human Disease

Virus	Disease in Humans	Vector	Where Found
Colorado tick fever	Fever, rarely pericarditis, encephalitis, or hemorrhage	Tick	Western North America
Kemerovo	Fever, meningitis	Tick	Western Siberia
Orungo	Fever	Mosquito	Nigeria, Uganda, Senegal, Central African Republic
Changuinola	Fever	Phlebotomine sandfly	Panama, northern South America

Pathogenesis

Colorado tick fever replicates in *Dermacentor andersoni* ticks that are infected in the larval stage when they feed on blood of the golden-mantled ground squirrel or other small rodents. After a period of days or weeks, the virus appears in the tick's saliva. The tick, which remains infectious for life, feeds on humans during its adult stage. The virus does not pass transovarially in the tick.

In humans, Colorado tick fever virus, possibly after infecting the regional lymph nodes, replicates in the bone marrow cells, causing maturation arrest of the polymorphonuclear leukocytes, eosinophils, and basophils and, in some instances, severe thrombocytopenia. Erythrocytes presumably are infected as erythroblasts and are later detected in large numbers as antigen-containing red blood cells in the peripheral blood. The virus is found only briefly in the serum of patients. Antibody appears about 2 weeks after onset of symptoms, but virus can still be isolated from peripheral blood cells for up to 6 weeks.

In about 15% of infected children under 10 years of age, Colorado tick fever virus invades the central nervous system and causes encephalitis. Virus has been isolated from the cerebrospinal fluid in these cases.

Host Defenses

Almost no studies exist of the host defenses against Colorado tick fever. Nonimmune persons appear to be uniformly susceptible. Symptoms subside when humoral antibody appears, although exacerbations are reported; the role of cell-mediated immunity is not known. The virus induces interferon; whether interferon is important in host defense, however, is not known.

Epidemiology

The distribution of Colorado tick fever is the same as that of its principal tick vector, *D andersoni*. This infrequent disease is found in California, Colorado, Idaho, Montana, Nevada, Oregon, Utah, Washington, Wyoming, British Columbia, and Alberta. Campers, hikers, and foresters are commonly infected. Infections occur in April, May, and June, when ticks are abundant. The virus winters in the nymphal ticks that feed on and infect small rodents in the spring. The rodents become viremic and in turn infect larval ticks. The larvae metamorphose during the summer; they winter as infected nymphs, and do not transmit virus to humans until the adult stage, which may be 1 or 2 years after infection. Foci of infected ticks occur primarily in ecologic zones favorable to large populations of the golden-mantled ground squirrel.

Diagnosis

Colorado tick fever should be suspected in individuals with diphasic fever, leukopenia, and a history of exposure to ticks in the western United States 3–6 days before onset of disease. Diagnosis of Colorado tick fever depends on isolation of the virus, demonstration of antigen in the red blood cells, or demonstration of a fourfold rise or fall in antibody titer. Virus is readily isolated from erythrocytes by inoculating tissue culture or baby mice intracerebrally. Trypsin treatment of red cells to remove antibody enhances the chance of isolation; red cells may still be positive up to 6 weeks after infection. Antigen also can be shown in the red blood cells by the immunofluorescence technique. Within one week after onset of symptoms, antibody appears in the serum as determined by indirect immunofluorescence. Neutralizing antibody appears somewhat later. The complement-fixation test does not become positive until about 3 weeks after onset of illness. A travel history can aid the physician and the laboratory in diagnosis. Because of the long duration of viremia, definitive diagnosis of Colorado tick fever has been made in persons returning home far from the endemic area where the infection was acquired.

Control

Colorado tick fever can be prevented by avoiding tick-infested areas, by checking the body for ticks every 3 hours while camping or hiking and removing them, and by using tick repellants such as diethyltoluamide. Theoretically, campgrounds should be located away from the habitat of the golden-mantled ground squirrel; however, this creature is a favorite of campers and such a measure would not be popular. An experimental killed vaccine for Colorado tick fever was developed but is not now in use. No specific treatment for the disease exists.

References

Barnes, G., et al.: A randomized trial of oral gamma globulin in low-birth-weight infants infected with rotavirus. *Lancet* 1982; 1:1371-1373.

Barnett, B.: Viral gastroenteritis. *Med Clin North Am* 1983; 67:1031-1058.

Bishop, R.F., et al.: Clinical immunity after neonatal rotavirus infection. A prospective longitudinal study in young children. *N Engl J Med* 1983; 309:72-76.

Ebina, T., et al.: Prevention of rotavirus infection by cow colostrum containing antibody against human rotavirus. *Lancet* 1983; 2:1029-1030.

Estes, M.K., Palmer, E.L., Obijeski, J.F.: Rotaviruses: A review. *Curr Top Microbiol Immunol* 1983; 105:123-184.

Gerna, G., et al.: Rapid serotyping of human rotavirus strains by solid-phase immune electron microscopy. *J Clin Microbiol* 1984; 19:273-278.

Gorman, B.M., Taylor, J., Walker, P.J.: Orbiviruses. In: *The Reoviridae*, Joklik, W.K. (editor). New York: Plenum Publishing Corp, 1983.

Holmes, I.H.: Rotaviruses. In: *The Reoviridae*. Joklik, W.K. (editor). New York: Plenum Publishing Corp, 1983.

Hoshino Y., et al.: Serotypic similarity and diversity of human and animal rotaviruses as studied by plaque reduction neutralization. *J Inf Dis* 1984; 149:694-702.

Hung, T., et al.: Waterborne outbreak of rotavirus diarrhoea in adults in China caused by a novel rotavirus. *Lancet* 1984; 1:1139-1142.

Kapikian, A.Z., et al.: Approaches to immunization of infants and young children against gastroenteritis due to rotaviruses. *Rev Infect Dis* 1980; 2:459-469.

Kapikian, A.Z., Yolken, R.H.: Rotavirus. In: *Principles and practice of infectious diseases,* 2nd ed. Mandell, G.L., Douglas, R.G. Jr., Bennett, J.E., (editors). New York: John Wiley and Sons, 1984.

Kapikian, A.Z., et al.: Gastroenteritis viruses. In: *Diagnostic procedures for viral, rickettsial, and chlamydial infections,* 5th ed. Lennette, E.H., Schmidt, N.J. (editors). Washington, D.C.: American Public Health Association, 1979.

Kapikian, A.Z., Chanock R.M.: Rotavirus. In: *Virology.* Fields, B.N. (editor). New York: Raven Press, 1985.

Rodriguez, W.J., et al.: Clinical features of acute gastroenteritis associated with human reovirus-like agent in infants and young children. *J Pediatr* 1977; 91:188-193.

Sack, D.A., et al.: Oral hydration in rotavirus diarrhea: A double blind comparison of sucrose with glucose electrolyte solution. *Lancet* 1978; 2:280-283.

Sato, K., et al.: Isolation of human rotavirus in cell cultures. *Arch Virol* 1981; 69:155-160.

Saulsbury, F.T., Winkelstein, J.A., Yolken, R.H.: Chronic rotavirus infection in immunodeficiency. *J Pediatr* 1980; 97:61-65.

Tan, J.A., Schnagl, R.G.: Inactivation of a rotavirus by disinfectants. *Med J Austrl* 1981; 1:19-23.

Vesikari, T., et al.: Protection of infants against rotavirus diarrhea by RIT 4237 attenuated bovine rotavirus strain vaccine. *Lancet* 1984; 1:977-981.

Yolken, R.H, et al.: Infectious gastroenteritis in bone marrow transplant recipients. *N Engl J Med* 1982; 306:1009-1012.

84 Parvoviruses

○

Neil R. Blacklow, MD

George Cukor, PhD

Neil R. Blacklow, MD

George Cukor, PhD

1 + or −

C = 12
18-26nm

General Concepts
ADENO-ASSOCIATED VIRUSES
Distinctive Properties
Pathogenesis
Host Defenses
Epidemiology
Diagnosis
Control

SERUM PARVOVIRUSLIKE VIRUS
Distinctive Properties
Pathogenesis
Host Defenses
Epidemiology
Diagnosis
Control

General Concepts

The parvoviruses (*parvo* meaning small) are a group of very small DNA viruses that are ubiquitous and infect many species of animals. Some parvoviruses that infect humans are known as adeno-associated viruses because of their dependence on concomitant adenovirus infection. The small amount of DNA contained in the virus appears to carry only sufficient genetic information to code for the capsid protein of the virus. As a result, parvoviruses have unusual requirements for replication, such as a helper virus or rapidly dividing cells. The parvoviruses are divided into two general groups on the basis of these requirements. One group contains the **defective parvoviruses,** which multiply only in cells coinfected with a helper adenovirus; these viruses are therefore called **adeno-associated viruses** (AAV). Humans are commonly infected with AAV, apparently always in association with adenovirus infection. As far as is known, the

---

The diagram of the virion morphology is derived from Chapter 62.

presence of AAV does not affect the disease expression of adenovirus infection nor does AAV produce disease by itself.

The second group of parvoviruses are autonomous and do not require a helper virus for their multiplication; however, they only multiply in cells that are in S phase (that is, cells in the process of replicating their own DNA). The disease caused by **autonomous parvoviruses** in animals often reflect their requirement for infecting tissues that contain rapidly dividing cells. For example, the H-1 hamster virus is teratogenic. The human serum parvoviruslike virus (SPLV) affects maturing red blood cells in the bone marrow, and thus produces bone-marrow aplastic crises in predisposed individuals who have disorders in which the survival of the red blood cell is shortened, such as sickle-cell anemia.

ADENO-ASSOCIATED VIRUSES

Distinctive Properties

The AAV are 20–25 nm in diameter, are nonenveloped, and possess icosahedral symmetry. They contain a small amount (1.5×10^6 daltons) of single-stranded linear DNA as their genome. Complementary strands of the DNA are separately encapsidated so that one-half of the virions contain a strand of positive polarity and the remainder of the virions possess a negative DNA strand. During viral replication, the strands from different virions that are infecting the same cell combine to form a double-stranded intermediate. Viral RNA transcription can occur only when cells are coinfected with a helper adenovirus, which is presumed to provide an adenovirus-specific enzyme to aid in this step of AAV replication. The resultant AAV mRNA is translated to form polypeptides of three size classes, which comprise the AAV capsid.

Four serotypes of AAV have been identified on the basis of antigenicity of the capsid. The AAV are not related to adenoviruses antigenically or genetically; that is, AAV DNA is not related to adenovirus DNA. Because of their strict dependence on the presence of a helper virus, AAV are found as contaminants of adenovirus in nature and in the laboratory. AAV have been termed **superparasites**—they are parasitic on another parasite. Any of the adenovirus serotypes can provide the complete helper function required for AAV growth. It is interesting that herpesviruses can act as incomplete helpers for AAV, in contrast to the complete helper effect provided by adenoviruses. During coinfection of cells with a herpesvirus and AAV, AAV-specific polypeptides are synthesized, but infectious AAV virions are not assembled. This difference between adenovirus and herpesvirus helper effects suggests that at least two defective steps occur in AAV replication, only one of which is aided by herpesviruses. One recent report, however, indicates that herpes simplex virus, like adenoviruses, can act as a complete helper for AAV in cell culture.

Pathogenesis

Human infection with AAV is common but occurs only in association with adenovirus infection. Thus, AAV may be isolated from clinical specimens such as feces, throat washings, and conjunctival swabs that frequently contain adenovirus. Outbreaks of AAV infection (coincident with adenovirus) have not been associated with any unique acute disease manifestations. In addition, AAV infection does not appear to modify the symptomatology or severity of adenovirus respiratory tract disease in children.

Host Defenses

The factors that eradicate adenovirus infection (see Chapter 86) presumably also lead to the elimination of AAV. Little more is known about host defenses to AAV except that serum antibodies specific for AAV are produced during infection.

Epidemiology

The person-to-person transmission of AAV infection is novel in that the virus appears to travel with its helper adenovirus. Human infection with AAV types 1, 2, and 3 is common; serum antibody to these viruses is found in approximately 50% of American adults. These antibodies are acquired, for the most part, during childhood, the peak age for adenovirus infection. AAV type 4 is a simian virus that rarely infects humans. An interesting finding in animal models shows that AAV infection abrogates tumors produced by adenovirus- or herpesvirus-transformed cells. That the same phenomenon occurs in humans is suggested by the lower incidence of AAV antibody (and therefore infection) reported among patients with genital malignancies in comparison with controls.

Diagnosis

The clinical manifestations of AAV infection (see Chapter 86) are merely those produced by its helper adenovirus. AAV may be isolated from stool, throat, or conjunctival specimens that are inoculated into adenovirus-infected cell cultures. The presence of AAV in these cultures is then ascertained by identification of AAV-specific complement-fixing antigens. Neutralization, complement-fixation, and fluorescent antibody techniques may be used to measure serum antibodies to AAV.

Control

Adeno-associated viruses are hardy, heat-stable organisms that have been found occasionally as contaminants of human and simian tissue cultures. Thus, their potential presence should be considered in selecting cells to be used for production of various viral vaccines.

SERUM PARVOVIRUSLIKE VIRUS

Distinctive Properties

The human serum parvoviruslike virus (SPLV) is 23 nm in diameter, nonenveloped, and spherical. It has been observed by electron microscopy only in human serum and is not related to the small viruslike particles occasionally seen in human stools. Originally called B-19 virus, SPLV is not related immunologically to AAV and is not found in association with adenovirus or herpesviruses.

SPLV has yet to be cultivated in cell culture or laboratory animals, and therefore it is not known if it is autonomous. Nothing is known about its nucleic acid, but its morphology, buoyant density, and propensity for infecting rapidly dividing bone marrow cells in humans are consistent with those of a parvovirus. The number of serotypes of SPLV is unknown.

Pathogenesis

SPLV was first associated with human illness in 1981. It produces bone marrow aplastic crises in individuals with chronic hemolytic anemias such as sickle cell anemia, hereditary spherocytosis, and pyruvate-kinase deficiency. These patients are no more susceptible to infection with SPLV than are normal persons; however, when they are infected, they are at high risk for developing an aplastic crisis, during which red blood cell production ceases for 5-7 days. Because of the shortened life span of erythrocytes in patients with chronic hemolytic anemias (10-15 days compared to 120 days in normal persons), lack of red blood cell production results in a sharp decrease in blood hemoglobin levels and patients present in acute distress.

The results of laboratory studies with SPLV correlate well with the pathogenesis of human disease. Human sera containing SPLV show a selective suppressive effect on the growth of erythroid cell precursors of the bone marrow in culture; this effect is not seen on the granulocytic cell series.

Recent preliminary evidence suggests that SPLV is also the cause of erythema infectiosum (fifth disease). This mild illness occurs in epidemic fashion, usually among children, and is characterized by the acute onset of an erythematous rash. Affected individuals seem to produce IgM antibody directed against SPLV; such antibody is seldom seen in controls.

Host Defenses

The primary risk factor in developing aplastic crises due to SPLV is the presence of underlying hematologic disease in which the red blood cells have a shortened life span. Serum antibodies, including those of the IgM class, are produced after infection with SPLV, but their role in recovery from infection is unknown. Other mechanisms of SPLV immunity have not been studied.

Epidemiology

The mechanism of person-to-person transmission of SPLV infection is unknown. The virus is present in blood but has yet to be detected in tissues. However, spread of infection in the community via a hematogenous route seems unlikely. A respiratory or fecal-oral route of transmission would be most consistent with the epidemiology of infection, but to date there is no virologic evidence for such a route.

Serologic assays indicate that approximately one-third of individuals possess serum antibody to SPLV by age 16 years. The peak time for acquisition of antibody is between the second and sixth year of life. In fact, the true incidence of infection with SPLV may be greater than one-third of individuals because the serologic assay used to derive this figure was relatively insensitive. Infections with SPLV appear to occur in 3–5 year cycles. An increased prevalence of antibody to SPLV has been observed among hemophiliacs who are receiving clotting factor concentrates, but not among those who are receiving blood transfusions. The clinical consequences of this observation are not known.

Diagnosis

Clinical and laboratory manifestations of aplastic crises in patients with chronic hemolytic anemia should suggest infection with SPLV. The virus can be detected in sera of affected patients by immune electron microscopy and by counterimmunoelectrophoresis. Development of antibody seroconversions to SPLV, which indicates recent infection, can be evaluated by counterimmunoelectrophoresis and radioimmunoassay. Because SPLV-specific IgM antibody also is produced for a short time after infection, its presence in a single serum specimen also indicates a recent infection.

Control

Attempts at control of SPLV infection will likely await propagation of the virus in cell culture. Culture of the virus may make it possible to develop a vaccine that prevents aplastic crises due to SPLV in patients with chronic hemolytic anemias.

References

Anderson, M.J.: The emerging story of a human parvovirus-like agent. *J Hyg* 1982; 89:1–8.

Anderson, M.J., et al.: An outbreak of erythema infectiosum associated with human parvovirus infection. *J Hyg* (Cambridge) 1984; 93:85–93.

Blacklow, N.R., et al.: A seroepidemiologic study of adenovirus-associated virus infection in infants and children. *Am J Epidemiol* 1971; 94:359–366.

Hoggan, M.D.: Adenovirus associated viruses. In: *Progress in medical virology,* vol 12. Melnick, J. (editor). New York: Karger, 1970.

Mortimer, P.P., et al.: A human parvoviruslike virus inhibits haematopoietic colony formation in vitro. *Nature* 1983; 302:426–429.

Serjeant, G.R., et al.: Outbreak of aplastic crises in sickle cell anaemia associated with parvovirus-like agent. *Lancet* 1981; 2:595–597.

Ward, D.C., Tattersall, P., (editors). *Replication of mammalian parvoviruses.* Cold Spring Harbor, N.Y.: Cold Spring Harbor Laboratory, 1978.

85 Caliciviruses and Norwalk Virus

○

1 +

C = 32 (holes)
35-40nm

Neil R. Blacklow, MD

General Concepts

The caliciviruses are small, nonenveloped RNA viruses that have characteristic cup-shaped depressions on a spherical capsid surface; hence their name, which is derived from *calyx* or chalice. These viruses were previously thought to be picornaviruses; however, caliciviruses differ from picornaviruses in their distinctive structure, sometimes described as a star of David, as well as in their larger diameter (35–40 nm), single major polypeptide composition, and single-stranded RNA genome functions. Caliciviruses produce mucocutaneous and respiratory tract lesions in several animal species, including swine, pinnipeds, and cats, and they have been grown in cell culture, purified, and characterized.

Few human caliciviruses have been cultivated in vitro and thus no human strains are as well characterized as the animal caliciviruses. Human viruses with morphologic and biophysical features similar to those of animal caliciviruses, however, are observed often in patients with diarrheal illness; but no one has yet reported conclusive proof that these

---

The diagram of the virion morphology is derived from Chapter 62.

human viruses are indeed caliciviruses. The best known of the human agents is Norwalk virus, which is a major cause of epidemics of self-limited diarrhea and vomiting in school children and adults. Resistance to the infection is unrelated to serum antibody. Another caliciviruslike agent also has been detected in some young children with diarrhea.

NORWALK VIRUS

Distinctive Properties

The Norwalk virus is round, somewhat smaller than the other caliciviruses (27 nm in diameter), and featureless—it lacks the distinctive substructure of the animal caliciviruses. It was previously described as "parvoviruslike." The change in designation occurred because Norwalk virus was found to contain a single major polypeptide with a molecular weight similar to that of the caliciviruses that have been characterized. In addition, the Norwalk viruses and caliciviruses have been found to have similar buoyant densities. Because it has not been cultivated in any cell culture or laboratory animal model system, Norwalk virus is recognized only in human stool specimens by immune electron microscopic or radioimmunoassay techniques. It is possible that the reason its morphologic characteristics may be different from those of animal caliciviruses is because the virus can only be visualized in feces as nonpurified aggregated particles. The nucleic acid of Norwalk virus is not known because not enough virus is present in feces for definitive analysis. Several serologically unrelated 27 nm Norwalklike viruses exist, such as Hawaii, W-Ditchling, and Snow Mountain; these agents also have been observed during outbreaks of gastroenteritis, but their medical importance is not known.

Pathogenesis

Norwalk virus produces nearly 50% of all outbreaks of acute infectious nonbacterial gastroenteritis that occur in the United States. This common syndrome is characterized by 1-2 days of diarrhea or vomiting or both, and is second only to acute respiratory tract disease as the most common cause of illness in American families. Although it is normally a self-limited, acute illness, Norwalk infection has been known to cause occasional deaths in elderly or debilitated persons. In developed areas, the illness typically occurs in older children and adults, and spares preschool children.

The virus was first discovered in diarrheal stool specimens from patients infected during an epidemic of gastroenteritis that occurred in Norwalk, Ohio, in 1968. The disease was reproduced in adult volunteers, who developed a transient mucosal lesion of the proximal small intestine. Norwalk infection seems to spare the large intestine, and thus fecal leukocytes are not present. Delayed gastric emptying occurs during this infection, which predominantly affects the small intestine.

Host Defenses

Although most adults have serum antibodies to Norwalk virus, the antibodies do not protect them from the disease. In fact, they may be a marker or risk factor for illness.

When Norwalk virus was given to volunteers, one of two types of immune responses occurred. One group of individuals, who lacked appreciable serum or intestinal antibodies, persistently failed to develop illness or to mount antibody responses on initial exposure to the virus and after rechallenge up to 3 years later. A second group of volunteers, who had systemic or local antibodies, developed gastroenteritis on initial exposure and were again susceptible when rechallenged 3 years later. After the illness, these individuals usually developed a short-term immunity that lasted for about 12 weeks. Further studies are needed to ascertain whether genetic susceptibility plays a role in Norwalk virus infection.

Epidemiology

Seroprevalence studies indicate that Norwalk virus infection occurs worldwide. Two-thirds of Americans have serum antibodies, which are uncommon in children, and are acquired during early adulthood. The results of antibody studies correlate with the rarity of Norwalk virus infection as a cause of gastroenteritis in infants and young children in the United States. Disease outbreaks among older children and adults occur in camps, schools, nursing homes, cruise ships, and areas with contaminated drinking or swimming water. The ingestion of raw shellfish or other uncooked foods, such as salads or cake frosting, that have been handled in an unsanitary manner may lead to the disease. Norwalk-virus outbreaks occur at all times of the year.

Infection is transmitted by the fecal–oral route. Although no evidence indicates that it is also spread by the respiratory route, it is conceivable that the virus may be transmitted via aerosolized virus-containing vomitus, in light of the very rapid secondary spread of infection during outbreaks.

Diagnosis

Norwalk virus may be identified in stool specimens, and antibody can be measured in serum samples by immune electron microscopic or solid-phase radioimmunoassay techniques. Because these diagnostic methods unfortunately require the use of human clinical materials (stools and sera), they can be performed in only a few research laboratories that possess the needed reagents. The radioimmunoassay is preferable to immune electron microscopy for the examination of large numbers of specimens that is required for epidemiologic studies.

Control

Prospects for vaccine development seem poor because of the complex pattern of clinical immunity to the virus. The development of a vaccine that produces long-lasting immunity seems unlikely because such immunity has been found to be absent in rechallenged volunteers. The inability to cultivate Norwalk virus and to purify it extensively from feces also precludes vaccine development. Hand washing and careful monitoring of water purification are the most important measures in the control of infection.

HUMAN CALICIVIRUSLIKE VIRUS

Caliciviruslike virus is recognized in human feces on the basis of its characteristic morphology, size, and buoyant density. It is 31-35 nm in diameter and round; it has characteristic cup-shaped indentations on its surface. Unlike Norwalk virus, it has been cultivated recently in the laboratory; however, its nucleic acid and definitive classification are not established. The virus has been detected in stools by electron microscopy and immune electron microscopy, particularly in samples from young children who have gastroenteritis. Serum antibodies to the virus are rapidly acquired during 6-24 months of age, and most older children and adults are seropositive. The recent development of a solid-phase radioimmunoassay technique to study this virus should permit an assessment of its medical importance in human disease.

No data are available on any potential relatedness of the human caliciviruslike virus and Norwalk virus. The reported sizes of these two viruses obtained in different laboratories vary, although Norwalk virus is described as slightly smaller. The featureless surface structure of Norwalk virus argues for the distinctness of the two viruses. The two agents also seem to differ in that antibody prevalence levels rise at later ages for Norwalk virus in populations residing in developed areas.

References

Blacklow, N.R., Cukor, G.: Viral gastroenteritis. *N Engl J Med* 1981; 304:397-406.

Cukor, G., Blacklow, N.R.: Human viral gastroenteritis. *Microbiol Rev* 1984; 48:157-179.

Greenberg, H.B., Valdesuso, J.R., Kalica, A.R., et al.: Proteins of Norwalk virus. *J Virol* 1981; 37:994-999.

Kaplan, J.E., et al.: Epidemiology of Norwalk gastroenteritis and the role of Norwalk virus in outbreaks of acute nonbacterial gastroenteritis. *Ann Int Med* 1982; 96:756-761.

Nakata, S., et al.: Microtiter solid-phase radioimmunoassay for detection of human calicivirus in stools. *J Clin Microbiol* 1983; 17:198-201.

Schaffer, F.L., et al.: Caliciviridae. *Intervirology* 1980; 14:1-6.

86 Papovaviruses

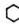

Janet S. Butel, PhD

1 ±

C = 72
45-55nm

General Concepts   Papillomaviruses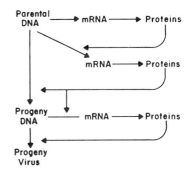
Distinctive Properties   **Host Defenses**
  Polyomaviruses   **Epidemiology**
  Papillomaviruses   **Diagnosis**
Pathogenesis   **Control**
  Polyomaviruses

General Concepts

Papovaviruses are small, nonenveloped, icosahedral viruses that contain circular, double-stranded DNA. The term papovavirus was derived from the first two letters of the names of three members of this group: *pa*pillomavirus, mouse *po*lyoma virus, and simian *va*cuolating virus (SV40). Members of this group can induce tumors in susceptible hosts, transform the morphologic characteristics of cells in culture, or both. The important members of the group are characterized in Table 86-1.

Papovaviruses are divided into two genera on the basis of physicochemical and biologic properties (see Table 86-1). The polyomaviruses, the smaller viruses, are about 45 nm in diameter and have a genome of approximately 3×10^6 daltons (approximately 5200 base pairs). These viruses tend to induce persistent, apparently harmless, infections in their natural hosts. They have attracted the attention of research scientists because they induce tumors when injected into rodents. In addition, because of their small

---

The diagrams of the virion morphology and the multiplication scheme are derived from Chapters 62 and 63, respectively. The multiplication scheme applies only generally as indicated in Chapter 63.

Table 86-1 Properties of Representative Papovaviruses

Characteristics	Subgroup (Genus)						
	Polyomavirus				*Papillomavirus*		
Virion							
Capsid symmetry	Cubic				Cubic		
No. of capsomeres	72				72		
Presence of envelope	No				No		
Size in diameter	45 nm				55 nm		
Genome							
Type of nucleic acid	DNA				DNA		
Structure	Circular, double-stranded				Circular, double-stranded		
Size	3×10^6 d				5×10^6 d		
Oncogenic							
Tumors in natural hosts	No				Yes		
Persistence of infectious virus in tumors	No				Yes		
Transform cells in vitro	Yes				Some (bovine)		
Individual members	Polyoma	SV40	BK	JC	Human	Bovine	Rabbit
Host of origin	Mouse	Monkey	Human	Human	Human	Cow	Rabbit
No. of types	1	1	1	1	>15	5	1

genetic content (only six or seven polypeptides can be encoded), the polyomaviruses have served as simple model systems for exploring the molecular events involved in transformation and other mammalian cell biologic processes. One of the SV40 early gene products, the tumor antigen, has been shown to be required for viral DNA replication during productive infection and for initiation and maintenance of the transformed phenotype. Two papovaviruses, BKV and JCV, have been found in humans.

The papillomaviruses are slightly larger, 55 nm in diameter, with a more complex circular DNA genome of 5×10^6 daltons (approximately 8000 base pairs) (see Table 86-1). In contrast to the polyomaviruses and many other DNA tumor viruses, the papillomaviruses induce tumors in their natural hosts. Papillomaviruses have been found in many species, including humans, rabbits, cows, and dogs. They are associated with a variety of benign papillomatous lesions of the skin and squamous mucosa. Analysis of their unique type of virus-host interaction at the molecular level has been impeded by the lack of a tissue culture system able to support papillomavirus replication in vitro.

Distinctive Properties

Polyomaviruses

Genome Organization. The genome of the polyomaviruses consists of about 5200 base pairs of double-stranded, circular DNA. The organization of the SV40 genome is

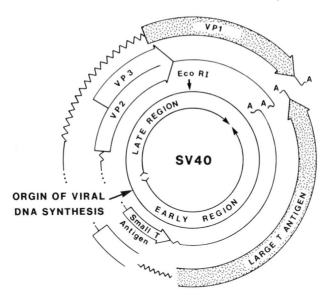

Figure 86-1 Physical and functional map of the SV40 genome. Arrowheads point in the direction of transcription. The boxed arrows indicate the coding regions of messenger RNA, with the encoded protein designated within each arrow. Stippled areas within boxed arrows indicate that viral-specified polypeptides or portions thereof are coded in different reading frames. Heavy black arrow at lower left marks the origin of viral DNA synthesis.

diagrammed in Figure 86-1. The genetic structure of other viruses in this genus, for example, JCV and BKV, resembles closely that of SV40. Polyoma virus differs only in that it codes for an additional early gene product. The entire nucleotide sequences of several papovavirus DNAs have been determined. About one-half of the SV40 genome encodes nonstructural proteins that are expressed before viral DNA synthesis begins. The products of that region are designated **early functions.** The early proteins are also referred to as **tumor antigens** because they were first detected in virus-induced tumors by using sera from tumor-bearing animals.

The other half of the viral genome codes for virion structural proteins, which are called **late functions** because they are expressed after viral DNA synthesis begins. The late proteins are required to construct the icosahedral capsid that packages the genomic DNA. The major capsid protein (VP1) has a mass of approximately 45,000 daltons and constitutes 70% of the virion protein. Two other polypeptides, with calculated molecular weights of 38,500 and 27,000 daltons, respectively, are minor components of the capsid. Cellular histones are also incorporated into the virions in close association with the viral DNA. The histones probably aid in packaging the DNA inside the capsid.

Maximum use is made of the limited amount of genetic information carried by these viruses. Some of the viral-coded proteins are encoded partly by shared regions of the DNA (for example, VP2 and VP3; small t and large T antigens). Other proteins are translated from different reading frames from overlapping regions of the DNA (for example, VP2 and VP1) (see Figure 86-1).

Productive Infections.   Polyomaviruses undergo two types of interactions with host cells (Figure 86-2). Permissive cells support virus replication, which results in the

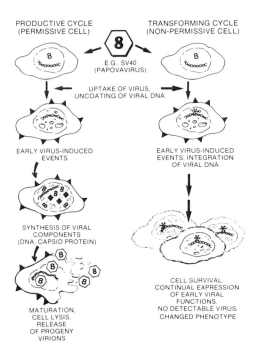

PRODUCTIVE CYCLE (PERMISSIVE CELL)　　　TRANSFORMING CYCLE (NON-PERMISSIVE CELL)

E.G., SV40 (PAPOVAVIRUS)

UPTAKE OF VIRUS, UNCOATING OF VIRAL DNA

EARLY VIRUS-INDUCED EVENTS

EARLY VIRUS-INDUCED EVENTS, INTEGRATION OF VIRAL DNA

SYNTHESIS OF VIRAL COMPONENTS (DNA, CAPSID PROTEIN)

CELL SURVIVAL, CONTINUAL EXPRESSION OF EARLY VIRAL FUNCTIONS, NO DETECTABLE VIRUS, CHANGED PHENOTYPE

MATURATION, CELL LYSIS, RELEASE OF PROGENY VIRIONS

Figure 86-2 Schematic comparison of two types of interaction between a papovavirus and a host cell. The productive cycle that results in synthesis of progeny virions is diagrammed on the left. The transforming cycle that is characterized by partial viral gene expression and cellular phenotypic changes is represented on the right. Modified from Benyesh-Melnick, M., Butel, J. *The Molecular Biology of Cancer.* New York: Academic Press, 1974.

synthesis of progeny virus and cell death. Nonpermissive cells do not support virus replication but can, on occasion, be transformed. When cells are transformed, the cells survive, the cellular phenotype is altered, and no progeny virus is produced. The expression of SV40 viral-specific events in lytic and in transforming infections is compared in Table 86-2.

The polyomaviruses have a narrow host range. Permissive cells are derived from the natural host of each isolate (monkey cells for SV40, mouse cells for polyoma, and human cells for BKV and JCV). Not all cell types from the susceptible species will support virus replication.

The infecting virion first attaches to specific receptors on permissive cells, then penetrates through the plasma membrane and is transported to the nucleus where the viral DNA is uncoated and released. During the early phase of the lytic cycle, the virus drives the cell into S phase, thereby increasing the amount of the cellular enzymes associated with DNA metabolism, such as thymidine kinase and DNA polymerase. The virus uses cellular enzymes for its own replication. The mechanism by which the virus activates cellular DNA synthesis is unclear, but that effect may be related to the transforming ability of the virus because tumor cells are continuously stimulated to grow and divide.

The early proteins (tumor antigens) are synthesized soon after infection and reach detectable levels about 10 hours after infection. Viral DNA synthesis begins shortly after that time. The large-tumor (T) antigen is a prerequisite for viral DNA replication; it

Table 86-2   Expression of Viral-Induced Events in Productive and Transforming Infections by Papovavirus SV40

Event	Cytolytic Cycle*	Transformed Cells*
Synthesis of viral mRNA—early	+	+
Synthesis of tumor antigens	+	+
Synthesis of transplantation antigen	+	+
Induction of host cell enzymes	+	+
Stimulation of host cell DNA synthesis	+	+
Integration of viral DNA into cellular chromosome	?	+
Synthesis of viral DNA	+	−
Synthesis of viral mRNA—late	+	−
Synthesis of virus capsid antigens	+	−
Formation of virus particles	+	−
Cell death	+	−

*+, present; −, absent.

binds to viral DNA at the site of initiation of DNA synthesis and is essential for virus replication in permissive cells. The expression of late viral genes occurs after DNA synthesis begins. Structural proteins VP1, 2, and 3 are made, and then particles are assembled and accumulate in the nucleus. Progeny virus can be detected by 24 hours after infection. The host cells are killed eventually. The papovaviruses have the longest (slowest) growth cycle among the viruses that contain DNA.

Transforming Infections.   Nonpermissive cells do not support virus growth, but may be transformed (see Figure 86-2). The viral-induced early events that are expressed in permissive cells also occur in nonpermissive cells. Host enzymes are induced, tumor antigens are synthesized, and cellular DNA synthesis is stimulated. However, no free viral DNA synthesis occurs, and late viral genes that encode capsid proteins are not expressed. The viral genome becomes integrated in the cellular chromosome. Integration of viral sequences into host cell DNA is random and can occur at many different sites. In general, only one or a very few viral DNA copies are present in an individual transformed cell. The entire viral genome need not be retained in transformed cells, but an intact early region is required because the transforming protein (the large-tumor antigen) must be synthesized continuously for a cell to remain transformed.

Transformation is a stable, inherited change in cell properties. The most prominent phenotypic modifications associated with SV40-transformed cells include: altered morphology (cells become more rounded); altered growth patterns (increased rate of growth, decreased requirement for serum growth factors, loss of contact inhibition, and enhanced ability to grow in semisolid medium [anchorage independence]); biochemical changes (increased metabolic rate, increased glycolysis, changes in properties of the cell membrane, synthesis of new antigens in the cell); and tumorigenicity (production of tumors when transformed cells are injected into appropriate test animals).

The molecular basis of cellular transformation mediated by papovaviruses is still not clear, despite intensive investigations. The large-tumor antigen is the critical gene product in the SV40 system. In transformed cells, the tumor antigen localizes predominantly in the nucleus, although a small fraction ($\leq 5\%$) is associated with the plasma membrane, where it is involved in virus-specific transplantation antigen reactions. The individual roles of the nuclear and membrane forms of T-antigen in the maintenance of transformation are not known. Papovavirus-transforming proteins mediate all the necessary events rapidly so that intermediate stages of phenotypic changes are not observed easily.

SV40 large-tumor antigen is one of the most thoroughly characterized of the known transforming proteins from viruses. Properties and functions attributed to the large-tumor antigen are presented in Table 86-3. The great diversity illustrated may be important in promoting the many cellular changes associated with the transformed phenotype. The functions of small-t-antigen have not been determined. However, deletion mutants that are unable to synthesize small-t–antigen are viable, which indicates that the protein is not needed for virus replication.

Another phenomenon that occurs in polyomavirus systems is **abortive transformation.** Many infected nonpermissive cells exhibit properties typical of the transformed phenotype transiently, but most cells revert rapidly to the normal cell phenotype. Only a few infected, nonpermissive cells are transformed permanently. If conditions are

Table 86-3   Properties and Functions Attributed to SV40 Large Tumor Antigen, a Papovavirus Transforming Protein

Biochemical characteristics
Size—calculated molecular weight, 82,000 d; apparent molecular weight, 90,000–100,000 d
Modifications—phosphorylation; N-acetylation; glycosylation; ADP-ribosylation; acylation
ATPase activity
Tightly associated with protein kinase activity

Role in virus replication
Sequence specific binding to origin of replication on viral genome
Initiation of viral DNA replication
Autoregulation of viral early transcription
Induction of viral late transcription

Effects on host cell
Binds to cellular DNA
Binds to cellular protein, p53
Initiation of cellular DNA replication
Induction of cellular enzyme synthesis
Activation of ribosomal DNA transcription
Expression of adenovirus helper function
Initiation and maintenance of oncogenic transformation
Target for cytotoxic T cells

Other
Induction of immunity to SV40 tumor cells
Localization in nucleus and plasma membrane

manipulated to prevent virus replication, however, transformation of permissive cells can be achieved.

In summary, the major hallmarks of cells transformed by the polyomaviruses are the presence of viral DNA that is integrated covalently into cellular chromosomal DNA, the expression of viral-coded tumor antigens, and the lack of production of virus particles.

Papillomaviruses

The papillomaviruses share certain physicochemical features with the polyomaviruses, but their biologic properties are quite different (see Table 86-1). Although the papillomavirus genome is larger (approximately 8000 base pairs) and fewer specific details about it are known, its structure and genetic organization appear to resemble that of the SV40 genome.

Papillomaviruses are highly tropic for epithelial cells of the skin and mucous membranes. Replication of the viruses depends strongly on the differentiated state of the cell; when present, progeny virions can be detected only in nuclei of cells in the upper layers of the infected epidermis. This dependence of virus replication on cell differentiation probably is responsible for researchers' failure to obtain a reproducible tissue culture system that is permissive for papillomavirus replication or transformation. Since several human and animal papillomavirus isolates have been cloned in bacterial plasmids by use of recombinant DNA technology, certain molecular analyses of the genomes have been accomplished in the absence of a system able to propagate infectious virus.

The papillomaviruses induce benign tumors (warts) of the epithelium in their natural hosts. This expression of oncogenic potential in natural hosts is in marked contrast to the actions of the polyomaviruses. The papillomaviruses have a narrow host range; no interspecies transmission has been documented.

Virus particles can be detected easily in some types of warts (for example, hand and plantar), but may not be found in other types of lesions (for example, larynx, external genitalia, and cervix). There is currently no evidence for integration of viral DNA into the host chromosome of the papillomatous lesion; transformation appears to be mediated by free episomal DNA molecules. These characteristics are also in contrast to the state and expression of polyomavirus genomes in transformed cells. Estimates of the number of episomal copies of the viral genome have ranged from 10-500 per cell. Because papillomavirus genomes remain extrachromosomal, scientists are interested in their potential usefulness as eukaryotic cloning vectors. Although molecular analyses of papillomavirus genomes have suggested similarities to that of SV40, putative papillomavirus transforming proteins have not yet been identified.

Widespread heterogeneity exists among the papillomaviruses. The isolates from different species are serologically distinct, although denatured structural polypeptides from them exhibit some common antigenic determinants. Antisera prepared against intact virus particles are type-specific and will not react with tissues infected by another type of papillomavirus, but antisera against virions disrupted by detergent cross-react with capsid antigens of all papillomaviruses, including those from other species. This indicates that there are shared amino-acid sequences in the structural proteins of the papillomaviruses that are not exposed on the surface of virus particles.

It has become apparent that surprising diversity exists among human papillomaviruses. Classical neutralization tests cannot be done because of the lack of an infectivity assay for papillomaviruses, so molecular criteria have been used as a basis of classification. Two different virus types share less than 50% DNA homology; two isolates are considered as subtypes if DNA homology exceeds 50% but the restriction enzyme cleavage patterns of the respective DNAs differ.

In summary, outstanding features of the papillomaviruses are the induction of tumors in natural hosts, the presence of virus particles in some tumor tissue, and the presence of viral DNA in infected and transformed cells that is maintained as episomal copies.

Pathogenesis

Polyomaviruses

The polyomaviruses establish persistent, yet harmless, infections in their natural hosts. The subclinical infections elicit virus-specific antibodies that can be detected by serologic tests. Although wild mice harbor polyoma virus, tumors do not result from natural infections. The virus probably is transmitted through urine, feces, and saliva. SV40 seems to localize in the urinary tract of its natural host, the rhesus monkey, but tumor induction in the monkey has not been observed. Early lots of live poliomyelitis vaccines that had been produced in monkey cells were contaminated by SV40. Although many persons inadvertently received such SV40-contaminated vaccines 20 years ago, none of them have been reported to develop SV40-related tumors. The oncogenic potential of the polyomaviruses can be demonstrated only by experimental inoculation of certain heterologous newborn animals (hamsters for SV40; mice, rats, and hamsters for polyoma virus).

Two human papovaviruses have been studied extensively. BK virus was isolated from the urine of a recipient of a renal allograft who was undergoing immunosuppressive therapy, whereas JC virus was recovered from the brain tissue of a patient with progressive multifocal leukoencephalopathy (PML), a rare demyelinating disease characterized by multiple foci of degeneration that sometimes accompanies chronic debilitating diseases. Both viruses are ubiquitous among humans, with the initial infection occurring during childhood. Available evidence suggests that both BKV and JCV may persist in the kidneys of healthy individuals after the primary infection, and may reactivate when the host's immune response is impaired. The two viruses are antigenically distinct from each other and from other members of the polyomavirus genus, but the early proteins (tumor antigens) induced by BKV and JCV have some of the same antigenic determinants as those of SV40.

BKV has not been proven to cause any clinical disease, although it has been implicated in acute respiratory tract disease. BKV is often activated in renal transplant patients and others who have received immunosuppressive agents, and is excreted in the urine. Several cases of papovavirus-associated obstruction of the ureter have been described. In addition, BKV has been recovered from the urine of patients with hereditary immunodeficiency diseases, such as the Wiskott-Aldrich syndrome. BKV may also be activated during normal prengancies.

JCV is presumed to cause PML. It has been identified in about 30 cases of progressive multifocal leukoencephalopathy. Large numbers of virus particles are present within the nuclei of glial cells in the brain lesions of patients with progressive multifocal leukoencephalopathy. In addition, JCV has been found to be disseminated widely in the extraneural tissue (for example, kidney, liver, lung, and spleen) of patients with PML. Apparently, the viral DNA is not integrated into the genome of the host cell in either the brain or kidneys of progressive multifocal leukoencephalopathy patients. Like BKV, JCV has been recovered from the urine of immunosuppressed individuals and may be reactivated and excreted in the urine during normal pregnancies. JCV has such a highly restricted host range that cultivation in vitro requires brain cells from human fetuses.

Both BKV and JCV are able to transform cells in vitro and induce tumors in newborn hamsters, but no evidence has indicated that either agent is involved in the etiology of any type of human cancer.

Papillomaviruses

A variety of benign papillomatous lesions of the skin and squamous mucosa are believed to be caused by human papillomaviruses, including common and plantar warts, flat warts, anal and genital condyloma acuminata, cervical flat warts, macular pityriasislike lesions in patients with epidermodysplasia verruciformis, oral papillomas, and juvenile laryngeal papillomas. The laryngeal papillomas can be dangerous because they occur in young children and tend to cause acute respiratory obstruction, and because they often recur. Anecdotal and epidemiologic evidence indicates that warts are contagious. Individual types of human papillomaviruses tend to induce particular kinds of clinical lesions (Table 86-4), although exceptions do occur.

Table 86-4   Association of Human Papillomavirus Types with Clinical Lesions*

Human Papillomavirus Type	Clinical Lesion	Suspected Oncogenicity†
1	Plantar warts	None
2	Common warts	None
3, 10	Flat warts	EV cancers, genital cancers
5, 8	Macular lesions in EV‡	Bowen's disease; squamous cell cancers
6	Anogenital condylomas; laryngeal papillomas	Buschke-Löwenstein tumors (giant condylomas)
7	Hand warts in butchers	None
11	Laryngeal papillomas; flat cervical condylomas	Cervical cancers
16	Anogenital condylomas	Genital cancers

*Modified from Lutzner M. A. *Arch Dermatol* 1983; 119:631-35.
†Based on presence of related sequences in tumor tissue.
‡EV, epidermodysplasia verruciformis.

The genomes of some types of papillomavirus, especially 6, 11, and 16, have been associated with malignant neoplasms of the skin and mucosa. Although the role played by the virus in those malignancies has not been clarified, research suggests that the human papillomaviruses may be involved in the development of those malignant neoplasms, in addition to their ability to induce benign warts. Some benign lesions (epidermodysplasia verruciformis, laryngeal papillomatosis, and condyloma acuminata) have been reported to progress to squamous cell carcinoma. Synergistic external factors, such as irradiation, often seem to promote this progression. Papillomavirus types 6 and 11 are both associated with genital condylomas and laryngeal papillomas. It has been observed that infants with laryngeal papillomas are often born to mothers with genital condylomas of the birth canal.

Host Defenses

The polyomavirus members of the papovavirus group produce asymptomatic, persistent infections in their natural hosts. They elicit an antibody response that can be detected serologically by, for example, neutralization or hemagglutination inhibition assays. BKV and JCV have been isolated often from immunosuppressed individuals, indicating that the expression of those viruses may be under the control of the immunologic system.

The immune response of animals with tumors induced by polyoma or SV40 has been studied extensively. Tumor-bearing animals develop antibodies against the virus-specific tumor antigens involved in the maintenance of the transformed phenotype. In addition, cellular immunity develops against virus-induced, tumor-specific transplantation antigens that are located at the cell membrane. This immunity renders the animals resistant to challenge with tumor cells. The transplantation antigen induced by each virus is unique and is related to the tumor antigens in the nuclei of the tumor cells. These rodent model systems afford an opportunity to understand more about the immune response to neoplastic cells in humans.

Host immune responses to papillomavirus infections have not been well described. In general, warts persist for variable periods of time and then regress. The host is probably immune to reinfection with the same virus. The respective roles of humoral and cellular immunity in this response are not known. Papovaviruses are generally poor inducers of interferon and vary greatly in their susceptibility to its antiviral action.

Epidemiology

Seroepidemiologic studies have shown that BKV and JCV are ubiquitous throughout the world. Infections occur early in childhood, and 70%–90% of adults have antibodies to these viruses. Occurrence of SV40 infection in humans is rare, even though many persons were exposed to the virus when they received contaminated poliovirus vaccines. Papillomaviruses also are widely distributed in humans, but antibody surveys have not been done.

Diagnosis

JC virus can be identified in the brain lesions of patients with progressive multifocal leukoencephalopathy by electron microscopy or by immunofluorescence using virus-specific antiserum.

Immunocytologic techniques can be used to detect the presence of papillomavirus antigens in wart specimens. Antibodies that are directed against detergent-disrupted virions, which detect genus-specific antigenic cross-reactivity, can be conjugated to an enzyme marker (such as peroxidase) and be used in a screening test to detect papillomavirus antigens, even in fixed and embedded wart tissue. Specific virus types can be identified by using type-specific antisera, conjugated with fluorescein, on frozen sections of warts. The technique of nucleic acid hybridization, which can detect viral-specific sequences when no virus particles are present, should be especially useful in determining whether papillomaviruses are associated with human malignancies.

Control

Because BK and JC viruses are ubiquitous in the human population, and apparently produce only asymptomatic infections, no control measures are necessary. No specific therapy has been developed for the rare cases of progressive multifocal leukoencephalopathy.

Warts are treated by destruction of the lesions by freezing, cauterization, or surgery. The treatment of choice for multiple laryngeal papillomas is repeated laser vaporizations. Recently, interferon was shown to be effective against warts and juvenile laryngeal papillomas.

References

Danos, O., Yaniv, M.: Structure and function of papillomavirus genomes. In: *Advances in viral oncology*, vol. 3. Klein G (editor). New York: Raven Press, 1983.

Howley, P.M.: The human papillomaviruses. *Arch Pathol Lab Med* 1982; 106:429-32.

Rigby, W.J.P., Lane, D.P.: Structure and function of simian virus 40 large T-antigen. In: *Advances in viral oncology*, vol. 3. Klein, G., (editor). New York: Raven Press, 1983.

Tevethia, S.S.: Immunology of simian virus 40. In: *Viral oncology*, Klein G., (editor). New York: Raven Press, 1980.

Tooze, J.: *DNA tumor viruses: Molecular biology of tumor viruses, part 2*, 2nd ed. New York: Cold Spring Harbor Laboratory, 1980.

87 Adenoviruses

Lennart Philipson, MD, Dr Med Sci

1 ±

C = 252
70-90nm

General Concepts

Distinctive Properties
- Structure
- Chemical Composition
- Classification of Human Adenoviruses
- Antigenic Composition

Pathogenesis
- Susceptible Host Cells
- Clinical Manifestations

Host Defenses

Epidemiology

Diagnosis

Control

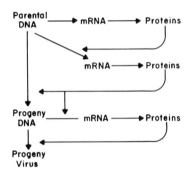

General Concepts

Adenoviruses, constitute a family of viruses originally isolated from the respiratory tract of humans and other animals. They cause mild respiratory infections and conjunctivitis in humans. Adenovirus infections occur frequently in children and military recruits, particularly during winter. Adenoviruses are nonenveloped icosahedral viruses with DNA genomes of intermediate size (20-30 × 10⁶ daltons). The Adenoviridae family has been subdivided into two genera, *Mastadenovirus* and *Aviadenovirus*, referring to viruses isolated from mammalian and avian hosts, respectively. There is no cross-reacting antigen between these two genera. Of the at least 80 different species that comprise the mastadenoviruses, 40 have been isolated from human sources. The aviadenovirus contains 14 distinct species.

The diagrams of the virion morphology and the multiplication scheme are derived from Chapters 62 and 63, respectively. The multiplication scheme applies only generally as indicated in Chapter 63.

Precise biochemical tools to characterize adenovirus genomes have become available. These include separated strands of DNA, genomic and cDNA recombinant DNA clones, and the messenger RNAs to detect the viral transcription products. In addition, proteins encoded by the adenovirus genome have been characterized by structure and function. This chapter describes properties of adenoviruses and their role in infectious human diseases.

A new vaccine based on virus protein components is being evaluated for respiratory infections; interferon is being tested for treatment of conjunctivitis.

Distinctive Properties

Structure

Adenoviruses are nonenveloped and have a diameter of 70-80 nm. The capsid is composed of 252 capsomers arranged into an icosahedron as shown in Figure 87-1. Of the 252 capsomers, 240 have six neighbors called **hexons,** whereas the 12 capsomers at the vertices have five neighbors called **pentons.** Each penton unit consists of a penton base anchored in the capsid and a rodlike projection, the fiber, attached to each penton. Inside the capsid is a core with a diameter of 40-45 nm, which contains the DNA and additional proteins. A circular protein-DNA complex has been observed after degradation of virions, and it has been established that the two termini of DNA in the virion are linked by proteins.

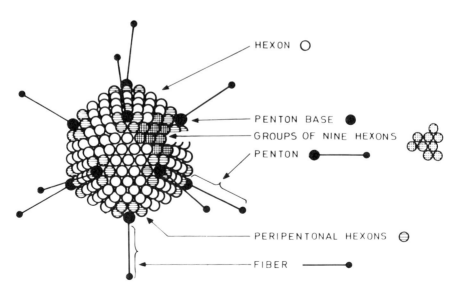

Figure 87-1 Structure of adenovirus capsid. Schematic drawing showing the icosahedral outline of the adenovirus capsid and the location of various components. From Philipson, L., Petterson, U., Lindberg, U. *Virol Monogr* 1975; 14:6.

Chemical Composition

The human adenovirus type 2 (ad2), which is the preferred model virus, has an estimated particle weight of 175×10^6 daltons. The virion contains 13% DNA, corresponding to 23×10^6 daltons, and several protein components. The virion of all adenoviruses analyzed contains a minimum of nine polypeptides, which range in size from 7500-120,000 daltons. Eight of these are antigenically distinct and reside in different structures after sequential degradation of the virion. Five of the polypeptides are integral parts of the capsomers or the core. They are shown in Figure 87-2.

The DNA of human adenoviruses has been characterized. Base composition differs among the various subgenera of human adenoviruses (Table 87-1). In addition, considerable homology of the DNA sequence exists within each subgenus, but only 10%-20% homology exists among DNA of members of different subgenera. The DNA for several species is infectious, but the specific infectivity is at least 10^6 times lower than for virions measured as number of infectious units per microgram of DNA. The protein associated with the termini of viral DNA appears to enhance infectivity of viral DNA. Specific fragments of DNA representing the left 8%-17% of the total genome can transform cells. The majority of the mRNA has been mapped on the viral DNA (Figure 87-3), and the total DNA sequence of the human ad2 genome comprising 35,000 base pairs has recently been determined.

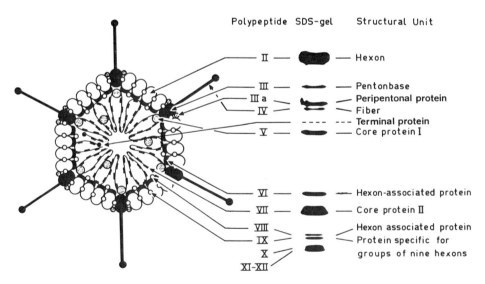

Figure 87-2 A tentative model of the location of different proteins in the ad2 virion. The core protein V may be located inside at the vertices since it is partially released with the peripentonal region. The core protein VII neutralizes around 50% of all phosphate residues in the DNA. Protein VI exists as a dimer on the internal surface of the capsid. Protein IX appears to be cementing substance between hexons from the facets, because it is associated with the ninemers of hexons. Protein VIII also is associated with the hexons and may reside at the inner surface of triangular facets. Polypeptide IIIa is located in the peripentonal region. The localization of the other protein is unknown. The polypeptide composition of the virion proteins as identified in a stained exponential (10%–16%) SDS-polyacrylamide gel are also shown. From Philipson, L., Petterson, U., Lindberg, U.: *Virol Monogr* 1975; 14:9).

Table 87-1   Classification of Human Adenoviruses*

Subgenus† (Subgroup)	Species (Serotypes)	Percent GC in DNA	Hemagglutination Subgroup‡	Length of Fibers (nm)	Oncogenicity in vivo§
A	12, 18, 31	47–49	IV	28–31	High
B	3, 7, 11, 14, 16, 21, 34, 35	50–52	I	9–11	Weak
C	1, 2, 5, 6	57–59	III	23–31	None
D	8, 9, 10, 13, 15, 17, 19, 20, 22–30, 32, 33, 36, 37	57–60	II	12–13	None
E	4	57	III	17	None

*Adapted from Wigand et al. *Intervirology* 1982; 18:169.
†Two additional subgenera, F and G, have recently been described (Wadell et al. *Ann NY Acad Sci* 1980; 354:16).
‡Group I agglutinate monkey and group II rat erythrocytes in a tight lattice forming a complete pattern. Group III and IV agglutinate rat erythrocytes in an incomplete pattern.
§Almost all nononcogenic serotypes have been shown to transform rodent cells in vitro.

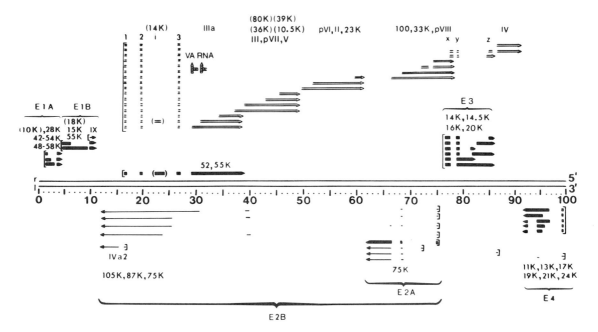

Figure 87-3 A genomic map of ad2-coded proteins and their mRNAs. The mRNAs shown in heavy lines can be detected early in the infection in the absence of protein synthesis. Thin lines indicate intermediate mRNAs; they can be expressed in the absence of viral DNA replication, but are most easily detected late in the infection. Arrowheads show the 3′ end, and tentative promoter sites are indicated with brackets. Proteins unequivocally identified in an early region are also indicated. Minor species are given in parentheses. All late mRNAs shown with double lines originate from the major promoter at coordinate 16.3; they contain triparite leader segments derived from coordinates 16.4, 19.6, and 26.6 joined to the body of each mRNA. The late transcripts belong to five different families having coterminal 3′ ends (arrowheads). A fraction of all late mRNA also contain a fourth leader segment, the i leader. The polypeptides located in the virion are designated with Roman numerals and nonvirion proteins with mol. wt. $\times$ 10^{-3} (K). From Persson H, Philipson L. *Current Topics Immunol Microbiol* 1982; 97:157.

Classification of Human Adenoviruses

Human adenoviruses have been separated into seven subgenera based on their ability to agglutinate monkey or rat erythrocytes. Members of each subgroup have fibers of a characteristic length (see Table 87-1). Classification based on oncogenicity into subgenera A–D has also been proposed. This classification correlates well with the DNA homology.

Antigenic Composition

Most antigens of adenoviruses reside in the outer capsid (Table 87-2). The hexons contain at least two different antigenic determinants, one group-specific (α) and the other type-specific (ϵ). The penton base contains a dominant group-specific antigenic determinant (β). The fiber contains a type-specific determinant (γ) residing in the distal knob that probably anchors the virus to the cell at infection. An intrasubgroup determinant (δ) also is present in the proximal part of the fiber of subgroups A, C, and D.

All human species display hemagglutinating capacity. The type-specific part of the fiber interacts with the red cell surface. The several vertex projections carried by the intact virion can establish a bridge between the erythrocytes and give a complete hemagglutination pattern.

Adenoviruses evidently carry a mosaic of antigenic specificities on their surfaces. By definition all species are distinct by neutralization, so species-specific antigens should induce neutralizing antibodies. Both the fiber (γ) and the hexon (ϵ) contain type-specific antigenic determinants, and both have been claimed to induce neutralizing antibodies. The mechanism for adenovirus neutralization is controversial. Antisera against crude hexon preparations induce neutralizing antibodies; purified hexons from subgenus B and D viruses give rise to neutralizing antibodies; but hexons from subgenus C virions

Table 87-2 Antigens Associated with the Major Structural Proteins

Protein	Corresponding* Polypeptide	Designation	Antigen Specificity	Remarks
Hexon	II	α	Group	Oriented toward inside of virion
		—	Intersubgroup and intrasubgroup	
		ϵ	Type	Available at surface of virion from serotypes belonging to subgroups B and D
Penton base	III	β	Group	Carries toxin activity
		—	Intersubgroup and intrasubgroup	
Fiber	IV	γ	Type	Reacts with HI-antibody
		—	Intersubgroup	Shared between members of subgroups C and D
		δ	Intrasubgroup	At the proximal part of the fiber only present in subgroups A, C, and D

*See Figure 87-2.

contain no or few exposed determinants of this sort. In general, antisera prepared against disrupted virions are more efficient in neutralization than antisera against purified capsid components. The neutralizing antigen of adenoviruses may therefore have escaped detection. The multiplication of the virus of this group is depicted on the first page of the chapter and described in detail in Chapter 63.

Pathogenesis

Susceptible Host Cells

All human adenoviruses produce cytopathic changes when propagated in primary or continuous cell lines of human origin. Characteristic cytopathic changes manifest themselves as rounding, enlargement, increased opacity, and aggregation of the cells into irregular clusters. Incomplete replication may occur in cells from other species. For example, monkey cells support the early and most of the late gene expression of human adenoviruses, but virions fail to assemble. The block may be overcome by concurrent infection with the unrelated monkey DNA virus SV40.

Figure 87-4 shows the time course of infection with adenovirus type 2. When cells are infected at high multiplicity, a synchronous response is observed with two functionally different phases of the infectious cycle. During the early phase, which precedes viral DNA replication, about 40% of the viral genome is expressed.

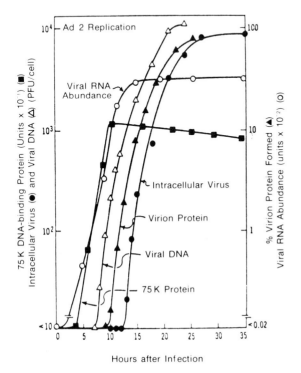

Figure 87-4 The replication cycle of adenovirus type 2. Time course of synthesis of viral RNA, early viral 75K protein, viral DNA, virion protein, and intracellular virus. From Wold, W.S.M., Green, M., Buettner, W. In: *The Molecular biology of animal viruses,* vol 2. Nayak, D.P., (editor). New York: Marcel Dekker, Inc., 1978.

Among the early products is the DNA-binding protein (mol. wt. 75,000 daltons). In the late phase, beginning with the onset of viral DNA synthesis around 6 hours after infection, about 90% of the genome is expressed, and the amount of viral RNA increases by a factor of about 10. About 14 hours after infection, synthesis of host cell proteins is largely replaced by fabrication of viral products—mostly viral structural proteins. New virus particles begin to appear at 15 hours, and the infectious cycle for ad2 and ad5, both members of subgroup C, is completed within 20-25 hours.

Several human adenoviruses as well as adenoviruses from other species can transform cells in vitro irrespective of their oncogenic capacity in vivo. Cells that are nonpermissive for virus replication are more susceptible to transformation. Events leading to transformation may occur even in permissive cells, but the transformation escapes detection because infected cells do not survive. Frequency of transformation is low for adenoviruses, with only one tranforming focus per 10^6 cells or more. Only 17% of the genome of ad5 is required for transformation as revealed by transformation with DNA fragments. Accordingly, several cells transformed with ad2 and ad5 contain a limited amount of the viral DNA integrated in the host cell genome. With ad12, on the other hand, most of the viral genome appears to be integrated in the host genome of the transformed cell.

Clinical Manifestations

Spread of adenovirus infection is almost always by droplet transfer. The respiratory tract is the main target organ. Human adenoviruses are almost exclusively pathogenic for humans. A single species of adenovirus may cause different clinical syndromes and, conversely, more than one species may be responsible for the same clinical pattern. Four different syndromes of respiratory infection have been associated with adenovirus.

Acute febrile pharyngitis appears to be the most common clinical manifestation, especially in infants and children. Individual cases of the disease are difficult to distinguish from infections caused by influenza and parinfluenza viruses, respiratory syncytial virus, certain enteroviruses, and members of the rhinovirus group. Subgenus C viruses appear mainly responsible for infection in early life. Most children show serologic evidence of prior exposure to one or more of these antigenic types by the time they reach school age.

Pharyngeal-conjunctival fever is an infection usually observed in children. This syndrome, which may occur in epidemic form, manifests itself as an acute febrile pharyngitis with concurrent conjunctivitis. Ad3 has been most frequently implicated as the etiologic agent, although ad7 and ad14 have also been involved. All three types belong to subgenus B. In exceptional cases, subgenus C viruses may cause this syndrome.

Acute respiratory disease is prevalent in military recruits, and may be observed among other institutionalized young adults of similar age. Ad4 and ad7 are most frequently associated with this syndrome in recruit populations, but other species within subgenus B may periodically be involved as the responsible agent.

Adenovirus pneumonia is usually seen as a complication of acute respiratory disease in patients infected with ad4 or ad7. The clinical course resembles that of pneumonia caused by *Mycoplasma pneumoniae,* but the disease does not respond to treatment with antibiotics. Pneumonia also is observed occasionally in infants, and several adenovirus species have been isolated from fatal cases in infants.

Adenoviruses may also cause nonrespiratory diseases. Infection of the eye may appear as an acute follicular conjunctivitis mainly seen in adults; it is principally caused by ad3 and ad7, although other species have been implicated as well. Ad8 is known as the major cause of epidemic keratoconjunctivitis of the classical type with corneal infiltrates. Intraocular inoculation in human volunteers has demonstrated that several adenovirus types may cause conjunctivitis.

Adenoviruses may be associated with still other nonrespiratory syndromes such as gastroenteritis and intussusception in infants and young children. Acute mesenteric lymphadenitis also may be associated with adenoviruses, although a causal relationship has not been established. Systemic infections by adenoviruses involving several organs have been observed mostly in infants or young children.

Host Defenses

The susceptibility or resistance to clinical infection was originally thought to correlate directly with the absence or presence of circulating neutralizing antibodies. Recent studies in an animal system show that adenovirus-infected cells are destroyed early in the infection cycle by sensitized, cytotoxic T lymphocytes that must share histocompatibility antigens with the virus-infected cell. This mechanism of defense probably also operates early in virus infection to terminate the disease before viral antibodies are developed. Adenovirus replication in cell culture is exceptionally resistant to interferon inhibition, possibly because the virus utilizes several pathways for macromolecular synthesis inherent in the uninfected cell. The reported prophylaxis of adenovirus conjunctivitis with interferon indicates that some strains are susceptible.

Epidemiology

Adenovirus infections have been studied extensively in many parts of the world. The clinical pattern is similar wherever they have been found. Serologic surveys indicate that infections with low-number species occur frequently in children before the age of 6 months, increase to a maximum in preschool years, remain frequent from 5 to 9 years of age, and diminish thereafter. The species most often involved in these childhood infections are, in order of frequency, 2,1,3,5,7, and 6, with species 2 and 1 from subgenus C accounting for about 60% of the isolates. In spite of this massive rate of infection, adenoviruses appear to account for only about 2%-5% of acute febrile respiratory illness among children in the whole population.

The other major group of subjects from whom adenoviruses are isolated is the population of military recruits. The species responsible for adenovirus disease in military recruits are different from those accounting for childhood disease. Most cases of acute respiratory disease and pneumonia due to adenovirus in military recruits in the United States are caused by adenovirus 4 and 7 and, to a lesser extent, by 3.

Adenoviruses tend to produce disease predominantly during the winter season, but they can be isolated throughout the year. Most adenoviruses do not cause epidemic illness, except for the species responsible for acute respiratory disease among military recruits (and occasionally among children) and ad8, which is responsible for epidemic keratoconjunctivitis.

Adenoviruses also may be responsible for a number of other syndromes, such as acute conjunctivitis, pharyngoconjunctival fever, keratoconjunctivitis, and hemorrhagic cystitis. In many cases, it appears that the infection is predominantly enteric, whereas illness is chiefly respiratory and often febrile. Viral transmission occurs mostly by person-to-person spread by respiratory or ocular secretions. Virus is often found in stools, but transmission by this route has not been documented.

Diagnosis

The agent responsible for an adenoviral infection may be identified by isolation of the virus or serologic techniques or both. Throat and feces samples are inoculated in susceptible cell cultures. Primary cultures of human cells are considered most advantageous to detect adenovirus infection. Rapid diagnosis by immunofluorescence of nasopharyngeal cells also has been used.

Serologic response is measured by several different techniques. The complement-fixation test is the single most useful procedure for serologic diagnosis of infection. A single group antigen can detect antibodies to all human adenovirus species, and the antibodies increase significantly in titer (fourfold or greater) in the sera of adult patients within 2 weeks of infection.

Provisional classification by subgenus may be made by determining whether the new isolate will agglutinate monkey or rat red blood cells. Hemagglutination-inhibition tests then may be performed with type-specific rabbit antisera to establish the virus species. Results should be controlled by neutralization test with specific antisera. To establish that a species-specific antibody rise occurs in patients, both hemagglutination-inhibition and neutralization tests should be performed on acute-phase and convalescent sera. In general, heterologous reactions occur more frequently in hemagglutination inhibition than in neutralization. Heterologous reactions observed with the neutralization test appear to be based more on the presence of overlapping intertypic antigenic determinants than on an anamnestic antibody response.

Control

Because adenoviruses cause only mild respiratory disease in most cases, they do not require containment or passive immunization. Adenoviruses are exceptionally good antigens; a single injection of vaccine gives almost maximal antibody response. Successful vaccination also has been achieved by oral administration of live virus enclosed in capsules that decompose only in the intestinal tract. Several studies have demonstrated reductions from 85%–90% in the attack rate of adenovirus in immunized groups. The low incidence of adenovirus infection in the civilian population, however, raises questions concerning the advisability of indiscriminant use of an adenovirus vaccine. When adenoviruses were shown to transform cells and induce tumors in hamsters, use of adenovirus vaccines was abandoned. Recently, new types of adenovirus vaccines have been introduced that contain only purified protein components from infected cells. Purified hexon or fiber preparations induce high levels of neutralizing antibodies in volunteers, and a vaccine produced from these components was effective in a field trial. Interferon has been reported to prevent adenovirus conjunctivitis.

References

Douglas, G.R., Jr.: Respiratory diseases. In: *Antiviral agents and viral diseases of man.* Galasso, G.J., Merigan, T.C., Buchanan, R.A., (editors). New York: Raven Press, 1984.

Fox, J.P., Call, C.E., Cooney, M.K.: The Seattle virus watch. VII. Observations of adenovirus infections. *Am J Epidemiol* 1977; 105:362-386.

Ginsberg, H.S.: Adenovirus structural proteins. In: *Comprehensive Virology,* vol 13. Fraenkel-Conrat, H., Wagner, R.R. (editors). New York and London: Plenum Press, 1979.

Knight, V., Kasel, J.A.: Adenoviruses. In: *Viral and mycoplasmal infections of the respiratory tract.* Knight, V., (editor). Philadelphia: Lea & Febiger, 1973.

Norrby, E., et al.: Adenoviridae. *Intervirology* 1976; 7:117-125.

Persson, H., Philipson, L.: Regulation of adenovirus gene expression. *Curr Top Immunol Microbiol* 1982; 97:157-203.

Philipson, L., Pettersson, U., Lindberg, U.: Molecular biology of adenoviruses. *Virology Monographs,* vol 14. Gard, S., Hallaver, C., (editors). Vienna and New York: Springer Verlag, 1975.

Potter, C.W.: The association of adenovirus infection with disease of the intestinal tract. In: *Modern trends in medical virology,* vol 1. Heath, R.B., Waterson, A.P., (editors). London: Butterworth, 1967.

Rose, H.M.: Adenoviruses. In: *Diagnostic procedures,* 4th ed. Lennette, E.H., Schmidt, N.J., (editors). Washington, D.C.: American Public Health Association, 1969.

Wadell, G., et al.: Genetic variability of adenoviruses. *Ann NY Acad Sci* 1980; 354:16-42.

Wigand, R., et al.: Adenoviridae, second report. *Intervirology* 1982; 18:169-176.

Wold, W.S.M., Green, M., Büttner, W.: Adenoviruses. In: *The molecular biology of animal viruses,* vol 2. Nayak, D.P., (editor). New York: Marcel Dekker, Inc, 1978.

88 Herpesviruses

André J. Nahmias, MD, MPH
Virginia A. Merchant, DMD

1 ±

C = 162
150-200nm

General Concepts	Host Defenses
Distinctive Properties	**Epidemiology**
Pathogenesis	**Diagnosis**
Herpes Simplex Viruses	**Control**
Varicella-Zoster Virus	Prevention
Cytomegalovirus	Therapy
Epstein-Barr Virus	

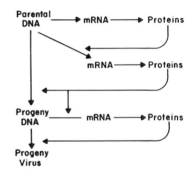

General Concepts

Herpesviruses are enveloped DNA viruses consisting of a core in which the linear double-stranded DNA is enclosed; this core is surrounded successively by a capsid, a globular tegument, and a bilayered envelope with surface projections derived primarily from the host cell nuclear membrane (Figure 88-1). The capsid (approximately 100 nm in diameter) appears as an icosahedron with five capsomeres on each edge and contains 150 hexameric and 12 pentameric capsomeres.

More than 70 herpesviruses have been identified so far in eukaryotic hosts ranging from fungi to humans. All these viruses have been found to cause acute infections, to be

---

The diagrams of the virion morphology and the multiplication scheme are derived from Chapters 62 and 63, respectively. The multiplication scheme applies only generally as indicated in Chapter 63.

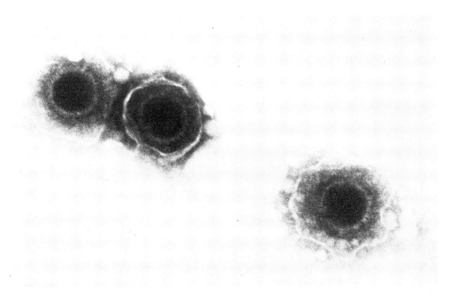

Figure 88-1 Electron microscopy of cytomegalovirus in urine. (×200,000.) Similar virus particles with a nucleocapsid measuring 100 nm surrounded by envelope are observed with all human herpesviruses.

capable of persisting in a noninfectious form (latency) throughout the host's life, and to cause recurrent infections. These recurrent infections are important sources of host-to-host transmission. In animals, several herpesviruses cause cancer; in humans, a weak-to-strong association with several cancers has been shown. Humans are the natural host for five herpesviruses: herpes simplex virus type 1 (HSV-1), herpes simplex virus type 2 (HSV-2), varicella-zoster virus (VZV), Epstein-Barr virus (EBV), and cytomegalovirus (CMV). Herpesviruses often spread in the body within cells (for example, in leukocytes) or cell processes (for example, axons or dendrites). The human herpesviruses are medically important because they produce many diseases, some of which are fatal or cause debilitating neurologic, ocular, or hearing sequelae (Table 88-1). Some recurrent infections, particularly of the genital tract with herpes simplex virus, may induce severe psychosocial problems. Humans can also be accidentally infected with the B herpesvirus of macaques, which causes an almost invariably fatal encephalitis. For some of the human herpesviruses, passive immunization and/or antivirals are useful in prevention and treatment. Several vaccines are also under current investigation.

Distinctive Properties

Although morphologically similar, human herpesviruses have many differences. HSV-1 and HSV-2 are the most closely related, with approximately 50% homology in their genome. Recently, similar nucleotide sequences have been detected in the short arm of the DNA molecules of HSV-1 and VZV. The molecular weight of HSV-1 and HSV-2 DNA is 96×10^6; of Epstein-Barr virus, 114×10^6; and of cytomegalovirus, 150×10^6. Although approximately 50 herpes simplex virus proteins have been identified, the DNA is large enough to code for a substantially greater number.

Table 88-1 Diseases Associated with the Human Herpesviruses

HSV-1	HSV-2	VZV	EBV	CMV
Common or characteristic diseases				
Stomatitis*	Urogenital lesions (penis, vulva, vagina, cervix)*	Varicella (chicken pox)	Infectious mononucleosis	Cytomegalic inclusion disease
Pharyngitis		Zoster (shingles)		Hearing defects
Cold sores*	Cutaneous lesions (below waist)*	Postherpetic neuralgia		Disseminated disease, particularly immunocompromized individuals
Keratoconjunctivitis*	Finger whitlows			
Cutaneous lesions* (above waist)*				Mononucleosis
Finger whitlows				
Infrequent diseases				
Encephalitis*	Meningitis*	Meningoencephalitis	Meningeoencephalitis	Encephalitis
Neuralgia	Myelitis*	Disseminated disease		Pneumonia
Disseminated disease	Neuralgia	Pneumonia	Pneumonia	Chorioretinitis
Pneumonia	Neonatal herpes*	Keratitis	Immunoproliferative disease	Fever of unknown origin
Eczema herpeticum*	Disseminated disease	Congenital defects	Fever of unknown origin	Arthritis
Laryngitis	Pneumonia	Ramsay-Hunt syndrome		
Esophagitis	Cystitis*	Reye's syndrome		
Arthritis	Urethritis*			
	Prostatitis*			
	Proctitis*			
Associated but still unproven				
Head and neck cancers	Cervical cancer		Burkitt's lymphoma	Kaposi's sarcoma
Bell's palsy	Vulvar cancer		Nasopharyngeal carcinoma	Prostatic cancer
Psychiatric disorders			Congenital defects	Guillain-Barré syndrome
Duodenal ulcers			Guillain-Barré syndrome	Ulcerative colitis
Arteriosclerosis			Bell's palsy	Hemolytic anemia
			Rheumatoid arthritis	Adenocarcinoma of the colon
				Alzheimer's disease
				Arteriosclerosis
				Acquired immune deficiency syndrome (AIDS)

*Occasionally may be caused by the other HSV type.

The structural and nonstructural proteins coded by the DNA of the five human herpesviruses are immunologically unrelated, except for those of HSV-1 and HSV-2, which share several common proteins. As a result of these type-common proteins, many cross-antigenic reactions can be elicited between the two HSV types. The cross-reactivity noted in complement-fixation tests between herpes simplex and varicella-zoster viruses is most likely related to common antigens.

Besides the major differences noted among the various human herpesviruses, human isolates within a virus group also have been shown by restriction analyses to differ in their DNA. These strain differences have been demonstrated with all the human herpesviruses and have already been found useful in defining more clearly the clinicopathology and epidemiology of these viruses.

The multiplication of this virus group is depicted on the first page of the chapter and described in detail in Chapter 63.

Pathogenesis

HSV-1 and HSV-2 have a wide host range, both in tissue culture and in experimental animals, whereas the other human herpesviruses have a much more limited host range. The herpes simplex viruses and varicella-zoster have a shorter replication cycle than the other two human herpesviruses and produce intranuclear inclusions and sometimes multinucleated giant cells. Besides intranuclear inclusions, cytomegalovirus can also produce intracytoplasmic inclusions. The plasma membranes of human-herpesvirus-infected cells contain virus-specified antigens; such cells can then be recognized as foreign by the host immune systems.

Primary infections with all of the human herpesviruses are most often asymptomatic, except for varicella-zoster virus infection, which is almost always clinically manifested as chickenpox. Infections with varicella-zoster virus, HSV-1, and HSV-2 usually involve the skin and mucous membranes, whereas cytomegalovirus and Epstein-Barr virus involve internal organs; Epstein-Barr virus has a particular tropism for B lymphocytes. In general, when clinically manifest, primary human herpesvirus infections tend to be more severe than recurrent infections.

The mechanism of latency of human herpesvirus is incompletely understood. Studies with HSV-1 and HSV-2 in animal models indicate that during the acute infection the viruses spread through local nerves and reach sensory or autonomic nervous system ganglia, where viral replication apparently ends. Shortly thereafter, infectious virus becomes undetectable but can be demonstrated again by explant cultures of the ganglia. In human cadavers, the herpes simplex viruses have been detected in explant cultures of sensory and autonomic nervous system ganglia. Clinically, a variety of stresses, such as fever, ultraviolet light, and trigeminal neurectomies or other types of surgery involving ganglia are known to reactivate herpes simplex virus. Recurrent infections tend to be more localized and less clinically severe than primary infections.

The site of latency in varicella-zoster virus also appears to be ganglia. In Epstein-Barr virus, the site is the B lymphocytes and, perhaps, epithelial cells. Cytomegalovirus seems to persist in various organs, including the salivary and breast glands, kidneys, and endocervix, and in semen and peripheral blood leukocytes. Asymptomatic virus shedding is common with all the human herpesviruses—except, apparently, varicella-zoster virus—and is increased severalfold in immunosuppressed hosts. Recurrent infections with cytomegalovirus and varicella-zoster virus in immunosuppressed hosts are often life threatening; they are less so with HSV-1 and HSV-2, in which the lesions tend to be more chronic. Recurrent infections with Epstein-Barr virus are almost always not clinically apparent. In immunosuppressed patients receiving kidney transplants that may contain latent or infectious cytomegalovirus, infection may occur. Kidneys from cytomegalovirus-negative donors are preferred because they are less likely to harbor virus.

Also striking is the dissimilarity between the clinical recurrences of the herpes simplex viruses and of varicella-zoster virus. Clinically manifest recurrences with herpes simplex virus tend to be frequent in many individuals (sometimes as often as once a month), to be limited in their localization, and to be associated usually with only one or a few lesions (for example, cold sores or genital ulcers). On the other hand, recurrence of a varicella-zoster virus infection is less commonly clinically manifested; it rarely occurs more than once in a lifetime, but causes large numbers of lesions along a particular dermatome.

Some animal herpesviruses have been causally related to solid or lymphoreticular tumors: a frog (Lucké) herpesvirus with adenocarcinoma of the kidney; a chicken (Marek's disease) and a rabbit herpesvirus with lymphomas or leukemias. In addition, two monkey herpesviruses (*H ateles* and *H saimiri*) have been found to cause lymphoreticular tumors in foreign hosts. Four of the five human herpesviruses have been associated with several types of human cancer (see Table 88-1). Evidence for the association has been obtained with one or more epidemiologic and laboratory approaches that have demonstrated: that those infected with the virus have a higher rate of the cancer; that cancer patients have a higher frequency or higher titers of antibodies to herpesviral antigens than do controls; that the herpesvirus could transform cells in culture and cause tumors in experimental animals; and that viral genetic information (DNA and RNA) and viral proteins could be detected in experimentally produced tumors and in associated human neoplasms. It is most likely that some of the human herpesviruses, particularly Epstein-Barr virus, are involved in human carcinogenesis. Because of the large numbers of individuals infected with these viruses and the infrequency of some of the related cancers, it is also apparent that other factors, such as genetic or immunologic characteristics of the host, must be operational.

The wide range of clinical diseases that can be produced by the human herpesviruses is indicated in Table 88-1. Some of the more important ones are described in the following sections.

Herpes Simplex Viruses

HSV-1 **gingivostomatitis** is a frequent disease that occurs most often in young children but can affect adults. The vesicles and ulcers, which may be confluent or discrete and involve any part of the oral cavity, are usually self-limiting, persisting up to 2 weeks. Cervical lymphadenopathy and fever are commonly present. Less frequently, the virus also causes pharyngitis or laryngitis. Recurrent infections are most often seen as herpes labialis (cold sores) and are commonly found on the vermillion border of the lower lip or the skin of the upper lip. Recurrent intraoral herpes infections occur infrequently; are usually limited to the attached mucosa (gingivae and hard palate); and are often confused with aphthous stomatitis (canker sores).

Herpetic keratitis, which can be accompanied by conjunctivitis, produces typical branched dendritic ulcers, best detected by fluorescein staining. Deeper stromal involvement also can occur, and the superficial corneal disease can become more severe with administration of corticosteroids. Such severe acute conditions, as well as recurrences of superficial infections leading to irreversible corneal scarring, can cause loss of vision.

Skin lesions may be associated with oral or ocular herpes, but more often HSV-1 vesicles and ulcers occur independently on the face or on the arms and trunk above the waist. Lesions on the fingers (**herpetic whitlows**) are noted particularly in medical, nursing, and dental personnel. Contact sports, particularly wrestling, may also lead to skin lesions on many parts of the body (**herpes gladiatorum**).

Genital herpes, a particularly recurrent infection, is usually caused by HSV-2. In women, the virus may involve the vulva, vagina, and cervix, the cervical infection often being asymptomatic. Men usually have lesions on the glans penis, prepuce, or penile shaft, and homosexual men may develop a severe proctitis. In both sexes, the urethra and bladder may be involved, and whitlows and skin lesions on other skin below the waist are not uncommonly associated. Primary infections may be accompanied by fever, pelvic pain, and inguinal adenopathy and meningitis. Clinically apparent recurrent infections are frequent in both sexes and subclinical genital infections are common in both sexes.

Neonatal herpetic diseases range from a localized infection of the skin, mouth, eyes, or brain to a disseminated infection of visceral organs and, often, the brain. Untreated, at least one-half the infected neonates die, and about one-half of the survivors develop neurologic or ocular sequelae or both.

Severe herpes simplex virus infections can disseminate to visceral organs, such as the liver, or cause pneumonia. They can occur also in older individuals who are severely malnourished, are immunosuppressed, or have severe burns. Patients with chronic dermatoses, particularly eczema, may have a disseminated skin infection (eczema herpeticum) and occasionally have internal organ involvement.

Another form of herpes simplex virus infection is encephalitis, which has a fatality rate of 70% if untreated. Encephalitis is rarely associated with HSV-2, which is more likely to cause meningitis and, occasionally, myelitis. HSV-2 has also been implicated as a cause of cervical carcinoma; HSV-1 has been related to head and neck cancers.

Varicella-Zoster Virus

Varicella-zoster virus is primarily responsible for two diseases: **varicella** (chickenpox) and **zoster** (shingles). Varicella is usually a relatively mild infection of children, infrequently affecting adults in whom the infection is more likely to cause pneumonia. The rash usually begins on the head and trunk, later involving the extremities. The maculopapular rash progresses through vesicular and pustular stages to crusting and subsequent healing, infrequently leaving scars. Because the lesions occur in crops, all stages can be seen simultaneously. Immunocompromised individuals such as leukemic children can develop fatal pneumonia and disseminated visceral disease.

Zoster, a manifestation of latent varicella-zoster virus acquired from a prior varicella infection, is occasionally noted in children but is more frequent in older patients, in whom severe postherpetic neuralgias can occur. The lesions are usually confined to areas of the skin innervated by the sensory nerves of a dorsal root ganglion and are most common in the thoracic and lumbar regions. The ophthalmic division of the trigeminal nerve may be involved, and keratitis can result. Zoster in the immunocompromised host occasionally causes disseminated skin lesions, pneumonia, or visceral organ involvement. Meningoencephalitis may be associated with either varicella or zoster.

Cytomegalovirus

Cytomegalovirus most often produces an asymptomatic infection, but infection in utero may produce **cytomegalic inclusion disease** with jaundice, hepatosplenomegaly, thrombocytopenia, and central nervous system disorders. One to ten percent of congenitally infected neonates demonstrate such clinical findings in the neonatal period, and at least another 10% develop sequelae, primarily hearing defects and sometimes mental retardation.

Cytomegalovirus also can produce a type of infectious mononucleosis characterized by fever, fatigue, and atypical peripheral lymphocytes; unlike Epstein-Barr mononucleosis, pharyngitis and cervical lymphadenopathy usually are absent and hepatitis occurs only occasionally. Cytomegalovirus mononucleosis can be distinguished from Epstein-Barr mononucleosis in that the patient with the former fails to develop antibodies against heterologous red cells (negative heterophile antibody test).

Cytomegalovirus infections may be severe in immunosuppressed individuals and are an important problem in renal, bone marrow, liver or cardiac transplant patients. Interstitial pneumonitis, disseminated disease, or chorioretinitis usually result from a primary infection but also may be due to a reactivated infection.

Epstein-Barr Virus

Epstein-Barr virus infection in childhood usually is asymptomatic, although it can cause infectious mononucleosis. Most often observed in adolescents and young adults, this self-limiting disease is characterized by fatigue, malaise, pharyngitis, fever, cervical lymphadenopathy, and splenomegaly. Epstein-Barr infections are infrequently associated with central nervous system involvement and with a familial immunoproliferative syndrome, which may include immunodeficiencies and lymphoreticular neoplasms. More recently, this viral infection has been related to a chronic fatigue syndrome.

Epstein-Barr virus has been strongly implicated as the cause of Burkitt's lymphoma, a malignancy noted most frequently in African children, and of nasopharyngeal carcinoma, which is most prevalent in adults in some Oriental and North African countries.

Host Defenses

A primary infection with any human herpesvirus produces short-lasting IgM-specific antibodies to the virus, followed by IgG antibodies, which are more long lasting; however, despite these antibodies, recurrent infections occur spontaneously and are increased by immunosuppression. IgM antibodies also can be demonstrated in the serum during recurrent infections. The role of IgA antibodies, which can be detected in some human herpesvirus infections, has not been elucidated. However, the demonstration of serum IgA antibodies to Epstein-Barr virus has been found useful to detect individuals prone to develop nasopharyngeal carcinoma.

The protective role of antibodies has been demonstrated most convincingly for varicella in that hyperimmune serum protects chickenpox contacts from expressing the disease. Individuals with Epstein-Barr virus antibodies do not experience infectious mononucleosis. Those with antibodies to HSV-1 or 2 or both are unlikely to demonstrate the severe clinical findings associated occasionally with a primary HSV-1 or HSV-2 infection. Maternally acquired antibody to HSV and CMV may not protect the newborn; the disease may be attenuated, although infection may still occur. Kidney, bone marrow, or cardiac transplant recipients may develop severe cytomegalovirus infections despite the presence of serum antibodies.

The more severe diseases observed with some herpesviruses in newborns, immunodeficient children, or immunosuppressed patients suggest that cellular immunity plays an important role in host defense. Many immunologic studies have been conducted in humans and, when possible (with HSV-1 and HSV-2), in experimental animals. These include studies of specific cell-immune T cell systems and their lymphokines (including interferon) and of nonspecific systems (for example, macrophages, natural killer cells, and nonimmune interferon). Furthermore, antibodies and complement as well as antibodies in conjunction with K lymphocytes, monocytes, or polymorphonuclear leukocytes from seronegative donors can lyse herpes-simplex-virus–infected cells. Although effects on the herpesvirus infection can be demonstrated with all of the systems studied, to date it is not possible to pinpoint the form of immunity that is critical in controlling a primary or recurrent herpesvirus infection. Current evidence suggests the greater likelihood that cooperation between various immune and nonspecific defenses aids in controlling the infections.

Genetic factors may influence susceptibility to herpesvirus infections. Best appreciated is the X-linked immunoproliferative syndrome associated with EB virus infection. With herpesvirus 1 and 2, several reports (such as of infections in patients with burns or eczema) indicate that the integrity of the skin serves as a barrier to these viruses.

Epidemiology

Prevalence of the herpesvirus infections depends on several variables. In lower socioeconomic populations, most adolescents are found to have experienced HSV-1, Epstein-Barr, or cytomegalovirus infections, usually subclinically. In higher socioeconomic populations, only about one-half have been infected by adolescence. This pattern is not observed with varicella-zoster virus infection in that the frequency of chickenpox appears to be as common in children of either socioeconomic group. Because HSV-2 infection is usually transmitted sexually (genital-genital, genital-oral, genital-anal), its prevalence is greatest in more sexually promiscuous adolescents or adults and in their sexual contacts. HSV-1 can also be transmitted occasionally to the genitals, usually by oral-genital contact; however, this virus is more often transmitted by saliva or kissing, one of the means by which Epstein-Barr virus and probably cytomegalovirus are also spread. In addition, HSV-1 can be transmitted by close body contact (as in wrestlers), as can varicella-zoster virus, for which aerosol spread has been also implicated. Cytomegalovirus, which is commonly recovered from the cervix and semen, may also be sexually transmitted.

Cytomegalovirus is often transmitted transplacentally to the fetus, and 0.5%–2.5% of newborns are found to have the virus in the urine at birth. Some evidence exists that other herpesviruses also may be infrequently transmitted transplacentally. Chickenpox, when acquired from a mother with the disease within 3 days of delivery, can be particularly serious in the newborn. In addition, a few babies born to mothers who had chickenpox in early pregnancy have developed a characteristic syndrome with several birth defects. Most often, newborns acquire their HSV-2 or HSV-1 infection at the time of delivery, when the mother has an asymptomatic or clinically manifest genital HSV infection. Cytomegalovirus is also frequently acquired intrapartum by an infant from a maternal asymptomatic cervical infection and by breast-feeding.

Nosocomial spread of the herpesviruses has been best substantiated for HSV-1, HSV-2 (including neonatal herpes), and varicella-zoster virus (chickenpox or zoster). Although nosocomial spread is possible for Epstein-Barr virus and cytomegalovirus, evidence for this route is still uncertain. The latter virus, however, can be transmitted by blood transfusion and in kidney transplant tissues. Many of the herpesviruses are transmitted readily in day care centers, providing an excellent mechanism for significant immunity to infection at an older age.

The incubation period for most cases of HSV-1 and HSV-2 averages 6 days, although in newborns the disease may take up to 4 weeks to become manifest. The incubation period for varicella is 10–23 days (average 15 days) and for Epstein-Barr virus (mononucleosis), 30–50 days. Information on cytomegalovirus is sparse, but intrapartum and blood-transmitted cases suggest a long incubation period of 3 or more weeks. It is of interest that in organ transplant patients, there is a sequence of reactivation of herpesviruses; in the first month: HSV-1 and/or HSV-2; from 1–6 months: cytomegalovirus; after 6 months, zoster.

Recent information obtained by use of restriction enzyme analysis of viral DNA strongly suggests that recurrent herpes simplex or cytomegalovirus infection can also result from exogenous reinfection with a different strain of the same virus group.

Diagnosis

Diagnosis of chickenpox, zoster, and several herpex simplex infections (for example, keratitis and cold sores) can be made clinically in most cases; at times, the clinical picture may resemble noninfectious or other infectious conditions, resulting in an erroneous diagnosis. Although not differentiating between HSV-1, HSV-2, or varicella-zoster infection, the characteristic cytologic findings obtained with a Tzanck smear or, preferably, a Papanicolaou scraping of the lesion can substantiate the clinicoepidemiologic findings (Figure 88-2). Cytomegalovirus inclusions are less likely to be found in the urine of infected patients, but in all four herpesvirus infections, histopathologic examinations of infected tissues, preferably fixed in Bouin's solution, will demonstrate inclusions.

Rapid methods of diagnosis by detecting herpesvirus particles with the electron microscope or by demonstrating viral nucleic acids or viral antigens in clinical specimens by newer methods appear promising. These techniques may obviate the time required for currently standard methods of virus isolation and identification in tissue culture: 1–4 days for HSV-1 and HSV-2; up to 4 weeks for varicella-zoster and cytomegalovirus. Care should be taken in ensuring definiteness of the specificity and sensitivity of any rapid test before its routine use. Although Epstein-Barr virus can be demonstrated by inoculating specimens in human cord blood lymphocyte cultures, this is a laborious test that is not readily available. Diagnosis of herpes simplex encephalitis requires a brain biopsy and demonstration of the virus.

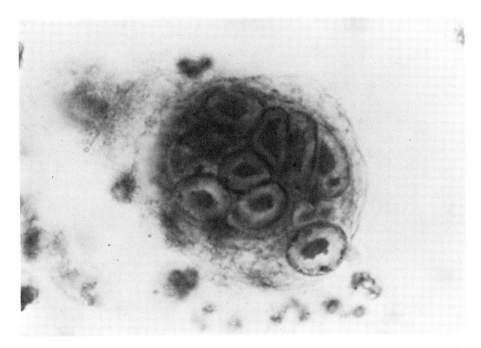

Figure 88-2 Multinucleated giant cells and intranuclear inclusions observed from scrapings of the margin of a herpes simplex virus vesicle (Papanicolaou stain). Similar cytologic findings can be noted with varicella-zoster infection.

Most helpful in diagnosing Epstein-Barr mononucleosis are the presence of atypical lymphocytes and a positive heterophile antibody test with differential absorptions with guinea pig kidney tissue and beef red cells, a microtest using horse red blood cell agglutination (mono spot), or an ox cell hemolysin test. Demonstrating a rise in titer in IgG antibodies to the Epstein-Barr capsid antigens or, in a single serum, IgG antibodies to the viral capsid without antibodies to the nuclear antigens, *or* IgM antibodies to the viral capsid antigen, is particularly helpful in diagnosing an acute Epstein-Barr infection without the mononucleosis syndrome. Serologic tests infrequently offer clinical assistance in diagnosing the other herpesvirus infections, but they are particularly useful in epidemiologic studies.

Control

Prevention

Vaccines for all of the human herpesviruses are at various stages of development. A serious problem with live attenuated herpesvirus vaccines has been latency. In the case of those herpesviruses associated with human cancers, concern has centered not only on attenuated vaccines but also on inactivated vaccines still containing viral DNA. Nevertheless, an attenuated varicella-zoster virus vaccine has already received extensive clinical testing in Japan; good evidence of protection and an apparent lack of complications have been reported. A similar type vaccine is under trial in the United States for target populations at high risk for developing severe varicella-zoster infections. An attenuated cytomegalovirus vaccine is also under evaluation for certain target populations, such as transplant recipients. Subunit HSV-1 and HSV-2 preparations containing viral proteins but no DNA have already undergone successful animal trials and are being tested in humans. Epstein-Barr virus membrane antigen preparations are at a more primitive stage of evaluation. With current genetic engineering, many other approaches to producing herpesvirus vaccines are under current study. This includes: a) inserting herpes genes coding for specific proteins in vaccinia virus; b) deleting "virulence" genes; c) inserting herpes genes in bacteria, yeast or mammalian cells.

Hyperimmunoglobulin for varicella-zoster virus (zoster immunoglobulin) has been shown to be protective when administered to susceptible individuals within the first few days of exposure and is used for high-risk patients (for example, leukemic children) exposed to varicella-zoster infection. Hyperimmunoglobulins for HSV-1 and HSV-2 are undergoing animal experimentation; hyperimmunoglobulin for cytomegalovirus, as well as plasma with high cytomegalovirus antibody titers, has been found to be useful in high-risk patients.

Prevention of neonatal herpes simplex virus is possible in many cases if a mother with an identified genital herpes simplex infection at the time of delivery undergoes a cesarean section, preferably before membranes are ruptured. Herpes simplex finger infections can be prevented if gloves are worn by medical, nursing, and dental personnel whose hands come in contact with patients' saliva. Hospitalized patients with varicella-zoster diseases or with herpes simplex infections, particularly eczema herpeticum or neonatal herpes, should be isolated. Transfusion-acquired cytomegalovirus disease may be prevented by administering only cytomegalovirus antibody-negative blood products to particularly susceptible hosts, such as newborn infants.

Therapy

Many therapeutic regimens have been attempted to treat human herpesvirus infections, particularly recurrent HSV-1 and HSV-2 infections. Unfortunately, controlled trials have been performed using only a few of these modalities. Those undergoing controlled study and found to be effective so far are topical iododeoxyuridine, trifluorothymidine, and adenine arabinoside for ocular herpes simplex infections; and systematically administered adenine arabinoside for herpes simplex encephalitis, neonatal herpes simplex infections, and cutaneous varicella-zoster infections in the immunocompromised host. Systematically administered interferon also has been found helpful in those with varicella-zoster infections and is under trial for several other herpesvirus infections. Topical, oral, or intravenous acyclovir is helpful for primary genital infections and for herpes simplex infection of the compromised host. Intravenously administered acyclovir is also useful for varicella-zoster infection in the compromised host; it is being compared to adenine arabinoside for herpes simplex encephalitis and neonatal herpes.

Although some progress has been made in controlling human herpesviruses, much remains to be done to alleviate these common and occasionally fatal viral infections. The knowledge being gained at the virologic, cellular, and immunologic levels, particularly regarding viral persistence and oncogenesis, is providing the necessary foundation.

References

Evans, A.S., (editor): *Viral infections of humans—epidemiology and control,* 2nd ed. New York: Plenum Press, 1982.

Epstein, M.A., Achong, B.G. (editors): *The Epstein-Barr virus.* New York: Springer-Verlag, 1979.

Henle, W., Rapp, F., de Thé, G. (editors): *Herpesviruses and oncogenesis.* Lyon: International Agency for Research on Cancer, 1978.

Jordan, M.C., et al.: Latent herpesviruses of humans. *Ann Intern Med* 1984; 100:866-880.

Kaplan A.S., (editor): *The herpesviruses.* New York: Academic Press, 1973.

Nahmias, A.: The evolution (evovirology) of herpesviruses. In: *Viruses, evolution and cancer.* Kurstak, E., Mamamarosch, K., (editors). New York: Academic Press, 1974.

Nahmias, A. O'Reilly, R., (editors): *Immunology of human infection,* vol 2, *Immunology of viral and parasitic infection.* New York: Plenum Press, 1981.

Nahmias, A., Dowdle, W., Schinazi, R., (editors): *The human herpesviruses—an interdisciplinary perspective.* New York: Elsevier-North Holland, 1981.

Rapp, F.: The challenge of herpesviruses. *Cancer Res* 1984; 44:1309-1315.

89 Poxviruses

Derrick Baxby, PhD

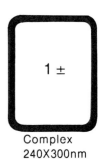

Complex
240X300nm

General Concepts
Distinctive Properties
Pathogenesis
Host Defenses
Epidemiology
Diagnosis
Control

General Concepts

The family Poxviridae (Table 89-1) contains large, complex, double-stranded DNA viruses that replicate in the cytoplasm. They cause localized and generalized skin infections in a variety of animal species. Although some animal poxviruses occasionally infect humans, only one serious human infection, smallpox, is caused by a poxvirus (Table 89-2). Historically important as a scourge of humans for centuries, smallpox was the first viral disease for which vaccines and chemoprophylaxis became available. It is also the first disease to be eradicated. The World Health Organization (WHO) eradication campaign started in 1967 and the last endemic case occurred in October 1977. Eradication was considered complete 2 years after the last case occurred.

Smallpox was acquired through the respiratory route, then spread through a transient viremia to internal organs, and through a second viremia to the skin to produce the characteristic lesions. Both cellular and humoral immunity appeared to be important in recovery from smallpox; immune globulin was used successfully to prevent disease in contacts. Available data indicate that smallpox did not have an animal reservoir and,

---

The diagram of the virion morphology is derived from Chapter 62.

Table 89-1 Poxviruses of Vertebrates*

Genus	Species/Members
Orthopoxvirus*	Smallpox,† monkeypox, vaccinia, cowpox,‡ buffalopox, camelpox, mousepox
Avipoxvirus	Fowlpox, canarypox, pigeonpox, sparrowpox, and others
Capripoxvirus	Sheeppox, goatpox, lumpy skin disease
Parapoxvirus	Orf (contagious pustular dermatitis), milker's nodes (pseudocowpox), bovine papular stomatitis
Leporipoxvirus	Myxoma, hare fibroma, rabbit fibroma, squirrel fibroma
Suipoxvirus	Swinepox

*Poxviruses not yet officially assigned to genera: elephant and carnivore poxviruses (both variants of cowpox?) and raccoonpox. These are orthopoxviruses. Tana and Yaba poxviruses are serologically related. Molluscum contagiosum virus is also not yet assigned to a genus. Viruses morphologically similar to parapoxviruses have been isolated from camels, squirrels, and kangaroos.
†Viruses (whitepox) indistinguishable from smallpox and thought to have been isolated from animals are probably laboratory contaminants.
‡Viruses resembling cowpox have been isolated from zoo animals in Europe.

Table 89-2 Poxviruses Pathogenic for Humans

Virus and Reservoir	Disease and Mortality Rate	Comments
Smallpox (human)	Generalized infection with pustular rash (1%–50%)	Total eradication confirmed in 1980
Monkeypox (not known)	Clinical human smallpox (15%)	167 cases reported in West Africa since 1970; little evidence of spread
Vaccinia (no natural host)	Rare complications of vaccination: Encephalitis (40%) Eczema vaccinatum (40%) Vaccinia gangrenosa (80%–100%)	Should disappear as vaccination is discontinued
Cowpox (not known)	Localized hemorrhagic skin ulcer with pyrexia	Restricted to Europe; buffalopox, camelpox, and elephantpox viruses may cause similar disease
Orf (sheep, goats)	Skin lesions similar to cowpox but painless	Occupational infection; sheeppox and goatpox viruses may cause similar disease
Milker's nodes (cattle)	Resembles orf; lesions may be nodular	Occupational infection
Tanapox (monkey)	Localized skin nodules with pyrexia	Incidence affected by environment?
Molluscum (human)	Multiple skin nodules; long-lasting	Often sexually transmitted

prior to its eradication, it spread in endemic areas (Asia, India, Africa, and South America) from person to person. Clinical diagnosis was based on the observation of pustular lesions, centrifugal rash, and synchronous development of lesions. Control and eradication of smallpox was achieved by prompt detection and isolation of cases and vaccination and isolation of contacts (surveillance-containment).

Scientists are assessing the significance of animal poxviruses as potential agents of human disease; monkeypox virus has caused some clinical human "smallpox" in West Africa.

Poxviruses are placed in genera according to genetic and serologic relationships (see Table 89-1). Since 1965, new orthopoxviruses have been isolated from various animals, but attempts to assess their interrelationships by traditional methods have had only limited success. For instance, viruses called whitepox isolated from monkeys and rodents in Africa and indistinguishable from smallpox virus are receiving urgent attention. Much current work is concentrated on vaccinia DNA, and the nucleotide sequence of some genes is known. One exciting development is the insertion of the gene coding for Hepatitis B surface antigen and a rabies glycoprotein into the vaccinia genome.

Distinctive Properties

Poxviruses are large, brick-shaped particles of complex symmetry. Orthopoxviruses are approximately 200×250 nm with small surface tubules 10 nm wide (Figure 89-1). Internally they have a dumbbell-shaped core and two lateral bodies (Figure 89-2). Parapoxviruses are narrower (160 nm) and have one long tubule winding round the virion. In micrographs of whole virions (Figure 89-3), this gives a criss-cross effect caused by superimposition of top and bottom surfaces.

The genome is one molecule of double-stranded DNA, mol. wt. $80-240 \times 10^6$. Genetic recombination within genera occurs readily. Poxviruses have a virion-associated DNA-dependent RNA polymerase and therefore can replicate in the cytoplasm. Other virus-coded enzymes also are found in the core. These complete the uncoating of infecting virions and initiate early stages of replication. Poxvirus DNA alone is not infectious, although it will produce infectious progeny in cells infected with a closely related poxvirus. Replication occurs in intracytoplasmic, acidophilic inclusions. Some poxviruses (cowpox, but not smallpox) also produce eosinophilic inclusions in which mature virions accumulate. The multiplication of the virus of this group is depicted on the first page of this chapter and described in detail in Chapter 63.

Poxviruses are antigenically complex, and all poxviruses are thought to share a common internal antigen. There is extensive cross-reaction with surface and soluble antigens within a genus, but not between genera. Some orthopoxviruses produce a hemagglutinin that is easily separable from the virion.

Pathogenesis

Smallpox is a systemic infection with a characteristic rash (Figure 89-4). Infection is transmitted via the respiratory tract. During the 12-day incubation period, the virus spreads to internal organs by a transient viremia. The onset of illness coincides with a

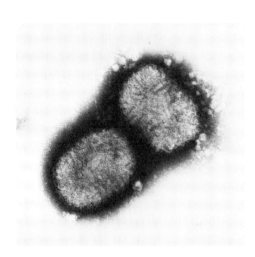

Figure 89-1 Orthopoxvirus (vaccinia). Whole virion negatively stained to show surface tubules (× 100,000).

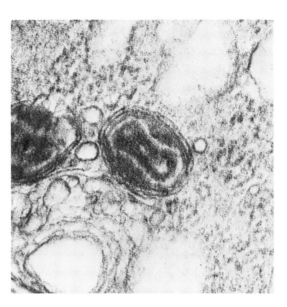

Figure 89-2 Orthopoxvirus (vaccinia). Thin section showing internal structure (× 100,000).

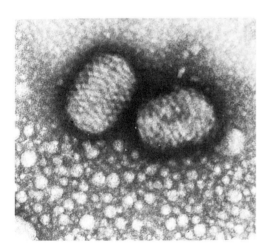

Figure 89-3 Parapoxvirus (orf). Whole virion showing surface structure (× 100,000). (Courtesy R.C. Jones, Liverpool Veterinary Faculty.)

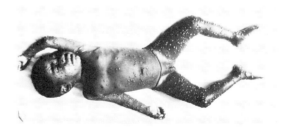

Figure 89-4 Smallpox in a child demonstrating the characteristic centrifugal distribution of the eruption. Courtesy WHO Smallpox Eradication Unit.

second, more marked viremia that spreads virus to the skin and other target organs. Lesions first appear in the mouth and throat and then on the skin as macules, then papules, vesicles, pustules, and, finally, crusts. The severity in individuals infected with the same strain may vary considerably. In addition, different strains of smallpox virus differ in virulence. Strains causing variola major, with a case fatality rate of up to 50%, and variola minor (or alastrim), with a case fatality rate of less than 1%, represent opposite ends of a spectrum spanned by strains of intermediate virulence. Infection from exhaled virus or from skin lesions is transmitted by close contact or fomites. Smallpox is not very communicable, and epidemics developed slowly. The pathogenesis and clinical features of human monkeypox are essentially the same as for smallpox.

Human infection with poxviruses other than smallpox and monkeypox is contracted through superficial scratches and, except for molluscum, usually remains localized. Recovery usually is straightforward; however, serious generalized infections with vaccinia and cowpox sometimes occur in people with eczema or immune deficiencies. Reduced immunity leads to enlargement of the primary lesion, and viremia leads to production of secondary lesions in skin and internal organs. The prognosis is grave in untreated cases.

Host Defenses

The value of humoral antibody in smallpox has long been assumed and was confirmed by successful use of γ-globulin to prevent disease in contacts. The importance of cellular immunity is indicated by recovery of vaccinees with hypo-γ-globulinemia who have normal T cell responses. An important finding is that virus released naturally from cells acquires an antigen not present on virus artificially extracted from within the cell. Antibody to this antigen is protective. Inactivated vaccines prepared from intracellular virus lack this antigen and do not elicit protective antibody. Live virus vaccines prepared from intracellular virus are protective because the antigen-deficient virus replicates and the progeny virus is naturally released from the cell, thereby acquiring the antigen necessary for protective antibody production.

Among the nonimmune defenses, interferon is stimulated by poxviruses and inhibits their replication. When interferon is removed, replication of poxviruses increases and more severe disease occurs. Also, interferon protects against experimental poxvirus disease in animals and humans. Thus, interferon and probably other nonimmune mechanisms are important defenses against poxvirus infections.

Epidemiology

Before eradication, the main endemic areas of smallpox were Asia and India for variola major, South America for alastrim, and Africa for intermediate strains. Isolation of whitepox strains from African animals led to reexamination of the question of animal reservoirs for smallpox. The strains were isolated in areas that remain free from human smallpox and may have been laboratory contaminants. They do not appear to represent an animal reservoir for smallpox.

Human poxvirus infections other than vaccinia (a laboratory virus with no natural host) and molluscum are contracted accidentally from animal reservoirs; molluscum is often sexually transmitted. In some cases the reservoirs are known (for example, for *Parapoxvirus,* buffalopox, and camelpox), and human infection is a minor occupational hazard. In other cases, such as cowpox and monkeypox, the true reservoirs are unknown, although domestic cats have been shown to be natural hosts of cowpox. Over 100 cases of human monkeypox have occurred in West Africa since 1970. Although the mortality rate is high (15%), most patients are unvaccinated, many are children, and nutritional and other environmental factors may affect the outcome; person-to-person spread is rare. Although the situation is being closely monitored by WHO, human monkeypox is not considered to be a serious threat.

Human Tanapox epidemics have occurred in Kenya, probably caused by overcrowding of human and simian populations during floods. Although monkeys in Malaysia have Tanapox antibody, no human infection has been reported there.

Some infections (for example, pigpox and myxomatosis) are spread by insects; it is possible that insects may transmit other pox infections to humans.

Although not important in human medicine, goatpox, sheeppox, and camelpox are important veterinary pathogens, and require further study.

Diagnosis

The chance of a patient having smallpox is extremely remote; *if smallpox is suspected, expert help must be sought immediately.* Clinical diagnosis is based on the combination of pustular lesions, centrifugal rash (see Figure 89-4), and synchronous development of lesions. Modification by previous vaccination used to be common. Virus, from vesicle fluid or crusts, can be recognized by electron microscopy, which rapidly eliminates chickenpox (the commonest cause of confusion), but does not differentiate smallpox from monkeypox, vaccinia, or Tanapox. This distinction is made by culture, particularly at restrictive temperatures; for example, monkeypox, but not smallpox, will replicate at 39 C. Orthopoxviruses can be isolated easily, and most of them can be identified without much difficulty. Parapoxviruses are not cultured routinely; diagnosis is made by electron microscopy.

Appropriate tests are used to detect antibody. Neutralizing antibody is long lasting; complement-fixing and, in *Orthopoxvirus,* hemagglutinin-inhibiting antibodies are less long lasting. Consequently, the presence of complement-fixing and hemagglutinin-inhibiting antibodies confirms recent poxvirus infection in cases where virus is not isolated.

Control

Smallpox was the first disease to be controlled by vaccination. Mass vaccination has been practiced in the past, but control of smallpox in nonendemic countries was based on isolation of cases and vaccination and isolation of contacts. Control in countries with poor vaccination levels was helped by the low communicability and the fact that cases are not infectious before the illness starts. Vaccination is regarded as successful if a vesicle forms at the inoculation site. With primary vaccination, this result is unequivocal. With revaccination, response is accelerated and vesicle formation is an important indicator of success; erythema alone may indicate a nonspecific or allergic reaction.

Immunoglobulin or methisazone had prophylactic value if given early in the incubation period. The serious effects of vaccinial complications could also be reduced by these means. Vaccination has only limited effect in preventing local *Orthopoxvirus* infections.

Certain features made smallpox an ideal candidate for eradication: ease of containment by isolation, effective vaccine, no animal reservoir, no latent infections, no subclinical carrier state, antigenic homogeneity, and antigenic stability. The last case of natural smallpox occurred in Somalia in 1977, and the WHO general assembly in May 1980 officially declared smallpox to be eradicated. No further cases have been reported. This is a remarkable achievement and a tremendous monument to international cooperation in preventive medicine.

The remaining poxviruses, although of only minor human medical importance, still pose veterinary problems; in addition, these viruses require constant monitoring to detect any possible changes in their relationship with humans.

References

Baxby, D.: Poxvirus hosts and reservoirs. *Arch Virol* 1977; 55:169–179.

Baxby, D.: Poxviruses. In: *Topley and Wilson's principles of bacteriology, virology and immunity,* 7th ed., vol 4. Wilson, G.S., Brown, F., (editors). Baltimore: Williams and Wilkins Co. 1984.

Brown, S.T., Nalley, J.F., Kraus, S.J.: Molluscum contagiosum. *Sex Transm Dis* 1981; 8:227–234.

Dales, S., Pogo, B.G.T.: *Biology of poxviruses.* Vienna: Springer-Verlag, 1981.

Dumbell, K.R., Kapsenberg, J.G.: Laboratory investigation of two 'whitepox' viruses and comparison with two variola strains isolated from India. *Bull WHO* 1983; 60:381–387.

Hoare, C.M., Bennett, M.: Cowpox in the cat. In: *The veterinary annual,* 25th ed. Grunsell, C.S.G., Hill, F.W.G., Raw, M.-E. (eds.). Bristol: Scientechnica, 1985.

Robinson, A.J., Petersen, G.V.: Orf virus infection of workers in the meat industry. *NZ Med J* 1983; 96:81–85.

Smith, G.L., Moss, B.: Uses of vaccinia virus as a vector for the production of live recombinant vaccines. *Bioessays* 1984; 1:120–124.

World Health Organization: *The global eradication of smallpox.* Geneva: WHO, 1980.

World Health Organization: The current status of human monkeypox. *Bull WHO* 1984; 62:703–713.

90 Hepatitis Viruses

A. J. Zuckerman, MD, DSc

General Concepts

Viral hepatitis has emerged as a major public health problem, occurring endemically in all parts of the world. The general term *viral hepatitis* refers to infections caused by viruses from several groups (Table 90-1): hepatitis type A, now classified taxonomically as enterovirus (picornavirus) type 72, type B (an unclassified 42 nm double-stranded DNA virus), hepadnavirus, and non-A:non-B. Hepatitis A virus is transmitted by the fecal-oral route, and hepatitis B is transmitted mainly by body fluids (for example, blood). The specific laboratory diagnosis of viral hepatitis has progressed to such an extent that it has revealed a new form of viral hepatitis called non-A:non-B. One non-A:non-B hepatitis is similar in its epidemiology to hepatitis B and is caused by at least 2 viruses. Another form is epidemiologically similar to hepatitis A and is called epidemic non-A hepatitis.

Acute viral hepatitis is a generalized or systemic infection, characterized particularly by inflammation and necrosis of the liver. The clinical picture of hepatitis ranges from

Table 90-1 Distinguishing Characteristics of Viral Hepatitis

Virus	Classification	Transmission	Mean Incubation Period	Disease
Hepatitis A	Enterovirus*	Fecal-oral	4 weeks	Acute or inapparent
Epidemic nonA	Unclassified	Fecal-oral	About 6 weeks	Acute or inapparent
Hepatitis B	Hepadnavirus	Blood	3 months	Acute or persistent
NonA : NonB	Unclassified	Blood	2 weeks–6 months	Acute or persistent
Delta agent	RNA genome, hepatitis B capsid	Blood	Not known and variable	Acute or persistent

*Picornavirus family.

inapparent or subclinical infection, slight malaise, mild gastrointestinal symptoms, and the anicteric form of the disease to acute icteric illness, severe prolonged jaundice, acute fulminant hepatitis, and chronic liver disease. The incidence of individual symptoms and signs varies in different epidemics and in sporadic cases.

The two clinically and pathologically similar forms of hepatitis can now be differentiated by specific laboratory tests for antigens and antibodies associated with these infections. However, hepatitis A is a self-limited infection, whereas hepatitis B and non-A:non-B may become chronic infections.

HEPATITIS A

Distinctive Properties

Hepatitis A virus contains a linear genome of single-stranded RNA. On the basis of its physicochemical and other properties, the virus has been classified as enterovirus type 72. Limited studies have shown hepatitis A virus to be relatively resistant to inactivation by ether, heating at 60 C for 1 hour, and pH 3, but the virus was inactivated by formaldehyde solution (0.25 mL/L) at 37 C for 72 hours and by chlorine (1 mg/L) for 30 minutes. Propagation of hepatitis A virus has been performed in primary and continuous cells of primate origin. Both live attenuated and killed hepatitis A vaccines are under clinical evaluation.

The multiplication of this virus group is described in detail in Chapter 63.

Pathogenesis

The clinical expression of infection with hepatitis A virus varies considerably, ranging from subclinical, anicteric, and mild illnesses in children to the full range of symptoms with jaundice in adults. The ratio of anicteric to icteric illnesses varies widely, both in individual cases and in outbreaks.

Hepatitis A virus enters the body by ingestion and intestinal infection. The virus then spreads, probably by the bloodstream, to the liver, a target organ. Large numbers of virus particles are detectable in feces during the incubation period in experimental infection in chimpanzees, beginning as early as 9 days after exposure and continuing, in general, until peak elevation of serum aminotransferases. Similar observations have been made in the course of natural infection in humans; virus also is detected in feces early in the acute phase of illness but relatively infrequently after the onset of clinical jaundice. Interestingly, antibody to hepatitis A virus that persists also is detectable late in the incubation period, coinciding approximately with the onset of biochemical evidence of liver damage. Hepatitis A antigen has been localized by immunofluorescence in the cytoplasm of hepatocytes after experimental transmission to chimpanzees. The antigen has not been found in any tissue other than the liver following intravenous inoculation.

Pathological changes produced by hepatitis A appear exclusively in the liver. Several such changes occur: conspicuous focal activation of sinusoidal lining cells; accumulations of lymphocytes and more histiocytes in the parenchyma, often replacing hepatocytes lost by cytolytic necrosis predominantly in the periportal areas; occasional coagulative necrosis in the form of acidophilic bodies; and focal degeneration.

Host Defenses

Antibody to hepatitis A virus develops late in the incubation period. Specific hepatitis A IgM is found in the serum within 1 week from the onset of dark urine, reaching maximum levels about 1 week later and declining slowly during the next 40-60 days. Specific IgG antibody appears shortly after IgM is detectable, reaching maximum titer after 60-80 days. This antibody is protective and persists for many years.

Epidemiology

Viral hepatitis type A (infectious or epidemic hepatitis) occurs endemically in all parts of the world, with frequent reports of minor and major outbreaks. The exact incidence is difficult to estimate because of the high proportion of subclinical infections and infections without jaundice, differences in surveillance, and differing patterns of disease. The degree of underreporting is believed to be very high.

The incubation period of hepatitis A is 3-5 weeks, with a mean of 28 days. Subclinical and anicteric cases are common and, although the disease has in general a low mortality rate, patients may be incapacitated for many weeks. There is no evidence of progression to chronic liver damage.

Hepatitis A virus is spread by the fecal-oral route, most commonly by person-to-person contact; infection occurs readily under conditions of poor sanitation and overcrowding. Common source outbreaks are most frequently initiated by fecal contamination of water and food, but waterborne transmission is not a major factor in maintaining this infection in industrialized communities. On the other hand, many food-borne outbreaks have been reported. This can be attributed to the shedding of large quantities of virus in the feces during the incubation period of the illness in infected food handlers; the source of the outbreak often can be traced to uncooked food or food that has been handled after cooking. Although hepatitis A remains endemic and common in the developed countries, the infection occurs mainly in small clusters, often with only few identified cases.

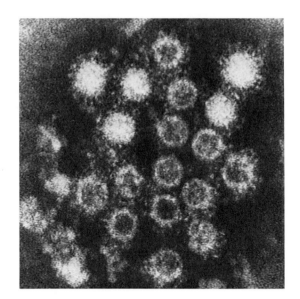

Figure 90-1 Hepatitis A virus particles found in fecal extracts by immune electron microscopy. Both full and empty particles are present. Particles are surrounded by a halo of hepatitis A antibody. The virus measures 27–29 nm diameter ($\times$ 300,000).

In 1973, immune electron microscopy led to the identification of virus particles in extracts of feces (Figure 90-1) during the early acute phase of illness, providing the long-awaited lead to further studies of this infection. Availability of viral antigen permitted, in turn, identification of specific antibody, development of serologic tests for hepatitis A, and determination of susceptibility to infection in human and nonhuman primates. Human hepatitis A has been transmitted to certain species of marmosets and to chimpanzees shown to be free of homologous antibody, thereby providing a model for experimental infection and, initially, also a source of reagents.

Availability of specific serologic tests for hepatitis A made possible the study of the incidence and distribution of hepatitis A in various countries. These studies have shown that infections with hepatitis A virus are widespread and endemic in all parts of the world, chronic excretion of hepatitis A virus does not occur, the infection is rarely transmitted by blood transfusion, and no evidence of progression to chronic liver disease has been found.

Diagnosis

Various serologic tests are available for hepatitis A, including immune electron microscopy, complement-fixation, immune adherence hemagglutination, radioimmunoassay, and enzyme immunoassay. Immune adherence hemagglutination, which had been widely used, is moderately specific and sensitive. Several methods of radioimmunoassay have been described; of these, a solid-phase type of assay is particularly convenient, very sensitive, and specific. Very sensitive enzyme immunoassay techniques also have been developed.

Only one serotype of hepatitis A virus has been identified in volunteers infected experimentally with the MS-1 strain of hepatitis A, in patients from different outbreaks of hepatitis in different geographic regions, in random cases of hepatitis A, and in naturally and experimentally infected nonhuman primates (certain species of marmosets and, particularly, chimpanzees). Because isolation of the virus in tissue culture requires prolonged adaptation, it is not yet suitable for diagnosis.

Control

Control of the infection is difficult. Spread of hepatitis A is reduced by simple hygienic measures and the sanitary disposal of excreta. Normal human immunoglobulin (a 16% solution in a dose of 0.02–0.12 mL/kg body weight), administered before exposure to the virus or early during the incubation period, prevents or attenuates a clinical illness. It will not always prevent infection, however, and inapparent or subclinical hepatitis may develop, excretion of virus in feces may occur, and active immunity may follow. Hepatitis A vaccines are being evaluated in clinical studies.

HEPATITIS B

Distinctive Properties

The discovery of Australia antigen in the circulation in 1965 and, subsequently, its association with hepatitis type B resulted in rapid advances in this field. Infection with hepatitis B virus (serum hepatitis) results in the appearance in serum of at least three serologic markers. The first is hepatitis B surface antigen (originally called **Australia antigen**) (Figure 90-2), which stimulates the homologous antibody, the surface antibody. The second antigen, located in the core of the 42-nm hepatitis B particle (Figure 90-3), gives rise to the core antibody. The third marker of hepatitis B virus infection, the **e antigen,** correlates closely with the number of virus particles and the relative infectivity of serum containing hepatitis B surface antigen. The e antigen is a distinct soluble antigen specifically associated with hepatitis B, but its precise location in the core of the virus particle is not yet established. Serum antibody to e indicates relatively low infectivity of serum. The sequence of development of these antigens and their corresponding antibodies is illustrated in Figure 90-4.

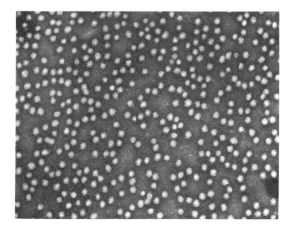

Figure 90-2 Purified preparation of approximately 22-nm spherical hepatitis B surface antigen particles. Such preparations are being used as subunit small particle hepatitis B vaccines. (× 126,000.)

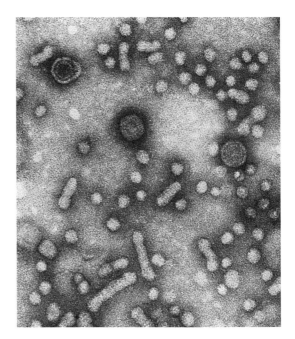

Figure 90-3 Electron micrograph of serum containing hepatitis B virus after negative staining. The three morphologic forms of antigen are shown: (a) Small pleomorphic spherical particles 20–22 nm in diameter. (b) Tubular forms. (c) 42 nm double-shelled virus. (×252,000.) From Zuckerman, A.J.: *Human viral hepatitis*. Amsterdam: North-Holland/American Elsevier, 1975.

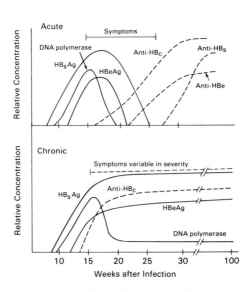

Figure 90-4 Sequence of development of viral antigens and antibodies in acute and chronic hepatitis B.

All these serologic markers can be detected by sensitive techniques such as radioimmunoassay and enzyme immunoassay. These serologic markers have proved extremely useful for unraveling the epidemiology of hepatitis B, established the global dissemination and public health importance of this infection, led to the routine screening of blood donors for the surface antigen, and resulted in remarkable advances in the knowledge of the virology and pathogenesis of hepatitis B and its associated chronic liver disorders.

The 42-nm particle is the hepatitis B virus. The core has a subunit structure organized according to the principles of icosahedral symmetry. It contains an endogenous, DNA-dependent DNA polymerase in close association with a DNA template. Double-stranded DNA has been isolated from circulating virus particles and also from cores extracted from the nuclei of infected hepatocytes. The DNA consists of circular nucleic acid molecules with a mean contour length of 0.79 ± 0.09 μm, corresponding to a molecular weight of approximately 1.6×10^6; however, more recent studies suggest a molecular weight of about 2.3×10^6. The DNA has been characterized by gel electrophoresis and restriction enzyme cleavage as approximately 3200 nucleotides in length, containing a single-stranded gap of 600-2100 nucleotides. The endogenous DNA polymerase reaction appears to repair the gap, but the relevance of the gapped circular DNA to the mode of viral replication is not clear.

Pathogenesis

Infection with hepatitis B virus may be followed by the persistent carrier state, which may be associated with liver damage. Infection early in life usually produces a carrier state, whereas only 5-10% of infections in adults produce carriers. If HBsAg persists for more than 6 months, the diagnosis is persistent hepatitis B infection (see Figure 90-3). Two chronic disease patterns may occur—chronic persistent or chronic active hepatitis; both are HBsAg positive. Patients who have chronic persistent hepatitis are usually asymptomatic but may have mild elevation of serum alanine transaminase (ALT). This syndrome, which occurs in 8%-10% of cases, is apparently not followed by liver fibrosis. In chronic active hepatitis, jaundice may be present, ALT levels are elevated, and the course of disease varies. Liver biopsy shows cell damage and cirrhosis. Liver failure occurs in a high percentage of patients.

Why chronic infections develop is unknown; however, factors found to be associated with chronicity are mild infection, a long incubation period, immunosuppression, and genetic predisposition. About 25% of chronically infected persons exhibit liver cell necrosis, which may progress to cirrhosis and liver failure. This predisposes the infected person to liver cell cancer. Whether hepatitis B virus acts alone or as a cocarcinogen for the development of cancer is not known. Survival of hepatitis B virus is ensured by the reservoir of carriers, estimated to number between 150-200 million. The prevalence of carriers, particularly among blood donors, appears to be 0.1% or less in North America and in Northern Europe, up to 5% in Central Eastern Europe; above 5% in Southern Europe and the countries bordering the Mediterranean; and, in as many as 20%-35% of the population in some parts of Africa, in Asia, and in the Pacific regions. The importance of the parenteral (direct inoculation into the tissues) and inapparent parenteral routes of transmission of hepatitis B virus are now well established.

Host Defenses

Antibody and cell-mediated immune responses to various types of antigens are induced during the infection; however, these do not always seem to be protective and, in some instances, may cause autoimmune phenomena that contribute to disease pathogenesis. The immune response to infection with hepatitis B virus is directed toward at least three antigens: hepatitis B surface antigen, the core antigen, and the e antigen. The view that hepatitis B exerts its damaging effect on hepatocytes by direct cytopathic changes is inconsistent with the persistence of large quantities of surface antigen in liver cells of many apparently healthy persons who are persistent carriers. Additional evidence suggests that the pathogenesis of liver damage in the course of hepatitis B infection is related to the immune response by the host.

The surface antigen appears in the sera of most patients during the incubation period, 2-8 weeks before biochemical evidence of liver damage or onset of jaundice. The antigen persists during the acute illness and usually clears from the circulation during convalescence. Next to appear in the circulation is the virus-associated DNA polymerase activity, which correlates in time with damage to liver cells as indicated by elevated serum transaminases. The polymerase activity persists for days or weeks in acute cases and for months or years in some persistent carriers. Antibody to the core antigen is found in the serum 2-10 weeks after the surface antigen appears, and it is frequently detectable for many years after recovery. The titer of core antibody appears to correlate with the amount and duration of virus replication. Finally, antibody to the surface antigen component appears.

During the incubation period and during the acute phase of the illness, surface antigen-antibody complexes may be found in the sera of some patients. Immune complexes have been found by electron microscopy in the sera of all patients with fulminant hepatitis, but are seen only infrequently in nonfulminant infection. Immune complexes also are important in the pathogenesis of other disease syndromes character-ized by severe damage of blood vessels (for example, polyarteritis nodosa, some forms of chronic glomerulonephritis, and infantile papular acrodermatitis).

Immune complexes have been identified in variable proportions of patients with virtually all the recognized chronic sequelae of acute hepatitis. Deposits of such immune complexes have also been demonstrated in the cytoplasm and plasma membrane of hepatocytes and on or in the nuclei; why only a small proportion of patients with circulating complexes develop vasculitis or polyarteritis is, however, not clear. Perhaps complexes are critical pathogenic factors only if they are of a particular size and of a certain antigen-to-antibody ratio.

Cellular immune responses are known to be particularly important in determining the clinical features and course of viral infections. The occurrence of cell-mediated immunity to hepatitis B antigens has been demonstrated in most patients during the acute phase of hepatitis B and in a significant proportion of patients with surface-antigen-positive chronic active hepatitis, but not in asymptomatic persistent hepatitis B carriers. These observations suggest that cell-mediated immunity may be important in terminating the infection and, under certain circumstances, in promoting liver damage and in the genesis of autoimmunity. Also, evidence suggests that progressive liver damage may result from an autoimmune reaction directed against hepatocyte membrane antigens, initiated in many cases by infection with hepatitis B virus. Although exogenous interferon may be effective in treating some patients with chronic hepatitis, as yet endogenous interferon production has not been detected during the natural infection. More studies to define the role of interferon are needed.

Epidemiology

Although various body fluids (blood, saliva, menstrual and vaginal discharges, seminal fluid, and breast milk) have been implicated in the spread of infection, infectivity appears to be especially related to blood. The epidemiologic propensities of this infection are therefore wide; they include infection by inadequately sterilized syringes and instruments, transmission by blood transfusion and blood products, by close contact, and venereally, and possibly mechanically by blood-sucking arthropods. Antenatal (rarely) and perinatal (frequently) transmission of hepatitis B infection from mother to child may take place; in some parts of the world (Southeast Asia and Japan), perinatal transmission is very common.

Diagnosis

Direct demonstration of virus in serum samples is feasible by visualizing the virus (Dane) particles by electron microscopy, by detecting virus-associated DNA polymerase, and by assay of viral DNA. All these direct techniques are impractical under normal laboratory conditions, and specific diagnosis must therefore rely on serologic tests.

Hepatitis B surface antigen first appears during the late stages of the incubation period and is easily detectable by radioimmunoassay or enzyme immunoassay. The antigen persists during the acute phase of the disease and sharply decreases when antibody to the surface antigen becomes detectable. Antibody of the IgM class to the core antigen is found in the serum after the onset of the clinical symptoms and slowly declines after recovery. Its persistence at high titer suggests continuation of the infection. Core antibody of the IgG class persists for many years and provides evidence of past infection.

Control

Groups that are at increased risk for hepatitis B urgently require a vaccine. These groups include persons who require multiple transfusions of blood or plasma, injection of blood products, or prolonged inpatient treatment; those who require frequent tissue penetration or need repeated access to the circulation; those with natural or acquired immune deficiency; and those with malignant disease. Viral hepatitis is an occupational hazard among health care personnel and residents and staff of institutions for the mentally retarded and, perhaps, other closed institutions. High rates of infection have been reported in drug abusers, prostitutes, and particularly among homosexual males. Individuals working in high endemic areas also suffer an increased risk of infection. Some authors also include military personnel and women of child-bearing age in areas of the world where the carrier state in that group is excessive. A more practical approach to control in these areas would be to immunize newborns in high endemic areas. Consideration must also be given to persons living in certain tropical and subtropical areas, where present socioeconomic conditions are poor and prevalence of hepatitis B infection is very high.

The repeated failure to grow and passage hepatitis B virus serially in tissue culture has hampered progress toward development of a conventional vaccine. Attention has therefore been directed toward the use of other preparations for active immunization. The foundations for such hepatitis B immunogens were laid by the demonstration of the relative efficacy of diluted serum containing hepatitis B virus heated to 98 C for 1 min in preventing or modifying the infection in susceptible persons.

Because the separated viral coat material (in this instance, hepatitis B surface antigen) leads to production of protective antibody, the possibility of using purified 22-nm spherical hepatitis B surface antigen particles (Figure 90-3) as a vaccine seems feasible. Such vaccines have been prepared from the plasma of apparently healthy carriers of this antigen. Human hepatitis B infection has been successfully transmitted to chimpanzees and, although the infection is mild, the biochemical, histologic, and serologic responses in these primates are very similar to those in humans. Limited numbers of susceptible chimpanzees have now been shown to be protected by the 22-nm particle immunogen treated with formalin. Small-scale safety tests in volunteers of such experimental subunit vaccine were followed by successful protective efficacy trials in several countries. Although it is generally accepted that the viral subunit preparations, when pure, are free of nucleic acid and are therefore noninfectious, the fact that the starting material for their preparation is human plasma obtained from persons infected with hepatitis B virus means that extreme caution must be exercised to insure that the vaccine is free from all harmful, contaminating material. Indeed, the plasma is collected from individuals who are persistent carriers of hepatitis B surface antigen, which is a marker of hepatitis B virus. The preparation and inactivation of the vaccine must guarantee inactivation of representatives of all groups of infectious agents, including the virus(es) causing acquired immunodeficiency syndrome (AIDS). Some concern has been expressed that the host components (including liver antigens) that may be present in the vaccine may induce harmful immunologic responses; however, such responses have not been observed in the chimpanzees and individuals immunized to date.

In addition to the development of hepatitis B vaccines composed of intact 22-nm spherical forms of the surface antigen, vaccines are being prepared from the constituent polypeptides. Vaccines prepared from polypeptides in micelle form have been shown to be highly immunogenic. Vaccines prepared by recombinant DNA techniques and by chemical synthesis are under evaluation.

NON-A:NON-B HEPATITIS

The specific laboratory diagnosis of hepatitis A and hepatitis B has revealed a previously unrecognized form of hepatitis, clearly unrelated to either type and referred to as non-A:non-B hepatitis. This is now the most common form of hepatitis occurring after blood transfusion and the administration of certain blood products in some areas of the world. The infection also has been transmitted experimentally to chimpanzees. Although specific laboratory tests for identifying this new type of hepatitis are not yet available, evidence indicates that this infection is not uncommon, that a carrier state exists, and that in a significant proportion of patients the infection progresses to chronic liver disease. At least two different types of parenterally transmitted non-A:non-B hepatitis have been implicated.

Several reports have been published on the identification of an antigen, in patients with non-A:non-B; however, none of these tests has proved reproducible. Many laboratories are now attempting to identify the viral antigens involved in these new forms of hepatitis.

EPIDEMIC NON-A HEPATITIS

Although only one serotype of hepatitis A virus has been identified in patients affected in different outbreaks of hepatitis A (in different geographic regions), in sporadic cases of hepatitis A, and in naturally and experimentally infected nonhuman primates, considerable evidence now indicates the existence of an epidemic form of a hepatitis-A-like illness, particularly in the subcontinent of India, the eastern Soviet Union, and other parts of Asia. This epidemic and endemic strain(s) of virus usually is transmitted by water contaminated with sewage, but other modes of fecal-oral transmission are possible. The epidemic form of non-A hepatitis is an acute, self-limiting disease that affects mostly young adults. The illness is more severe in pregnant women, among whom it produces a high mortality rate, especially during the last trimester of pregnancy. Significant fetal deaths occur. Ample serologic evidence indicates that this form of hepatitis is not caused by the recognized serotype of hepatitis A, which is not surprising considering that this illness occurs in regions in which most individuals are infected with hepatitis A during the first few years of life and are thus immune. Indeed, no serologic evidence for reinfection of patients with hepatitis A virus has been found. It is not known whether the epidemic hepatitis is caused by a distinct, but previously unrecognized, serotype or serotypes of hepatitis A. Specific laboratory tests are not available, although a serologic test against one type of infection is being developed, following preliminary characterization of virus particles in studies conducted during an outbreak of the infection in the eastern Soviet Union.

δ-ANTIGEN–ASSOCIATED HEPATITIS

δ-antigen is associated with hepatitis B infection and appears to be a defective transmissible agent that is dependent on a helper function of hepatitis B virus for its replication. The δ-agent consists of a particle 35–37 nm in diameter that resembles the hepatitis B virus and indeed shares the surface antigen protein coat of hepatitis B virus. It contains an internal component, the δ-antigen, and a very small RNA molecule, mol. wt. approximately 5×10^5 daltons. This RNA does not hybridize with the DNA of hepatitis B virus. Only one serotype of the δ-agent has been recognized.

Epidemiologic studies of δ-hepatitis infection indicate that it occurs in many countries and is most common in persistent carriers of hepatitis B surface antigen or those who are at risk of repeated exposure to hepatitis B infection. The infection is transmitted by contaminated blood and blood products, and serologic evidence of infection is found most often in patients with hemophilia and other persons who are exposed to blood, and drug addicts who use the parenteral route. It is possible that the infection also is transmitted by nonpercutaneous routes.

The δ-agent has been associated with both acute and chronic hepatitis, always in the presence of infection with hepatitis B virus. δ-antigen–associated infection is generally more severe than that of hepatitis B in the absence of the δ-agent. Severe, rapidly progressive, chronic active hepatitis often is associated with combined infection with hepatitis B virus and the δ-agent. A sudden exacerbation of severe hepatitis in a carrier of hepatitis B virus is suggestive of superinfection with the δ-agent. Furthermore, 5%–10% or more of patients with fulminant hepatitis B have serologic evidence of coinfection with the δ-agent.

Sensitive laboratory techniques have been developed for detection of the δ-antigen and anti-δ-antibody, including immunofluorescence, radioimmunoassay, and enzyme immunoassay. Seroepidemiologic studies to determine the distribution and effect of δ-infection in different parts of the world are in progress.

References

Deinhardt, F., Gust, I.D.: Viral hepatitis. *Bull WHO* 1982; 60:661–691.

Gerety, R.J., (editor): *Non-A, non-B hepatitis.* New York: Academic Press, 1981.

McCollum, R.W., Zuckerman, A.J.: Viral hepatitis: Report on a WHO informal consultation. *J Med Virol* 1981; 8:1–29.

Szmuness, W., Alter, J.H., Maynard, J.E. (editors): *Viral hepatitis. 1981 international symposium.* Philadelphia: Franklin Institute Press, 1982.

Zuckerman, A.J.: Viral hepatitis. In: *The liver annual 1/1981, 2/1982, 3/1983, 4/1984.* Arias, I.M., Frenkel, M., Wilson, J.H.P., (editors). Amsterdam: Excerpta Medica, 1984.

Zuckerman, A.J.: Priorities for immunisation against hepatitis B. *Br Med J* 1982; 1:686–688.

Zuckerman, A.J., et al.: Prevention of primary liver cancer. Report on a meeting of a WHO group. *Lancet* 1983; 1:463–465.

91 Scrapie-Kuru Group: Subacute Spongiform Virus Encephalopathies

C. J. Gibbs, Jr., PhD

General Concepts
Distinctive Properties
Pathogenesis
Host Defenses
Epidemiology
Diagnosis
Control

General Concepts

Subacute progressive degenerative diseases of the central nervous system of humans and animals are important because most of these diseases are of unknown etiology and have been categorized as noninfectious. Few, if any, of these diseases are curable. Although some are genetically determined, most of these disorders occur sporadically, and a history of the disease does not appear in close relatives. Thus, it was surprising to discover that two of these chronic idiopathic disorders of humans, kuru (a heredofamilial disease restricted in distribution to the Eastern Highlands of Papua New Guinea) and the sporadic and familial types of Creutzfeldt-Jakob disease (a presenile dementia with worldwide distribution) were shown to be caused by infection.

The transmissible agents of kuru and Creutzfeldt-Jakob disease are indistinguishable from the etiologic agent of scrapie, a subacute progressive degenerative disease of the central nervous system of sheep and goats. Scrapie, like Creutzfeldt-Jakob disease, appears to occur worldwide. One of the most challenging aspects uncovered in the study of the agents of kuru, Creutzfeldt-Jakob disease, and scrapie is their sharing of biologic, physical, and chemical properties that are so unusual they are called the **unconventional viruses** and classified within a new group of microorganisms, those that cause the subacute spongiform virus encephalopathies. These agents are unconventional in the following ways: they do not induce inflammatory lesions; they are highly resistant to ultraviolet light and gamma radiation; they have not yet been shown to induce an immune response; their morphologic structure has not yet been recognized by electron microscopy; and they have not yet been associated with a nucleic acid type. Such properties suggest the involvement of a subviral pathogen such as the unique filamentous structures observed in cells from infected animals. An alternate etiologic agent might be a naked nucleic acid similar to the *viroids* that infect plants.

The unconventional viruses have been called "slow viruses," although this term is misleading; there are no "slow" viruses. *Slow* modifies *infection*, not *virus*.

There are, however, other persistent infections of the human central nervous system that have been shown to be caused by classical viruses. These viruses can be visualized as distinct morphologic structures by electron microscopy; they induce specific antigen-antibody reactions; they usually induce histopathologic lesions more generally associated with virus infections; and they have an RNA or DNA type of nucleic acid. The infections produced are described in Chapters 79 and 86. In fact, both conventional and unconventional viruses are capable of inducing subacute progressive degenerative diseases of the central nervous system many months to years after initial infection.

This chapter describes two human slow infections (kuru and Creutzfeldt-Jakob disease) and one slow infection of animals (scrapie of sheep and goats). These illnesses, together with transmissible mink encephalopathy and chronic wasting disease of mule deer and captive elk, form the subacute spongiform virus encephalopathies (Table 91-1). This chapter also reviews the mechanisms of virus–host cell interactions in these diseases.

Distinctive Properties

The nature of the transmissible agents isolated from the tissues of human patients with kuru and Creutzfeldt-Jakob disease and from the tissue of animals with scrapie and

Table 91-1 Subacute Spongiform Virus Encephalopathies

Human
Kuru
Creutzfeldt-Jakob disease
Gerstmann-Straussler-Scheinker's disease

Animals
Scrapie
Transmissible mink encephalopathy
Chronic wasting disease of mule deer
Chronic wasting disease of elk

related diseases remains to be determined. The unusual biological, physical and chemical properties, including the stability of the subacute spongiform encephalopathy viruses, have formed the basis for numerous hypotheses concerning their nature. They have been referred to as classical viruses, unconventional viruses, agents lacking nucleic acids, replicating membrane, replicating polysaccharide, a proteinaceous infectious particle (PRION), a fibrillar virion (SAF—scrapie associated fibril), a naked nucleic acid (VIROID), and a small informational molecule of nucleic acid protected by host protein (VIRINO).

The unconventional viruses of the scrapie-kuru group have unusual resistance to ultraviolet radiation and to ionizing radiation. However, this should not be taken as proof that no genetic information exists in these viruses as nucleic acid molecules, since work with the smallest RNA viruses (called viroids) indicates a similar resistance to ultraviolet inactivation in crude preparations of infected plant sap. Ultraviolet resistance also depends greatly on small RNA size, as shown by the high resistance of the purified, very small (80,000 daltons) tobacco-ring-spot satellite virus RNA. Partial purification of scrapie virus by fluorocarbon increases only slightly its ultraviolet sensitivity at 254 nm. Kuru and Creutzfeldt-Jakob disease viruses also show enormous resistance to inactivation by ^{60}Co radiation in high dosage. A dosage as high as 20×10^6 rads does not appear to reduce the infectivity titer more than one $\log_{10}$ or to influence the incubation period of the disease in nonhuman primates. Although the resistance to radiation and to the UV action spectrum suggests a nonnucleic acid genome, it also is compatible with the concept of a small nucleic acid genome embedded within a chemical complex.

In addition, these viruses have unusual resistance to heat, to various enzymes such as carbohydrases, lipases, proteases, and nucleases, and to formaldehyde, β-propiolactone, and sodium deoxycholate. In contrast, they are moderately sensitive to a number of organic solvents, including acetone, acetone ether, 2-chloroethanol, chloroform-butanol and chloroform-methanol, ether, fluorocarbon (Arcton 113), and 90% phenol. Although stable over a range of pH of 2.0 to 10.4, when exposed to 1 N sodium hydroxide, scrapie infectivity is destroyed. Inactivation has been obtained with relatively low concentrations of chaotropic ions of the hydroxal group.

On electron microscopic examination, density-gradient fractions of high infectivity of the scrapie virus (10^7–10^8 mouse LD_{50}/mL) reveal only smooth vesicular membranes with mitochondrial and ribosomal debris and no structures resembling recognizable virions.

Recently, however, abnormal fibrils, which have been designated as **scrapie associated fibrils (SAF)** have been observed in synaptosomal preparations of scrapie-infected brain. These fibrils may be composed in part of a protein of 26,000 daltons. SAF also are present in scrapie-infected hamsters and monkeys; in humans with Creutzfeldt-Jakob disease; and in kuru-infected monkeys. SAF never have been found in other encephalopathies with similar histopathologic findings, ultrastructural features, or disease symptoms. Infectivity studies indicate a correlation between the presence of SAF and virus titers: the time of appearance and the quantity of SAF in brain and spleen have been found to coincide with an increase in infectivity within these organs. Thus, SAF may be the etiologic agent of the spongiform encephalopathies; if this hypothesis is proven, the SAF will represent a new class of filamentous animal viruses.

All attempts to induce antibody formation in laboratory animals and to show immune responses in infected patients or animals with the spongiform encephalopathies have failed. In contrast, sera from some patients and animals infected naturally with the subacute spongiform virus encephalopathies contain a high titer of an autoantibody that is directed against the normal fibrillar protein (mol. wt. 200,000 and 150,000 daltons) within the axon of the mature central neurons of rodents (in culture) or cryostat sections of rodent spinal cords. This autoantibody can be detected by immunoflourescence staining or by the more sensitive Western blot technique, which employs a partially purified preparation of neurofilaments as the antigen substrate. The role of this heterospecific autoantibody in the pathogenesis of the transmissible spongiform encephalopathies, as well as the clinical value of assessment of the antibody during the course of these diseases, is not clear, because the antibody is occasionally detected in sera from patients with other neurologic diseases, particularly familial Alzheimer's disease, and (to a much lesser degree) in healthy subjects.

In addition to their natural hosts, unconventional viruses have been shown to be transmissible to various rodents and nonhuman primate species. The typical and atypical properties of these agents are summarized in Tables 91-2 and 91-3. Recent studies have shown that many different strains of these types of viruses infect humans and animals and induce a variety of host reactions.

Pathogenesis

Slow infections have the following criteria: a long initial period of latency, lasting from several months to several years; a protracted course of illness following the appearance of clinical signs with progression to death; primary anatomic lesions limited to a single organ system; and a limited range of susceptible hosts (in natural infections).

Clinically, kuru runs an afebrile course and is characterized by the insidious onset of ataxia, which becomes progressively more severe and is soon accompanied by a fine tremor involving the trunk, head, and extremities. Both involuntary tremor and ataxia increase and progress until the patient is unable to walk or stand without considerable support (Figure 91-1).

Table 91-2 Classic Virus Properties of Unconventional Viruses

Filterable to 25-nm average pore diameter (APD) (scrapie, mink encepalopathy), 100-nm APD (kuru, Creutzfeldt-Jakob disease)

Titrate "cleanly" (all individuals succumb to high LD_{50} in most species)

Replicate to titers of 10^8/g-10^{12}/g in brain

Pathogenesis: first replicate in spleen and elsewhere in the reticuloendothelial system; later in brain

Specificity of host range

"Adaptation" to new host (shortened incubation period)

Genetic control of susceptibility in some species (sheep and mice for scrapie)

Strains of varying virulence and pathogenicity

Clonal (limiting dilution) selection of strains from "wild stock"

Interference of slow-growing strain of scrapie with replication of fast-growing strain in mice

Table 91-3 Atypical Properties of Unconventional Viruses

Physical and Chemical Properties	*Biologic Properties*
Resistant to:	Long incubation period (months to years; decades)
Formaldehyde	
β-propiolactone	No inflammatory response
EDTA	Chronic progressive pathology (slow infections)
Proteases (trypsin, pepsin)	No remissions or recoveries: always fatal
Nucleases (ribonucleases A and III, deoxyribonuclease I)	Degenerative histopathology: amyloid plaques, gliosis
Heat (80 C); incompletely inactivated at 100 C	No visible viruslike structures by electron microscopy
Ultraviolet radiation: 2540Å	No inclusion bodies
Ionizing radiation (γ-rays): equivalent target 150,000 daltons	No interferon production or interference with interferon production by other viruses
Ultrasonic energy	No interferon sensitivity
Atypical ultraviolet action spectrum: 2370Å = 6 × 2540Å inactivation	No virus interference (with more than 30 different conventional viruses)
Invisible as recognizable virion by electron microscopy (only plasma membranes, cord, and coat)	No infectious nucleic acid demonstrable
	No antigenicity
No nonhost proteins demonstrated	No alteration in pathogenesis (incubation period, duration, course) by immunosuppression or immunopotentiation:
	ACTH, cortisone
	Cyclophosphamide
	X-ray
	Antilymphocytic serum
	Thymectomy or splenectomy
	Nude athymic mice
	Adjuvants
	Immune B cell and T cell functions intact in vivo and in vitro
	No cytopathic effect in infected cells in vitro
	Varying individual susceptibility to high infection dose in some host species (as scrapie in sheep)

Intelligence remains normal during the early months of illness, but speech slowly becomes slurred and ultimately becomes unintelligible. This dysarthria is associated with progressive slowing of intellectual functions. In the advanced stage, swallowing and chewing are no longer possible and the patient succumbs from rapid starvation, decubitus ulcerations, and terminal static bronchopneumonia.

Pathologically, no significant morphologic changes are found in organs other than the CNS. Grossly the brain appears normal, but in some cases the frontal lobes or cerebellum show atrophy. Microscopically, widespread neuronal degeneraton and loss are seen with subsequent overgrowth of astroglial cells. The degenerating neurons may be swollen and vacuolated. This status spongiosis becomes pathognomonic in the

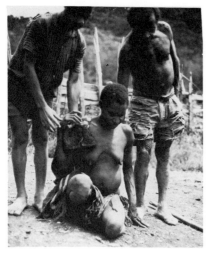 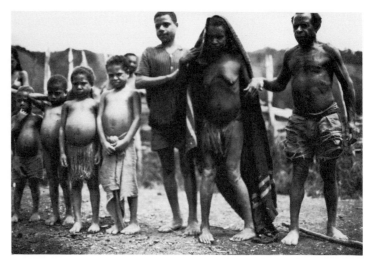

Figure 91-1 A woman with stage II kuru. The patient had marked tremor and severe cerebellar ataxia. Although able to sit, she could not rise, stand, or walk without full assistance. Unlike patients with Creutzfeldt-Jakob disease, this patient did not manifest signs of dementia or myoclonic jerking. She is shown in her village with her husband and her children.

human disease. The pathologic lesions are found throughout the cortical gray matter, particularly affecting the cerebellum, pons, thalamus, and basal ganglia and are diffuse in the cerebral cortex and anterior horns of the spinal cord.

The clinical and pathologic course of Creutzfeldt-Jakob disease is similar, although some variability has been reported; this has led to a variety of synonyms appearing in the literature (Table 91-4). In most cases, Creutzfeldt-Jakob disease appears as a process primarily of the cortical gray matter of the brain. The disease usually presents as a variable period of vague psychic disturbances, progressing in a few weeks or months to frank dementia that is complicated by cerebellar, extrapyramidal, or pyramidal symptoms, and finally to mutism, rigidity, and death. It is associated with myoclonic jerking and electroencephalographic changes consisting of periodic spiking slow waves. (See Figure 91-2.)

Scrapie is a natural disease of sheep and occasionally of goats. Like Creutzfeldt-Jakob disease, scrapie has been described in the literature under a wide variety of

Table 91-4 Synonyms for Creutzfeldt-Jakob Disease

Disseminated encephalomyelopathy	Subacute vascular encephalopathy with
Spastic pseudosclerosis	mental disorder, focal disturbances, and
Creutzfeldt-Jakob disease	myoclonus epilepsy
Cortico-pallido-spinal degeneration	Subacute spongiform encephalopathy
Cortico-striato-spinal degeneration	Subacute progressive encephalopathy
Jakob's syndrome	Subacute presenile spongiosus atrophy
Presenile dementia with cortical blindness	Nevin-Jones disease
Heidenhain's syndrome	Brownell-Oppenheimer syndrome

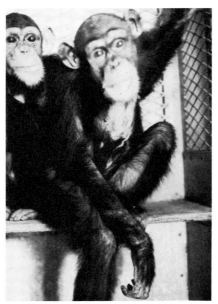

Figure 91-2 A female chimpanzee that developed Creutzfeldt-Jakob disease 12.5 months after inoculation with brain suspension from a chimpanzee who died of the disease. The chimpanzee showed tremor, incoordination, myoclonic jerking, fasiculation, right-sided neglect of limbs and confusion (as manifested by inattention, listlessness, lethargy, and irritability).

Table 91-5   Synonyms for Scrapie

Tremblante (France)	Lumbar neuralgia
Polioencephalomyelitis	Jumping disease
Convulsive disease	Enzootic peripheric neuritis
Crazy disease	Traberkrankheit (Germany)
Nervous disease	Guubberkrankheit (Germany)
Disease of the nerves	Wetzkrankheit (Germany)
Vertigo	Surlokozjanka (Hungary)
Lumbar prurigo	Rida (Iceland)

synonyms (Table 91-5). The clinical picture and histopathologic findings of scrapie closely resemble those of kuru.

In the natural disease, onset is insidious and without any recognizable antecedent fever or other acute manifestations. Early signs are apprehension, restlessness, hyperexcitability, and aggressiveness, and some animals even manifest apparent dementia. Early in the disease, fine tremors of the head and neck are observed; as the disease progresses, the tremors become more generalized, involving the whole body and producing a shivering effect as disturbances in locomotion become evident; in advanced stages of the disease, animals become stuporous and manifest visual impairment, excessive salivation, urinary and fecal incontinence, and wasting lassitude. Pathologic alterations are similar to those occurring in kuru.

Apart from an increase in the amount of cerebrospinal fluid in some animals, the significant changes are microscopic, found only in the CNS, and notably destructive of gray matter.

Host Defenses

None of the defense mechanisms known to control conventional viral diseases has been shown to play a role against spongiform encephalopathy viruses. Antibody is not produced during the infection, and the course of the infection is not altered by suppression or potentiation of the host immune response (see Table 91-3). Also, interferon is undetectable, and administration of exogenous interferon or interferon inducers is not protective.

Epidemiology

Kuru, now nearing extinction, had a heredofamilial distribution among people of the Eastern Highland region of Papua New Guinea. Transmission of the virus occurred through ritual cannibalism (devouring of the brain of deceased tribesmen, mostly by women and children). Elimination of cannibalism is apparently eradicating the disease, and new cases occur only in older members of the population—people known to have participated in cannibalism.

Creutzfeldt-Jakob disease, first described in the early 1920s by Creutzfeldt and subsequently by Jakob, occurs throughout the world with a prevalence of about one death per year per million population; this rate is approximately the same on all six continents. The mean age of onset is 57 years, ranging from the second to the ninth decade; age, however, should not be a determining factor in diagnosis, since cases now have been recognized in patients as young as 16 and 20 years of age and in some over 80 years of age. Men and women are equally affected. About 16% of the cases are of the familial form, in which occurrence is characterized by a single autosomal-dominant gene pattern, even though the disease is caused by a virus. This is the first example of an autosomal-dominant, single-gene inheritance controlling the appearance of an infectious disease in humans. Remissions and relapses have not been recorded.

Transmission mechanisms for most cases of Creutzfeldt-Jakob disease have not been established. The only proven mechanism of person-to-person transmission is by iatrogenic means. In 1974, Duffy et al discovered Creutzfeldt-Jakob disease in a patient who had undergone corneal transplantation surgery in which the donor cornea was from a patient who had died from the disease. In two other cases, patients with the disease had undergone stereotactic electrode implantation for study of chronic focal epilepsy. The silver electrodes used in these two patients had been implanted previously into the brain of a patient with Creutzfeldt-Jakob disease. Both of the patients with chronic epilepsy developed Creutzfeldt-Jakob disease within 2 years of the implantation of the electrodes.

Scrapie is widely distributed in Europe, America, and Asia. The first recorded attempt to transmit scrapie was in 1899; however, not until 1936 were transmission studies successful and later extended to show its filterable nature and other viruslike properties. This has permitted scrapie to be more intensely studied than either of the transmissible human spongiform encephalopathies; nevertheless, the mechanism of scrapie spread in nature remains obscure. It may spread from naturally infected sheep to uninfected sheep and goats, although such horizontal transmission has not been observed in experimentally infected sheep or goats. Sheep, goats, mice, hamsters, mink, and nonhuman primates have been infected experimentally by intracerebral and peripheral routes of inoculation, as well as by the oral route. The disease appears to pass from ewes to lambs, even without suckling; the contact of the lamb with the infected ewe at birth appears to be sufficient because the placenta itself is infectious. Transplancental versus oral, nasal, optic, or cutaneous infections in the perinatal period are unproved possibilities. Older sheep are infected only after long contact with diseased animals; however, susceptible sheep have developed the disease in pastures previously occupied by sheep with scrapie. Interestingly, in a flock of naturally infected Suffolk sheep, scrapie virus was detected (by inoculation of mice with tissues from asymptomatic lambs) at 10-14 months of age and was limited to lymphatic tissues and intestine. Virus was not detected in the central nervous system until the onset of clinical symptoms at about 25 months of age.

Diagnosis

Clinical diagnosis of the human diseases may be confirmed by brain biopsy or early autopsy. Virus isolation may be attempted in chimpanzees, squirrel monkeys, capuchin monkeys and, in some instances, in guinea pigs and mice from brain samples obtained from biopsy or autopsy.

Control

As already mentioned, kuru apparently is being eradicated by discontinuing cannibalistic practices. No specific control measures are available for Creutzfeldt-Jakob disease. Scrapie in the United States is controlled through condemnation and slaughter of propositus and all other sheep that have been exposed, including progeny.

References

Bernoulli, C., et al.: Danger of accidental person-to-person transmission of Creutzfeldt-Jakob disease by surgery. *Lancet* 1977; 1:478-479.

Diringer, H., et al.: Scrapie infectivity, fibrils and low molecular weight protein. *Nature* 1983; 306:476-478.

Gibbs, C.J. Jr., Gajdusek, D.C.: Atypical viruses as the cause of sporadic, epidemic, and familial chronic diseases in man: Slow viruses and human diseases. In: *Perspectives in virology,* Vol. 10. Pollard, M., (editor). New York: Raven Press, 1978.

Masters, C.L., et al.: Creutzfeldt-Jakob disease: patterns of worldwide occurrence and the significance of familial and sporadic clustering. *Ann Neurol* 1978; 5:177-188.

Merz, P.A., et al.: An infection specific particle from the unconventional slow virus diseases. *Science* 1984; 225:437-440.

Prusiner, S.B., Hadlow, W.J., (editors): *Slow transmissible diseases of the nervous system.* Volume 1. *Clinical, epidemiological, genetic and pathological aspects of the spongiform encephalopathies.* New York: Academic Press, 1979.

Prusiner, S.B., Hadlow, W.J., (editors): *Slow transmissible diseases of the nervous system.* Volume 2. *Pathogenesis, immunology, virology and molecular biology of the spongiform encephalopathies.* New York: Academic Press, 1979.

Sotelo, J., Gibbs, C.J. Jr., Gajdusek, D.C.: Autoantibodies against axonal neurofilaments in patients with kuru and Creutzfeldt-Jakob disease. *Science* 1980; 210:190-193.

V PARASITOLOGY

Introduction

L. J. Olson, PhD

Medical parasitology traditionally has included the study of three major groups of animals: parasitic protozoa, parasitic helminths (worms), and those arthropods that directly cause disease or act as vectors of various pathogens. A **parasite** is a pathogen that simultaneously injures and derives sustenance from its host. Some organisms called parasites are actually **commensals,** in that they neither benefit nor harm their host (for example, *Entamoeba coli*). Although parasitology had its origins in the zoologic sciences, it is today an interdisciplinary field, greatly influenced by microbiology, immunology, biochemistry, and other life sciences.

Parasitic infections of humans number in the billions and range from relatively innocuous to fatal. The diseases caused by these parasites constitute major human health problems throughout the world (approximately 30% of the world's population is infected with the nematode, *Ascaris lumbricoides*). Many of these problems (for example, schistosomiasis, malaria) have increased rather than decreased in recent years.

A misconception about parasitic infections is that they occur only in tropical areas. Although the prevalence rates of most of these infections are higher in such regions, many people who live in temperate and subtropical areas also become infected. In addition other people return to nontropical areas with infections acquired in the tropics.

The unicellular (protozoa) and multicellular (helminths, arthropods) parasites are antigenically and biochemically complex, as are their life histories and the pathogenesis of the diseases they cause. These parasites undergo several developmental stages during their life history; these stages involve changes not only in structure but also in biochemical and antigenic composition. Certain of the larval stages of the helminths have little resemblance to the adult stages (for example, those of tapeworms and flukes). Some of the protozoa also differ greatly throughout their life history; for example, *Toxoplasma gondii* is an intestinal coccidian in cats, but in humans it takes on a different form and localizes in deep tissues. Certain of these infections can convert from a well-tolerated or asymptomatic infection to life-threatening disease. Many parasitic infections are transmitted from animals to humans (zoonotic) and cause a disease in humans that may or may not resemble that in the lower animal host. This section has two types of chapters. Several general chapters deal with the structure and classification of parasites and the mechanisms of parasitic diseases. Most of the chapters in the section, however, describe specific parasites and the diseases they cause. Throughout, emphasis has been placed on the basic biology of the pathogens and their host–parasite relationships. Thus, descriptions of the basic properties of the pathogens, the pathogenesis of the diseases they cause, host defenses, and epidemiology are highlighted. Practical information on diagnosis and control has been included in the chapters on specific pathogens.

In most chapters, pathogens that are closely related have been grouped together (for example, trematodes, cestodes, enteric nematodes, intestinal protozoa, hemoflagellates). The common characteristics of these parasites are discussed, as are the specific characteristics of each parasite. Other chapters are more limited in scope (for example, Toxoplasmosis, Malaria, *Pneumocystis*) because of the expertise of the authors and the difficulty involved in including these species within the groups discussed in the other chapters.

Collectively, the chapters in this section give the reader a broad, in-depth coverage of medically important parasites. Without such comprehensive coverage, students may—on the basis of the superficial attention given to parasitology in most microbiology texts—fail to gain the awareness and understanding necessary for proper diagnosis, treatment, and prevention of the parasitic infections. On the other hand, medical scientists who understand the biology of these parasites are well prepared to make appropriate medical decisions. This basic understanding also serves as a foundation for the addition of new knowledge in the future.

The most important element in diagnosing a parasitic infection is the physician's suspicion that a parasite may be the cause of a patient's disease, an etiologic possibility that often is not considered. Prerequisite to this consideration is knowledge of the biology of parasitic pathogens. For example, familiarity with a parasite's life cycle in the human host and its transmission among hosts generates useful questions and facilitates proper decisions regarding diagnostic procedures, treatment, and prevention.

Diagnosis of parasitic infections requires, in most instances, laboratory support, since clear-cut pathognomonic signs and symptoms often do not appear. A variety of methods and specimens are used for diagnosis. Since the most common group of parasites is the enterics, microscopic examination of fecal specimens is done more often than any other laboratory procedure in the diagnosis of parasitic disease. In some patients with certain enteric infections of the small intestines (for example, *Strongyloides stercoralis, Giardia lamblia*), an examination of a sample of duodenal contents may be positive when fecal specimens are negative. The specimens that are used in the diagnosis of the extraintestinal parasites are selected on the basis of the organotropisms of the pathogens. For example, stained blood smears are used in the diagnosis of *Plasmodium* spp infections, since these pathogens invade red cells. Other specimens that may be collected for microscopic assessment of extraintestinal parasites include sputum, vaginal exudate, skin scrapings, lymph, and various biopsy specimens. Culture has little practical application in the diagnosis of most parasitic infections, although culture has been employed (for example, in the diagnosis of *Trichomonas vaginalis* and *Entamoeba histolytica*). Culture of fecal specimens from patients with *Strongyloides* will sometimes yield positive results when microscopic examination of fecal specimens is negative. Immunodiagnostic tests are useful in several infections, including extraintestinal amebiasis, visceral larva migrans, and trichinosis.

Because the laboratory is so important in diagnosis, laboratory personnel must be well trained. Continuing training and refresher courses should be encouraged and supported. In the United States, excellent short courses in diagnostic parasitology are available in various state and federal health laboratories and at the Centers for Disease Control in Atlanta. These laboratories also offer a variety of diagnostic services in parasitology, including certain serologic tests. Medical scientists in the United States should be aware of the Parasitic Disease Drug Service at the Centers for Disease Control, from which drug information and certain drugs not readily available may be obtained.

92 Protozoa: Structure, Classification, Growth, and Development

Edith D. Box, ScD

General Concepts
Structure
Classification
Nutrition and Cultivation
Life Stages and Reproduction

General Concepts

Protozoa are defined as one-celled (or acellular) eukaryotes with nucleus and cytoplasm enclosed by a membrane. As in the case of many other groups of organisms, the taxonomy of protozoa has changed over the years. Currently, they are regarded as a subkingdom with seven phyla (Levine et al, 1980). Several thousand of a total of more than 30,000 existing protozoan species are parasitic. All of these species have been identified since the seventeenth century when Antony van Leeuwenhoek, using microscopes of his own construction, first saw *Giardia* in his own stools. Relatively few species of parasitic protozoa are of importance in human disease, but some of these few can be very devastating or very common. Species of *Plasmodium*, which cause malaria, have added to human suffering and death throughout recorded history, and the disease is becoming more prevalent in many areas of the world. One form of trypanosomiasis is a cause of morbidity and mortality in much of Africa; another trypanosome infection is an important cause of sickness and death in Central and South America. In the United

States, protozoan infections are less pathogenic than in the examples above, but some species are extremely common. Giardiasis (*Giardia lamblia* infection) has become an important infection in such diverse groups as children in day care centers, back-packers, and tourists. Trichomoniasis, caused by *Trichomonas vaginalis,* is one of the most common venereal infections; toxoplasmosis is acquired by more than one-half of the people in the United States during their lifetime.

New human diseases caused by protozoa are still being discovered. One example, babesiosis, is an infection of the erythrocytes long known as an important disease of cattle. A species of *Babesia* was discovered infecting persons living in Martha's Vineyard, Nantucket Island, and Long Island. Healy et al (1976) found that it is actually a zoonosis transmitted by ticks and maintained in rodents.

Another zoonosis called cryptosporidiosis was described by Current et al (1983). It is a cause of self-limited diarrhea in normal people, but causes an intractable diarrhea in immunodeficient persons. A species of *Cryptosporidium* infecting cattle, which was formerly thought to be host-specific, can apparently infect humans as well as a number of other animals.

Structure

Parasitic protozoa range in size from about 1–100 μm. The nuclei of protozoa are **vesicular** or **compact**. The compact type has a dense homogeneous distribution of chromatin, whereas the vesicular nuclei are characterized by more or less central bodies called nucleoli, endosomes, or karyosomes.

Included in the cytoplasm are a variety of organelles such as the Golgi apparatus, mitochondria, microtubules, and endoplasmic reticulum. Specialized structures are present in some groups; for example, hemoflagellates have kinetoplasts containing extranuclear DNA and the malaria, and *Toxoplasma* organisms have an apical complex.

Most protozoa also have organelles for locomotion that are useful in classification.

Classification

Three of the seven phyla of protozoa contain species of medical importance (Table 92-1). The phylum Sarcomastigophora contains amebas and flagellates that are characterized by possession of pseudopodia or flagella or both; members of the phylum Ciliata have cilia for motility. The phylum Apicomplexa, formerly called Sporozoa, contains protozoa with no permanent organelles for motility. After development of electron microscopy, it was discovered that members of this group of protozoa possessed a complex of organelles at the anterior end (Figure 92-1), presumably for attaching to and entering cells. This feature gave rise to the name Apicomplexa and helped elucidate some uncertain relationships among the protozoa.

Nutrition and Cultivation

Protozoa parasitizing a host can obtain food in a variety of ways. Food may be taken in through the outer membrane by pinocytosis, engulfed by phagocytosis, or obtained by use of a special structure called a cytostome (Figure 92-2).

Table 92-1   Classification and Characteristics of Parasitic Protozoa

Phylum	Subphylum	Representative Genera	Disease Produced in Human Beings	Chapter Title and Number
Sarcomastigophora (with flagella and/or pseudopodia)	Mastigophora (flagella)	Leishmania	Kala-azar, espundia	Hemoflagellates (97)
		Trypanosoma	Sleeping sickness Chagas' disease	
		Giardia	Diarrhea	Other Intestinal Protozoa and Trichomonas vaginalis (95)
		Trichomonas	Vaginitis	
	Sarcodina (pseudopodia)	Entamoeba	Dysentery	Intestinal Protozoa: Amebas (94)
		Dientamoeba	Colitis	
		Naegleria	Meningoencephalitis	Naegleria and Acanthamoeba (96)
		Acanthamoeba		
Apicomplexa (apical complex)	—	Babesia	Babesiosis	Malaria (98)
		Plasmodium	Malaria	
		Isospora	Diarrhea	Other Intestinal Protozoa and Trichomonas vaginalis (95)
		Cryptosporidium	Diarrhea	
		Toxoplasma	Toxoplasmosis	Toxoplasmosis (99)
Ciliophora (with cilia)	—	Balantidium	Dysentery	Other Intestinal Protozoa and Trichomonas vaginalis (95)
Unclassified	—	Pneumocystis	Pneumonia	Pneumocystis carinii (100)

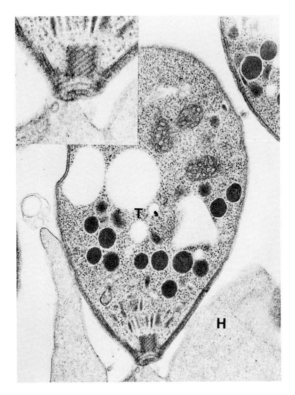

Figure 92-1 *Toxoplasma* organism (T) entering a host cell (H) (×27,000). Inset: higher magnification of apical complex with some of the associated organelles (×52,000). From Aikawa, M., et al.: *Am J Path* 1977; 87:285–290.

The parasitic protozoa are more difficult to culture in vitro than are bacteria. Usually culture is not a rewarding diagnostic procedure, and few parasites can be grown in defined media; however, many are cultured for research purposes. As an example, Trager and Jensen's (1976) development of a comparatively simple method of in vitro culture of erythrocytic stages of the malaria parasite *Plasmodium falciparum* was a significant advance in malaria research.

Life Stages and Reproduction

In the simplest life cycles of parasitic protozoa, there are only two major stages: **trophozoites** and **cysts** (see Figures in Chapters on intestinal protozoa). Trophozoites are active, multiplying, and invasive, whereas cysts are quiescent, are comparatively resistant to environmental factors outside the host, and are the usual transmission stage. Types of cysts important in medical protozoology include *fecal cysts* of intestinal protozoa, *tissue cysts* of *Toxoplasma,* and *oocysts* resulting from sexual reproduction in the Apicomplexa.

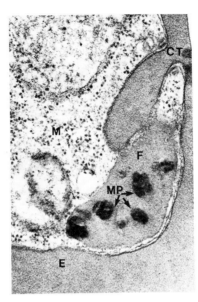

Figure 92-2 Malarial parasite (M) with cytostome (CT) in an erythrocyte (E), showing formation of food vacuole (F) containing malarial pigment (MP) (×70,000). From Aikawa, M., et al.: *J Cell Biol* 1966; 28:355–373.

Trophozoites usually multiply by binary fission (asexual reproduction). In the Apicomplexa, however, reproduction is more complex; parasites in this group may divide into multiple organisms by a process called schizogony (merogony). The Apicomplexa also reproduce sexually, forming gametes (gamogony), and after fertilization form oocysts containing sporozoites (sporogony).

Specialized trophozoites of *Toxoplasma* are sometimes given a name to indicate whether they are the rapidly multiplying forms, **tachyzoites,** present in the acute stages of an infection, or the slowly multiplying **bradyzoites** in tissue cysts.

The hemoflagellates also have special names for trophozoite forms that develop in the life cycle. The names refer to the flagellum (Greek: *mastig,* whip). Hence *amastigote* means without flagellum, *promastigote* means flagellum originating anterior to the nucleus, *epimastigote* means flagellum originating on the upper surface, and *trypomastigote* refers to a form with the flagellum originating posteriorly. In the latter two forms, the flagellum extends along an undulating membrane (see Figure 92-1).

References

Beaver, P.C., Jung, R.C., Cupp, E.W.: *Clinical parasitology,* 9th ed. Philadelphia: Lee and Febiger, 1984.

Current, W.L., et al.: Human cryptosporidiosis in immunocompetent and immunodeficient persons. *N Engl J Med* 1983; 308:1252–1257.

Healy, G.R., Spielman, A., Gleason, N.: Human babesiosis: Reservoir of infection on Nantucket Island. *Science* 1976; 192:479–480.

Levine, N.D., et al.: A newly revised classification of the Protozoa. *J Protozool* 1980; 27:37–59.

Trager, W., Jensen, J.B.: Human malaria parasites in continuous culture. *Science* 1976; 193:673–675.

93 Protozoa: Pathogenesis and Defenses

John Richard Seed, PhD

General Concepts

Immunity to parasitic protozoa appears to be similar to that observed with other infectious agents, although the mechanisms in protozoa are not yet as well understood. In recent years, there has been considerable interest in the genetic factors that influence the hosts' resistance to parasitic infections. In visceral leishmaniasis, a single gene appears to control susceptibility in mice, whereas, in African trypanosomiasis, resistance appears to be under polygenic control. The relationship between this gene or genes and the histocoompatibility loci seems to vary according to the particular parasitic protozoan. Similarly, depending on the parasite, different humoral and/or cellular immune responses have been observed. For example, in malaria and African trypanosomiasis, antibody appears to play a major role in immunity; in both *Trypanosoma cruzi* and *T brucei gambiense* infections, antibody-dependent cytotoxicity reactions against the parasite have been reported. In contrast, cellular immunity is believed to be a most important defense mechanism in leishmaniasis and toxoplasmosis. Also, in animals infected with *Toxoplasma*, the activated macrophage has been found to play an important role in resistance to this organism.

Differences between protozoans and other infectious agents appear to be due to the chronic nature of the diseases they produce—diseases often lasting from many months to years. This chronicity of protozoan infections in association with a strong host immune response appears to lead to a high incidence of immunopathology. It also raises the question of how these parasites survive in an immunocompetent animal. Therefore, the major topics to be covered in this chapter are mechanisms responsible for pathology, particularly immunopathology, and mechanisms by which parasites escape from the immune responses of the host.

Pathology

Immunopathology has been described for a variety of parasitic protozoan diseases. For the most part, this pathology has been associated with the humoral responses, in which antigen-antibody complexes in the region of antibody excess activate Hageman blood coagulation factor (factor XII), which in turn activates the coagulation, fibrinolytic, kinin, and complement systems. This type of mechanism has been suggested to be responsible for various clinical syndromes in African trypanosomiasis, including blood hyperviscosity, edema, and hypotension. Similar mechanisms of disease would also be expected in other protozoan diseases in which a strong humoral immune response occurs.

Immune complexes have been found circulating in serum, as well as deposited in the kidneys and other tissues of humans and other animals infected with protozoans. These parasite antigens and antibodies, plus complement, have been eluted from kidney tissue in malaria and African trypanosomiasis. In addition, antigen and antibody have been localized in the glomeruli of infected animals by light and electron microscopic techniques. In cases in which such deposits are detected, signs of glomerulonephritis are usually seen. Because the African trypanosomes are also found in extravascular sites, antigens may be released at these sites; immune complexes have been found in these tissues as well as in the vascular bed.

An additional form of antibody-mediated pathology is **autoimmunity.** Autoantibodies to a number of different host antigens (for example, red blood cells and DNA) have been demonstrated. These autoantibodies may play a role in the pathology of parasitic diseases in two basic ways. The first is by the direct cytotoxic action of the antibody on the host cells (autoantibodies coat red blood cells, thereby producing hemolytic anemia); the second is through a buildup of the antigen-autoantibody complexes within the kidneys or other tissues, which leads to glomerulonephritis or other forms of immediate hypersensitivity.

Cellular hypersensitivity also is observed in protozoan diseases. For example, in leishmaniasis (*Leishmania tropica*), the associated lesions appear to be cell-mediated and have many, if not all, of the characteristics of granulomas observed in tuberculosis or schistosomiasis. Continued immune response to parasites that are able to escape the host's defense mechanisms causes further influx of inflammatory cells. This leads to sustained reactions and continued pathology at the sites of antigen (parasite) deposition.

Numerous authors have suggested that, in addition to immunopathology, the parasitic protozoa produce various toxic products, responsible for at least part of the pathology observed. For example, the glycoproteins on the surface of the trypanosomes have been found to fix complement. This activation of complement presumably results in the production of biologically active and toxic fragments. In addition, the trypanosomes are known to release proteases and phospholipases on cell lysis. These enzymes can produce host cell destruction, inflammatory responses, and gross tissue pathology. Furthermore, it has been hypothesized that the trypanosomes contain a B cell mitogen, which may alter the immune response of the host by including a polyclonal B cell response that leads to immunosuppression. Parasitic protozoa also have been reported to synthesize (or contain) low–molecular-weight toxins. For example, the trypanosomes produce several indole catabolites; at pharmacologic doses, some of these catabolites can produce pathologic effects such as fever, lethargy, and even immunosuppression. Toxins that are similar to the potent toxins produced by bacterial cells, as in cases of anthrax and botulism, have not been observed.

Immune Escape

Parasite escape mechanisms include a number of different phenomena: antigenic **mimicry** (or masking), in which the parasites are coated with host components and fail to be recognized as foreign; **blocking,** whereby noncytotoxic antibody combines with parasite antigens and inhibits the binding of cytotoxic antibodies or cells; parasites that reside in **intracellular locations** (RBCs and macrophages), which may be sheltered during parts of their life cycle from intracellular digestion and from the cytotoxic action of antibody or leukocytes; **antigenic variation,** in which a parasite alters its surface coat and evades the host's immune responses; and **immunosuppression,** in which a parasite reduces the immune response of its host specifically to itself or to foreign antigens in general.

Mimicry (Masking)

Various species of trypanosomes have host immunoglobulins associated with their cell surfaces. These antibodies are bound to the trypanosomes not through their variable regions but presumably through the Fc portion of their molecule. These antibodies may prevent immune recognition of the parasite by the host; however, other than the presence of immunoglobulins on the surface of the trypanosomes, no evidence currently supports this hypothesis. Mimicry, in which the parasite has the genetic information to synthesize antigens identical to those of its host, has not been demonstrated in the parasitic protozoa.

Blocking (Serum Factors)

One hypothesis holds that the binding of antigen-antibody complexes in serum of infected animals to the parasite's surface mechanically blocks the actions of cytotoxic antibodies or lymphocytes, or directly inhibits the actions of lymphocytes. This type of immune escape mechanism has been proposed for tumor cells and the parasitic helminths. Because the trypanosomes contain immunoglobulins on their cell surfaces, a similar mechanism could be suggested for them; however, the only evidence to support this idea is the demonstration of these immunoglobulins on the surface of the cell.

Intracellular Location

Many protozoan parasites grow and divide within host cells. This intracellular position may protect them from the lethal (or harmful) effects of antibody or cellular defense mechanisms. For example, *Plasmodium* may be susceptible to the actions of antibody only during extracellular phases of its life cycle.

A number of parasitic protozoa also reside within macrophages. Although the organisms found within these cells are protected from external environmental factors, these organisms must have an additional mechanism or mechanisms to allow them to escape from the normal digestive functions of the macrophage. Three ways in which this can occur are suggested. One is by preventing the fusion of the lysosomes to the phagocytic vacuole. This has been shown to occur in cells infected with *Toxoplasma*. A second mechanism is the ability of *Trypanosoma cruzi* to escape from the phagocytic vacuole into the cytoplasm of the macrophage. Finally, some parasites conceivably are able to survive in the presence of lysosomal enzymes, as is the case with the leprosy bacillus.

Antigenic Variation

At present, at least two major groups of the parasitic protozoa appear to be capable of changing the antigenic properties of their surface coat. The African trypanosomes can completely replace the antigens within their glycocalyx each time their host responds with a new humoral response. The best evidence to date suggests that these changes in surface coat are phenotypic, possibly induced by an external environmental factor (antibody). These alterations in the serotype of the African trypanosomes are at least one important way in which these organisms escape from their host's defense mechanisms. Although not as well characterized, similar changes are reported to occur in *Plasmodium* and *Babesia*, and have been suggested for other protozoans that cause chronic infections.

Immunosuppression

Immunosuppression of the host has been observed in infections of almost every parasitic organism examined. In some cases, this suppression is specific and involves only the host's response to the parasite. In other host-parasite relationships, the suppression is much more general, involving the response to various heterologous and nonparasitic antigens. That this suppression allows the parasites to survive within a normally immunocompetent host has been hypothesized but not proved for any of the parasitic protozoans. Experimentally induced immunosuppression of the host by various extraneous agents has been shown to produce higher parasitemia levels, greater incidence in infection rates, or both. Therefore, the hypothesis that parasite-induced immunosuppression increases the chance for a parasite to complete its life cycle appears to be logical, although the mechanisms responsible for immunosuppression are only beginning to be understood.

References

Cohen, S.: Plasmodium—mechanisms of survival. In: *The host-invader interplay*. van den Bossche, H., (editor). Amsterdam: Elsevier/North-Holland Biomedical Press, 1980.

Damian, R.T.: Molecular mimicry in host-parasite adaptations. In: *Host-parasite interfaces*. Nickol, B.B., (editor). New York: Academic Press, Inc, 1979.

Goodwin, L.G.: Vasoactive amines and peptides: Their role in the pathogenesis of protozoal infections. In: *Pathophysiology of parasitic infection*. Soulsby, E.J.L., (editor). New York: Academic Press, Inc, 1976.

Jones, T.C., Masur, H.: Survival of *Toxoplasma gondii* and other microbes in cytoplasmic vacuoles. In: *The host-invader interplay*. van den Bossche, H., (editor). Amsterdam: Elsevier/North-Holland Biomedical Press, 1980.

Mansfield, J.M., (editor): *Parasitic Diseases: The Immunology*. New York: Marcel Dekker, 1981.

Sher, A., Scott, P.A.: Genetic factors in influencing the interaction of parasites with the immune system. *Clinics in Immunology and Allergy* 1982; 2:489–510.

Tizard, I., et al.: Biologically active products from African trypanosomes. *Microbiol Rev* 1978; 42:661–681.

Turner, M.J.: Antigen variation. In: *The molecular basis of microbial pathogenicity*. Smith, H., Skehel, J.J., Turner, M.J., (editors). Deerfield Beach, Fla.: Verlog Chemie (Life Science Research report No. 16), 1980.

Wallach, D.F.H., (editor): The membrane pathobiology of tropical disease. Tropical diseases research series no. 2. Basel: Schwabe & Co. A.G, 1979.

94 Intestinal Protozoa: Amebas

William A. Sodeman, Jr., MD

General Concepts
ENTAMOEBA HISTOLYTICA
Distinctive Properties
Pathogenesis
Host Defenses
Epidemiology
Diagnosis
Control

DIENTAMOEBA FRAGILIS
Distinctive Properties
Pathogenesis
Host Defenses
Epidemiology
Diagnosis
Control

General Concepts

Amebas are unicellular organisms common in the environment; many are parasitic in vertebrate and invertebrate life forms. Relatively few species inhabit the human intestine (Table 94-1) and only two, *Entamoeba histolytica* and *Dientamoeba fragilis*, are identified as human intestinal pathogens. Because *D fragilis* does not invade tissues, the mechanism by which it produces symptomatic diarrhea remains obscure. *E histolytica*, on the other hand, although often living as a harmless commensal in the digestive tract, harbors the capacity to penetrate intestinal mucosa and to invade tissues and cause ulceration. After tissue invasion occurs, progression of infection to other organs, such as the liver or the lung, by direct extension or metastatic spread is possible.

ENTAMOEBA HISTOLYTICA

Distinctive Properties

E histolytica has a relatively simple life cycle that consists of *trophozoite* (actively metabolizing and motile) and **cyst** (dormant, resistant) stages. Most diagnostic concern

Table 94-1 Intestinal Amebas of Humans

	Size (μm)		Trophozoite			Cyst		Remarks
	Trophozoite	Cyst	Motility (Fresh)	Nuclei (Stained)		Nuclei (Numbers)	Chromatoidals	
Entamoeba histolytica	10–60	10–20 Round	Active	Karyosome small, central; chromatin fine, peripheral		1–6	Ends round or square	Pathogen
Entamoeba hartmanni	4–12	5–10 Round	Active	Karyosome small, central; chromatin fine, peripheral		1–4	Ends round or square	Nonpathogen
Entamoeba gingivalis	5–35	—	—	Karyosome small, central; chromatin fine, peripheral		—	—	Mouth-dwelling nonpathogen
Entamoeba polecki	10–20	5–10 Round	Sluggish	Karyosome small, central; chromatin variable		1	Ends pointed	Rare in humans; nonpathogen
Entamoeba moshkovskii	10–60	5–20 Round	—	Karyosome small, central; chromatin fine, peripheral		1–4	Ends rounded	Nonpathogen
Entamoeba coli	10–50	10–35	Sluggish	Karyosome large, eccentric; chromatin clumps, peripheral		1–8	Ends jagged	Nonpathogen
Dientamoeba fragilis	3–20	—	Active	Karyosome central; chromatin granules central 4-8		—	—	Pathogen
Endolimax nana	6–15	4–14 Oval	Sluggish	Karyosome large, variable; chromatin little or none		1–4	None	Nonpathogen
Iodamoeba buetschlii	6–25	6–20	Active	Karyosome large, central; chromatin clumps, central		1	None	Nonpathogen

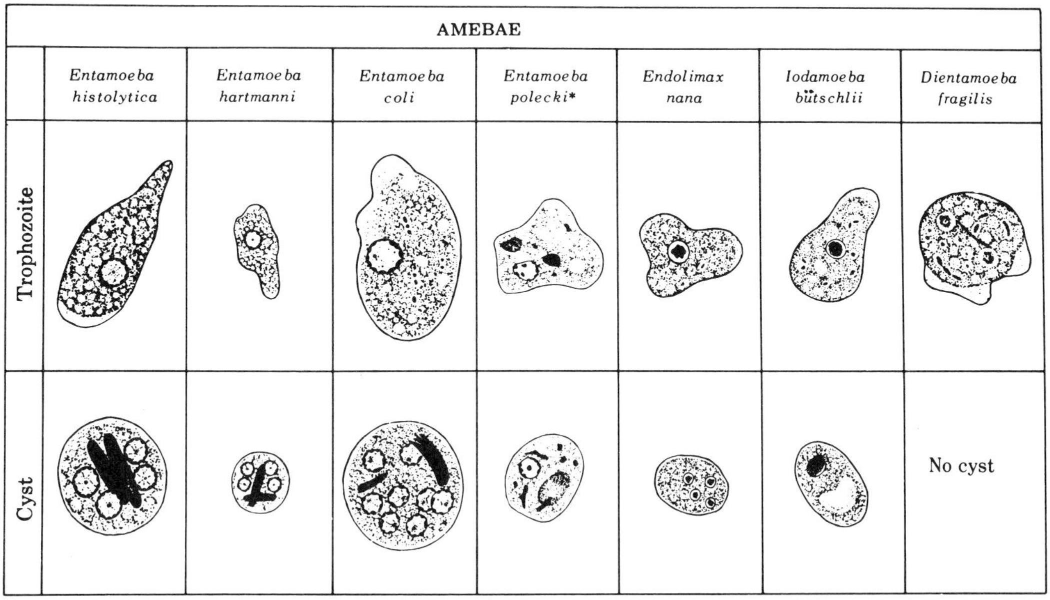

*Rare, probably of animal origin

Figure 94-1 Amebas found in stool specimens of humans. From Brooke, M.M., Melvin, D.M.: *Morphology of diagnostic stages of intestinal parasites of man.* Public Health Service Publication No. 1966, 1969.

centers on the trophozoite and the cyst (Figure 94-1). Trophozoites vary remarkably in size (10-60 μm or greater in diameter) and, when alive, are actively motile. Amebas are anaerobic organisms that do not have mitochondria. The endoplasm is finely granular and contains the nucleus and various food vacuoles, which hold bacteria and red cells. The trophozoite is sheathed by a clear outer ectoplasm. In permanent stained preparations, the characteristic nuclear morphology becomes evident, with a distinctive central karyosome and finely beaded chromatin lining the nuclear membrane. The cyst is a spherical structure, 10-20 μm in diameter, with a thin, transparent wall. When fully matured or ripe, the cyst contains four nuclei of the characteristic morphology. Rodlike structures (**chromatoidal bars**) are variably present, but are usually more common in the immature cyst. Inclusions in the form of glycogen masses also may be present. Replication of the nucleus occurs during the maturation of the cyst. Following excystment, the quadrinucleate form undergoes a further division process that produces eight small amebas, which initiate the infection.

Pathogenesis

When cysts of *E histolytica* are ingested, they excyst in the small intestine. Trophozoites are carried to the colon, where they mature and reproduce. The parasite may lead a commensal existence in the crypts of the colonic mucosa. Successful colonization depends on a number of factors, including inoculum size, intestinal motility, the presence of specific intestinal flora, and the host's diet. These amebas encyst as the colonic contents undergo desiccation, and they are evacuated with the stool.

E histolytica is the only intestinal ameba of humans that can invade tissue. The factors that lead to tissue invasion are not well understood, but they do seem largely dependent on some intrinsic characteristic of the parasite itself. Strains of *E histolytica* can be characterized as having low or high pathogenicity, usually by standardized testing in an animal model, or by concanavalin A agglutination, which does not affect avirulent strains. Debility and immunosuppression can promote tissue invasion.

The initial lesion is in colonic mucosa, most often in the cecum or in the sigmoid colon. Slowing of the intestinal stream in these two locations seems an important factor in the formation of lesions. Slowing of transit of intestinal contents affords greater mucosal contact time for the ameba, as well as permitting changes in the intestinal milieu. Initially, a superficial ulceration forms, which may deepen into the submucosa and muscularis to become the characteristic flask-shaped, chronic amebic ulcer. Spread may occur by direct extension, including fistulous communication to the skin with the occurrence of amebiasis cutis. If the amebas gain access to the lymphatic or vascular circulation, metastases may occur; the amebas spread first to the liver, and by a combination of direct extension and vascular metastasis can then spread to the lung, brain, and other visceral organs.

Virulent *E histolytica* are capable of penetrating intact intestinal mucosa. The infection is not opportunistic and does not require preexisting mucosal damage to initiate penetration. Numerous proteases have been observed in *E histolytica;* however, the mechanism of mucosal damage remains poorly understood. Occasionally, a lesion evolves into a proliferative granulomatous mass called an **ameboma.** Metastatic foci present as abscesses, with a central zone of lytic necrosis surrounded by a zone of leukocytic infiltration. Metastatic abscesses behave as space-occupying lesions, unless they become secondarily infected or rupture.

Clinical presentation of intestinal infections depends on the degree of ulceration and mucosal damage. When ulcerations are small and infrequent, symptoms may be absent. As the involved area of mucosa increases in size, motility disturbances, primarily diarrhea with cramping pain, occur. Exudation from the denuded mucosa adds to this problem. When the mucosal involvement becomes extensive, diarrhea is replaced by dysentery with the passage of exudate, blood, and mucus. Toxic megacolon and perforation are recognized complications of extensive involvement. Systemic signs of infection include fever, rigors, and polymorphonuclear leukocytosis.

Host Defenses

Usually, amebas alone stimulate little or no direct cellular response. Primary intestinal lesions elicit little reaction until secondary bacterial infection occurs. Amebic abscesses similarly elicit only a mild leukocytic response, which may be largely a response to host cellular debris contained in the abscess. Amebas are antigenic and elicit an antibody response and cellular sensitivity. In vivo studies have yielded contradictory results regarding the response of amebas to exposure to humoral antibodies. The occurrence of progressive infection and of reinfection in the face of established immune sensitivity suggests that host immune mechanisms are relatively ineffective as a defense mechanism against established infection.

Epidemiology

The life cycle of the ameba is simple and does not involve intermediate hosts or nonhuman reservoirs. Cyst forms remain viable for days under mild environmental conditions if not desiccated. Fecal contamination with transmission of viable cysts by food or water may result from failure of sanitary sewage disposal or improper personal hygiene. Experimental trials suggest that ingestion of cysts must occur in substantial numbers (2,000 or more cysts) to ensure infection, although smaller inocula can sometimes produce infection. Accordingly, world distribution of *E histolytica* infection is more closely related to control of environmental contamination by feces than to climate. *E histolytica* is found in the Arctic as well as in temperate and tropical zones. Laboratory observations suggest that the rapid passage of parasites from individual to individual may enhance the intrinsic pathogenicity of the parasite. This may explain partly the minor clinical significance of amebiasis in the United States, even though a 1%–2% prevalence of infection appears to exist.

Diagnosis

Classification of the clinical syndromes caused by *E histolytica* adopted by the World Health Organization, and their related pathophysiologic mechanisms, appear in Table 94-2.

Definitive diagnosis of amebiasis depends on demonstration of the ameba in stool or exudate (see Figure 94-1). Under some circumstances, the physician must settle for a

Table 94-2   Classification of Amebiasis

WHO Clinical Classification of Amebiasis Infection (Modified)	*Pathophysiologic Mechanisms*
I. Asymptomatic infection	Colonization without tissue invasion
II. Symptomatic infection	Invasive infection
Intestinal amebiasis	
A. Amebic dysentery	Fulminant ulcerative intestinal disease
B. Nondysentery colitis	Ulcerative intestinal disease
C. Ameboma	Proliferative intestinal granuloma
D. Complicated intestinal amebiasis	Perforation, hemorrhage, fistula
E. Post-amebic colitis	Mechanism unknown
III. Extraintestinal amebiasis	
A. Nonspecific hepatomegaly	No demonstrable invasion accompanies intestinal infection
B. Acute nonspecific infection	Amebas in liver but without abscess
C. Amebic abscess	Focal structural lesion
D. Amebic abscess complicated	Direct extension to pleura, lung, peritoneum, pericardium
E. Amebiasis cutis	Direct extension to skin
F. Visceral amebiasis	Metastatic infection of lung, spleen, or brain

presumptive diagnosis based on serologic or clinical evidence alone. The ease or difficulty of diagnosis depends on the numbers of organisms shed in the stool. Effective methods exist for concentration of cysts, but not of trophozoites, in stool specimens. Fortunately, a direct relationship usually is seen between the severity of disease and the numbers of amebas shed in the stool; hence, as the infection becomes more severe, the diagnosis is made more readily. Unfortunately, a number of interfering substances may be administered to a patient in the course of diagnosis or for therapy. These compounds can suppress the shedding of amebas into the stool without necessarily interfering with the course of the invasive infection. Such compounds include barium, bismuth, kaolin, soap suds enemas, and antimicrobials that can reach the intestinal lumen. This suppression may be short-lived, as in the case of soap suds enemas, or prolonged for weeks or months, as in the case of some broad-spectrum antibiotics. These compounds render direct diagnosis unreliable and often impossible.

Amebas may be identified on direct smear, but specific diagnosis usually depends on obtaining a fixed stained preparation. Trophozoites rapidly deteriorate in stool specimens, so the use of preservatives, either polyvinyl alcohol or the merthiolate-iodine-formaldehyde (MIF) combination, is an important diagnostic aid. Finally, to search for trophozoites in formed stool is unrewarding. Cysts may be present in formed stool, but without diarrhea, most trophozoites will have undergone alteration to cyst forms by the time of stool passage. More infections are detected by examining three specimens passed over a 7-10 day period than by examining a single specimen. Trophozoites may be obtained by use of a purge or collected by scraping suspicious lesions at the time of sigmoidoscopy.

Amebas are difficult to demonstrate in aspirates of extraintestinal abscesses unless special precautions are taken because, in most amebic abscesses, the contents are relatively free of the organisms. Instead, a concentration of organisms is found adjacent to the walls of the abscess cavity. If care is taken during aspiration to separate serial aliquots, amebas may be found in the last syringeful of aspirate that empties the abscess cavity. Cysts or trophozoites may be absent from approximately one-half the stools of the patients with liver abscess.

Serologic studies may be useful, particularly when direct diagnosis is not possible. A variety of serologic methods have been used, including gel diffusion, immunoelectrophoresis, countercurrent electrophoresis, indirect hemagglutination, indirect fluorescent antibody, skin test, Elisa, and latex agglutination. Many of these methods are best suited for immunoepidemiology, but gel diffusion, countercurrent electrophoresis, and latex agglutination are also useful as diagnostic studies, because they can be run on a single sample of serum. All of these tests indicate only prior experience with invasive amebiasis. In environments in which amebiasis has a low prevalence, such as the United States, a positive titer warrants serious consideration of active disease, particularly if the clinical findings are appropriate. In areas of high prevalence, a single elevated antibody titer is relatively less significant. The physician rarely has the opportunity to observe a patient long enough to note an increase in the antibody titer as evidence of active ongoing invasive infection.

Amebas may be cultured from stool; however, because the techniques involved are somewhat more cumbersome than those routinely applied to bacterial organisms, they are not used widely as diagnostic tools.

Control

Preventive measures are limited to control of environmental and personal hygiene. Treatment depends on drug therapy. Effective drugs are available for liver abscess, but intestinal infection is less well treated. No completely effective drug is available for eradication of amebas from the gut, so reliance is placed on combination drug therapy.

Treatment of acute amebic dysentery involves combining a broad-spectrum antibiotic such as tetracycline or paromomycin with an amebicidal drug such as metronidazole. The antibiotic has its primary effect on enteric flora, which are necessary symbionts for amebas; thus, a drug such as metronidazole is necessary to eliminate amebas from the gut. Metronidazole is a relatively poor intestinal amebicide, even in doses of 750 mg three times daily for 10 days. Other more effective amebicides, such as diloxanide furoate and diiodohydroxyquin, are not licensed in the United States. The mutagenic potential of metronidazole, plus the known side effects of antibiotics in the gut, make this a less-than-satisfactory treatment; however, it is the best available.

Amebic liver abscess is best treated by metronidazole, although numerous cases of drug failure have been reported. Chloroquine and dehydroemetine are second-line therapy, to be used when metronidazole fails. Aspiration of liver abscesses may be of diagnostic importance, but it is of little therapeutic significance unless rupture is imminent. Amebic abscesses heal at the same rate, whether evacuated or not. Secondary bacterial infection may require surgical intervention in addition to chemotherapy.

No effective, nontoxic therapy is now available in the United States for the treatment of asymptomatic cyst passers. Diloxanide furoate would be the best drug if available, and paromomycin is probably the next best choice. When the need for therapy of amebiasis arises, the physician should contact the Parasitic Disease Drug Service of the CDC to ensure that the most effective drug available in this country is employed.

DIENTAMOEBA FRAGILIS

D fragilis is an ameboid parasite of the large intestine that has a disputed taxonomic status and has elicited some controversy concerning its role in human disease. Some authorities now regard this parasite as a flagellate, related to the trichomonads, because of its fine structure and antigenic composition; however, under a light microscope, it resembles an ameba and lacks flagella and certain other structures characteristic of the trichomonads. Most careful investigators have found it to be a significant human pathogen that produces disturbing, although hardly lethal, gastroenteritis. Of all human intestinal parasites, it is probably the most easily and commonly overlooked organism.

Distinctive Properties

D fragilis lacks a cyst form. The trophozoite is small (3-20 μm in diameter), and is actively motile (see Figure 94-1). Ectoplasm and endoplasm are differentiated. In stained preparations, the nuclear morphology shows characteristic clumping of chromatin around the central karyosome with otherwise clear nucleoplasm. *D fragilis* reproduces by binary fission, and the many binuclear forms may represent an incomplete reproduction.

Pathogenesis

The portal of entry is the mouth. Once in the gut, the parasite is lumen-dwelling, living in the crypts of the colon. The parasite is not known to be invasive; thus, the usual target organs are the colon and the appendix, although it has been recovered from the biliary tract, where it was also lumen-dwelling. The mechanism of disease is largely speculative. *D fragilis* infection is not lethal, and observations of it have been confined to material obtained at the time of appendectomy. Fibrosis of the appendix has been described regularly without evidence of mucosal invasion. Irritability coupled with increased mucus production has been the suggested mechanism of disease.

The primary symptomatology reported is related to disturbances in intestinal motility, which cause diarrhea, sometimes alternating with constipation, abdominal pain, nausea, belching, and flatus. Some studies suggest that abdominal pain is more common than diarrhea. The passage of bloody mucus has been reported but is uncommon, as are systemic symptoms, headaches, fever, and weight loss.

Host Defenses

Host defense mechanisms are unknown. Spontaneous remission of symptoms does occur. Reinfection after therapy has been reported, suggesting that little protective immunity can be acquired. Antigen has not been available to evaluate the occurrence of any other host response.

Epidemiology

Because *D fragilis* lacks a cyst form, the mechanism of its transmission and its epidemiology have been matters of substantial interest. *D fragilis* is a hardy organism, but it cannot resist gastric juice or desiccation. Eggs of *Enterobius vermicularis* may act as vectors for this protozoan.

D fragilis is widely distributed in the environment and is found in temperate and tropic zones. The best information suggests that it has a prevalence of greater than 2% in the United States. No nonhuman or reservoir host is known.

Diagnosis

Diagnosis is made by identifying the parasite in stools or tissue section. *D fragilis* may be cultured by methods used for *E histolytica;* however, this has not been used as a diagnostic tool. The small size of *D fragilis* and its regular occurrence in binucleate form make it easily confused with small nonpathogenic amebas, such as *E hartmanni,* and with host cells, particularly polymorphonuclear cells and macrophages. For this reason, permanent stained preparations as employed for *E histolytica* are important. Serologic studies for *D fragilis* are not available.

D fragilis infection presents clinically as a gastroenteritis, sometimes with mild systemic symptoms. It is distinguished only by its chronicity and the occurrence in some patients of a mild eosinophilia.

Control

Treatment with drugs suitable for intestinal *E histolytica* infection has been effective. No reports of the effectiveness of newer drugs, such as metronidazole or diloxanide furoate, have been published. The mainstay of therapy remains broad-spectrum antibiotics, tetracycline, or paromomycin.

References

Beaver, E.C., Jung, R.C., Cupp, E.W.: *Clinical Parasitology*, 9th ed. Philadelphia: Lea and Febiger, 1984.

Kean, B.H., Malloch, C.L.: The neglected ameba: Dientamoeba fragilis. *Am J Digest Dis* 1966; 11:735-46.

Kean, B.H.: The treatment of amebiasis. *JAMA* 1976; 235:501.

Millet, V., et al.: *Dientamoeba fragilis*, a protozoan parasite in adult members of a semicommunal group. *Dig Dis Sci* 1983; 28:335-339.

Sepulveda, B.: Amebiasis: host-pathogen biology. *Rev Infect Dis* 1982; 4:836-842.

Sepulveda, B., Diamond, L.S.: *International conference on amebiasis*. Mexico City: Instituto Mexicano Del Seguro Social, 1976.

Wilcocks, C., Manson-Bahr, P.E.C.: *Manson's Tropical Diseases*. Baltimore: The Williams & Wilkins Co, 1972.

Wolfe, M.S.: Nondysenteric intestinal amebiasis. *JAMA* 1973; 224:1601-1604.

World Health Organization: *Amoebiasis Report of a WHO Expert Committee*. WHO Technical Report Series, 1969.

Yang, J., Scholten, T.: *Dientamoeba fragilis:* A review with notes on its epidemiology, pathogenicity, mode of transmission, and diagnosis. *Am J Trop Med Hyg* 1977; 26:16-22.

95 Other Intestinal Protozoa and *Trichomonas vaginalis*

Ernest A. Meyer, ScD

General Concepts

These human protozoan parasites belonging to six different genera, *Giardia, Trichomonas, Chilomastix, Balantidium, Isospora,* and *Cryptosporidium,* are discussed in this chapter. Species of *Giardia, Trichomonas,* and *Chilomastix* are flagellates; *Balantidium coli* is a ciliate, and *Isospora* and *Cryptosporidium* are coccidians. All are intestinal parasites that are transmitted by the fecal-oral route, except for *T vaginalis,* which is usually spread by sexual contact. The intestinal parasite most likely to be encounterd is *Giardia lamblia.* Three trichomonads are discussed, only one of which, the common genitourinary tract inhabitant, *Trichomonas vaginalis,* causes disease. Of the remaining four genera, *Chilomastix* (*C mesnili*), an intestinal flagellate that parasitizes humans, is generally considered nonpathogenic, and representatives of the genera *Balantidium* and *Isospora*, although not commonly encountered in humans, are considered capable of causing disease. Observations indicate that protozoa in the genus *Cryptosporidium* may cause mild or severe gastroenteritis. (See diseases listed on Table 92-1, p. 997).

GIARDIA LAMBLIA

Distinctive Properties

The *G lamblia* trophozoite is easily recognizable by microscope. This organism, which is shaped like a pear cut in half lengthwise and is about 12-15 μm long, has two nuclei that resemble eyes, structures called **median bodies** that resemble a mouth, and four pairs of flagella that look like hair; these combine to give the stained trophozoite the eerie appearance of a face (see Figure 95-1). Their flagella enable these organisms to migrate to a given area of the small intestine, where an adhesive disk enables them to attach to epithelial cells and maintain their position despite peristalsis, which minimizes the numbers of other small intestinal microorganisms.

The *Giardia* life cycle involves two protozoan forms: the trophozoite and the cyst. The trophozoite, or actively metabolizing, motile form, lives in the upper two-thirds (duodenum and jejunum) of the small intestine, and multiplies by binary fission. Trophozoites that are swept into the fecal stream lose their motility, round up, and are excreted as dormant, resistant cysts.

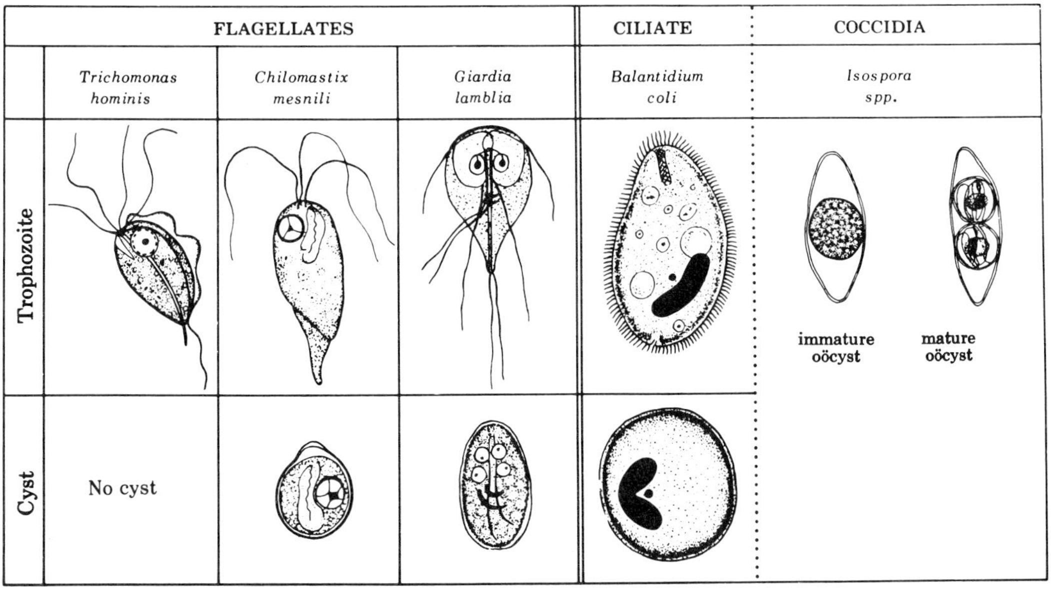

	FLAGELLATES			CILIATE	COCCIDIA
	Trichomonas hominis	*Chilomastix mesnili*	*Giardia lamblia*	*Balantidium coli*	*Isospora* spp.
Trophozoite					immature oöcyst mature oöcyst
Cyst	No cyst				

Figure 95-1 Protozoa found in human stool specimens. From Brooke, M.M., Melvin, D.M., *Morphology of diagnostic stages of intestinal parasites of man.* Public Health Service Publication No. 1966, 1969.

The trophozoite-to-cyst transformation takes place in the intestine; excreted trophozoites disintegrate. The cyst, although not as resistant as many bacterial endospores, is sufficiently hardy to survive host-to-host transfer under conditions in which the trophozoites cannot survive. For example, some *Giardia* cysts are capable of excystation after more than 2 months' storage in water at refrigerator temperatures.

Giardia infection is acquired by ingesting cysts. The exposure of cysts to host stomach acidity and body temperature triggers excystation, which is completed in the small intestine with emergence from the cysts of trophozoites that promptly attach to host intestinal epithelium.

Pathogenesis

Giardia infection may result in asymptomatic infection, diarrheal disease that is self-limiting, or a severe chronic disease syndrome. The length of the incubation period, usually 1-3 weeks, depends at least partly on the number of cysts ingested.

Most *Giardia* infections are asymptomatic. For this reason, and because these organisms are so widespread, it was earlier believed that *Giardia* was a commensal that was never pathogenic; enough evidence has now accumulated to show that *G lamblia* can cause disease. One type of evidence supporting *Giardia* pathogenicity is that in some cases of diarrheal disease, *Giardia* is the only known pathogen present; treatment with any of a number of antiprotozoal agents promptly results in the disappearance of disease and organisms. Reacquisition of infection is accompanied by return of symptoms.

The normal human hosts with giardiasis may have any or all of the following signs and symptoms: diarrhea or loose, foul-smelling stools, steatorrhea (a fatty diarrhea), malaise, abdominal cramps, or excessive flatulence; fatigue and weight loss also may occur.

The mechanisms that cause these signs and symptoms are not known. Ordinarily, the trophozoites remain in the intestinal lumen. That their mere presence, even in enormous numbers, in the intestine is sufficient to interfere mechanically with digestion seems unlikely. Rather, it seems more likely that symptoms result from an inflammation of the mucosal cells of the small intestinal wall known to be caused at times by these organisms; this results in an increased turnover rate of intestinal mucosal epithelium. The immature replacement cells offer reduced functional surface area and reduced digestive and absorptive ability. Additional mechanisms of pathogenesis may well exist.

Some patients with giardiasis have severe disease that is not self-limited; their signs and symptoms may include interference with the absorption of fat and fat-soluble vitamins, retarded growth, weight loss, or a celiaclike syndrome. Although most cases are seen in hosts with some concomitant condition, such as an immune deficit, protein-calorie malnutrition, or bacterial overgrowth of the small intestine, some cases of severe giardiasis occur in apparently normal hosts. Possibly some variation in virulence exists among different strains of *G lamblia*.

Host Defenses

The fact that many symptomatic *Giardia* infections in humans and experimental animals undergo spontaneous resolution is evidence for the presence of a host immune response to these organisms. The nature of this response is currently being studied. Evidence exists that humoral and cellular immune mechanisms operate in host resistance to *Giardia* infection. The fact that severe disease is likely to occur in hosts with γ-globulin deficiencies suggests that humoral immunity plays a role. Although the observed prevention of infection in suckling mice by milk from immune mothers seems to indicate a role for IgA, the precise nature of this protection requires clarification. Furthermore, experiments with nude (congenitally athymic) mice suggest that the thymus-dependent immune system also plays a role in control of these infections. In these mice, wasting and premature death may result when *Giardia* infection is present. Nude mice "reconstituted" with thymus transplants are able to reduce the numbers of infecting *Giardia*.

In vitro studies have found normal human milk (but not cow's milk or goat's milk) kills trophozoites of both *G lamblia* and *E histolytica* (see Chapter 94), and that this killing does not depend on secretory immunoglobulin A. This raises the possibility that even mother's milk that does not have antiprotozoal antibody may protect infants exposed to these parasites.

Epidemiology

Giardia infection occurs worldwide; its incidence usually is 1.5%–20%. Higher incidences are likely where sanitary standards are low. Although people of all ages may harbor these organisms, infants and children are more often infected than are adults. Carriers are probably more important in the spread of these organisms than symptomatic patients, because cysts are less likely to be present in diarrheic specimens. This disease, as well as others spread by the fecal-oral route, has been a problem in institutions, nurseries, and day-care facilities.

Recent outbreaks, some of epidemic proportions, have occurred, particularly in North America and the Soviet Union. Epidemiologic studies confirm that they are related to the drinking of water from community water supplies or directly from rivers or streams.

Many animal species harbor *Giardia* that are indistinguishable from *G lamblia*. In the past, these were assumed to be host-specific. Recent evidence suggests this is not always the case; at least some of the *Giardia* that parasitize lower animals may also infect humans and vice versa. Although this complicates the problem of defining species in this genus, what is more important is that it raises the possibility that animal reservoirs of *Giardia* may exist from which humans may be infected. The finding of *Giardia*-infected animals in watersheds from which humans acquired giardiasis, and the successful interspecies transfer of these organisms, strengthen the possibility that giardiasis is a zoonotic infection. Infected beaver are believed to be one source of waterborne giardiasis. The report that, experimentally, beaver *Giardia* were capable of infecting dogs and humans raises the possibility that canines may be another source of human giardiasis.

The fact that *Giardia* infection may be transmitted by sexual activity, particularly among homosexual men, has been recognized only recently. These organisms also may be transmitted by sexual activity among heterosexuals. Physicians should attempt to determine if giardiasis is being acquired in this way so that they can distinguish between failure of drug treatment and prompt reinfection. Perhaps more important, the likelihood of a *Giardia* infection acquired in this way should alert the physician to the possibility that the patient may have acquired other, more serious fecal-oral infections, including amebiasis, syphilis, gonorrhea, or hepatitis, in the same manner.

Diagnosis

The symptoms of giardiasis are not pathognomonic. Although a patient's history may indicate possible recent exposure to *Giardia* and thus increase the index of suspicion, definitive diagnosis (as in most parasitic infections) is made by identifying some form of the causative organism from the host. In giardiasis, the stool is the preferred specimen. Formed stools contain only the oval cysts, about 12 μm in length; longitudinal fibrils and the nuclei located at one end aid cyst identification (see Figure 95-1). Diarrheal specimens may contain cysts and trophozoites that, if still motile, have a typical "falling leaf" movement.

Because cysts are often shed intermittently, three stool specimens should be obtained at approximately 48-hour intervals; examination of these specimens permits detection of the organism in most cases. The chances of finding cysts in a light infection increase if the stool specimen is examined after being subjected to a concentration method, such as the zinc sulfate centrifugal flotation technique. When stools are negative and giardiasis is still suspected, diagnosis sometimes can be made by demonstrating trophozoites obtained directly from the small intestine. This can be done by duodenal intubation, capsule, or by the use of a long nylon thread, one end of which is swallowed. The trophozoites attach to the thread, which is then retrieved (the Enterotest capsule).

The finding of *Giardia* does not necessarily mean these organisms are responsible for the patient's symptoms. The infecting organisms should be treated and eliminated when found, but other pathogens should be sought as well.

Control

Attention to personal hygiene is the key to preventing the spread of this infection. Controlling the spread of *Giardia* in drinking water should be possible where community water treatment methods are available; it is known, for example, that the halogens iodine and chlorine will kill *Giardia* cysts under appropriate conditions. Destruction of *Giardia* cysts becomes more difficult, however, when the water is near freezing or contains considerable organic matter or both, because under such conditions so much halogen must be added to be effective that the water is not palatable. Heating water to boiling, when possible, probably is the best solution, because this treatment inactivates *Giardia* cysts promptly.

The drug of choice for treating *Giardia* infections is quinacrine hydrochloride. This drug frequently causes dizziness, headache, and vomiting. Metronidazole or furazolidone also may be used. Although metronidazole is highly effective, its use in treating *Giardia* infections has not been officially approved in the United States. One drawback is that it frequently causes headache and nausea; another is that it is believed to be carcinogenic in rodents and mutagenic in bacteria. Its use in pregnant women is generally contraindicated, particularly in the first trimester. Furazolidone is not quite as effective against *Giardia* as are the other two drugs, but its availability in liquid form makes it useful for treating young children. None of these drugs can cure all *Giardia* infections, and none is particularly well tolerated; an anti-*Giardia* agent without these drawbacks would be welcomed.

TRICHOMONAS VAGINALIS

Distinctive Properties

Trichomonads have the simplest kind of protozoan life cycle, in which the organism occurs only as a trophozoite. In the absence of a cyst form, transmission of these flagellated organisms from host-to-host must be relatively direct.

All the trichomonads are morphologically similar, having a pear-shaped body, a single anterior nucleus, three to five forward-directed flagella, and a single posteriorly directed flagellum, which forms the border of an undulating membrane. A hyaline rod-like structure, the **axostyle,** runs through the length of the body and exits at the posterior end (see Figure 95-1).

Of the three trichomonads considered common human parasites, only one, *T vaginalis*, causes disease. *T vaginalis* inhabits the vagina in women, the prostate and seminal vesicles in men, and the urethra in both sexes.

Pathogenesis

Although the incidence of *T vaginalis* infections varies widely, trichomoniasis is generally considered one of the commonest, if not the most common, of the sexually transmitted diseases. In some areas of the United States, incidence among women has been reported to be as high as 50%. More women than men are infected with *T vaginalis*. Most of these infections, in both sexes, are asymptomatic or accompanied by symptoms so minor that medical aid is not sought. Symptomatic infection occurs commonly in women, rarely in men.

Trichomoniasis in women is frequently chronic and is characterized by vaginitis, a vaginal discharge, and dysuria. The inflammation of the vagina is usually diffuse and is characterized by hyperemia of the vaginal wall (with or without small hemorrhagic lesions) and migration of polymorphonuclear leukocytes into the vaginal lumen. Although the mechanism that triggers this inflammatory response is not known, it may be caused by the mechanical irritation resulting from contact between the parasite and vaginal epithelium. However, inflammation can occur in areas where parasites are not found, suggesting that the explanation may be more complicated.

Host Defenses

Relatively little is known about the human immune response to *T vaginalis* infection. Studies employing experimental animals suggest that antibody may play a role in protecting against *T vaginalis* infection. Whatever protective antibodies are elicited by infection with these organisms are short-lived, however, and disappear completely in 6-16 months.

Epidemiology

Trichomoniasis is a common, worldwide infection. Although sexual intercourse is believed to be the usual transfer mechanism, some infections probably are acquired through fomites such as towels, toilet seats, and sauna benches; the organisms may spread in mud and water baths as well. Survival studies of *T vaginalis* in vaginal discharges have shown that these trophozoites can be cultured from toilet seats for 30 minutes or more.

It has been suggested that this organism is frequently transmitted from a woman, serving as a reservoir of infection, to a man, the carrier, and subsequently to another woman. Although the nonvenereal spread of *T vaginalis* has been the subject of conjecture, little hard evidence exists to indicate the relative importance of this means of transmission.

Diagnosis

A wet mount preparation of discharge from the patient should be examined microscopically as a first step in diagnosing *T vaginalis* infection. The presence of pear-shaped trophozoites, usually 10-30 μm in length, with "bobbling" motility and, on careful examination, the wavelike movements of the undulating membrane, are usually sufficient to characterize *T vaginalis*. Material that is negative by wet mount examination should be cultured because culture is a considerably more sensitive, although more time-consuming, method of diagnosis.

Control

Because of the frequent involvement of the asymptomatic male sex partner in spreading trichomoniasis, control of this infection necessitates examination of the man, and, if he is infected, treatment of him. Avoidance of sexual intercourse and the use of condoms are effective methods of preventing transmission of these trichomonads.

A number of 5-nitroimidazole compounds have been found to be effective antitrichomonal agents. The chemical in this group that is approved for treating these infections in the United States is metronidazole. (The potential drawbacks of this drug were discussed in the section on control of *Giardia*.) Treatment of both sexual partners at the same time is recommended to prevent the "ping-pong" spread of this infection.

OTHER TRICHOMONADS

Another member of the *Trichomonas* genus, *T tenax,* inhabits the human oral cavity; this organism occurs particularly in tartar, cavities, and at the gingival margins. It is a cosmopolitan parasite whose incidence is inversely proportional to the level of oral hygiene. Because it cannot survive intestinal passage, *T tenax* transfer must be by oral droplets, kissing, or fomites such as eating utensils. Although considered nonpathogenic, it has been reported rarely in lung or thoracic abscesses.

The third human trichomonad parasite inhabits the intestinal tract in the area of the cecum. This parasite may be referred to alternately as *T hominis* or, because most of these organisms in culture have five (rather than four) anterior flagella, as *Pentatricho-monas hominis*. There is no evidence that the parasite is pathogenic.

Each of these three trichomonads is a distinct species that is site-specific and demonstrably different from the other two organisms.

CHILOMASTIX MESNILI

C mesnili is a nonpathogenic intestinal commensal of humans. It exists as a pear-shaped trophozoite, usually 10-15 μm long, with a large anterior cytostome, three forward-directed flagella, and a sharply pointed posterior end, or as a lemon-shaped, uninucleate cyst, 7-9 μm long (see Figure 95-1).

BALANTIDIUM COLI

Balantidium coli, the only ciliate and by far the largest organism in this group, is an acknowledged pathogen. *B coli* trophozoites, which are ovoid, 40-70 μm or longer, and covered with cilia (see Figure 95-1), live in the large intestine of humans, swine, and perhaps other animals. Trophozoites can divide by transverse binary fission. They do, however, have a large, kidney-shaped macronucleus and a smaller ovoid micronucleus; conjugation has been described. *B coli* also exists in a resistant nonmotile, transfer form, the cyst usually being 50-55 μm in diameter. Although the usual diet of *B coli* is believed to consist of host intestinal contents (hence some infections are asymptomatic), at times these organisms attack the host large intestine (aided apparently by a boring action and the enzyme hyaluronidase) and cause ulcers. In contrast to *E histolytica, B coli* does not invade extraintestinal tissues. Balantidiasis often is accompanied by diarrhea or dysentery, abdominal pain, nausea, and vomiting. Diagnosis is made by demonstrating the cysts or trophozoites in stools or host tissue.

Balantidium infection is acquired by ingesting cysts in fecal material from another parasitized host; waterborne epidemics have been reported. The precise relationship between the *Balantidium* organisms, which have been rarely reported from humans, and those commonly parasitic in pigs, has been the subject of considerable unresolved debate and is worthy of clarification. Tetracyclines, the drugs recommended for treating *Balantidium* infections, are considered to be investigational drugs for this purpose in the United States.

ISOSPORA

Organisms in the genus *Isospora* are considered to be uncommon intestinal parasites of humans. *Isospora*, like *Cryptosporidium* and *Toxoplasma*, are coccidian parasites: protozoa whose complex life cycle includes both sexual and asexual stages occurring in association with host intestinal cells. The *Isospora* life cycle in the human host has been described from intestinal biopsy material obtained from chronically infected patients.

The diagnostic forms of the human *Isospora* are oocysts, inside of which are sporocysts (see Figure 95-1); they are transparent and not easily recognized in stool specimens. The immature oocyst has a single nucleus that divides once and secretes a cyst wall to become a sporocyst. Further division results in the formation of four elongate sporozoites in each sporocyst. The mature oocyst, usually 28–30 μm in length, thus contains two sporocysts, each with four sporozoites.

Most *Isospora* infections are believed to be asymptomatic. In experimental infections, these organisms may cause a diarrhea, usually mild and self-limited, with abdominal pain. Diagnosis is made by demonstrating oocysts in the feces. Although no animal reservoir host for these organisms has been identified, the rarity with which human infection is encountered and its wide distribution raise the possibility that humans are incidental hosts for these parasites. The treatment of choice is furazolidone; alternatively, trimethoprim-sulfamethoxazole is recommended.

CRYPTOSPORIDIUM

Distinctive Properties

The usual habitat of *Cryptosporidium* is the vertebrate host intestine, in which the protozoa grow attached to the epithelial cell membrane in the brush border. Both sexual and asexual forms are found in this area (Figure 95-2). Whether this organism should be regarded as an intracellular or an extracellular parasite is not resolved.

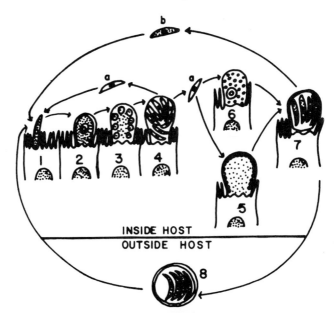

Figure 95-2 Diagrammatic representation of the life cycle of *Cryptosporidium*. (1 to 4) Asexual cycle of the endogenous stage: 1, sporozoite or merozoite invading a microvillus of a small intestinal epithelial cell; 2, a fully grown trophozoite; 3, a developing schizont with eight nuclei; 4, a mature schizont with eight merozoites. (5 and 6) Sexual cycle: 5, microgametocyte with many nuclei; 6, macrogametocyte. (7) A mature oocyst containing four sporozoites without sporocyst. (8) Oocyst discharged in the feces. a, Merozoite released from mature schizont; b, sporozoite released from mature oocyst. From Tzipori, S.: *Microbiol Rev* 1983; 47:84–96.

Members of this genus have been found in a variety of mammals, birds, and reptiles since their discovery in 1907, but they were not reported to be associated with human disease until 1976. Until recently, they received little attention because few diagnosticians were aware of their existence, they were not considered to be pathogenic, and they are not likely to be encountered in routine stool examinations.

Pathogenesis

It is now clear that *Cryptosporidium* may be pathogenic for humans; evidence from clinical studies indicates it can produce illness in some cases. *Cryptosporidium* oocysts, the form excreted in feces and used in diagnosing infection, were found in some patients with gastroenteritis, but were not found in patients without intestinal symptoms. The infection occurs most often in children and is characterized by an incubation period averaging 4-12 days, and a moderate-to-profuse diarrhea lasting 4-30 (average 10) days. Although the disease is self-limiting in normal persons, the diarrhea can become chronic and can cause death of a patient who is immunologically compromised.

Little is known about the mechanism by which these organisms cause disease. They are believed to be noninvasive. Examination of biopsy material from symptomatic patients has revealed a variety of changes in intestinal mucosa, including partial villous atrophy, crypt lengthening, low cuboidal surface epithelium, cellular infiltration of the jejunal and ileal lamina propria, and inflammation. The cause of one such fatal case was probably malabsorption that resulted from intestinal damage from the prolonged protozoal infection.

Although investigators can identify the host cells damaged in cryptosporidiosis, the means by which the organism creates such damage is not known; mechanical damage and damage produced by toxins, enzymes, or immune-mediated mechanisms, working alone or together, may be instrumental.

Host Defenses

Immune mechanisms of the host may be involved in eliminating cryptosporidial infection, given that the disease is self-limiting in normal persons and usually is severe and long-lasting in immunologically compromised humans (such as AIDs patients) and lower animals. Neonatal infections of calves and lambs can produce a severe, fatal, diarrhea. Serum antibodies to *Cryptosporidium* have been shown to develop during recovery from infection.

Epidemiology

Many questions about the epidemiology of cryptosporidiosis remain to be be answered. It is known that these organisms are not highly host specific; thus, human infections may be acquired from other humans or from animals. Infection probably is by ingestion of oocysts, although the identification of this infection in the upper respiratory tract of at least three animal species, including humans, raises the possibility that the respiratory route also may be involved.

Diagnosis

Traditionally, diagnoses of these infections have been established by microscopic observations of the developmental stages of the organism in an intestinal biopsy specimen. Because *Cryptosporidium* oocysts have been found to be shed in feces during infection, many researchers have compared techniques for recovery and demonstration of these forms in stool specimens. Several studies have found that formalin concentration techniques and a modified Ziehl–Neelsen acid-fast stain are effective (Figure 95-3). The development of diagnostic methods that employ antibody against these organisms would be a valuable contribution.

Control

Because so much remains to be learned about the epidemiology of cryptosporidiosis, the only recommendations for prevention of this infection are those usually made for avoiding any pathogens transmitted by the fecal-oral route.

Most persons with normal immunity recover spontaneously from cryptosporidiosis and thus do not require therapy directed at the parasite, although they may require supportive treatment. Because this infection may be life-threatening in immunologically compromised individuals, however, many antimicrobial agents have been tested for anticryptosporidial effects; no safe, effective therapeutic agent has been discovered yet.

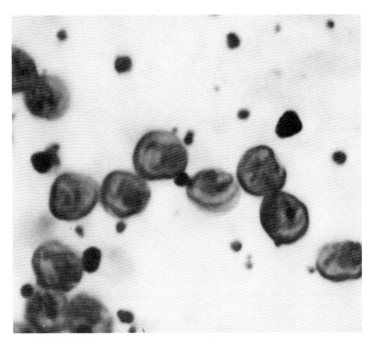

Figure 95-3 *Cryptosporidium* oocysts recovered from stool material and stained by the modified acid-fast technique (×2,700). From Garcia, L.S., et al.: *J Clin Microbiol* 1983; 18:185–190.

References

Beaver, E.C., Jung, R.C., Cupp, E.W.: *Clinical parasitology,* 9th ed. Philadelphia: Lea and Febiger, 1984.

Dubey, J.P.: *Toxoplasma, Hammondia, Besnoitia, Sarcocystis,* and other tissue cyst-forming coccidia of man and animals. In: *Parasitic protozoa,* Vol. III. Kreier, J.P., (editor). New York: Academic Press, 1978.

Erlandsen, S.L., Meyer, E.A. (editors): Giardia *and giardiasis. Biology, pathogenesis, and epidemiology.* New York: Plenum Press, 1984.

Gillin, F.D., Reiner, D.S., Wang, C.S.: Human milk kills parasitic intestinal protozoa. *Science* 1983; 221:1290-1291.

Honigberg, B.M.: Trichomonads of importance in human medicine. In: *Parasitic protozoa,* Vol II. Kreier, J.P., (editor). New York: Academic Press, 1978.

Jakubowski, W., Hoff, J.C., (editors): Waterborne transmission of giardiasis. *Proceedings of a Symposium.* Washington, D.C.: U.S. Environmental Protection Agency EPA-600/9-79-001, 1978.

Jarroll, E.L., Bingham, A.K., Meyer, A.E.: Effect of chlorine on *Giardia lamblia* cyst viability. *Appl Env Microbiol* 1978; 41: 483-487.

Kulda, J., Nohynkova, E. Flagellates of the human intestine and of intestines of other species. In: *Parasitic protozoa,* Vol. II. Kreier, J.P., (editor). New York: Academic Press, 1978.

Meyer, E.A., Radulescu, S.: *Giardia* and giardiasis. In: *Advances in Parasitology.* Lumsden W.H.R., (editor). London: Academic Press, 1979.

Tzipori, S.: Cryptosporidiosis in animals and humans. *Microbiol Rev* 1983; 47: 84-96.

Underdown, B.J., et al.: Giardiasis in mice: studies on the characteristics of chronic infection in C3H/He mice. *J Immunol* 1981; 126:669-672.

Zaman, V.: *Balantidium coli.* In: *Parasitic protozoa,* Vol. II. Kreier, J.P., (editor). New York: Academic Press, 1978.

96 *Naegleria* and *Acanthamoeba*

Clyde G. Culbertson, MD

General Concepts

Experiments and clinical observation have proved that isolates of several species of small, free-living amebas of *Naegleria* and *Acanthamoeba* are pathogenic for humans and for some domestic and wild animals. The natural infection is accidental, usually following introduction of amebic trophozoites (or possibly their cysts) into the nasal passage. Approximately 130 cases of fatal human amebic meningoencephalitis, and many fewer domestic and wild animal infections, have been reported. Most common is acute *Naegleria* meningoencephalitis, which usually occurs in healthy children who swim in water containing the amebas. One well-documented case occurred in Africa, where a patient was believed to have been infected with *Naegleria* by dust inhalation. *Acanthamoeba* has been found to cause a small number of more chronic infections in persons (usually adults) who lack normal defense mechanisms due to disease or immunosuppressive drugs.

Acanthamoeba often has been found unexpectedly in tissue cultures. In some cases, the amebas were airborne contaminants; the dry cysts are carried in dust. More often, the amebas were introduced into tissue cultures because they happened to be present in nasopharyngeal secretions that were inoculated into culture for virus isolation. Some species of *Acanthamoeba* produce changes that may be mistaken for virus damage to the cells; the degree of tissue damage produced frequently corresponds to the degree of animal pathogenicity. The more extensive studies support the view that the amebas exist in cystic form in the nasal secretions and excyst in the tissue cultures.

Distinctive Properties

The appearance of the amebas in stained tissue sections is deceivingly similar; *Naegleria* is smaller than *Acanthamoeba*. In the living state, however, marked differences appear between the two organisms (Figure 96-1).

Naegleria is a biphasic ameboflagellate. Actively mobile, the ameboid form consists of multiple "eruptive" lobate ectoplasmic pseudopods, often extending the ameba into elongated, sluglike structures. When rounded up and immobilized by toxic diluting fluid in a counting chamber, amebas in the spinal fluid can be mistaken for leukocytes; in the untreated fluid sediment preparations, their long-lasting motility calls them to attention. The flagellate form, unimportant in the pathologic process, is temporary; it can be produced by adding distilled water to the living amebas and incubating at 37 C

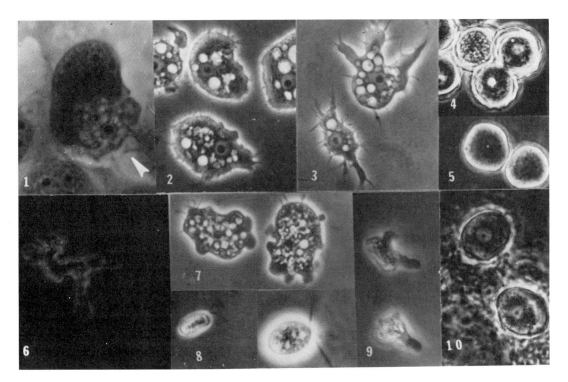

Figure 96-1 Some morphologic features of *Acanthamoeba* and *Naegleria fowleri*. **1,** Tissue culture. *Acanthamoeba* attacking cell nucleus (arrow). (H & E stain × 1000.) **2** and **3,** *A culbertsoni* from culture showing variation in form. (Phase × 1200.) **4,** Wrinkled cysts of *A polyphaga*. **5,** Smooth-walled cysts of *A culbertsoni*. **6,** Active larvalike form of *N fowleri* as sometimes appears in cerebrospinal fluid. (Phase × 1000.) **7,** *N fowleri* from agar surface culture. (Phase × 1200.) **8,** Two flagellate forms of *N fowleri*. (Phase × 1000). **9,** Two active *N fowleri* from liquid culture. (Phase × 1000.) **10,** Two cysts of *N fowleri* from culture on agar with *Escherichia coli*. (Phase × 1600.)

for several hours. Flagellates are small, actively motile, pear-shaped bodies having two or more flagellas.

Acanthamoeba usually are larger than *Naegleria* and move more sluggishly by extending broad ectoplasmic pseudopodia from which spinelike "acanthapodia" protrude.

Naegleria infections occur in healthy persons. *Acanthamoeba* has caused fatalities in patients with lowered resistance. Direct microscopic examination of cerebrospinal fluid, confirmed by culture, is used to identify either type of infection. In addition, *Acanthamoeba* infections have sometimes been diagnosed by autopsy, by brain biopsy or immunodiagnosis. Most of the known cases have been diagnosed at autopsy.

Pathogenesis

Naegleria meningoencephalitis in humans begins with infection of the nasal mucosa and extends to the brain. The nasal phase following experimental intranasal inoculation in mice lasts only 24-48 hours; how long this phase exists in humans is not known. Also not known is whether *Naegleria* ever produces a nasal infection that does not progress to fatal brain involvement. In experimental disease, the meningeal phase is reached rapidly, and amebas quickly invade the perivascular spaces and the brain substance. At death, the gray matter of the brain and spinal cord is devastated by amebic proliferation. The natural infection follows a similar course.

Acanthamoeba meningoencephalitis also is an acute disease in the experimental animal when highly virulent strains are used, but known human and animal fatalities appear to have been caused by less virulent types, because the observed lesions are subacute or chronic abscesses, granulomas, or both. A marked tendency to thrombosis and hemorrhage always is seen in these cases, which clinically resemble mycotic or chronic viral disease.

The discovery of *Acanthamoeba* in and around corneal ulcers and in the conjunctival fluid suggests that these amebas may cause the ulcers. At present, whether the amebas play a primary or secondary role in this process is uncertain; however, the presence of the amebas is considered at least to interfere with the healing process.

Animal diseases due to *Acanthamoeba* have included pulmonary, heart, nasal, and brain lesions; however, no systematic survey has been made of the general incidence of such diseases.

Host Defenses

Naegleria

As previously stated, almost all of the *Naegleria* infections have been found in healthy young persons. Attempts to immunize mice against *N fowleri* have been reported, with only marginal results. Some experiments using active or passive immunization showed no significant protection; thus, natural or induced immunity seems unlikely.

Acanthamoeba

In contrast to the *Naegleria* infection, reported *Acanthamoeba* fatalities occurred in patients with other medical problems characterized by general lowering of resistance. In healthy mice, intraperitoneal injections of formalin-killed *A culbertsoni* produced solid immunity to intranasal infection. In vitro studies of phagocytosis have shown that *A culbertsoni* is susceptible to neutrophilic attack, but *Naegleria* appear to be quite resistant under the same conditions.

Epidemiology

Naegleria infections have been reported in almost all parts of the world that have warm climates. The *Naegleria* infection has almost always attacked children, who usually have normal resistance to disease. Why a few contract fatal meningoencephalitis, whereas most do not, is unknown and may depend on the degree of nasal aspiration during swimming or diving.

The amebas in their cystic form are not killed by the low temperatures that prevail in water under the ice covering frozen streams and lakes; they certainly grow abundantly when the water becomes warm, if enough bacteria are present. An important discovery was made in a Czechoslovakian swmming pool outbreak; leaks in the pool wall allowed water to collect outside the pool, permitting the amebas to grow and feed back into the pool.

Acanthameoba infection is not known to be related to any geographic factors. Because only a few cases have been found, little information is available.

A relationship between Legionnaires' disease and the free-living amebas, *Acanthamoeba* and *Naegleria,* has been suggested. Rowbotham (1980) reported that certain *Legionella* organisms can infect the amebas present in air conditioning and cooling equipment and that the infected amebas could serve as the infective airborne particle for humans.

Diagnosis

Direct Microscopic Examination and Cultures

Accurate diagnosis can be made only when the ameba can be observed directly and cultured. This has been accomplished many times in *Naegleria* infection but not in *Acanthamoeba* cases. Awareness of the existence of the disease is important for timely collection of fresh tissue and fluid for study. Specimens should be processed promptly and must not be frozen.

Simple microscopic observation may be sufficient for cerebrospinal fluid sediments that require only a clean slide and cover glass. Culture in its simplest form requires a Petri plate containing 1½% agar made up in distilled water. A spot 1½-2 cm in diameter is covered with growth of a young culture of *Escherichia coli* from an agar slant. A drop of the suspected sediment or tissue suspension is placed on the spot. The plate is sealed with tape and incubated at 35-37 C, and the inverted plate is examined microscopically, daily at ×100 magnification, for small cells growing out from the inoculum. The differentiation of the free-living species from the parasitic *E histolytica* in fixed, stained tissue sections is made by examination of the morphology of the nuclei (Figure 96-2).

Immunologic Methods

Measurement of serum antibody to Acanthamoebae has been used to detect infection by this genus in both experimental animals and humans by means of such techniques as

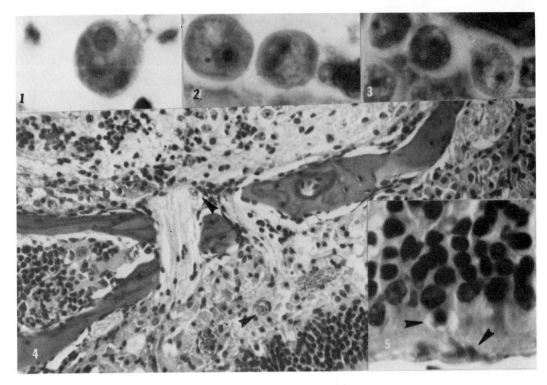

Figure 96-2 Pathomorphology and pathogenesis of amebic meningoencephalitis (**1, 2, 3**). Individual amebas as they appear in H & E stained sections, ×1000, for comparison. **1,** *Entamoeba histolytica* from an intestinal ulcer. **2,** *A culbertsoni* from a human brain abscess. **3,** *N fowleri* from human meningoencephalitis. **4** and **5,** Pathogenesis of free-living amebic meningoencephalitis. In **4,** cribriform plate of experimental mouse is traversed by olfactory nerve filaments by Acanthamoebas after penetration of nasal mucosa (arrows). (H & E stain ×250.) In **5,** a small area of normal olfactory mucosa of experimental mouse shows *Acanthamoeba* invading the superficial layer. Amebic nucleus is below surface, and remainder of amebic cell is flattened on the surface. (H & E stain × 1000.)

complement fixation and immunofluorescence. Comparable experimental results have been obtained by using formalinized, stained protein A staphylococci as "second antibody" after a specific immune serum has been applied to living amebas. A characteristic staphylococci coagglutinate on the amebic surface permits identification of amebic species in exudates and body fluids.

Treatment and Control

Almost all patients have succumbed to *Naegleria* meningoencephalitis despite treatment; only one exception has been reported. Amphotericin B is moderately active against experimental mouse infection, but results in humans have been disappointing. Recently, a patient whose illness was considered caused by *Naegleria* recovered after treatment with a combination of amphotericin B and an experimental drug, miconazole. The clinical course of *Naegleria* infection is so rapid and its early recognition so difficult that therapeutic efforts are fraught with great uncertainties.

As mentioned previously, *Naegleria* meningoencephalitis follows amebic infection of the nasopharynx, and thus is not a "primary" infection. At this early stage, a child who develops rhinitis after having been exposed by swimming in water of questionable purity should be suspected of having nasal infection by virulent amebas. The nasal and bronchial secretions available should be examined promptly; if amebas are identified, therapy with intravenous amphotericin B should be instituted.

Acanthamoebic meningoencephalitis, because it is such a rare entity, has not been recognized before death, and no specific treatment has been tried. Experimental therapeutic studies in mice have shown that at least some of the *Acanthamoeba* were susceptible to treatment by sulphadiazine.

The ubiquitous presence of these organisms is such that contact with humans is naturally universal. Large numbers of amebas may be present in water that contains coliform bacteria; therefore, use of such water for bathing and water sports must be avoided. Infections by *Naegleria,* usually prevalent in warm climates, can occur in cooler areas as a result of heated swimming pools or thermal pollution of streams by industrial discharge of hot water.

In view of the biologic information available, inhalation of dust and intranasal aspiration of water of unknown purity into the nares are risks of these and perhaps other afflictions. Although the risk is small, as evidenced by the limited number of reported cases, the high mortality rate suggests it should not be ignored.

References

Carter, R.F.: Primary amoebic meningoencephalitis. An appraisal of present knowledge. *Trans R Soc Trop Med Hyg* 1972; 66:193-213.

Cleland, P.G., et al.: Chronic amebic meningoencephalitis. *Arch Neurol* 1982; 39:56-57.

Culbertson, C.G., Harper, K.: Surface coagglutination with formalinized stained protein A staphylococci in the immunologic study of three pathogenic amebae. *Am J Trop Med Hyg* 1980; 29:785-794.

Culbertson, C.G.: The pathogenicity of soil amebas. *Ann Rev Microbiol* 1971; 25:231-254.

Culbertson, C.G.: Amebic meningoencephalitis. *Antibiot Chemother* 1981; 30:28-53.

Dorsch, M.M., et al.: The epidemiology and control of primary amoebic meningoencephalitis with particular reference to South Australia. *Trans R Soc Trop Med Hyg* 1983; 77:372-377.

Jager, B.V., Stamm, W.P.: Brain abscesses caused by free-living amoeba probably of the genus *Hartmannella* in a patient with Hodgkin's disease. *Lancet* 1972; 2:1343-1345.

John, D.T.: Primary amebic meningoencephalitis and the biology of Naegleria fowleri. *Ann Rev Microbiol* 1982; 36:101-23.

Kadlec, V., et al.: Virulent *Naegleria fowleri* in indoor swimming pool. *Folia Parasitol* (Praha) 1980; 27:11-17.

Kenney, M.: The micro-Kolmer complement fixation test in routine screening for soil ameba infection. *Health Lab Sci* 1971; 8:5-10.

Lawande, R.V., et al.: Recovery of soil amebas from the nasal passages of children during the dusty harmattan period in Zaria. *Am J Clin Pathol* 1979; 1:201-203.

Ma, P., et al.: A case of keratitis due to *Acanthamoeba* in New York, New York, and features of 10 cases. *J Infect Dis* 1981; 143:662-667.

Martinez, A.J.: Is *Acanthamoeba* encephalitis an opportunistic infection? *Neurology* 1980; 30:567-574.

Martinez, A.J., et al.: Granulomatous encephalitis, intracranial arteritis, and mycotic aneurysm due to a free-living ameba. *Acta Neuropathol (Berlin)* 1980; 49:7-12.

Page, F.C.: Taxonomic criteria for limax amoebae, with description of 3 new species of *Hartmannella* and 3 of Vahlkampfia. *J Protozool* 1967; 14:499-521.

Rowbotham, T.J.: Preliminary report on the pathogenicity of *Legionella pneumophila* for freshwater and soil amoebae. *J Clin Pathol* 1980; 33:1179-1183.

Seidel, J.S., et al.: Successful treatment of primary amebic meningoencephalitis. *N Engl J Med* 1982; 306:346-348.

Skočil, V., et al.: Epidemiological study of the incidence of amoebas of the limax group in military communities. V. Relation between the presence of amoebas of the limax group in nasal swabs and a pathological finding in nasal mucosa. *J Hyg Epidemiol Microbiol Immunol* 1972; 16:101-106.

97 Hemoflagellates

Rodrigo Zeledón, ScD

General Concepts

The flagellate family Trypanosomatidae has two genera (*Trypanosoma* and *Leishmania*) that include important pathogens for humans and domestic animals. The diseases caused by these protozoa are endemic or enzootic in different parts of the world and constitute serious medical and economic problems. Because these protozoa require hematin obtained from blood hemoglobin for aerobic respiration, they are called hemoflagellates. The digenetic (two-host) life cycles of these two genera involve an insect and a vertebrate. Other genera of the same family include the digenetic *Phytomonas,* which infects plants and some monogenetic (one-host) species, which infect only invertebrate hosts.

Morphology of the hemoflagellates varies among species and has been classified into seven types based on placement and origin of the flagellum. Several flagellated types are found only in the vector or in culture; in the vertebrate, two types can occur (amastigote and trypomastigote); in the invertebrate, promastigotes and epimastigotes (Figure 97-1) can also be found.

Besides the nucleus and the flagellum, a trypanosomatid cell has a unique organoid called the **kinetoplast.** The kinetoplast appears to be a special part of the mitochon-

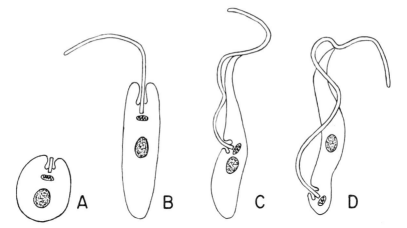

Figure 97-1 Four of the seven morphologic types of a trypanosomatid flagellate. **A,** Amastigote. **B,** Promastigote. **C,** Epimastigote. **D,** Trypomastigote.

drion, is rich in DNA, and apparently controls certain hereditary characteristics, particularly those related to morphogenesis. When stained by Giemsa, the kinetoplast is reddish purple and darker than the nucleus, in contrast to the pale blue cytoplasm.

Monogenetic species are more primitive and grow easily in synthetic culture media. Some digenetic species can be cultivated in complex synthetic media, but the results are not regularly reproducible, which poses an obstacle to the advance of basic knowledge of these parasites. The medium most commonly used is NNN, which has a solid phase of rabbit blood agar and a liquid phase of a physiologic salt solution. Liquid media are also available. Only the invertebrate phase is reproduced in such media, and the forms may or may not be infectious for the vertebrate hosts, depending on the species.

Replication of trypanosomatids occurs by single or multiple fission of the kinetoplast first, then the nucleus, and finally the cytoplasm.

The hemoflagellates attack a variety of organs, including the heart (*T cruzi*), and the central nervous system (African trypanosomes). The skin, nasal and oral mucosa, and various internal organs can be invaded by various species of *Leishmania*. The hemoflagellates are transmitted by insect vectors and hence control depends heavily on insecticides.

TRYPANOSOMES

Distinctive Properties

Trypanosoma (Schizotrypanum) cruzi produces Chagas' disease, which is named for its discoverer, Brazilian Carlos Chagas, and is found in only the western hemisphere. *T brucei gambiense* and *T b rhodesiense* cause African sleeping sickness, which can be distinguished from Chagas' disease on clinical, geographic, and epidemiologic grounds. All these species are present in blood as trypomastigotes, but *T cruzi* can be easily differentiated morphologically from the *T brucei* forms. *T cruzi,* whose mean length is 21 μm, has a large kinetoplast and a poorly developed undulating membrane; the African forms can reach more than 30 μm but have a smaller kinetoplast, a well-developed undulating membrane, and a more rounded posterior end. Pleomorphism is more common in the African forms. In the vertebrate host, *T cruzi* amastigotes multiply in reticuloendothelial or muscular cells; the blood trypomastigotes do not divide. The African forms do not produce intracellular amastigotes, but multiply as trypomastigotes while in the blood or cerebrospinal fluid.

Pathogenesis

American trypanosomiasis begins as a localized infection, followed by a parasitemia and a generalized infection. *T cruzi* enters the host through an abrasion in the skin. Infection may be evidenced by a small tumor (chagoma) at the site, or by Romaña's sign (unilateral palpebral edema) when the infective forms reach the conjunctiva of the eye (Figure 97-2). These are typical local inflammatory reactions, accompanied by swelling of satellite lymph nodes. The lesion may start 1-2 weeks after infection and persist for 1-2 months. The infective trypomastigotes from the insect penetrate local cells and multiply until the host cell ruptures. The amastigotes then give rise to the blood trypanosomes that invade other parts of the body, especially the heart muscle, and the disease enters the acute phase. After 1-3 months, the parasites, as a consequence of the action of immunologic mechanisms, gradually diminish to very low numbers in the bloodstream, and remain lodged in body tissues; the patient then enters an indeterminant period or early chronic phase.

Inflammatory phenomena produced mainly by the rupture of parasitized cells during the acute period lead to pathologic manifestations (for example, acute myocarditis and destruction of nerve cells, particularly of parasympathetic ganglia of the heart and the myenteric plexus) that are responsible for changes that occur in the chronic phase. Destruction of neurons, including some in the central nervous system, may be due to an autoimmune process. The histopathologic changes in chronic Chagas' myocardiopathy include focal myocarditis, fibrosis, and extensive myocytolysis. These changes usually occur in the absence of demonstrable parasites and can lead to sudden death. Thromboembolisms caused by heart damage can appear, and some authors consider the thinning of the apices of the ventricles a characteristic lesion.

In African trypanosomiasis, an initial chancre and regional lymphadenitis also may occur, and persist for several weeks. After a period of local multiplication, the trypanosomes enter the general circulation via the lymphatics, and fever appears. Even at this early stage, trypanosomes may invade the central nervous system. As the disease develops, inflammatory changes lead to a demyelinating encephalitis. This condition may also have an autoimmune basis; antibodies against myelin have been detected. The immune suppressive action of the parasites probably permits such concomitant infections as pneumonia.

Host Defenses

The host's response to trypanosomes includes an inflammatory reaction and various immunologic changes (discussed in Chapter 93). During the acute stage of Chagas'

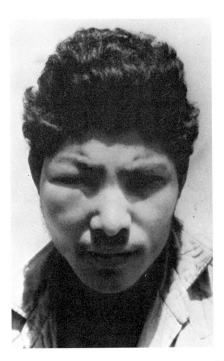

Figure 97-2 Romaña's sign in an acute case of Chagas' disease.

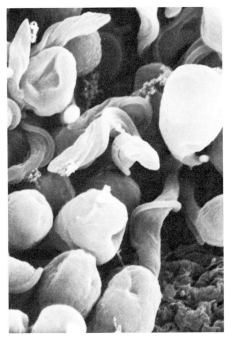

Figure 97-3 Metacyclic trypomastigotes and epimastigotes of *T cruzi* attached to the epithelium of the rectal gland of *Triatoma dimidiata*. (Scanning electron micrograph courtesy of the Electron Microscopy Unit, University of Costa Rica, ×7000.)

disease, rupture of the amastigote pseudocysts of *T cruzi* causes infiltration of polymorphonuclear neutrophils, monocytes, and lymphocytes, accompanied by edema, particularly in the heart. In African trypanosomiasis, mesenchymal inflammatory reactions in the brain are common in the early phase; these reactions are predominantly perivascular, with lymphocytes, histiocytes, and plasma cells. In both types of trypanosomiasis, the production of antibodies starts early during the acute period, but IgM reaches higher levels in the African cases. Evidence for cell-mediated immune mechanisms also has been observed.

Epidemiology

T cruzi is transmitted by hematophagus hemipteran bugs of several genera (*Triatoma*, *Rhodnius*, and *Panstrongylus*). While taking a blood meal from an infected host, the insect ingests trypomastigotes, which transform mainly into epimastigotes in the midgut of the insect and finally reach the posterior intestine. Here, the epimastigotes become attached by the flagellar sheath to the epithelium of the rectal gland, where they reproduce actively (Figure 97-3). In about 1 week, trypomastigote forms appear that can infect a vertebrate when they are flushed out of the gut with the urine or feces of the insect. Contact of the infected feces with the bite wound or other abrasion is necessary for initiation of the infection in the vertebrate; hence, transmission does not necessarily ensue after every blood meal. Congenital and blood transfusion transmission also can occur.

Natural foci of Chagas' disease exist among wild mammals and their associated triatomines. Humans and their domestic animals became involved in the epidemiologic chain several centuries ago when insects living under wild conditions began adapting to households. Opossums, armadillos, bats, and wild rats are reservoirs of the parasite, linking the wild and domestic cycles (Figure 97-4). Cases of human trypanosomiasis have been reported in almost all countries of the Americas, including the southern United States, but the main foci are located in poor rural areas of Latin America.

Epidemiologically, the two forms of African trypanosomiasis differ entirely from Chagas' disease. They are transmitted in the daytime by the bite of infected tsetse flies (*Glossina* sp), which inhabit the open savannah (*T b rhodesiense*) or riverine areas (*T b gambiense*). Trypanosomes ingested by the fly during a bite must reach the salivary glands within a few days, where they reproduce actively as epimastigotes until

WILD CYCLES   DOMICILIARY CYCLES

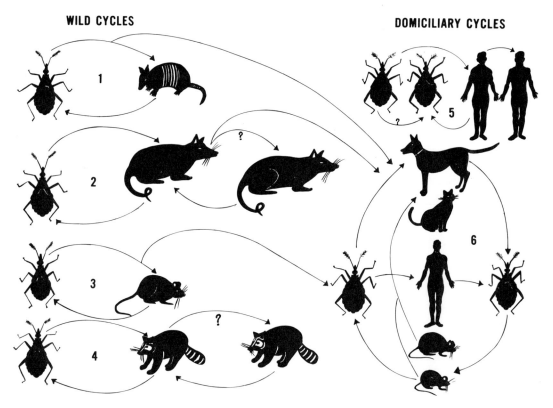

Figure 97-4 Wild and domestic life cycles of Chagas' disease. Triatomine bugs live with different wild animals to which they transmit *T cruzi* (**1–4**). On the other hand, insects adapted to houses transmit the parasite to humans and their domestic animals (**5** and **6**). Links between these cycles can be established when insects or reservoirs come to houses. From Zeledon, R.: In: *Trypanosomiasis and leishmaniasis*. Ciba Foundation Symposium, No. 20, New York: Elsevier, North Holland, Inc., 1974.

transformed into infective trypomastigotes. Wild game mammals (bushbuck, hartebeest, lion, hyena), as well as cattle, act as reservoirs of *T b rhodesiense*, but *T b gambiense* has been found in only domestic pigs and dogs, although some evidence that game animals in Upper Volta may carry the organism has been presented recently. Thus, the more virulent *T b rhodesiense* is maintained in the more resistant wild reservoirs, resulting in continuous selection of aggressive strains. The Gambian sleeping sickness covers a vast territory of tropical middle and west Africa; the Rhodesian type is confined mainly to the eastern part of that continent.

Diagnosis

In the acute phase of Chagas' disease, symptoms such as fever, edema, diarrhea, adenopathy, moderate hepatosplenomegaly, myocarditis, and sometimes meningoencephalitis may be observed; however, in most cases, this period is subclinical or mild, and many patients may become asymptomatic for the rest of their lives. After several years, enlargement and other alterations of the heart may appear and, in some areas of South America, enlargement of parts of the digestive tract (megaesophagus, megacolon) occurs. In the acute phase of Chagas' disease, demonstration of the parasite is relatively easy, by direct microscopic blood examination, by xenodiagnosis (feeding clean insects reared in the laboratory on a suspected person or an animal and later examining the insect feces), or by culture of the blood. In the chronic phase, xenodiagnosis and culture, alone or in combination, reveal the parasite in only 30%-60% of the cases, but serologic tests (complement-fixation, indirect hemagglutination, indirect immunofluorescence) can form a basis for diagnosis in most cases. Electrocardiograms are useful in revealing characteristic cardiac damage, such as right bundle branch block, particularly in young persons.

The clinical manifestations of African trypanosomiasis have common features regardless of the type of parasite involved; in general, however, the Rhodesian type evolves more acutely to a fatal resolution and its neurologic effects are less characteristic. The Gambian form is often subacute and can take several years to develop into typical sleeping sickness. Weakness, somnolence, cachexia, and coma may develop as the disease progresses. Parasites of African trypanosomiasis can be demonstrated in lymph nodes or in blood during the early stages, or later on in the cerebrospinal fluid. Culture or laboratory animal inoculations can be useful. Serologic tests are of limited value.

Control

The only practical measures to control American trypanosomiasis are insecticides directed against the insect vectors. Vaccination trials in animals have yielded only partial protection; live attenuated vaccines apparently are more effective, but are too risky for use in humans. An effective treatment for Chagas' disease has not been found; new drugs effective against the trypomastigotes and the amastigotes are needed, although nitrofurans (nifurtimox) and benznidazole are now used with good or partial success in acute cases.

Combating the vectors of African trypanosomiasis is more difficult. No reliable vaccine is available, and the variability in antigenic composition of the blood populations makes vaccination a difficult goal. Arsenicals and other organic chemical drugs are successful in treatment, particularly in an early phase, and some are useful for chemoprophylaxis.

LEISHMANIAS

Distinctive Properties

Organisms of the genus *Leishmania* are parasites present as intracellular amastigotes (3-6 by 1.5-3 μm) in humans or other vertebrates, and as promastigotes in the intestine of the sandfly vectors. Some species have become adapted to living in the human skin, the nasal and oral mucosa, or both; others, which can resist temperatures of 37 C, can invade internal organs and cause visceral leishmaniasis. The main species in the first group are, in the Old World, *L tropica* and *L major* (oriental sore); in the New World, *L mexicana* (Chiclero ulcer), *L peruviana* (uta), and *L braziliensis* (espundia, dermal leishmaniasis). Responsible for visceral leishmaniasis in the Old World are *L donovani* and *L infantum;* in the New World, *L chagasi*. Recently, researchers have divided some of the species into subspecies, but more work is needed before the species of *Leishmania* in both hemispheres can be properly identified and classified. Biochemical characterization is aiding this endeavor.

Pathogenesis

Several forms of disease have been described for the leishmanias. Promastigotes from the proboscis of an infected sandfly are injected during the biting act and taken up by local macrophages. After 2-3 weeks, a small cutaneous lesion or papule appears, grows, becomes indurated, and finally ulcerates (Figure 97-5). In the oriental sore form of the disease, the lesion normally evolves to spontaneous cure after a few months; in Chiclero ulcer, spontaneous cure also may occur, except when the lesions are in the ear, where they become chronic for many years. In the *L braziliensis* form, the parasites are more aggressive; lesions usually become chronic, and may disseminate to other areas of the skin or the lymphatics and sometimes to the nasopharyngeal and oral mucosa (*L b braziliensis*). In the Central American form, produced by *L b panamensis* (dermal leishmaniasis), the mucosae normally are spared and spontaneous cure may occur.

In visceral leishmaniasis, the initial nodule at the site of the bite rarely ulcerates. Instead, it usually disappears in a few weeks or months and a spontaneous cure may occur. In more serious visceral forms, the parasites disseminate to internal organs (liver, spleen, bone marrow, and lymphatic nodes), where they occupy the reticuloendothelial cells. The pathogenetic mechanisms are not fully understood, but clearly in those organs that exhibit marked cellular alterations, histiocyte hyperplasia leads to hypertrophy. Parasitized macrophages replace hematopoietic tissue in the bone marrow. Patients whose infections are in advanced stages are likely to be victims of other infections.

Host Defenses

The typical granuloma observed at the site of an early lesion consists of macrophages with intracellular parasites, lymphocytes, and plasma cells. In the disseminated form

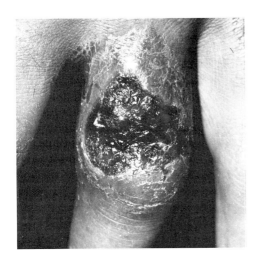

Figure 97-5 Ulcerative dermal leishmaniasis of central finger of the right hand produced by *L braziliensis panamensis.*

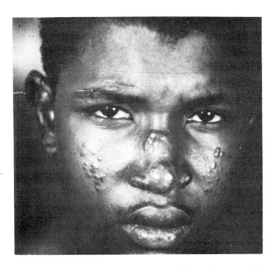

Figure 97-6 Diffuse cutaneous leishmaniasis attributed to *L mexicana pifanoi.* (Courtesy Jacinto Convit.)

(diffuse cutaneous leishmaniasis), the nodules are lepromatoid, consisting mainly of foamy histiocytes filled with parasites, a reaction typical of an impairment of the cell-mediated immune mechanisms of the host, specifically attributed to the presence of an adherent suppressor cell (Figure 97-6). Also, lesions of ear and nose cartilage can become chronic due to poor immunologic reaction; however, a tuberculoid picture normally develops with lymphocytes and plasma cells. In the tegumentary forms, cell-mediated immunity is important, and relatively low titers of antibodies are produced; in visceral leishmaniasis, high levels of IgG and other globulins are common. (See also Chapter 93.)

Epidemiology

When a female sandfly of the genus *Lutzomyia* in the New World or *Phlebotomus* in the Old World sucks the blood of an infected person or animal reservoir (rodents, carnivores, sloths), the parasites ingested pass into the stomach of the insect, transform into flagellates, and start multiplying. They may attach by the flagellum to the walls of the midgut and esophagus, but some eventually reach the proboscis and are inoculated into a new host (Figure 97-7).

The epidemiology of visceral leishmaniasis can vary from the village type of transmission without an extrahuman reservoir (as occurs in India) to that of rural, semiarid zones in Latin America, where the vector is abundant and lives close to houses, and both wild and domestic dogs enter the epidemiologic chain. Although cutaneous leishmaniasis can attack exposed persons of any age, some forms of visceral leishmaniasis, including the Latin American type, predominate in children.

Diagnosis

Tegumentary leishmaniasis may vary clinically from single or multiple ulcers to dry verrucous lesions. In some cases, metastatic, granulomatous oral or nasal lesions can be

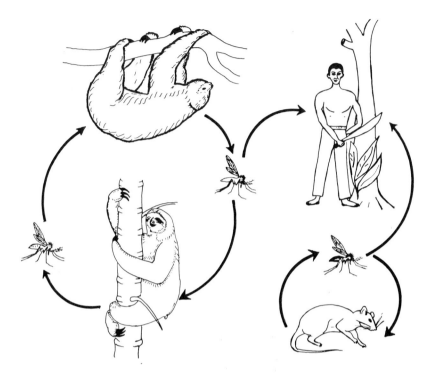

Figure 97-7 Simplified life cycle for *L braziliensis panamensis* (left) and *L mexicana* (right). At least two species of sloths are common reservoirs of *L b panamensis;* humans become victims when they enter the tropical forest and are attacked by infected arboreal sandflies. In the same way, *L mexicana* is maintained in rodents and is occasionally transmitted to humans by sandflies that live close to the floor of the forest.

observed, either concomitantly or several years after skin lesions have healed. The cartilaginous areas of the nasal septum and palate are slowly destroyed, and the process sometimes extends to the pharynx and larynx. These largely destructive forms (espundia) are more commonly observed in Brazil, but are also seen in Sudan, where they are usually less severe.

In visceral leishmaniasis, symptoms such as fever, splenomegaly, hepatomegaly, emaciation, and anemia are common. The disease may be acute, but it is more commonly chronic. In kala-azar, infiltrative or nodular lesions of the skin may appear after treatment (post-kala-azar dermal leishmaniasis), a condition seen frequently in India.

In cutaneous forms, parasites are easily demonstrated in scrapings of early skin lesions. Once the lesion becomes ulcerated and bacterial contamination is established, the parasites become scarce. Culture in blood agar media increases markedly the possibilities of isolation of the parasite, if material from direct puncture of the lesion borders or from lymph nodes or triturated biopsy tissue is used. Various immunodiagnostic tests, including immunofluorescence and immediate and delayed skin reactions, have been used for indirect diagnosis. The Montenegro skin test, in which an indurated area appears at the site of inoculation of the antigen after 72 hours, is always positive after 2-3 months of infection and remains so throughout the patient's lifetime. In visceral leishmaniasis, the parasite usually can be demonstrated in stained or cultured bone marrow or spleen material. Serologic reactions (for example, complement-fixation and immunofluorescence) are useful, particularly in surveys.

Control

Leishmaniasis transmitted in or near houses can be prevented with insecticides, but this procedure is not practical for the forest tegumentary type. Vaccination trials are in the experimental phase, and results have indicated that a reliable and effective human vaccine is still some distance away. Trivalent and pentavalent organic antimonials are available for treating leishmaniasis; these drugs act favorably in dermal and visceral forms but have some limitations due to their toxic effects. Certain aromatic diamidines act successfully in kala-azar. More research is needed to develop less toxic drugs that can be administered orally and that can be useful for prophylaxis and treatment.

References

Bray, R.S.: *Leishmania. Ann Rev Microbiol* 1974; 28: 189-217.

Brener, Z.: Immunity to *Trypanosoma cruzi. Adv Parasitol* 1980; 18: 247-292.

Brener, Z., Andrade, Z. (editors): *Trypanosoma cruzi e Doença de Chagas*. Rio de Janeiro: Guanabara Koogan, 1979.

Chang, K.P., Bray, R.S. (editors): *Leishmaniasis*. Amsterdam: Elsevier Biomedical Press, 1985.

Elliott, K., O'Connor, M., Wolstenholme, G.E.W., (editors): Trypanosomiasis and leishmaniasis with special reference to Chagas' disease. *Ciba Foundation Symposium 20, New Series*. North-Holland: Elsevier Exc. Med, 1974.

Hoare, C.A.: *The trypanosomes of mammals: A zoological monograph*. Oxford and Edinburgh: Blackwell Scientific Pub, 1972.

Lumsden, W.H.R., Evans, D.A., (editors): *Biology of the Kinetoplastida*, Vols. 1 and 2. London and New York: Academic Press, 1979.

Molyneaux, D.H., Ashford, R.W.: *The Biology of* Trypanosoma *and* Leishmania, *Parasites of Man and Domestic Animals*. London: Taylor and Francis, 1983.

Pan American Health Organization: New approaches in American trypanosomiasis research. *Proc Intl Symp* Belo Horizonte, Minas Gerais, Brasil. P.A.H.O. Sc. Publ. No. 318, 1976.

Petersen, E.A., et al.: Specific inhibition of lymphocyte-proliferation responses by adherent suppressor cells in diffuse cutaneous leishmaniasis. *N Engl J Med* 1982; 306: 387-390.

Zeledón, R., Rabinovich, J.E.: Chagas' disease: An ecological approach with special emphasis on its insect vectors. *Ann Rev Entomol* 1981; 26:101-133.

98 Malaria

Robin D. Powell, MD

General Concepts   **Epidemiology**
Distinctive Properties   **Diagnosis**
Pathogenesis   **Treatment and Prevention**
Host Defenses   **Control**

General Concepts

Malaria's domain of endemicity has been reduced, but this protozoan scourge continues to exact a substantial toll in human life and suffering, particularly in the tropics and subtropics. Clearly, this mosquito-borne disease will remain a formidable problem in some parts of the world for many years. Frequent and rapid travel to and from malarious areas necessitates alertness to malaria throughout the world.

The four species of the genus *Plasmodium* long known to cause human malaria are *Plasmodium falciparum, P vivax, P ovale,* and *P malariae.* Because these parasites invade and destroy red blood cells, definitive diagnosis depends on identification of malarial parasites by microscopic examination of stained blood smears. Falciparum and vivax infections are more common than ovale and quartan (*P malariae*) infections. Falciparum infections carry a high risk of serious complications, including death. Prompt diagnosis and treatment are especially important in falciparum malaria.

The diagnosis of malaria and selection of appropriate chemotherapy may be difficult. Antimalarial drugs vary in the effects they exert against different species, different stages in the life cycle of malaria parasites in humans, and different strains of the same species. Falciparum parasites resistant to widely used synthetic drugs have been an increasing problem. When a question of suspected or confirmed malaria arises, consultation with a qualified clinician is useful.

Distinctive Properties

Malaria parasites perpetuate their own kind through a remarkable series of morphologic transformations and host interactions (Figure 98-1). They reproduce in the mosquito host through a process termed **sporogony**, the end products of which are called **sporozoites.** They reproduce in hepatic cells and in red blood cells of the vertebrate host through a process termed **schizogony**, the end products of which are called **merozoites.**

Sporozoites are inoculated into humans when an infective mosquito obtains a blood meal. After a brief sojourn in the blood stream, some of the sporozoites invade parenchymal cells of the liver, where schizogony occurs. Parasitized hepatic cells rupture, releasing merozoites that invade circulating red cells. Schizogony then occurs in the red cells, the parasitized red cells rupture, merozoites are released and invade other red cells, and the sequence is then repeated over and over.

Some of the young erythrocytic parasites develop into gametocytes, the forms of the parasite that infect mosquitos. When mature gametocytes are ingested by a suitable anopheline vector, sporogony occurs, and oocysts form on the mosquito's gut wall.

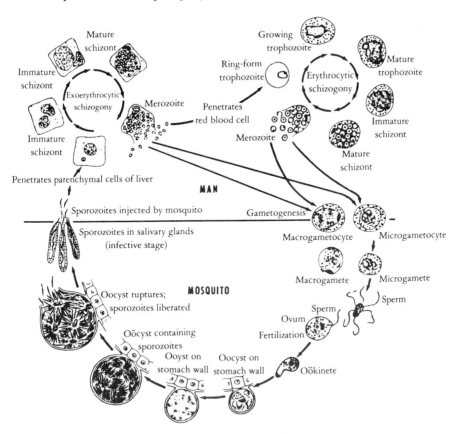

Figure 98-1 Life cycle of malaria. (From Melvin, D.M., Brooke, M.M., Healy, G.R. In: *Common blood and tissue parasites of man,* Public Health Service Publication No. 1234, 1965.)

Oocysts rupture, releasing sporozoites that migrate to the mosquito's salivary glands, setting the stage for transmission of the parasites to humans, and sustaining the mosquito-person-mosquito-person cycle when the mosquito obtains a blood meal from another person.

Parasites that undergo schizogony in red cells, termed **asexual erythrocytic forms** or **blood schizonts,** are the forms associated with symptoms of malaria. Schizogony in red cells requires about 3 days in quartan infections and about 2 days in infections with the other three species. If asexual parasites in different red cells undergo synchronous development, attacks of malaria may display an every-third-day periodicity in quartan infections, and an every-other-day periodicity in falciparum, vivax, or ovale infections.

Parasites that develop in the liver before red cells are invaded are termed **preerythrocytic forms, primary exoerythrocytic forms,** or **primary tissue schizonts.** Persisting or secondary tissue schizonts may develop, and periodic release of merozoites from the tissue reservoir may cause relapses in sporozoite-induced infections with *P vivax* or *P ovale.* Some strains of *P vivax* are characterized by early relapses; others are characterized by lengthy intervals between initial attacks and first relapses. Persisting or secondary tissue schizonts apparently do not develop in falciparum malaria. Whether they occur in quartan malaria is uncertain.

The asexual erythrocytic forms of *P vivax* and *P ovale* develop chiefly in young circulating red cells (reticulocytes). Those of *P malariae* develop in old red cells. Levels of parasitemia in infections with these species seldom exceed 50,000/mm³. Asexual erythrocytic forms of *P falciparum* thrive in red cells regardless of the age of the cell. As a result, high levels of parasitemia may occur in falciparum malaria.

Pathogenesis

Red cells parasitized by asexual erythrocytic forms of *P falciparum* stick to walls of small blood vessels. As levels of parasitemia increase, small blood vessels in virtually any part of the body may be occluded with resultant hypoxic damage. Massive hemolysis (destruction of circulating red cells), involving both parasitized and nonparasitized red cells, and disseminated intravascular coagulation may occur. The kidneys, lungs, brain, heart, or other vital organs may be affected. Acute renal failure, acute respiratory distress syndrome, coma, cardiac dysrhythmias, marked jaundice, gastrointestinal bleeding, or other complications may ensue. Anemia that reflects hemolysis and impaired red cell production is common, as is splenomegaly. The spleen removes from the circulation many parasites as well as deformed red cells or red cell fragments, thereby playing a major role in combating the infection.

Host Defenses

Humoral (IgG) and cellular immune mechanisms are mobilized in the body's efforts to check the infection and to dispose of the parasites. Acquired immunity, largely species- and strain-specific, is directed chiefly at asexual erythrocytic parasites. Over several weeks, as immunity or premunity in humans develops, levels of parasitemia previously associated with marked symptoms are tolerated increasingly well, levels of asexual parasitemia gradually decrease, and a state of asymptomatic or near-asymptomatic persisting parasitemia may develop. Gametocytes in such persons provide a source for transmission of the parasites by mosquitos.

Innate host resistance at times blunts asexual parasitemia or prevents establishment of schizogony in red cells. Examples are sickle cell hemoglobin and glucose-6-phosphate dehydrogenase (G6PD) deficiency, which may confer partial protection against falciparum malaria in some persons. Many blacks have innate Duffy blood-group–related resistance to vivax malaria.

Epidemiology

Children bear much of the brunt of malarial morbidity and mortality in areas of high endemicity. Useful malariometric or epidemiologic indicators include the percent incidence of overt splenomegaly (spleen rate) and of positive blood smears (parasite rate) in children of indigenous populations, as well as serologic studies for malaria antibodies and the numbers of cases of malaria reported. Case report data generally represent underestimates because many cases go unreported.

Degrees of endemicity differ from area to area and from one time to another in the same area. Rainfall, temperature, and vegetation influence mosquito breeding and thereby contribute to seasonal or other fluctuations in levels of malarial transmission. Other elements of the dynamics of malaria include its prevalence in the indigenous population, parasite species and strains, immunity level of the population, population housing and sleeping habits and mobility, degree to which environmental conditions are conducive to sporogony in the mosquito host, presence of susceptible new human hosts, and presence of suitable anopheline vectors. Not all species of anopheline mosquitos transmit malaria; the species principally responsible for transmission differ from area to area.

Persons who acquire considerable immunity to species and strains of malaria parasites in one area may be susceptible to species and strains in other areas. Movement of such persons from one malarious area to another may be associated with enhanced problems due to malaria. Only a small fraction of the population may have immunity in areas of low endemicity. Suitable vectors are present in many formerly malarious areas where the disease is no longer endemic. Effective systems for early detection and treatment of imported cases of malaria are critical to minimize the chances of reinstitution of transmission of malaria in such areas.

Malaria poses a threat to nonimmune persons who visit or reside temporarily in areas where transmission of malaria is occurring. Problems with malaria occupy a prominent position in the history of many armed conflicts. The steps that can be taken to prevent malaria in tourists or others who visit malarious areas warrant broad appreciation and use.

Diagnosis

Definitive diagnosis hinges on identification of malaria parasites by microscopic examination. Blood smears (thick and thin) stained with Giemsa or Wright's stain should be examined as promptly as possible when malaria is suspected. Examination should be repeated when initial smears are negative; levels of parasitemia may fluctuate, and smears may be intermittently negative. Accurate identification of the species is important.

Treatment and Prevention

The main initial therapeutic aims are to terminate the acute attack of malaria as soon as possible by eliminating asexual erythrocytic parasites, and to prevent and correct complications. Steps to combat dehydration, overhydration, anemia, renal failure, hypoxia, or electrolyte disturbances can be crucial elements of management, especially in severe falciparum infections.

A 4-aminoquinoline, notably chloroquine or amodiaquine, is the drug of choice for terminating acute attacks of vivax, ovale, or quartan malaria. Chloroquine should completely eliminate asexual erythrocytic forms of these species. Gametocytes of these three species are not long-lived. Blood smears usually prove negative for asexual parasites and gametocytes within several days after initiation of treatment with a 4-aminoquinoline. The 4-aminoquinolines do not eliminate persisting or secondary tissue forms of *P vivax* or *P ovale*. Primaquine, an 8-aminoquinoline, can be given orally to try to destroy such tissue forms and minimize chances of subsequent relapses of vivax or ovale malaria.

Quinine is at present the drug of choice to terminate acute attacks of falciparum malaria acquired by nonimmune persons in areas where chloroquine-resistant *P falciparum* is known to exist. Chloroquine-resistant strains are widespread in parts of Latin America, the Philippines, and Southeast Asia. Such strains often display resistance not only to other 4-aminoquinolines but to other widely used synthetic antimalarial agents as well. Chloroquine can be used to treat falciparum malaria acquired in Africa. Recently, however, chloroquine-resistant *P falciparum* has been documented in several parts of East Africa, and has been reported from a steadily increasing number of countries in other areas.

One should be wary of the possibility of a chloroquine-resistant infection when chloroquine is used to treat falciparum malaria. High degrees of chloroquine resistance are unusual. Resistance usually is manifested by a recrudescence of falciparum malaria several days to several weeks after treatment with a 4-aminoquinoline, reflecting a failure to eliminate all of the asexual erythrocytic parasites. Similar recrudescences may occur after treatment with quinine. A combination of quinine and one or two other agents has, at times, been employed to try to prevent such recrudescences. Several promising new prospective antimalarial agents (including a mefloquine-pyrimethamine-sulfadoxine combination) have been identified and may greatly enhance the arsenal of useful antimalarial drugs.

Mature falciparum gametocytes may persist in the circulation and remain infective for mosquitos for several weeks, despite treatment with agents such as chloroquine or quinine. A single dose of primaquine renders falciparum gametocytes noninfective and destroys them.

Chloroquine usually is well tolerated. The main adverse effect of primaquine is drug-induced hemolysis in persons who have G6PD deficiency or other disorders of the pentose phosphate pathway of erythrocytes. Quinine may cause tinnitus and other symptoms collectively referred to as **cinchonism.** Plasma quinine levels should be monitored and the dosage of quinine reduced in patients with renal failure.

A single oral dose of chloroquine or of amodiaquine can be ingested once a week to prevent malaria in adults who visit malarious areas. The regimen should begin 1–2 weeks before the person departs for a malarious area, and should be continued for 8 weeks after he or she leaves it. A 14-day course of primaquine can be administered at some point during the 8-week period to eliminate possible tissue forms of *P vivax* and *P ovale* and to reduce chances of subsequent attacks of vivax or ovale malaria. Such prophylactic regimens may not prevent overt infections with 4-aminoquinoline-resistant *P falciparum*. Tourists or others who plan to visit malarious areas should be advised to contact a physician promptly if they develop symptoms such as headaches, chills, and fever while in the malarious area or after departing from it. Steps that may reduce contact with mosquitos, such as the use of insect repellents and long-sleeved shirts, also merit emphasis.

Control

Malaria control and eradication efforts have been based largely on antimosquito measures, including the use of residual insecticides such as DDT. Case detection and treatment activities, mass administration of antimalarial drugs in some instances, or preventive steps by individuals or groups benefit those treated or protected and limit the gametocyte reservoir.

Behavioral characteristics of certain of the anopheline vectors render them invulnerable to residual insecticides. Some vectors have developed resistance to DDT or other insecticides. Drug resistance and other limitations of antimalarial agents have posed problems. Economic, social, and political factors have played a major role in limiting headway in malaria control and eradication programs.

Previous progress in malaria control and eradication activities represents a monumental achievement. Unfortunately, resurgences of malaria have occurred in parts of southern Asia, Latin America, and Turkey. The number of cases of malaria reported worldwide has been increasing. Available means to combat malaria are far from ideal. The need for basic and applied malaria research clearly remains substantial.

Recent basic research has concentrated on the following areas: identification of forms of the parasite termed **hypnozoites** that probably cause relapses, or delayed primary attacks, in infections with certain species of plasmodia; development of a malaria vaccine; elucidation of the fundamental mechanisms of the cell and molecular biology, and the immunology of malaria parasite-host interactions. New methods for the prevention, diagnosis, treatment, and control of human malaria no doubt will be developed. However, the health care systems in developing nations must be capable of using these tools if human malaria is to be eradicated. Basic and applied research must be conducted in tandem with development of health care delivery in malarious areas.

References

Bruce-Chwatt, L.J.: Transfusion malaria. *Bull WHO* 1974; 50:337–345.

Bruce-Chwatt, L.J.: Man against malaria: Conquest or defeat. *Trans R Soc Trop Med Hyg* 1979; 73:605–617.

Bruce-Chwatt, L.J., (editor): *Chemotherapy of malaria.* Geneva: World Health Organization, 1981.

Bruce-Chwatt, L.J.: Chemoprophylaxis of malaria in Africa: The spent "magic bullet." *Brit Med J* 1982; 285:674–676.

Clayman, C.B., Powell, R.D.: Malaria—are we prepared? *JAMA* 1981; 246:989.

Cohen, S., et al.: Acquired immunity and vaccination in malaria. *Am J Trop Med Hyg* 1977; 26:223-232.

Cox, F.E.G.: Oxidant killing of the malaria parasites. *Nature* 1983; 302:19.

Ellis, J., et al.: Cloning and expression in *E. coli* of the malarial sporozoite surface antigen gene from *Plasmodium knowlesi. Nature* 1983; 302:536-538.

Jungery, D., et al.: Lectin-like polypetides of *P. falciparum* bind to red cell sialoglycoproteins. *Nature* 1983; 310:704.

Harrison, G.: *Mosquitoes, malaria and man: A history of the hostilities since 1880.* New York: E.P. Dutton, 1978.

Kean, B.H., Reilly, P.C., Jr.: Malaria—the mime. *Am J Med* 1976; 61:159-164.

Krotoski, W.A., et al.: Demonstration of hypnozoites in sporozoite-transmitted *Plasmodium vivax* infection. *Am J Trop Med Hyg* 1982; 31:1291-1293.

Malaria prevention in travellers from the United Kingdom. *Br Med J* 1981; 283:214-218.

Miller, L.H., et al.: The resistance factor to *Plasmodium vivax* in blacks. *N Engl J Med* 1976; 295:302-304.

Miller, L.H., et al.: A monoclonal antibody to rhesus erythrocyte Band 3 inhibits invasion by malaria (*Plasmodium knowlesi*) merozoites. *J Clin Invest* 1983; 72:1357-1364.

Newmark, P.: What chance a malaria vaccine? *Nature* 1983; 302:473.

Peters, W.: Drug resistance in malaria—a perspective. *Trans R Soc Trop Med Hyg* 1969; 63:25-45.

Peters, W.: Chemotherapy of malaria. In: *Malaria, volume 1, epidemology, chemotherapy, morphology, and metabolism.* Kreier, J.P., (editor). New York: Academic Press, 1980.

Powell, R.D., McNamara, J.V., Rieckmann, K.H.: Clinical aspects of acquisition of immunity to falciparium malaria. *Proc Helminth Soc Wash* 1972; 39:51-66.

Schultz, M.G.: Imported malaria. *Bull WHO* 1974; 50:329-336.

Wernsdorfer, W.H., Kouznetsov, R.L.: Drug-resistant malaria—occurrence, control, and surveillance. *Bull WHO* 1980; 58:341-352.

World Health Organization: *Malaria control and national health goals.* Geneva: World Health Organization, 1982.

99 Toxoplasmosis

J. P. Dubey, MVSc, PhD

General Concepts
Distinctive Properties
Pathogenesis
Host Defenses
Epidemiology
Diagnosis
Control

General Concepts

Toxoplasma gondii is an intestinal coccidium of the cat family with an unusually wide range of intermediate hosts. Infection by this parasite is common in many warm-blooded animals, including humans. *T gondii* is considered one of the important pathogens for nearly all domestic animals and for humans. Although much progress was made in the diagnosis and treatment of toxoplasmosis between the years 1948 and 1965, its life cycle was described only in 1970, when cats were found to be the definitive host for this parasite.

Infection in humans can be congenital (mother infected during pregnancy) or acquired. Ocular disorders are the most common sequelae of congenital toxoplasmosis. An acquired infection generally produces lymphadenitis. Most natural infections are acquired by ingestion of meat containing cysts or of foods contaminated by cat feces. Diagnosis is based on serologic or histologic examination of tissues. Acute cases are treated with sulphonamides and pyrimethamine. Thorough cooking of meat and proper management of pet cats aid in the control of the disease.

Distinctive Properties

Cats, not only domestic but also wild Felidae, are the definitive hosts of *T gondii,* and various warm-blooded animals are the intermediate hosts. *Toxoplasma* is transmitted by three known modes: congenital, carnivorism, and fecal (Figure 99-1).

Cats can acquire infection by ingesting any of three infectious stages of *Toxoplasma:* rapidly multiplying forms called **tachyzoites** (Figure 99-2), cysts (Figure 99-3), or oocysts (see Figure 99-1). Prepatent periods (time to the shedding of oocysts after initial infection) vary according to the stage of *Toxoplasma* ingested. Fewer than 50% of cats shed oocysts after ingesting tachyzoites or oocysts, whereas nearly all cats shed oocysts after ingesting cysts. Only the cyst-induced cycle has been studied in detail.

After the ingestion of cysts by the cat, the cyst wall is dissolved by the proteolytic enzymes in the stomach and small intestine. The released organisms (slowly multiplying forms called **bradyzoites**) penetrate the epithelial cells of the small intestine and initiate formation of numerous asexual generations of *Toxoplasma* (Figure 99-4) before the sexual cycle (gametogony) begins. After the male gamete fertilizes the female gamete, two walls are laid around the fertilized gamete, and the oocytes are excreted in feces in an unsporulated stage. These unsporulated oocysts measure about 10 by 12 μm. Sporulation occurs outside the body, and oocysts become infectious within 1–5 days after excretion. The sporulated oocyst contains two sporocysts, and each sporocyst has

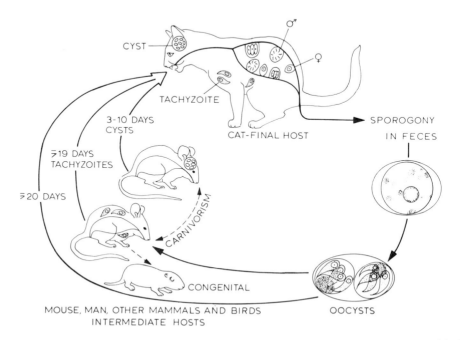

Figure 99-1 Cats, the definitive hosts of *T gondii,* can become infected by ingesting infected animals or sporulated oocysts. The oocysts are infectious to most mammals and birds. *Toxoplasma* can be transmitted to intermediate hosts through oocysts, by carnivorism, or transplacentally. Transplacental transmission is most important in humans and sheep. Cats probably become infected in nature mainly by preying on infected hosts. From Dubey, J.P.: *J Am Vet Med Assoc* 1976; 169:1071.

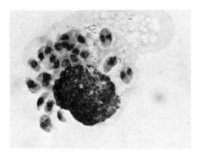

Figure 99-2 Tachyzoites in impression smears. (Giemsa stain × 1250.)

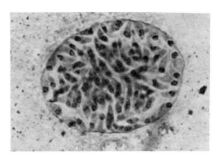

Figure 99-3 A cyst containing many bradyzoites, impression smear. (Giemsa stain × 1250.)

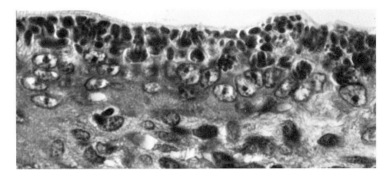

Figure 99-4 Numerous enteroepithelial stages of *Toxoplasma* in small intestine of a cat. (H & E stain × 1000.)

four sporozoites (see Figure 99-1). Sporulated oocysts are remarkably resistant structures that can survive in soil for several months.

At the same time that *Toxoplasma* multiplies in the surface epithelial cells of the feline intestine, the bradyzoites released from the cyst penetrate the lamina propria of intestine and multiply as tachyzoites. Within a few hours after infection, *Toxoplasma* may disseminate to extraintestinal tissues of cats through lymph and blood. Tachyzoites multiply in almost any type of host cell until the host cell is filled with parasites (see Figure 99-2). The released tachyzoites enter the new host cell, multiply, and kill the host cell. The host usually recovers from these microfoci of necrosis, and the parasite enters the "resting" stage, the tissue cyst. Cysts are formed most commonly in the brain, liver, and muscles. *T gondii* cysts are usually spherical and contain hundreds of bradyzoites (see Figure 99-3). Cysts usually cause no host reaction and may remain for the life of the host. The extraintestinal cycle of *Toxoplasma* in the cat is similar to the cycle in nonfeline hosts such as humans or mice, but sexual stages do not occur in humans, mice, or other nonfeline hosts.

Pathogenesis

Toxoplasma usually parasitizes the definitive and intermediate hosts without producing clinical signs; only rarely does it cause severe clinical manifestations. Most natural infections probably are acquired by the ingestion of cysts in infected meat or oocysts from food contaminated with cat feces. Bradyzoites from the cysts or sporozoites from oocysts penetrate the intestinal epithelial cells and multiply in the intestine. *Toxoplasma* may spread locally to mesenteric lymph nodes and to distant organs by invading lymphatics and blood. Necrosis (Figure 99-5) in intestinal and mesenteric lymph nodes may occur before other organs become severely damaged. Focal areas of necrosis may develop in many organs. The clinical picture is determined by the extent of injury to these organs, especially vital organs such as the eye, heart, and adrenals. Necrosis is caused by intracellular growth of tachyzoites. *Toxoplasma* does not produce a toxin.

Most human infections are asymptomatic, but at times the parasite can produce devastating disease. Infection may be congenitally or postnatally acquired. Congenital infection occurs only when a woman becomes infected during pregnancy. A wide spectrum of clinical disease occurs in congenitally infected children. Mild disease may consist of slightly diminished vision, whereas severely diseased children may have the full tetrad of signs: retinochoroiditis, hydrocephalus, convulsions, and intracerebral calcification. Of these, hydrocephalus is the least common (about 3% of congenital infections) but most dramatic lesion of toxoplasmosis. By far the most common sequela of congenital toxoplasmosis is ocular disease. Except for an occasional involvement of an entire eye, the disease almost always is confined to the posterior chamber.

Toxoplasma proliferates in the retina, which leads to inflammation in the choroid; the disease is correctly designated as retinochoroiditis. The lesions of ocular toxoplas-

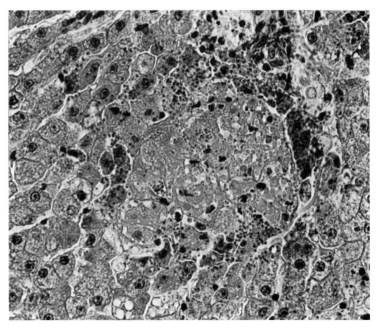

Figure 99-5 A focus of necrosis in the liver of a cat due to toxoplasmosis. More *Toxoplasma* than host cells appear. (H & E stain ×400.)

mosis are fairly characteristic in humans. Such lesions in the acute or subacute stage of inflammation appear as yellowish white, cottonlike patches in the fundus. The lesions may be single or multiple, and may involve one or both eyes. During the acute stage, inflammatory exudate may cloud the vitreous and may be so dense as to preclude visualization of the fundus by an ophthalmoscope. As the inflammation subsides, the vitreous clears, and the diseased retina and choroid can be seen through the ophthalmoscope. Retinal lesions may be single or multifocal small, gray areas of active retinitis with minimal edema and reaction in the vitreous humor. The punctate lesions usually are harmless, unless they are located in a macular area. Although severe infections may be detected at birth, milder infections may not flare up until adulthood.

Postnatally acquired infection may be localized or generalized. Lymphadenitis is the most frequently observed human clinical form of toxoplasmosis. Although any nodes can be infected, the most frequently involved are deep cervical nodes. When infected, these nodes are tender and discrete, but not painful; the infections resolve spontaneously in weeks or months. Lymphadenopathy is associated with fever, malaise, and fatigue in about one-half of patients, muscle pains in one-third, and sore throat and headache in one-fifth. Although the condition may be benign, its diagnosis is vital in pregnant women, because of the risk to the fetus. Encephalitis is an important manifestation of toxoplasmosis in immunosuppressed patients and in those with acquired immunodeficiency syndrome (AIDS). Clinically, patients may have headache, disorientation, drowsiness, hemiparesis, reflex changes, and convulsions, and many may become comatose.

Host Defenses

The host may die from toxoplasmosis, but much more often recovers and acquires immunity. Inflammation usually follows necrosis. By about the third week after infection, *Toxoplasma* tachyzoites begin to disappear from visceral tissues and may localize as cysts in neural and muscular tissues. *Toxoplasma* tachyzoites may persist longer in the spinal cord and brain, because immunity is less effective in neural organs than in visceral tissues. Chronic infections may be reactivated locally, for example, in the eye. Reactivation possibly results from the rupture of a cyst. Probably many tissue cysts rupture at different times during the life of the host, and released bradyzoites are destroyed by the host's immune responses (see Chapter 93). This reaction may cause local necrosis accompanied by inflammation. Hypersensitivity is said to play a major role in such reactions; however, infection usually subsides with no local renewed multiplication of *Toxoplasma* in an immunocompetent host. In immunosuppressed patients, rupture of a cyst may result in renewed multiplication of bradyzoites into tachyzoites, and the host may die from toxoplasmosis.

Epidemiology

Toxoplasma infection in humans is widespread throughout the world. Approximately one-half billion humans have antibody to *T gondii*. Infection in humans and animals varies in different geographic areas of a country, and the cause for these variations is not yet known. Environmental conditions, cultural habits of the people, and animal fauna are among factors that may determine the degree of natural spread of *Toxoplasma*. Only a small proportion (less than 0.1%) of people acquire infection congenitally. Mothers of congenitally infected children do not give birth to infected children in subsequent pregnancies. Unlike its occurrence in humans, repeated congenital infection can occur in mice, rats, guinea pigs, and hamsters without reinfection from outside sources.

The relative frequency with which postnatal toxoplasmosis is acquired by eating raw meat and by ingesting food contaminated by oocysts from cat feces is unknown and difficult to investigate. Both modes of infection are reported to cause toxoplasmosis. *Toxoplasma* infection occurs commonly in many animals used for food (for example, sheep, pigs, and rabbits). Infection in cattle is less prevalent than in sheep or pigs, at least in western Europe, the United States, New Zealand, and Denmark.

Oocysts are shed by cats—not only the domestic cat, but other members of Felidae like ocelots, marguays, jaguarundi, bobcats, and Bengal tigers. Oocyst formation, however, is greatest in the domestic cat. Widespread natural infection is possible because a cat may excrete millions of oocysts after ingesting one infected mouse. Oocysts are resistant to most ordinary environmental conditions, and can survive in moist conditions for months and even years. Invertebrates such as flies, cockroaches, and earthworms can spread oocysts mechanically.

Only a few cats may be involved in the spread of *Toxoplasma* because at any given time as little as 1% of the domestic cat population may be shedding oocysts in the United States. Whether cats shed oocysts only once or several times in nature is not known. Under experimental conditions, cats usually did not reshed oocysts after reinoculation of *Toxoplasma* cysts. Immunity to *T gondii* in cats may wane with time, and cats may reshed oocysts in nature.

Diagnosis

Diagnosis can be aided by serologic or histocytologic examination. Clinical signs of toxoplasmosis are nonspecific and cannot be depended on for a definite diagnosis, because toxoplasmosis clinically mimics several other infectious diseases.

Many serologic tests have been used for the detection of antibodies of *T gondii*. Of these serologic tests, the most reliable is the cytoplasm-modifying, or dye, test. Live virulent tachyzoites of *Toxoplasma* are used as antigen and are exposed to dilutions of the test serum and a complement accessory factor resembling complement that is obtained from *Toxoplasma* antibody-free human serum. This test is sensitive, and so far is the most specific test for toxoplasmosis. Its main disadvantages are its high cost and the human hazard due to the use of live organisms. The indirect fluorescent antibody test (IFAT) overcomes some disadvantages of the dye test. In IFAT, killed tachyzoites of *Toxoplasma*, which are available commercially, are used as antigen. Titers obtained by IFAT are comparable to those in the dye test. Disadvantages of the IFAT are that a microscope with UV light is required, fluorescent antispecies globulin is required for each species to be tested, and false-positive titers may occur in patients with antinuclear antibodies. Its suitability in animal diagnostic work is therefore limited, but it has proved useful in diagnosing acquired human toxoplasmosis. Other serologic tests—the indirect hemagglutination test, the agglutination test, ELISA, and the complement-fixation test—each offer some advantages. Indirect hemagglutination and agglutination tests are easy to perform, but need further evaluation for specificity of titers.

Antigens for indirect hemagglutination tests are now commercially available in several countries, including the United States. Although this test is easy to perform, it usually does not detect antibodies during the acute phase of toxoplasmosis. The agglutination test has disadvantages similar to those of the indirect hemagglutination test, but a recent modification of the agglutination test shows great promise. In the modified agglutination test, the test serum is treated with 2-mercaptoethanol to eliminate nonspecific agglutinins. The complement-fixation test is useful in diagnosing acute infection, because antibody measured in this test appears during acute infection and usually disappears soon after the acute infection ends. The results vary, depending on the antigenic preparation. The ELISA test appears to be specific and may be the test used most often in the future.

Examining one positive serum sample only establishes that the host has been infected at some time in the past. Serologic evidence for an acute acquired infection is obtained when antibody titers rise by a factor of four to eight in serum taken 2-4 weeks after initial serum collection, or when specific IgM antibody is detected. The finding of antibody in even undiluted serum is useful in the diagnosis of ocular toxoplasmosis because patients with this disorder usually have low *T gondii* antibody titers.

Diagnosis can be made by finding *Toxoplasma* in host tissue removed by biopsy or at necropsy. This procedure is particularly useful in immunosuppressed patients, or in patients with AIDS, whose antibody synthesis may be delayed or hampered. A rapid diagnosis can be made by making impression smears of lesions on glass slides. After drying for 10-30 minutes, the smears are fixed in methyl alcohol and stained with Giemsa. Well-preserved *Toxoplasma* are crescent-shaped and stain well with any of the Romanowsky stains (see Figure 99-2); however, degenerating organisms, commonly found in lesions, usually appear oval and their cytoplasm stains poorly as compared to their nuclei. Diagnosis should not be made unless organisms with typical structure are located, because degenerating host cells may resemble degenerating *Toxoplasma*. In sections, the tachyzoites are oval to round and usually do not stain distinctively from host cells (see Figure 99-5). In sections stained with hematoxylin and eosin, tachyzoites may be easily located by deeply staining the host tissue. Occasionally, cysts may be found in areas with lesions. Tissue cysts are usually spherical and have silver-positive walls; the bradyzoites are strongly PAS-positive (see Figure 99-3). Immunoperoxidase staining can be used to identify *Toxoplasma* cysts or tachyzoites in fixed impression smears and in tissues fixed in formalin. Computed tomography (CT) techniques are also useful in the diagnosis of human cerebral toxoplasmosis.

Control

Sulfonamides and pyrimethamine (Daraprim) are two drugs widely used for therapy of toxoplasmosis. They act synergistically by blocking the metabolic pathway involving *p*-aminobenzoic acid and the folic-folinic acid cycle, respectively. These two drugs usually are well tolerated, but sometimes thrombocytopenia, leukopenia, or both may develop. These effects can be overcome without interfering with treatment by administering folinic acid and yeast, because the vertebrate host can utilize presynthe-sized folinic acid whereas *Toxoplasma* cannot. The commonly used sulfonamides—sulfadiazine, sulfamethazine, and sulfamerazine—are all effective against toxoplasmosis. Generally, any sulfonamide that diffuses across the host cell membrane is useful in antitoxoplasma therapy. Although these drugs have beneficial action when given in the acute stage of the disease process, usually they will not eradicate infection when active multiplication of the parasite occurs. Sulfa compounds are excreted within a few hours of administration; therefore, treatment has to be administered in daily divided doses. No vaccine is currently available to reduce or prevent congenital infections in humans and animals, but research is being done on the development of such an agent. Certain drugs can minimize or prevent oocyst formation in the cat, but the feasibility of incorporating these agents in cat food is controversial.

To prevent *Toxoplasma* infection, the following precautions should be taken. Heat meat to 66 C throughout before eating. Wash hands with soap and water after handling meat. Never feed raw meat to cats; feed only dry or canned food or cooked meat. Keep cats indoors. Change litter boxes daily. Flush cat feces down the toilet or burn them. Clean litter pans by immersing in boiling water. Use gloves while working in garden. Cover children's sandboxes when not in use.

References

Beverley, J.K.A.: Some aspects of toxoplasmosis, a world wide zoonosis. In: *Parasitic zoonoses*. Soulsby, E.J.L. (editor). New York: Academic Press, 1974.

Beverley, J.K.A.: Toxoplasmosis in animals. *Vet Rec* 1976; 99:123-127.

Conley, F.K., Jenkins, K.A., Remington, J.S.: *Toxoplasma gondii* infection of the central nervous system. Use of the peroxidase-antiperoxidase method to demonstrate *Toxoplasma* in formalin-fixed, paraffin-embedded tissue sections. *Human Pathol* 1981; 12:690-698.

Desmonts, G., Couvreur, J.: A prospective study of 378 pregnancies. *N Engl J Med* 1974; 290:1110-1116.

Dubey, J.P.: *Toxoplasma, Hammondia, Besnoitia, Sarcocystis,* and other tissue cyst-forming coccidia of man and animals. In: *Parasitic protozoa,* Vol. III. Kreier, J.P., (editor) New York: Academic Press, 1977.

Feldman, H.A.: Toxoplasmosis. *N Engl J Med* 1968; 279:1370-1375. 1431-1437.

Frenkel, J.K.: Toxoplasmosis: Parasite life cycle, pathology and immunology. In: *The coccidia,* Hammond, D.M., Long, P.L., (editors). Baltimore: University Park Press, 1973.

Luft, B., et al.: Outbreak of central nervous system toxoplasmosis in western Europe and North America. *Lancet* 1983; 1:781-784.

O'Connor, G.R.: Ocular toxoplasmosis. *Jap J Ophthalmol* 1975; 19:1-24.

Post, M.J.D., et al.: Toxoplasma encephalitis in Haitian adults with acquired immunodeficiency syndrome: A clinical-pathologic-CT correlation. *Am J Neuroradiol* 1983; 4:155-162.

Siim, J.C., Biering-Sørensen, U., Moller, T.: Toxoplasmosis in domestic animals. *Adv Vet Sci* 1963; 8:335-429.

Teutsch, S., et al.: Epidemic toxoplasmosis associated with infected cats. *N Engl J Med* 1979; 300:695-699.

100 *Pneumocystis carinii*

Walter T. Hughes, MD

General Concepts
Distinctive Properties
Pathogenesis
Host Defenses
Epidemiology
Diagnosis
Control

General Concepts

Pneumocystis carinii is a cause of diffuse pneumonia in the immunocompromised host. Even in fatal cases, the organism and the disease remain localized to the lung. The pneumonia rarely, if ever, occurs in healthy individuals.

P carinii, an extracellular protozoan, has been observed in three forms. Diagnosis requires identification of *P carinii* in lung tissue obtained by invasive techniques. Experimental studies have shown that the organism can be transmitted by inhalation.

Distinctive Properties

The taxonomy of *P carinii* has not been established. The structural forms that have been recognized are the cyst, which is thick-walled; the sporozoite, an intracystic structure; and the thin-walled trophozoite. The cyst form is a spherical-to-ovoid structure measuring 4-6 μm in diameter (Figure 100-1). The cyst may contain as many as eight pleomorphic sporozoites (Figure 100-2). The trophozoite is a thin-walled extracystic cell representing the excysted sporozoite. Although the mode of replication has not been described, the organism can be propagated in embryonic chick epithelial lung cell

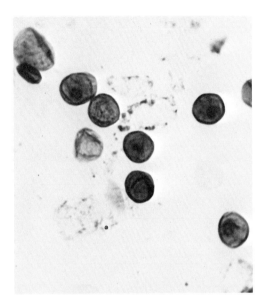

Figure 100-1 *Pneumocystis carinii* cysts stained with Gomori's methenamine silver nitrate method. Cysts stain brownish black and measure 4–6 μm in diameter. From Hughes, W.T. In: *Practice of pediatrics,* Vol. 2. Kelley, V.C., (editor). Hagerstown, Md.: Harper & Row Pub., Inc., 1977.

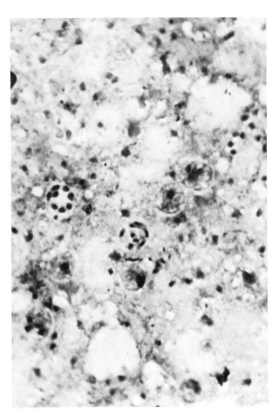

Figure 100-2 *Pneumocystis carinii* stained with polychrome methylene blue. Intracystic sporozoites are visualized, but the cyst wall is not stained. Sporozoites measure 1–2 μm in diameter. From Hughes, W.T. In: *Practice of pediatrics,* Vol. 2. Kelly, V.C., (editor). Hagerstown, Md.: Harper & Row Pub., Inc., 1977.

cultures or in Vero cell culture. The organism does not enter the host cell, but instead attaches to its surface during a phase in the replicative cycle.

Specific antigenic components have not been elucidated, but infection elicits IgG and IgM antibody responses. No evidence for toxin production exists.

Pathogenesis

The portal of entry for *P carinii* has not been firmly established; however because it has been found in only the lung, with rare exception, inhalation is a likely mode of transmission. In some individuals, the organism may be dormant and sparsely dispersed in the lung, with no apparent host response (latent infection). In others, such as the immunocompromised host, the organism occurs in massive numbers, filling the alveolar spaces and eliciting an active response of the alveolar macrophages and phagocytosis. In debilitated infants, the alveolar septum is thickened with an interstitial plasma cell and lymphocyte infiltration. The infection results in impaired ventilation and severe hypoxia.

Clinical features are to some extent age-dependent. In premature and debilitated infants, onset is subtle with mild tachypnea. Within a week or so, respiratory distress is apparent, with marked tachypnea, flaring of the nasal alae, retractions, and cyanosis. The illness may last 4-6 weeks and has a mortality rate of 25%-50%. In the immunodeficient child or adult, onset is abrupt, with fever, tachypnea, and respiratory distress. Deterioration progresses to fatality in almost all cases if no treatment is given. In both types, arterial oxygen tension is low, arterial pH usually increased, and carbon dioxide retention usually does not occur.

Host Defenses

Disease from *P carinii* occurs, with rare exceptions, only when natural mechanisms of host defense are compromised. Pneumonitis has occurred in patients with B or T cell deficiency, or both, and it is a major infection in patients with the acquired immune deficiency syndrome (AIDS). Severe protein-caloric malnutrition alone may provoke the disease. Immunosuppressive drugs used for cancer or organ transplantation render the individual susceptible to *P carinii* pneumonitis. Both IgG and IgM antibody responses occur with infection or experimental immunization; however, humoral antibody does not protect against the disease. In the alveoli, active phagocytosis and digestion occur with alveolar macrophages. In infected infants, extensive plasma cell infiltration occurs in the alveolar septae, but this is not found in the immunosuppressed child or adult.

Epidemiology

The life cycle of *P carinii* has been studied in vitro in embryonic chick epithelial cell lung cultures. Here the trophozoite attaches to the host cell, enlarges to the cyst form, and detaches without entry into the host cell. The cyst matures, and intracystic sporozoites develop. Excystment occurs through single or multiple breaks in the cyst wall, releasing the sporozoites, which are then referred to as trophozoites. The life cycle in animals has not been described.

P carinii has been found in the lungs of rats, rabbits, mice, dogs, sheep, goats, guinea pigs, horses, and monkeys. The organism has been reported in lower animals and humans from all continents. Animal-to-animal transmission by the airborne route has been demonstrated. Because up to 70% of healthy individuals may have humoral antibody to *P carinii,* subclinical infection must be highly prevalent.

Diagnosis

Tachypnea and fever are consistent features of the pneumonitis, and diffuse bilateral alveolar disease can be observed by radiography. Diagnosis requires the identification of *P carinii* in pulmonary tissue. An open lung biopsy, needle aspiration of the lung, or other invasive techniques are required to obtain a specimen. The Gomori, Giemsa, Gram-Weigert, or toluidine blue O stains may be used to identify the organism. Serum antibody titers provide little diagnostic aid. The possibility that *P carinii* antigen can be detected in sera is under study; so far, the method has not proven to be particularly helpful in the diagnosis of the pneumonitis.

Control

Experimental studies show that immunization with *P carinii* does not protect the animal from pneumonitis; however, the disease can be prevented by prophylactic administration of trimethoprim-sulfamethoxazole.

Drugs available for therapy of *P carinii* pneumonitis are pentamidine isethionate and trimethoprim-sulfamethoxazole. The two are equally effective, but trimethoprim-sulfamethoxazole is preferred because of its low toxicity.

References

Hughes, W.T.: A natural mode of aquisition for de novo infection with *Pneumocystis carinii*. *J Infect Dis* 1982; 145:842-848.

Hughes, W.T., et al.: Comparison of pentamidine isethionate and trimethoprim-sulfamethoxazole in the treatment of *Pneumocystis carinii* pneumonia. *J Pediatr* 1978; 92:285-291.

Hughes, W.T., et al.: Successful chemoprophylaxis for *Pneumocystis carinii* pneumonitis. *N Engl J Med* 1977; 297:1419-1426.

Meuwissen, J.H.E., et al.: Parasitologic and serologic observations of infection with *Pneumocystis carinii* in humans. *J Infect Dis* 1977; 136:43-49.

Pifer, L., Hughes, W.T., Murphy, M.: Propagation of *Pneumocystis carinii in vitro. Pediatr Res* 1977; 11:305-316.

Pifer, L., et al.: *Pneumocystis carinii* infection: Evidence for high prevalence in normal and immunosuppressed children. *Pediatrics* 1978; 61:35-41.

Ruskin, J., Hughes, W.T.: *Pneumocystis carinii.* In *Infectious diseases of the fetus and newborn infant,* 2nd ed. Remington, J.S., Klein, J.O., (editors). Philadelphia: W.B. Saunders, 1983.

Stagno, S., et al.: *Pneumocystis carinii* pneumonitis in young immunocompetent infants. *Pediatrics* 1980; 66:56-62.

Walzer, P.D., et al.: *Pneumocystis carinii* pneumonia in the United States. *Ann Intern Med* 1974; 80:83-93.

101 Helminths: Structure, Classification, Growth, and Development

Gilbert A. Castro, PhD

General Concepts
Flukes (Trematodes)
Tapeworms (Cestodes)
Roundworms (Nematodes)
Helminth Structure and Development in Host–Parasite Relationships

General Concepts

Helminth is a general term meaning *worm*. Its usage, however, connotes parasitic forms within several taxonomic categories; the most important from a medical point of view are the Platyhelminthes (flatworms) and the Nematoda (roundworms). The strict zoologic classification, which reflects phylogenetic and evolutionary relationships in addition to speciation, is of no significant medical interest. In medically oriented schemes, helminths are classified for convenience as flukes, tapeworms (both are flatworms), or roundworms and, more definitively within these groups, according to the host organ in which they reside (for example, blood flukes, liver flukes, and intestinal roundworms). Structurally, helminths are multicellular invertebrates with several organ systems. In comparison to other parasites, their antigenic characteristics and physiology are complex. The life history of helminths contain several developmental stages. In some species, asexual reproduction takes place in the larval stages; the sexual reproduction occurs in the adult stage. This chapter presents the structure, growth, and development of flukes, tapeworms, and nematodes.

Flukes (Trematodes)

The structure and development of flukes are summarized in Figures 101-1 and 101-2. A dorsoventrally flattened body, bilateral symmetry, and a definite anterior end are features of platyhelminths in general and trematodes specifically. Flukes are leaf-shaped, ranging in length from a few millimeters to 7–8 centimeters. The "skin," or **tegument,** of the fluke is morphologically and physiologically complex. As adhesive organs for attachment to host tissue, flukes possess an oral sucker around the mouth and a ventral sucker or acetabulum. A body cavity is lacking. Organs are embedded in specialized connective tissue or parenchyma. Layers of somatic muscle permeate the parenchyma and attach to the tegument.

A muscular pharynx and esophagus characterize a well-developed alimentary canal. The intestine usually takes the form of a branched tube (secondary and tertiary branches may be present) composed of a single layer of epithelial cells. The main branches usually end blindly or, in a few species, open into an excretory vesicle. The excretory vesicle also accepts the two main lateral collecting ducts of the excretory system. This system is the protonephridial type with flame cells, which are anchored in the parenchyma, directing tissue filtrate through canals into the two main collecting ducts. A **flame cell** is a hollow terminal excretory cell in certain invertebrates that contains a beating (flamelike) group of cilia.

Except for the blood flukes, trematodes have male and female reproductive organs in the same individual (**hermaphroditism**). The male reproductive system usually consists of two testes with associated accessory glands and ducts leading to a **cirrus,** or penis equivalent, that extends into the common genital atrium. The female reproductive system consists of a single ovary with a seminal receptacle and **vitellaria,** or yolk glands, that connect with the oviduct as it expands into an ootype. The tubular uterus

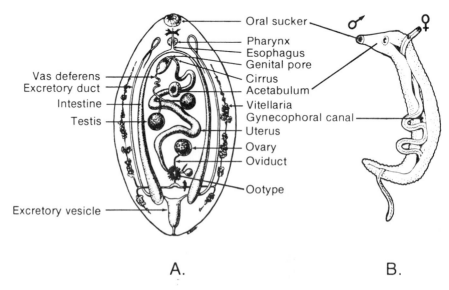

A.   B.

Figure 101-1 Structure of flukes. **A,** Hermaphroditic fluke. **B,** Bisexual fluke. From Hunter, G.W., Schwartzwelder, J.C., Clyde, D.F.: *A manual of tropical medicine,* 5th ed. Philadelphia: W.B. Saunders Co., 1976.

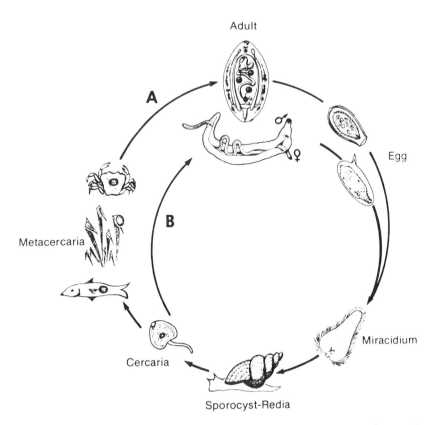

Figure 101-2 Generalized life cycle of flukes. **A,** Hermaphroditic fluke. **B,** Bisexual fluke. From Smyth, J.D.: *The physiology of trematodes.* Edinburgh: Oliver & Boyd Ltd., 1966; and from Hunter, G.W., Schwartzwelder, J.C., Clyde, D.F.: *A manual of tropical medicine,* 5th ed. Philadelphia: W.B. Saunders Co., 1976.

extends from the ootype and opens into a small cavity, the genital atrium. Both self- and cross-fertilization of ova take place. The components of the egg are assembled in the ootype. Eggs pass through the uterus into the genital atrium and exit ventrally through the genital pore. Fluke eggs, except for the schistosomes, are operculated.

The blood flukes, schistosomes, are the only bisexual flukes that develop in humans. Although the sexes are separate, the general structure is the same as that found in hermaphroditic flukes. Within the definitive host, the male and female worms inhabit the lumen of blood vessels and are found in close physical association. The female lies within a tegumental fold, or gynecophoral canal, on the ventral surface of the male.

Medically important flukes belong to the taxonomic category Digenea. This group of flukes has a developmental cycle requiring at least two hosts, the first being a snail. Depending on the species, other intermediate hosts may be involved before humans, the definitive hosts, become infected.

Flukes go through several larval stages, each with a specific name, before reaching adulthood. A generalized life cycle of digenetic flukes, taking into account the major variations among species, runs the following course. Eggs are passed in the feces, urine, or sputum of humans and reach an aquatic environment. The eggs either hatch, releasing ciliated larvae, **miracidia,** that penetrate a snail intermediate host, or they are eaten by a snail host. Either way, a nonciliated saclike sporocyst or redia stage develops from a miracidium within the tissues of the snail. The sporocyst gives rise to either rediae or to a daughter sporocyst stage. In turn, the redia or daughter sporocyst gives rise, asexually, to cercariae, which migrate out of snail tissues and enter the water.

The **cercariae,** which possess a tail for swimming, develop further in one of three ways: they penetrate the definitive host and transform directly into adults; they penetrate a second intermediate host, encyst, and develop as metacercariae; or they encyst on a substrate such as vegetation and develop as metacercariae. When a metacercarial cyst is ingested, the cyst wall is digested, liberating an immature fluke that migrates to a specific site and develops into an adult worm.

Tapeworms (Cestodes)

As members of the Platyhelminthes, the cestodes, or tapeworms, possess many basic structural characteristics of flukes, but also show striking differences. General features of structure and development of tapeworms are shown in Figure 101-3. Whereas flukes are flattened and generally leaf-shaped, adult tapeworms are flattened, elongated, and comprised of a few to numerous segments or proglottids. Tapeworms vary in length from 2-3 mm to 10 m, being made up of three to several thousand segments, or **proglottids.**

Anatomically, cestodes are divided into a **scolex,** or head, which bears the organs of attachment, a neck region immediately posterior to the scolex, and a chain of proglottids or the **strobila.** The **strobila** elongates with formation of new proglottids from the neck region. Proglottids nearest the neck are immature (sex organs not fully developed); those more posterior are mature. Terminal proglottids are gravid, with the egg-filled uterus as the most prominent feature.

Internally, the scolex contains the cephalic ganglion, the "brain" of the tapeworm nervous system. Externally, the scolex is characterized by holdfast organs. Depending on the species, these organs consist of bothria or acetabula, and in some cases a rostellum. **Bothria** are long, narrow grooves of weak muscularity, characteristic of the pseudophyllidean tapeworms. **Acetabula** (suckers like those of digenetic trematodes) are characteristic of cyclophyllidean tapeworms. A **rostellum** is a retractible, conelike structure located on the anterior end of the scolex that in some species is armed with hooks. Differential features of pseudophyllidean and cyclophyllidean tapeworms are listed in Table 101-1. Most human tapeworms are members of the cyclophyllidean group.

A characteristic feature of adult tapeworms is the absence of an alimentary canal, which is intriguing in view of the fact that all these adult worms inhabit the small intestine. The lack of an alimentary tract means that substances entering the tapeworm do so across the tegument. This structure appears well adapted for transport functions; it is covered with numerous microvilli resembling those lining the epithelial surface of the mammalian intestine. The excretory system is the flame cell type.

Cestodes are hermaphroditic, each proglottid possessing male and female reproductive systems similar to those of digenetic flukes. Differences are evident, however, between tapeworms and flukes in the mechanism of egg deposition. Eggs of pseudophyllidean tapeworms exit through a uterine pore in the center of the ventral

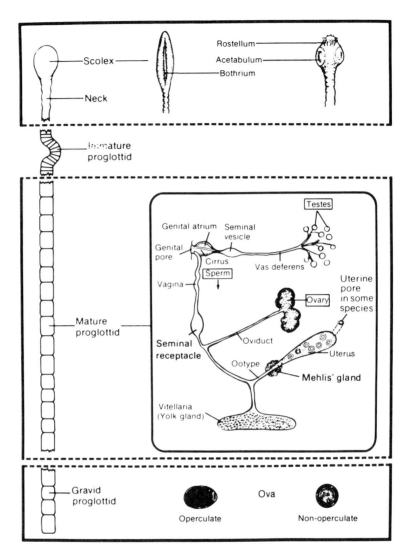

Figure 101–3 Structure of tapeworms. From Jeffrey, H.C., Leach, R.M.: *Atlas of medical helminthology and protozoology.* Edinburgh: Churchill Livingstone Ltd., 1968.

surface, rather than through the genital atrium as in flukes. In cyclophyllidean tapeworms, the female system includes a uterus without a uterine pore (see Figure 101-3). Thus, the cyclophyllidean eggs are released only when the tapeworms shed gravid proglottids into the intestine. Some proglottids disintegrate, releasing eggs that are voided in the feces, whereas others are passed intact.

The eggs of pseudophyllidean tapeworms are operculated, but those of cyclophyllidean species are not. Eggs of all tapeworms, however, contain at some stage of development an embryo with six hooks, that is, a hexacanth embryo, or **oncosphere**. The oncosphere of pseudophyllidean tapeworms is ciliated externally and is known as a

Table 101-1 Basic Differences Between Pseudophyllidean and Cyclophyllidean Tapeworms

Differentiating Feature	Pseudophyllidea	Cyclophyllidea
Scolex	Two sucking grooves (bothria)	Muscular suckers or acetabula
Genital pore	Located in center of each proglottid	Located at margin(s) of each proglottid; may be located on both sides in an irregular pattern (*Taenia* sp.), all on the same side (*Hymenolepis* sp.) or each proglottid may have a pore on each side (*Dipylidium caninum*).
Uterine pore	Located in center of proglottids on ventral surface	Absent; uterus ends blindly
Uterus (gravid)	Relatively long and coiled	Saclike, highly branched
Eggs (as voided from definitive host)	Operculate, immature	Nonoperculate, mature
Oncosphere	Ciliated (coracidium)	Nonciliated
Larvae	Procercoid and plerocercoid; both forms solid	Cysticercoid, cysticercus, hydatid; all forms cystic

coracidium. As the coracidium develops in its crustacean first intermediate host, it becomes a procercoid; and in its next intermediate host or hosts it becomes a plerocercoid larva, which develops into the adult worm in the definitive, final, host. The oncosphere of cyclophyllidean tapeworms, depending on the species, develops into a cysticercus larva, cysticercoid larva, coenurus larva, or hydatid larva (cyst) in specific intermediate hosts. These larvae, in turn, develop into adults in the definitive host. (See Chapter 104 for illustrations of these larval forms and representative life cycles.)

Roundworms (Nematodes)

Basic anatomic and developmental characteristics of nematodes are outlined in Figures 101-4 and 101-5. The nematode, in contrast to platyhelminths, is cylindrical rather than flattened. The body wall is composed of an outer cuticle (body covering) that is a noncellular structure, an underlying hypodermis, and musculature. The cuticle in some species has longitudinal ridges or alae. The copulatory bursa, a flaplike extension of the cuticle on the posterior end of male nematodes of certain species, is used to grasp the female during copulation.

The cellular hypodermis bulges into the body cavity or pseudocoelom to form four longitudinal cords—a dorsal, a ventral, and two lateral cords. The lateral cords may be seen on the surface as lateral lines. Nuclei of the hypodermis are located in the region of the cords. The somatic musculature lies beneath the hypodermis and is composed of a single layer of smooth muscle cells. These cells are separated, when viewed in cross-section, into four zones by the hypodermal cords. The musculature is innervated by extensions of muscle cells to nerve trunks running anteriorly and posteriorly from ganglion cells that ring the midportion of the esophagus.

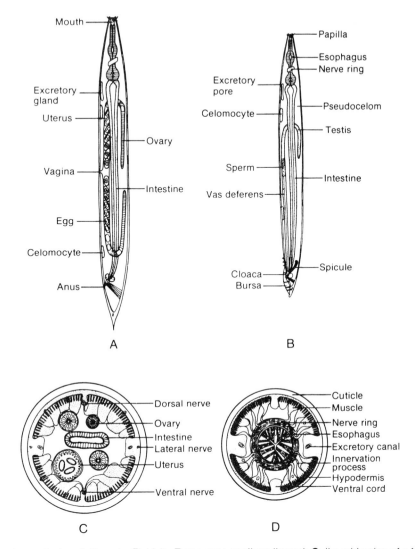

Figure 101-4 Structure of nematodes. **A,** Female. **B,** Male. Transverse sections through **C,** the midregion of a female worm, and **D,** the esophageal region. From Lee, D.L.: *The physiology of nematodes.* Edinburgh: Oliver & Boyd Ltd., 1965.

The space between the muscle layer and viscera is the pseudocoelom, which is unlined with mesothelium. This cavity contains fluid and fixed cells (celomocytes), which vary in number from two to six and are usually associated with the longitudinal cords. The function of celomocytes is not yet known.

The alimentary canal of roundworms is complete with mouth and anus. The mouth is surrounded by lips bearing sensory papillae, or bristles. The esophagus, a conspicuous feature of nematodes, is a muscular structure varying in shape with different species and functioning to pump food into the intestine. The intestine is a tubular structure

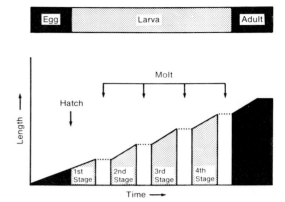

Figure 101-5 Generalized life cycle showing growth and development of a nematode. From Lee, D.L.: *The physiology of nematodes.* Edinburgh: Oliver & Boyd Ltd., 1965.

constituted of a single layer of columnar cells possessing prominent microvilli on their apical surface.

The excretory system of some nematodes usually consists of an excretory gland and pore located ventrally in the midesophageal region. In other nematodes, this structure is drawn into extensions that presumably give rise to the more complex tubular excretory system. This is usually H-shaped, with two anterior limbs and two posterior limbs located in the lateral cords. The gland cells and tubes are thought to serve as absorptive bodies, collecting wastes from the pseudocoelom, and to function in osmoregulation.

Nematodes usually are bisexual, males being distinguishable from females by their smaller size, curved posterior end, and (for some species) the presence of copulatory structures such as spicules (usually two) or a bursa, or both. The males have one (in most cases) or two testes. Each is at the free end of a convoluted or recurved tube leading into a seminal vesicle and eventually into the cloaca.

The female system is tubular also, and usually consists of two reflexed ovaries. Each ovary is continuous with an oviduct and tubular uterus. The uteri join to form the vagina, which in turn opens to the exterior through the vulva.

Copulation between a female and a male nematode is necessary for fertilization, except in the genus *Strongyloides,* in which parthenogenetic development occurs. **Parthenogenesis** is the development of an unfertilized egg into a new individual. Some evidence exists that sex attractants (pheromones) play a role in heterosexual mating. During copulation, sperm is transferred into the vulva of the female. The sperm enters the ovum and a fertilization membrane is secreted by the zygote. This membrane gradually thickens to form the chitinous shell. A second membrane, referred to as the vitelline membrane, is secreted by the zygote within the shell. This membrane makes the egg impervious to essentially all substances except carbon dioxide and oxygen. In some species, as the egg passes down the uterus, a third proteinaceous membrane may be secreted by the uterine wall and deposited outside the shell.

The life cycle of nematodes consists of egg, larval, and adult stages. Most nematodes parasitic in animals lay eggs that, when voided, may contain an uncleaved zygote, a group of blastomeres, or a completely formed larva. Some nematodes such as the filariae and *Trichinella spiralis* produce larvae that are deposited in host tissues.

As in arthropods, the growth process in nematodes is accompanied by molting.

Each of the four larval stages is followed by a molt. After the first molt, larvae are called second-stage larvae, and so on (see Figure 101-5). The nematode formed at the fifth stage is the adult.

Helminth Structure and Development in Host–Parasite Relationships

Sustenance, growth, and development of helminths depend on food: an energy source, carbon source, nitrogen source, minerals, and growth factors such as vitamins. The dependency of a helminth on its host apparently is related to some physiologic or biochemical inadequacy that prevents growth and development in a free-living state. It is axiomatic that to remain healthy the host must adapt to any parasite-induced nutritional drain or stress. If it does not, homeostasis is altered, and disease ensues. Knowledge of structural and functional adaptations evolved by helminths to sustain themselves, and knowledge of growth and developmental patterns, provide a basis for definitive diagnosis and give insight into the pathogenic nature of helminths.

References

Ash, L., Orihel, T.C.: *Atlas of human parasitology.* Chicago: American Society of Clinical Pathology, 1980.

Fairbairn, D.: Biochemical adaptations and loss of genetic capacity in helminth parasites. *Biol Rev* 1970; 45:29-72.

Hunter, G.W., Swartzwelder, J.D., Clyde, D.F.: *A manual of tropical medicine,* 5th ed. Philadelphia: W.B. Saunders Co., 1976.

Jeffrey, H.C., Leach, R.M.: *Atlas of medical helminthology and protozoology.* Edinburgh: Churchill Livingstone Ltd., 1968.

Lee, D.L.: *The physiology of nematodes.* Edinburgh: Oliver and Boyd Ltd., 1965.

Rogers, W.P.: *The nature of parasitism.* New York: Academic Press, 1962.

Smyth, J.D.: *The physiology of trematodes.* Edinburgh: Oliver and Boyd Ltd., 1966.

Smyth, J.D.: *The physiology of cestodes.* Edinburgh: Oliver and Boyd Ltd., 1969.

Schmidt, G.D., Roberts, L.S.: *Foundations of parasitology,* 2nd ed. St. Louis: The C.V. Mosby Co., 1981.

Zaman, V.: *Atlas of medical parasitology.* Philadelphia: Lea and Febiger, 1979.

102 Helminths: Pathogenesis and Defenses

Norman F. Weatherly, PhD

General Concepts
Host–Parasite Factors
  Host Factors Influencing Susceptibility
  Parasite Factors Influencing Susceptibility
Pathogenic Mechanisms
  Harmful Effects Related to Host Nutrition
  Harmful Effects on Host Blood and Blood
    Formation

Destruction of Host Tissues
Tissue Damage from Migrations
Damage Caused by Toxic Secretions and
  Excretions
Abnormal Growths Associated with Helminth
  Infections
Insusceptibility to Host Response

General Concepts

Helminths, like microbes, can gain entrance into the human body, survive, and cause disease. The mechanisms of pathogenesis and host defense probably are similar in most helminthic infections. Peculiarities of helminths are their large size, methods of host penetration, and migrational ability, which are not found in other infectious agents. These differences may account for some of the more unusual pathologic effects, such as intestinal blockage and some of the apparent inefficiencies of the host defense system. Many helminths can reside in human tissues and intestines for long periods, even though the individual may be found immunocompetent by various in vivo and in vitro tests. Infections range from a symptomatic to lethal. Several host-derived factors influence the course of these infections.

    Factors that determine whether a helminth can cause disease are often unclear. All stages in the development of the organisms may cause disease. The migratory pathways and feeding habits of the parasite also play a role in production of disease. The pathogens damage or destroy tissues and organs by physical trauma, toxic secretions, or immunologic injury. Until those factors that make an individual helminth species pathogenic for its particular host are understood, complete control of these infections will not be possible.

Host–Parasite Factors

Host Factors Influencing Susceptibility

Helminthic infections can be harmless and asymptomatic in one host, yet lead to disease and even death in another. The results of an infection depend on the interaction between the host and the helminth, with characteristics of both partners contributing to the outcome of an infection. The number of worms present in the host also is a factor in the severity of the infection. This interaction should not be viewed as static, but rather as dynamic and constantly changing. If the host gains the advantage, the parasite dies and is expelled from the intestine or it is walled off and destroyed in a tissue site. On the other hand, if the parasite wins the conflict, disease and death may ensue, even though demise of the host is disadvantageous to the parasite. Fortunately, most human helminthic infections are thought to be asymptomatic; only when the parasites have gained the upper hand are the infections brought to the attention of the physician. It is not known what proportion of severe infections seen by clinicians are due to some host genetic deficiency or compromised state. The recent increase in disseminated and overwhelming *Strongyloides stercoralis* infections illustrates this point dramatically. Some host factors that influence susceptibility to infection and disease are age, sex, diet and nutritional status, stress—emotional as well as the physiologic stressful conditions of pregnancy and lactation—prior medical treatment, and genetics. In general, susceptibility is greater in the young and in men than it is in women, except for those who are pregnant and lactating; also, susceptibility is greater in those who are malnourished and stressed. These various conditions of increased susceptibility (immunosuppression) are considered to be mediated by corticosteroids (for stress), sex hormones, protein shortages (for malnutrition), and, possibly, prolactin or other lactogenic hormones (during pregnancy and lactation).

Parasite Factors Influencing Susceptibility

The student of infectious diseases must know as much as possible about the properties of helminths to appreciate their success. Helminthic factors affecting pathogenesis are genetics, virulence, reproductive pattern, host contact history, habitat in humans, size, feeding method, migrational ability, and length of life. The last four factors are somewhat peculiar to helminth parasites and should be emphasized. The size of adult helminths ranges from millimeters (*Enterobius, Trichinella, Strongyloides, Clonorchis*) to centimeters (*Trichuris, Ascaris, Hymenolepis, Fasciolopsis*) and even to meters (*Taenia, Diphyllobothrium*). Although some exceptions occur, size is related to longevity; larger worms survive longer. Possibly, the host's immune response cannot deal as effectively with large organisms as it can with small organisms.

The body sometimes walls off the parasites in an attempt to localize and destroy the invader. This is difficult if not impossible to do to many helminths, because of their migrational abilities. Also, many nematode and trematode parasites ingest inflammatory cells and exudates. Thus, size, migrational abilities, and the ingestion of host tissues including inflammatory exudates, may partially account for the abilities of many helminths to reside for long periods in humans. The pathogenesis of helminthic infections largely results from these long periods of residency, during which tissues sustain continuing damage from feeding, migrations, and a continual outpouring of antigenic material.

The larval and juvenile stages of helminths also contribute significantly to pathology. For example, a number of nematode larvae, after penetrating through the skin or the intestinal wall, use a migratory pathway that includes the liver, heart, and lungs. Some of these larvae may reside in the liver and lungs for days before completing their migrations to the final habitat. Other larvae become lodged in tissues, such as the brain, eye, bones, and other vital organs, where, depending on the site, they may cause serious and even lethal damage.

Pathogenic Mechanisms

Harmful Effects Related to Host Nutrition

Much has been written about the interactions between infection and nutrition; however, little is understood about this relationship. Controversy therefore arises over whether parasitism causes malnutrition or whether the malnourished become more susceptible to infection. Whatever the etiology, the association is commonly observed, especially in the lower socioeconomic groups in developing countries.

Some researchers think that helminths may "rob" their hosts of food. This idea most likely arose from the observation that the severely malnourished persons may harbor large worm burdens, and the size of some of the helminths suggests that they are competing with the host for nutritional substance. Most research does not support this concept; on the contrary, inappetence (or going "off feed") appears to be a factor contributing to malnourishment, in addition to nausea, vomiting, and diarrhea.

Malabsorptive states frequently are associated with helminthic infections. A number of nematodes, such as *Strongyloides* and *Trichinella*, are true tissue parasites; they live embedded in the intestinal mucosa. Because of burrowing and feeding activities, cellular infiltration, edema, atrophy of the mucosal layer, and blunting of the villi occur. Other nematodes, such as the hookworms, reside in the lumen of the small intestine, where they live attached to the intestinal villi. Villi are damaged, blood and fluid accumulate, and the intestinal folds widen and thicken. Chronic inflammation, caused by the action of the nematode alone or, frequently, by secondary microbial infection, may lead to impaired absorption of materials. In addition to adult helminths, eggs and larvae of helminths can also contribute to malabsorptive states. Two examples are the newborn larvae of *Trichinella* on their way to entering the vascular system, and the eggs of schistosomes in various tissues. The latter condition, in which granulomatous reactions occur around the eggs, results in hyperplasia, fibrosis, and scarring, which most likely interfere with proper absorption.

Numerous helminths in the adult, larval, or egg stage, reside in the liver for short or long periods of time. Depending on the parasite and its stage, mechanical destruction of liver tissues, hyperplasia, hypertrophy, and inflammatory responses alter the liver's capacity to function normally. Granulomatous reactions, fibrosis, cirrhosis, jaundice, and fatty degeneration are not uncommon manifestations. At times, as in *Echinococcus*-induced disease, an entire lobe may be rendered useless. Any or all of these may exacerbate the harmful effects of malabsorption.

Harmful Effects on Host Blood and Blood Formation

The feeding habits of many helminths, especially *Fasciola, Trichuris,* and hookworms, can produce anemia, the degree of which depends on such factors as worm burden, size and age of host, and the general state of host nutrition.

The chronic loss of erythrocytes due to feeding activity of helminths such as hookworms may deplete iron stores and cause iron deficiency anemia. *Diphyllobothrium latum,* if attached high in the small intestine of some individuals, may interfere with normal vitamin B_{12} absorption, causing vitamin B_{12} deficiency and megaloblastic anemia. The cestode, by elaborating releasing factor, causes the uncoupling of vitamin B_{12} from intrinsic factor, so that the vitamin cannot be absorbed by the host. Although the cestode accumulates relatively large amounts of vitamin B_{12}, the biologic function of this vitamin in the helminth is not known.

Destruction of Host Tissues

Helminths often damage or destroy a wide variety of host tissues. This destruction can be caused by feeding activities, mechanical blockage, pressure atrophy, migrational activities, and toxic secretions. More often than not, a single helminthic species may cause tissue destruction by more than one of these means.

Helminths can be generally classified into those that are **absorbers, chyme ingesters, browsers,** or **tissue liquifiers.** All cestodes (adults as well as larvae), some trematodes (such as schistosomes), and some nematodes (filariae) are thought to absorb all or significant amounts of their nutritional materials. This type of feeding results in little, if any, direct damage to host tissues. Chyme ingesters, such as adult *Ascaris* and *Enterobius,* also do not produce much pathology, because they feed on the semidigested food in the intestinal tract.

Browsers and tissue liquifiers, on the other hand, can cause considerable tissue destruction. Many trematodes found in the liver and bile ducts actually feed on liver parenchyma or bile duct mucosa. This provokes inflammation, hyperplasia, and fibrotic changes. Hookworms browse on the mucosa of the intestinal villi. While the helminth is feeding, it secretes histolytic enzymes and anticoagulants that add to the damage. Tissue liquifiers, those helminths such as *Trichinella* and *Strongyloides* that invade tissues, damage tissue by their penetration activities and by the secretion of histolytic enzymes. In general, cells are damaged mechanically or enzymatically; the liquified material is then taken up by the helminth.

Host tissue also may be damaged or altered as a result of mechanical blockage. In addition to the tissue damage, organ dysfunction may occur, as illustrated by the following examples. Blockage of the small bowel may result from heavy *Ascaris* infections, or infections with *Diphyllobothrium latum.* Numerous reports in the literature indicate that aberrant *Ascaris* migrations can cause blockage of the bile and pancreatic ducts. *Fasciola* and *Clonorchis* infections also are known to be associated with blocked bile ducts; in these situations, hyperplasia of the bile duct epithelium is thought to contribute to the blockage. Elephantiasis of limbs, scrotums, and breasts may result from blockage of various parts of the lymphatic system by the nematode *Wuchereria*. In this infection, adult worms become lodged in lymphatic sites and, in hypersensitive individuals, a striking proliferation of connective tissue assists in the blockage of lymph flow, causing massive edema, hypertrophy, and hyperplasia.

Pressure atrophy is characteristic of some larval cestode infections in humans. Unilocular hydatid disease, seen most commonly in sheep raisers, usually manifests itself as primary cysts in the liver. As these cysts grow, liver tissue undergoes atrophy and pressure necrosis. Secondary cysts, usually in the lung and brain, cause increased pressure that produces jacksonian epilepsy; renal cysts cause hematuria and kidney dysfunction. Multilocular hydatid cyst, the larval stage of *Echinococcus multilocularis*, also may be present in humans. Rather than being restricted by a strong cyst wall, cyst growth is neoplastic, and metastases frequently occur by direct extensions or through the lymph and blood vessels. Although multilocular cysts usually are present in the liver, where damage is due to pressure necrosis, untreatable osseous infections also occur. In the bone, the parasite replaces the hemopoietic tissue in the marrow.

An especially dangerous infection is cysticercosis, caused by the larval stage of *Taenia solium*. Cysticerci may develop in any organ of the body, including the eye and brain. Eye infections may result in loss of vision, and brain cysts may produce cerebral edema, obstruction of the flow of cerebrospinal fluid, and other devastating effects. Convulsions resembling those of epilepsy, severe headache, and local paralysis usually precede death.

Tissue Damage from Migrations

Many helminths gain entrance into the body by larvae penetrating through the skin or mucous membranes of the oral cavity. Also, in many orally acquired infections, larvae must first penetrate the intestinal tissues and then make a vascular or somatic migration before reaching the site required by the adult worm. These migrations damage tissue directly and initiate hypersensitivity reactions. Organs most affected during such migrations are the liver, lungs, and intestines. Petechial hemorrhages, pneumonitis, eosinophilia, pruritus, hepatomegaly, splenomegaly, granulomatous lesions, urticaria, myositis, and numerous other pathologies and signs and symptoms are produced during helminthic infections. These migrations, which disrupt the integrity of various tissues, allow a wide variety of secondary microbial infections to become established. Indeed, some helminths act as vectors of various pathogenic microbes.

Damage Caused by Toxic Secretions and Excretions

Many helminthic parasites elaborate substances that may interfere with the normal physiologic activities of the host, as well as cause cellular and tissue destruction, suggested by the observation that clinical manifestations of infections include vomiting, anorexia, bed wetting, fretfulness, and various neurologic disorders. Tissue and cellular damage results from the excretion or secretion of various enzymes.

Abnormal Growths Associated with Helminth Infections

Hyperplasia usually occurs after any inflammatory reaction and repair of damaged tissue. Because helminths cause extensive damage, the fact that hyperplasia is a common response during many of these infections is not surprising. Hyperplasia of the bladder and intestinal walls is caused by the presence of schistosome eggs, of bile ducts (from *Fasciola* and *Clonorchis*), and of the lymphatic endothelium (from *Wuchereria*).

Metaplasia is reported as a consequence of lung fluke (*Paragonimus*) infection in humans. In this infection, the columnar ciliated epithelium of the bronchi changes to a cuboidal, nonciliated, replicating type.

Both benign and malignant types of neoplasia frequently are associated with helminthic infections. Colonic papilloma and liver granulomas in patients infected with schistosomes are examples of benign neoplasias. Lymphomas have been seen in patients infected with *Strongyloides;* other malignant neoplasias (sarcomas and squamous cell carcinomas of the bladder) have been reported in some patients infected with *S haematobium*. Numerous hypotheses such as carcinogenic excretion, enhancing antibody, and chronic irritation have been proposed to explain this association between helminth and neoplasms; however, no definitive answers are yet available, and no cause-effect relationship has been convincingly demonstrated between the helminths of humans and cancer.

Insusceptibility to Host Response

Long periods of worm survival in otherwise immunocompetent hosts is one of the peculiarities of many helminthic infections. The worms' large size and migrational behavior may account for this characteristic as may some other evasion mechanisms. One that has received considerable attention is the ability of some helminths, such as the schistosomes, to acquire or develop body surfaces that are similar in nature to host proteins, thus making the worm's surface nonantigenic (antigenic mimicry). According to another theory, helminths, being metazoan animals, secrete and excrete large quantities of antigenic materials, and thus large volumes of antibodies are produced by the host. These antibodies, being defective or incapable of killing the helminth, coat and, in effect, mask the parasite (enhancing antibody). Anticomplementary secretions by young cestode cysticerci, cytotoxic secretions by *Trichinella,* and change of metabolic pathways by nematode parasites also have been reported to contribute to long survival times. Finally, some nematode larvae may migrate to fatty tissues and remain dormant until the density of adult organisms decreases in the intestine before completing their life cycle; immunosuppression of the host also can trigger the maturation process. This phenomenon is known to occur in hookworm and some *Strongyloides* infections of domestic animals, but it has not been investigated fully in humans. It may account for the isolated reports in the literature of, for example, intestinal infections with hookworms in babies 1-2 months old. In these situations, dormant larvae, triggered by some stimulus during lactation, may enter the nursing baby through the milk of a nursing mother.

References

Binford, C.H., Connor, D.H.: *Pathology of tropical and extraordinary diseases: An atlas,* Vol 2. Washington, D.C.: Armed Forces Institute of Pathology, 1976.

Brown, H.A., Neva, F.A.: *Basic clinical parasitology.* Norwalk, Connecticut: Appleton-Century-Crofts, 1983.

Manson-Bahr, P.E.C., Apted, F.I.C.: *Manson's tropical diseases,* 18th ed. London: Bailliere Tindall, 1982.

Mims, C.A.: *The pathogenesis of infectious disease,* 2nd ed. New York: Academic Press, 1982.

Soulsby, E.J.L., (editor): *Pathophysiology of parasitic infection.* New York: Academic Press, 1976.

Strickland, G.T.: *Hunter's tropical medicine,* 6th ed. Philadelphia: W. B. Saunders Co., 1984.

Warren, K.S., Mahmoud, A.A.F.: *Tropical and geographical medicine.* New York: McGraw-Hill Book Co., 1984.

103 Schistosomes and Other Trematodes

Kenneth S. Warren, MD

General Concepts
Distinctive Properties
Pathogenesis
Host Defenses
Epidemiology
Diagnosis
Control

General Concepts

Trematodes, or flukes, are parasitic flatworms with unique life cycles involving sexual reproduction in mammalian and other vertebrate definitive hosts, and asexual reproduction in snail intermediate hosts. These organisms are characterized by their final habitats in humans according to the following four anatomic categories: (1) the hermaphroditic liver flukes, which reside in the bile ducts and infect humans on ingestion of watercress (*Fasciola*) or raw fish (*Clonorchis* and *Opisthorchis*); (2) the hermaphroditic intestinal fluke (*Fasciolopsis*), which infects humans on ingestion of water chestnuts; (3) the hermaphroditic lung fluke (*Paragonimus*), which infects humans on ingestion of raw crabs or crayfish; and (4) the bisexual blood flukes (*Schistosoma*), which live in the intestinal or vesical venules and infect humans by direct penetration through the skin.

Fascioliasis is a cosmopolitan zoonosis; sporadic cases in humans have appeared in most parts of the world. The remainder of the hermaphroditic fluke infections of humans are confined largely to Asia. Schistosomiasis occurs in South America, the Caribbean, Africa, the Middle East, and Asia and is spreading in many areas due to the introduction of dams and irrigation systems.

Note that flukes do not multiply in humans, that intensity of infection is related to degree of exposure to the infective larvae, that in most endemic areas the majority of cases have light or moderate worm burdens, and that overt disease occurs largely in the relatively small proportion of those with heavy worm burdens, although genetic predisposition may also play a role. Pathogenicity may be due to the worms themselves (as with liver flukes, which damage the bile ducts) or their eggs (for example, schistosome eggs, which induce granulomatous inflammation in the venules or tissues). Treatment of all fluke infections has been greatly improved by the introduction of praziquantel.

Distinctive Properties

The flukes of medical importance undergo two different modes of reproduction: sexual, in the definitive host (humans); and asexual, in the intermediate host (snails). This complex life cycle was first worked out for *Fasciola hepatica*, a liver fluke, which predominantly infects ruminants and incidentally infects humans. This inch-long, hermaphroditic flatworm resides in the bile ducts of the liver, where it produces large numbers of eggs daily over a period of many years. The eggs pass into the lumen of the small intestine and out of the body in the feces. If deposited in fresh water, the eggs hatch into ciliated miracidia, which on penetration into certain species of snails, undergo several developmental stages that produce large numbers of cercariae. These tailed, free-swimming organisms leave the snail and encyst as metacercariae on the leaves of freshwater plants. When ingested by the definitive host, the larvae excyst, penetrate through the gut wall into the peritoneal cavity, enter the liver capsule, and begin to wander through the hepatic tissues. This migratory phase continues for about 7 weeks, after which the half-grown flukes penetrate the bile ducts, where they mature and begin to produce eggs.

Clonorchis sinensis, Opisthorchis felineus, and *O viverrini* are also liver flukes (Figure 103-1); in their case, the eggs hatch only after ingestion by certain species of snails, and the cercariae penetrate under the scales or into the flesh of certain freshwater fish, where they encyst as metacercariae. After they are ingested in raw or inadequately cooked fish, the organisms excyst within the duodenum and, in contrast to *F hepatica*, pass directly into the bile ducts through the ampulla of Vater.

Figure 103-1 Life cycle of liver fluke.
A. Final host: Human, cat, dog, and household and farm animals
  1. Sexually mature liver fluke
  2. Egg (with miracidium) of *Clonorchis sinensis*

B. 1. Intermediate hosts: snails of the genus *Bulimus* (= *Bythinia*) and others
  3. (a) Young sporocyst
     (b) Mother redia
     (c) Daughter redia with rudiments of cercariae
  4. Cercariae that have become free

C. 2. Intermediate host: chiefly Cyprinidae
  5. Fish with cercariae
  6. Metacercariae (greatly magnified)

  I. *Clonorchis sinensis* (magnified about 5:1)
  II. *Opisthorchis felineus* (magnified about 7:1)
  IIa. Egg of *O felineus* with miracidium
  III. Free miracidium from snail
  IV. Cercaria as it typically appears when swimming

From Piekarski, G.: *Medical parasitology*. Heidelberg: Springer Verlag, p. 68.

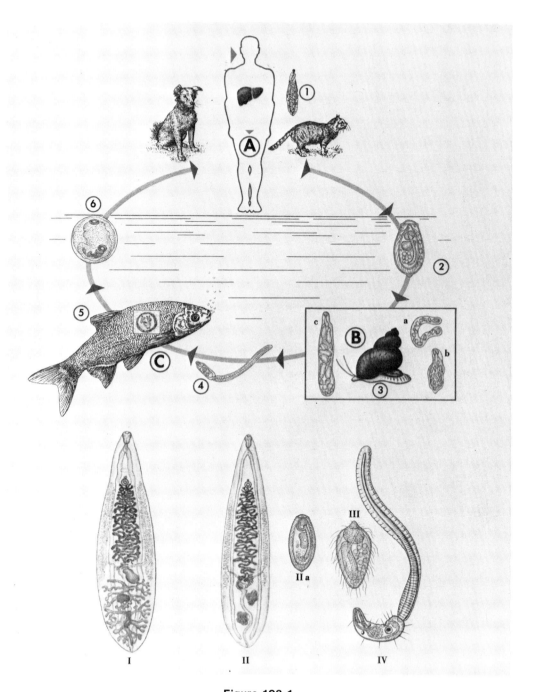

Figure 103-1

(See legend on facing page)

The cercariae of *Fasciolopsis buski*, the intestinal fluke, encyst on certain species of water plants. When ingested, the metacercariae excyst within the duodenum, attach to the nearby intestinal wall, develop into adult worms, and begin egg production. The eggs pass out in the feces into fresh water, where the hatched miracidia penetrate into snails within which the cercariae develop.

The eggs of *Paragonimus westermani*, the lung fluke, pass into the bronchioles, are coughed up, and are voided in the sputum or swallowed and passed in the feces. After undergoing a period of embryonation, the eggs hatch and the miracidia penetrate into certain species of freshwater snails. Cercariae develop within the snails, and then pass out and penetrate into crustaceans where they encyst. When inadequately cooked freshwater crayfish and crabs are ingested, the metacercariae excyst in the duodenum, penetrate the intestinal wall, and enter the peritoneal cavity from whence they migrate through the diaphragm and pleural cavity into the lungs.

Three major species of schistosomes infect humans: *S mansoni, S japonicum,* and *S haematobium* (Figure 103-2). The adult schistosomes are flukes of both sexes that reside in human mesenteric and vesical venules. The fertilized female worms produce large numbers of eggs, which pass out of the blood vessels, through the tissues, and into the lumen of the gut (*S mansoni* and *S japonicum*) or the urinary bladder (*S haematobium*). After a period of asexual multiplication in snails, the cercariae pass out into water, from which they directly penetrate into human skin. The young schistosomes migrate from the skin to the lungs and then to the hepatoportal system, where they mature, mate, and pass down into the mesenteric or vesical venules.

Pathogenesis

Fascioliasis in humans and animals has two distinct clinical phases. The first occurs in the initial 6-9 weeks of infection, when the larvae are migrating within the liver; the second begins when the larvae enter the bile ducts. The acute clinical syndrome is characterized by prolonged fever, pain in the right hypochondrium, and sometimes hepatomegaly, asthenia, and urticaria; a marked eosinophilia usually is seen during this period. Asymptomatic acute infection has been reported in England and seems to be common in Peru. After the flukes enter the bile ducts, the symptoms appear to decline and disappear completely. Although animals with particularly heavy worm burdens may

Figure 103-2 Life cycle of schistosome.
A. Final host: Humans. Site of the worms: the mesenteric vessels
1. (a) Sexually mature pair of flukes of *S mansoni*
   (b) Mature egg of *S mansoni* (lateral spine)
2. Miracidium
B. Intermediate host: aquatic snails (Planorbidae, for example, *Planorbis boissyi, Australorbis glabratus*)
3. (a) Sporocyst of the first order (mother sporocyst)
   (b) Sporocyst of the second order (daughter sporocyst)
4. Free cercaria (forked-tail cercaria)

I. *S haematobium*: egg with miracidium (terminal spine); shells of the intermediate hosts of the species:
   a. *Bulinus truncatus* (North Africa)
   b. *Bulinus globosa* (West Africa)
II. *S japonicum*: egg with miracidium (very small lateral spine); shells of intermediate hosts of the genera:
   a. *Schistosomophora*
   b. *Oncomelania*
   c. *Katayama*
From Pierarski, G.: *Medical parasitology.* Heidelberg: Springer-Verlag, p. 80.

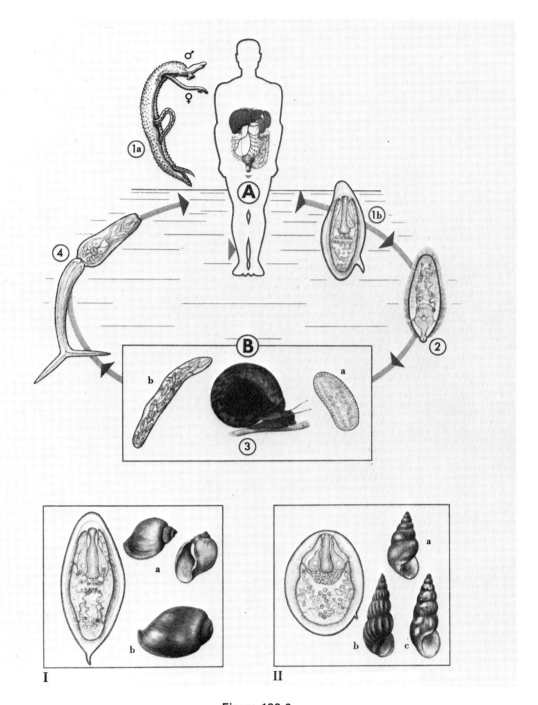

Figure 103-2

(See legend on facing page)

develop chronic biliary tract disease, this condition has been rarely reported in humans, usually as an incidental finding at surgery or autopsy.

In contrast, clonorchiasis and opisthorchiasis do not cause an acute syndrome, as the larval flukes enter directly into the bile ducts. Most individuals with *Clonorchis* and *Opisthorchis* infections show no significant signs or symptoms of disease when compared with uninfected matched control groups. Pathologic studies have revealed no gross changes in the liver in milder early infections. Despite these generally negative findings, patients with severe chronic disease—cholangitis, cholangiohepatitis, and cholangiocarcinoma—may filter through to hospital centers.

Fasciolopsiasis also appears to be associated with few or no manifestations of disease in individuals examined in field environments. In a controlled study involving clinical examination, evaluation of growth and development, hematologic studies, and screening tests for intestinal malabsorption, no significant differences from uninfected subjects were found. Cases of severe clinical illness characterized by diarrhea, abdominal pain, edema (often facial), and passage of undigested food in the feces have been reported, however, in patients with heavy infections.

Paragonimiasis usually comes to the attention of the physician when the patient complains of cough or intermittent hemoptysis. Profuse expectoration and chest pain of a pleuritic type are also found. Nevertheless, clinical studies of groups of individuals indicate that, in most endemic areas, the majority of infections are light or moderate and are associated with few signs or symptoms. Cerebral paragonimiasis is encountered in highly endemic regions and is manifested as jacksonian epilepsy, tumors, or embolism of the brain.

Three major disease syndromes occur in schistosomiasis: schistosome dermatitis, acute schistosomiasis, and chronic schistosomiasis. The first is a pruritic rash that appears after repeated exposure to cercariae, usually those of birds and small mammals. Acute schistosomiasis or Katayama fever begins between 4-8 weeks after primary exposure and lasts for just a few weeks. It appears most commonly in *S japonicum* infection, is much less common in *S mansoni* infections, and is seen rarely in patients with schistosomiasis haematobia. This syndrome is an acute febrile illness with cough, hepatosplenomegaly, lymphadenopathy, and eosinophilia; it may be fatal.

A wide variety of symptoms has been associated with chronic schistosomiasis; these include fatigue, abdominal pain, and intermittent diarrhea or dysentery in *S japonicum* and *S mansoni* infection, and dysuria in *S haematobium* infection. Recent field studies of schistosomiasis mansoni and japonica, however, have demonstrated few symptoms even in patients with heavy infections. Nevertheless, in a significant proportion of patients (usually those with heavy worm loads), the chronic stage may reveal itself eventually by the development of significant disease. In areas of high prevalence and intensity of schistosomiasis haematobia, intravenous pyelography reveals renal (hydronephrosis), ureteral, and bladder lesions in large proportions of school children.

Fewer than one-half the schistosome eggs pass out of the body; the rest remain in the local tissues or pass through the bloodstream into other organ systems, where they are sieved out as the veins decrease in caliber. These eggs elicit a marked granulomatous reaction, which results in considerable destruction of tissue and fibrosis. In schistosomiasis japonica and mansoni, egg embolization of the liver may result in an intrahepatic presinusoidal block that leads to portal hypertension and esophageal varices. The liver parenchymal cells are not harmed directly by the disease process; therefore, liver function tests are usually within or close to normal limits, and no stigmata of chronic hepatic disease are seen. Clinically, the earliest sign of involvement of the liver is hepatomegaly, which may be followed by the development of an enlarged, firm spleen. The major complication of hepatosplenic schistosomiasis is bleeding esophageal varices as manifested by hematemesis.

In schistosomiasis haematobia, disease is due to obstruction to urine flow that results from florid granuloma formation around masses of *S haematobium* eggs, and from fibrosis in the ureters and bladder. This may lead to hydronephrosis and, eventually, uremia. Symptoms may also be related to reduced distensibility of the bladder because of calcification of the eggs and scarring. Incidence of cancer of the bladder is said to be increased.

Patients with severe hepatosplenic schistosomiasis and portal systemic collateral circulation may develop pulmonary involvement as eggs bypass the liver and are trapped in the lungs, leading to pulmonary hypertension and cor pulmonale. Involvement of the central nervous system, although rare, is a major complication; it seems to be caused by the large masses of eggs laid by ectopic worm pairs. *S japonicum* tends to localize within the brain and is associated with the development of focal epilepsy or diffuse cerebral disease, whereas *S mansoni* and *S haematobium* usually are found in the spinal cord and are associated with a syndrome resembling transverse myelitis.

Host Defenses

Little is known about host defenses in the hermaphroditic fluke infections. In schistosomiasis, delayed hypersensitivity and a wide variety of antibodies have been demonstrated in experimental animals and in humans. Immunity has been demonstrated in some primates and laboratory animals, but resistance to reinfection has not been shown in humans. Although various mechanisms of acquired resistance have been seen in experimental animals, antibody-dependent cellular cytotoxicity, principally by eosinophils, has been demonstrated in animals in vivo and humans in vitro.

Schistosomiasis appears to be an immunologic disease caused by cell-mediated granulomatous hypersensitivity around the parasite eggs. An ameliorating factor is modulation of granuloma formation, which occurs naturally in chronic infection. This modulation is caused by antibody and suppressor cells.

Epidemiology

F hepatica infection occurs worldwide in ruminants and can cause significant morbidity and mortality in domesticated animals such as sheep and cattle. For the most part, human infection is sporadic, and only a few hundred cases have been reported in the world literature, usually associated with ingestion of wild watercress. Fascioliasis in humans has almost always been identified during the acute migratory stage of infection; occasionally, worms are found in the bile ducts at surgery or autopsy. Foci of chronic human fascioliasis have been found in rural areas of Peru.

C sinensis, O felineus, and *O viverrini* are common liver flukes of cats and dogs; they also infect many other mammalian hosts. Although humans are incidental hosts, millions of individuals are infected with these organisms. Clonorchiasis is prevalent in China, Hong Kong, Vietnam, Korea, and Taiwan. Infection with *O felineus* has been reported in many parts of Southeast Asia and Asia as well as Eastern Europe and the Soviet Union; infection with *O viverrini* is widespread in Thailand. Infection occurs after ingestion of raw or inadequately cooked or pickled freshwater fish (saltwater fish do not carry these parasites). *F buski* is a common parasite of humans and pigs in the Far East and Southeast Asia. Infection results from consumption of raw pods, roots, stems, or bulbs of certain water plants and is related to peeling of the metacercaria-infested hull of these vegetables with the teeth before consumption.

P westermani has a cosmopolitan distribution among mammals; human infection is found in the Far East. Closely related species have been reported in humans in Africa and South and Central America. Dietary habits are a major factor, because paragonimiasis is transmitted by eating uncooked freshwater crayfish or crabs.

Three different species of human schistosome parasites are responsible for 200 million infections. *S mansoni* occurs in South America, the Caribbean, and Africa; *S haematobium,* in Africa and the Middle East; and *S japonicum,* in the Far East. *S japonicum* is the only species that has significant animal reservoirs. Frequency and duration of water contact appear to be major influences on the prevalence and intensity of infection in schistosomiasis.

Within humans, the trematodes do not undergo direct replication, but produce large numbers of eggs that pass out of the body in the feces, urine, or sputum. Thus, humans have different intensities of infection, related largely to exposure to infective larvae—that is, the frequency of consumption of contaminated foods or of water exposure. Mathematical models suggest that the intensity of infection in mammalian populations follows a negative binomial distribution; the largest proportion of individuals have light-to-moderate infections. In recent years, controlled studies have revealed that most infected individuals show no overt signs or symptoms of disease. Significant disease, whether hepatic, intestinal, pulmonary, or vesical, occurs largely in the small proportion of individuals who are infected with large numbers of flukes.

Diagnosis

The anatomic locations of the symptoms and signs provide obvious means of deciding whether liver, intestinal, lung, or urinary fluke infection is possible. Except in the case of fascioliasis, the geographic history should be of particular value, because all other fluke infections of humans have relatively specific distributions. A careful dietary history is important in the case of the hermaphroditic flukes, and provides relatively clear-cut evidence. In schistosomiasis, significant contact with fresh water is important.

Demonstrating the eggs of the parasite in the feces provides a definitive diagnosis in all cases of fluke infection. Because the characteristic ova may be scanty, a concentration procedure is necessary. One method is the formol-ether technique involving mixture of feces with saline, centrifugation, decantation, addition of formalin and then ether, further centrifugation, and examination of the sediment. For schistosomiasis mansoni and japonica, the Kato thick-smear method (50 mg of feces placed on a slide covered with a plastic cover slip soaked in glycerol and allowed to clear for 24 hours) provides a quantitative estimate of egg output. For *S haematobium* infection, Nuclepore filtration of 10 mL of urine is the simplest and most rapid method. Most immunodiagnostic methods are not specific or sensitive enough to assess these infections.

Control

Fascioliasis can be prevented by using only watercress from protected commercial sources. Liver and lung fluke infection can be avoided by thorough cooking of freshwater fish and crustacea. The risk of these infections can be diminished by reduction of fecal contamination. For schistosomiasis, water contact should be reduced; molluscicides to kill the snail intermediate host may also be of value.

Treatment of all fluke infections has been revolutionized by the drug Praziquantel, which is administered orally for only 1 day.

References

Facey, R.V., Marsden, P.D.: Fascioliasis in man: an outbreak in Hampshire. *Br Med J* 1960; 2:619-625

Mahmoud, A.A.F., et al.: Effect of targeted mass treatment on intensity of infection and morbidity in schistosomiasis. *Lancet* 1983; 1:849-851.

Plaut, A.G., Kamapanart Sanyakorn, C., Manning, G.S.: A clinical study of *Fasciolopsis buski* infection in Thailand. *Trans R Soc Trop Med Hyg* 1969; 63:470-478.

Strauss, W.G.: Clinical manifestations of clonorchiasis: a controlled study of 105 cases. *Am J Trop Med Hyg* 1962; 11:625-630.

Upatham, E.S., et al.: Morbidity in relation to intensity of infection in opisthorchiasis viverrini: Study of a community in Khon Kaen, Thailand. *Am J Trop Med Hyg* 1982; 31:1156-1163.

Warren, K.S.: The kinetics of hepatosplenic schistosomiasis. *Sem Liver Dis* 1984; 4:293-300.

Wykoff, D.E., Chittayasothorn, K., Winn, N.M.: Clinical manifestations of *Opisthorchis viverrini* infections in Thailand. *Am J Trop Med Hyg* 1966; 15:914-918.

Zhong, et al. Recent progress in studies of *Paragonimus* and paragonimiasis control in China. *Chinese Med J* 1981; 94:483-494.

104 Cestodes

Donald Heyneman, PhD

General Concepts
Distinctive Properties
Pathogenesis
Host Defenses
Epidemiology
Diagnosis
Control

General Concepts

Tapeworms are ribbon-shaped multisegmented flatworms that dwell as adults entirely in the human small intestine. The larval forms lodge in skin, liver, muscles, the central nervous system, or any of various other organs. Their life cycles involve a specialized pattern of survival and transfer to specific intermediate hosts, by which they are transferred to another human host. Each pattern is characteristic of a given tapeworm species.

In general, the common gut-dwelling adult cestodes are well adapted to the human host, induce few symptoms, and only rarely cause serious pathology. This reality belies innumerable fearsome and largely apocryphal stories of tapeworms stealing food and causing ravenous hunger (far more commonly, the appetite is depressed). Larval cestodes, however, develop in human organs or somatic tissues outside of the gut and are therefore far more pathogenic.

The adult cestodes elicit little host inflammatory or immune response in contrast to the strong responses elicited by the larval stages in tissues. Adult cestodes are often acquired by ingestion of meat from intermediate hosts. Extraintestinal infection with larvae results from ingestion of eggs of fecal origin. Diagnosis of infection with adult cestodes is based on identification of eggs and segments (proglottids) in feces. Larval infections are more difficult to assess; serology and biopsy are helpful. Control depends on sanitation, personal hygiene, and thorough cooking of meat and fish.

Distinctive Properties

Adult cestodes can be characterized as ribbonlike, flattened, segmented, hermaphroditic flatworms consisting of scolex, neck, and immature, mature, and ripe segments in linear sequence extending from a few inches to many feet. The distinctive morphologic and physiologic properties of adult tapeworms are a reflection of their remarkably specialized characteristics for survival in the vertebrate intestine combined with their massive reproductive powers, made possible by multiple sexual units, or segments. This ensures the worm species against the enormous rate of loss of the segments (proglottids) or eggs passed in the feces, with only the most remote probability of any one egg succeeding in reaching its next host and being transferred to another human (the structure of adults is described in Chapter 101).

Larval cestodes of humans (Figure 104-1) are nonsegmented. They usually consist of scolex and neck enclosed in a minute, tailed, tissue-lined capsule (cysticercoid larva of *Hymenolepis nana* in the human villus); a fluid-filled, pea-sized sac (cysticercus larva of *Taenia solium*); a larger sac with several to a hundred or so larval heads (coenurus larva of *Multiceps*); or a far larger membrane-lined, fluid-filled sac with thousands of floating and attached heads on the inner membrane surface, and floating daughter colonies containing additional masses of scoleces (hydatid larva of *Echinococcus granulosus*). The rare and usually fatal alveolar hydatid of *Echinococcus multilocularis* is not enclosed in a confining membrane and therefore grows cancerlike, spreading through the organ infected, usually the liver. Another aberrant larval cestode of humans is the wormlike sparganum (or plerocercoid) larva of *Spirometra*, a relative of the broad fish tapeworm of humans.

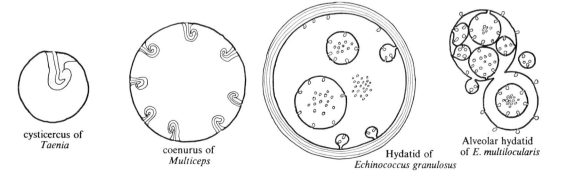

cysticercus of
Taenia

coenurus of
Multiceps

Hydatid of
Echinococcus granulosus

Alveolar hydatid
of *E. multilocularis*

Figure 104-1 Larval types found in the taeniid tapeworms. From Muller, R.: *Worms and disease: a manual of medical helminthology.* London: William Heinemann Medical Books, Ltd., 1975.

Pathogenesis

Clinical manifestations of adult worms are confined to occasional queasiness, nausea, or vomiting, appetite loss, epigastric or umbilical pain, and weight loss. Moderate eosinophilia may develop. A disturbing manifestation of *T saginata* infection is the active crawling of the muscular segments out the anus. Rarely, intestinal perforation may occur from the scolex of *Taenia,* or proglottids may be vomited and then aspirated. The broad fish tapeworm, *Diphyllobothrium latum,* sometimes is associated, chiefly among the Finns, with a megaloblastic pernicious anemia caused by competitive absorption of the host's vitamin B_{12}, perhaps only in persons already suffering from a B_{12} deficiency.

Larval worms may induce serious pathology, chiefly by mechanically obstructing or directly damaging sensitive organs such as those of the central nervous system. Infection with *T solium,* the pork tapeworm, carries the dual threat of larval infection (cysticercosis) as well as adult worm infection—a condition apparently absent in *T saginata* infection. Ripe segments of *T solium* that chance to be carried anteriorly into the duodenal region by reverse peristalsis may be digested open, permitting the release of eggs, which hatch and release their six-hooked larvae (the oncosphere or hexacanth). These larvae can then penetrate the gut and pass through the circulation into various parts of the body, including subcutaneous tissues, muscles, the central nervous system, and the eye, where each larva forms a cysticercus. Cysticercosis is acquired primarily from ingestion of infective eggs through contamination with egg-bearing human feces (including autoreinfection by an infected individual through the anus-to-mouth route).

Other serious larval infections of humans are coenurus (rare) and hydatid infections (see Epidemiology section for discussion of life cycle). Because cysts in hydatid infections may reach massive proportions and occupy critical sites in viscera, brain, or even within the long bones, damage can be severe. Cysts also can induce anaphylactic shock if the hydatid bursts from trauma or surgery, releasing the highly allergenic hydatid fluid and scoleces, each of which can then reattach in a nonimmunized host and initiate production of a new hydatid cyst.

Host Defenses

Because of its limited contact with the epithelial lining, the gut-dwelling adult tapeworm induces little host inflammatory, allergic, cell-mediated, or humoral response. The sucking action of the scolex and even the attachment of rostellar hooks appear to have relatively limited immunogenic effect; however, the tissue phase of the direct cycle of *Hymenolepis nana* infection (Figures 104-2 and 104-3) does initiate a profound cellular and humoral response, rendering most hosts immune to subsequent infection (as demonstrated experimentally in rodents). In contrast, the indirect cycle through infected insects lacks mucosal embryogenesis in humans and induces little or no immunity, even permitting occasional massive internal reinfection to occur. In general, larval infections induce a strong immunogenic response against a challenge infection, but it is seldom effective against the inducing infection itself because the tissues have already been invaded by that time, a protective cyst has been formed, and the damage has been done. Skin tests and serologic diagnostic tests usually are strongly positive following tissue invasion by larval cestodes. Occasionally, old infections are destroyed—even large hydatid cysts—indicating that a strong host response has been elicited.

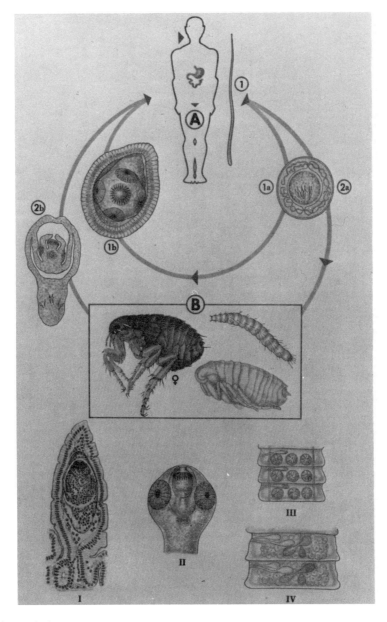

Figure 104-2 *Hymenolepis nana.*

A. Final host: humans (also dog, rodents)
    1.   *Hymenolepis nana,* sexually mature worm, about natural size
    1a–1b.   Development without an intermediate host
    1a.   Egg with 6-hooked larva (oncosphere)
    1b.   Cysticercoid from the intestinal mucosa (compare with I below)
B. Intermediate host: for example, a rodent flea (including larva and pupa)
    2a.   Development within intermediate host, in which the flea larva takes up the egg of the tapeworm, to a
    2b.   Cysticercoid from the body cavity of the flea (tail appendage with the hooks left in it)—longitudinal section
    I.   Villus of the small intestine of a mouse with cysticercoid (transverse section)
    II.   Scolex of *Hymenolepis nana*
    III.   Immature }
    IV.   Mature   } segments of the tapeworm

From Piekarski, G.: *Medical parasitology*. Heidelberg: Springer-Verlag.

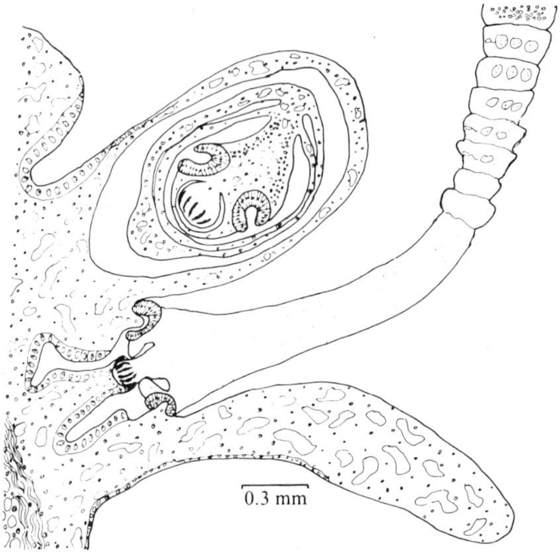

Figure 104-3 Diagrammatic section of adult and larval *H nana* in the gut of a mouse. In heavy infections in this host, much of the mucosal lining is abraded. From Muller, R.: *Worms and disease: a manual of medical helminthology.* London: William Heinemann Medical Books, Ltd., 1975.

0.3 mm

Epidemiology

In humans, cestodes are found as adult tapeworms (*H nana*, Figures 104-2 and 104-3; *Taenia* sp, Figure 104-4; *Dipylidium caninum;* and *Diphyllobothrium latum*, Figure 104-5) or as larval forms (see Figure 104-1) (*Echinococcus* sp, Figure 104-6; *Multiceps*, *T solium*, and *Spirometra*).

T saginata, the commonest large tapeworm of humans, is transmitted to humans as cysticerci in beef ("measly beef"). Partially cooked, smoked, or pickled beef can still be infective, although raw beef (steak tartar) is the commonest mode of infection, as witnessed by the frequency of taeniasis in countries like Ethiopia and Argentina where raw or undercooked beef often is eaten. The scolex of the cysticercus is released in the small intestine through the action of digestive enzymes; it attaches and grows rapidly. In about 3 months, a 4-5 m or longer worm develops, gradually extending through much of the small bowel. Terminal segments break loose and pass—or crawl actively— through the large bowel and out the anus. The worm may reach up to 9 m in length, growing 20-30 cm a day, and conveying up to a million eggs daily into the environment. Passed segments tend to crawl away from the fecal mass and attach to grass stalks, where they contract and release eggs are readily available to cattle or other herbivores. Eggs may also be present in pastures following pollution by sewage or the use of sewage sludge. After ingestion by cattle, the eggs hatch to release the oncospheres, which penetrate the gut wall and eventually encyst in various muscle tissues, ready for another human host.

T solium has a similar cycle but passes through pork instead of beef. Its segments are not active and ordinarily do not crawl away from the fecal bolus; hence, they are readily available to pigs, which are coprophagic. Humans are the only known final hosts of *T saginata* and *T solium*.

Adult *H nana* are threadlike, 5-15 cm long, and probably the commonest human cestode. The ingested eggs hatch in the duodenum, and the oncospheres penetrate only

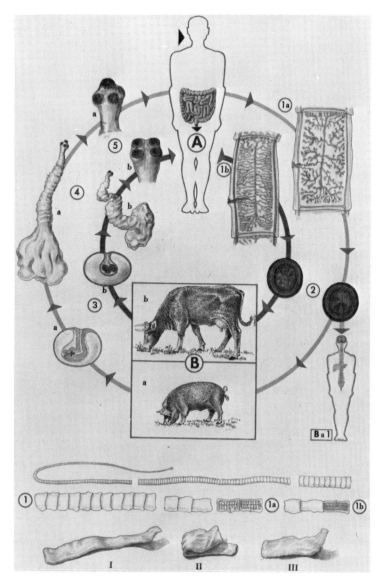

Figure 104-4 *Taenia solium* and *T saginata. a,* The pork (pig) tapeworm (outer developmental cycle); *b,* the beef (cattle) tapeworm (inner developmental cycle).

A. Final host: humans only. Tapeworm in the small intestine

    1. Tapeworm with its head (see **B**-5 below)

    1a. Mature segment of *T solium*

    1b. Mature segment of *T saginata*

    2. Tapeworm egg (= embryophore with 6-hooked larva), (the species cannot be morphologically differentiated)

B. Intermediate host

    a. Pig; humans rarely (Ba₁) (cysticercosis)

    b. Cattle

  3–4. Cysticercus (measle) in different stages of evagination of the scolex

3a. *Cysticercus cellulosae* of *T solium* (with its crown of hooklets and 4 suckers); commencing evagination

3b. *Cysticercus bovis* of *T saginata* (with four suckers only)

4.   Evaginated cysticercus stage of *T solium* (a) and *T saginata* (b)

5.   Head: a. of the pork tapeworm (with its crown of hooklets)

              b. of the beef tapeworm (without a crown of hooklets)

I-III. Phases of the movements of freshly detached tapeworm segments

From Piekarski, G.: *Medical parasitology.* Heidelberg: Springer-Verlag.

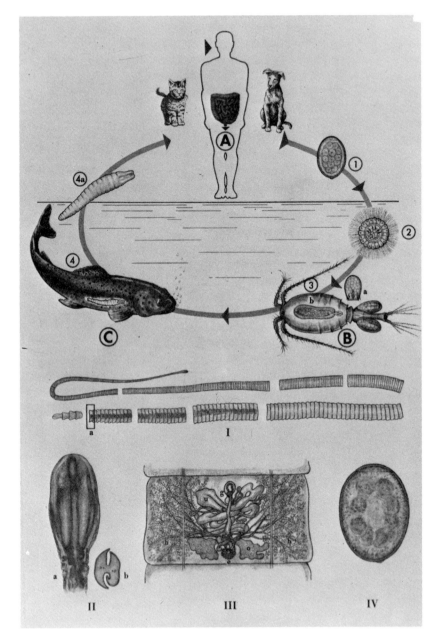

Figure 104-5

(See legend on facing page)

into the villi. There, each oncosphere forms a cysticercoid larva that emerges, 4-5 days later, into the gut lumen as a young scolex with attached neck; this scolex attaches to the mucosa, the neck proceeds to strobilate, and the worm reaches full size in 5-10 days (see Figure 104-2). The adult worm sheds its terminal segments, which are delicate and disintegrate in the intestine, releasing eggs that are found in the feces. When these eggs are ingested by another (nonimmune) human, the life cycle begins again. Worms live only a short time, perhaps 4-6 weeks. Rodents also can harbor these worms and may serve as reservoir hosts, infecting humans by their pellets or, remarkably, by grain beetles, fleas, or other insects that feed on contaminated rodent droppings (see Figure 104-2). Insects that ingest the *H nana* eggs can therefore serve as hosts for the cysticercoid larvae. Humans who accidentally ingest infected grain beetles (some, such as *Tribolium,* may be only 2-3 mm long) digest free the cysticercoids; digestive enzymes act on the cysticercoid to release the scolex, which attaches and develops by this indirect cycle into an adult worm (which appears to be exactly the same as an adult derived from an egg infection by the direct life cycle). *H diminuta,* the 20-30 cm rat tapeworm, and *Dipylidium caninum,* a 15-18 cm dog and cat tapeworm, are also transmitted through insects and can infect humans by this route. Both are rare in humans because they use only the indirect cycle, and not the direct egg-borne cycle.

D latum, the broad fish tapeworm of humans, is the only adult cestode of humans that has an aquatic life cycle (see Figure 104-5). Eggs are passed in feces of an infected human (or bear, dog, cat, wolf, raccoon, or other freshwater-fish-eating mammal). If passed into lake or pond water, the eggs will develop in 2 or more weeks (varying with the temperature) and hatch, releasing a round ciliated larva (the coracidium) that contains the oncosphere. When ingested by an appropriate water flea (copepods such as *Cyclops* or *Diaptomus*), the coracidium sheds the ciliated coat, penetrates into the hemocoel, and changes in 2-3 weeks into a 0.5 mm, tailed, second-stage larva (the procercoid). If the infected copepod is then ingested by a minnow or other fish,

Figure 104-5 *Diphyllobothrium latum.*
A. Final host: humans, dogs, cats (and other fish-eating domesticated and wild animals). Site of the tapeworm: small intestine.
  1. Egg after it is passed in feces
  2. Ciliated larva, the coracidium, containing the embryo with six hooklets (oncosphere)
B. 1. First intermediate host: small crustacean (copepod such as *Cyclops*)
  3a. 6-hooked larva emerged from coracidium in gut of a *Cyclops*
  3b. Procercoid in body cavity of *Cyclops*
C. 2. Second intermediate host: predatory fish or fish such as the carp.
  4. Trout with a plerocercoid (sparganum); final larval stage
  4a. Isolated plerocercoid
  I. Sexually mature *D latum;* pieces of tapeworm composed of proglottids in different stages of maturity;

  a. Mature proglottid with rosette-shaped uterus (see III)
  IIa. Scolex, spatula-shaped
  b. Transverse section of a scolex; the suctorial grooves on the two sides are seen clearly
  III. Mature tapeworm segment (proglottid)
  e. Mehlis' gland
  h. Testes
  o. Ovary
  g. Sexual opening
  u. Uterus
  IV. A single egg from the stool

From Piekarski, G.: *Medical parasitology.* Heidelberg: Springer-Verlag.

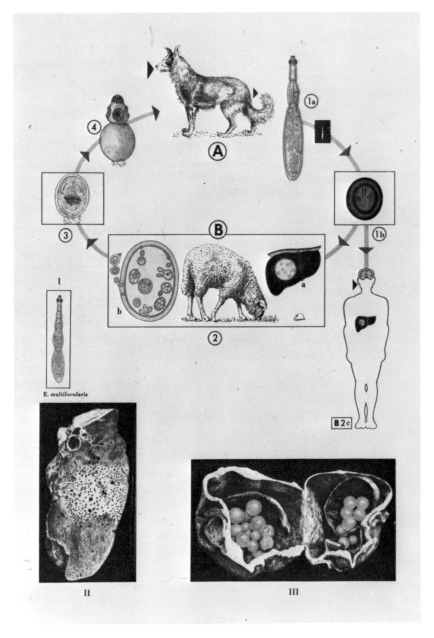

E. multilocularis

Figure 104-6

(See legend on facing page)

the procercoid penetrates the fish gut in a few hours and later develops into a third-stage larva (the plerocercoid or sparganum). Usually, these small infected fish are eaten by larger ones; in each new fish host, the plerocercoid penetrates into the fascia or muscles. Eventually, a large game fish, such as a perch or pike, is infected; after being eaten by a human, the fish releases its tapeworm passenger to begin adult life. The young worm attaches by its scolex with a pair of longitudinal sucking grooves and growth begins. In a few months, the worm is 5-10 m long and produces many hundreds of thousands of eggs a day.

Echinococcus is the chief larval cestode that infects humans. (*T solium,* as noted before, has a cycle identical in principle to that of *T saginata,* except for the rare, but dangerous, possibility of cysticercosis.) *H nana* also has a larval stage in humans, but it is followed quickly by emergence of the scolex into the gut lumen and rapid maturation of the worm.

E granulosus causes a zoonosis; the adult is a parasite of the domestic dog and is involved in a dog-sheep cycle. Wild animal cycles, such as wolf-caribou or coyote-deer, also are found (see Figure 104-6). The canid predator is the final host, harboring hundreds or even thousands of the tiny adult worms in its small intestine. Eggs passed by the dog can be ingested by sheep or other herbivores, or by humans who have close contact with fecally contaminated dog fur. Within the sheep or human intermediate host, the eggs hatch, the oncospheres penetrate the gut, and ultimately one forms the enormous hydatid cyst with many thousands of future worms in the form of multiple floating scoleces. Because they resemble grains of sand, these scoleces are often called hydatid sand. *Only* the hydatid cyst from an ingested egg forms in humans, who cannot serve as a final host for the adult worm (even if hydatid fluid were to be consumed). Yet a broken cyst within the human body cavity can result in dozens of new cysts—limited, in most cases, by a strong cellular immunologic response of the host.

E multilocularis normally infects foxes in a fox-field-mouse or fox-vole cycle. Occasionally, a fur trapper handling fox fur may ingest eggs and develop the alveolar or multiloculate hydatid cyst of this worm. The multilocular cyst is unimpeded by a membranous sheath, as in the *E granulosus* hydatid (unilocular cyst), and continues to grow and spread, usually causing death by liver failure after destroying most of the organ.

Figure 104-6 *Echinococcus granulosus* and *E multilocularis.*

A. Final host: dog (and other Canidae)
1a. *Echinococcus granulosus* (beside it the worm is reproduced in its natural size)
  b. Embryophore, the so-called egg with its 6-hooked larva (oncosphere)
B. Intermediate host: sheep (for *E granulosus*); mouse (for *E multilocularis*)
2a. Liver with *Echinococcus* cyst (hydatid stage)
  b. Diagram of an *Echinococcus* hydatid with daughter cysts and scoleces (compare with III)
2c. Humans as the accidental intermediate host

(echinococcosis); organs most often infected: liver, brain
3,4. Isolated scoleces: invaginated (3), evaginated (4) on which the crown of hooklets and the suckers can be seen
  I. *Echinococcus multilocularis,* sexually mature worm
 II. Human liver infected by the hydatid of *E multilocularis*
III. Hydatid cyst of *E granulosus* opened up; daughter cysts visible

From Piekarski, G.: *Medical parasitology.* Heidelberg: Springer-Verlag.

Multiceps, a taenioid related to *Echinococcus,* has a similar life cycle and pattern of human infection. *Multiceps* is much rarer in humans and produces a smaller cyst, the coenurus, seldom more than 3 cm in circumference; however, the coenurus tends to develop in the spinal cord, brain, or eye, and is consequently a dangerous parasite for humans, as it is for its normal intermediate hosts (sheep and other herbivores).

Sparganosis is a tissue infection with the sparganum (or plerocercoid) of *Spirometra,* a genus related to *Diphyllobothrium.* These two genera have similar life cycles, but usually *Spirometra* utilizes frogs, reptiles, or various mammals as intermediate hosts, whereas *Diphyllobothrium* uses fish. In the Far East, frog flesh (rather than beef steak) is used as a poultice over a wound or black eye, which allows the sparganum to crawl into the wound or orbit, initiating a severe inflammatory response. Human infection also can occur from drinking water containing infected *Cyclops* and possibly from undercooked snake or other infected meat. The procercoids from *Cyclops* invade the gut wall of its human or animal intermediate host and usually migrate to subcutaneous tissues to form a sparganum, which induces, in humans, formation of a fibrous nodule that encloses and destroys the worm.

Diagnosis

Adult tapeworm infections can be diagnosed by identifying eggs or segments in the feces. *Taenia* sp can be identified only by the segments because the eggs are identical. The uterus of *T saginata* usually forms 12–20 branches on each side of the main uterine stem, and 7–10 in the smaller and relatively wider *T solium* segment (see Figure 104-4). *H nana* and *D latum* produce eggs that are readily distinguished in the feces by microscopic examination. *Echinococcus* eggs from dogs are indistinguishable from those of *Taenia* and because dogs can also harbor species of *Taenia,* the worms must be purged (by arecoline or other drugs) to identify the parasite positively and to reduce the danger of the dog infecting humans when *Echinococcus* is present.

Diagnosis of larval tapeworm infections of humans is difficult and usually requires serologic and clinical assessments. Indirect hemagglutination, indirect fluorescence, various flocculation tests, and other serologic procedures are available; these tests are strongly indicative, but cross-reactions and false-negatives may be produced under some conditions. The Casoni skin test for hydatid disease indicates past exposure, but is chiefly an epidemiologic tool and not a reliable diagnostic test. Old infections that show calcification (as may occur in cysticercosis) have a characteristic rice grain appearance on roentgenograms, and hydatidosis produces characteristic lung or liver shadows. Clinical manifestations, such as central nervous system symptoms or eye involvement, may suggest cysticercosis, although the manifestations are variable, depending on the number and precise localization of the cysticerci. Hydatid disease also can often be diagnosed by tapping an abdominal cyst (never by needle biopsy!).

Control

Proper cooking of meat or fish is the best way to prevent taeniasis or diphyllobothriasis. Pickling and salting are usually not reliable for *Taenia* cysticerci in beef or pork, although thorough pickling and complete drying of fish will kill *D latum* plerocercoids.

Freezing at -7 to -10 C for 4 days usually is lethal to *Taenia* cysticerci, but they can withstand 70 days at 0 C. Plerocercoids in fish can be killed in 15 minutes at -10 C.

The eggs of *Echinococcus* are particularly resistant, surviving $2\frac{1}{2}$ years at 2 C or 54 days at -26 C. Hence, they can overwinter readily and infect a sheep herder by aerial spread a year or two later as well as directly from contaminated dog fur. Many cases of pulmonary hydatidosis probably result from aerial infection. Control is difficult and requires a well-organized campaign of regular treatment of sheep dogs and prevention of access of dogs to sheep carcasses or the viscera of slaughtered animals. Fur trappers of wild predators are in particular jeopardy.

Treatment is readily available for the intestinal adult worms. Niclosamide, the drug of choice, is a nonabsorbed oxidative phosphorylation inhibitor that kills the scolex and anterior segments on contact, after which the worm is expelled. The broad-spectrum antibiotic paromomycin sulfate also is effective and is not readily absorbed in the gastrointestinal tract. A new drug, praziquantel, is said to be a highly effective and nontoxic cestodicidal compound. One caution about these newer drugs: the scolex usually is destroyed, but assurance of complete elimination of the worm (which can regenerate a complete new worm if the scolex and a minute portion of the neck survive) requires routine followup for several months.

For larval cysts, such as hydatid, surgery is the only recourse. The surgeon must take great care not to spill the scolex-bearing fluid into the abdominal cavity because this can result in an anaphylactic reaction and possible generation of new cysts. Frequently, hypertonic glucose or saline, 50% ethanol, 10% formalin, or 2% sodium hypochlorite is injected repeatedly into the cyst after surgical exposure and aspiration of some of the fluid, until the hydatid fluid has been replaced. The cyst can then be removed safely. Mebendazole in very high doses has also been used with limited success to reduce the size of hydatid cysts or to destroy their contents before surgery.

References

Abdussalam, M.: *The problem of taeniasis—cysticercosis. PAHO* Sci. Publ. No. 295, Washington, D.C.: World Health Organization, 1975.

Arambulo, P., Steele, J.H., (editors): *Handbook series in zoonoses, section C: parasitic zoonoses.* Boca Raton, Fla.: CRC Press, 1982.

Araujo, F.P., et al.: Hydatid disease transmission in California. A study of the Basque connection. *Am J Epidemiol* 1975; 102:291-302.

Arme, C., Pappas, P.W. (editors): *Biology of the Eucestoda,* 2 vols. London: Academic Press, 1983.

Binford, C.H., Connor, D.H., (editors): *Pathology of tropical and extraordinary diseases,* vol 2. Washington, D.C.: Armed Forces Institute of Pathology, 1976.

von Bonsdorff, B.: *Diphyllobothriasis in man.* London: Academic Press, 1977.

Burridge, M.J., Schwabe, C.W., Fraser, J.: Hydatid disease in New Zealand: Changing patterns in human infection, 1872-1972. *N Z Med J* 1977; 85:173-177.

Cho, C., Patel, S.P.: Human sparganosis in the northern United States. *NY State J Med* 1978; 78:1456-1458.

Eckert, J., Muller, B., Partridge, A.J.: The domestic cat and dog as natural definitive hosts of *Echinococcus (Alveococcus) multilocularis* in southern Federated Republic of Germany. *Tropenmed Parasitol* 1974; 25:334-337.

Gemmell, M.A., Soulsby, E.J.L.: The development of acquired immunity to tapeworms and progress towards active immunization, with special reference to *Echinococcus* sp. *Bull WHO* 1968; 39:45-55.

Gemmell, M.A., et al.: Effect of metronidazole against *Echinococcus granulosus* and *Taenia hydatigera* infections in naturally infected sheep and its possible relevance to larval tapeworm infections in man. *Z Parasitenkd* 1981; 64:135-147.

Markell, E.K., Voge, M.: *Medical parasitology.* Philadelphia, W.B. Saunders Co, 1981.

Mueller, J.F.: The biology of *Spirometra. J Parasitol* 1974; 60:3-14.

Rausch, R.L.: Taeniidae. In: *Diseases transmitted from animals to man,* Hubbert, W.T., McCulloch, W.F., Schnurrenberger, P.R. (editors). Springfield, Ill.: C.C. Thomas, 1975.

Schwabe, C.S.: Epidemiology of echinococcosis. *Bull WHO* 1968; 39:131-135.

Smyth, J.D., Heath, D.D.: Pathogenesis of larval cestodes in mammals. *Helminthol Abstr* 1970; 36:1-23.

Templeton, A.C.: Anatomical and geographical location of human coenurus infection. *Trop Geograph Med* 1971; 23:105-108.

Webbe, G.: The hatching and activation of taeniid ova in relation to the development of cysticercosis in man. *Zeitschrift fur Tropenmedizin and Parasitologie* 1967; 18:354-369.

Williams, J.F.: Cestode infections. In: *Immunology of parasitic infections,* Cohen, S., Warren, K.S. (editors). Boston: Blackwell Scientific, 1982.

World Health Organization. Echinococcosis. *Bull WHO* 1968; 39:1-136.

105 Enteric Nematodes of Humans

John H. Cross, PhD

General Concepts

Enteric nematodes are among the most common and widely distributed animal parasites of humans. In his classic address to the American Society of Parasitologists in 1946, entitled "This Wormy World," Stoll estimated 2.3 billion helminthic infections in a human population of 2.2 billion. Since 1946, the world population has doubled and, by all indications, enteric nematode infections of humans have maintained the pace. The most common intestinal roundworms are those transmitted through contact with the soil (for example, *Ascaris lumbricoides*, *Trichuris trichiura*, the hookworms, and *Strongyloides stercoralis*); these, with *Enterobius vermicularis*, accounted for three-quarters of all helminthic infections in Stoll's estimations.

Most enteric nematodes have established a well-balanced host–parasite relationship with the human host; humans tolerate these parasites well. Little disease is associated with light infection, but when the worm load increases, a corresponding increase in disease usually occurs. The worms may irritate the intestinal mucosa, causing inflammation and ulceration. Some may produce toxic substances; the larger worms may become entangled and block the intestinal tract. Larval worms, which must migrate through the tissue to complete their life cycle, may lose their way in traversing the body, end up in the wrong organ, and cause severe disease. Nutritional problems may also be associated with the intestinal parasitosis, and persons with deficient diets often suffer from polyparasitism.

Diagnosis usually is based on microscopic examination of feces for eggs and larvae, except in the case of pinworm infections, which are diagnosed by examination of samples taken with perianal swabs. Many anthelmintics are available to treat patients with these infections. Control depends largely on proper disposal of human feces and personal hygiene.

Enteric nematodes to be discussed in this chapter are *A lumbricoides*, the hookworms *Necator americanus* and *Ancylostoma duodenale*, *S stercoralis*, *T trichiura*, and *E vermicularis*. *A suum*, *Capillaria philippinensis*, and *Trichostrongylus* sp are mentioned briefly.

ASCARIS LUMBRICOIDES

Distinctive Properties

A lumbricoides is the largest and most common intestinal nematode of humans. It is creamy-to-pinkish-white, elongated, and tapers at each end. Sexually mature males are smaller than females; the latter are approximately 30 cm long. Females produce as many as 200,000 eggs per day, and 25 million in a lifetime. Mated females produce fertile eggs, which are oval-to-subspherical, thick-shelled with a light brown outer mamillated albuminous coat, and measure 45–75 by 35–50 μm (Figure 105-1A, B). When passed in feces, the eggs are unsegmented. Unmated females, for example, in single-sex infection, produce unfertilized eggs that are thin-shelled, are ellipsoidal, and measure 78–105 by 38–55 μm (Figure 105-1C). The mamillated coat is irregular and the inner contents are granular and disorganized. Some eggs are passed without the outer mamillated coat (decorticated) (Figure 105-D) and can be confused with hookworm or eggs from other worms.

A lumbricoides is found in the small intestine, particularly the jejunum. Adult females produce unsegmented eggs that are passed in the feces. In moist, warm (20–30 C), and shady soil, an infected larva develops within the egg in about 3 weeks. After being ingested by a human being, the eggs pass to the duodenum; there, the larvae

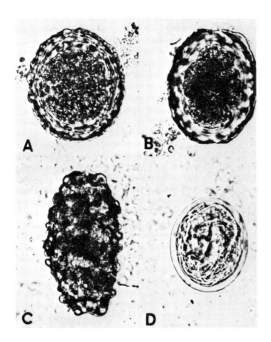

Figure 105-1 *Ascaris lumbricoides* eggs. **A** and **B,** Fertile eggs. **C,** Unfertile egg. **D,** Decorticated egg with outer coat lost. From Juniper, K. In: *Gastroenterologic medicine.* Paulson, M., (editor). Philadelphia, Lea & Febiger, 1969.

hatch, penetrate the intestinal mucosa, enter the lymphatics and portal system, and are carried to the liver, heart, and lungs. This requires only a few days. The larvae break out of the capillaries into the alveoli, pass up the respiratory tree, and are swallowed. They reach the intestines, continue their development, and, 8-12 weeks after infection, become sexually mature adults. The adults may live for 1 year or more, and are subsequently passed in the feces.

Pathogenesis

Adult *A lumbricoides* infections involving only a few worms are usually asymptomatic, but as the worm load increases, symptoms of abdominal discomfort, nausea, vomiting, weight loss, fever, and diarrhea develop. Large numbers of worms may form a bolus and cause intestinal obstruction. Stimulation causes adult worms to become erratic and invade the appendix and the biliary and pancreatic ducts. Migrating adult worms have been vomited and passed from nose and mouth, anus, umbilicus, and lacrimal gland. They can perforate the intestines and enter the peritoneal cavity, the respiratory tract, urethra, and vagina, and even invade the placenta and fetus. The reasons for these abnormal migrations are not known; febrile illness may cause such migrations.

Excessive worm loads, especially among malnourished children, may lead to further nutritional impairment due to malabsorption of proteins, fats, and carbohydrates.

Initial pathology is associated with migrating larvae; severity depends on the number of invading organisms, the sensitivity of the host, and the host's nutritional status. Larvae migrating through the lungs of a sensitized person may cause a pneumonitis with cough, low-grade fever, chest pain, and eosinophilia.

Host Defenses

Persons with ascariasis can manifest allergic manifestations of urticaria, asthma, fever, conjunctivitis, and eosinophilia. Some parasitologists, through years of contact with the parasite, have become sensitized and develop severe reactions when exposed to *A lumbricoides* antigens. Further work with the worm becomes almost impossible. Ascariasis often leads to increased serum IgE levels, especially in children.

Epidemiology

A lumbricoides is distributed widely in tropical and subtropical areas, especially in the developing countries in South America, Africa, and Asia. More than 600 million infections are estimated to exist at any given time; in a rural area of Asia, to find 85% of the population passing eggs is not unusual. The parasite is found in all age groups, with the highest prevalence rates in younger groups. Prevalence rates are much lower in the United States. In a 1978 CDC report, 1.5% of more than 300,000 stools examined at state health laboratories were positive for *A lumbricoides* eggs.

The parasite retains high endemicity in an area by the continuous seeding of the soil with eggs by indiscriminant defecation. Human excrement used as fertilizer (night soil) has been incriminated as an important source of infection; however, in rural areas of the Philippines and Indonesia where night soil is not used, the prevalence of *A lumbricoides* and other soil-transmitted helminths is often as high, if not higher, than in areas where night soil is used.

Infections are acquired by ingesting eggs in contaminated water or dirt, on raw vegetables, or on inanimate objects. The eggs are susceptible to dryness, developing best in warm, moist soil. Cold climates inhibit development of larvae, and high temperatures kill them. Eggs are resistant to disinfection, can survive sewage treatment, can remain viable in night soil, and can live for years in dilute formalin.

Diagnosis

Clinical diagnosis of ascariasis is unusual because pneumonitis, eosinophilia, and intestinal symptoms are difficult to distinguish from those caused by other helminthic infections. Infections before eggs appear in the feces, infections with only male worms, and extraintestinal infections are difficult to diagnose. Radiologic examinations may reveal adult intestinal infections, but definitive diagnosis requires finding characteristic eggs in feces. Eggs are usually so numerous that simple direct smear microscopic examination of the feces is all that is necessary. Concentration techniques by flotation or sedimentation also may be used. Techniques are available to estimate the intensity of an infection on the basis of number of eggs in a stool sample.

Control

The most effective method to control ascariasis, as well as other soil-transmitted helminthiasis, is sanitary disposal of feces. In some areas, this requires changing century-old habits and educating the population. Mass treatment programs have been initiated in many parts of the world and, in some Asian countries, efforts are being made to deworm all school children. In a pilot program in the Philippines to eradicate the soil-transmitted helminths by periodic mass treatment of a barrio population, the prevalence of ascariasis decreased from 78% to less than 1% over a 3-year period. Mebendazole (Vermox), the drug used, is effective in treating numerous intestinal nematode infections and causes few side effects. Levamisole (Ketrax) also is useful, as are pyrantel pamoate (Combantrin), piperazine citrate (Antepar), thiabendazole (Mintezol), and albendazole (Zentel).

Care must be taken in treating mixed helminthic infections involving *A lumbricoides*, because an ineffective ascaricide may stimulate the parasite to migrate to another location. Persons in whom asymptomatic ascariasis is detected incidentally should be treated to prevent the future possibility of an abnormal migration of these large worms into extraintestinal sites.

ASCARIS SUUM

The large intestinal roundworm of pigs, *A suum*, is difficult to distinguish morphologically from *A lumbricoides*. On occasion, this parasite is known to infect humans and cause disease (see Chapter 106).

HOOKWORMS

Distinctive Properties

Two major hookworm species infect humans; the Old World hookworm (*A duodenale*) and the New World hookworm (*N americanus*). The worms are cylindrical and grayish white. Females (approximately 1 cm long) are larger than males. The major differentiating characteristics between the two species are the buccal capsule and male bursa. The bell-shaped bursa, used for attachment to the female during copulation, is membranous and symmetrical and has fingerlike rays, arranged differently for each species. The most prominent difference in these buccal capsules is the presence in *N americanus* of two ventral semilunar cutting plates, as compared to the four ventral teeth in *A duodenale*.

Female *A duodenale* produces 10,000–20,000 eggs per day compared to 5,000–10,000 for *N americanus*. The eggs are ovoidal, thin-shelled, and transparent; in fresh stools, they are in the four- or eight-cell stage. The eggs from these species are indistinguishable from each other and measure 55–79 by 35–47 μm (Figure 105-2).

The newly hatched first-stage (rhabditiform) larva that develops within the eggs (see Figure 105-2) has a thick-walled, long, and narrow buccal cavity. The muscular esophagus is flask-shaped and occupies the anterior one-third of the body. Slender third-stage (filariform) larvae are 500–700 μm long. The mouth is closed, and the elongate esophagus occupies one-third of the body. The tail is sharply pointed. Rhabditiform larvae of the two species cannot be differentiated, but the filariform larvae of *N americanus* have dark, prominent buccal spears and a striated cuticle seen more clearly at the posterior end; these characteristics are not seen in *A duodenale*.

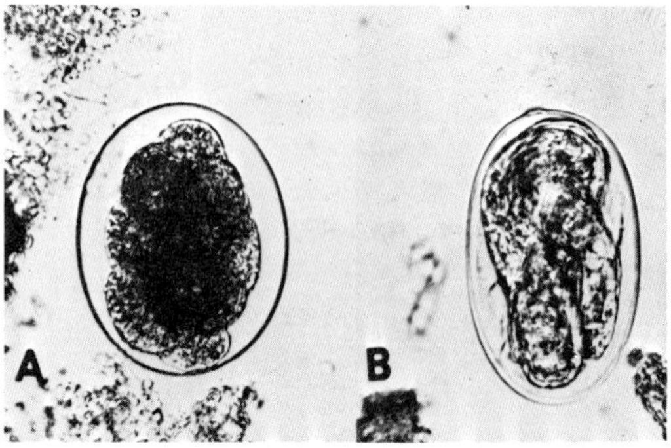

Figure 105-2 Hookworm eggs. **A,** In eight-cell stage. **B,** With developing larva. From Juniper, K. In: *Gastroenterologic medicine.* Paulson, M., (editor). Philadelphia, Lea & Febiger, 1969.

Adult hookworms generally attach to mucosa in the jejunum, and the female deposits eggs that pass in the feces. In the proper soil, under ideal conditions, the eggs hatch in 1-2 days. These larvae (rhabditiform) feed on bacteria and organic debris, molt twice, and develop into slender, infective (filariform) larvae in 5-8 days. These larvae do not feed; if they are unable to penetrate a host, they die within a few weeks. Once in the skin, they enter the venules and are carried to the heart and lungs, where they grow; eventually, they break out into the alveoli and pass up the respiratory tree. After they are swallowed, they attach to the intestinal mucosa and become sexually mature in 5-6 weeks. Although infections are known to persist for as long as 14 years, most terminate in 2-6 years. Infection by ingestion of larvae may also occur; *A duodenale* is well adapted to this route.

Pathogenesis

Hookworm larvae usually gain access to the body by penetrating the skin. At the invasion sites, usually feet and hands, local reactions called ground itch may result, particularly in sensitized individuals. Secondary bacterial infection may also occur at these sites. Large numbers of larvae migrating through the lungs at the same time may cause pneumonitis. In the small intestine, worms attach to the mucosa by the buccal capsule. The worms' feeding on the mucosa produces a considerable amount of blood loss. The worm ingests mucosal tissue with blood; much of this blood is excreted into the lumen of the host's intestine. Blood also is lost by seepage around the attachment site. When the worm changes attachment sites, the wound oozes blood for several days. One *A duodenale* is estimated to be responsible for the loss of 0.15-0.26 mL blood per day and *N americanus* for 0.03 mL per day. An anticoagulant secreted in the buccal capsule of these worms also contributes to blood loss. Excessive blood loss can lead to anemia. Infections involving a few worms usually are asymptomatic, but in heavy infections, hookworm disease (including anemia) results, especially if accompanied by concomitant infections and malnutrition. Infections with *A duodenale* are considered more pathogenic.

Ground itch, pneumonitis, cough, dyspnea, and, occasionally, hemoptysis are early symptoms. Symptoms associated with the intestinal phase of infection include anorexia or a huge appetite with pica (desire to eat unusual substances such as dirt), fever, diarrhea, abdominal discomfort, weight loss, nausea and vomiting, spleen and liver enlargement, and edema. Children may suffer from mental, physical, and sexual retardation. Eosinophilia is usually marked; iron-deficiency anemia and hypoalbuminemia can result. Hemoglobin levels as low as 2% often are seen. Although hookworm infection is common in some areas, infection does not necessarily lead to hookworm disease.

Host Defenses

Immunity to hookworm develops in dogs, but no strong evidence suggests that it occurs in humans. Ground itch is thought to be an allergic reaction, but the response is minimal unless accompanied by bacterial infection.

Seasonal fluctuation in hookworm egg production has been reported and is thought to be due to host resistance. In some persons, a "self-cure" or a spontaneous reduction of worms may occur and may be attributed to immediate hypersensitivity reactions in the intestinal wall. IgE antibody (high in persons with hookworm), mast cells, and worm allergens are thought to provide the necessary ingredients for the reaction.

Epidemiology

More than 600 million infections are estimated to exist at any time; in surveys conducted in Asia, prevalence rates of 60%–70% were not unusual. Infections are found equally in males and females, with the lowest prevalence rates in younger age groups. Once highly endemic in the southern United States, hookworm has decreased dramatically. The 1978 CDC report indicated infections in only 0.6% of the stools examined at state health laboratories.

Both *N americanus* and *A duodenale* are endemic in tropical areas that have warm, moist climates, and where people defecate in the soil. Places where individuals defecate collectively, such as homes and schools with outhouses and coal and other underground mines, are frequent sites of infection. *N americanus* is not confined to the Americas, but is the most common species in Asia, Central and South Africa, and Central and South America. *A duodenale* is found in these areas to a lesser degree, but is more prominent in India, China, the Soviet Union, and North Africa. Surveys using Harada-Mori cultures in the Philippines from 1975–1978 showed 30% of the stools positive for *N americanus*, 5% for *A duodenale*, and less than 1% positive for both.

Temperatures between 25 C and 35 C and a shady, sandy, or loamy soil with vegetation are most favorable for larval development. A population that does not wear shoes also facilitates maintenance and spread of the parasite.

Diagnosis

Hookworm infection is difficult to differentiate clinically from other parasite infections and certain other diseases. Diagnosis is made by demonstrating the egg in stool specimens, although these two species cannot be distinguished on the basis of their eggs. Direct microscopic examination of the stools may suffice in heavy infection, but a concentration method should be used in most cases (for example, zinc sulfate flotation or formalin-ether concentration). An estimate of the intensity of the infection can be made on the basis of the number of eggs in the fecal sample. Specimens should be examined quickly, since rhabditiform larvae may develop and hatch from the egg within a few hours. When larvae are present in the feces, they must be differentiated from those of other nematode species.

Control

Hookworm can be controlled in a population by sanitary disposal of feces, treatment of infected persons, wearing of shoes, health education, and improved nutrition. In the Philippines, the prevalence rate was decreased from 33% to less than 1% in 3 years by a control program of mass treatment with mebendazole.

Mebendazole is an effective treatment. Also effective are thiabendazole, pyrantel pamoate, albendazole, and levamisole. Older preparations such as tetrachlorethylene and bephenium hydroxynaphtholate also can be used, although the former is not effective against *A duodenale*. Antihelminthic treatment should be supplemented with an improved diet, including administration of iron.

STRONGYLOIDES STERCORALIS

Distinctive Properties

S stercoralis is unique in that it may have both parasitic and free-living adults, and that it may utilize three different life cycles: direct, indirect, and autoinfection. In the direct life cycle, parasitic females (approximately 2 mm long) are found in the epithelium of the duodenum or upper jejunum, where they reproduce by parthenogenesis. Thin-shelled, oval eggs are laid in the mucosa. Eggs mature rapidly and hatch in the mucosa. First-stage (rhabditiform) larvae (Figure 105-3) pass in the feces, and develop on the soil into infective (filariform) larvae, which can penetrate the skin of humans, enter cutaneous blood vessels, migrate to the lung, and finally mature in the small intestine. Females lay eggs about 1 month after infection of the host. In the indirect life cycle,

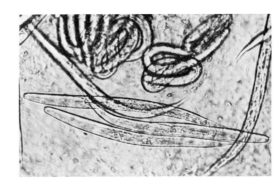

Figure 105-3 *Strongyloides stercoralis* rhabditiform larvae. From Juniper, K. In: *Gastroenterologic medicine.* Paulson, M., (editor). Philadelphia, Lea & Febiger, 1969.

larvae passed in the feces develop on the ground into free-living adult males and females; the eggs that are laid hatch and give rise to a generation of infective larvae, which can penetrate skin and develop as in the direct life cycle. In autoinfection, first-stage larvae transform into infective larvae while they are in the intestine or on the skin of the perianal region; these larvae penetrate the wall of the large intestine or the perianal skin. Some eventually develop into adults in the small intestine. Thus, autoinfection results in a replacement or an increase of the patient's intestinal worm burden, and accounts for the presence of this infection in patients who no longer live in endemic areas.

Pathogenesis

When infective larvae from the soil penetrate the skin in large numbers, they may cause pruritus or ground itch. Pneumonitis can result from larval lung invasion. In heavy infections, damage to the intestines may be severe, with edema, inflammation, and increased secretion of mucus. Epigastric pain, mucous diarrhea, and eosinophilia may occur. A malabsorption syndrome has been reported. In patients with autoinfection, the parasite may be found in all parts of the body. Disseminated strongyloidiasis sometimes occurs in persons receiving immunosuppressive drugs. Autoinfection may increase the worm burden of the intestine greatly, leading to severe ulceration of the mucosa and sloughing of intestinal tissue, as well as functional changes of the gut. Linear skin lesions of the lower abdomen and buttocks may also develop in patients with autoinfection due to penetration of the perianal skin by infective larvae. (See discussion of cutaneous larva migrans in Chapter 106.)

Host Defenses

Immunity in strongyloidiasis is not well understood, but autoinfection generally occurs in persons with suppressed cell-mediated immunity. Infected patients with lymphocytic leukemia, malignancy, malnutrition, leprosy, or systemic lupus erythematosus who are receiving immunosuppressive therapy are most susceptible. Serum IgE levels usually are elevated in persons with this parasite. In severe strongyloidiasis, some patients may have significantly decreased IgG levels and low levels of IgA and M. Eosinophil counts also may be lower in patients with massive infections. These findings indicate that eosinophils and antibodies may be important in the defense mechanism against *S stercoralis* larvae.

Epidemiology

S stercoralis may coexist with hookworm; both require similar soil and climatic conditions for development. Heavy contamination of soil results from warm and moist conditions that foster reproduction of the free-living stages. Because of autoinfection, persons who have contracted this infection in endemic areas may remain infected for years after leaving such areas.

Strongyloidiasis is more common in tropical and subtropical areas, but is much less prevalent than hookworm infection. Stoll estimated approximately 35 million *S stercoralis* infections; recent surveys in Southeast Asia rarely found the parasite, even with the use of filter paper cultures. Parts of Africa, however, report prevalences as high as 21%. In the United States, infections are more common in the South and in institutionalized populations; in the 1978 CDC survey, the parasite was found in 0.2% of the stools examined at state health laboratories.

Dogs have been found infected with *S stercoralis;* but although dogs are considered a source of human infections, the primary source continues to be human.

Diagnosis

Eosinophilia, epigastric pain, and mucus diarrhea suggest *S stercoralis* infection, but definitive diagnosis requires finding larvae in the stool or, on rare occasions, in sputum or urine. Eggs are not found except in cases of severe dysentery. Direct smear or concentration methods of stool examination usually suffice, but cultivation is recommended when infection is suspected but unconfirmed. Free-living stages can be seen easily in cultures after a few days. Larval stages must be distinguished from hookworm larvae. The first-stage (rhabditiform) larvae (see Figure 105-3) are 225–250 μm long; they resemble those of hookworm, but can be distinguished by the shorter buccal capsule and larger genital primordium. The infective (filariform) larvae, 550–700 μm, also resemble those of hookworm, but the tail is notched and the esophagus is about one-half the length of the body. Duodenal intubation and examination of aspirates, or a string-test (Enterotest) and examination of intestinal mucus, is recommended in suspected cases even when serial stool examinations are negative.

Control

Strongyloidiasis, like other soil-transmitted nematodes, can be controlled by improving sanitary conditions and by proper disposal of feces. Patients with this infection should be treated, even if they are asymptomatic, to preclude possible onset of autoinfection. Steroids are contraindicated in these patients.

Thiabendazole, the most effective therapeutic agent, can cause side effects of vertigo, nausea, and vomiting. Prolonged or repeated treatment may be required in patients receiving immunosuppressive drugs. Pyrvinium pamoate (Povan) and albendazole, have also been found to be effective.

TRICHURIS TRICHIURA

Distinctive Properties

T trichiura is known as whipworm because the long, narrow anterior end and the shorter, more robust posterior end give the worm a whiplike appearance (Figure 105-4A). The pinkish white worms are threaded through the mucosa and attach by their anterior ends. Females (approximately 45 mm long) are larger than males; they are bluntly rounded posteriorly, whereas the males have a coiled posterior. Females lay 2000–10,000 eggs per day for several years. The eggs are in the single-cell stage when passed in the feces, and are brown and barrel-shaped with prominent bipolar, blisterlike protuber-

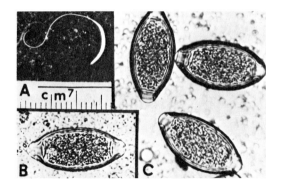

Figure 105-4 *Trichuris trichiura.* **A,** Adult worm. (Scale in centimeters.) **B** and **C,** eggs in unstained and iodine-stained wet preparations. From Juniper, K. In: *Gastroenterologic medicine.* Paulson, M., (editor). Philadelphia, Lea & Febiger, 1969.

ances; they measure 22 by 52 μm (Figure 105-4B, C). Eggs require about 3 weeks to become infective under favorable conditions. After being ingested, the embryonated eggs hatch in the small intestine; the infective larvae penetrate the villi and continue development. The young worms move to the cecum, penetrate the mucosa with their anterior ends, and complete their development. The females lay eggs about 3 months after infection of the host.

Pathogenesis

The parasite lives primarily in the cecum and appendix; when present in large numbers it can also be found in the colon and rectum. Petechial hemorrhage, edema, inflammation, and mucosal bleeding develop and, when infections are heavy, prolapsed rectum can result. Small amounts of blood (0.005 mL per worm) are lost each day by seepage at the attachment site. Patients may have diarrhea, anemia, weight loss, abdominal pain, nausea, vomiting, and eosinophilia.

Host Defenses

Little information is available on the immunologic responses to *T trichiura* infection. In some endemic areas, equal occurrence of infection in all age groups suggests little age-related resistance.

Epidemiology

Whipworm infections are prevalent in tropical and subtropical countries with moist, shaded, and warm soil. More than 500 million infections (including two million in the United States) are estimated to exist. In Asia, surveys indicate *T trichiura* is more common than *A lumbricoides*. In the United States, the parasite was found in 1.8% of more than 300,000 stools examined in 1978 at state health laboratories.

No reservoir hosts for *T trichiura* are known to exist. Most infections are acquired by eating contaminated soil, foods, or drink. A single infection may last for several years.

Diagnosis

Symptomatic diagnosis of trichiuriasis is difficult to make, but the parasitologic diagnosis is made easily by identification of eggs in the feces. In heavy infections, the stools are frequently mucoid and contain Charcot-Leyden crystals. Concentration methods are required for diagnosis in light infections, and the intensity of infection can be estimated by the Stoll or Kato-Katz techniques. In heavy infections, the parasite can be seen in the rectal mucosa by sigmoidoscopy.

Control

Sanitary disposal of feces is the best control measure. Mass treatment with mebendazole has shown promise in the Philippines, where administration of the drug periodically over 3 years has reduced the prevalence rate from 88% to 2%. Mebendazole is presently the drug of choice for treating trichiuriasis. Oxantel and albendazole have also been reported to be effective.

ENTEROBIUS VERMICULARIS

Distinctive Properties

It is safe to say that everyone, at one time or another, has had pinworms. The whitish, spindle-shaped worms, pointed at both ends, have characteristic cephalic swellings and a muscular esophagus with a large posterior bulb. Females are approximately 1 cm long and larger than males (Figure 105-5B). The male's posterior end is curved ventrad. Males die after copulation and females, when gravid, migrate out of the anus at night and lay eggs on the perianal skin. One female can lay as many as 10,000 eggs. The eggs are thin-shelled, ovoidal, and flattened on one side; they measure 50–60 μm by 20–30 μm (Figure 105-5A). The eggs mature and are infective within hours after being deposited on the perianal skin. The eggs are ingested and hatch in the small intestine, each releasing an infective larva. The parasite moves to the cecum, becoming an adult 2–4 weeks after infecting the host. Infections are self-limiting, unless reinfection occurs.

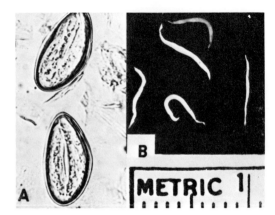

Figure 105-5 *Enterobius vermicularis.* **A,** unstained eggs on cellulose tape preparation. **B,** Adult worms. (Scale in centimeters.) From Juniper, K. In: *Gastroenterologic medicine.* Paulson, M., (editor). Philadelphia, Lea & Febiger, 1969.

Pathogenesis

Enterobiasis usually causes little disease. The most common symptom is pruritis ani, which may disturb sleep and, in children, may cause loss of appetite and irritability. The parasite has been suspected as a cause of appendicitis, and gravid female worms have been known to migrate into the vagina, uterus, fallopian tubes, and peritoneal cavity and become encapsulated. Pinworm urinary tract infection and vaginitis in young girls are being recognized more often.

Host Defenses

Little is known about immune responses to pinworm infection. Infections are more common in children than in adults, suggesting acquired immunity or age-related resistance. IgE serum levels in patients are reported to be within normal limits.

Epidemiology

Pinworm is a cosmopolitan parasite found most often in families and in institutionalized children. Pinworm is transmitted hand-to-mouth after scratching the perianal region, by handling contaminated bedding and night clothing, or by inhaling eggs in airborne dust. Eggs will not embryonate at temperatures below 23 C, but embryonated eggs remain viable for several weeks under moist and cool conditions.

Prevalence rates for *E vermicularis* are highest in temperate regions and are estimated at more than 200 million infected persons. In the United States, pinworm is considered the most common helminthic infection, with the highest prevalences in children. Only 1.3% of 300,000 stools examined in 1978 at state health laboratories were positive; however, examination of feces is not the recommended means of diagnosis.

No animal reservoirs exist for *E vermicularis,* although dogs and cats have been incriminated erroneously.

Diagnosis

Children suffering sleepless nights because of perianal itching often have pinworms. Eggs are rarely found in the feces, and the diagnosis is made by finding eggs in perianal swabs made of scotch tape. The tape is presented onto the perianal region, adhered to a microscope slide, and examined microscopically. Perianal specimens are best obtained in the morning before bathing or defecation. Three specimens should be taken on consecutive days before pinworm infection is ruled out.

Control

When an infection is recognized, efforts should be made to improve personal hygiene. Fingernails should be cut short, the perianal region washed in the morning, and bedding and sleeping garments washed daily. Other members of a patient's family should be checked; the entire household may need treatment to eliminate infection. Although several antihelminthics are effective in treating enterobiasis, the drugs presently recommended are pyrvinium pamoate, pyrantel pamoate, mebendazole, and albendazole.

CAPILLARIA PHILIPPINENSIS

Intestinal capillariasis is a relatively new disease, first recognized in 1967 in the Philippines and then in Thailand. More than 1800 cases have been reported. The parasite is small (females approximately 4 mm, males smaller) and lives in the jejunum. Infections are characterized by diarrhea, gurgling stomach, malabsorption, and a protein-losing enteropathy. Untreated patients usually die. Infections are acquired from eating uncooked freshwater fish that contain infective larvae. These larvae mature in the human intestine. In experimental animal infections, the larvae develop into adults in 12–14 days, and the females produce larvae. The second generation larvae mature in 2 weeks, and the females produce eggs that pass in the feces. The eggs that reach water embryonate in 10 days and, after being ingested by fishes, these eggs hatch in the intestine and develop into infective forms. Autoinfection is part of the life cycle, and several hundred thousand worms have been recovered from one body at autopsy.

Mebendazole is the drug of choice. Thiabendazole also is effective, but is less desirable because of side effects.

The eggs can be confused with *T trichiura,* and the parasite may be more widely spread than reports indicate. The fish serving as intermediate hosts are reported from many areas of Asia. Although none is known, a reservoir host, such as a fish-eating bird, is suspected.

TRICHOSTRONGYLUS SP

Trichostrongylus sp are related to hookworms, but lack a buccal capsule and are smaller. Most are parasites of herbivores, but human infections have been reported from several areas, including the Middle East, South America, Asia, and the Soviet Union. *T orientalis* is the most common species in Korea and Japan. Larvae develop in the soil, and infection is acquired by ingestion of vegetation contaminated with infective third-stage larvae. Only heavy infections are clinically important. Thiabendazole and pyrantel pamoate are effective against the parasite. Eggs are similar in appearance to hookworm, but are larger and the ends are more pointed. Hookworm infections that fail to respond to routine treatment may prove to be trichostrongyliasis. Rhabditiform larvae have been cultured from feces and can be differentiated from hookworm by a minute knob at the tip of the tail.

References

Carvalho, E.M., et al.: Immunological features in different clinical forms of strongyloidiasis. *Trans R Soc Trop Med Hyg* 1983; 77:346–349.
Centers for Disease Control. Intestinal parasite surveillance annual summary 1978. Atlanta: US Public Health Service. 1979.

Cross, J.H., et al.: Biomedical survey in North Samar Province, Philippine Islands. *Southeast Asian J Trop Med Pub Hlth* 1977; 8:464-475.

Cross, J.H., Banzon, T., Singson, C.N.: Further studies on *Capillaria philippinensis:* Development of the parasite in the Mongolian gerbil. *J Parasitol* 1978; 64:208-213.

Juniper, K.: Parasitic diseases of the intestinal tract. In: *Gastroenterologic medicine.* Paulson, M., (editor). Philadelphia: Lea and Febiger, 1969.

Rabbani, G.H., et al.: Comparison of string-test and stool examination in the diagnosis of strongyloidiasis and giardiasis in gastroenteritis patients. *Asian Med J* 1982; 25:695-700.

Stoll, N.: This wormy world. *J Parasitol* 1947; 33:1-18.

Whalen, G.E., Rosenberg, E.B., Strickland, G.T., et al.: 1969. Intestinal capillariasis. A new disease in man. *Lancet* 1:13-16.

World Health Organization: Intestinal protozoan and helminth infections. *WHO Tech Rpt Ser 666.* Geneva: WHO, 1981.

106 Enteric Nematodes of Lower Animals: Zoonoses

Doris S. Kelsey, MD

General Concepts

The more common zoonoses caused by enteric nematodes of lower animals will be reviewed in this chapter. Humans are not natural hosts for these parasites. Human infections are accidental, and the disease may or may not resemble that of the animal host. Understanding the epidemiology and pathogenesis of these zoonoses requires basic knowledge of the life cycle of the involved nematode in its natural animal host and in humans. If the parasite is not able to complete its life cycle in a human, as it does in the animal host, the disease process will differ accordingly. This is exemplified by the syndrome of visceral larva migrans, which is caused by the ascarids of dogs and cats. The adult worms cannot mature in the human host, so developmental arrest occurs in the larval stage. The larvae persist in tissue producing the clinical symptomatology associated with this syndrome. Other enteric nematodes such as *Trichinella spiralis* can complete their life cycle in humans, and produce disease similar to that in other mammalian hosts.

VISCERAL AND OCULAR LARVA MIGRANS

Visceral larva migrans (VLM) and ocular larva migrans (OLM) are clinical syndromes occurring primarily in children as a result of the systemic migration of the larval forms of animal helminthic parasites. *Toxocara sp*, the common roundworms of dogs and cats, are usually implicated.

Distinctive Properties

Toxocara canis, the dog roundworm, is the most frequent etiologic agent of VLM and OLM; *Toxocara cati*, the cat roundworm, is less frequently responsible. During their tissue phase, several other animal nematodes and human helminths may produce VLMlike syndromes.

The mature *Toxocara canis* worms live in the small intestine of the dog, their natural host. They have an average life span of about 4 months. A single female can produce 200,000 eggs per day. Heavily infected animals can pass millions of eggs per day in feces. Under appropriate environmental conditions in the soil, the eggs become infective after a few weeks, and remain infective for many months.

The VLM and OLM syndromes are caused by extraintestinal migration of larvae after ingestion of infective eggs by humans. The *Toxocara canis* larvae (20 μm in diameter and 400 μm in length) and their secretory-excretory products contain many antigens, including stage-specific antigens, that are not found in adult worms. The immunologic response of the human host to these antigens provides the basis for the currently available serodiagnostic tests. *Toxocara* larvae also contain surface antigens that stimulate isohemagglutin production.

Pathogenesis

Human infection caused by *Toxocara* results from ingestion of embryonated eggs. The larvae hatch in the small intestine, invade the mucosa, and enter the portal system. Some are trapped in the liver, but others proceed to the lungs and into the systemic circulatory system, from which they may be disseminated to virtually any organ.

Clinical manifestations are dependent on the magnitude of tissue damage produced by the invading larvae, and the associated immune-mediated inflammatory response. Two distinct patterns of infection are recognized: VLM and OLM. Infections not involving the eye that are caused by few parasites may be asymptomatic and hence may not be recognized clinically.

The classic VLM syndrome usually occurs in preschool children with a history of geophagia. Patients who have severe infections often present with eosinophilia, persistent fevers, and marked hepatomegaly; there may be associated respiratory symptoms with wheezing and coughing. Pulmonary infiltrates on chest roentgenograms usually are transient. Pruritic rashes are common. Seizure activity may occur in association with neurologic involvement. Death has been associated with myocarditis, encephalitis, and respiratory syndromes.

The ocular form of the disease usually occurs in children who are between school age and young adulthood. Ocular invasion by the larva may produce retinal granulomas or endophthalmitis, leukokoria (white pupillary reflex), decreased visual acuity, strabismus, or eye pain. Clinical resemblance to retinoblastoma has resulted in unnecessary enucleation of the involved eye. Patients with OLM rarely have a history of pica. It has been suggested that OLM is associated with fewer larvae than is VLM; the larvae thus fail to stimulate the magnitude of the host reaction seen in VLM. The host usually is asymptomatic until ocular involvement becomes apparent. This view is generally supported by the finding of higher serum titers in patients with VLM than in those with OLM. Rarely, the two forms of the disease coexist, which is presumably related to massive infection.

Host Defenses

VLM is associated with marked hematologic and immunologic host response in contrast to OLM, in which, presumably, the fewer parasites cause less host reactivity. Serum toxocara antibody titers usually are elevated to diagnostic levels in both syndromes. In VLM, leukocytosis with eosinophilia occurs. Peripheral leukocyte counts exceeding 100,000 per mm^3, with a predominance of eosinophils, are seen. Hypergammaglobulinemia is common, with IgE being markedly elevated. In addition to developing antibodies specific for larvae and their secretory-excretory products, a number of nonspecific antibodies may be produced, including IgM antibodies to IgG (rheumatoid factors) and elevated antibody titers to human A and B blood group substances.

Epidemiology

Approximately 20% of adult dogs are actively infected with *Toxocara canis*. Dogs commonly acquire infection transplacentally, but may also be infected by the transmammary route or by ingestion of embryonated eggs. When infective eggs are ingested by a canine host, the larvae hatch in the small intestine, invade the intestinal mucosa, and undergo an extraintestinal migratory phase. In older dogs, many larvae remain trapped in body tissues. In puppies, the majority of the larvae migrate through the bronchioles to the trachea and pharynx where they are swallowed, and complete maturation to the adult form in the intestine. Young puppies between 3 weeks and 3 months of age excrete a large number of eggs, which become infective in a few weeks under appropriate environmental conditions in the soil. Backyards, children's sandboxes, public parks, and beaches accessible to dogs are often contaminated with *Toxocara* ova, which may retain their infectivity for many months. These areas are potential sites of exposure for young children or others who accidentally ingest the infective eggs. Subsequently, larvae ingested by humans hatch in the small intestine; although they are not able to complete their life cycle in the human, an unnatural host, they persist in extraintestinal sites, causing the syndromes of VLM and OLM.

Diagnosis

The diagnosis of VLM usually is based on the clinical findings of visceral involvement in association with hypergammaglobulinemia, leukocytosis, and eosinophilia. Liver biopsy may be diagnostic, although the larvae are difficult to find even in the presence of eosinophilic granulomas (Figure 106-1 and Figure 106-2). Elevated titers of the anti-A

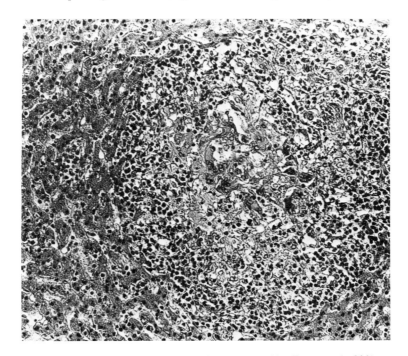

Figure 106-1 Liver biopsy from child with visceral larva migrans caused by *Toxocara* (×200).

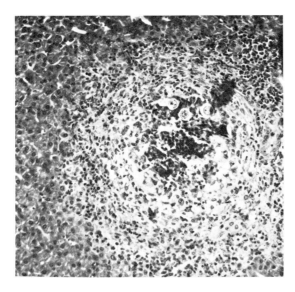

Figure 106-2 *Toxocara canis* larva in a liver lesion from an experimental animal (×200).

and anti-B isohemagglutinins support the diagnosis. An ELISA that uses larva-specific antigen has proven to be a reliable serologic test. It is especially useful in evaluation of ocular infections, which do not characteristically exhibit the peripheral eosinophilia and other host responses of VLM.

Control

Prevention of human infection centers on appropriate treatment of *Toxocara* infections in dogs and cats, and sanitary disposal of pet feces. Public education about the necessity of these preventive measures is needed. Many responsible pet owners are unaware of the health hazards imposed on humans by animal roundworm infections. Once the soil has become contaminated, infective eggs persist for months.

There is no treatment of proven efficacy for disease caused by *Toxocara* sp in humans. The antihelminthic drugs, diethylcarbamazine and thiabendazole, are of uncertain benefit. Corticosteroids have been used to decrease the inflammatory response in ocular infections and in severe respiratory or cardiac disease.

CUTANEOUS LARVA MIGRANS

Cutaneous larva migrans (creeping eruption) is a dermatitis caused by the larvae of *Ancylostoma braziliense*, the dog and cat hookworm, which penetrate human skin and migrate in the subcutaneous tissue. *Ancylostoma caninum* and other species of hookworms also can cause this infection. A similar cutaneous eruption may occur in patients with intestinal infection with *Strongyloides stercoralis* when autoinoculation of the perianal skin occurs by infective larvae passed in the stool. This syndrome is called larva currens (racing larva) because of the rapid migration of this larva in the skin.

Distinctive Properties

The third-stage hookworm larvae, which can penetrate unbroken human skin, are found in soil contaminated with excreta from infected animals. As the larvae invade the skin, a "tingling" sensation may be felt at the site of involvement. Proteolytic enzymes present in larval secretions may cause an inflammatory reaction associated with intense pruritis as the lesion progresses.

Pathogenesis

At the site of skin penetration by the *Ancylostoma* larva, an erythematous pruritic papule usually develops within a few hours. This intensifies over the next few days, and develops into a slightly raised erythematous serpiginous tract that usually progresses at the rate of 1-2 cm/day. The larvae migrate in the epidermis just above the basal layer and rarely penetrate into the dermis. Skin lesions may be single or numerous in massively infected persons. The most frequent areas of skin involvement are the feet, hands, buttocks, and genital areas. Lesions may become secondarily infected from scratching. Although the larvae cannot reach the intestine to complete their life cycle in their unnatural human host, they do occasionally migrate to the lungs where they produce pulmonary infiltrates. Both larvae and eosinophils have been demonstrated in the sputum of patients with pulmonary involvement.

Host Defenses

Hypersensitivity to the parasite can occur. Peripheral eosinophilia is common. However, protective immunity does not develop, and repeated infections may occur with subsequent exposure.

Epidemiology

Cutaneous larva migrans is primarily a disease of the southern United States, Central and South America, and other subtropical climates. The common etiologic agent, *Ancylostoma braziliense,* is an enteric parasite of dogs and cats. Humans acquire the infection when eggs are passed on to the soil from infected animals. Under favorable conditions of moisture and temperature, they develop within a few days into rapid-growing preinfective (rhabditoid) larvae, which feed on organic matter in the soil, molt, and then develop into nonfeeding infective (filariform) larvae. These larvae, infectious for man, remain in the upper one-half inch of soil, where contact with a new host can be established easily.

The disease is an occupational hazard for construction workers, plumbers, and electricians who are exposed to contaminated soil under buildings and crawlspaces. Children who go barefoot or play in backyards or sandboxes accessible to infected dogs and cats and sunbathers on the beach are other prime candidates for acquiring the infection. However, anyone who has skin contact with damp soil contaminated with the excreta of infected dogs or cats is subject to infection.

Diagnosis

Visual inspection of the classic serpiginous eruption is the usual method of diagnosis. Biopsy of the leading edge of the tract may demonstrate the larva.

Control

Control of human infections is dependent on periodic examination of dogs and cats for intestinal parasites, appropriate treatment, and sanitary disposal of animal excreta.

Treatment of cutaneous larva migrans topically with thiabendazole (available in a 10% suspension) usually is effective and without the side effects of oral therapy. In multiple or persistent infections, a combination of oral and topical thiabendazole can be given.

OTHER LARVAL MIGRATORY DISEASES

Several other animal parasites have been associated with VLMlike syndromes. These include *Ascaris suum*, *Capillaria hepatica*, *Angiostrongylus cantonsensis*, and *Angiostrongylus costaricensis*. The tissue phase of human helminths such as *Strongyloides stercoralis* and *Ascaris lumbricoides* also can produce similar clinical syndromes. Larvae of species of *Anisakis* and closely related nematodes of marine mammals have been reported to invade the stomach and other areas of the gastrointestinal tract of humans.

Ascaris suum, the common intestinal roundworm of domestic swine, is morphologically very similar to the human roundworm, *Ascaris lumbricoides*. Human infections with *Ascaris suum* are uncommon, but have been associated with a visceral larva migrans syndrome in children. The larvae invade the liver and lungs, but usually do not develop to maturity in the intestine.

Capillaria hepatica is a rat liver parasite. If the rat (the natural host) is eaten by a predator, the eggs found in the liver are released by the digestive process and passed in feces to soil. Human infection is acquired by ingestion of the infective eggs through contaminated food or water. The larvae hatch in the intestine and migrate to the liver, where maturation is completed. Clinical manifestations usually are those of an acute or subacute hepatitis. Eosinophilia and massive hepatomegaly may develop. Diagnosis is made by liver biopsy (Figure 106-3). There is no proven drug therapy.

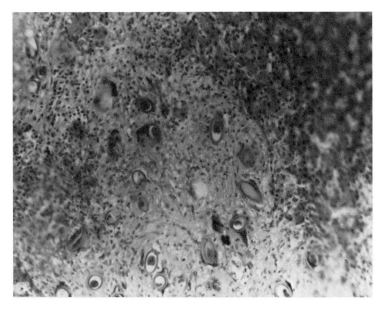

Figure 106-3 Human liver showing lesions containing eggs of *Capillaria hepatica*. Courtesy G.M. Ewing and I.L. Tilden.

Gnathostoma spinigerum are nematodes that reside in the stomach wall of dogs and cats. Most human infections occur in Thailand and other Asian countries. Infective larvae develop in copepods and are transferred through the food chain. Human infection results from consumption of improperly cooked fish or other foods that contain infective larvae. The larvae migrate in the tissues and may invade eye, brain, or any organ. They may cause eosinophilic meningitis. The immature worm may be demonstrated in subcutaneous nodules. Surgical removal of the larvae from eye lesions may be indicated to prevent migration to the central nervous system, which may result in death. Treatment with mebendazole is recommended.

Angiostrongylus cantonensis, the rat lungworm, may be the cause of eosinophilic meningitis and ocular disease in Southeast Asia, the Pacific Islands, and Cuba. In the United States, Hawaii is the only endemic site. Human infections are caused by ingestion of infected mollusks, the intermediate host, snails or slugs, or other members of the food chain containing infective larvae from these hosts. The larvae migrate to the brain, producing an eosinophilic meningitis. Paresthesias and ocular palsies are common. There is no specific treatment, but the prognosis usually is favorable.

Angiostrongylus costaricensis is a parasite of the mesenteric arteries of wild rats. Distribution is reported to be widespread in regions from Mexico to Brazil; the parasite is found even in cotton rats in Texas. Most reported cases of human disease have occurred in children from Costa Rica. Humans become infected by consumption of raw vegetables contaminated by a slug (the intermediate host) with infective third-stage larvae. The larvae mature in the mesenteric arteries, and produce a granulomatous inflammatory reaction. Abdominal pain and a mass in the right iliac fossa are the usual clinical manifestations, simulating appendicitis. The diagnosis usually is made by surgical exploration. A VLM syndrome has been reported with migration of the parasite to the liver. Thiabendazole has been used for treatment.

Species of *Anisakis* and certain members of related genera have been reported in the stomach and other areas of the alimentary tract of humans. Several hundred cases have been reported in various countries, particularly Japan; cases also have been reported from the East and West Coasts of the United States. Humans acquire this infection by eating raw fish, which contain the larvae of these nematodes. Following ingestion, these larvae penetrate the gastric mucosa and elicit an intense inflammatory response, gastric pain, vomiting, and diarrhea. Diagnosis is by surgery, gastroscopic examination, examination of vomitus, and histologic sections. In nature, these species develop to adults in the stomach of marine mammals; eggs, passed in the feces, hatch and are ingested by crustaceans in which larvae develop into an infective stage for fish. Ingestion of infected fish by marine mammals completes the life cycle.

TRICHINOSIS

Trichinosis is acquired by eating raw or inadequately cooked meat that contains the encysted larvae of the nematode, *Trichinella spiralis.* Any carnivorous mammal can be infected. The distribution of *Trichinella* is worldwide except for Australia and a few Pacific Islands.

Distinctive Properties

Trichinella spiralis completes its life cycle within one animal host. The infective larvae are about 1 mm in length, encyst in striated muscle, and retain their variability and infectivity for years. When ingested by a carnivorous host, they are released by gastric acid and peptic enzymes to mature and reproduce in the small intestine of the host. This enteric phase usually ends within 1 month. The adult viviparous female is about 3 mm in length, and is larger than the male. She may produce 1000 larvae during her life span. The larvae migrate throughout the body of the host and become encysted (encapsulated) in striated muscle to complete the life cycle.

Pathogenesis

Trichinosis is acquired by eating raw or inadequately cooked meat containing the encysted larvae of *Trichinella spiralis*. In humans, pork is the primary vehicle, although bear meat and wild carnivorous game are minor sources of infection. The severity of the disease is proportionate to the number of larvae ingested. In heavy infections, the clinical symptomatology may be correlated with the biologic stages of *Trichinella* as it completes its life cycle. Initially, the encysted larvae are released in the small intestine, where maturation to the adult stage occurs within 2-6 days. The adult worms burrow into the intestinal mucosa, where the viviparous female delivers the larvae. Early in the enteric phase, the host may experience gastrointestinal symptoms including abdominal pain, vomiting, and diarrhea. Within 1 week to 10 days after infection, fever, eosinophilia, muscle edema, and myalgias usually occur, because there is a diffuse inflammatory and allergic response with larval migration. The larvae are disseminated throughout the body via the circulatory system. Any organ may be involved, but survival and encapsulation occur in only striated muscle. The diaphragm, intercostal muscles, tongue, and facial muscles often are involved. An elevation of muscle enzymes (creatine kinase and serum glutamic oxalo-acetic transaminase) may develop during this stage. Serious complications may be related to invasion of the heart, lung, or central nervous system. Larval encystment in muscle usually begins about 3 weeks after the female delivers the larvae; calcification of cysts may take place within 6-9 months. This completes the life cycle. Humans usually are an end-stage host.

Host Defenses

Many immunologic responses may play a role in decreasing the severity of *Trichinella* infections. Massive eosinophilia, or hypergammaglobulinemia with markedly elevated IgE and circulating immune complexes, may accompany infection. Activated macrophages also appear to be involved in host defense. Although the mechanism is poorly understood in humans, animal experiments suggest that the rate of expulsion of the adult worms from the intestine is dependent on B and T lymphocyte function. Serum antibodies (IgM, IgG, and secretory IgA) also have been shown to inhibit larval production by mature worms. Other defenses are targeted toward the migratory larvae, which do not possess the thick cuticle of the adult. These may be exposed to or elicit a variety of humoral and cellular effector mechanisms during the migratory phase. Host resistance also has been shown to be enhanced by cell-mediated immunity.

Epidemiology

The incidence of *Trichinella* infections has declined; an average of less than 150 cases per year have been reported in the United States during the last decade. Most cases are acquired from infected pork that is inadequately cooked. Certain ethnic groups whose culinary preferences include raw pork are at special risk. The custom of sampling raw homemade sausage for flavor during the addition of seasonings and spices is another recognized cause of infection in the United States. Many consumers are unaware that the stamp "US Inspected and Passed" on raw pork products does not include inspection for *Trichinella*—inspection for *Trichinella* larvae is not included under the United States Department of Agriculture (USDA) specifications for pork products. Although cattle are herbivorous and consequently are not a reservoir of *Trichinella*, beef products may be contaminated by meat grinders also used for pork. Wild game is another minor source of *Trichinella* infection in humans.

Diagnosis

A history of ingestion of undercooked pork and the distinctive clinical features in association with eosinophilia suggest the diagnosis. If available, any leftover, suspect meat should be examined for *Trichinella* larvae. Serum antibodies are not usually detectable before 3 weeks after infection. A number of serodiagnostic tests, including the bentonite flocculation test, ELISA, fluorescent antibody, and complement fixation tests, have facilitated diagnosis. The bentonite flocculation test is a reliable serodiagnostic method and is positive in over 90% of cases; serum specimens may be submitted through State Public Health Departments for transmittal to the CDC for performance of the test. Definitive diagnosis is made by biopsy of striated muscle (Figure 102-4). To find the greatest concentration of larvae, the site should be near a tendinous insertion of an

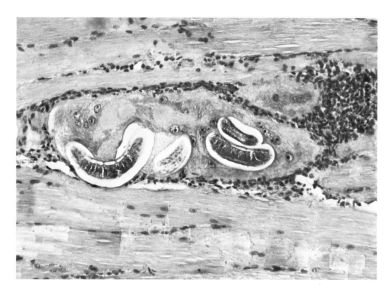

Figure 106-4 Encapsulated *Trichinella spiralis* larva in muscle from experimental animal (×200).

involved muscle. Histopathologic examination for larvae should be done. Also, a specimen of muscle should be examined fresh; compressing the specimen between two slides may reveal larvae on microscopic examination. Treatment of a portion of the muscle specimen for several hours with pepsin and hydrochloric acid to liberate the encysted larvae, followed by microscopic examination of the concentrated sediment for larvae, may improve the diagnostic yield.

Control

Trichinosis in humans can be prevented by adequate cooking of pork and wild game. According to USDA specifications, *Trichinella* larvae in pork products are killed when the latter are heated to an internal temperature of at least 58.3 C, or when frozen at −15 C for 20 days. However, freezing may not kill cold-resistant strains of *Trichinella*.

There is no proven effective therapy for trichinosis, but thiabendazole is thought to be an effective prophylactic agent for persons known to have ingested infected meat. In serious infections, thiabendazole and corticosteroids have been used. Some of the benefits of thiabendazole may be attributed to its antiinflammatory effects.

References

Bathrick, M.E., Mango, C.A., Mueller, J.F.: Intraocular gnathostomiasis. *Opthalmology* 1981; 99:1293-1295.

Beaver, P.C., Jung, R.C., Cupp, E.W.: *Clinical parasitology,* 9th ed. Philadelphia: Lea and Febiger, 1984.

Cypess, R.H., et al.: Larva-specific antibodies in patients with visceral larva migrans. *J Infect Dis* 1977; 135:633-640.

Edelgass, J.W., et al.: Cutaneous larva migrans in northern climates: A souvenir of your dream vacation. *J Am Acad Dermatol* 1982; 7:353-358.

Glickman, L.T., Schantz, P.M.: Epidemiology and pathogenesis of zoonotic toxocariasis. *Epidemiol Rev* 1981; 3:230-250.

Huntley, C.C., Costas, M.C., Lyerly, A.D.: Visceral larva migrans syndrome: Clinical characteristics and immunologic studies in 51 patients. *Pediatrics* 1966; 36:523-536.

Kazura, J. W.: Host defense mechanisms against nematode parasites: Destruction of newborn trichinella spiralis larvae by human antibodies and granulocytes. *J Infect Dis* 1981; 143:712-718.

Morera, P., et al. Visceral larva migrans-like syndrome caused by *Angiostrongylus costaricensis. Am J Trop Med Hyg* 1982;31:67-70.

107 Filarial Nematodes

Adam Ewert, PhD

General Concepts

Filariasis is a major public health problem infecting up to one-half of the adult human population in many tropical and subtropical areas. These infections are transmitted by arthropod vectors. Adult filariae are elongated, threadlike nematodes that, depending on the species, affect various parts of the body. Some are located in the lymphatics, where blockage and host reaction produce lymphatic dysfunction, edema, and fibrosis. Others are located in subcutaneous tissues, where they induce nodule formation. In some species, the microfilariae (juvenile stage) circulate in the blood, apparently causing little morbidity. In other species, microfilariae are present in tissue fluids of the skin, where they may produce dermatitis, or from which they may migrate to the eyes, causing loss of vision due to trauma and hypersensitivity reactions. Before the parasite can be transmitted, microfilariae must be ingested by arthropod intermediate hosts, in which they develop to the infective stage. (See Table 107-1 for a summary of major filarial infections of humans.)

LYMPHATIC FILARIAE (*WUCHERERIA BANCROFTI* AND *BRUGIA MALAYI*)

Distinctive Properties

Adults of *W bancrofti* and *B malayi* are elongated and slender (30–100 mm by 100–300 μm); thus they are adapted to living in lymphatic vessels, where they produce microfilariae that gain access to the blood. Both species are transmitted by mosquitoes. *W bancrofti* is endemic in many tropical areas of the world, whereas *B malayi* generally is restricted to Southeast Asia. Except for strains in the South Pacific, *W bancrofti* microfilariae show a strong nocturnal periodicity: the number of microfilariae in peripheral blood increases at night. Microfilariae are sequestered in capillaries, especially in the lungs, during the day. *B malayi* also may show microfilarial periodicity, but it is not as marked as in *W bancrofti*.

Pathogenesis

Infective larvae that have emerged from feeding vector mosquitoes enter a puncture wound in the skin. These larvae then migrate to the regional lymphatic vessels, causing the eventual blockage and edema characteristic of *W bancrofti* and *B malayi* infections.

Pathology varies greatly from one individual to another, and the exact mechanism is not completely understood. Considerable host reaction to the parasite occurs, especially when the worms molt, when the females first begin to deposit microfilariae, and when the worms die and degenerate. Lymph thrombi and masses of dead worms with granulomatous reactions often induce lymphatic dysfunction as vessels become partially or completely blocked. Static lymph favors secondary bacterial and mycotic infection. Figures 107-1 and 107-2 show the effect of filariae on the lymphatics of experimentally infected animals.

Elephantiasis, a grotesque enlargement of the infected area, may occur in some individuals after recurring attacks of lymphangitis (Figure 107-3). The initial inflammation of regional lymph nodes or of major lymphatic vessels may be followed by a prolonged asymptomatic period, and by recurring attacks of lymphangitis and "filarial fever" over a period of years. The exact cause of elephantiasis is not understood; however, repeated exposure appears to lead to production of abnormally large amounts of collagenous material and fibrosis of the tissue around the affected lymphatics.

Host Defenses

An inflammatory response causes the endothelial lining of the lymphatic vessels to thicken; a chronic inflammatory reaction is seen as the disease progresses. Information

Table 107-1   Summary of Major Filarial Nematodes that Infect Humans

Species	Location of Adults	Major Pathology	Location of Microfilariae	Major Vectors	Geographic Distribution
Wuchereria bancrofti	Lymphatics	Lymphangitis; elephantiasis	Blood; may exhibit nocturnal periodicity	Species of *Culex*, *Aedes*, and *Anopheles* mosquitoes	Widespread in tropical and subtropical countries
Brugia malayi	Lymphatics	Lymphangitis; elephantiasis	Blood	Species of *Mansonia* mosquitoes	Southeast Asia
Onchocerca volvulus	Subcutaneous nodules	Loss of vision; dermatitis	Tissue fluid in the skin	*Simulium* sp (blackflies)	Africa; Mexico; Guatemala; foci in Central and South America
Loa loa	Subcutaneous nodules	Transient swelling; temporary loss of vision	Blood; exhibit diurnal periodicity	*Chrysops* sp (deer flies)	Tropical Africa
Mansonella ozzardi	Subcutaneous and connective tissue (based on experimental animal studies)	Not well defined	Blood	Small biting flies in genera *Simulium* and *Culicoides*	West Indies; Central and South America
Dirofilaria sp	None in humans	Subcutaneous nodules; lung lesions	None in humans	Many species of mosquitoes	Cosmopolitan

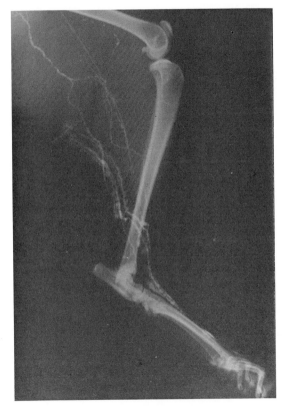

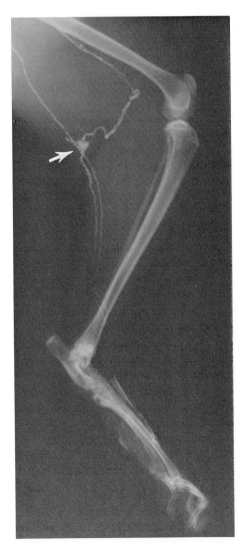

Figure 107-1 Lymphogram of *B malayi*-infected limb of laboratory animal. Note dilated, tortuous lymphatic vessels and presence of small, newly formed collateral vessels. Compare to lymphogram of a normal uninfected limb in Figure 107-2.

Figure 107-2 Lymphogram of uninfected limb of experimental animal. Note relatively fine, straight lymphatic vessels leading to the popliteal lymph node at arrow.

on specific immune responses of human filariasis is still limited, and has been accumulated mostly from serologic studies. Development of animal models in which long-term, controlled studies can be carried out may further understanding of the wide spectrum of clinical syndromes associated with lymphatic filariasis.

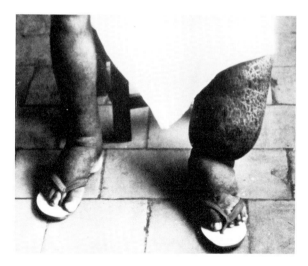

Figure 107-3 Elephantiasis of leg caused by chronic infection with the filarial nematode, *Wuchereria bancrofti.* (Photo courtesy of Shoyei Yamauchi.)

Epidemiology

W bancrofti is prevalent in many parts of the tropics and subtropics. Species from three major genera of mosquitoes that serve as vectors are the common house mosquito *Culex pipiens quinquefasciatus (C fatigans)* in many urban centers, *Aedes* sp in the South Pacific islands, and *Anopheles* sp in more isolated rural areas. Severe disease such as elephantiasis results from repeated exposure. The effect that the degree and frequency of infection has on development of the disease is still not fully understood. Circulating microfilariae may persist for many years in the absence of specific symptoms. Periodicity of microfilariae levels in the blood usually coincides with peak biting times of the vector mosquitoes prevalent in the area.

Humans previously were assumed to be the only hosts for *W brancrofti;* however, studies have shown several species of monkeys can be infected experimentally with *W bancrofti* larvae recovered from mosquitoes fed on human volunteers. To date, no naturally infected reservoirs other than humans have been identified.

B malayi and *W bancrofti* are similar in many ways, but some differences can be noted. Whereas *W bancrofti* is prevalent in tropical areas all over the world, *B malayi* is found mainly in Southeast Asia. In contrast to *W bancrofti*, which is transmitted by mosquitoes of the three major genera, the principal mosquito vectors of *B malayi* belong to the genus *Mansonia. B malayi* is less host-specific than *W bancrofti;* it has been recovered from naturally infected monkeys, cats, and dogs, and has been maintained in several laboratory animals.

Diagnosis

Enlarged and tender lymph nodes, especially in the inguinal region, or inflammation of lymphatic vessels of the extremities, should alert physicians in an endemic area to consider filariasis in their differential diagnosis. Definitive diagnosis may be accomplished by identifying microfilariae in thick blood smears. Species identification is based on the presence of a sheath and positioning of terminal nuclei. Because of nocturnal periodicity, blood smears are better made at night. Light infections may be detected by using one of several concentration methods.

Unfortunately, microfilariae may not be present in the blood during the early and late stages of the disease. When microfilariae are not detectable, a history of recurrent episodes of lymphangitis and lymphadenitis may form the basis for a presumptive diagnosis. Skin tests have been largely unsatisfactory, and commercial antigen is not widely available. Serologic tests are useful in epidemiologic studies, but have limited value in the management of individual cases.

Control

Attempts to reduce the prevalence of lymphatic filariae include vector control and mass treatment campaigns using diethylcarbamazine citrate. This drug reduces the microfilariae level in the blood significantly; however, it must be given over a prolonged period, and side effects such as fever, vertigo, headaches, nausea, and lymphatic inflammation occur frequently. Consequently, patient cooperation needed to complete the necessary series of treatments is often difficult to obtain.

ONCHOCERCA VOLVULUS

Distinctive Properties

Onchocerciasis is a nonfatal, filarial infection characterized by subcutaneous nodules formed in response to adult worms, chronic dermatitis caused by microfilariae in the skin, and impaired vision due to microfilariae in the eye. Humans become infected when vector blackflies bite and infective larvae gain entrance to the skin. Developing larvae and adult worms (up to 60 cm long) remain in subcutaneous tissue. Microfilariae produced by adult female worms migrate through the skin and subcutaneous tissues, but do not circulate in the blood.

Pathogenesis

Adult worms in the subcutaneous tissues cause varying degrees of inflammation and may induce subcutaneous nodules. These nodules may be seen 3-4 months after infection, but the microfilariae are not generally detectable until 1 year after infection. Adult worms may be surrounded by an inflammatory response that progresses to granuloma formation and fibrosis or calcification, depending on the condition of the worm and age of the nodule.

Microfilariae appear to move upward and, in chronic heavy infections, may be seen in the eye. Ocular damage is thought to be due to trauma caused by living microfilariae and a hypersensitivity reaction to dead ones. Therefore, treatment must include attention to eyes.

Host Defenses

Nodules containing adult worms are surrounded by inflammatory cells that are replaced by fibrotic tissue, thereby localizing the worms. Degenerating microfilariae may evoke increased infiltration of eosinophils and granulomatous reactions that ultimately destroy the microfilariae.

Epidemiology

Transmission occurs through bites of vector blackflies in the family Simuliidae. Although a few vector species breed in slow-moving streams, the majority require fast-flowing streams that provide adequate oxygenation. For this reason, the ocular disease is often called river blindness.

Onchocerciasis is prevalent in many parts of tropical Africa and has been reported in a few places in the Middle East. In the Western hemisphere, it is an important and widespread infection in Guatemala and the southern states of Mexico. It also appears in other areas of Central America, and a few foci have been found in Venezuela, Colombia, Surinam, Brazil, and Ecuador.

Diagnosis

Onchocerciasis is suggested by subcutaneous nodules or a characteristic scaly skin in individuals living in endemic areas. Positive diagnosis is usually made by identifying microfilariae from a superficial skin biopsy made with a scalpel or an appropriate punch. Biopsies, usually taken from the shoulder, are placed in a drop of saline or distilled water on a microscope slide, incubated for 30 minutes, and examined.

Removal of adult worms from nodules and observations of microfilariae in the eye also constitute definitive diagnosis. Serologic tests are being developed to aid in diagnosis when microfilariae cannot be detected, but onchocerciasis is suspected.

Control

Three main measures—vector control, nodule removal, and drug treatment—provide limited control of onchocerciasis. Control of blackfly vectors is difficult, because most species breed in fast-flowing streams where insecticides cannot be applied easily. Nodules harboring adult worms are commonly removed, presumably reducing the source of microfilariae, thereby reducing damage to the eyes as well as decreasing the number of microfilariae available to vectors. Mass treatment poses difficulties because suramin, the drug of choice for killing adult worms, must be given intravenously and is toxic. Diethylcarbamazine, which kills microfilariae but has limited efficacy against adult worms, has the disadvantage that some patients experience severe reaction to dying microfilariae, resulting in increased eye damage. Newer filaricides that eventually may replace current therapy are being evaluated.

LOA LOA

Distinctive Properties

Loiasis is a filarial infection in which the adult form of *L loa* may cause transitory subcutaneous swellings. The disease is restricted to tropical Africa, where it is transmitted by a biting fly of the genus *Chrysops*. Because adult *L loa* are seen frequently in the eyes, this organism has been known for many years as the African eye worm. Adult females are approximately 60 mm long; males are somewhat smaller. Microfilariae are sheathed but, in contrast to *W bancrofti*, exhibit a diurnal periodicity.

Pathogenesis

Humans become infected when vector *Chrysops* bite and the infective stage larvae gain access to the skin, developing to the adult stage in the subcutaneous tissue. Migration of adult worms in the subcutaneous tissue may cause transient large, discrete Calabar or fugitive swellings. These swellings in the skin generally regress in a few hours to a few days. Localized reactions such as swelling, itching, and pain occur as the worm migrates beneath the conjuctiva. Central nervous system involvement may occur, but it is less common.

Host Defenses

Host defenses are not well understood. It is not known whether the transient subcutaneous swelling characteristic of *L loa* infections is a reaction to the migrating worm, to toxins produced by the worms, or to the shedding of many microfilariae.

Epidemiology

Loiasis is restricted to West and Central African rain forest areas. Day-biting flies of the genus *Chrysops* transmit the disease.

Diagnosis

Diagnosis usually is based on identification of the sheathed microfilariae in blood smears. *L loa* must be differentiated from *W bancrofti* in geographic areas where the two infections overlap. Because the microfilariae are diurnally periodic, blood smears can be made during the day. Occasionally, diagnosis can be made by removing an adult worm from the skin or from the eye.

Control

Control consists of eliminating *Chrysops* breeding sites and treating infected individuals with diethylcarbamazine.

MANSONELLA OZZARDI

Distinctive Properties

Mansonella ozzardi is restricted to the Western hemisphere. Studies in animal models have suggested that the filaria typically inhabits the subcutaneous tissues. Unsheathed microfilariae are present in peripheral blood, especially in superficial capillaries of the skin.

Pathogenesis and Host Defenses

Documented information about pathology and host reactions is still very limited. Recent success in infecting experimental animals should result in additional information.

Epidemiology

M ozzardi is found in numerous countries in Central and South America and the West Indies. Depending on the geographic location, it is transmitted by biting flies of the genus *Simulium* or *Culicoides*.

Diagnosis

No set of clinical symptoms has yet been identified that suggests infection with *M ozzardi*. Diagnosis usually is based on demonstrating unsheathed microfilariae in blood. Because the microfilariae level is often relatively low, concentration methods are useful. Skin biopsies such as those used for detection of *Onchocerca* may show microfilariae, but histologic examination of these biopsies shows that most microfilariae do in fact come from superficial vessels rather than from tissue fluid as in *Onchocerca*.

Control

Control measures consist of eliminating breeding sites of small, biting flies that are usually found in rivers and streams.

DIROFILARIA SP

Dirofilaria immitis (dog heartworm) is a worldwide filarial parasite of dogs; adult worms (up to 30 cm long) usually are located in the dog's heart. In heavy infections, or when adult worms die, the parasites may be carried to the pulmonary vessels, where they may produce emboli. In humans, adult worms are not seen, but larval stages have been reported in cutaneous nodules, which may be confused with tumors, and have sometimes produced lesions in the lung (coin lesions) or breast tissue. Pulmonary lesions may be asymptomatic or may cause symptoms of coughing or chest pains. Roentgenograms frequently show a discrete mass suggestive of a tumor. Larvae of other *Dirofilaria* sp found in lower animals occasionally may be found in the skin or eyes of humans.

References

Beaver, P.C., Jung, R.C., Cupp, E.W.: *Clinical Parasitology*, 9th ed. Philadelphia: Lea and Febiger, 1984.

Orihel, T.C., Eberhard M.L.: *Mansonella ozzardi:* A redescription with comments on its taxonomic relationship. *Amer J Trop Med Hyg* 1982; 31:1142-1147.

Palmieri, J.R., et al: Animal model of human disease: Bancrofti filariasis. *Wuchereria bancrofti* infection in the silvered leaf monkey (*Prechytis cristatus*). *Am J Pathol* 1983; 112:383-386.

Sasa, M.: *Human filariasis. A global survey of epidemiology and control.* Baltimore: University Park Press, 1976.

Strickland, G.T.: *Hunter's tropical medicine*, 6th ed. Philadelphia: W.B. Saunders Co., 1984.

VI MICROBIOLOGY OF ORGAN SYSTEMS

Introduction

Johnny W. Peterson, PhD

C. P. Davis, PhD

Up to this point, this textbook has emphasized principles and concepts of microbiology. The goal of education, however, goes beyond the learning of discrete principles and concepts; ultimately, the student must pull these unrelated pieces of information together and be able to use them in an integrated manner. Therefore, this section provides a different perspective on the infectious disease process in the human host. Unlike earlier chapters, which approached the subject from the standpoint of the microbe, each chapter in this section takes a major organ system as its starting point and then describes various infections and their clinical implications for a particular organ system.

The student will be presented with numerous clinical syndromes that may be caused by multiple microbial genera. The student then is presented with the information about specimen collection, organism characteristics, host manifestations and laboratory tests that allow the investigator to differentiate one etiologic agent from another. The chapters offer help in deciding what sequences one may either follow or design to implicate a certain agent in disease. In addition, the chapters frequently give clues about the pathophysiology of a particular organ system that is infected by certain agents.

Viewing microbiology in this way should promote the student's grasp of the subject's medical relevance. The chapters included here correlate specific mechanisms of infection with disease manifestations in human organ systems, providing an overview of clinical problems in relation to the unique characteristics of the offending pathogens. By thus emphasizing the relative clinical importance of particular microorganisms, this section is a final step in preparing the student to bridge the gap between basic science and clinical medicine.

108 Microbiology of the Respiratory System

Chien Liu, MD

General Concepts

Acute respiratory infection is the most common acute illness bringing patients to their physicians. Respiratory diseases are grouped primarily by clinical symptoms and anatomic involvement of the respiratory tract without specific etiologic consideration. All upper respiratory tract infections (rhinitis, sinusitis, pharyngitis, and tonsillitis) are commonly grouped together. Upper respiratory infections are usually benign, transitory, and self-limited illnesses. Most are caused by viral agents and require no specific antimicrobial therapy. On the other hand, lower respiratory tract infections, especially pneumonia, are potentially life threatening because progressive inflammatory changes of the bronchial and alveolar spaces may compromise gas exchanges across the alveolar membranes, resulting in hypoxia. Pneumonia remains a leading cause of death in the United States today.

Etiologic agents associated with these diseases are viruses, mycoplasmas, bacteria, and fungi. Important variables include age, patient condition, time of year, and prevalence of microorganisms. The etiologic agents are identified by specific laboratory tests.

Methods for Laboratory Diagnosis

Collection of Specimens

Specimens for microscopic examinations and cultures can be collected easily from the respiratory tract by swabbing the nasopharynx or oropharynx. Expectorated sputum from patients with lower respiratory infections should be fresh. If no sputum is available, needle puncture and aspiration of tracheal fluids may be necessary, particularly in getting specimens for anaerobic cultures. If sputum samples cannot be obtained from tuberculous patients, collections of gastric contents by lavage may be necessary. When pleural effusion or empyema is present, specimens should be obtained by needle aspiration. In patients in whom a pneumonic process is not following the usual course of a bacterial pneumonia, perhaps because the patients are immunocompromised, a definitive etiologic diagnosis cannot be established by use of such traditional collection procedures. Under such circumstance, invasive procedures, including lung biopsy, should be pursued to achieve a correct diagnosis so that an appropriate therapy may be instituted.

Examination of Smears

Diagnosis of pharyngitis does not generally depend on microscopic examinations of smears prepared from pharyngeal secretions. Some reports indicate early diagnosis of streptococcal pharyngitis can be made by examining gram-stained smears from pharyngeal secretions for the presence of polymorphonuclear neutrophils and streptococci.

Sputum smears may be helpful in diagnosing acute bacterial pneumonia. Patients with anaerobic pulmonary infections usually produce putrid sputums. Sputum should be obtained by having the patient cough deeply, which will produce secretions from the lower respiratory tract. If the smear contains few or no polymorphonuclear neutrophils, or if the more than 10 squamous epithelial cells per high-power field are seen, the specimen is contaminated by oropharyngeal secretions and is considered unsatisfactory. The presence of predominant organisms in appropriately prepared smears, such as gram-positive, lancet-shaped diplococci, gives a presumptive diagnosis of pneumococcal pneumonia and allows early institution of antimicrobial therapy. Acid-fast stains are used to detect tuberculous and nocardial organisms.

Cultures

Except for some medical centers and state laboratories, most hospital clinical laboratories do not have facilities to perform viral cultures. Routine bacterial throat or sputum cultures should be inoculated onto sheep blood agar and chocolate agar plates and incubated at 35–37 C in a 5% CO_2 incubator or candle jar. If tuberculosis or fungal infections are suspected, specimens are inoculated in Lowenstein-Jensen medium or sabouraud agar and incubated accordingly.

Serologic Tests

For most bacterial infections involving the respiratory tract, serologic tests to confirm the diagnosis are rarely needed; however, serologic tests are helpful in confirming diagnosis of viral, mycoplasmal, fungal, and rickettsial infections. The quelling test (see Chapter 29) in typing pneumococci and the immunofluorescent staining for identification of group A β-hemolytic streptococci are valuable. Immunofluorescent staining provides the most useful procedure for diagnosis of Legionnaires' disease by visualizing *Legionnella pneumophila* organisms in infected lungs and by showing antibody response to the infection.

Normal Bacterial Flora in the Upper Respiratory Tract

The respiratory tract is contiguous to the outside environment and therefore is not sterile. Various microorganisms, often termed normal flora, reside in the nasopharynx and oropharynx. The predominant bacteria in the normal throat are α-streptococci, *Branhamella catarrhalis, Haemophilus hemolyticus,* some coagulase-negative staphylococci, and, to a lesser extent, pneumococci, diphtheroid bacilli, nonhemolytic streptococci, coliform organisms, and occasionally β-hemolytic streptococci. Although not considered a part of the respiratory tract, the mouth is continuous with the oropharynx. Various microorganisms, including many anaerobic organisms, are found in the buccal mucosa and gingiva. When these normal flora contaminate cultures, diagnostic interpretation is difficult.

Upper Respiratory Infections

The anatomic region above the larynx is considered the upper respiratory tract. Actually, the fact that only a short distance separates the nose from the larynx explains why upper respiratory infections are rarely confined to one specific area. Therefore, categorizing these infections clinically into common cold, pharyngitis, and laryngitis is highly artificial but useful. Viruses are the major etiologic agents. More than 150 members of different respiratory viruses have shown to be associated with upper respiratory infections (Table 108-1).

Common Cold

The cold is the most prevalent of all respiratory infections. Rhinitis, nasal obstruction, and watery discharge are the usual clinical manifestations. Viruses almost always cause an uncomplicated common cold; bacterial agents are rarely repsonsible. Rhinoviruses, with more than 100 different serotypes, are the largest single etiologic group of agents. Coronavirus follows, accounting for 10%–20% of colds in adults. Although parainfluenza viruses, adenoviruses, and respiratory syncytial virus are most often associated with other forms of respiratory illnesses, they can also induce a common cold syndrome, particularly in adults.

Table 108-1 Common Etiologic Agents Associated With Respiratory Infections

		Etiologic Agents		
Clinical Illness	Bacteria	Viruses	Fungi	Others
Common cold (rhinitis, coryza)	Rare	Rhinoviruses Coronavirus Parainfluenza viruses Adenoviruses Respiratory syncytial virus	Rare	Rare
Pharyngitis and tonsillitis (tonsillopharyngitis)	Group A β-hemolytic strepto- coccus Corynebacterium diphtheriae Neisseria gonorrhoeae Mycoplasma pneumoniae Mycoplasma hominis ?	Adenoviruses Coxsackieviruses A Herpesvirus hominis Influenza viruses Parainfluenza viruses	Candida albicans	Rare
Epiglottitis and laryngo- tracheitis (croup)	Haemophilus influenzae, type B Corynebacterium diphtheriae	Respiratory syncytial virus Parainfluenza viruses	Rare	Rare
Bronchitis and bronchiolitis	Haemophilus influenzae Streptococcus pneumoniae Mycoplasma pneumoniae	Parainfluenza viruses Respiratory syncytial virus	Rare	Rare
Pneumonia	Streptococcus pneumoniae Staphylococcus aureus β-hemolytic streptococcus Haemophilus influenzae Klebsiella pneumoniae Escherichia coli Pseudomonas aeruginosa Mycoplasma pneumoniae Legionnella pneumophila Anaerobic bacteria Mycobacterium tuberculosis and other species Coxiella burnetti Chlamydia psittaci Chlamydia trachomatis	Adenoviruses Parainfluenza viruses Respiratory syncytial virus Influenza viruses Varicella-zoster virus Measles virus Cytomegalovirus	Histoplasma capsulatum Blastomyces dermatitidis Paracoccidioides brasiliensis Coccidioides immitis Candida albicans Filobasidiella (Cryptococcus) neoformans Aspergillus fumigatus and other species	Pneumocystis carinii

Pharyngitis

Pharyngeal irritation, pain, and redness of the throat occur in pharyngitis. In tonsillitis, exudates and membranes over the tonsils are seen. Ulcers with an erythematous base on the pharyngeal wall may be present. Viral, bacterial, and fungal agents can be etiologic agents, but the second two groups of microbes probably account for fewer than 10% of the total infections. Of the bacterial agents, group A β-hemolytic streptococcus (*Streptococcus pyogenes*), *Corynebacterium diphtheriae*, and *Neisseria gonorrhoeae* are significant causes of pharyngitis. No evidence has shown staphylococcus, pneumococcus, or *H influenzae* to be responsible for acute bacterial pharyngitis. *Candida albicans* normally inhabits the human alimentary tract and the mucocutaneous regions. Poor oral hygiene, chronic debility, and impaired host defenses promote overgrowth of *Candida* organisms leading to oral candidiasis, which frequently also involves the pharynx. Incidence of oral candidiasis in newborns has been reported to be 4%-18%.

Herpes simplex virus frequently causes mucocutaneous ulcers in the oral cavity and pharynx. Many type A coxsackieviruses can also produce painful ulcerated lesions in the pharyngeal areas (herpangina), mainly in young children during summer months. Adenoviruses, parainfluenza, and influenza viruses can all cause pharyngitis. To differentiate various forms of viral or bacterial pharyngitis on clinical grounds alone is difficult, if not impossible. Epidemiologic surveillance of outbreaks helps. In sporadic cases, an etiologic diagnosis can only be established by isolation and serologic studies. *Mycoplasma pneumoniae* is a well-known cause of pneumonia; however, 10% of individuals infected with *M pneumoniae* may have pharyngitis rather than pneumonia. *M hominis*, type 1, has caused acute pharyngitis in human volunteer studies, but its role in naturally occurring human disease is uncertain.

Epiglottitis and Laryngotracheitis

Inflammatory changes and edema from infection of the epiglottis and larynx often cause hoarseness and upper airway obstruction. Acute epiglottitis usually begins with an abrupt onset of fever, sore throat, malaise, and marked difficulty in swallowing. It is most prevalent in young children between 2 and 5 years of age. The responsible organism is almost always *H influenzae* type b. This condition is a medical emergency requiring early diagnosis, establishment of a patent airway, and institution of appropriate antimicrobial therapy.

Laryngotracheitis, or croup, is characterized by hoarseness, a brassy cough, and fever. Pathologically, subglottic inflammation and swelling occur, which may progress to airway obstruction. Viruses are the most common etiologic agents, with parainfluenza viruses and respiratory syncytial virus predominating. *C diphtheriae* is the bacterial agent that should be considered, particularly in an unimmunized individual.

Lower Respiratory Infections

In contrast to the upper airway, the lower respiratory tract is generally sterile; thus, any microorganisms that multiply in the lower tract may cause infection. Nearly 50% of lower respiratory infections may be bacterial.

Bronchitis and Bronchiolitis

Acute bronchitis is usually preceded by an upper respiratory infection, or it can be a part of certain specific infections such as pertussis, scarlet fever, typhoid fever, measles, or influenza. Cough, sputum production, substernal discomfort, and coarse, moist rales on auscultation are common clinical manifestations. Etiologic diagnosis may be difficult because throat or sputum cultures from these patients often yield a variety of bacteria, including pneumococcus, *Streptococcus* sp, *Haemophilus* sp, and *Staphylococcus* sp. The etiologic significance of such cultural results is difficult to assess, as these organisms normally inhabit the upper respiratory tract. Viruses associated with upper respiratory infections and *M pneumoniae* generally are believed capable of causing bronchitic infections.

Chronic bronchitis, a condition characterized by cough with excessive sputum production, usually is associated with other chronic obstructive pulmonary diseases. Etiologically, environmental factors, such as air pollution and cigarette smoking, are important contributors, with microbial agents perhaps playing only a secondary role. Pneumococcus and *H influenzae* are the most commonly isolated organisms from sputum of symptomatic patients with chronic bronchitis, but their roles remain unclear. *Pseudomonas* may also be recovered, particularly in patients with serious obstructive lung disease, including cystic fibrosis. A study of acute exacerbations of chronic lung disease showed 64.2% associated with nonbacterial agents: rhinoviruses (42.8%), respiratory syncytial virus (11.9%), and *M pneumoniae* (9.5%).

Bronchiolitis, an acute respiratory infection of young infants, is characterized by obstruction of the terminal bronchial tree. Viral agents usually are the causative organisms; respiratory syncytial virus and type 3 parainfluenza virus are the most important. Other viruses (including adenoviruses, rhinoviruses, and influenza viruses) may also contribute to this clinical syndrome.

Pneumonias

When an imflammatory disease involves the parenchymal lung tissues and leads to consolidation detectable by physical examination and roentgenogram, it becomes pneumonia. Although chemical and physical agents can cause pneumonia, only microbial agents are discussed in this chapter. Invading microorganisms may reach the lungs by droplet inhalation, aspiration, or the blood. Virtually any bacterial or nonbacterial organism can be an etiologic agent. Chronically debilitated, unconscious, or immunosuppressed patients are more prone to develop pulmonary infections.

Bacterial Pneumonia   *S pneumoniae* is by far the most common organism responsible for acute bacterial pneumonia. Sixteen serotypes, as classified by capsular polysaccharides (1, 3, 4, 5, 6, 7, 8, 9, 11, 12, 14, 18, 19, 20, 22, and 23) have been shown to account for 85% of all bacteremic pneumococcal infections in the United States. *Staphylococcus aureus* pneumonia usually results from staphylococcal bacteremia, but also occurs as a complication of influenza viral infection. Group A β-hemolytic streptococcus sometimes causes pneumonia that is commonly hemorrhagic and accompanied by empyema.

Gram-negative organisms do not often cause pneumonia in healthy individuals; however, in chronically debilitated patients (those with obstructive lung disease and those requiring mechanical ventilation for sustaining pulmonary functions), nosocomial gram-negative pneumonia is a hazardous complication with significant mortality rates. *Klebsiella pneumoniae, Escherichia coli, Pseudomonas aeruginosa,* and other gram-negative organisms are the etiologic agents. *Francisella tularensis,* the causative agent of tularemia, can produce pneumonia. *Yersinia pestis,* which is transmitted to humans by fleas on rodents, usually produces bubonic plague or septicemia. Pneumonia can be a complication, however, and droplet inhalation can allow pneumonic plague to spread from person to person directly.

Anaerobic bacterial pleuropulmonary infections occur mostly in patients with altered consciousness as a result of aspiration. The infections often lead to extensive necrosis, abscess formation, bronchopleural fistula, and empyema. Various organisms, including *Peptococcus, Peptostreptococcus, Veillonella, Propionibacterium, Bacteroides,* and *Fusobacterium* are isolated from such pleuropulmonary specimens. Frequently, a mixed culture with several species of organisms (including aerobes) is found. *Actinomyces,* often considered a fungus, but actually an anaerobic bacterium, can be another causative agent.

M pneumoniae, which lacks a cell wall, produces pneumonia clinically quite different from those previously described. *M pneumoniae* infection occurs most commonly in the young (5-19-year-old age group). The agent spreads slowly from person to person. Most outbreaks are reported in military recruits and college students. *M pneumoniae* is a fastidious organism requiring special enriched medium and prolonged incubation for cultural growth.

L pneumophila is the etiologic agent responsible for the Legionnaires' disease that occurred in members attending the American Legion Convention held in Philadelphia in 1976. Although the original Philadelphia outbreak involved a rather serious pneumonia with characteristic symptomatology and a mortality rate of 17%, studies on other outbreaks showed more protean manifestations. *L pneumophila* and Legionellalike organisms including the Pittsburg pneumonia agent have been implicated in nosocomial pneumonias. Legionella organisms survive well in water, and their presence in aerosolized tap water of respiratory devices, air conditioners, and showers has been reported to cause pneumonia in hospital patients. Laboratory diagnosis is difficult. The bacterium is rarely demonstrable in sputum specimens, but is found in lung tissues or pleural fluid by using immunofluorescent staining and culture with enriched media. Serologic diagnosis also is available by employing the indirect immunofluorescent staining technique for antibody titration on acute and convalescent serums.

The incidence of tuberculosis in developed countries has declined steadily, but this disease still contributes significantly to morbidity and mortality in the general population. A total of 25,520 cases of active tuberculosis in the United States were reported to the CDC in 1982, with higher case rates in older age groups. The atypical mycobacteria can produce pulmonary infections indistinguishable from those caused by *M tuberculosis.* Pulmonary tuberculosis is usually a chronic disease; however, in occasional cases, acute pneumonia with pleural effusion can occur.

Confirmatory laboratory diagnosis of tuberculous infection of the respiratory system rests on the demonstration of mycobacteria in sputum with acid-fast stain or fluorescent microscopy and on culture of the organisms. Because tubercle bacilli grow slowly, 4-6 weeks are required for cultivation. A positive skin test with PPD tuberculin preparation is helpful; however, a negative test may be seen in early tuberculosis infections, in disseminated military tuberculosis, and in anergic patients.

Viral Pneumonia   Among the 33 serotypes of adenoviruses, fatal pneumonias in infants have been associated with types 1, 2, 3, 7, and 7a. Necrotizing bronchitis and pneumonitis seen at autopsy with intranuclear inclusion bodies in infected cells are the major findings. Incidence of adenoviral infections in civilian populations is relatively low; however, in military recruits, adenoviral acute respiratory disease (ARD) is common and types 2, 4, and 7 have been associated with pneumonias.

Respiratory syncytial viral pneumonia in infants occurs most often in winter months. A study over an 8-year period at the Children's Hospital in Washington, D.C., showed that respiratory syncytial virus was isolated in 29.6% of infants wtih bronchiolitis, and in 9.5% of those with pneumonia.

Influenza viruses usually cause self-limited diseases with tracheobronchitis and constitutional symptoms. A serious complication is pneumonia from secondary bacterial infections due to staphylococcus or pneumococcus. Primary influenza viral pneumonia with a high mortality rate also can occur, particularly in geriatric patients and in patients with underlying chronic pulmonary, cardiovascular, renal, or metabolic diseases.

Cytomegalovirus, which is known to cause congenital infections in neonates and an illness resembling mononucleosis in adults, has now been recognized as a significant etiologic agent of pneumonias in patients whose immunologic capacity has been compromised congenitally, through disease, or as a consequence of immunosuppressive therapy. Clinically, cytomegalovirus pneumonia is impossible to differentiate from other nonbacterial pneumonias.

Varicella-zoster virus classically causes cutaneous lesions seen in chicken pox and herpes zoster. Primary varicella pneumonia rarely occurs in children; more than 90% of cases are seen in persons over 19 years old. When pneumonia complicates varicella, the mortality rate is significant (10%-30%).

Measles (rubeola) patients almost always have cough and signs of acute bronchitis. Although bacterial pneumonia is a serious complication, primary measles pneumonia also can occur in certain patients. Children with immunodeficiency disorders or with malignant diseases should not receive live measles vaccine because giant-cell pneumonia due to attenuated measles vaccine has been reported in such hypervulnerable children.

Fungal Infection   Pneumonia caused by fungi may be acute; however, many fungal organisms produce pulmonary infections that usually are chronic and may or may not be clinically apparent. Pathologically, the characteristic lesion is a chronic granuloma.

The systemic pathogenic fungi (*Histoplasma capsulatum, Blastomyces dermatitidis, Paracoccidioides brasiliensis*, and *Coccidioides immitis*) may cause pulmonary diseases in normal as well as in immunologically compromised patients. Diagnosis based on clinical grounds alone is difficult; however, these diseases usually have a specific geographic distribution that can help in differentiation. Confirmatory diagnosis can be obtained by finding the organisms by microscopic examinations, by cultures from sputum specimens and lung tissues, or both.

Filobasidiella (Cryptococcus) neoformans, Candida albicans, Aspergillus fumigatus, and other species are generally opportunistic organisms more prone to produce disease in compromised patients. *Actinomyces* and *Nocardia* actually are not fungal agents, but are often discussed under mycology in many medical and microbiology textbooks. They too can produce pulmonary disease.

Other Agents   *Coxiella burnetii* is a rickettsia responsible for Q fever. The disease is an acute systemic infection characterized by sudden onset of fever, malaise, headache, chills, and pneumonitis that is usually mild and self-limiting; however, chronic Q fever with endocarditis is a frequently fatal illness.

Chlamydia is a group of obligate intracellular parasites that reproduce by binary fission in living cells. The two main species, *C psittaci* and *C trachomatis*, each contain subtypes. Many birds and nonprimate animals are the natural hosts of *C psittaci*. Humans are only occasionally accidental hosts. Infections may cause systemic disease with pneumonia. *C trachomatis* is an almost exclusively human parasite, responsible for trachoma-inclusion conjunctivitis, lymphogranuloma venereum, and nongonococcal urethritis. In addition, *C trachomatis* has been shown to be an important agent responsible for pneumonitis in newborns and young infants.

Pneumocystis carinii is a protozoanlike organism that caused epidemics of interstitial plasma cell pneumonia in premature, debilitated babies in Europe and Asia during World War II. *P carinii* has been found to produce a potentially life-threatening pneumonia in infants with immunodeficiency, in compromised hosts (with hematologic malignancies or collagen vascular disease), and in patients with organ transplants who are receiving corticosteroids and other immunosuppressive therapy. *P carinii* pneumonia is a major problem in acquired immune deficiency syndrome (AIDS). Confirmatory diagnosis of *P carinii* pneumonia is not easy because the organism is rarely detectable in sputum smears and cannot be cultivated. Aggressive invasive diagnostic procedures such as open lung biopsy to obtain tissues for histologic examinations usually are necessary.

References

Anderson, L.J. et al.: Viral respiratory illnesses. *Med Clin North Am* 1983; 67:1009-1030.

Cherry, J.D.: Acute epiglottitis, laryngitis, and croup. In: *Current clinical topics in infectious diseases 2.* Remington, J.S., Swartz, M.N., (editors). New York: McGraw-Hill, 1981.

Christie, A.B.: Acute respiratory infections. In: *Infectious diseases,* 3rd ed. Christie, A.B., (editor). Edinburgh: Churchill Livingston, 1980.

Donowitz, G.R., Mandell, G.L.: Acute pneumonia. In: *Principles and practice of infectious disease,* 2nd ed. Mandell, G.L., Douglas, R.G., Jr, Bennett, J.E., (editors). New York: John Wiley and Sons, 1985.

Gulick, P., Hall, G., McHenry, M.C.: Office microbiology. *Med Clin North Am* 1983; 67:39-57.

Liu, C.: Nonbacterial pneumonias. In: *Infectious diseases,* 3rd ed. Hoeprich, P.D., (editor). Hagerstown, MD: Harper and Row, 1983.

Murray, P.R., Washington, J.A.: Microscopic and bacteriologic analysis of expectorated sputum. *Mayo Clin Proc* 1975; 50:339-344.

Ogra, P.L., Fishaut, M., Welliver, R.C.: Mucosal immunity and immune response to respiratory viruses. In: *Seminars in infectious diseases 3.* Weinstein, L., Fields, B.N., (editors). New York: Thieme-Stratten, Inc, 1980.

Rubin, R.H., Greene, R.: Etiology and management of the compromised patient with fever and pulmonary infiltrates. In: *Clinical approach to infection in the compromised host.* Rubin, R.H., Young, L.S., (editors). New York: Plenum Medical Book Co, 1981.

Yoshikawa, T.T.: Collection, handling, and processing of specimens for the laboratory. In: *Infectious diseases.* Yoshikawa, T.T., Chow, A.W., Guze, L.B., (editors). Boston: Houghton Mifflin Professional Publishers, 1980.

109 Microbiology of the Circulatory System

Lawrence L. Pelletier, Jr., MD

General Concepts

The circulatory system, comprised of the blood, blood vessels, and the heart, is normally free of microbial organisms. Isolation of bacteria or fungi from the blood of ill patients usually signifies serious and uncontrolled infection that may result in death. The presence of bacteria (bacteremia) and fungi (fungemia) in the blood occurs in more than 250,000 individuals per year in the United States and causes at least 50,000 deaths annually. Because rapid isolation, identification, and performance of antimicrobial susceptibility tests may lead to initiation of lifesaving measures, the culturing of blood to detect microbemia is one of the most important clinical microbiology laboratory procedures.

Clinical Syndromes

Asymptomatic Microbemia

Microbes enter the circulatory system via lymphatic drainage from localized sites of infection or mucosal surfaces that are subject to trauma and are colonized with normal bacterial flora. Organisms may also be introduced directly into the bloodstream by infected intravenous needles or catheters or contaminated intravenous infusions. Small numbers of organisms or nonvirulent microbes are removed from the circulation by fixed macrophages in the liver, spleen, and lymph nodes. The phagocytes are assisted by circulating antibodies and complement factors present in serum. Under certain conditions, antibodies and complement factors may kill gram-negative bacteria by lysis of the cell wall. Also, they may promote phagocytosis by coating bacteria (opsonization) with antibody and complement factors that have receptor sites for neutrophils and macrophages.

When defense mechanisms effectively remove small numbers of organisms, clinical signs or symptoms of microbemia (asymptomatic microbemia) may not be present. Asymptomatic bacteremias caused by endogenous bacterial flora have been observed in normal individuals after vigorous chewing, dental cleaning or extraction, insertion of urinary bladder catheters, colon surgery, and other manipulative procedures. Asymptomatic bacteremias may occur if localized infections are subjected to trauma or surgery.

Most asymptomatic bacteremias are of no consequence; however, occasionally virulent organisms causing a localized infection (such as a *Staphylococcus aureus* skin boil) may produce infection at a distant site (for example, bone infection) by means of asymptomatic bacteremia. Similarly, artificial or damaged heart valves may be colonized by viridans streptococci during asymptomatic bacteremia induced by dental manipulation. Infection of the heart valve (infective endocarditis) is fatal if not treated. Therefore, individuals with known valvular heart disease who undergo dental work or other procedures that produce asymptomatic bacteremias are given antibiotics to prevent colonization of the heart.

Symptomatic Microbemia

When a sufficient number of organisms is introduced into the bloodstream, an individual will develop an elevated temperature (fever), cold sensation (chills), shivering (rigors), and sweating (diaphoresis). Patients with microbemias usually look and feel ill. As macrophages and polymorphonuclear leukocytes phagocytize microbes, they synthesize and release interleukin 1 into the circulation. This small molecular weight protein acts on the temperature regulatory center in the brain and sets the body thermostat at a higher level. The thermoregulatory center acts to decrease heat loss by reducing peripheral blood flow to the skin (pale appearance) and increases heat production by muscular activity (shivering), resulting in a rise in body temperature. When either a high body temperature level is attained or the microbemia terminates, the central nervous system thermostat becomes reset at a lower level and acts to reduce body temperature by increased peripheral blood flow to the skin (flushed appearance) and by sweating.

Symptomatic microbemias are most commonly caused by the organisms listed in Table 109-1. In recent years, the incidence of gram-positive coccal bacteremias resulting from intravascular access infections in debilitated patients with serious underlying conditions has increased steadily, but gram-negative bacillary infection still predominates. Hospitalized patients frequently have had surgery, severe trauma, or neoplasms that predispose to complicated local infections; also, these individuals' host defenses have been compromised by malnutrition, age, and corticosteroid or cancer chemotherapy. Granulocytopenia due to leukemia, cancer, or cancer chemotherapy is a frequent

Table 109-1 Common Causes of
Symptomatic Microbemia*

BACTERIA

Gram-positive

Streptococcus pneumoniae

S aureus

Enterococcus

Nonenterococcal group D streptococci

Streptococci (viridans)

Group B streptococcus

Group A streptococcus

Microaerophilic and anaerobic cocci

Clostridia sp

Listeria monocytogenes

Gram negative

Escherichia coli

Klebsiella-Enterobacter-Serratia sp

Bacteriodes fragilis

Pseudomonas aeruginosa

Proteus sp

Haemophilus influenzae

Neisseria sp

Acinetobacter sp

Salmonella sp

FUNGI

Candida sp

Torulopsis glabrata

*See chapters 64, 67, and 71 for discussions of the pathogenesis of virus
infections for viruses that cause viremia.

predisposing cause of microbemia and a reason for poor response to antimicrobial
therapy. Occasional outbreaks of gram-negative bacteremia have been related to
contaminated respirators, infected intravenous solutions, and indwelling urinary catheters. Table 109-2 lists a number of conditions predisposing to symptomatic microbemia
and the organisms most commonly associated with those conditions. Organisms other
than those listed in Table 109-1 may produce microbemia in severely compromised
hosts. Skin contaminants, such as *Staphylococcus epidermidis* and diphtheroid species,
may cause significant microbemias if isolated from multiple blood cultures and are
associated with intravenous catheters or prosthetic heart valves.

A number of disseminated virus infections are spread through the body via the
bloodstream. These viruses include polioviruses, hepatitis viruses, the scrapie-kuru
group, rubella virus, measles virus, smallpox virus, and arboviruses (mainly togovirus).
Signs and symptoms of disease may or may not accompany viremia. Most viremias are
acute and last for several days. Viremias due to serum hepatitis virus, the scrapie-kuru
group, and rubella virus may persist for weeks, months, or years.

Table 109-3 presents a classification of symptomatic microbemia based on
persistence and recurrence of microbemia. **Transient microbemias** are self-limited

Table 109-2 Conditions Predisposing to Symptomatic Microbemia

Condition	Mechanism	Organisms
Urinary tract catheter	Microbial colonization of urinary tract	Gram-negative enteric bacilli, *P aeruginosa, Serratia* sp, Enterococcus
Intravenous catheter	Direct access of skin flora to circulatory system	*S aureus, S epidermidis*, gram-negative bacilli, *Candida* sp
Endotracheal intubation or tracheotomy	Microbial colonization of lower respiratory tract	*S aureus*, gram-negative enteric bacilli, *P aeruginosa*
Extensive burns	Loss of skin barrier function with burn wound infection	Group A streptococcus, *P aeruginosa*, gram-negative enteric bacilli, *Candida* sp
Granulocytopenia	Loss of polymorphonuclear leukocyte phagocyte function	*P aeruginosa, Klebsiella* sp other gram-negative enteric bacilli, *Candida* sp, *S aureus*
Hypogammaglobulinemia	Loss of opsonization of microbes by antibodies	Pneumococcus, *H influenzae*, meningococcus
Splenectomy	Loss of fixed macrophages and antibody-producing lymphocytes	Pneumococcus, *H influenzae*, meningococcus
Newborns	Immature host defense mechanisms; colonization by maternal and hospital organisms	Group B streptococci, *E coli*, other gram-negative enteric bacilli, *S aureus, L monocytogenes*
Contaminated intravenous infusions	Direct intravascular infusion of microbes that grow at room temperature or below	*Klebsiella-Enterobacter* sp, *Candida* sp
Abnormal heart valve	Increased likelihood of colonization of heart valve during transient bacteremias	Viridans streptococci, enterococci, nonenterococcal group D streptococci, *S aureus*, microaerophilic streptococci, *Haemophilus* sp.
Prosthetic heart valve (within 2 months of surgery)	Foreign body providing site of intravascular colonization at or after surgery	*S aureus, S epidermidis*, gramnegative bacilli, *Candida* sp, group D streptococci, diphtheroids
Prosthetic heart valve (more than 2 months after surgery)	Focus of colonization for transient bacteremias	Streptococci, enterococci, *S aureus, S epidermidis, Haemophilus* sp

and often due to manipulation of infected tissues, such as incision and drainage of an abscess; early phases of localized infection, such as pneumococcal bacteremia in pneumoccal pneumonias; or bacteremias associated with trauma to mucosal surfaces colonized by normal host flora. When multiple blood cultures are positive over a period of 12 hours or more, a **continuous microbemia** is present. The presence of continuous microbemia suggests a severe spreading infection that has overwhelmed host defenses. A continuous microbemia may originate from an intravascular site of infection in which

Table 109-3 Types and Causes of Microbemia

Transient Microbemias
    Manipulation of infected tissues
    Early phases of localized infection
    Trauma to mucosal surfaces
Continuous Microbemias
    Severe generalized infections
    Intravascular foci of infection
        Infective endocarditis
        Endarteritis
        Septic thrombophlebitis
        Infected intravenous catheter or device
        Contaminated intravenous infusions
    Specific infections
        Typhoid fever
        Tularemia
        Brucellosis
        Plague
        Glanders
        Melioidosis
        Rat bite fever
        Leptospirosis
Intermittent Bacteremias
    Undrained abscess or closed space infection
    Repeated manipulation of infected tissues
    Recurrent obstruction of infected urinary or
      biliary tracts
    Specific infections
        Chronic meningococcemia
        Chronic gonococcemia
        Brucellosis

organisms are shed directly into the bloodstream (e.g., infective endocarditis or an infected intravascular catheter), or from an early phase of specific infections characterized by a continuous microbemia (e.g., typhoid fever).

Microbemias may persist despite treatment with antimicrobial agents to which the organisms are susceptible. Thus, repeated blood cultures should be performed in patients who do not appear to respond to treatment, even though antimicrobial administration is continued. During the first 3 days of treatment, positive blood cultures often are associated with inadequate antimicrobial dosage. Microbemias that persist longer than 3 days may be caused by organisms resistant to multiple antimicrobial agents, undrained abscesses, or intravascular foci of infection. When positive blood cultures with the same organism are separated by negative cultures, an **intermittent microbemia** is present. Common causes of intermittent microbemias are listed in Table 109-3.

Septic Shock

Septic shock occurs in approximately 40% of patients with gram-negative bacilli bacteremia and 5% of patients with gram-positive bacteremia. The septic shock syndrome consists of a fall in systemic arterial blood pressure with resultant decreased effective blood flow to vital organs. Septic shock patients frequently develop renal and pulmonary insufficiency and coma as part of a generalized metabolic failure caused by inadequate blood flow. Survival depends on rapid institution of broad-spectrum antimicrobial therapy, intravenous fluids, and other supportive measures. Elderly patients and those with severe underlying surgical or medical diseases are less likely to survive. Mortality for gram-negative septic shock ranges from 40%–70%. Septic shock may also occur with rickettsial, viral, and fungal infections.

Septic shock due to gram-negative rod bacteremias constitutes the most common serious infectious disease problem in hospitalized patients. The high frequency of septic shock in gram-negative bacillary infection is attributed to the toxic effect on the circulatory system of lipopolysaccharides (endotoxin) found in the cell wall of gram-negative organisms. Endotoxin within the circulatory system has multiple and complex effects on neutrophils, platelets, complement, clotting factors, and other substances in the blood. The symptoms of bacteremia and septic shock can be reproduced when purified cell-wall endotoxin is injected into the circulation.

Infective Endocarditis

Heart valve infections generally are classified as acute endocarditis, subacute endocarditis, and prosthetic valve endocarditis. If they are untreated, these infections are fatal. With treatment, mortality averages 30% and is higher in acute and prosthetic valve infections.

Acute endocarditis usually occurs when heart valves are colonized by virulent bacteria in the course of microbemia. The most common cause of acute endocarditis is *S aureus;* other less common causes are *Streptococcus pneumoniae, Neisseria gonorrhoeae, Streptococcus pyogenes,* and *Streptococcus faecalis* (enterococcus). Patients with acute endocarditis usually have elevated temperature, marked prostration, and signs of infection at other sites. Infected heart valves may be destroyed rapidly, leading to heart failure from valve leaflet perforation and acute valvular insufficiency. Infected pieces of fibrin and platelet vegetations on the valves may break loose into the circulation and lodge at distant sites, producing damage to target organs. Metastatic infection due to emboli may involve arterial walls (mycotic aneurysm) or produce abscesses.

Patients with **subacute endocarditis** usually have underlying valvular heart disease and are infected by less virulent organisms such as viridans streptococci, enterococci, nonenterococcal group D streptococci, microaerophilic streptococci, and *Haemophilus* sp. Frequently, the source and onset of infection are not clear, and patients consult physicians with complaints of fever, weight loss, or symptoms related to embolic phenomenon and congestive heart failure.

Prosthetic valvular endocarditis may present either acute or subacute in onset, and the infecting organisms differ, depending on whether endocarditis develops within 2 months of surgery or later (Table 109-2). Whereas infections on nonprosthetic valves usually are eradicated by antimicrobial therapy alone, prosthetic valve infections frequently require surgical removal of the infected valve before the infection is eliminated. Antimicrobial therapy of endocarditis is prolonged and should be guided by susceptibility studies. Fungal endocarditis is rare, but *Candida* sp infections occur in those with prosthetic valves and drug addicts. *Aspergillus* sp endocarditis may occur after cardiac valve surgery.

Blood Cultures

The presence of microbemia is demonstrated by blood cultures. Blood cultures should always be obtained prior to institution of antimicrobial drug therapy for suspected microbemia, since that therapy may interfere with the ability to isolate and identify the infecting agent. When antimicrobial therapy is to be instituted immediately in critically ill patients, two or three blood cultures should be drawn by separate venipunctures at 5-10 minute intervals. Isolation of the same organism from multiple cultures obtained at different venipuncture sites helps to discriminate true microbemias from false-positive blood culture results due to skin contaminants. In less critically ill patients, spacing of blood cultures several hours apart may help to discriminate transient from continuous microbemias. With the techniques outlined here no less than two and no more than three blood cultures should be obtained in a 24-hour period. More frequent cultures do not increase the likelihood of detecting microbemia.

Cultures should be obtained when symptoms suggest the presence of microbemia or septic shock. Although drawing blood cultures 1 hour before the onset of fever offers a theoretical advantage, fever is the most common initial symptom that alerts the physician to order blood cultures. Thus, in practice, blood cultures are drawn when microbemia is suspected.

Specimen Collection

Blood for culture should be collected by venipuncture and not through indwelling catheters, because catheter cultures have been shown to increase the rate of false-positive results. Once a suitable vein is identified, the skin should be disinfected. Tincture of iodine (2%) or povidone iodine solution is applied with saturated swabs starting over the vein and working outward from the venipuncture site in a concentric area. Two of three swabs should be used and the iodine left in contact with the skin 1-2 minutes. The iodine may then be removed by a sponge saturated with isopropyl alcohol. If the vein is missed, the needle should be replaced with a new sterile needle prior to a second attempt at venipuncture to decrease the likelihood of contamination. Povidone iodine solutions contaminated with *P cepacia* have caused epidemics of false-positive blood cultures. For patients allergic to iodine, isopropyl alcohol should be used for skin disinfection.

In adults, 20-30 mL of blood should be withdrawn using either 10-mL vacutainers containing sterile saline and 0.35% polyanethol sulfonate (SPS) as an anticoagulant or needle and syringe with direct inoculation of blood culture bottles at the bedside. If vacutainers are used, a sterile plastic hub should be used, the vacutainer tops swabbed with iodine or isopropyl alcohol, and the blood mixed with saline and anticoagulant to prevent clotting. The vacutainer is then sent to the laboratory for inoculation of blood culture media bottles. The liquid in the vacutainer should not be allowed to enter the bloodstream because bacteremias have been induced by contaminated vacutainer tubes. If blood culture bottles are inoculated directly at the bedside, 10 mL of blood should be injected into each bottle containing 100 mL of broth media. In small children, 1-5 mL of blood is sufficient for blood cultures. The most important aspect of collection is to reduce the incidence of positive blood cultures due to skin contaminants. Even with optimal technique, 1%-5% of cultures may be contaminated with *Corynebacterium* sp, *Micrococcus* sp, and *S epidermidis* originating from the skin.

Culture Media

Many laboratories use commercially prepared blood culture bottles containing 100 mL of tryptic or trypticase soy broth with 0.03% polyanethol sulfonate (SPS) overlaid by a partial vacuum and 10% carbon dioxide. SPS is a polyanionic anticoagulant that inactivates serum lysozyme, inhibits the bactericidal effect of complement, prevents phagocytosis by neutrophils, and partially inactivates aminoglycoside antibiotics. SPS also may inhibit the growth of *Peptostreptococcus anaerobius, Gardnerella vaginalis, M hominis, N gonorrhoeae,* and *N meningitidis.*

In the laboratory, two or three blood culture bottles are inoculated with 10 mL of blood each to produce 10:1 dilution of the blood. The dilution of blood is important to reduce the bactericidal effect of blood and to dilute any residual antibiotics below their inhibitory concentrations. The vacuum is released in one bottle by venting with a sterile needle plugged with cotton. After releasing the vacuum, the needle is removed so that the carbon dioxide is not dissipated. This bottle becomes an aerobic culture, yielding higher isolation rates for absolute aerobes such as *Pseudomonas aeruginosa* and *Candida* sp. The unvented bottle provides an oxygen-free environment with higher yields of anaerobic organisms.

It is not clear whether an antimicrobial withdrawal device or the incorporation of resin into the incubation bottle increases the isolation of organisms from individuals previously treated with antimicrobial agents by inactivation or absorption of antibiotics. Resins may absorb bacteria, and thereby produce false-negative results.

Standard blood culture media permit growth and isolation of a wide range of organisms; however, specific organisms and certain clinical situations require special techniques for isolation of pathogens. Both clinicians and laboratory personnel should be alert to the need for special techniques outlined in Table 109-4. The BACTEC system detects *Candida* sp and other yeasts faster and more often than the biphasic bottles used in the past. When penicillinase is added to blood culture media, the penicillinase should be subcultured to ensure that it is sterile and does not produce a false-postive culture. Most laboratories should not attempt cultures of blood for *Francisella tularensis* or *Yersinia pestis,* because risk of laboratory-acquired infections is great. Specimens should be sent to state public health laboratories or the CDC.

Culture Processing

Inoculated bottles should be incubated at 35-37 C and examined for signs of growth once or twice daily. After inoculation, blood will settle into a bottom layer beneath the broth. Positive cultures usually show one or more signs of growth: turbidity and gas bubbles in the broth layer, hemolysis with release of hemoglobin into the broth layer, or cotton ball colonies on the top of the blood layer. Certain organisms may not

Table 109-4 Organisms and Situations Requiring Special Blood Culture Techniques

Situation	Altered Technique
Prior administration of cell wall–active antibiotics (e.g., penicillins and cephalosporins)	Add penicillinase to inactivate β-7 lactam antibiotics present in serum
	Pass blood through an antimicrobial withdrawal device before inoculating the blood culture bottle, or incubate in a bottle that contains resin
	Add 10%–30% sucrose to produce hyperosmolar solution that promotes growth of cell-wall-defective bacteria
	Prolonged incubation (2 weeks)
Suspected infective endocarditis	Incubate negative cultures 2 weeks
	Hold negative bottles for 4 weeks before discarding
Suspected fungemia (e.g., *Candida* sp, *Torulopsis* sp, Histoplasmosis, *Cryptococcus* sp)	Inoculate BACTEC bottle or inoculate biphasic bottle with brain heart infusion broth and agar slant that is vented to air and is incubated 3-4 weeks at 30 C
	Inoculate buffy coat cultures of venous blood on Sabouraud dextrose agar and brain heart infusion agar; incubate at 30 C for 3-4 weeks
Brucellosis	Inoculate at bedside biphasic brucella broth bottle (Castenada) with agar slant under 5%-10% CO_2; incubate 4 weeks; perform serologic test
Contaminated blood or intravenous-infusion-related microbemias	Inoculate third bottle and incubate at 25 C to isolate psychrophilic bacteria that may grow better at lower temperatures
Franciscella tularensis	Inoculate 0.5 mL on multiple cystine-glucose blood agar slants with control slant; incubate 3 weeks (laboratory hazard); perform serologic test
Yersinia pestis	Laboratory hazard; perform serologic test
Leptospirosis	Inoculate one to three drops of fresh blood into tubes containing Fletcher's medium enriched with ≤14% vol/vol rabbit serum; incubate at 30 C for 4 weeks; examine surface growth by dark field technique; results positive only during the first week of illness; perform serologic test
L monocytogenes	Inoculate an extra bottle and store at 4 C for 4 weeks; subculture periodically
M intracellulare in patients with acquired immunodeficiency syndrome	Inoculate Middlebrook 7H11 agar and Lowenstein-Jensen medium with lysed blood
M hominis in genitourinary tract infections	Stain with acridine orange and not gram stain. Subculture to Columbia sheep blood agar; incubate 3 days at 37°C in 5% CO_2; examine plate with stereoscopic microscope

demonstrate gross changes and will be discovered only by routine subculture. These organisms include *Haemophilus influenzae, Neisseria* sp, *P aeruginosa, Streptococcus pneumoniae,* and rarely *Bacteroides* sp or *Fusobacterium* sp.

Some laboratories prefer an automated commercial radiometric BACTEC system to detect bacterial growth in blood culture bottles rather than rely on visual inspection. Special culture bottles containing nutrients in the liquid phase labeled with radioactive carbon 14 are used. As bacteria or fungi grow, they metabolize the carbon 14 to carbon dioxide, which is released into the gaseous phase, where it may be detected by aspirating a small amount of the atmosphere and testing for the presence of radioactivity. Automation permits more frequent examination of blood culture bottles and often results in earlier detection of growth, although sometimes contamination of the sampling device may lead to false-positive blood cultures because of inoculation of adjacent bottles.

Once growth is identified by inspection or radiometric techniques, a Gram stain is performed, and subcultures are made onto both chocolate and blood agar plates incubated in 10% carbon dioxide. An inoculated blood agar plate is incubated anaerobically; MacConkey or EMB agar plates also are inoculated if gram-negative rods are present. Subcultures should be incubated 72 hours before discarding plates without growth. Susceptibility and commercial biochemical identification tests may be set up directly from the positive blood culture bottles to provide information to clinicians, but these results must be confirmed with properly standardized tests.

Subcultures of bottles that do not show signs of growth are made 6-17 hours and 48 hours after inoculation onto chocolate agar plates incubated in 10% carbon dioxide. Routine anaerobic subcultures of bottles that do not show signs of growth are seldom positive, and therefore are not usually done. Acridine orange fluorochrome stains are used by some laboratories to detect rapidly the presence of bacteria during subcultures of bottles that do not show signs of growth because they are more sensitive than the Gram stain. Negative cultures are reported to physicians as no growth after 4 days' incubation (preliminary report), and as no growth after 7 days' incubation (final report). Negative bottles may be discarded after 7 days, but if fastidious organisms or infective endocarditis are suspected, bottles should be held 2-4 weeks. Prolonged incubation will result in more frequent isolation of *Corynebacterium* sp, *S epidermidis,* and *Propionibacterium acnes* skin contaminants.

When a positive culture is obtained, more than one organism may be present; multiple organisms are isolated in 6%-15% of positive blood cultures. Care should be taken to isolate and identify all organisms present. A second subculture of positive-culture bottles, begun 3 days after the first subculture, may detect additional bacterial species and enhance the detection of polymicrobial bacterias. *Corynebacterium* sp must be differentiated from *L monocytogenes.* Group D streptococci isolated from blood must be separated into enterococcal and nonenterococcal organisms by appropriate tests because enterococci require combination antimicrobial therapy.

Organisms that will not grow on subculture may be seen on Gram stain of the blood culture. If gram-positive cocci are seen, inoculation of media containing pyridoxine may permit growth of fastidious streptococci (viridans) mutants. Blood culture media may contain organisms killed during preparation that may be seen on Gram stain. If this is suspected, Gram stain should be made from uninoculated media from the same lot. Rarely, blood culture bottles may be contaminated with viable organisms due to inadequate sterilization or defects in the bottles (usually *Bacillus* sp).

References

Bryan, C.S., Reynolds, K.L., Brenner, E.R.: Analysis of 1,186 episodes of gram-negative bacteremia in non-university hospitals: The effects of antimicrobial therapy. *Rev Infectious Dis* 1983; 5:629-38.

Hansen, S.L., Hetmanski, J.: Enhanced detection of polymicrobic bacteremia by repeat subculture of previously positive blood cultures. *J Clin Microbiol* 1983; 18:208-10.

Kelly, M.T., Buck, G.E., Fojtasek, M.F.: Evaluation of a lysis centrifugation and biphasic bottle blood culture system during routine use. *J Clin Microbiol* 1983; 18:554-57.

Kiehn, T.M., et al.: Infections caused by *mycobacterium avium* complex in immunocompromised patients: Diagnosis by blood culture and fecal examination, antimicrobial susceptibility tests, and morphological and senoagglutination characteristics. *J Clin Microbiol* 1985; 21:168-173.

Maki, D.G.: Nosocomial bacteremia. *Am J Med* 1981; 70:719-32.

McCabe, W.R., Treadwell, T.L. De Maria, A., Jr.: Pathophysiology of bacteremia in body fluids and infectious diseases. Balows, A., Tilton, R.C., (editors). *Am J Med* [suppl] 1983; S7-18.

Plorde, J.J., Carlson, L.G., Dau, M.E.: Lack of clinical relevance in routine final subcultures of radiometrically negative bactec blood culture vials. *Am J Clin Pathol* 1982; 78:753-55.

Prevost, E., Bannister, E.: Detection of yeast septicemia by biphasic and radiometric methods. *J Clin Microbiol* 1981; 13:655-60.

Reller, J.B., et al.: *Cumitech IA: Blood cultures II*. Washington, D.C.: American Society for Microbiology, 1982.

Smaron, M.F., Angoor, S., Zierdt, C.H.: Detection of *mycoplasma hominis* septicemia by radiometric blood culture. *J Clin Microbiol* 1985; 21:298-301.

Weinstein, M.P., et al.: The clinical significance of positive blood cultures: A comprehensive analysis of 500 episodes of bacteremia and fungemia in adults. I. laboratory and epidemiologic observations. *Rev Infectious Dis* 1983; 5:35-53.

110 Microbiology of the Gastrointestinal Tract

Sherwood L. Gorbach, MD

General Concepts
Toxin-Mediated Diarrheas
  Cholera
  Toxigenic *Escherichia coli*
  Other Diarrheal Toxins

Invasive Bacterial Pathogens
  Salmonella
  Shigella
Viral Diarrhea
Clinical Diagnosis of Diarrheal Disease
Parasitic Diarrheas

General Concepts

Gastrointestinal infectious diseases may be caused by toxin-producing and invasive bacteria, viruses and parasites. The proximal gastrointestinal tract (which includes the stomach, duodenum, jejunum, and upper ileum) normally has a sparse microflora with bacterial concentrations of fewer than 10^4 organisms per milliliter. Most of the organisms are derived from the oropharynx, as each meal passes through the upper intestine in a wavelike fashion. Colonization of the upper intestine by coliform organisms is an abnormal event, characteristic of certain infectious pathogens such as *Vibrio cholerae* and toxigenic *Escherichia coli*. In contrast, the large intestine normally contains a luxuriant microflora with total concentrations of 10^{11} bacteria per gram. Anaerobes such as *Bacteroides*, anaerobic streptococci, and clostridia outnumber aerobic bacteria such as coliforms by a factor of 1000.

Not only are bacteria distributed longitudinally in the gastrointestinal tract, but they are also arranged cross-sectionally with regard to the mucosal surface. The microflora is found within the lumen, overlying the epithelial cells, and occasionally adhering to the mucous layer. Penetration of bacteria through the mucosal surface is an abnormal event that can be caused by infectious agents such as *Shigella, Salmonella,* and *Yersinia.*

The same mechanisms that control the normal flora also protect the bowel from invasion by pathogens. At the portal of entry, gastric acid suppresses most organisms that are swallowed. Individuals with reduced or absent gastric acid have a high incidence of bacterial colonization in the upper small bowel and are more susceptible to bacterial diarrheal diseases. Bile has antibacterial properties and thus may be another factor in controlling flora. Forward propulsive motility is a key element in maintaining the sparse flora of the upper bowel. Finally, the microflora itself, by producing its own antibacterial substances (for example, fatty acids), maintains stability of the normal populations and prevents implantation of pathogens.

Toxin-Mediated Diarrheas

Several toxin-producing bacteria may cause diarrheal disease (Table 110-1). Diarrheal disease caused by *V cholerae* and toxin-producing *E coli* has three main characteristics. First, the disease is characterized by intestinal fluid loss that is related to the action of the enterotoxin on the small bowel epithelial cell. Second, the organism itself does not invade the mucosal surface; rather, it colonizes the upper small bowel, "sticking" to the epithelial cells and elaborating an enterotoxin. The mucosal architecture remains intact with no evidence of cellular destruction. Bacteremia does not occur. Third, the fecal effluent is watery and often voluminous producing clinical features of dehydration. The fluid originates in the upper small bowel, where the enterotoxin is most active.

Cholera

The archetype of toxigenic diarrhea is cholera, a disease in which stool volume can exceed 1 liter per hour with daily fecal outputs of 15–20 liters if parenteral fluid replacement therapy is maintained. Cholera begins as vibrios are taken in by mouth, usually with contaminated water. The vibrios proceed to colonize the small intestine in

Table 110-1   Toxin-Producing Bacteria Associated With Diarrheal Disease

Microorganism	Action of Toxin		
	Adenylate Cyclase	Cytotoxic	Guanylate Cyclase
Vibrio cholerae	+		
E coli (heat-labile toxin)	+		
E coli (heat-stable toxin)			+
Shigella		+	
Staphylococcus aureus		+	
Clostridium perfringens		+	

large numbers. The enterotoxin (known as "entero" because its major activity takes place in the small intestine) is elaborated by the vibrios, which themselves adhere to the epithelial surface. The enterotoxin interacts with the mucosal cell at a receptor site, identified as GM_1 ganglioside.

Cholera toxin is a protein with a molecular weight of 84,000. It has two types of subunits: one is responsible for binding to the cell membrane and the other activates membrane-bound adenylate cyclase. The mucosal cell has increased levels of cyclic AMP, which appears to activate a kinase system; the final event is secretion of fluid and electrolytes from the epithelial cell to the lumen of the gut. The areas most sensitive to the toxin are the duodenum and upper jejunum. The ileum is less affected and the colon, which is insensitive to the toxin, remains in a state of absorption. Thus, cholera is a form of "overflow" diarrhea in which large volumes of fluid produced in the upper intestine overwhelm the reabsorptive capacity of the lower bowel.

The visual appearance of cholera stool is "rice water" (a fecal effluent that has lost all of its pigment and becomes a clear fluid with small flecks of mucus). The electrolyte composition of the stool is isotonic with plasma and the stool has a low protein concentration. Microscopy reveals no inflammatory cells in the fecal effluent; all that can be seen are small numbers of shed mucosal cells.

Toxigenic *Escherichia coli*

Certain strains of *E coli* can cause diarrheal disease by elaborating enterotoxins. *E coli* produces two types of toxin. The first type, known as heat-labile toxin (LT), is destroyed by heat and acid and has a molecular weight of approximately 80,000 daltons. It acts physiologically like cholera toxin by activating adenylate cyclase and causing secretion of fluid and electrolytes into the intestinal lumen. The LT toxin also shares antigenic components with cholera toxin. The second toxin, known as heat-stable toxin (ST), is stable to heat at 100 C, has a low molecular weight of approximately 4500 daltons, fails to activate adenylate cyclase, and has no biochemical similarity to cholera toxin. Recent evidence suggests that guanylate cyclase is activated by ST. Both LT and ST can cause diarrhea in humans and in domestic animals such as sheep, cows, and pigs. Toxigenic *E coli* pose a particular threat to travelers, since 75% of "turista" (travelers' diarrhea) is caused by these organisms.

Other Diarrheal Toxins

Many strains of *Shigella* produce an enterotoxin that causes secretion of fluid from the small intestine. Although first noted with the Shiga bacillus, this toxin has now been identified with *S flexneri* and *S sonnei* as well. The toxin has a destructive or cytotoxic effect on the small-bowel epithelium, causing gross injury to the bowel surface. It does not activate adenylate cyclase. Another organism that produces a cytotoxin is *V parahaemolyticus,* a bacterium associated with seafood and shellfish. The food poisoning strains of *Staphylococcus aureus* and *Clostridium perfringens* both produce toxins that are directly cytotoxic. The staphylococcal toxin also acts as a neurotoxin.

Invasive Bacterial Pathogens

Distinct from the toxigenic group, the invasive organisms have their main impact on the host by causing gross destruction of the epithelial architecture; histologic findings include mucosal ulceration and an inflammatory reaction in the lamina propria. The principal pathogens in this group are *Salmonella, Shigella, Campylobacter,* invasive *E coli,* and *Yersinia.* Some invasive organisms also produce enterotoxin; for example, *Shigella* and *Campylobacter.* Viruses are also invasive agents, although the degree of mucosal destruction is considerably less than that caused by the bacterial pathogens.

Salmonella

Salmonella, a large group of organisms, now consists of nearly 2000 serotypes, widely disseminated among animals and occasionally infecting humans. The main portal of entry is the mouth through contaminated food and drink. The site of attack is the lower ileum, where the salmonellae cause mild musocal ulceration. They make their way rapidly through the epithelial surface to the lamina propria and then to the lymphatics and blood stream.

At least two microbial virulence factors are involved in the intestinal infection: one is associated with mucosal invasion; the other causes fluid and electrolyte secretion into the lumen of the bowel. The invasive factor destroys the mucosa and produces bacteremia, whereas the other factor causes fluid secretion and diarrhea.

Shigella

Shigella organisms cause dysentery, a diarrhea stool containing blood and inflammatory exudate composed of polymorphonuclear leukocytes. The exudate is derived from the invasion of the colonic epithelium. This invasive process is determined by two genetically controlled virulence mechanisms within the microorganism. The first mediates initial penetration of the mucosal surface by destroying the brush border, which is followed by engulfment of the pathogen by invagination of the epithelial cell membrane. The second virulence mechanism is the organism's ability to multiply within the mucosal tissue. Mucosal ulceration is produced, as well as an intensive inflammatory response in the lamina propria. The infectious process in bacillary dysentery, however, usually is restricted to the intestinal mucosa; lymph node involvement and bacteremia seldom occur.

The precise mechanism of fluid production in invasive diarrhea is unknown. Three theories currently exist.

The first theory suggests that many *Shigella* strains elaborate an enterotoxin that causes fluid secretion. In addition, some evidence suggests that a similar toxin contributes to the pathogenesis of *Salmonella.* Such toxins are thought to be responsible for the watery diarrhea that occurs in patients with salmonellosis and bacillary dysentery.

Second, evidence exists that invasive organisms increase local synthesis of prostaglandins at the site of the intense inflammatory reaction. In experimental animals, for instance, fluid secretion can be blocked by prostaglandin inhibitors such as indomethacin and aspirin. This theory suggests that prostaglandins are responsible for fluid secretion and subsequent diarrhea.

Third, current evidence suggests that transudation from the colon is not a significant factor in the production of diarrhea, but that it may result from damage to the epithelial surface that prevents reabsorption of fluid entering the colon from the small intestine.

Viral Diarrhea

An agent resembling reovirus is now thought to cause most cases of infantile diarrhea. Known as rotavirus, this agent is approximately 70 nm in diameter and has a single capsid type. Clinical disease occurs almost exclusively in children under the age of 2 years. Epidemiologic studies have suggested that 30%-60% of children with acute diarrhea in this age group are infected by this agent. Although adults can shed the organism, they rarely develop the disease. The virus is visualized in fecal effluent of infected individuals with the aid of electron microscopy. Viral replication in organ cultures has been observed, but no convenient tissue culture system to propagate this virus exists.

Another group of viruses can produce diarrheal disease in all age groups and have been recognized to cause major epidemics (as in Norwalk, Ohio, for which this organism was named "the Norwalk agent"). Following infection with the Norwalk agent, the initial lesion occurs in the proximal small bowel. The mucosal architecture is damaged, with shortening of the villi and hyperplasia of the crypts. An inflammatory exudate then appears in the lamina propria.

The mechanisms of fluid secretion in viral diarrhea have not been elucidated. It is known that infection with the Norwalk agent can produce steatorrhea and xylose malabsorption, as well as direct damage to brush border enzymes. Adenylate cyclase activity in the epithelial cells is not altered in the acute illness.

Clinical Diagnosis of Diarrheal Disease

A pathophysiologic approach can be used to make a presumptive etiologic diagnosis in patients with infectious diarrhea. Perhaps the most convenient approach is to separate pathogens that involve the small intestine from those that attack the large bowel. Toxigenic bacteria (*E coli, V cholerae*), viruses, and the parasite *Giardia* are examples of small bowel pathogens. These organisms produce watery diarrhea, which may lead to dehydration. Abdominal pain, although often diffuse and poorly defined, is generally periumbilical. Microscopic examination of the stool fails to reveal formed cellular elements such as erythrocytes and leukocytes.

A large bowel pathogen, the major ones being *Shigella* and *Campylobacter,* is an invasive organism that causes the clinical syndrome of dysentery. Characteristic rectal pain, known as tenesmus, strongly suggests colonic involvement. Although the fecal effluent may be watery at first, by the second or third day of illness it becomes a relatively small volume stool that is often bloody and mucoid. Microscopic examination almost invariably reveals abundant erythrocytes and leukocytes. Proctoscopy shows a

Table 110-2 Clinical Features of Diarrheal Diseases

	Location of Infection	
	Small Bowel	*Large Bowel*
Pathogens	*V cholerae*	*Shigella*
	E coli (LT/ST)	*Campylobacter*
	Reovirus	*E coli* (invasive)
	Parvovirus	*Entamoeba histolytica*
	Giardia	
Location of pain	Midabdomen	Lower abdomen, rectum
Volume of stool	Large	Small
Type of stool	Watery	Mucoid
Blood in stool	Rare	Common
Leukocytes in stool	Rare	Common (except in amebiasis)
Proctoscopy	Normal	Mucosal ulcers, hemorrhagic, friable mucosa

diffusely ulcerated, hemorrhagic, and friable colonic mucosa. These features are summarized in Table 110-2.

Salmonella does not fit into the simple schema presented in Table 110-2, because this organism has features of both groups. *Salmonella* is invasive for the mucosa of the small intestine, particularly the ileum, and it causes fluid secretion, often in voluminous quantities. In addition, septicemia and metastatic spread of the pathogen to other organs occur in some cases.

Parasitic Diarrheas

Several species of protozoa and helminths, particularly the enterics, are known to cause diarrheal disease. Thus, parasites also should be considered in the differential diagnosis of patients with diarrheal diseases. Several of these infections may be acquired within the United States, although the risk of exposure to parasites is greater in less developed countries. Clinical diagnosis of the parasitic diseases is detailed in the chapters devoted to parasitology. Some of the more common parasitic causes of diarrhea include *Entamoeba histolytica*, *Giardia lamblia*, *Strongyloides stercoralis*, and the intestinal flukes.

References

Brown, K.H., MacLean, W.C., Jr.: Nutritional management of acute diarrhea: an appraisal of the alternatives. *Pediatrics* 1984; 73:119-125.

DuPont, H.L.: Enteropathogenic organisms: New etiologic agents and concepts of diseases. *Med Clin North Am* 1978; 62:945.

Gertler, S., et al.: Management of acute diarrhea. *J Clin Gastroenterol* 1983; 5:523-534.

Gorbach, S.L., Haskins, D.W.: Travelers' diarrhea. *Disease-a-Month* 1982; 27:1.

Guerrant, R.L., et al.: Campylobacteriosis in man: pathogenic mechanisms and review of 91 bloodstream infections. *Am J Med* 1978; 65:584.

Sprinz, H.: Pathogenesis of intestinal infections. *Arch Pathol* 1969; 87:556.

Schreiber, D.S., et al. Recent advances in viral gastroenteritis. *Gastroenterology* 1977; 73:174.

111 Microbiology of the Nervous System

Neal Nathanson, MD

Richard Moxon, MD

John R. Martin, MD

General Concepts

An infectious agent must meet several requirements to produce disease in the nervous system. First, the agent must gain entry into the nervous system. Second, because the number of infectious units initially gaining entry is usually small, the agent must undergo replication. Third, the agent must damage a significant number of cells or, alternatively, the host response may cause cellular injury. This chapter describes some of the more important anatomic and functional features of the central and peripheral nervous systems (CNS and PNS) that influence infection in the nervous system, and then considers the pathogenesis of bacterial and viral infections.

Several special features characterize CNS infections. The blood-brain barrier protects the CNS from blood-borne bacteria or viruses, and penetration requires a high agent titer in the circulation over a considerable time, or a physical break in the barrier. Once within the CNS, bacteria usually are confined to the membranes of the brain and cause meningitis. Less frequently, bacteria may replicate focally in the brain parenchyma, causing an abscess. Viruses that have penetrated the brain spread widely within the parenchyma. Different agents replicate preferentially in neurons or supporting cells, accounting for a diversity of pathologic and clinical diseases. A few viruses, such as herpes and measles, may persist in the nervous system, with consequent acutely recurrent or chronic illness.

Nervous System Features that Affect Infection

Blood–Central Nervous System Barrier

The most important route of entry for most organisms is from blood into the CNS across the blood-brain barrier. The barrier concept arose from the observation that tracer molecules in cerebral vessels did not freely enter the neural compartment and that a large concentration gradient could be maintained between them.

The anatomic basis of this barrier is three-fold (Figure 111-1). The first barrier site is the vascular endothelium of the central and peripheral nervous systems (PNS). Adjacent endothelial cell margins are bound to one another by continuous tight junctional bands. These junctions are sufficient to prevent the spread of even small tracer molecules from the vessel lumen between adjacent endothelial cells. Neither the thin basement membrane that surrounds the endothelial layer nor the layer of astrocyte processes that surrounds this membrane in cerebral capillaries and venules forms a barrier to the passage of proteins from the lumen into the brain if the integrity of the endothelial barrier is lost.

In certain regions of the nervous system, however, the barrier to tracers is incomplete. These include the pineal gland, posterior pituitary, median eminence, the tuber cinereum, area postrema, paraphysis, walls of supraoptic recess, eminentia saccularis, the optic nerve as it penetrates the sclera of the eye, and the region of terminations of receptor neurons in the olfactory mucosa. In the PNS, the barrier is similarly incomplete in sensory ganglia and at the peripheral terminations of axons. Whether the increased permeability of tracers at these sites is due to transendothelial transport of macromolecules in cytoplasmic vesicles or to penetration via fenestrations, both of which are characteristic of the endothelium in these regions, is not known.

The second anatomically distinct site at which a barrier has been demonstrated is the choroid plexus. Here the vascular endothelium is fenestrated by pores that are closed by thin diaphragms and that measure 20-100 nm in diameter. Macromolecules and tracers can pass readily across the endothelium and its basement membrane into the underlying connective tissue stroma, but the choroidal epithelium prevents any further penetration. These epithelial cells have continuous apical bands of tight junctions that surround each cell, joining it to its neighbors and thus forming a barrier to the passage of tracer into the CSF. Substances that enter the CSF may then pass readily across the

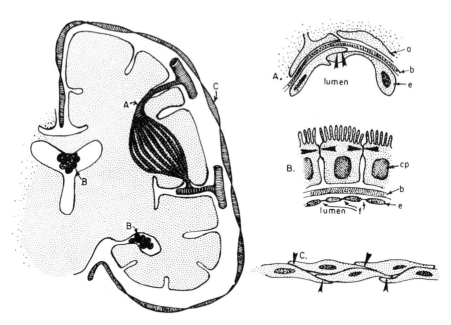

Figure 111-1 The blood-brain barrier. The three barrier sites (left) are subarachnoid and parenchymal blood vessels (A), choroid plexus (B), and arachnoid membrane (C). A sleeve of pial membrane surrounding each vessel as it enters the brain is separated from it by the Virchow–Robin space, which is continuous with the subarachnoid space. In blood vessels (A), junctions (at arrowheads) between adjacent endothelial cells (e) prevent passage of macromolecules from vessel lumen. If the integrity of endothelium is altered, macromolecules pass across basement membrane (b) and between astrocytic foot process (a). In the choroid plexus (B), macromolecules from the lumen cross the fenestrated (f) endothelium, basement membranes, and intervening stroma. Choroid plexus epithelial cells (cp) joined at their apices by tight junctions (arrowheads), prevent passage into the ventricle (top). Cells of the arachnoid membrane (C) are joined to one another by junctional complexes (arrowheads) forming the third barrier component.

ependymal epithelium into the extracellular space of the brain, since the ependyma does not form an effective barrier.

The arachnoidal membrane, which is separated from the pial covering of the CNS by the subarachnoid space, is the site of the third barrier to free exchange of macromolecules into and out of the CNS. The arachnoidal cells are joined to one another by junctional complexes that do not permit passage of tracers between cells.

Peripheral Nerves

Peripheral nerves are important in certain infectious diseases of the nervous system because their axons provide a continuous cytoplasmic tract from periphery into the CNS. Furthermore, a flow of axoplasm in both centipetal and centrifugal directions provides a potential conduit for viruses. Infectious agents, if introduced by trauma into the vicinity of peripheral axons, may be transported passively into the CNS. In the olfactory mucosa, naked nerve endings are exposed to the external milieu, offering a particularly vulnerable point of access.

Bacterial Infections of the Central Nervous System

Bacterial infections of the CNS take the form of generalized leptomeningeal inflammation or abscess formation. The abscesses may involve brain parenchyma, the spaces between the meningeal layers (epidural, subdural, or subarachnoid), or the ventricular cavities. During the last four decades, antibiotics have reduced dramatically the frequency and case fatality rate of bacterial infections of the CNS. On the other hand, the fraction of the population with high susceptibility to bacterial infections of the CNS is increasing. Morbidity and mortality from bacterial meningitis in the United States currently exceed that occurring from diseases such as poliomyelitis and measles, now preventable by immunization.

Routes of Entry

Foci of infection in parameningeal or otolaryngeal structures may erode through the skull and dura. This is particularly common in the pathogenesis of brain abscess. Direct implantation of bacteria into the CNS may occur as a sequal to trauma, neurosurgery, or in persons with severe congenital defects such as myelomeningocele; however, hematogenous dissemination of bacteria is the major pathway for leptomeningeal infections and also accounts for many instances of abscess formation.

Pathogenesis

The site and mechanism by which bacteria invade the basement membrane of the vascular endothelial cells of the CNS are not known. Bacteremias, especially transient ones, are extremely common, yet CNS infections ensue rarely. It is thus assumed that bacteria do not readily localize to the endothelium of CNS vessels. Experimental studies support this contention in that the CNS is not readily infected following systemic inoculation of large numbers of bacteria; however, CNS localization can be demonstrated if bacteria circulate in the bloodstream long enough and in high enough concentrations, or if prior damage to the blood-brain barrier has occurred.

Rats inoculated with *H influenzae* develop leptomeningitis after several hours of intense bacteremia (more than 1000 organisms per mL); however, if infection is initiated after passive systemic administration of immune serum, bacteremia is prevented or diminished and meningitis does not result (Figure 111-2). On the other hand, following splenectomy—the spleen being a major determinant of intravascular bacterial clearance—rats have more severe bacteremia and increased incidence of meningitis. Taken together, these observations suggest that an important factor in the proclivity of certain bacteria to cause meningitis resides in their capacity to evade intravascular clearance. Note that more than 90% of bacterial meningitis cases are caused by three species of bacteria: *H influenzae, Neisseria meningitidis,* and *Streptococcus pneumoniae.* Furthermore, more than one-half these infections occur in infants. These facts are in accord with the observations that strains of these bacteria isolated from CSF are encapsulated (a property associated with increased resistance to phagocytosis) and that infants lack serum bactericidal antibodies to the capsular antigen of these three bacteria.

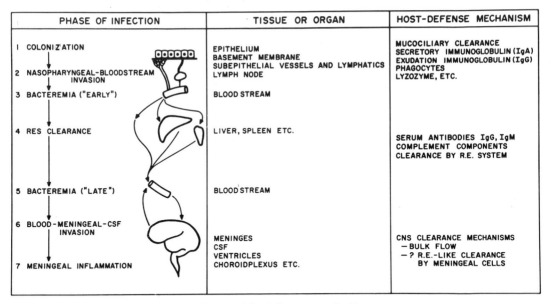

PHASE OF INFECTION	TISSUE OR ORGAN	HOST-DEFENSE MECHANISM
1 COLONIZ'ATION 2 NASOPHARYNGEAL-BLOODSTREAM INVASION 3 BACTEREMIA ("EARLY") 4 RES CLEARANCE 5 BACTEREMIA ("LATE") 6 BLOOD-MENINGEAL-CSF INVASION 7 MENINGEAL INFLAMMATION	EPITHELIUM BASEMENT MEMBRANE SUBEPITHELIAL VESSELS AND LYMPHATICS LYMPH NODE BLOOD STREAM LIVER, SPLEEN ETC. BLOOD STREAM MENINGES CSF VENTRICLES CHOROIDPLEXUS ETC.	MUCOCILIARY CLEARANCE SECRETORY IMMUNOGLOBULIN (IgA) EXUDATION IMMUNOGLOBULIN (IgG) PHAGOCYTES LYZOZYME, ETC. SERUM ANTIBODIES IgG, IgM COMPLEMENT COMPONENTS CLEARANCE BY R.E. SYSTEM CNS CLEARANCE MECHANISMS —BULK FLOW —? R.E.-LIKE CLEARANCE BY MENINGEAL CELLS

Figure 111-2 Pathogenesis of experimental *Haemophilus influenzae* meningitis.

Experimental and clinical observations indicate that brain abscess occurs in sites of brain injury. Thus, systemic inoculation of large numbers of virulent organisms does not result in brain abscess in normal animals; however, cauterization of small areas of brain facilitates localization of bacteria to the site of injury, and abscess formation may result.

As elsewhere in the body, bacterial infection of the CNS involves a classic inflammatory response; capillaries dilate and neutrophils and monocytes accumulate in neural tissue (brain abscess) or in the pia-arachnoid and subarachnoid space (leptomeningitis). In brain abscess, damage to the CNS may be due to direct cytotoxicity of the in situ bacteria; however, in leptomeningitis, the pia is rarely penetrated by bacteria, so that white and gray matter are damaged by indirect mechanisms. The pathophysiology of this injury is complex and poorly understood. Three possible mechanisms include diffusion of cytotoxic bacterial substances or products of inflammation or both into neural tissues; impairment of circulation due to inflammation of vessels in the subarachnoid and Virchow-Robin spaces; and impaired production, circulation, or absorption of CSF, resulting from inflammation of the choroid plexus, of subarachnoid space and arachnoid granulations, or of the ventricles.

The antibacterial defenses of the CNS itself are poorly understood. A minimal number of virulent bacteria are necessary to establish meningitis, although the entire population of bacteria within the CNS of an experimentally infected animal may result from survival of a single organism. This indicates the existence of a vigorous set of defenses.

Bacteria that have penetrated the CNS may be removed by phagocytosis and some may be cleared during CSF adsorption through the arachnoid granulations. Concentrations of antibody and complement in the CNS are low, but they increase following generalized inflammation. The production of local antibody and its possible role in bacterial infection of the CNS has not been adequately investigated.

Viral Infections of the Central Nervous System

Entry

The specialized anatomy of the nervous system offers special barriers to invasion of the CNS by viruses and unique routes of entry.

The most common source of invading virus is the blood. Most viruses (for example, picornaviruses and togaviruses) circulate in the plasma phase. Some agents may also be associated with leukocytes and a few such as Colorado tick fever virus replicate in rodent and human erythrocytes. To enter the neural parenchyma, circulating virus must traverse the capillary endothelium and the basement membrane that limits the perivascular or Virchow–Robin space. The mechanism by which this occurs remains poorly understood, although, in many instances, passive transport of mature virions may be involved. Consistent with this presumption, the probability of CNS invasion is correlated with the duration and intensity of viremia, and passive systemic administration of neuralizing antibody can prevent neural invasion. A few agents can replicate in endothelial cells, and others may be transported by infected leukocytes that can actively migrate across the blood-brain barrier.

An alternative route into the CNS is centripetal transport up peripheral nerves. This route is utilized by a few agents, notably, rabies virus and some herpesviruses. Good evidence exists that following entry of these viruses into axoplasm at a peripheral site, the viral genome is transported passively by axoplasmic flow, with replication occurring in cytoplasm (with rabies) or in neuronal nuclei (in herpes). A variation on this route is transit through the olfactory nerve, with initial entry of virus into the naked processes of first-order sensory neurons in the olfactory mucosa. The occasional laboratory-acquired, aerosol-transmitted infection of the CNS with rabies or other more exotic agents probably involves the olfactory route.

Target Cells

Within the CNS, various cells are available as potential hosts for virus replication, including neurons, oligodendrocytes, astrocytes, vascular endothelium, and the membranous linings (meninges and ependyma). The wide variety of patterns of localization of virus replication has been dramatically documented by immunofluorescent and ultrastructural observations (Table 111-1).

Among neuronal populations, differences in susceptibility are evidenced by the contrast between poliovirus (lower motoneurons) and the encephalitic togaviruses (forebrain neurons). Rabies virus preferentially infects the hippocampus and other limbic structures, whereas parvoviruses select the proliferating granule cell populations in postnatal animals.

Table 111-1 Examples of Diverse Localization of Virus Infections of the Central Nervous System

Example/Host	Pathology or Disease	Target Cells	Common or Rare
Poliomyelitis/human	Cytolysis	Motoneurons	Common
Herpes simplex 1/human	Fever blister; encephalitis	Neurons	Common
JHM coronavirus/mouse	Focal demyelination	Oligodendrocytes	Rare
Creutzfeldt-Jakob/human	Vacuolation; astrogliosis	Neurons; astrocytes	Rare
Paramyxovirus/mouse	Ependymitis; hydrocephalus	Ependyma	Rare
Lymphocytic choriomeningitis/mouse	Inflammation	Choroid plexus	Rare
Rat virus/rat	Hemorrhage	Endothelium	Rare

Some agents such as poliovirus are almost exclusively neuronotropic, whereas others (for example, herpes simplex) infect glia as well as neurons. The selective ability to replicate in oligodendrocytes can produce unusual pathologic changes, such as the demyelination seen with persistent coronavirus infection (JHM virus in mice). Other agents infect astrocytes, which show morphologic changes in certain persistent infections such as progressive multifocal leukoencephalopathy (a polyomavirus) or scrapie (a spongiform encephalopathy).

Endothelial infections are unusual but may be striking, as in the hemorrhagic encephalopathy exhibited by selected strains of rat virus. Ependymal infections are produced by numerous agents, including many orthomyxoviruses and paramyxoviruses, which are poorly adapted to replicate in CNS tissues. In young animals, such ependymal infections can destroy the aqueduct of Sylvius and produce a striking internal hydrocephalus. Another unusual but dramatic localization is exhibited by lymphocytic choriomeningitis and other arenaviruses, which replicate in the choroid plexus and pia mater and produce a convulsive pathophysiologic syndrome.

The basis for selective virus replication is not understood; however, a few pioneering models are under exploration and these may provide prototypes. For example, the use of recombinant reoviruses indicates that marked differences in CNS localization of different reovirus types are associated with a single structural polypeptide in the viral capsid.

Pathogenesis

The great diversity of pathologic pictures produced by viruses in the CNS is to a considerable extent a reflection of the sites of virus replication (Table 111-1); however, within the CNS, the same variety of virus cell interactions that occurs elsewhere can be seen. Thus, polioviruses, togaviruses, and herpesviruses destroy neural cells during replication and release. Many paramyxoviruses may destroy cells during cycles of abortive replication with little production of infectious virions. On the other hand, the arenaviruses can persist as long-term productive infections in cells that are morphologically intact. Such persistently infected cells may exhibit alterations in their specialized neural functions. Persistent CNS infections with tumor viruses can induce various tumors from transformed neuronal or glial elements. Quasitransformation is seen with other agents, as exemplified by the altered morphology of astrocytes in progressive multifocal leukoencephalopathy or scrapie. Other cytologic responses include induction of intracellular vacuoles by the spongiform agents and by certain strains of murine leukemia and paramyxoviruses.

Viruses may also initiate various immune-mediated lesions in the CNS. Lymphocytic choriomeningitis is the classical example, but several arenaviruses can also produce lytic lesions of neuroparenchyma. Certain demyelinating lesions associated with persistent infection (Theiler's virus, visna virus, and canine distemper virus) are almost certainly immune-mediated, as are some other chronic degenerations of white matter such as those caused by the paramyxovirus 6/94.

One special feature of cell destruction in the nervous system is the inability of mature neurons to regenerate, so that cell losses are permanent. This accounts for residua that follow severe poliomyelitis and encephalitis; also, this inability to regenerate enhances the clinical implications of sublethal virus infections that involve the CNS. Glia, on the other hand, can regenerate, and some degree of remyelination often is seen in chronic infections of white matter.

Variables in Pathogenesis

That most neurotropic virus infections vary in severity from inapparent to fatal has been well recognized. This variation reflects numerous virus and host parameters, which can be clearly delineated in experimental models. Among well-described factors of importance are virus virulence (neuroinvasiveness and neurovirulence), virus dose and route of infection, genetic susceptibility, age, and immunologic competence of the host. These variables have a dramatic effect on the consequences of infection; a virus that is lethal under one set of conditions can be innocuous under other circumstances. The mechanisms that underlie virus and host genetic determinants are only beginning to be explained.

Host Defenses

It has been established that the immune response plays a critical role in the outcome of many primary viral infections. This is particularly true in the CNS, because the interval from beginning of infection to CNS invasion (3–10 days) is similar to the period required for immune induction. The immune response may prevent CNS invasion altogether or limit the spread of virus within the brain.

Both B and T effector cells are involved in recovery from CNS infections. Plasma cells can be identified readily in the inflammatory response produced by many virus infections, and CSF often contains impressive levels of virus-specific antibody. Because the blood-brain barrier usually remains intact during a virus infection, local antibody production can be inferred.

Evidence for the presence of T effector cells in the virus-infected CNS has not yet been developed as thoroughly. Cytolytic T cells have been detected in the CSF in lymphocytic choriomeningitis, and it may be inferred that they are present in other viral infections as well. Also, there is good evidence in lymphocytic choriomeningitis that T cells can mediate clearance of virus from the CNS and other tissues Undoubtedly, cellular immunity constitutes an important adjunct to antibody by providing a mechanism for destruction of virus-infected cells. Furthermore, in certain instances, the immune response may play a dual role, capable of protecting the host or of mediating a pathologic response.

In reinfections, in which a neurotropic virus is introduced into an immune animal, antibody probably plays a preeminent role by clearing the blood of circulating virus and thus preventing neuroinvasion. Administration of passive antibody has demonstrated the importance of this mechanism for poliomyelitis and the encephalitic arboviruses. Cellular immunity and immune interferon responses also play a role in protection against reinfection with some viruses.

Persistent Infections and Chronic Neurologic Diseases

Persistent virus infections often involve the nervous system (Table 111-2). Although relatively rare in humans, such infections have elicited interest because of their unusual biologic and pathologic features and because they may be associated with certain enigmatic chronic neurologic diseases such as multiple sclerosis. The following brief account refers to human and animal prototypes.

Numerous strategies can be used by a virus to escape the host's immune mechanisms. In some instances, the viral genome is latent (herpesvirus infection of sensory ganglia or visna infection of the CNS) and presents no antigenic target. In other cases, the agent is present at high titer but is relatively nonantigenic (scrapie) or produces a state of quasitolerance (arenaviruses). Intermediate strategies occur in persistent myxovirus infections (as in subacute sclerosing panencephalitis), in which a defective genome spreads to adjacent cells through intercellular bridges.

The pathologic features of persistent CNS infections often differ from their acute counterparts. Focal demyelination is produced by certain coronavirus (mouse hepatitis virus) and picornavirus (Theiler's murine encephalitis virus) infections of mice. Other

Table 111-2 Examples of Persistent Virus Infections of the Nervous System: Genome Expression and Immune Response*

Example/Host	Associated Disease	Genome Expression	Immune Response
Kuru/human	Spongiform encephalopathy	+	0
Rubella/human	Fetal anomalies	+	±
LCM/mouse	Immune complex glomerulonephritis	+	±
Visna/sheep	Chronic encephalitis	±	+
TME/mouse	Focal demyelination	±	+
SSPE/human	Panencephalitis	±	+ +
VZ/human	Herpes zoster	0	+

*LCM, lymphocytic choriomeningitis; TME, Theiler's murine encephalomyelitis; SSPE, subacute sclerosing panencephalitis; VZ, varicella zoster. ±, partial or minimal; +, normal; + +, supranormal.

agents can produce nondemyelinating white matter degeneration (6/94 virus), neuronal vacuolation (neurotropic murine leukemic virus and scrapie), or panencephalitis (canine distemper and subacute sclerosing panencephalitis). In general, persistent infections frequently are associated with white matter pathology, a hallmark of certain chronic neurologic diseases.

Persistent infection may be the cause of numerous chronic neurologic diseases of unknown pathogenesis, including multiple sclerosis, amyotrophic lateral sclerosis, and senile dementia of the Alzheimer type. This suggestion is based on the study of animal models and on the documentation during the last 10-15 years that certain chronic neurologic diseases of humans are caused by viruses or viruslike agents. This group includes subacute sclerosing panencephalitis (measles and rubella viruses); progressive multifocal leucoencephalopathy (JC polyomavirus); and kuru and Creutzfeldt-Jakob disease (spongiform agents). Whether additional chronic diseases of the nervous system are virus-induced is now under intensive investigation in many laboratories.

References

Bell, W.E., McCormick, W.F.: *Neurologic infections of children.* Philadelphia: W.B. Saunders Co., 1975.

Johnson, R.T.: *Viral infections of the nervous system.* New York: Raven Press, 1982.

Kimberlin, R.H., (editor): *Slow virus diseases of animals and man.* Amsterdam: North Holland Publishing Co., 1976.

Moxon, E.R., et al.: Haemophilus influenzae meningitis in infected rats following intranasal inoculation. *J Infect Dis* 1974; 129:154.

Nathanson, N., Cole, G.A.: Immunosuppression and virus infections of the central nervous system. *Adv Virus Res* 1970; 16:397.

Notkins, A.L., (editor): *Viral immunology and immunopathology.* New York: Academic Press, 1975.

Schlessinger, D., (editor): Symposium on persistent virus infections. In: *Microbiology—1977.* Washington, D.C.: American Society for Microbiology, 1977.

Swartz, M.N., Dodge, P.R.: Bacterial meningitis: A review of selected aspects. *N Engl J Med* 1965; 272:725.

112 Microbiology of the Genitourinary System

Erwin Neter, MD†

General Concepts

Infection of the urinary tract (caused by several species of bacteria, notably *Escherichia coli* and viruses such as herpes type 2; Table 112-1) may lead to overt disease with such symptoms as fever, discomfort on urination, and pain. Such an infection also may result in asymptomatic bacteriuria, a condition that is not accompanied by symptoms observed by the patient, and that cannot be diagnosed by the physician on the basis of a physical examination alone. Genitourinary infections may be due to microorganisms acquired from outside (for example, sexually transmitted *Neisseria gonorrhoeae* or herpesvirus, type 2) or from the endogenous normal flora of the patient (for example, from the fecal flora). Infections such as syphilis may be transmitted from mother to newborn through the placenta during pregnancy. In contrast, *N gonorrhoeae* and *C trachomatis* usually are transmitted during delivery.

†Deceased.

Table 112-1   Infectious Agents of the Genitourinary Tract

General Group	Distinctive Property or Subgroup	Specific Agents
Bacteria	Bacilli	*Escherichia*
		Enterobacter
		Klebsiella
		Citrobacter
		Serratia
		Pseudomonas
		Proteus
		Haemophilus
		Listeria
	Cocci	*Staphylococcus aureus*
		S. epidermidis
		Streptococcus faecalis
		Neisseria gonorrhoeae
	Spiral	*Treponema pallidum*
	Intracellular	*Chlamydia trachomatis*
		Calymmatobacterium granulomatis
	Cell wall-deficient	*Ureaplasma urealyticum*
	Anaerobic	*Bacteroides*
		Peptococcus
		Peptostreptococcus
Fungi	Yeast	*Candida albicans*
Viruses	Adenovirus	Several serotypes
	Herpesvirus	Varicella-zoster
		Herpes simplex
	Paramyxovirus	Mumps virus
		Measles virus
	Picornavirus	Poliovirus
		Coxsackievirus
	Myxovirus	Influenza virus
	Togavirus	Rubella virus
Parasites	Trematodes	*Schistosoma haematobium*
	Protozoa	*Trichomonas vaginalis*

Urinary tract infection also depends on predisposing factors. The disease is far more common in women than in men because of the differing lengths of the urethra. Manipulation, such as the introduction of an indwelling catheter or other interference with excretion of urine, also increases the risk of infection.

Because diseases of the genitourinary tract may be caused by several microbial species, microbial etiology cannot be determined on clinical grounds alone. As a corollary, susceptibility patterns to antimicrobial agents may differ from species to species, and identification of the etiologic agent and its antibiogram may thus aid the physician in selecting a suitable drug. Relapse occurs after an apparent cure when infection from the same microorganism recurs; reinfection occurs when the species or

Table 112-2 Infectious Diseases of the Genitourinary Tract

Tract	Disease
Urinary	Cystitis
	Pyelonephritis
	Bacteriuria
	Renal abscessses
Genital	Skin ulcer
	Vulvovaginitis
	Urethritis
	Cervicitis
	Uterine infections
	Salpingitis
	Orchitis
	Oophoritis
	Prostatitis
	Epididymitis
	Warts

types of microorganisms causing the two attacks differ. Untreated chronic or recurrent infection involving the kidney may produce significant tissue injury, which may lead eventually to loss of renal function, which necessitates dialysis or kidney transplant. Besides causing infection of the genitourinary tract, herpesvirus is also important because it may be related to development of malignancy. Education can help in the control of diseases of the genitourinary tract that are transmitted sexually. Common diseases of the genitourinary tract appear in Table 112-2.

Urinary Tract Infections

Cystitis, Pyelonephritis, and Asymptomatic Bacteriuria

Microorganisms may cause infection of various parts of the urinary tract, from the urethra to the bladder to the kidney. Infection of the bladder is called cystitis; infection of the kidney is pyelonephritis. (Urethritis is discussed under Genital Infections.) Urinary tract infections may be acute or chronic.

Relapses and recurrences differ distinctly from each other and require different therapeutic approaches. To prevent a relapse, treatment of the original infection must be effective; to prevent a recurrence, elimination of factors predisposing to infection by another microorganism, usually from the intestinal tract or the periurethral area, must be accomplished. The microorganisms usually enter the urinary tract from the urethra (ascending infection). Occasionally, the kidneys become infected from bacteremia. Conversely, ascending infection reaching the kidney may invade the blood stream. Bacteria often invade the urinary tract and are present within the lumen; however, they do not cause an inflammatory response of the tissues that leads to overt manifestations. This entity is called asymptomatic bacteriuria. Because no inflammation occurs, pus cells and other components of the inflammatory process (for example, proteins) may be absent. However, under certain circumstances the disorder becomes an active and clinically overt disease. For example, pyelonephritis develops more frequently in pregnant women with asymptomatic bacteriuria than in nonpregnant subjects or in pregnant women without bacteriuria. Thus, the definitive diagnosis of asymptomatic bacteriuria can be accomplished only by bacteriologic examination including microscopy and culture.

Infection is facilitated by interference with excretion of the urine caused by congenital anomalies; acquired obstruction such as that associated with pregnancy, enlarged prostate, or stones; paralytic disease affecting bladder function; or the presence of indwelling catheters or other manipulations. Diagnosis of congenital anomalies sometimes is made when infection of the urinary tract leads to a symptomatic illness and a complete examination. Correcting an obstruction may prevent serious or complete destruction of renal tissue due to the development of hydronephrosis (retention of urine in the kidney pelvis without pus) or pyonephrosis (retention of urine in the kidney pelvis with pus).

Etiologic Agents.   Of the bacteria responsible for urinary tract infection (Table 112-1), *E coli* is found most often. Certain serogroups are encountered more frequently than others. Thus, of more than 140 serogroups of *E coli*, serogroups 01, 02, 04, 06, 07, 011, 015, 062, and 075 account for 40%–70% of infections. Other members of the family Enterobacteriaceae (*Klebsiella, Enterobacter, Citrobacter, Serratia,* and *Proteus* sp) as well as *Pseudomonas aeruginosa*, are encountered less often. Streptococci, particularly of the enterococcus variety, are seen frequently; in chronic infection, they are often encountered with gram-negative bacilli. Sometimes urinary tract infection is caused by *Staphylococcus aureus* and, rarely, by *S epidermidis*. Under certain circumstances, such as in diabetic patients, fungal infection (usually that caused by *Candida albicans*) is seen.

Microbiologic Diagnosis.   Voided specimens for microbiologic diagnosis must be obtained aseptically and examined within 2–3 hours, because urine is an excellent culture medium and voided specimens can become contaminated easily with the normal flora of the urethra. If necessary, urine may be refrigerated at 4 C for 24–48 hours. Under these conditions, the microorganisms remain viable and counts remain stable. If voided urine is not available, or if a definitive diagnosis has to be made, urine obtained by suprapubic aspiration yields the best results. Alternatively, specimens may be obtained by means of a properly used catheter. Voided urine specimens from healthy individuals are sterile or contain only a few microorganisms per milliliter of urine (up to about 10^4). In contrast, voided urine from most patients with definitive infection of the urinary tract has many microorganisms, usually exceeding 10^5 per milliliter of urine. For this reason, quantification is used widely to differentiate contamination from infection. Numerous methods available for the quantification include pour plates or inoculating agar plates with minute (for example, 0.001 mL) amounts of urine by means of a special bacteriologic loop. Automated instruments are being devised to enumerate and identify bacteria in urine specimens.

Antibodies directed againt *E coli* and other etiologic agents may be produced locally in the urinary tract. These antibodies become attached to the homologous bacteria in the urine and can be demonstrated with fluorescein-labeled antibodies against human immunoglobulins. Antibody-coated bacteria are found more frequently in pyelonephritis than in cystitis or asymptomatic bacteriuria, a factor that may aid in the identification of the site of infection.

Chemotherapy.   Antibacterial agents are employed frequently in the management of urinary tract infection; the physician is aided by information on the susceptibility or resistance of the etiologic agent or agents to various chemotherapeutic drugs, including antibiotics. The laboratory determines the antibiograms using standardized in vitro tests.

Renal and Perinephritic Abscesses

Occasionally, large lesions with pus develop inside the kidney (renal abscesses) or adjacent to it (perinephritic abscesses). Renal abscesses are usually hematogenous in origin and commonly are caused by *S aureus*. Only if the lesion communicates with the excretory system is the microorganism present in the voided urine. Perinephritic abscesses also may be hematogenous in origin, but they can develop as an extension of a renal lesion. Staphylococci, as well as other etiologic agents of pyelonephritis, are responsible for this infection. Examination of the surgically obtained pus by Gram stain and culture clarifies the microbiologic diagnosis.

Tuberculosis

Tuberculous infection of the urinary tract in the United States is far less common today than it was some decades ago. Kidney involvement usually occurs because of hematogenous spread of *Mycobacterium tuberculosis*. Usually, one or a few lesions develop in the kidney. When hematogenous spread is rather massive, as in miliary tuberculosis, numerous lesions develop in both kidneys. From the kidney, the infection may spread to lower parts of the urinary tract. For purposes of microbiologic diagnosis, the physician should remember that the number of microorganisms in the urine usually is rather low and clearly not comparable with the number found in *E coli* infection. Thus, for diagnosis to be valid, larger amounts of urine should be collected and the microorganisms concentrated. The microorganisms are recognized on the basis of their acid-fastness by means of a special staining procedure such as the Ziehl-Neelsen method. Because some saprophytic mycobacteria (for example, *M smegmatis*) colonize the urinary tract, acid-fast stains of urine are of limited diagnostic value. Special media are required to culture mycobacteria from urine, as well as to determine their susceptibility to antituberculous drugs. Because tubercle bacilli, even under the best of conditions, grow only slowly, recovery of the microorganism may take weeks. Determining the susceptibility of the isolate to various chemotherapeutic agents provides the clinician with important information applicable to therapy. Because tuberculosis occurs much less frequently in the United States today than in past decades, tuberculosis often can be excluded by a negative tuberculin skin test (absent cellular immunity), provided that immunosuppressive events, such as measles infection or treatment with certain drugs have not occurred recently.

Viral Infections

Surprisingly, acute and chronic infections of the urinary tract are caused only rarely by viruses, which play such a predominant role in infections of the respiratory and digestive tracts. Cystitis or urethritis may be due to adenoviruses, certain herpesviruses (varicella-zoster), and mumps virus; however, viruses are frequently present in the urinary tract in systemic viral infections such as those caused by poliovirus, coxsackievirus, influenza, mumps, measles, and rubella viruses, herpesviruses, and poxviruses. Clinicians must be aware of possible excretions when dealing with a virus such as rubella that may transmit infections to exposed, nonimmune, pregnant women, thus posing serious danger to the fetus.

Parasitic Infection

Even parasites can produce inflammation of the urinary tract; for example, a serious tropical disease, schistosomiasis, is caused by a fluke (*Schistosoma haematobium*). In this disease, the female *S haematobium* tends to deposit eggs in the bladder mucosa, causing acute hemorrhagic cystitis (see Chapter 103).

Genital Infections

Veneral diseases have become more prevalent in recent years. In 1978, according to the CDC, more than a million cases of gonorrhea were reported in the United States alone, as well as about 64,000 cases of syphilis, 500 cases of chancroid, 72 cases of granuloma inguinale, and 284 cases of lymphogranuloma venereum. Venereal disease is caused by microorganisms of various categories: namely, cocci (*Neisseria gonorrhoeae*), bacilli (*Haemophilus ducreyi*), spirochetes (*Treponema pallidum*), intracellular pathogens (*Chlamydia trachomatis*), and viruses (herpesvirus).

Neisseria gonorrhoeae Infections

Clinical Entities.   An interesting relationship exists between the site of clinical illness and the pathogen *N gonorrhoeae*. In young girls, the gonococcus causes inflammatory disease of the vulva and vagina, resulting in vulvovaginitis. In contrast, following puberty, the vagina is not the site of inflammation; rather, the inflammatory process is localized in the urethra and the cervix of the uterus, which produces exudate that may be found in the vagina. In males, urethritis occurs. The infection may spread to the endometrium, salpinx, and pelvis in women, and to the epididymis and prostate in men. Gonococci also may be present in the pharynx or anal canal. Occasionally, they reach other organs through the bloodstream. Gonococcal conjunctivitis of the newborn has now become rare.

Etiologic Agent. *N gonorrhoeae* is a gram-negative diplococcus with flat, adjacent sides; the organism is fastidious, requiring special culture media and increased CO_2 in the atmosphere to facilitate its growth. The genus to which it belongs also includes *N meningitidis,* as well as the nonpathogenic *N lactimica* and *N catarrhalis.*

Mode of Transmission. Gonorrhea usually is acquired through sexual intercourse from individuals with overt disease and notably from women with subclinical infection. Conjunctivitis of the newborn results from the infant's exposure, during birth, to a mother harboring gonococci. Only rarely is the infection acquired through indirect means.

Microbiologic Diagnosis. Presumptive microbiologic diagnosis of gonorrhea in men is made by microscopic examination of the gram-stained urethral exudate. Definitive diagnosis of gonorrhea, in men and women, is made by culture. The gonococcus is isolated far more frequently today than previously because of the availability of the Thayer-Martin medium, which suppresses the growth of most microorganisms, yet supports that of *N gonorrhoeae* and the meningococcus. Isolation of the microorganism is facilitated also by the suitable transport media that are available. The microorganism is identified on the basis of typical enzymatic activities.

Therapy and Prophylaxis. Penicillin, in the absence of allergy to this antibiotic, is the drug of choice; however, because of increasing resistance of recent and current isolates, larger doses or other drugs have to be employed. Treatment of carriers and patients prevents spread of the infection. The routine use of silver nitrate or penicillin applied to the conjunctiva of the infant shortly after birth prevents gonococcal conjunctivitis. In the past, this infection frequently caused blindness.

Syphilis

Syphilis usually begins as a seemingly innocuous, nonpainful localized lesion; unless it is treated, it spreads readily to other parts of the body and may produce severe pathologic changes over many years. Therefore, early diagnosis and therapy are crucial, although prophylaxis is more desirable.

Etiologic Agent. *T pallidum,* the only causative agent of syphilis, is one of the relatively few microorganisms that still cannot be grown on artificial culture media in its virulent form. Its characteristic morphology (dark-field or phase-contrast examination) permits diagnosis in specimens obtained from active lesions.

Mode of Transmission. The infection is transmitted from person to person, usually by sexual intercourse. It also may be acquired by the fetus from the syphilitic mother. When the microorganism is present in the blood, it may be transmitted through blood transfusion.

Microbiologic Diagnosis.   Diagnosis in the first stage of the disease is made by finding *T pallidum* in the primary lesion. The lesion usually is present on the genitalia in the form of ulcers (hard chancre), accompanied by involvement of the regional lymph nodes. Dark-field examination of a specimen obtained from the ulcer establishes the diagnosis. As the microorganism spreads, the patient develops a characteristic immune response. Wassermann first detected syphilis antibodies by means of a complement-fixation test that bears his name (Wassermann test). The reactive antigen has been identified as cardiolipin. Numerous precipitation tests were developed to demonstrate this antibody. Because cardiolipin is not unique to *T pallidum* but is part of tissues as well, antibodies are produced occasionally under other conditions; nonetheless, these tests are excellent tools for screening purposes. Specific antibodies against the spirochete itself can be demonstrated by several recently developed procedures including TPI (*T pallidum* immobilization), FTA-ABS (fluorescent treponemal antibody absorption), and *T pallidum* complement-fixation tests.

Therapy.   In 1910, Ehrlich developed the first "magic bullet" designed to kill an infectious agent and still be relatively harmless to the host. Arsphenamine, which resulted from these extensive studies, was used early in the twentieth century; today, penicillin is the drug of choice. When the patient is allergic to this antibiotic, other antimicrobial agents, such as a tetracycline or an erythromycin, must be used. Effective treatment of syphilis during the early stages of pregnancy prevents the disease in the newborn child. Because prevention is far better than later treatment, a routine diagnostic blood test for syphilis during pregnancy is mandated in many parts of the world.

Lymphogranuloma Venereum

A third venereal disease is lymphogranuloma venereum, also called lymphogranuloma inguinale. It is caused by members of the species *C trachomatis,* a group of organisms that, as the name indicates, is responsible also for trachoma, an eye infection. A genital lesion is the primary site of infection; subsequent enlargement of the inguinal lymph nodes gives the disease its name. Microbiologic diagnosis requires isolating the microorganism or demonstrating the immune response of the patient, or both. The immune response can be demonstrated by the Frei test, a skin test for delayed-type hypersensitivity to the antigen. Because of the variable incidence of false-negative reactions, this test has limited usefulness. The diagnosis also can be made by demonstrating specific antibodies in the patient's serum. Chemotherapeutic agents such as tetracycline and sulfonamides have been used to treat this infection. For an overview of *Chlamydia* infections, see Chapter 54.

Nongonococcal Urethritis

As the availability of highly selective culture media has improved bacteriologic diagnosis of gonorrhea, it is now frequently possible to diagnose nongonococcal urethritis. Two microorganisms have been identified as causes of this entity. *C trachomatis* belongs to the group of microorganisms that also causes lymphogranuloma venereum. The other microorganism is a mycoplasma, *Ureaplasma urealyticum,* which is also referred to as T-strain mycoplasma. In practice, microbiologic diagnosis of nongonococcal urethritis is made primarily by excluding gonorrhea on the basis of microscopic or cultural examination or both. Tetracycline is used frequently to treat this disease.

Chancroid

Another venereal disease, encountered only rarely in this country, is chancroid. It is also referred to as soft chancre (ulcer), in contrast to syphilis, which yields a lesion characterized as hard chancre. The disease is caused by a member of the *Haemophilus* group, *H ducreyi,* a gram-negative, rather fastidious bacillus. The microorganism may be demonstrated in specimens from the lesion by microscopic and cultural examinations. Sulfonamides are effective in treating this condition.

Granuloma Inguinale

Granuloma inguinale is a rare venereal disease in the United States. This disease is characterized by formation of an ulcerative lesion in the genital or perianal areas. Infection may spread to the regional lymph nodes through the lymphatics. In its early stages, this disease may be mistaken for syphilis. The causative agent is a gram-negative bacillus called *Calymmatobacterium granulomatis,* formerly *Donovania granulomatis.* Bacteria may be present inside of host cells and are referred to as Donovan bodies. Various antibiotics (tetracyclines, gentamicin, and streptomycin) have been used successfully to treat this infection.

Chlamydia Infections

Chlamydia trachomatis is an important cause of sexually transmitted infections of the urogenital tract, including nongonococcal urethritis. *C trachomatis* is responsible for epididymitis and prostatitis in men, and cervicitis, endometritis, and pelvic inflammatory diseases in women. The microbiologic diagnosis is made by demonstrating characteristic inclusions in infected cell cultures. The microorganism may be transmitted during delivery and cause infections in newborns including conjunctivitis and respiratory illness. In adults the infection can be treated successfully with antibiotics such as tetracycline.

Herpes Infections

Herpes infection of the genital tract has gained special attention because of its relative frequency and possible relationship to malignancy. Because it is not a reportable disease, accurate data on its occurrence are not available. It is estimated that some 400,000 subjects contract this infection a year and that between 5–20 million individuals in the United States have the infection. The infection may be clinically overt or silent and, as in herpetic infections of other sites, relapse is encountered frequently. The majority of genital infections are caused by type 2, but a significant proportion is caused by type 1. Transfer of the virus to the fetus during delivery may result in serious and even fatal infection. The microbiologic diagnosis is based on pathologic findings, including electron microscopy and demonstration of characteristic inclusion bodies, cultivation of the virus, and/or antibody response of the patient. A highly effective, nontoxic, specific chemotherapeutic agent is not available.

Trichomoniasis

The protozoan *Trichomonas vaginalis* is responsible for genitourinary tract infection in women and men; it is symptomatic far more often in women than in men. The microorganism usually is transmitted during sexual intercourse. The microbiologic diagnosis is made by identifying the motile parasite, either by microscopic examination of discharge or by culture. The disease is widespread and can be treated effectively with metronidazole.

Infection of the Female Genital Tract

Vaginitis or vulvovaginitis and related infections of the female genital tract may be caused by a large variety of microorganisms other than those mentioned previously. These microorganisms include certain bacteria, chlamydiae, mycoplasma, fungi, proto- zoa, and viruses. The protozoan *Trichomonas vaginalis* is a flagellated protozoan that can be identified readily by its characteristic features, including motility in properly prepared wet specimens from secretions. Numerous species of bacteria that are responsible for vaginitis include streptococci, staphylococci, gonococci in children, and *H vaginalis*. Group B hemolytic streptococci in the vagina may or may not be associated with inflammation and clinical manifestations; yet, on transfer to the newborn during delivery, these streptococci may be responsible for sepsis or meningitis or both, which usually are fatal unless treated with suitable antibiotics. Thus, this infection in the adult and the newborn represents an instructive example of the role of the host in the relationship between microorganism and its possible victim. *Listeria monocytogenes* also may be present without overt illness in the genital tract of pregnant women, who then give birth to infants with serious listeriosis. Among the fungi, *Candida albicans* and other *Candida* sp play a significant role in vaginitis.

Infection of the cervix, uterus, salpinges, and ovaries often is due to spread of the microorganisms from the vagina. Anaerobic bacteria (notably *Bacteroides fragilis* and *Peptostreptococcus*), as well as numerous faculative aerobic bacteria (for example, *N gonorrhoeae* and streptococci), are among the etiologic agents. In the days before aseptic practice in obstetrics, ascending infection of the uterus and complications such as bloodstream infection occurred frequently following manual procedures. Semmelweis and Oliver Wendell Holmes, Sr. proved independently that such infection was iatrogenic and could be avoided, as it often resulted from contamination of the physician's hands.

Infection of the Male Genital Tract

Prostatitis is an acute or chronic infection of the prostate gland that may be caused by various microorganisms, which also play a major role in cystitis and pyelonephritis. Gram-negative bacilli (notably *Escherichia coli,* as well as *Klebsiella, Enterobacter, Proteus,* and *Pseudomonas* sp) are most commonly encountered. Staphylococci and other gram-positive bacteria play a lesser role. Bacteriologic examination of appropriately obtained urine specimens may identify the etiologic agents. When the inflammatory process results in enlargement of the gland, obstruction of the urethra may follow and thus predispose the urinary tract to infection.

Infrequently, virus infections may manifest themselves in the male genital tract. For example, orchitis and epididymitis are well-known complications of mumps.

References

de la Maza, L.M., Peterson, E.M.: Genital infections. *Med Clin North Am* 1983; 67:1059-73.

Feigin, R.D., Cherry, J.D., (editors): *Textbook of pediatric infectious diseases.* Philadelphia: W.B. Saunders Co., 1981.

Gabre-Kidan, T., Lipsky, B.A., Plorde, J.J.: Hemophilus influenzae as a cause of urinary tract infections in men. *Arch Intern Med* 1984; 149:1623-1627.

Lennette, E.H., et al., (editors): *Manual of clinical microbiology,* 3rd ed. Washington, D.C.: American Society for Microbiology, 1980.

Rose, N.R., Friedman, H., (editors): *Manual of clinical immunology,* 2nd ed. Washington, D.C.: American Society for Microbiology, 1980.

Wehrle, P.F., Top, F.H., Sr., (editors): *Communicable and infectious diseases,* 9th ed. St. Louis: The C.V. Mosby Co., 1981.

Youmans, G.P., Paterson, P.Y., Sommers, H.M.: *The biologic and clinical basis of infectious diseases,* 2nd ed. Philadelphia: W.B. Saunders Co., 1980.

113 Microbiology of Skin and Nails

Raza Aly, PhD

General Concepts

The skin is one of the largest organs of the human body; it has an average area of 1.75 m^2 and weighs about 5 kg. The skin is rarely sterile; microbes are abundant, especially in moist areas such as body folds. Skin infections due to bacteria may be divided into primary and secondary types, a distinction that is useful clinically. **Primary bacterial infections** have characteristic morphologies and courses, are initiated by a single organism, and usually arise in normal skin. They are most frequently caused by *Staphylococcus aureus*, β-hemolytic streptococci, or coryneforms.

Secondary infections originate in diseased skin as superimposed conditions resulting in acute or chronic intermingling of the underlying skin disease and the infection; thus, they do not follow a characteristic course. The role of bacteria in these conditions often is difficult to assess. The most common organisms in secondary infections are the same as those in primary infections and gram-negative organisms (*Proteus, Pseudomonas,* and *Escherichia coli*).

Etiologic agents associated with skin diseases are viruses, bacteria, and fungi. Specific laboratory media and tests are required to identify these agents.

Methods for Laboratory Diagnosis

Specimen Collection

Bacteria.   Specimens are collected with a blade or by swabbing the involved areas of the skin. When pustules or vesicles are present, the roof or crust is removed with a sterile Bard–Parker No. 11 blade. The pus or exudates are spread as thinly as possible on a clear glass slide for Gram staining. Cultures in cellulitis and erysipelas are performed by injecting preservative-free physiologic saline into the involved skin and culturing the withdrawn fluid as soon as possible. Even when meticulous techniques are used, bacteria are rarely cultured from these lesions.

For actinomycetes, the skin is rubbed with swabs soaked in 70%-90% ethyl or isopropyl alcohol. Pus is collected from closed lesions by aspirations with sterile needle and syringe. Material is collected from draining sinuses by holding a sterile test tube at the edge of the lesion and allowing the pus to run into the tube. The cotton fibers of gauze covering the lesions should be examined for the presence of granules. Granules are aggregates of inflammatory cells, debris, proteinaceous material, and delicate branching filaments. Pus and other exudates are examined microscopically for the presence of granules. A granule is placed in a drop of water on a glass slide, crushed under a microscopic cover slip, and examined under the microscope for the presence of branching filaments.

Viruses.   Vesicles are cleaned with 70% alcohol or sterile saline. Viruses are obtained by unroofing a vesicle with a needle or a scalpel blade. The fluid is collected with a swab or with a tuberculin syringe with a 26-27 gauge needle. The fluid obtained from fresh vesicles may contain a sufficient number of viruses for culture. Direct smears are prepared by scraping cells from the base of the lesions. The cells are smeared on a slide, fixed, and stained with Giemsa or Wright stains. The specimens from ulcers are collected by rubbing the lesions firmly with a swab moistened with nutrient broth.

Fungi.   Cutaneous samples are obtained by scraping skin scales or clipping infected nails into a sterile Petri dish or a clean envelope. The areas to be sampled are washed with soap and water or 70% alcohol. Samples should be collected from the peripheral margins of typical ringworm infections. In the presence of suppurative lesions of deep skin and subcutaneous tissues, aspiration with a sterile needle and syringe is recommended. Direct mounts are made by mixing a small portion of the sample in two to three drops of physiologic saline or KOH on a microscope slide. Ten percent or 20% KOH is recommended for skin or nail scrapings. The mounting fluid (KOH) clears out background debris and keratinous material, making the hyphal forms easier to see. A glass coverslip is placed over the preparation before microscopic examination.

Microscopic Examination

When the pus or exudate is obtained from an intact pustule, bulla, or abscess, demonstration of organisms in such fluids strongly suggests a pathogenic relationship. Morphologic arrangement of individual cells, shapes, and Gram stain reactions are helpful hints for presumptive diagnosis. Cultures allow complete identification of the organism. Acid-fast stains are used to detect tuberculosis and nocardial organisms.

The KOH mount is examined with bright-field illumination by lowering the condenser (to reduce the amount of incident light) for the presence of hyphal or other fungal structures. A single, carefully performed microscopic examination identifies up to 90% of dermatophyte infections, whereas a culture identifies the remaining 10%.

Cultures

Most pathogenic skin bacteria grow on artificial media, and selection of the medium is important. For general use, blood agar plates (preferably 5% defibrinated sheep blood) are recommended. In many situations, a selective medium combined with a general purpose medium is recommended. For example, *Staphylococcus aureus* may overgrow *Streptococcus pyogenes* in blood agar medium when both organisms are present. When crystal violet (1 μg/mL) is added to blood agar, *S pyogenes* is selected over *S aureus*. Cultures for meningococci, gonococci, and brucellae must be incubated in a CO_2 atmosphere. For *Propionibacterium acnes*, trypticase soy agar or brain heart infusion agar with 1% glucose are satisfactory media. *P acnes* grows anaerobically. If tuberculosis or fungal infection is suspected, specimens are collected on appropriate media and incubated aerobically. Except for some medical centers, state health laboratories, or commercial laboratories, most hospital clinical laboratories do not have facilities for viral cultures.

Bacterial Skin Infections

The classification of skin infections is an attempt to integrate various clinical entities in an organized manner. An arbitrary but useful classification for primary and secondary infections is presented in Table 113-1. The list is not complete and includes only the more common skin diseases.

Primary Infections

Impetigo.   Three forms of impetigo are recognized on the basis of clinical, bacteriologic, and histologic findings. The lesions of common or superficial impetigo may contain group A β-hemolytic streptococci, *S aureus*, or both, and controversy exists about which of these organisms is the primary pathogen. The lesions have a thick, adherent, recurrent, dirty yellow crust with an erythematous margin. This form of impetigo is the most common skin infection in children. Impetigo in infants is highly contagious and requires prompt treatment because it may lead to poststreptococcal glomerulonephritis.

The lesions in bullous (staphylococcal) impetigo, which are always caused by *S*

Table 113-1 Classification of Selected Bacterial Skin Infections

Infection Classification	Common Etiologic Agents
Primary	
Impetigo	*Staphylococcus aureus*, group A streptococci
Cellulitis and erysipelas	Group A streptococci
Staphylococcal scalded skin syndrome	*S aureus*
Folliculitis	*S aureus*
Superficial folliculitis	
Staphylococcal folliculitis	*S aureus*
Gram-negative folliculitis	*Klebsiella pneumoniae*, *Enterobacter aerogenes*, and *Proteus vulgaris*
Propionibacterium acnes folliculitis	*Propinonibacterium acnes*
Deep folliculitis	
Sycosis barbae	*S aureus*
Furuncles or carbuncles	*S aureus*
Pitted keratolysis	Gram-positive coryneforms
Erysipeliod	*E rhusiopathiae*
Erythrasma	*Corynebacterium minutissimum*
Trichomycosis	*Corynebacterium tenuis*, bacteria resembling *C minutissimum*, and lipophilic coryneforms
Secondary	
Intertrigo	Overgrowth of resident and transient bacteria
Acute infectious eczematoid dermatitis	*S aureus*
Pseudofolliculitis of the beard	Resident flora (gram-positive cocci)
Toe web infection	Fungi, coryneforms, *Brevibacterium*, and gram-negative rods
Other Skin Diseases	
Mycobacteria	*Mycobacterium tuberculosis*, *M marinum*, and *M ulcerans*
Actinomycetes	*Actinomyces israelii*

aureus, are superficial, thin-walled, and bullous. When a lesion ruptures, a thin, transparent, varnishlike crust appears, which can be distinguished from the stuck on crust of common impetigo. This distinctive appearance of bullous impetigo results from the local action of the epidermolytic toxin (exfoliation). The lesions most often are found in groups in a single region.

Ecthyma is a deeper form of impetigo. Lesions usually occur on the legs and other areas of the body that are generally covered, and often occur as a complication of debility and infestation. The ulcers have a punched-out appearance when the crust or purulent materials are removed. The lesions heal slowly and leave scars.

Cellulitis and Erysipelas. β-hemolytic streptococci are the most common etiologic agents in cellulitis, a diffuse inflammation of loose connective tissue, particularly subcutaneous tissue. Cellulitis occurs generally through a breach in the skin surface, especially if tissue edema is present. Cellulitis, however, may arise in normal skin. The lesion of cellulitis is erythematous, edematous, brawny, and tender, with borders that are poorly defined.

No absolute distinction can be made between streptococcal cellulitis and erysipelas. Clinically, erysipelas is more superficial, with a sharp margin as opposed to the undefined border of cellulitis. Lesions usually occur on the cheek.

Staphylococcal Scalded Skin Syndrome (SSSS).   SSSS (Lyell's disease or toxic epidermal necrolysis) starts as a localized lesion, followed by widespread erythema and exfoliation of the skin. This disorder is caused by phage group II staphylococci, which elaborate an epidermolytic toxin. The disease is more common in infants than in adults.

Folliculitis.   Folliculitis can be divided into two major categories, based on histologic location: superficial and deep.

The most superficial form of skin infection is staphylococcal folliculitis, manifested by minute erythematous follicular pustules without involvement of the surrounding skin. The scalp and extremities are favorite sites. Gram-negative folliculitis occurs mainly as a superinfection in acne vulgaris patients receiving long-term, systemic antibiotic therapy. These pustules are often clustered around the nose. The causative agent is found in the nostril and the pustules. *P acnes* folliculitis has been misdiagnosed as staphylococcal folliculitis. The primary lesion is a white-to-yellow follicular pustule, flat or domed. Gram stain of pus reveals numerous intracellular and extracellular gram-positive pleomorphic rods. The lesions are seen more often in men than in women. The process may start at the age when acne usually occurs, yet most cases occur well past this age.

In deep folliculitis, infection extends deeply into the follicle, and the resulting perifolliculitis causes a more marked inflammatory response than that seen in superficial folliculitis. In sycosis barbae (barber's itch), the primary lesion is a follicular pustule pierced by a hair. Bearded men may be more prone to this infection than shaven men.

A furuncle (or boil) is a staphylococcal infection of a follicle with involvement of subcutaneous tissue. The preferred sites of furuncles are the hair parts or areas that are exposed to friction and macerations. A carbuncle is a confluence of boils, a large indurated painful lesion with multiple draining sites.

Erysipeloid.   This benign infection, which occurs most often in fishermen and meat handlers, is characterized by redness of the skin (usually on a finger or the back of a hand) which persists for several days. The infection is caused by *Erysipilothrix rhusiopathiae.*

Pitted Keratolysis.   Pitted keratolysis is a superficial infection of the plantar surface producing a punched-out appearance. The pits may coalesce into irregularly shaped areas of superficial erosion. The pits are produced by a lytic process that spreads peripherally. The areas most often infected are the heels, the ball, the volar pads, and the toes. Humidity and high temperature are frequent aggravating factors. Gram-positive coryneforms have been isolated from the lesions.

Erythrasma.   Erythrasma is a chronic, superficial infection of the pubis, toe web, groin, axilla, and inframammary folds. Most lesions are asymptomatic, but lesions may be mildly symptomatic with burning and itching. The patches are irregular shaped, dry and scaly, initially pink, and later turning brown. The widespread, generalized form is more common in warmer climates. *Corynebacterium minutissimum* is the etiologic agent. Because of its small size, the organism is difficult to observe in KOH preparations of infected scales; however, it is readily demonstrable by Gram staining of stratum corneum.

Trichomycosis.   Trichomycosis involves the hair in the axillary and pubic regions and is characterized by development of nodules of varying consistency and color. The condition is generally asymptomatic and not contagious. Underlying skin is normal. Infected hairs obtained for microscopic examination are placed on a slide in a drop of 10% KOH under a coverslip. The nodules on the hairs are composed of short bacillary forms. Three types of coryneforms are associated with trichomycosis; one resembles *C minutissimum*, one is lipolytic, and the third is *C tenuis*.

Secondary Infections

Intertrigo.   Intertrigo is most commonly seen in chubby infants or obese adults. In the skin fold, heat, moisture, and rubbing produce erythema, maceration, or even erosions. Overgrowth of resident or transient flora may produce this problem.

Acute Infectious Eczematoid Dermatitis.   Actue infectious eczematoid dermatitis arises from a primary lesion such as a boil or a draining ear or nose, which are sources of infectious exudate. A hallmark of this disease is a streak of dermatitis along the path of flow of the discharge material. Coagulase-positive staphylococci are the organisms most frequently isolated.

Pseudofolliculitis of the Beard.   Pseudofolliculitis of the beard, a common disorder, occurs most often in the beard area of black people who shave. The characteristic lesions are usually erythematous papules or, less commonly, pustules containing buried hairs. This occurs when a strongly curved hair emerging from curved hair follicles reenters the skin to produce an ingrown hair. Gram-positive microorganisms that are resident flora are associated with this disorder—a clear illustration of the opportunism of nonpathogenic bacteria when the host defense is impaired.

Toe Web Infection.   The disease commonly referred to as athlete's foot has traditionally been regarded as strictly a fungal infection. This assumption has been revised, however, because fungi often cannot be recovered from the lesions throughout the disease course. Researchers now believe that the dermatophytes, the first invaders, cause skin damage that allows bacterial overgrowth, which promotes maceration and hyperkeratosis. The fungi, through the production of antibiotics, then create an environment that favors the growth of certain coryneforms and *Brevibacterium*. Proteolytic enzymes, which are produced by some of these bacteria, may aggravate the condition. If the feet become superhydrated, resident gram-negative rods become the predominant flora, and the toe webs incur further damage. The fungi are then either eliminated by the action of antifungal substances of bacterial origin or by their own inability to compete for nutrients with the vigorously growing bacteria.

Other Bacterial Skin Diseases

Skin Tuberculosis (Localized Form). Localized skin tuberculosis follows inoculation of *mycobacterium tuberculosis* into a wound in individuals with no previous immunologic experience with the disease. The course starts as an inflammatory nodule (chancre) and is accompanied by regional lymphangitis and lymphadenitis. The course of the disease depends on the patient's resistance and the effectiveness of treatment. In an immune or partially immune host, two major groups of skin lesions are distinguished: tuberculosis verrucosa and lupus vulgaris.

Mycobacterium marinum **Skin Disease.** Many cases of *M Marinum* skin disease occur in children and adolescents who have a history of using swimming pools or cleaning fish tanks. Often, they present a history of trauma, but even in the absence of trauma, the lesions appear frequently on the sites most exposed to injury. The usually solitary lesions are tuberculoid granuloma that rarely show acid-fast organisms, but the skin tuberculin test is positive.

Mycobacterium ulcerans **Skin Disease.** Lesions in *M ulcerans* skin disease usually occur on the arms or legs, but they may occur elsewhere (except palms and soles). Most patients have a single, painless cutaneous ulcer with characteristic undermined edges. Geographic association of the disease with swamps and water courses has been reported. In some tropical areas, chronic ulcers by this organism are common.

In scrofuloderma, tuberculosis of lymph nodes or bones is extended into the skin, resulting in the development of ulcers.

A disseminated form of the disease occurs when bacteria are spread through the bloodstream in patients who have fulminating tuberculosis of the skin. When hypersensitivity to tubercle bacilli is present, hematogenously disseminated antigen produces tuberculids, such as lichen scrofulosus.

Actinomycetoma. Several etiologic agents cause actinomycetoma. About one-half of the cases are due to actinomycetes (actinomycetoma) and the other one-half, to fungi (eumycetoma). The most common causes of mycetoma in the United States are *Pseudallescheria* (Petriellidium) *boydii* (a fungus) and *Actinomyces israelii* (a bacterium). Regardless of the organism involved, the clinical picture is the same. Causative organisms are introduced by trauma into the skin. The disease is characterized by cutaneous swelling that slowly enlarges and becomes softer. Tunnellike sinus tracts form in the deeper tissues, producing swelling and distortion of the foot. The draining material contains granules of various sizes and colors, depending on the etiologic agent.

Actinomycosis. *Actinomyces israelii* usually is the etiologic agent for human actinomycosis; *Arachnia propionica* (*Actinomyces propinicus*) is the second most common cause of the disease. The characteristic appearance of the lesion in actinomycosis is a hard, red, slowly developing swelling. The hard masses soften and eventually drain, forming chronic sinus tracts with little tendency to heal. The sinus tract discharges purulent material containing "sulfur" granules. In about 50% of actinomycosis cases, the initial lesion is cervicofacial, involving the tissues of the face, neck, tongue, and mandible. About 20% of the cases show thoracic actinomycosis, which may result from direct extension of the disease from the neck or from the abdomen or as a primary infection from oral aspiration of the organism. In abdominal actinomycosis, the primary lesion is in the cecum, the appendix, or the pelvic organs.

Viral Skin Diseases

Viral diseases can produce localized and generalized skin infections (Table 113-2). There are several major groups of viruses responsible for skin lesions.

Herpes Simplex

Herpes simplex infection is probably the most common viral skin disease. Almost the entire adult population has sustained this infection at one time or another. Herpes simplex, a DNA virus, is the etiologic agent.

Poxviruses

The smallpox virus is transmitted from person to person and has no known animal reservoir or vector. Cowpox is an infection of cattle and is acquired by handling infected cows. Lesions may occur on the hands, arms, and faces of those handling infected animals. Vaccinia viruses are vaccine strains developed in the laboratory and adapted to grow in the skin of humans, rabbits, and calves. Several clinical manifestations may

Table 113-2   Viruses Associated With Skin Infections

Infection Classification	Virus Group
Localized infections	
Cold sores and genital lesions	Herpes simplex
Shingles	Vaccinia-zoster (herpes)
Eczemia vaccinatum	Vaccinia
Molluscum contagiosum	Pox
Warts	Papova
Generalized infections	
Measles	Measles (paramyxovirus)
Picornavirus	Several picornaviruses
Rubella	Rubella (togavirus)
Herpesviruses	Several, but especially varicella virus
Smallpox	Pox

occur in individuals who are vaccinated with vaccinia virus against smallpox. The main problem with vaccinia arises when it becomes desirable to vaccinate a person already suffering from eczema or other skin diseases; vaccination may produce eczema vaccinatum. The viruses of smallpox, vaccinia, and cowpox are closely related; all are large DNA viruses.

Molluscum Contagiosum

Molluscum contagiosum is characterized by numerous small, pink nodules, most often seen on the face, genitalia, or the rectal area. Lesions on the back, arms, buttocks, and inner thighs are also seen. The disease is generally harmless and self-limiting. Due to its size and shape, the etiologic agent belongs to the pox group.

Warts

Verruca vulgaris.   Verruca vulgaris occurs commonly on hands and fingers as single or multiple lesions. These warts are generally painless, firm, dry, and rough to the touch. They may remain stable or regress spontaneously. The etiologic agent is a papovavirus.

Plantar Warts.   Verruca plantaris is a clinical variety of verruca vulgaris on the sole of the foot. Because of body pressure, they grow in depth and may be painful. Genital warts appear as large lesions of red, soft masses that may coalesce.

Verruca Plana Juvenilis.   Juvenile warts (also known as flat warts) occur most commonly in children. The lesions are in groups and may appear on the face, neck, back of the hands, and arms. Although children are most frequently infected, these warts also occur in adults. Warts are caused by the papovavirus group, composed of small DNA viruses.

Fungal Skin Diseases

Several genera of fungi are responsible for diseases of the skin. This group of fungi, known collectively as dermatophytes, is discussed in detail in Chapter 59. Some nondermatophytes, including yeasts, can also cause skin infections.

Nail Infections

The nail consists of four epidermal components: matrix, proximal nailfold, nailbed, and hyponychium (Figure 113-1). The matrix is close to the bony phalanx. The horny end product of matrix is the nail plate, which moves distally over the nailbed. Only the distal portion, the lunula, is visible as a white, crescent-shaped structure. The proximal nailfold is a modified extension of the epidermis of the dorsum of the finger, which forms a fold over the matrix; its horny end product is the cuticle. The nail bed is an epidermal structure beginning at the distal margin of the lunula and terminating in the

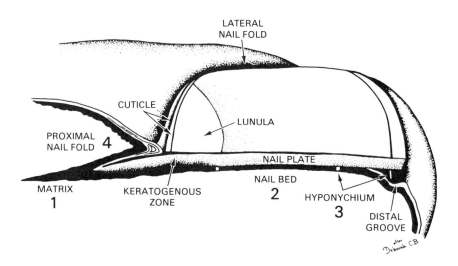

Figure 113-1 Longitudinal section (diagrammatic sketch) of fingernail showing 1, matrix, 2, nail bed, 3, hyponichium, and 4, proximal nail bed. Adapted from Zaias N: *Arch Dermatol* 1972; 105:263.

hyponichium, which is the extension of the volar epidermis under the nail plate and ends adjacent to the nailbed.

Fungal Infections

Onychomycosis is defined as infection of the nail by fungi. Universally recognized etiologic agents are species of *Trichophyton, Microsporum* (rarely) and *Epidermophyton* (Table 113-3). These dermatophytes are commonly called ringworm fungi.

Nondermatophytic fungi also exist; they rarely have been reported to cause onychomycosis. This type of fungi usually causes a toenail problem and is rarely seen in the fingernail.

Conventionally, onychomycosis is classified into four types:

1. Distal subungual onychomycosis primarily involves the distal nailbed and hyponichium, with secondary involvement of the underside of the nail plate. *Trichophyton rubrum* is one of the organisms that causes this clinical type.

2. White superficial onychomycosis involves the toenail plate on the surface of the nail. It is produced by *T mentagrophytes,* species of *Cephalosporium, Aspergillus,* and *Fusarium.*

3. Proximal subungual onychomycosis is an invasion of the nail plate from the proximal nailfold producing a specific nail condition. It is produced by *T rubrum* and *T megninii.* This is a rare type of onychomycosis.

4. Candida onychomycosis involves all of the nail plate. It is caused by *C albicans* and is seen in patients who have chronic cutaneous candidiasis, a syndrome associated with cellular and humoral abnormalities.

Table 113-3   Fungi Associated With Onychomycosis

Dermatophytes	Nondermatophytes
Trichophyton rubrum	Aspergillus sp
T mentagrophytes	Cephalosporium sp
T violaceum	Fusarium oxysporum
T schoenleini	Scopulariopsis brevicaulis
T tonsurans	
T megninii	
T concentricum (rare)	
T soudanense (rare)	
T gourvilii (rare)	
Epidermophyton floccosum	
Microsporum gypseum (rare)	
M audouini (rare)	
M canis (rare)	

Bacterial Infections

Pseudomonas aeruginosa is associated with green nail syndrome, which is essentially a greenish discoloration of the nail plate. Attempts to culture *Pseudomonas* from the deep section of the nail have not been successful; however, *P aeruginosa* has been isolated on paronychia (inflammatory lesion around the margin of a nail) cultures. Whether there is a true invasion of the nail plate by the bacteria or just the diffusion of the pigment into the nail plate is not certain. Black-colored paronychia is associated with *Proteus* sp.

References

Aly, R., Maibach, H.I.: *Clinical skin microbiology.* Springfield, Ill.: Charles C Thomas, 1978.

Aly, R., Maibach, H.I.: In: *Recent advances in dermatology.* Rook, A.J., Maibach, H.I., (editors). London: Churchill-Livingston, 1983.

Lennette, E.H., et al., (editors): *Manual of clinical microbiology,* 3rd ed. Washington, D.C.: American Association for Microbiology, 1980.

Maibach, H.I., Aly, R., (editors): *Skin microbiology: relevance to clinical infection.* New York, Heidelberg, Berlin: Springer-Verlag, 1981.

Noble, W.C.: *Microbiology of human skin.* London: Lloyd-Luke, 1981.

Rogers, D.E., Schaffner, W.: Rickettsial and viral diseases with cutaneous involvement. In: *Dermatology in general medicine.* Fitzpatrick, T.B., et al., (editors). New York: McGraw-Hill Book Co., 1971.

Sutton, R.L., Jr., Waisman, M.: Dermatoses due to bacteria. *Cutis* 1975; 16: 695-729.

Zaias, N.: Onychomycosis. *Arch Dermatol* 1972; 105: 263-273.

114 Microbiology of Dental Decay and Periodontal Disease

Walter J. Loesche, DMD, PhD

General Concepts

The tooth surfaces are unique in that they are the only body part not subject to metabolic turnover. Once formed, the teeth are essentially indestructible, as witnessed by their importance in fossil records and forensic medicine. Yet in the living individual, the integrity of the teeth is assaulted by a microbial challenge so great that dental infections rank as the most universal affliction of humankind. The discomfort caused by these infections and their enormous cost (dental infections rank third in medical costs, behind heart disease and cancer, in the United States) gives dental diseases prominence despite their non-life-threatening nature.

This chapter reviews the bacterial aspects of dental caries and periodontal disease and suggests that future treatment will be directed toward eliminating or suppressing certain bacterial species that appear to be overt pathogens in plaque.

Dental infections include tooth decay and periodontal disease and, to a lesser extent, overt abscesses and yeast infections. Decay and periodontal disease are initiated and mediated by dental plaque, the dense aggregation of bacteria found on the tooth surfaces. Plaque often is defined according to its tooth location. Thus, supragingival

---

plaque is present on tooth surfaces above the gingiva or gum margin. Subgingival plaque is present on tooth surfaces below the gingival margin. At one time, all plaques were considered to have equal disease potential and to contain essentially similar organisms. Studies of the pathogenesis of dental decay and periodontal disease have revealed that different bacteria are associated with each clinical entity.

Decay is the acid dissolution of the tooth mineral. The microbes capable of effecting this decalcification have to be both acidogenic and aciduric (acid resistant), as most of the demineralization occurs at a plaque pH value of 5 or below. Periodontal disease does not involve demineralization but, in fact, often is associated with an ectopic mineralization of the tooth surface known as dental calculus. Periodontal disease includes an array of "infections" that cause an inflammatory response in the gingival and periodontal tissues. These infections are unusual in that bacterial invasion of the tissues is rarely encountered. Rather, bacteria in the plaque touching the tissue elaborate various compounds such as H_2S, NH_3, amines, endotoxins, and enzymes such as collagenases and antigens, all of which penetrate the gingiva and elicit an inflammatory response. This inflammatory response, although overwhelmingly protective, appears responsible for a net loss of periodontal supporting tissue, and leads to periodontal pocket formation, loosening of the teeth, and eventual tooth loss. The bacteriologic culturing of plaques associated with dental decay and the various forms of periodontal disease led to the demonstration that different microbial combinations were associated with various clinical entities.

Available information indicates that a measurable amount of decay may be due to a sucrose-dependent *Streptococcus mutans* infection. Individuals at risk for this infection can be treated by frequent mechanical intervention, by intensive application of prescription levels of fluorides, by restriction of ingestion of sucrose between meals, or by use of products that contain sucrose substitutes (such as xylitol). Gingivitis and periodontitis are the host response to a variety of noxious bacteria in the subgingival plaque. These bacteria tend to be gram-negative anaerobes. Individuals with periodontal disease also can be treated by frequent mechanical intervention or by the judicious use of systemic antimicrobials such as metronidazole or tetracyclines.

Oral Ecosystems

The mucous membranes of the oral cavity and especially the teeth harbor the same microbial density as is generally found in the large intestine and in feces (approximately 10^{11} bacteria per gram wet weight of plaque). Saliva has a microbial density about 0.001% that of plaque, but even so, 1 mL of saliva contains about 10^8 bacteria. An average person swallows about 10^{11} bacteria per day. These large quantities of bacteria could not be conveniently isolated and enumerated until quantitative culturing procedures were employed. Even then, the recovery of viable organisms was only a small fraction (10%) of what could be observed under the microscope.

In the 1960s, several investigators demonstrated that the indigenous oral flora consisted of anaerobic and facultative bacteria. When plaque was cultured in the absence of oxygen, as many as 70% of the bacteria present in plaque could be isolated.

Saliva, like feces, can be collected conveniently and its bacteriologic profile used to provide insights on disease prevalence; however, most salivary organisms are derived

Table 114-1   Microbial Ecosystems on the Tooth Surface*

	Teeth			
Streptococcal Species	*Supragingival*	*Subgingival*	*Soft Tissue*	*Saliva*
S salivarius	−	−	+ +	+ +
S sanguis	+ +	+	+	+
S mitis	+ +	+	+	+
S mutans	+	−	−	±

*−, not usually detected; ±, found in less than 1% of flora if present; +, in less than 10% of flora; + +, in greater than 10% of flora.

from the oral soft tissues such as the tongue and the palate and do not quantitatively reflect the plaque flora. This was demonstrated by the distribution of various oral streptococcal species. (Table 114-1). *Streptococcus salivarius*, the predominant streptococcus in the saliva, is rarely present in plaque but is found regularly on the tongue and soft tissue. Prominent supragingival plaque species such as *S sanguis* and *S mitis* are present in the saliva at lower levels than *S salivarius*. *S mutans* is found only on certain tooth surfaces, especially those that are decayed. Subsequent studies established the importance of selective adhesion in explaining this localization of the oral streptococci on the various oral surfaces. Adhesion is now regarded as the dominant factor in mucous membrane microbial ecology; it is considered especially important as a virulence factor for certain enteropathogenic organisms.

Bacterial Succession and Periodontal Plaques

Emphasis shifted away from the culturing of saliva to the culturing of plaque, especially plaque removed from discrete anatomic sites on the tooth surface. The bacterial succession that occurred in plaque formation was documented by cultural and microscopic means. Immediately after the teeth are mechanically cleaned, their surfaces selectively adsorb an acidic glycoprotein from the saliva, forming a bacteria-free layer called the acquired enamel pellicle. Most bacteria in the saliva apparently cannot bind to this pellicle; therefore, most of the smooth tooth surfaces, especially the most coronal or top aspects, have a very low bacterial density.

The initial colonizers invariably include *S sanguis* and *S mitis*, indicating that these organisms have a special affinity for sites on the pellicle. These streptococci proliferate and in turn become colonized by other bacteria present in saliva (for example, *Actinomyces* and *Veillonella* sp). The greatest growth occurs at the gingival margin, where plaque accumulations usually are clinically visible after several days. This plaque may, in some instances, provoke a bleeding gingivitis. At the time that gingivitis is detected, spirochetes and *Actinomyces viscosus* are prominent members of the plaque flora. If this plaque remains undisturbed, the flora gradually shifts toward an anaerobic, gram-negative flora that includes a greater variety of spirochetes, *Bacteroides melaninogenicus*, and *B gingivalis*. The increase in these organisms can be explained by the low oxidation-reduction potential of the aged plaque and by nutrients derived from the inflammatory exudate at the site. These nutrients include serum proteins such as α-2-globulin used by *Treponema dentium;* also included are hemin, vitamin K, estradiol, and progesterone, all of which are involved in electron transport for the two *Bacteroides* species.

The gingivitis may resolve itself or fester subclinically for an indeterminant period; however, potential for the formation of a periodontal pocket (periodontitis) exists at any time. A pocket is a 3-15 mm pathologic extension of the space normally found at the gingiva-tooth interface. It probably forms as a tissue retraction from the noxious products elaborated by the plaque bacteria. When pockets are detected clinically, they usually have hardened plaque deposits called calculus present on the tooth surfaces. For many years, calculus was thought to be the etiologic agent of periodontitis, because inflammation usually subsided when it was removed and the tooth surfaces were mechanically cleaned. However, calculus is always colonized by plaque, and removal of calculus would be synonymous with debridement of plaque.

Recently, the subgingival plaque taken from pockets has been shown to vary with different clinical entities (Table 114-2). If the pocket is without symptoms (no bleeding or exudate present on clinical probing), the proportions of *B melaninogenicus, B gingivalis, A viscosus, Capnocytophaga ochracea,* and the various spirochetes are less than 10% of the flora. If, however, probing elicits bleeding, or if evidence exists that the pocket has recently elongated, or both, the proportions of *B gingivalis* or spirochetes or both can comprise a significant percent of the flora. Shifts in proportions of the cultivable flora have been recognized in plaque removed from the deep pockets found in juvenile periodontitis. In this instance, the scant flora is dominated by gram-negative organisms such as *Capnocytophaga (Bacteroides) ochracea* and *Actinobacillus actinomycetemcomitans.* The presence of high proportions of an organism during active disease has been interpreted as evidence for the involvement of that organism in the disease process; however, this type of evidence is circumstantial because the increased proportions could be secondary to other events such as *B gingivalis* proliferating in response to the greater nutrient availability of hemin, vitamin K, or the steroids. The

Table 114-2   Bacterial Differences in Healthy and Disease-Associated Plaques*

Bacterial Species	Supragingival		Subgingival		
	Health	*Caries*	*Health*	*Gingivitis*	*Periodontitis*
S. sanguis	+ +	+	+ +	+	−
S. mutans	±	+ +	−	−	−
Lactobacilli sp.	±	+	−	−	−
A. viscosus	±	+	+	+ +	+
B. gingivalis	−	−	±	±	+ +
Spirochetes	−	−	−	+	+ +
Capnocytophaga sp.	−	−	−	±	+
B. melaninogenicus	−	−	±	+	+
A. actinomycetemcomitans	−	−	−	−	+ (J.P.)

*−, not detected; ±, found in less than 1% of flora, if present; +, in less than 10% of flora; + +, in greater than 10% of flora; J.P., juvenile periodontitis.

pathogenic potential of an isolate can be assayed by inoculation into a germ-free rat. Many of the cited species (*A viscosus, B gingivalis, A actinomycetemcomitans,* and *C ochracea*) cause extensive periodontal pathology simply by colonizing the dentogingival surfaces in this gnotobiotic model. Thus, this animal pathogenicity combined with increased proportions in the clinical lesion argue strongly for the specific involvement of these organisms in the various periodontal pathologies. If this is so, diagnosis and treatment should be geared toward these organisms.

Cariogenic Plaque

The scenario previously described does not include dental decay as a possible consequence of plaque accumulation (Figure 114-1), because the bacteria that normally colonize the tooth surfaces do not cause appreciable amounts of decay. Historically, individuals in the West did not experience decay until sucrose became an important component of their diet. Today, most adult residents of the third world nations have not experienced decay because sucrose is relatively scarce in their foods; however, in some of these countries (such as Nigeria), new affluence has introduced sugar products and the incidence of dental decay in children has become almost epidemic.

The relationship between sucrose ingestion and dental caries is reasonably well understood. The supragingival plaque flora derives its nutrients from various sources that include diet, saliva, sloughed epithelial cells, dead microbes, and gingival crevice fluid or exudate. All sources except the foods in the diet provide only small amounts of

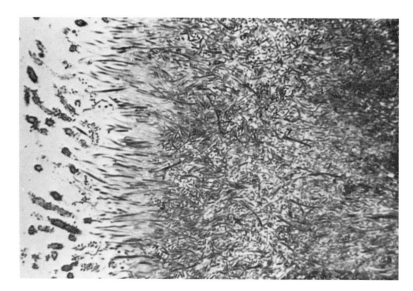

Figure 114-1 Plaque accumulation on tooth surface. Note dense bacterial accumulations at enamel surface. At saliva surface, long filamentous forms are oriented perpendicular to tooth surface. From Listgarten, M.A.: *J Periodont* 1976; 47:8.

nutrients. Dietary components are normally high-molecular-weight polymers (such as starch and proteins) that are in the mouth for short periods. They have a minimal effect on plaque growth except in those instances when food is retained between and on the teeth. Sucrose, however, changes this pattern because it is a low-molecular-weight disaccharide that can be rapidly sequestered and utilized by the plaque flora. Plaque organisms capable of fermenting sucrose have a decided advantage over the nonsucrose fermenters in that they can proliferate during periods of sucrose ingestion and thereby become the dominant plaque organisms. Sucrose fermentation produces an acute drop in the pH, to 5.0 or lower, at the point of interface between plaque and enamel. When sucrose is ingested during meals, sufficient saliva is secreted to buffer the plaque pH and decay does not occur. In fact, studies show that as much as a one-half a pound of sucrose consumed daily at meals for two years was not associated with an increase in dental decay; however, when the same or lesser amounts of sucrose were ingested between meals, subjects developed new decay at the rate of about three to four tooth surfaces per year. The frequent ingestion of sucrose has been shown to increase the levels of salivary sugar, and to increase the lengths of time that sucrose could be detected in the saliva. This means that if sucrose would be available for microbial fermentation for long periods each day, low plaque pH results. When the plaque pH value falls below 5.0–5.2, the salivary buffers are overwhelmed and tooth enamel begins to dissolve, releasing Ca and PO_4 ions from sites beneath the surface enamel. Normally, the bathing saliva replenishes these minerals, but if the length of the flux from the enamel is great, repair does not occur and cavitation results. Thus, sucrose consumption per se does not cause decay, but the frequent ingestion of sucrose is cariogenic.

Plaque bacteria that ferment sucrose produce acids, which in vitro lower the pH value to below 5.0; however, most of these plaque bacterial species do not cause decay in germ-free animals fed a high-sucrose diet. This suggests that microbial acid production is not the exclusive determinant of decay. One organism, *S mutans*, caused extensive destruction of the teeth in the germ-free rat. This organism previously had been shown by Keyes to cause a transmissible caries infection in hamsters. In fact, Koch's postulates have been fulfilled with *S mutans* in the hamster model. *S mutans* was isolated from a carious lesion and made resistant to the antibiotic streptomycin, so as to facilitate its identification. This streptomycin-resistant *S mutans* was then introduced into the mouths of young caries-free hamsters ingesting a sucrose diet. Within several months, caries developed and the streptomycin-resistant *S mutans* were isolated from the carious lesions.

S mutans was subsequently shown to metabolize sucrose in a remarkably diverse fashion that is not matched by any other known plaque organism. The major pathway is concerned with energy metabolism; in this process, the enzyme invertase splits sucrose into its component glucose and fructose molecules, which are then converted to lactic acid by the glycolytic pathway. Other enzymes, called glucosyltransferases, split sucrose but transfer the glucose moiety to a glucose polymer know as a glucan. Several glucans are formed by *S mutans*, differing in their core linkage, amount of branching, and molecular weight. The first glucan identified had a core linkage consisting of an α 1-6 bond that classified it as a dextran. Later, another glucan having an α 1-3 core linkage was identified. This glucan appears to be unique to *S mutans* and has been given the name mutan. Neither of these glucans consists of a linear molecule; rather, both have varying amounts of branching and varying lengths. *S mutans* also has enzymes that split sucrose and transfer the fructose moiety to a fructose polymer know as a fructan. At least two fructosyltransferases are present, as levan (a β 2-6 fructose core linkage), and inulin can be found in *S mutans* cultures. Other plaque bacteria can form from sucrose one or more of these polymers with the exception of mutan. Only *S mutans* can form all these polymers, a fact that led to an inquiry into the relationship between caries formation and polymer production.

All the polymers are extracellular and account for about 20% of the sucrose utilized by *S mutans*. It seems unlikely that an organism would invest energy and enzyme machinery into the formation of these polymers unless they had some survival value. Several oral organisms, especially *S salivarius*, have been shown to form levan during a period of nutrient excess and then to degrade the levan during a period of nutrient depletion. In this regard, the levan served as a reserve energy compound much as glycogen and lipids serve as energy-storing compounds in animals. Thus, the formation of a reserve energy compound enables a plaque organism to maintain itself and possibly to grow during the relatively long periods of famine that occur between meals and at night. But no reserve energy functions could be readily shown for dextran and mutan. Then, in an observation made by Gibbons, *S mutans* was observed to adhere to the walls of glass culture vessels in the presence of sucrose. The adhering substance was shown to be the extracellular glucans. These adhesive polymers confer upon *S mutans* a great in vivo survival value because *S mutans* can adhere tenaciously to the tooth surface and not be washed away by and swallowed with the saliva.

Animal experiments have shown that treatment with the enzymes dextranase or mutanase, or both, which degrade the extracellular polymers, reduces the incidence of caries. Other investigations, in which rodents were infected with mutants of *S mutans* that lacked the ability to form either one of these two glucans, indicate mutan is more caries conducive than dextran. In particular, absence of mutan is associated with greater reduction in smooth surface decay than is absence of dextran. In each instance, the amount of pit and fissure decay is not significantly affected by these mutations. This has been a recurring observation from animal studies in that procedures that reduce decay by *S mutans* usually do so primarily by reducing smooth surface decay. Decay on smooth surfaces seems to depend on the retentive polymers formed by *S mutans*, whereas in sites where retention is provided by the anatomy of the teeth (pits, fissures, and contact points between teeth), these polymers are not as important. Accordingly, pit and fissure decay may be caused simply by any acidogenic organism that happens to colonize these retentive sites.

This nonspecific explanation does not seem completely satisfactory, because in animal models and in human caries *S mutans* again is the dominant organism involved or associated with pit and fissure decay; however, a few other organisms such as *Lactobacillus casei* and *Streptococcus faecalis* can cause fissure decay in germ-free rats. *S faecalis* is an uncommon plaque organism in the human and has never been associated with human tooth decay. Lactobacilli species, however, long been associated with human decay. These three organisms have in common that they are relatively aciduric compared to other plaque bacteria. That is, they not only produce acids, but they are relatively resistant to the resulting low pH caused by acid accumulation. Lactobacilli are the most aciduric of the plaque bacteria, but these organisms only predominate by the time the carious lesion has extended into the dentin. At the time the earliest carious lesion is detected, only *S mutans* has reached significant levels and proportions. When *S mutans*, lactobacilli, and other plaque species were compared in vitro for their ability to ferment sucrose at different pH values, *S mutans* was found to be more active than the other bacteria at pH 5.0. In fact, *S mutans* produced more lactic acid at pH 5.0 than it did at pH 6.5; thus, it is probably most active at the very pH at which teeth regularly begin to demineralize.

The degree of aciduricity seems to explain best the involvement of both *S mutans* and lactobacilli in human decay. A retentive site is colonized by those organisms present in saliva. *S mutans*, although present in low numbers in the initial inoculum (fewer than 0.1% of the initial colonizers), is selected for if the pH value in the site is not well buffered by saliva. Frequent ingestion of sucrose-containing products predisposes toward a lower pH value and, thus, selects for *S mutans*. As long as the pH remains in the vicinity of 5.0-5.5, tooth mineral is solubilized, thereby buffering the plaque and maintaining an environment suitable for growth of *S mutans*. Eventually, the cavitation extends into the dentin, forming a semiclosed system in which the pH value drops below 5.0. Under these acidic conditions, growth of lactobacilli is favored, and these organisms succeed as the predominant flora in the carious lesion.

Treatment of Dental Caries and Periodontal Disease

The prior discussion indicates that plaque frequently exposed to sucrose invariably is dominated by *S mutans* and lactobacilli, which creates a pathologic situation. Also, plaques that are left undisturbed due to poor oral hygiene habits develop a complex anaerobic flora, which may harbor one or more bacterial species uniquely capable of eliciting an inflammatory response in the periodontal tissue. Treatment strategy should be oriented toward preventing these specific plaque infections.

Conventional dental therapy, however, has not yet incorporated any microbiologically based strategy into its armamentarium. Instead, a treatment based on response to symptoms has prevailed. The bankruptcy of this approach, which depends on a turn-of-the-century biologic base, has been demonstrated in the Scandinavian countries, where a socialized dental delivery system has made quality dentistry available to everyone. Because of the emphasis on treatment rather than prevention, the result has been only prolonged (approximately 10 years) life span of the tooth, a rather poor therapeutic result. In England, where the health care system also emphasized treatment rather than prevention, one-half the people over 35 years of age are edentulous. The Scandinavians, especially in Sweden, have changed their approach and have instituted plaque prophylactic programs for children and in adults. Thorough dental cleaning with a 5% fluoride paste given at 2-4 week intervals combined with oral hygiene education has lowered dental decay in children by about 80%-90% compared to youngsters receiving symptomatic treatment. (Symptomatic treatment involves placing dental restorations in an obviously carious tooth, and pulling teeth.) Similar success has been achieved in adults with and without periodontal disease.

Thorough cleanings with fluoride apparently have prevented formation of the complex anaerobic plaque that can elicit gingival and periodontal inflammation. This treatment selects for the more desirable bacterial types such as *S sanguis* and *S mitis*, which are capable of rapidly colonizing the tooth surfaces. *S mutans* presumably does not have an opportunity to become dominant, because the frequent debridement neutralizes its ability to adhere to the tooth surfaces and to be selected for by the low pH values that characterizes an undisturbed plaque. Also, the 5% fluoride paste has an immediate bactericidal effect on the plaque organisms and possibly a delayed effect, because of the ability of the fluoride ion to be taken up by the enamel and then to be slowly released. This antibacterial effect of fluoride may enable dentists in the United States to achieve similar reductions in dental decay without the enormous investment in clinics and time that characterizes the dental programs that are oriented toward relief of symptoms.

Fluoride as an Antimicrobial Agent in Plaque

The mechanisms by which fluoride prevents decay are not fully understood. The 30%-50% reduction in decay that follows water fluoridation is generally attributed to the fluoride replacing hydroxyl groups in the tooth crystal, thereby forming fluorapatite. Fluorapatite is less soluble in acid than hydroxyapatite, which means that a tooth containing fluorapatite dissolves slowly in the low pH value found in plaque and, accordingly, remineralizes faster in the intervals between sugar ingestion. This explanation does not completely account for the proved efficacy of topically applied fluorides and raises questions about other modes of fluoride action.

The fluoride ion (F^-) inhibits the bacterial enzyme enolase, thereby interfering with production of phospho-enol-pyruvate (PEP). PEP is a key intermediate of the glycolytic pathway and, in many bacteria, is the source of energy and phosphate needed for sugar uptake. In the presence of 10-100 ppm of F^-, most plaque bacteria are inhibited. These levels are delivered easily by most prescription fluoride preparations such as were used in the Swedish studies. Of equal interest is the finding that at acidic pH values (5.5 or below), low levels of F^- (1-5 ppm) inhibit the oral streptococci. These levels are found in plaque, especially in individuals who drink fluoridated water or who have been treated with topical fluorides. If this plaque fluoride is derived from the tooth, an antibacterial mode of action, which involves a depot effect, can be postulated for systemic (water) and topical fluoride administration.

The depot effect comes about in this manner. Water fluoridation causes fluorapatite, whereas topical fluorides cause a net retention by the enamel of fluoride as fluorapatite or as more labile calcium salts. Microbial acid production in the plaque may solubilize this fluoride, which at the prevailing low pH in the plaque microenvironment could be lethal for the acid-producing microbes. Such a sequence would discriminate against *S mutans* and lactobacilli because they, as a result of their aciduric nature, are most likely the numerically dominant acid producers at the plaque–enamel interface. The fluoridated tooth thus contains a depot of a potent antimicrobial agent that is not only released at an acid pH value but is most active at this pH value. This hypothesis then attributes some of the success of water fluoridation and most of the success of topical fluorides to an antimicrobial effect. It further suggests that judicious use of topical fluorides in patients with highly active caries would be effective.

The most effective dose schedule and fluoride preparation have not been determined. Neutral 1.0% sodium fluoride given daily to adults who normally would experience rampant caries secondary to a xerostomia following irradiation for jaw cancer has resulted in few or no caries. Controls, who were given a placebo as well as the best available hygiene instruction, averaged 2.5 new decayed surfaces per postradiation month. When they were placed on the daily fluoride regimen, their decay rate dropped almost to zero. Five- to 6-year-old children who had ten or more carious tooth surfaces were given the necessary dental restorations and either 1.2% F$^-$ as a neutral sodium fluoride gel or a placebo gel. The gels were taken unsupervised at home, twice a day for 1 week. Retreatment for 1 week was repeated at approximately 6-month intervals. After 2 years, the fluoride group had about 40% less decay than the placebo group. Eleven of 20 of these subjects with formerly rampant caries had no new decay in their permanent teeth. In the xerostomia and the child patients, the initially high proportions of *S mutans* were reduced by the fluoride treatments.

Sucrose Substitutes that Aid in Caries Control

Eating foods that contain sucrose between meals can be highly cariogenic. Dietary counseling that instructs patients to avoid between meal snacks may help to decrease the incidence of dental decay, but only if the patients are compliant. Another dietary approach to caries control is to recommend that patients eat snack foods that contain compounds that provide the hedonistic appeal of sucrose, but are not fermented by the plaque flora to the low pH levels associated with enamel demineralization.

The least acidogenic sucrose substitutes are the polyols, such as sorbitol, mannitol, and xylitol. Few plaque bacteria can ferment these substances, and those that can (*S mutans* and *L casei* ferment sorbitol and mannitol) exhibit a slow fermentation because glucose catabolite repression keeps the necessary degradative enzymes to minimum levels. Xylitol, the only polyol with a sweet taste comparable to that of sucrose, and the only one that cannot be fermented by *S mutans,* has been shown to be noncariogenic, and possibly anticariogenic, when substituted for sucrose in either foods or chewing gum. In the chewing gum study, young adults who consumed about 6 to 7 g of xylitol gum per day had, after one year, an 80% reduction in caries increment compared to a control group who consumed 6 to 7 g of sucrose gum per day.

In later studies, this type of intensive use of a xylitol chewing gum was shown to decrease salivary and plaque levels of *S mutans. S mutans,* the plaque organism that is most efficient in promoting sucrose metabolism, is most active at the acidic pH levels found in plaques after sucrose ingestion. When the between-meal sucrose supply is reduced, the levels of *S mutans* will decline, as the low plaque pH values that selected for it are not as dominant a factor in the plaque microecology. However, xylitol can satisfy the craving for sweets without serving as an energy source for *S mutans.*

Antimicrobials in Periodontal Disease

Gingivitis and periodontitis reflect the host response to a complex, anaerobic flora that has accumulated on the tooth and root surfaces. The Scandinavian studies demonstrate that if this plaque is disrupted periodically by mechanical debridement of the tooth surfaces, periodontal health is restored and maintained. Health maintenance can be facilitated by antimicrobial adjuncts such as fluoride and chlorhexidine. Chlorhexidine is a bis-biguanide, which because of its net positive charge is adsorped to the oral and dental surfaces following its application as a mouth rinse or gel. The chlorhexidine is released slowly over the next several hours by salivary cations, thereby exerting an antimicrobial effect that dramatically reduces plaque formation, even in the absence of toothbrushing. This agent is currently used worldwide for plaque control. Frequent use often is associated with tooth staining, a cosmetic disadvantage that has discouraged the over-the-counter marketing of chlorhexidine in the United States. Accordingly, chlorhexidine seems to have a limited future in the United States.

Mouth rinses and gels are not likely to penetrate the periodontal pocket and inhibit the bacterial species contributing to periodontitis. Antimicrobial agents must be directly introduced into the pocket or delivered systemically. The agents used should affect an extremely broad spectrum of bacterical agents, as do chlorhexidine or fluoride, or should be effective against anaerobes. An active infection requires treatment for only a short time if current findings that a limited number of species are involved are correct. Persons in whom a clinical or bacterial diagnosis of active infection can be made should be treated. The systemic agent metronidazole (Flagyl) has been used to treat individuals with an anaerobic periodontitis, which is evident when pockets bleed on probing and when high proportions of *B gingivalis* and spirochetes exist in the pocket plaque. A 1-week treatment has resulted in pocket reduction of 2 or more mm in the most diseased sites and a suppression of *B gingivalis* and the spirochetes for up to 6 months after treatment. The microaerophilic organism *A actinomycetemcomitans* has been postulated to cause deep pockets and bone loss in localized juvenile periodontitis. In patients with this condition, therefore, mechanical debridement of the root surfaces, in addition to 2-3 weeks of systematic tetracycline therapy, may result in pocket reduction that coincides with the disappearace of *A actinomycetemcomitans*. These findings suggest that judicious usage of antimicrobials could presage a new era in the treatment and management of periodontal disease.

References

Genco, R.J., Mergenhagen, S.E., (editors): *Host-parasite interactions in periodontal disease*. Washington, D.C.: American Society for Microbiology, 1982.

Gibbons, R.J., van Houte, J.: On the formation of dental plaque. *J Periodont* 1973; 44:347-360.

Gustafsson, B.E., et al.: The Vipeholm dental caries study. The effect of different levels of carbohydrate intake on caries activity in 436 individuals observed for five years. *Acta Odont Scand* 1954; 11:232-364.

Keyes, P.H.: Research in dental caries. *J Am Dent Assoc* 1968; 76:1357-1373.

Listgarten, M.A.: Structure of surface coatings on teeth: a review. *J Periodont* 1976; 47:139-147.

Löe, H.: A review of the prevention and control of plaque. In: *Dental plaque*. McHugh, W.D., (editor). Edinburgh: E & S Livingstone, 1970.

Loesche, W.J.: *Dental caries: a treatable infection*. Springfield, Ill: Charles C Thomas, 1982.

Loesche, W.J., et al.: Treatment of periodontal infections due to anaerobic bacteria with short-term treatment with metronidazole. *J Clin Periodontol* 1981; 8:29-44.

Scheinin, A., Makinin, K.K.: Turku sugar studies I-XXI. *Acta Odont Scand* [Suppl 70] 1975; 33:1-348.

Socransky, S.S.: Microbiology of periodontal disease: Present status and future considerations. *J Periodont* 1977; 48:497-504.

115 Bone and Necrotizing Soft Tissue Infections

Jon T. Mader, MD

General Concepts
Necrotizing Soft Tissue Infections
  Crepitant Anaerobic Cellulitis
  Necrotizing Fasciitis
  Nonclostridial Myonecrosis
  Clostridial Myonecrosis
  Fungal Necrotizing Cellulitis
  Miscellaneous Necrotizing Infections in the
    Immunocompromised Host

Bone Infections
  Hematogenous Osteomyelitis
  Contiguous Focus Osteomyelitis
  Chronic Osteomyelitis
  Diagnosis of Bacterial Osteomyelitis
  Skeletal Tuberculosis
  Fungal Osteomyelitis

General Concepts

Necrotizing infections of the soft tissues considered in this chapter are characterized by extensive tissue necrosis and the production of tissue gas. These infections may extend through tissue planes and are not well contained by usual inflammatory mechanisms. They usually occur in traumatic or surgical wounds, in patients with diabetes mellitus or vascular insufficiency, or in combinations thereof. The vast majority of cases are caused by anaerobes and are facilitated by hypoxic tissue conditions. Infections may develop and progress with dramatic speed and extensive surgery and systemic antibiotics are required to eradicate them.

Bone infections are termed **osteomyelitis** (*osteo* means bone, *myelitis* means inflammation of the marrow). **Hematogenous** and **contiguous focus** osteomyelitis are the two major types of bone infections. Both types can progress to a chronic bone infection characterized by large areas of dead bone. Most cases of osteomyelitis are

Table 115-1 Systemic and Local Factors that Adversely Affect the Host Response

Systemic Factors	Local Factors
Malnutrition	Major vessel compromise
Renal, liver failure	Chronic lymphoedema
Diabetes mellitus	Arteritis
Malignancy	Extensive scarring
Immunosuppressive therapy	Radiation fibrosis
Chronic hypoxia	Small vessel disease
Immune deficiency	Venous stasis
Extremes of age	
Alcohol abuse	

caused by *Staphylococcus aureus,* although a significant number of cases involve group B streptococci and gram-negative bacilli.

Bone and soft tissues, except the skin, are normally sterile areas. Bacterial organisms reach these sites by either hematogenous spread or spread from an exogenous or endogenous contiguous focus of infection. The host plays a major role in containing these infections. A systemically or locally compromised host (Table 115-1) is more likely to develop and handle poorly these types of infections.

Necrotizing Soft Tissue Infections

An exact classification of necrotizing subcutaneous, fascial, and muscle infections is difficult because the distinctions between many of the clinical entities are blurred. Useful clinical divisions are: (1) crepitant anaerobic cellulitis, (2) necrotizing fasciitis, (3) nonclostridial myonecrosis, (4) clostridial myonecrosis, (5) fungal necrotizing cellulitis, and (6) miscellaneous necrotizing infections in the immunocompromised host. These types of infections, summarized in Table 115-2, usually occur in traumatic or surgical wounds and around foreign bodies, and affect patients who are medically compromised by either diabetes mellitus, vascular insufficiency, or both. In the traumatically, surgically, or medically compromised patient, local tissue conditions consisting of hypoxia and decreased oxidation reduction potential (Eh) promote the growth of anaerobes. The vast majority of necrotizing soft tissue infections have an endogenous anaerobic component. Because anaerobes are the predominant microflora on mucous membranes, there is a plethora of potential pathogens. Hypoxic conditions also allow the proliferation of facultative aerobic organisms because polymorphonuclear leukocytes function poorly under decreased oxygen tensions. The growth of aerobic organisms further lowers the Eh, more fastidous anaerobes become established, and the disease process rapidly accelerates.

Discernible quantities of tissue gas are present in most of these infections. Carbon dioxide and water are the natural end products of aerobic metabolism. Carbon dioxide rapidly dissolves in aqueous media and rarely accumulates in tissues. Incomplete

Table 115-2   Differentiation of the Common Necrotizing Bacterial Soft Tissue Infections

	Crepitant Anaerobic Cellulitis	*Necrotizing Fasciitis*	*Nonclostridial Myonecrosis*	*Clostridial Myonecrosis*
Incubation	<3 days	1-4 days	3-14 days	<3 days
Onset	Gradual	Acute	Acute	Acute
Toxemia	None or slight	Moderate to marked	Marked	Marked
Pain	Absent	Moderate to severe	Severe	Severe
Exudate	None or slight	Serosanguinous	"Dishwater" pus	Serosanguinous, profuse
Odor to exudate	+/− Foul	Foul	+/− Foul	Sweet
Gas	Abundant	Usually not present	Not pronounced	Not pronounced
Muscle	No change	Viable	Marked change	marked change
Skin	Little change	Pale red cellulitis	Minimal change	Tense, dusky bullae
Mortality	5%-10%	30%-40%	75%	15%-30%

oxidation of energy sources, by anaerobic and facultative bacteria, can result in the production of gases that are less water soluble and therefore accumulate in tissues. Hydrogen is presumably the major tissue gas found in mixed aerobic-anaerobic soft tissue infections. Its presence indicates that rapid bacterial multiplication is occurring at a low Eh.

Clinically, the hallmarks of mixed aerobic-anaerobic soft tissue infections are tissue necrosis, a putrid discharge, gas production, the tendency to burrow through soft tissue and fascial planes, and the absence of classical signs of tissue inflammation. The differentiation between the common bacterial necrotizing soft tissue infections is shown in Table 115-2.

Crepitant Anaerobic Cellulitis

Nonclostridial and clostridial cellulitis are similar clinically and are known as crepitant anaerobic cellulitis. Crepitant anaerobic cellulitis manifests as a necrotic soft tissue infection with abundant connective tissue gas. The condition usually occurs after local trauma in patients with vascular insufficiency of the lower extremities. Multiple aerobic and anaerobic organisms have been isolated, including *Bacteroides, Peptostreptococcus,* and *Clostridia* spp, as well as the Enterobacteriaceae. Crepitant anaerobic cellulitis can be differentiated from more serious soft tissue infections by the abundance of soft tissue gas, the lack of marked systemic toxicity, gradual onset, less-severe pain, and an absence of muscle involvement.

Necrotizing Fasciitis

Necrotizing fasciitis is a relatively rare infection with a high mortality rate (40%). The infection was originally labeled as hemolytic streptococcal gangrene, but better culturing techniques have demonstrated that organisms other than *Streptococcus pyogenes* more commonly cause these infections. Clinical manifestations include extensive dissection and necrosis of the superficial and often the deep fascia. The infection leads to the undermining of adjacent tissue and marked systemic toxicity. Necrosis of the overlying skin occurs secondarily to the thrombosis of the subcutaneous blood vessels. Initial local pain is replaced by numbness or analgesia as the infection involves the cutaneous nerves. Most cases of fasciitis occur following minor trauma or surgery. The highest incidence is seen in patients with small vessel diseases, such as those with diabetes mellitus. With careful bacteriologic technique, anaerobes, particularly *Peptostreptococcus*, *Bacteroides*, and *Fusobacterium* spp, have been found in 50%–60% of the cases. Aerobic organisms, especially *Streptococcus pyogenes*, *Staphylococcus aureus*, and the Enterobacteriaceae also have been isolated. Most infections are mixed aerobic-anaerobic infections, but a type of necrotizing fasciitis caused solely by *Streptococcus pyogenes* has been reported.

Nonclostridial Myonecrosis

Nonclostridial myonecrosis, also termed synergistic necrotizing cellulitis, is a particularly aggressive soft tissue infection. This infection is similar to clostridial myonecrosis in that there is widespread involvement of soft tissue with necrosis of muscle and fascia. The prominent involvement of muscle differentiates this infection from necrotizing fasciitis. The subcutaneous tissue and the skin are secondarily involved. Clinically, exquisite local tenderness with minimal skin changes and drainage of foul-smelling pus that resembles dishwater from small skin ulcers are present. Severe systemic toxicity is found in the majority of patients. Nonclostridial myonecrosis occurs most frequently in the perineal area as a result of an extension of a perirectal abscess and in the lower extremities of patients with vascular insufficiency. Multiple organisms have been isolated including *Peptococcus*, *Peptostreptococcus*, and *Bacteroides* spp, and the Enterobacteriaceae. The mortality rate from this infection approaches 75%.

Clostridial Myonecrosis

Clostridial myonecrosis, or gas gangrene, is an infection primarily of muscle tissue caused by clostridial organisms. *Clostridium perfringens* is isolated in 95% of these infections. Other clostridial species frequently isolated are *C novyi* (8%), *C septicum* (4%), *C histolyticum*, *C fallax*, and *C bifermentans*. Usually, clostridial myonecrosis has an acute presentation and a fulminant clinical course. The infection usually occurs in areas of major trauma or surgery, or as a complication of thermal burns. However, clostridial myonecrosis also has been reported following minor trauma, including intravenous administration of drugs, intramuscular injections of epinephrine, insect bites, and nail punctures. In the absence of recent trauma, this infection may occur by activation of dormant clostridia spores present in old scar tissue.

The diagnosis of clostridial myonecrosis is made mainly on a clinical basis. The infection may progress so rapidly that any delay in recognition or treatment may be fatal. The onset is sudden, often occurring within 4 to 6 hours after an injury. Sudden, severe pain in the area of infection is an early clinical finding. Early in the course of infection the skin overlying the wound appears shiny and tense, and then it becomes dusky. Within hours, the skin color may progress to a bronze discoloration, which can advance at a rate of 1 inch every hour. Vesicles or hemorrhagic bullae appear near the wound. A thin, brownish, often copious fluid exudes from the wound. Bubbles may occasionally appear in the drainage. This exudate has often been described as having a sweet "mousy" odor. Swelling and edema in the area of infection are pronounced. Within hours the skin overlying the lesion can rupture and the muscle herniate. At surgery, the infected muscle appears dark red to black, is noncontractile, and does not bleed when cut. Crepitus, although not prominent on examination, can at times be detected. Tissue gas may be seen on X-ray examination outlining fascial planes and muscle bundles.

The rapid tissue necrosis of clostridial myonecrosis is caused by the clostridial toxins. Clostridial species are capable of producing multiple toxins, each with its own mode of action. *C perfringens* produces at least 12 different extracellular toxins. The most prevalent toxin, a lecithinase termed α-toxin, is hemolytic, histotoxic, and necrotizing. Other toxins act as collagenases, proteinases, deoxyribonucleases, fibrinolysins, and hyaluronidases. The systemic toxic reaction cannot be fully explained by a single circulating exotoxin. The "toxic factor" may be produced by the interaction of the clostridia toxins with infected tissue. The mortality from clostridial myonecrosis ranges from 15% to 30%.

Fungal Necrotizing Cellulitis

Phycomycetes spp and *Aspergillus* spp may cause a gangrenous cellulitis in the compromised host. The hallmark of these infections is blood vessel invasion by hyphae followed by thrombosis and subsequent necrosis extending to all soft tissue compartments. Spores from these fungi are ubiquitous.

The *Phycomycetes* spp are characterized by broad-base nonseptate hyphae. *Rhizopus, Mucor,* and *Absidia* are the major pathogenic genera within the class of Mucoraceae. Serious pulmonary, rhinocerebral, or disseminated infections have been found in patients with diabetes, lymphoma, or leukemia. Phycomycotic gangrenous cellulitis usually occurs in patients with severe burns or diabetes mellitus. The characteristic dermal lesion is a black anesthetic ulcer or an area of necrosis surrounded by a purple edematous margin. There is no gas or exudate, and the infection may show rapid progression.

Aspergillus spp are characterized histologically by branched, septate hyphae. These fungi can cause serious pulmonary or disseminated infections in compromised hosts. *Aspergillus* grangrenous cellulitis may be primary or from a disseminated infection. The dermal lesion is an indurated plaque that leads to a necrotic ulcer. Gas and exudate are not present.

Miscellaneous Necrotizing Infections in the Immunocompromised Host

A variety of organisms may produce a gangrenous cellulitis in the immunocompromised host. *Pseudomonas aeruginosa* sepsis may be complicated by metastatic gangrenous cellulitis. Skin and subcutaneous necrosis may be present. Ecthyma gangrenosum represents a specific morphologic form of *Pseudomonas aeruginosa* infection. Rarely, other gram-negative aerobic bacteria may cause similar lesions.

Necrotic dermal plaques and ulcers have been described for *Aeromonas hydrophilia* and cryptococcal infections. Crepitant cellulitis has been reported for *A hydrophilia* and *B cereus* infections. A fulminant myonecrosis has been described for *Klebsiella pneumoniae* and nocardial infections.

Bone Infections

Based on clinical and pathologic considerations, osteomyelitis may be classified as either hematogenous or secondary to a contiguous focus of infection. Contiguous focus osteomyelitis can be further subdivided into bone infection with relatively normal vascularity and bone infection with generalized vascular insufficiency. Either major class of osteomyelitis may progress to a chronic bone infection.

Hematogenous Osteomyelitis

Hematogenous osteomyelitis occurs mainly in infants and children, but is being found with an increasing frequency in the adult population. In infants and children the metaphysis of the long bones (tibia, femur) is most frequently involved. The anatomy in the metaphyseal region of long bones seems to explain this clinical finding. Nonanastomosing capillary ends of the nutrient artery make sharp loops under the growth plate and enter a system of large venous sinusoids where the blood flow becomes slow and turbulent. Any end capillary obstruction would lead to an area of avascular necrosis. Minor trauma probably predisposes the infant or child to infection by producing a small hematoma and subsequent bone necrosis, both of which can be infected by a transient bacteremia. The infection produces a local cellulitis which results in increased bone pressure, decreased pH, and a breakdown of leukocytes. All these factors contribute to bone necrosis. The infection may proceed laterally through the haversian and Volkmann canal systems, perforate the cortex, and lift up the periosteum. The infection may also extend into the intramedullary canal. Extension of the infection leads to further vascular compromise and bone necrosis. In the infant, some capillaries still penetrate the growth plate. Thus, the infection can also spread to the epiphysis and into the joint space. In the child over 1 year of age, the growth plate is not penetrated by capillaries and the epiphysis and joint space are protected from infection. In adults, the growth plate has reabsorbed and joint extension of a metaphyseal infection can again occur. However, in adults the diaphysis of the long bones and the lumbar and thoracic vertebral bodies of the axial skeleton are the sites most frequently involved. Adults with axial skeletal osteomyelitis often have a history of preceding urinary tract infections or intravenous drug abuse.

In hematogenous osteomyelitis, a single pathogenic organism is usually responsible for the infection (Table 115-3). Polymicrobic hematogenous osteomyelitis is rare. *Staphylococcus aureus* is the most frequent organism isolated, but *Streptococcus pyogenes* and *Streptococcus agalactiae* are responsible for a significant number of bone infections, especially in infants. Aerobic gram-negative organisms are responsible for an increasing number of bone infections. Many adults with vertebral osteomyelitis in whom *Pseudomonas aeruginosa* is isolated are also intravenous drug abusers.

Table 115-3   Osteomyelitis: Commonly Isolated Organisms

Hematogenous Osteomyelitis (Monomicrobic Infection)			Contiguous Focus Osteomyelitis (Polymicrobic Infection)
Infants, up to 1 year	*Childhood, 1–16 years*	*Adults, 16 years and older*	
Group B streptococcus	*Staphylococcus aureus*	*Staphylococcus aureus*	*Staphylococcus aureus*
Staphylococcus aureus	Group B streptococcus	*Staphylococcus epidermidis*	*Staphylococcus epidermidis*
Escherichia coli	*Haemophilus influenzae*	Gram negative bacilli	Group A streptococcus
		Pseudomonas aeruginosa	Enterococcus
		Serratia marcescens	Gram-negative bacilli
		Escherichia coli	Anaerobes

Patients with hematogenous osteomyelitis usually have normal soft tissue around the infected bone. If antimicrobial therapy directed at the responsible pathogen is begun prior to extensive bone necrosis, the patient has an excellent chance of being cured of the infection.

Contiguous Focus Osteomyelitis

In contiguous focus osteomyelitis with no generalized vascular insufficiency, the organism is directly inoculated into the bone at the time of surgical or other trauma or extends from adjacent infected soft tissue. Common predisposing conditions include open fractures, surgical reduction and internal fixation of fractures, and wound infections. In contrast to hematogenous osteomyelitis, multiple bacterial organisms are isolated from the infected bone. The bacteriology is diverse (see Table 115-3), but *S aureus* remains the most commonly isolated pathogen. In addition, aerobic gram-negative bacilli and anaerobic organisms are frequently isolated. Bone necrosis, soft tissue damage, and loss of bone stability occur regularly, making this form of osteomyelitis very difficult to manage.

The small bones of the feet, principally the metatarsal bones and phalanges, are commonly involved in osteomyelitis secondary to contiguous focus of infection with generalized vascular insufficiency. Usually, the infection develops as an extension of a local infection, either from cellulitis or a trophic skin ulcer. The inadequate tissue perfusion predisposes to the infection by blunting the local inflammatory response. Multiple aerobic and anaerobic bacteria are usually isolated from the infected bone. Although cure is desirable, a more attainable goal of therapy is to suppress the infection and maintain functional integrity of the involved limb. Recurrent bone infection or a new bone infection occurs in a large number of patients. In time, amputation of the infected area is almost always necessary.

Chronic Osteomyelitis

Both hematogenous and contiguous focus osteomyelitis can progress to a chronic bone infection. No exact criteria separate acute from chronic osteomyelitis. Clinically, newly recognized bone infections are considered acute, whereas a relapse of the infection represents chronic disease. However, this simplistic classification is clearly inadequate. The hallmark of chronic osteomyelitis is the presence of large areas of dead bone (*sequestra*). *Involucrum* (reactive bony encasement of the sequestrum) and persistent drainage via a sinus tract(s) are usually present. In chronic osteomyelitis, multiple species of bacteria are usually isolated from the necrotic infected bone (see Table 115-3), except in chronic hematogenous osteomyelitis, in which a single organism is usually recovered. Unless the necrotic infected bone can be removed, antibiotic therapy of chronic osteomyelitis is usually unsuccessful. The prognosis for arresting the infection is reduced in the presense of poor soft tissue integrity surrounding the infection, sclerosis of the involved bone, or bone instability.

Diagnosis of Bacterial Osteomyelitis

The laboratory diagnosis of bacterial osteomyelitis rests on the isolation of the causative bacteria from the bone or the blood. In hematogenous osteomyelitis, positive blood cultures can often obviate the need for a bone biopsy when there is associated radiographic or radionuclide scan evidence of osteomyelitis. In chronic osteomyelitis, sinus tract cultures are not a reliable means of predicting which organism(s) will be isolated from the infected bone, and antibiotic treatment of osteomyelitis should not be based on the results of such cultures. In most instances, bone biopsy cultures are mandatory to guide specific antimicrobial therapy in osteomyelitis.

Skeletal Tuberculosis

Skeletal tuberculosis is the result of hematogenous spread of the tuberculosis bacillus early in the course of a primary infection. Rarely, skeletal tuberculosis may be a contiguous infection from an adjacent caseating lymph node. The primary bone infection, if not initially arrested, or reactivation of a quiescent bone focus produces an inflammatory reaction followed by the development of granulation tissue. The granulation tissue erodes and destroys the cartilage and cancellous bone. Eventually the infection causes bone demineralization and necrosis. Protolytic enzymes, which can destroy cartilage, are not produced in skeletal tuberculosis. Cartilage is destroyed slowly by granulation tissue, thus preserving the joint or disc space for considerable periods. Healing of the infection involves deposition of fibrous tissue. Pain is the most frequent clinical complaint.

Any bone may be involved in skeletal tuberculosis, but the infection is generally limited to one site. In children or adolescents, the metaphysis of the long bones is most frequently infected. In the adult, the axial skeleton followed by the proximal femur, knee, and small bones of the hands and feet are most often involved. In the axial skeleton, the thoracic vertebral bodies are most frequently infected followed by the lumbar and cervical vertebral bodies. Vertebral infection usually begins in the anterior portion of a vertebral body and is adjacent to an intervertebral disc. The infection produces destruction of the nearby bone and the intervertebral disc. Adjacent vertebral bodies may become infected and a paravertebral abscess may develop. Of the patients with skeletal tuberculosis, 60% have evidence of extraosseous tuberculosis.

Tissue for culture and histology is almost always required for the diagnosis of skeletal tuberculosis. Cultures for tuberculosis are positive in approximately 60% of the cases, but 6 weeks may be required for growth and identification of the organism. Histology showing granulomatous tissue compatible with tuberculosis and a positive tuberculin skin test are sufficient to begin therapy. However, a negative skin test does not rule out skeletal tuberculosis. Therapy for skeletal tuberculosis involves prolonged chemotherapy and, in some cases, surgical debridement.

Fungal Osteomyelitis

Bone infections may be caused by a variety of fungal organisms, including coccidioidomycosis, blastomycosis, cryptococcus, and sporotrichosis. The most common presentation is a cold abscess overlying an osteolytic lesion. Joint space extension may occur in coccidioidomycosis and blastomycosis. Treatment for fungal osteomyelitis involves surgical debridement and antifungal chemotherapy.

References

Cierny, G., Mader, J.T.: Management of adult osteomyelitis. In: *Surgery of the musculoskeletal systems.* Evarts, C.M., (editor). New York: Churchill Livingston, 1983.

Finegold, S.M., et al.: Management of anaerobic infections. *Ann Intern Med* 1975; 83:375-389.

Mackowiak, P.A., Jones, S.R., Smith, J.W.: Diagnostic value of sinus tract cultures in chronic osteomyelitis. *JAMA* 1978; 239:2772-2775.

Meleney, F.L.: Hemolytic streptococcal gangrene. *Arch Surg* 1924; 9:317-364.

Stone, H.H., Martin, J.D., Jr.: Synergistic necrotizing cellulitis. *Ann Surg* 1972; 175:702-711.

Waldvogel, F.A., Medoff, G., Swartz, M.N.: Osteomyelitis: A review of clinical features, therapeutic considerations, and unusual aspects. *N Engl J Med* 1970; 282:198-206, 260-266, 316-322.

Glossary

ABO blood group system   Alloantigens of the major human blood group system.

abortive infection   Virus infection in which usually only a few viral genes are expressed and no infectious virus is produced.

accessory cells   Lymphoid cells of the monocyte/macrophage lineage that cooperate with T and B cells in immune responses.

acid-fastness   Property of retaining dye following decolorization with acidic ethanol.

actinomycetomata   Localized swollen lesions at a site of traumatic inoculation of *Nocardia* where skin, subcutaneous tissue, fascia, and bone become involved.

actinomycosis   Infection occurring when actinomyces organisms normally found in the mouth are introduced into the tissues and cause chronic, granulomatous, suppurative disease.

active immunization   Specific acquired immunity resulting from disease or immunization with microorganisms or their products.

active immunotherapy   Administration of or immunization with specific antigens (eg, vaccines) or nonspecific immunostimulating agents to stimulate immune resistance.

adjuvant   Substance administered with antigen that increases the immune responsiveness.

adoptive immunotherapy   Transfer of histocompatible immunocompetent lymphocytes to a nonimmune recipient.

adsorption   Specific binding of virion attachment protein (antireceptor) to a cell surface constituent (receptor).

affinity constant (for antigen-antibody complex)   Measure of the avidity that an antibody has for an antigen.

agglutination   Antigen-antibody reaction in which a particulate antigen forms a visible clump when mixed with specific antibody.

airborne transmission   Method of spread of infection by droplet nuclei or dust.

allele   Alternative form or duplicate of a gene present at the same locus on the homologous chromosomes.

allergen   Any substance that induces an allergic reaction.

allergy   Unusually high immune reactivity of an individual after exposure to a foreign substance (eg, antigen), which can have an adverse effect on the host.

alloantibody   Antibody produced against an alloantigen.

alloantigen   Antigen eliciting an immune response in an allogeneic situation.

allogeneic   Describes the relatedness between individuals that are genetically and antigenically dissimilar but of the same species.

allograft   Graft between two genetically dissimilar individuals of the same species.

allotype   Variation in antigenic determinants on immunoglobulins from members of the same species.

alternative complement pathway   Activation pathway of complement that involves the direct stimulation of C3 without previous activation of C1, C4, and C2.

amphibolic   Describes a biochemical pathway that serves the dual functions of catabolism and anabolism.

amphotropic viruses   Retroviruses that share the host range of both ecotropic and xenotropic viruses: they productively infect original host species cells and also cells from heterologous species.

anaerobic   1. Lacking O_2. 2. Use of an electron acceptor other than O_2 in an electron-transport oxidation.

anamnestic response   Rapid rise in antibody or immune cells following a second exposure to antigen.

anaphylatoxin   Substance produced by complement activation that causes the release of histamine from basophils and mast cells.

anaphylaxis Acute hypersensitivity reaction (local or systemic) resulting from an antigen-antibody reaction, often involving IgE antibody and mast cells or basophils.

anaplerotic Describes a reaction that replenishes intermediates of a biosynthetic pathway.

anergic Lowered or absent responsiveness to specific antigens.

anergy Inability to respond to specific antigens.

antibody A soluble protein (immunoglobulin) produced in response to an antigen, which has the ability to specifically combine with that antigen.

antibody combining site The part of an antibody molecule that binds to an antigenic determinant.

antibody-dependent cellular cytotoxicity (ADCC) Cell-mediated cytotoxicity in which an effector cell kills an antibody-coated target cell via recognition of the Fc receptor.

antigen Substance that can induce a detectable immune response when introduced into an individual.

antigenic determinant Area of an antigen that determines the specificity of antigen-antibody binding (same as **epitope**).

antigenic drift Minor antigenic change in the (influenza) virus hemagglutinin or neuraminidase antigens, resulting in new but serologically related antigens; responsible for epidemics.

antigenic mimicry Process in which parasites are coated with host components to escape the host immune mechanisms.

antigenic shift Major change in one or both (influenza) virus surface antigens (hemagglutinin, neuraminidase) resulting in new antigens with no demonstrable antigenic relationship to earlier antigens; responsible for pandemics.

antireceptor Virion attachment protein on virus surface used for binding to a specific receptor on cell surface.

arthrospore Spore resulting from the separation of a hypha and released by fragmentation of the hypha.

Arthus phenomenon Local necrotic lesion resulting from injection of antigen into a previously sensitized animal, mediated by an antigen-antibody reaction.

atopy Immediate hypersensitivity characterized by hereditary transmission and eosinophilia.

attenuated Describes a less virulent strain of a pathogen capable of immunizing a host against a virulent pathogen.

attenuation Selection of a less virulent strain of a pathogen.

autoimmunity Immunologic attack that occurs against the body's own tissue.

autoinfection Reinfection of a host by the progeny of a parasite while still within the host.

autologous referring to self (eg, antigens or antibodies).

autotroph Organism able to utilize CO_2 as its sole source of carbon.

axenic culture Culture consisting of a single species.

B lymphocyte (B cell) Bursa-derived or bursa-equivalent derived lymphocyte that is the precursor to antibody-producing plasma cells.

bacteremia Presence of bacteria in the blood.

bacteriocin Protein produced by certain bacteria that exert a lethal effect on closely related bacteria.

bacteriophage Virus that infects bacteria.

bacteriophage typing Distinguishing strains of bacteria by the pattern of susceptibility to lysis by specific bacteriophages.

bacteriostatic Property of inhibiting bacterial growth without killing.

bactericidal Property of killing bacteria.

basophil Granulocyte characterized by a pale lobate nucleus and large dense granules containing mediators of hypersensitivity reactions, such as histamine and leukotrienes.

Bence-Jones proteins Immunoglobulin light chains found in urine or blood of patients with myeloma tumors.

blast cell Lymphocyte that has been stimulated to become a large metabolically active cell capable of proliferation.

blocking factors Substances (antibodies) present in the serum that are capable of blocking the ability of lymphocytes to kill tumor cells.

booster Second dose of vaccine given to enhance antibody production.

bradyzoite Slowly multiplying forms of the toxoplasma parasite.

Braun's lipoprotein Small lipoprotein with one end embedded in the bacterial outer membrane and the other end linked to the peptidoglycan.

bronchopleural fistula Hole through the bronchial membrane allowing communication between a bronchus and a collection of exudate in the pleural cavity.

bursa of Fabricus Hindgut organ in the cloaca of birds that controls the ontogeny of B lymphocytes.

capping   Movement of cell surface antigen molecules (eg, Ig) to form a cluster of molecules that are cross-linked by ligands (eg, antigens or antibodies).

capsid   Highly regular, shell-like protein structure, composed of aggregated subunits, that encloses the nucleic acid component of viruses (eg, protein coat of a virus).

capsomere   Individual protein subunit of the capsid (or virus protein coat).

carrier   1. Substance to which a hapten is coupled to induce an immune response. 2. An asymptomatic individual releasing infective organisms.

carrier-culture infection   Persistent infection in which only a fraction of a cell population is productively infected at any given time.

catabolite repression   Effect of catabolites to repress the synthesis of catabolic enzymes by repressing transcription of their genes.

cell-mediated immunity   Immunity effected predominantly by T lymphocytes and macrophages.

cell-mediated lymphocytotoxicity (CML) reaction   Reaction of specific cytotoxic T lymphocytes against target cells.

cellulitis   Diffuse inflammation of loose connective tissue (particularly subcutaneous tissue).

central unresponsiveness   Tolerant state in which immunocompetent cells specific for a given antigen are absent or nonfunctional.

cercarciae   Free-swimming stage in the development of trematodes within the molluscan host.

chagoma   Small subcutaneous tumor at the site of initial *Trypanosoma cruzi* infection.

chemotactic factor   Substances (eg, lymphokines) that attract phagocytic cells to the vicinity of the factor.

chemotaxis   Attraction of leukocytes or other cells by chemical stimuli.

chimera   Animal composed of both foreign and autologous cells.

chromomycosis   General term for any infection involving fungi with dark pigment in their walls.

chronic infection   Continued presence of infectious virus in a host following clinical recovery from a primary infection.

classical complement pathway   Series of sequential enzyme–substrate interactions activated by immune complexes in which all components of complement are activated.

clonal selection theory   Theory of antibody formation that suggests an antigen selectively stimulates a lymphocyte clone bearing the receptor for (and capable of producing antibodies to) that antigen only.

clone   Set of cells derived from a single precursor cell and thus having the same genetic constitution.

cloning vector   Plasmid or bacteria phage DNA into which foreign DNA may be inserted to be propagated using recombinant DNA techniques.

coagglutination   Clumping by a particulate antigen and the homologous antibody.

coat proteins   External structural proteins of a virus that surround the nucleic acid (ie, capsid proteins).

cold agglutinins   Antibodies, mostly of the IgM type, that bind to red blood cells at 4° C and dissociate at 37° C.

colony-forming units (CFU)   Organisms or cells capable of multiplying to form distinct colonies.

colony-stimulating factor (CSF)   Glycoprotein derived from monocytes that controls the production of granulocytes by the bone marrow.

commensal   Symbiont that neither benefits nor harms the host but derives benefit from the host.

common vehicle transmission   Method of transmitting infective agents by a common inanimate vehicle resulting in multiple cases of disease.

competence   Ability to act in a process (eg, ability of bacteria to take up extracellular DNA to become genetically transformed).

complement   Group of serum proteins that bind to antigen-antibody complexes causing lysis of microorganisms and cells and also causing chemotaxis.

complementation   Introduction of a gene whose functional product substitutes for a defective product.

conditional-lethal mutants   Class of mutants whose viability is dependent on environmental conditions, with growth occurring only under permissive conditions (eg, temperature-sensitive mutants are inhibited by conformational changes in the mutant gene product at nonpermissive conditions).

congenic   Describes a strain of animal genetically identical to another strain except at one genetic locus.

conidia   Nonmotile asexual spores produced at the sides or tips of hyphae.

conjugation   Transfer of genetic information from one bacterium to another by cytoplasmic connections.

conjunctivitis Inflammation of the conjunctiva of the eye.

constant region Region of an immunoglobulin (heavy or light chain) whose amino acid sequence is shared among molecules of the same antibody class (isotypes) irrespective of antigenic specificity.

contagious Refers to a transmissible (or communicable) disease.

continuous antigenic sites Antigenic sites whose amino acid residues are directly linked by peptide bonds.

continuous microbemia Condition in which blood cultures are positive longer than 12 hours.

cord factor Surface component of diphtheria bacilli and *Mycobacterium tuberculosis* capable of impairing the mitochondrial membrane of mammalian cells.

cuffing Perivascular infiltration of lymphocytes in response to certain infection.

cutaneous larva migrans Pruritic eruption of the skin caused by the subcutaneous migration of the larvae of animal hookworms and other metazoan parasites.

cystitis Infection of the bladder.

cytolytic infection Virus infection resulting in lysis of infected cell, releasing new progeny virus and virus-specified antigens.

cytopathic effects (CPE) Morphological changes in cells resulting from virus infection.

cytotoxic hypersensitivity (Type III) Reaction initiated by antibodies combining with the surface of cells or with antigens attached to tissues.

cytotoxic T cell (T$_{CTL}$ or CTL) T cell, referred to as effector or killer cell, capable of lysing other cells in an antigen-specific manner.

defective interference Genetic interaction between viruses in which one virus bearing a lethal mutation can block or alter the replication of a second wild-type virus.

defective viruses Viruses that cannot replicate in cells without the presence of a second (helper) virus because they lack essential genetic information.

delayed-type hypersensitivity (DTH) (Type IV) T cell mediated hypersensitivity reaction not requiring antibodies and whose manifestations appear 18–48 hours after antigen challenge.

demyelination Destruction of the myelin from the medullary sheath of Schwann cells in the peripheral nerves or oligodendria in the brain.

denitrification Reduction of nitrate ($NO_3{}^-$) into nitrogen and ammonia gases.

dermatomycoses Fungal infections of keratinized body areas.

dermatophytes Infection of the stratum corneum, hair, or nails by fungi belonging to the genera *Trichophyton*, *Microsporum*, or *Epidermophyton*, and which are able to utilize keratin.

dermatophytids ("ids") Sterile lesions on the skin distant to the infected area that develop on patients sensitized to dermatophyte products.

diapedesis Passage of blood cells through the intact walls of blood vessels.

diaphoresis Sweating.

diauxic growth Growth in two separate phases.

dimorphism Phenomenon in which a fungus may exist as either a yeast or a mold in response to temperature or nutrition.

diphtheroids Wide range of bacteria that morphologically resemble *Corynebacter diphtheriae*.

discontinuous antigenic sites Antigenic sites whose amino acid residues are not directly linked but are located on different parts of the primary protein structure.

dissemination Movement of an infectious agent throughout an organ or the body.

domain Segments of a protein (eg, immunoglobulin) that are folded into a loop and usually stabilized by disulfide bonds; in some cases, each segment may be the site for one of the activities of an antibody (eg, antigen binding, complement fixation, Fc receptor).

eclipse phase Interval between viral penetration and detection of virus by electron microscopy during which viral biosynthesis is occurring.

ecotropic viruses Retroviruses that replicate only in cells from the original host species.

Embden-Meyerhof-Parnas (EMP) pathway Glycolytic pathway.

empyema Condition of pus in the pleural cavity.

encephalitis Inflammation of the brain.

endemic Describes a low level of disease that is constantly present in a population; ongoing occurrence of disease in a population.

endocarditis Inflammation of a heart valve.

endocytosis Uptake of exogenous material by a cell, consisting of pinocytosis and phagocytosis.

endodyogeny Asexual multiplication by certain protozoa in which two daughter cells are formed within the parent cell.

endogenous viruses 1. Viruses normally present in a population. 2. Viruses that have all or part of their genome(s) in a proviral state that is stably integrated into the host cell DNA and that can be transmitted from parent to daughter cells via normal cell division.

endospore Dehydrated resting cell formed within the bacterium.

endotoxin The lipopolysaccharide of gram-negative bacteria.

enteritis Inflammation of the intestines.

enteropathogenic Describes an organism causing intestinal disease.

enterotoxigenic Describes an organism producing an enterotoxin.

Entner-Doudoroff pathway Glucose catabolizing pathway almost exclusively found in obligate aerobic bacteria.

eosinophils White blood cells that contain cytoplasmic granules with affinity for acid dyes and are mobile, phagocytic cells; often associated with immediate hypersensitivity and parasitic infections.

epidemic Disease occurring in an unusually high number of individuals in a community at the same time.

episome Nonchromosomal, self-regulating genetic element also capable of existing as a part of a chromosomal segment.

epitope Synonym for **antigenic determinant.**

equilibrium dialysis Technique for measuring the affinity of molecules, such as an antibody for an antigen.

erythrocyte-antibody-complement (EAC) rosette Assay used to detect complement receptors on lymphocytes, in which red blood cells with antibody and complement bound to their surfaces form a cluster around a lymphocyte that has complement receptors.

exogenous viruses 1. Viruses not normally present in a population. 2. Viruses that replicate in and are released from infected cells of a host but are not demonstrable in normal cells of the same host.

Fab fragment Univalent antigen-binding fragment produced by papain digestion of an IgG molecule that consists of one light chain and one-half of the heavy chain.

F(ab′)₂ fragment Bivalent antigen-binding fragment that consists of two Fab fragments and is produced by pepsin digestion of an IgG molecule.

Fc fragment Crystallizable fragment obtained by papain digestion of an IgG molecule that does not bind antigen and contains the constant portion of heavy chains.

Fc receptor Receptor present on various leukocytes and some virus infected cells that binds the Fc portion of immunoglobulins.

fastidious Requiring specific growth factors.

fermentation Microbial oxidation of organic compounds by an anaerobic process.

fimbria (pili) Short proteinaceous filamentous structures, generally present in many copies on the surface of some bacteria and used for attachment to a substrate.

flagellum (flagella) Motility organelle found on an extremity of a bacterium.

flagellins Protein subunits composing flagella.

frank pathogens Infectious agents of disease that do not require strict conditions (eg, host debilitation) to cause disease.

functional complementation Cooperative coinfection by two different mutant viruses whereby each possess a normal counterpart of the other's defective gene, thus producing normal gene products that support the replication of both parents.

GALT (gut-associated lymphoid tissue) Subepithelial lymphoid cell layer of the lamina propria of the intestine responsible for synthesis of IgA.

gamma globulins Serum proteins that migrate in the gamma electrophoretic region and that comprise the majority of immunoglobulins.

genome Complete set of genes of an organism.

genotype Genetic complement or constitution of an organism.

glomerulonephritis Renal disease characterized by an inflammation of the glomeruli, often preceeded by a β-hemolytic streptococcal infection; also associated with deposition of antigen-antibody complex within the glomeruli.

graft-vs-host (GVH) reaction Reaction resulting from the attack by immunocompetent cells in a graft against the host.

gram-negative staining Losing the crystal violet stain and retaining the color of the counterstain (red) in the Gram stain.

gram-positive staining Retaining the blue color of the crystal violet in the Gram stain.

granuloma Focal inflammatory response with accumulation of epitheloid and lymphoid cells.

granulopoietin   See colony-stimulating factor.

gumma   Highly destructive lesion of tertiary syphilis, usually in skin and bones.

H-2 locus   MHC complex in the mouse, located on chromosome 17.

haplotype   Designation of a particular combination of alleles of an individual organism.

haptens   Small molecules that react with antibodies but cannot induce antibody production.

hapten-carrier effect   Phenomenon in which B lymphocytes react with the hapten determinant and T helper lymphocytes react with the carrier in order to produce an antibody response.

helical symmetry   Molecular configuration in which the nucleic acid and protein subunits of a viral nucleocapsid are arranged in a helix.

helper T cells (T_H)   T cells, stimulated by antigen in association with Class II MHC molecules, that are able to enhance the function of other lymphocytes.

hemagglutination   Agglutination of red blood cells.

hemagglutinin   Viral surface glycoprotein so named because of its ability to agglutinate red blood cells; One of the viral antigens used for classification and immunization (ie, influenza).

hemolysis   Lysis of red blood cells.

heterofermentation   Fermentation of glucose or other sugars to a mixture of products.

heterogonic   Alternating parasitic and free-living generations in a life cycle.

heterologous   Referring to nonself (foreign) antigen or antibody from members of other species (also xenogeneic).

heterotrophs   Organisms using organic compounds as a carbon source.

hexons   In an icosahedral capsid, the capsomers having six neighboring capsomers.

hexose monophosphate shunt   Oxidative pathway bypassing glycolysis (pentose phosphate pathway).

hinge region   Region of the antibody molecule in which disulfide bonds form between the two heavy chains of an immunoglobulin; the site of papain and pepsin attack.

histamine   Chemical substance produced by basophil and mast cells that mediates smooth muscle contraction, vasodilation, and mucous secretion.

histiocyte   Macrophage found in connective tissue.

histocompatibility antigens (H antigens)   Alloantigens found on virtually all cells that determine the compatibility of transplanted tissues.

holozoic nutrition   Feeding of actively ingested food.

homofermenter (homofermentation)   Fermentation of glucose or other sugar leading to virtually a single product, lactic acid.

homologous   Referring to nonself but derived from members of the same species (eg, serum or tissues).

horizontal transmission   Transfers of infectious virus from one individual to another by nongenetic means such as direct contact, droplet transfer, feces, urine, or indirect contact.

host   Organism susceptible to infection by a parasite.

host cell   Cell whose metabolism may be utilized by a virus or other microorganism for replication.

host range   Variety of cells and species of animals susceptible to a particular virus or other microbe.

human leukocyte antigens (HLA)   MHC complex in the human.

humoral immunity   Immunity mediated by antibodies.

Hutchinson's triad   Three common manifestations of late congenital symphilis: interstitial keratitis, notched incisors, eighth-nerve deafness.

hybridoma   Antibody-secreting cell line formed by the fusion of myeloma tumor cells with normal B lymphocytes.

hydronephrosis   Condition in which urine is retained in the kidney pelvis in the absence of exudate.

hypersensitivity   Inappropriate or excessive activation of the immune system, which can be harmful to the host.

hypervariable region   Region of extreme structural variability on antibodies that is responsible for antibody diversity (forms the antigen binding site).

hyphae   Microscopic filaments that compose the colony of a fungus.

Ia antigens   Glycoproteins coded for by genes in the I region of the MHC that are involved in the genetic regulation of the immune response.

icosahedral symmetry   Molecular configuration in which protein subunits of a virus capsid are assembled into a symmetrical polyhedron having 20 equilateral triangular faces and 12 vertices.

icteric   Jaundiced.

idiotope   Single antigenic determinant (epitope) within an idiotype of antibody.

idiotype Antigenic determinants of the variable region of an immunoglobulin that is linked to the antibody having specificity to an antigen.

Ig class switching Change in the class of antibody synthesized by a B cell due to transposition of the heavy chain variable genes (V, D, and J) from the original constant region gene to the new constant region gene.

IgA Serum immunoglobulin that may occur as a dimer, possessing alpha (α) heavy chains, and is often secreted into body surface fluids.

IgD Immunoglobulin possessing delta (δ) heavy chains whose apparent function is to serve as receptor for antigen on the lymphocyte surface.

IgE Serum immunoglobulin possessing the epsilon (ϵ) heavy chain; most often elicited in hypersensitivity reactions.

IgG Major immunoglobulin class in normal serum, possessing gamma (γ) heavy chains, and most often elicited during the secondary antibody response.

IgM Serum immunoglobulin consisting of five Ig units, possessing mu (μ) heavy chains, and most often elicited in the primary antibody response.

immediate hypersensitivity (Type I) Reaction starting within minutes after the antigens interact with appropriate antibodies.

immune adherence Agglutination between C3b-coated cells and indicator cells bearing C3b receptors.

immune complexes Formation of antigen-antibody complexes.

immune complex hypersensitivity (Type III) Occurs when antigens combine with antibodies in circulation, forming aggregates called immune complexes.

immune surveillance Theory that the immune system recognizes and rejects newly formed small clones of malignant cells.

immunoglobulin All serum and extravascular proteins that are antibodies (IgM, IgG, IgA, IgD, and IgE).

inclusion bodies Morphologic lesions in the nucleus and/or cytoplasm of infected cells.

incubation period Interval between the time of infection and the onset of clinical symptoms.

infecting dose Number of parasites necessary to cause infection.

infection Multiplication of organisms or infectious agents in the cells or tissues of a host body.

infectious dose 50 (ID$_{50}$) Smallest quantity of an inoculum required to infect 50% of inoculated hosts.

infectivity Potential of a microorganism to infect and replicate in a host.

inoculum Material used to start a microbial culture.

integrated-virus infection Integration of all or part of the viral genome into the host cell DNA. When this occurs, viral progeny may or may not be produced (eg, retroviruses) and new virus-specified antigens may appear on the cell surface. See **transformation.**

interference See **viral interference.**

interferon (IFN) Family of cellular proteins produced and secreted in response to foreign nucleic acids (eg, viral), cells, or antigens that confer antiviral and other properties to cells they contact.

interleukin 1 Substance produced by macrophages that stimulate proliferation of lymphocytes; formerly *LAF* (lymphocyte activating factor).

interleukin 2 Factor produced by sensitized T cells that stimulate proliferation of other T cells; formerly *TCGF* (T-cell growth factor).

interleukins Soluble substances produced by leukocytes that stimulate the growth or activities of other leukocytes ("acting between leukocytes").

intermediate host Required host in which only partial development of a parasite occurs.

intermittent microbemia Condition in which blood cultures alternate between positive and negative for the presence of an infecting microbe.

internal image Antibody variable region that crossreacts (corresponds) with epitopes of an antigen; for every antigenic determinant (epitope), there is a corresponding antibody variable region (idiotype).

intracellular obligate parasite Microorganism unable to multiply outside of a host cell.

invasiveness Degree to which an organism is able to spread through the body from a focus of infection.

Ir genes Immune response genes that map within the major histocompatibility complex genetic locus.

isotype Characteristic markers shared by all immunoglobulins of the same class; the 5 classes are μ, γ, α, δ, or ϵ.

J chain Protein joining chain found in oligomers of IgA and IgM.

junctional diversity Generation of different amino acid sequences due to the somatic recombination of gene segments during the production of an immunoglobulin.

K cell   Cytotoxic cell responsible for ADCC.

kappa chain   Antigenically distinct light chain of an immunoglobulin.

keratitis   Inflammation of the cornea.

kinin system (kinins)   Formation of vasoactive peptides (prototype: bradykinin) that activate neutrophils, involved in inflammation and in the pathogenesis of shock, arthritis, burn injury, etc.

lambda chain   Antigenically distinct light chain of an immunoglobulin.

larva   Juvenile stage of helminths and arthropods.

latent infection   Little or no infectious virus detectable, despite its presence, between episodes of recurring disease; a virus present in a cell not yet causing any detectable effects.

lavage   Cleaning out of a hollow organ (eg, stomach or lower intestine) by copious flushing with liquids.

lectin   Plant substance with the ability to induce some aspects of an immune response, such as lymphocytic blast transformation or erythrocyte agglutination.

leptospiremia   Bacteremia during acute phase of leptospirosis.

leptospiruria   Leptospira multiplying in the convoluted tubules of the kidneys and shed into the urine.

lethal dose 50 (LD$_{50}$)   Amount of an inoculum required to cause mortality in 50% of infected animals.

leukemia   Type of cancer of the blood caused by extensive proliferation of immature leukocytes.

leukocyte   All white blood cells and their precursors.

leukosis   Abnormal proliferation of one or more of the leukopoietic tissues (bone marrow, reticuloendothelial and lymphoid tissues).

leukotrienes   Bioactive molecules synthesized from cell membrane lipids in response to a specific allergen and that mediate hypersensitivity reactions.

logarithmic phase   Period in the multiplication of cells or microorganisms characterized by an exponential increase in their number.

lymphocyte   Leukocyte associated primarily with all aspects of specific immunity.

lymphokines   Soluble mediators produced by lymphocytes that influence the function of other cells (eg, MIF, MAF).

lymphoma   Cancer of lymphatic tissue.

lysogeny   Ability of bacteriophage to survive in a bacterium as a stable prophage integrated into the bacterial genome.

lysosome   Granules that contain hydrolytic enzymes.

lytic infection   Viral infection resulting in lysis of infected host cells.

lytic virus   Viruses whose multiplication leads to host cell lysis.

macrophage   Phagocytic mononuclear cell derived from monocytes.

macrophage-activating factor (MAF)   Lymphokine produced by T cells that enhances macrophage function.

maduromycosis   Fungal infection resulting in granulomatous lesions that have draining sinuses and "grains" of microorganisms in the drainage.

major histocompatibility complex (MHC)   Short chromosomal region containing the genes for histocompatibility antigens and the genes involved in the immune response.

mantoux test   Intracutaneous injection of tuberculin or PPD to determine sensitivity to *Mycobacterium tuberculosis.*

mast cell   Cell containing numerous basophilic granules that release histamine during a hypersensitivity reaction (ie, basophiles).

maturation phase   Period when viral progeny are assembled and can be detected by infectivity.

membranous epithelial cells (M cells)   Specialized epithelial cells that may provide a pathway for the direct access of intestinal antigens to lymphoid tissues.

meningitis   Inflammation of the membranes of the spinal cord or brain.

merogony   Asexual reproduction of certain parasitic protozoa.

merozoite   Stage of the malarial parasite that invades red blood cells.

mesophiles   Organisms living in the temperature range around that of warm-blooded animals (20–40 C).

mesosomes   Membrane structures formed by the invagination of the plasma membrane.

MHC restriction   Property of T cells to recognize only the antigens that are in molecular complex with MHC products on a cell surface.

microbemia   Presence of microorganisms in the blood.

miracidium   Ciliated larval stage of trematodes.

microaerophilic   Requiring O_2 for multiplication but at a lower level than atmospheric O_2 (5% instead of 20%).

migration inhibition factor   Lymphokine that prevents the movement of macrophages away from an area of infection.

missense mutation   Mutation that results in the replacement of one amino acid for another within a polypeptide chain.

Mitchell hypothesis   Theory explaining the conservation of free energy in biologic systems by the chemiosmotic coupling of oxidative phosphorylation.

mitogens   Substances that stimulate DNA synthesis in lymphocytes (and other cells).

mixed lymphocyte reaction (MLR)   In vitro test in which two populations of allogeneic cells are mixed to determine their histocompatibility.

mold   Mycelial form of a fungus.

monokine   Interleukin or cytokine produced by macrophages.

monomer   Basic unit of a protein, which may be composed of multiple polypeptide units.

monomeric antibodies   Immunoglobulins that consists of a single basic monomeric unit: two L (light) chains and two H (heavy) chains.

monopartite   All genes linked in a single DNA molecule.

monotrichous   Having a single polar flagellum.

monovalent antigens   Antigens possessing only one antigenic site.

monocyte   White blood cell that is the precursor to macrophages.

mosaics   Phenotypic mixing of viral structural proteins from two different but structurally analogous co-infecting viruses (viruses may or may not be related).

multipartite   Distribution of genes among several DNA molecules that together constitute the entire genome.

multivalent antigens   Antigens having more than one antigenic site.

mutant   Variant strain of an organism differing from the parental or wild type.

mutation   Heritable change in the nucleotide sequence of the genome of an organism.

mycelia   Mass of filaments (hyphae) in a fungus.

mycelium   Mass of hyphae constituting the colony of a fungus.

mycetoma   Term used to describe swollen, supperative, granulomatous lesions with multiple draining sinuses, containing granules composed of the etiologic agent usually found on hands and feet.

mycology   Study of fungi.

myeloma   Cancer of a single B lymphocyte clone producing a single or monoclonal immunoglobulin.

myiasis   Invasion of body tissues or cavities by fly larvae.

natural killer (NK) cells   Lymphocyte that can destroy virus-infected or tumor cells without prior sensitization.

nephritic factor   Autoantibody-like serum protein that may activate the alternative complement pathway in some patients with glomerulonephritis.

network theory   Theory proposed by Neils Jerne according to which there would normally exist an immunoregulatory equilibrium of antibodies (with idiotypic determinants) and anti-idiotypic antibodies.

neuraminidase   Viral capsid antigen demonstrating enzymatic activity disrupting or preventing the formation of viral aggregates. One of the antigens used for classification and immunization of orthomyxoviruses and paramyxoviruses.

neutrophil   Polymorphonuclear phagocytic leukocyte with granules.

nonsense codon   Chain-terminating codons for polypeptide synthesis.

nosocomial   Hospital-acquired.

nucleocapsid   Particle consisting of viral nucleic acid within its protein capsid.

nucleoid   Inner core of an RNA tumor virus particle, consisting of RNA surrounded by an icosahedral protein shell.

nude mouse   Hairless mouse that is congenitally without the thymus gland.

null cells   Lymphocyte lacking B or T cell markers.

oncofetal antigens   Antigens present on fetal tissue that are reexpressed on the surface of neoplastic cells.

oncogene   1. Gene of a cancer-inducing virus that is responsible for transformation. 2. Gene in the host cell that when mutated or produced in excess may lead to transformation.

oncogenicity   1. Ability of transformed cells to produce tumors when injected back into the animal of origin. 2. Ability of a virus to produce transformed cells.

oncogenic virus   Virus able to transform cells and to induce tumors when inoculated into laboratory animals.

operator   Site on DNA where specific regulatory proteins bind to restrict the binding of RNA polymerase.

operon   Cluster of genes whose expression is controlled by a single operator.

opsonin   Antibodies that bind to microorganisms and facilitate phagocytosis.

opsonization   Action of opsonins to facilitate phagocytosis.

opportunistic pathogen   Organism causing disease in host with an impaired physiological state.

otitis media   Inflammation of the middle ear.

palindrome   Sequence in DNA with adjacent reverse repeats, which is the same when one strand is read left to right or the other is read right to left.

pandemic   Worldwide epidemic.

parasite   Organism that injures its host while deriving sustenance from the host.

paratope   Antigen-binding site of the antibody molecule.

passive immunization   Transfer of antibodies from an immune individual to a nonimmune individual.

passive immunotherapy   Protective administration of immunological end-products, such as specific antibody.

pasteurization   Process using mild heat to reduce the viability of the microbial population (eg, used for milk).

patching   Stage in which originally diffusely distributed cell surface molecules (eg, Ig or B cells) group into small aggregates due to cross-linking with a ligand.

pathogen   Infectious agent able to inflict damage to a host organism.

pathogenicity   Ability to cause disease.

penetration   Entry of a viral particle into a host cell, which occurs following adsorption.

pentons   In viruses having icosahedral symmetry, the 12 capsomers located at the vertices that have 5 neighboring capsomers.

peptidoglycan   Rigid layer of bacterial walls; a thin sheet composed of N-acetylglucosamine, N-acetylmuramic acid, and a few amino acids.

periodic trend   Pattern of changing occurrence of a disease over time, usually indicating a change in antigenic characteristics of the disease agent.

peripheral inhibition   Tolerant state in which immuno-competent cells are present but unable to produce an immune response.

peritrichous   Having flagella attached to many places on the cell surface.

persistent infection   Condition in which there is the continued presence of virus in a host for longer than one month after the primary infection.

Peyer's patch   Lymphoid tissue found mostly in the submucosa of the ileum near its junction with the colon.

phagocytosis   Engulfment of a cell or other particulate matter by phagocytic leukocytes or other cells.

phenotype   Appearance or characteristics of an organism.

phylogeny   Ordering of species into higher taxa.

piedra   Superficial fungal infection growing as nodules on the external hair shaft.

pili (fimbriae)   Short filamentous structures on a bacterial cell.

pinocytosis   Uptake of liquid by a cell from the surrounding environment without the release of lysosomal enzymes.

plasma cells   Antibody-secreting cells derived from B lymphocytes.

plasmid   Self-replicating extrachromosomal circular DNA genetic element.

plasmin   Fibrinolytic enzyme capable of digesting proteins, such as complement factor C1.

plaque   Localized region of cell lysis induced by a virus or other microbes on a cell monolayer.

pleomorphic   Existing in more than one form and able to undergo change.

pleural effusion   Escape of fluid from blood vessels or lymphatics into the pleural cavity.

polykaryocyote   Cell with multiple nuclei.

polymeric antibodies   Immunoglobulins that consist of more than a single basic monomeric unit (eg, dimeric IgA and pentameric IgM), which are held together by the J chain.

polymorphonuclear leukocytes (PMNs)   White blood cells with a multilobed nucleus that are very active in phagocytosis.

porin   Outer membrane proteins forming a channel that allows only small (600 mol. wt.) hydrophilic molecules across the outer membrane.

primary antibody response   Antibody formation that occurs following the first contact of an individual with an antigen.

prion   Infectious protein.

productive infection Infection of a permissive cell by a virus resulting in the production of infectious progeny virus.

prokaryote Cell or organism lacking a true nucleus.

promoter Sequence of DNA to which RNA polymerase and other regulatory proteins bind; site for the initiation of transcription.

properdin pathway Alternative complement pathway.

prophage Bacteriaphage genome covalently integrated into the host genome.

protomer Identical protein units comprising the helical capsid of a virus.

provirus Virus genome covalently integrated into a host cell chromosome that can be transmitted from one cell generation to the next.

pseudotype Progeny genome of one parent virus that is enclosed by the capsid specified by a second co-infecting parent virus.

psychrophiles Organisms able to grow at low temperatures.

pyelonephritis Infection of the kidney.

pyogenic Pus-forming; causing abscesses.

pyonephrosis Condition in which urine is retained in the kidney pelvis with the presence of exudate.

pyrogen Fever-inducing.

Quellung reaction Capsular swelling (opacity) procedure often used to type *Haemophilus influenzae*.

R factor Plasmid coding for resistance to antibiotics.

radioimmunoassay Sensitive assay to detect antigen using antibody labelled with a radioisotope (eg, ^{125}I).

reagin IgE antibody. Historically, serum antibody to syphilis.

recombination Process by which genetic elements in two separate genomes are brought together in one unit.

recrudescence of malaria Relapse of malaria due to the survival of erythrocytic plasmodia.

replica plating Technique of transferring bacterial colonies from a master plate to other agar plates using a sterile velveteen surface.

replicon Discrete unit of DNA replication.

respiration Oxidation of organic compounds (such as glucose) in which molecular oxygen serves as the terminal electron acceptor.

reservoir Repository source of infectious organism; site where organism resides, metabolizes, and multiplies.

restriction endonuclease Enzyme (bacterial in origin) capable of cleaving double-stranded DNA at sequence specific locations.

restrictive infection Infection by a virus in nonpermissive cells or in cultures where only a few susceptible cells in a population produce viral progeny.

reticuloendothelial system (RES) Mononuclear phagocytic system found in lung, liver, spleen, and lymph nodes.

reverse transcriptase DNA polymerase coded by certain RNA viruses (retroviruses) that makes complementary DNA strands from viral RNA templates.

revertant Organism derived by the reversal of a mutant to parental type phenotype.

Rh antigens Human blood group antigens responsible for a hemolytic disease in the newborn.

rheumatoid factor Antibody (IgM) directed against IgG and usually found in patients with rheumatoid arthritis.

rickettsiae Small obligate intracellular bacteria (responsible for typhus and Rocky Mountain spotted fever).

rigors Shivering.

Romana's sign Unilateral edema of the eyelids due to recent infection with *Trypanosoma cruzi*.

salpingitis Inflammation of the fallopian tube.

saprophytic Living in decaying or dead matter.

sarcoma Cancer of connective tissue.

Schick test Absolute test designed to determine the degree of immunity to diphtheria toxin by injecting dilute diphtheria toxin into the forearm.

schizogony Asexual reproduction of certain protozoa by multiple fission (eg, *Plasmodium* in red cells).

Schwartzman reaction or phenomenon Necrotic reaction, either local or systemic, produced in response to administered endotoxin.

secretory IgA (sIgA) Dimer of IgA joined by a J chain, produced by plasma cells located close to the epithelial surface and secreted by the epithelial cells.

secretory piece Nonimmunoglobulin glycoprotein associated with the secretory IgA during its secretion into mucosal fluids.

secondary antibody response Anamnestic antibody response.

secular trend Occurrence of disease over a prolonged period (years).

septicemia　Presence of pathogenic microorganisms in the blood.

serum sickness　Anaphylactic reaction that occurs after administration of a heterologous antigen, usually a heterologous serum.

siderophores　Microbial substances that chelate iron in competition with the host.

sigla　Names that are abbreviations formed from a few or initial letters of descriptive words (eg, *Reo*viridae = *r*espiratory, *e*nteric, *o*rphan viruses).

slow infection　Infectious process in which a prolonged incubation period is followed by progressive disease; an acute primary infection that is usually not evident.

slow reacting substance (SRS)　Substance released during an anaphylactic reaction that causes slow or prolonged contractions of smooth muscle.

sporogony　Reproduction by multiple fission of a protozoan zygote (eg, plasmodium).

sporotrichosis　Chronic granulomatous fungal infection usually involving the skin and superficial lymph nodes.

sporozoite　Stage of the malarial parasite transmitted to the host via mosquito bite.

stationary phase　Period during the growth cycle of cells or microbes in which replication slows.

steady-state infection　Persistent infection in which all cells of a culture are infected and produce noncytolytic virus.

stem cell　Undifferentiated cell from which effector cells are derived.

subcutaneous mycoses　Chronic fungal diseases of subcutaneous tissues following traumatic implantation.

succession　Replacement of populations in a habitat through a regular progression to a stable state.

suppressor mutation　Compensating mutation that restores wild-type phenotype without affecting the mutant gene, arising by mutation in another gene.

suppressor T cell (T$_s$)　Subclass of T lymphocytes that exerts an inhibitory control on B cells, helper T cells, and effector T cells.

suppurative　Producing exudate.

susceptibility　Sensitivity of a host cell or organism to infection.

syncytia　Fusion of adjacent cells resulting in polykaryocytes (multinucleated giant cells).

syngeneic　Describes the relatedness of individuals that are genetically identical.

T lymphocyte　Thymus-derived lymphocyte responsible for cell-mediated immunity or for immune regulation.

tachyzoite　Rapidly multiplying form of the toxoplasma parasite.

thermophile　Organism living at high temperature (40-70 C).

thymocyte (thymic lymphocytes)　Progenitor T cell that has migrated into the thymus and differentiated.

thymopoietin　Hormone that stimulates thymocyte differentiation.

tine test　Multiple puncture skin test for tuberculosis.

tineas　Superficial fungal infections of the skin caused by dermatophytes.

tissue culture infectious dose 50 (TCID$_{50}$)　Smallest quantity of inoculum required to infect 50% of cell cultures; infection is usually determined by cytopathology.

tolerance　Specific refractory state (unresponsiveness) to a given antigen.

toxinoses　Bacterial infections in which the major manifestations of disease are caused by secreted toxic proteins.

trachoma　Infection of conjunctival epithelial cells by *Chlamydia trachomatis*.

transduction　Transfer of genetic information from one organism or cell to another by a virus or bacteriaphage.

transfection　Process by which a bacteria or other cell takes up an intact bacteriophage, plasmid, or viral DNA.

transfer factor　Dialyzable factor from lymphocytes that is capable of transferring cell mediated immunity to a nonsensitized host.

transformation　1. Transfer of genetic information via free DNA. 2. Infectious process in which a virus does not kill the host cell, but induces morphological, biochemical, and biological changes in the host cell that may lead to malignancy.

transforming protein　Specific viral protein whose constant production is required to maintain a transformed state.

transient microbemia　Self-limiting microbial infection that is transiently detectable in a blood culture.

transition　Substitution of a pyrimidine for another pyrimidine or a purine for another purine within a single DNA strand.

transovarial transmission　Transmission from one generation to the next through the egg.

transplantation antigens　Major histocompatibility antigens.

transposon Segment of DNA able to replicate and insert one copy at a new place in the genome.

transversion Substitution of a purine for a pyrimidine or vice versa in a single strand of DNA.

trophozoite Motile stage of protozoa.

tubercle Tuberculous granuloma consisting of central giant, epithelioid, and lymphocytic cells characteristized by caseating necrosis.

tumor (T) antigens Viral specific proteins associated with transformed cells. Some appear to be required to maintain transformation; others do not.

tumor associated antigen (TAA) Antigens found on tumor cells that are undetectable on normal cells of adult individuals.

tumor-specific antigens (TSA) Antigens that are uniquely present on tumor cells.

tumor-specific transplantation antigens (TSTA) Antigens found on the surface of tumor cells that induce immune-specific resistance to tumor growth in animals.

turbidimetric determinations Indirectly measuring growth of a bacterial culture by its turbidity.

uncoating Viral replicatory event involving the removal of viral capsid, thus freeing the viral genome for expression of its functions.

vagility The ability of arthropods to move through space.

variable region N-terminal region of an immunoglobulin that determines immunospecificity. The region varies greatly in amino acid sequence from one antibody species to another.

vector 1. Intermediate host (eg, arthopod) that transmits the causative agent of disease from infected to noninfected hosts. 2. Vehicle of transfer of genetic material from one bacterium to another (eg, phage or plasmid).

vertical transmission Transmission of virus from parent to progeny through the genetic material or extracellularly (eg, through milk or across the placenta).

viral core Viral nucleic acid and associated basic proteins.

viral interference Infection by one virus rendering host cells highly resistant to another superinfecting virus.

virion Complete virus particle.

virogenes Virus derived genes incorporated in somatic (host) cell DNA and carried by the cell as part of its normal genome.

viroid Naturally infectious RNA that does not require a protective protein coat (capsid).

virulence Measure of the ability of an infectious agent to inflict damage on a host.

virus Infectious agent whose genetic element may be either DNA or RNA and which alternates between intracellular and extracellular states. The extracellular form (virion) of a virus contains nucleic acid and protein.

visceral larva migrans Invasion of and migration in the visceral tissues by larval helminths of animal origin.

Wasserman antibody (Reagin) antibody to cardiolipin utilized in a serological test for syphilitic infection.

Weil-Felix reaction Agglutination of *Proteus* organisms due to the development of cross-reacting *Proteus* antibodies in certain rickettsial diseases.

xenogeneic Describes the relatedness between organisms belonging to different species.

xenograft Tissue or organ graft between members of different species.

xenotropic viruses Retroviruses that replicate only in cells from animals other than the host species.

zoonosis Infectious disease transferred from animals to humans.

Index

NOTE: A small "f" following a page number refers to a figure; a "t" refers to a table.